Medical-Surgical Nursing

Medical-Surgical Nursing

BT Basavanthappa
MSc (N) PhD

Professor
Government College of Nursing, Bangalore
PhD Guide for Research Work

Member
Faculty of Nursing, RGUHS, Karnataka

Member
Academic Council RGUHS, Karnataka

Examiner
UG and PG, Courses on Nursing Various Universities

Ex-programme Incharge
IGNOU, BSc N. Course, Karnataka and Goa

Life Member
Nursing Research Society of India, New Delhi

Life Member
Trained Nurses Association of India, New Delhi

President
RGUHS, Nursing Teachers Association, Karnataka

Winner
Bharat Excellence Award and Gold Medal

Winner
Vikas Ratan Gold Award

Winner
UWA Lifetime Achievement Award

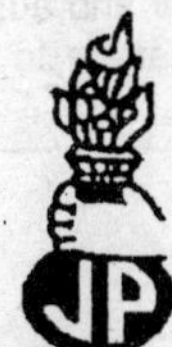

JAYPEE BROTHERS
MEDICAL PUBLISHERS (P) LTD
New Delhi

Published by

Jitendar P Vij
Jaypee Brothers Medical Publishers (P) Ltd
EMCA House, 23/23B Ansari Road, Daryaganj
New Delhi 110 002, India
Phones: 23272143, 23272703, 23282021, 23245672, 23245683
Fax: 011-23276490
e-mail: jpmedpub@del2.vsnl.net.in
Visit our website: http://www.jpbros.20m.com

Branches

- 202 Batavia Chambers, 8 Kumara Kruppa Road
  Kumara Park East, **Bangalore** 560 001, Phones: 2285971, 2382956
  Tele Fax : 2281761
  e-mail: jaypeebc@bgl.vsnl.net.in
- 282 IIIrd Floor, Khaleel Shirazi Estate, Fountain Plaza
  Pantheon Road, **Chennai** 600 008, Phone: 28262665 Fax: 28262331
  e-mail: jpmedpub@md3.vsnl.net.in
- 4-2-1067/1-3, Ist Floor, Balaji Building, Ramkote Cross Road,
  Hyderabad 500 095, Phones: 55610020, 24758498 Fax: 24758499
  e-mail: jpmedpub@rediffmail.com
- 1A Indian Mirror Street, Wellington Square
  Kolkata 700 013, Phone: 22451926 Fax: 22456075
  e-mail: jpbcal@cal.vsnl.net.in
- 106 Amit Industrial Estate, 61 Dr SS Rao Road
  Near MGM Hospital, Parel, **Mumbai** 400 012
  Phones: 24124863, 24104532 Fax: 24160828
  e-mail: jpmedpub@bom7.vsnl.net.in

Medical-Surgical Nursing

First Edition : **2003**

Reprint : **2005**

ISBN 81-8061-173-6

Typeset at JPBMP typesetting unit

Printed at Gopsons Papers Ltd, A-14, Sector 60, Noida

To

My parents,

My nursing profession

and

My dear students

Preface

It gives me immense pleasure and satisfaction to introduce *Medical-Surgical Nursing* to nursing community. In offering this text, I remain grateful for the support given to my earlier titles, i.e. Community Health Nursing, Nursing Research, Nursing Administration and Fundamentals of Nursing.

The book you are holding is the first text on Medical-Surgical Nursing written by an Indian author. I have carefully preserved the aspects of the book, that have met with such universal acceptance—its state-of-the-art, scientific based information, its string, its logical and uses-friendly organization and its easy reading style.

Medical-Surgical Nursing was developed to provide nursing students with the knowledge and skill they need to become competent, think critically and possess the sensitivity they need to become caring nurses. Professional nursing practice continues to evolve and adapt to society's changing health priorities. The rapidly changing health care delivery system offers new opportunities for nurses to alter the practice of *Medical-Surgical Nursing* and to improve the way nursing care is given.

In this changing world on health care delivery system, nurses will need a broad knowledge from which to provide the expert care needed in nursing profession. New efforts to reform health care and guarantee with high quality and cost-effective care are radically transforming the culture of care-giving. I believe that the changes in health care present exciting challenges to nurses and it is felt that there is a need for good nursing texts of Indian origin to assist nurses to meet these challenges in the Indian context, since there is obvious need for nursing text to fit the Indian situation. Nursing education must reflect these changes.

In view of the above changes the text *Medical-Surgical Nursing* is organized into 19 chapters, ideally, the text is flowed sequentially, but every effort has been made to respect the differing needs of diverse curricula and students. Thus, each chapter stand on its own merit and may be read independently of others. This work is designed to meet the nursing students requirement as per their respective universities, boards and also Indian Nursing Council.

I am aware of manifold reasons, errors might have crept in. I shall feel obliged, if such errors are brought to my notice. I sincerely, welcome constructive criticism from both teachers and students that would help me to enrich myself and good suggestions will be incorporated in next revised edition.

BT Basavanthappa

Acknowledgements

Any author who has interest for writing any book needs help and encouragement of other persons is very essential. The author is indebted to so very many persons that it is impossible to acknowledge every one who has given such help and encouragement. However, there are a few individuals who have given much encouragement and help that acknowledgement is due them.

It is my bounden duty to express at the outset heartiest gratitude to Shri G Basavannappa, Former Minister of Karnataka, during his tenure in 1960s initiated me to take up this Noble Profession "Nursing".

I also take this opportunity to express my sincere gratitude to Dr (Mrs) Manjula K Vasundhra, Former Professor and Head of the Department of Preventive and Social Medicine, Bangalore Medical College, for constant guiding spirit throughout and consistent encouragement for writing books on Nursing.

I also take this opportunity to express my deep sense of gratitude to my parents, Shri Thukkappa and Smt Hanumanthamma, my wife Smt Lalitha, and my children Mr BB Mahesh and Ms BB Gaanashree for their unselfish love, endless patience, quiet understanding that allow me to devote such a large part of my life to my career and support throughout what is inevitably a continuing but exciting experience.

I express my warm appreciation to the M/s Jaypee Brothers Medical Publishers (P) Ltd, New Delhi and Bangalore branch for sharing my vision for this book *Medical-Surgical Nursing* and giving me the chance to turn vision into reality. My sincere thanks go to Mr Jitendar P Vij, Chairman and Managing Director, Mr R K Yadav (Publishing Director) and staff of the 'Jaypee House' for their untiring exceptional efforts and cooperation.

Contents

Brief History of Medicine and Nursing in India

The history of medicine in India goes back through the centuries to about 3000 BC. The beginnings are shrouded in the mist of ancient myths. The experience and concern in health development date back to vedic period between 3000 BC-1400 BC. The Indus Valley Civilization showed relics of planned cities and practice of environmental sanitation. According to Dr. Wheeler on the basis of his research studies from South, Arikamedu (Pondicherry) to North Mohenjodaro and Harappa, only one culture had been followed. An ideal healthful living of the people, such as every house of Mohenjodaro and Harappa had separate good water supply. In every backguard of the houses, there was a wide royal street and by the side of the street there was an arrangement of some drinking water. Actually, this was followed by Dravidians who lived at that time. After the invasion of Aryans, the Dravidian got relegated to South. The specialist of pictograph reader, FATHER HERAS says that it was a fact that ancient people of Mohenjodaro were proto-Dravidians, a fact also hinted by Sir John Marshall that there was a link between all that is the Dravidian culture, including Mohenjodaro and Karnataka. The AYURVEDA and other system of medicine practised during this time suggests the development of comprehensive concept of health by the ancient sages of India.

TRADITIONAL MEDICINE AND SURGERY IN INDIA

Indian medicine is ancient. Its earliest concepts are set out in the sacred writings called the Vedas, especially in the metrical passages of the Atharvaved, which may possibly dates as far back as the second millennium BC. According to a later writer, the system of medicine called Ayurveda was received by a certain Dhanvantari from Brahma, and Dhanvantari was defined as the god of medicine. In later times, his status was gradually reduced, until he was credited with having been an earthly king who died of snakebite. Legends tell of Dhanvantari's relations with snakes and illustrates the skill with which early Indian practitioners treated snakebite.

The period of Vedic medicine lasted until about 800 BC. The Vedas are rich in magical practices for the treatment of diseases and in charms for the expulsion of the demons traditionally supposed to cause diseases. The chief conditions mentioned are fever, cough, consumption, diarrhea, dropsy, abscesses, seizures, tumors and skin diseases (including leprosy). The herbs recommended for treatment are numerous.

GOLDEN PERIOD OF INDIAN MEDICINE

The golden age of Indian medicine, from 800 BC until about AD 1000 may be termed the Brahmanistic period. It is marked especially by production of the medical treatises knwon respectively as the CHARAKA-SAMHITA and SUSHRUTA-SAMHITA, attributed respectively to the physician Charaka and Susruta, traditionally a surgeon. Both these works were formerly regarded as being of great antiquity, and hence claims arose for the priority of Indian scientific medicine over its Greek counterpart. Another school asserted that these works were written many centuries after the beginning of the Christian Era. The most recent estimates place the CHARAKA SAMHITA its present form as dating from the Ist century AD, and there were earlier versions. The SUSHRUTA-SAMHITA probably originated in the last centuries of the pre-Christian Era and became fixed in its present form in the 7th century AD at the latest. Other medical treatises of lesser importance are those attributed to Vagbhata (c.8th century). All later treatises were based on these works.

Because the Hindus were prohibited by their religion from cutting the dead body, their knowledge of anatomy was limited. The SUSHRUTA-SAMHITA recommends that a body be placed in a basket and sunk in a river for seven days. On its removal, the parts could be easily separated without cutting. As a result of these crude methods, the emphasis in Hindu anatomy was given to the bones, and then to the muscles, ligaments and joints. The nerves, blood vessels and internal organs were very imperfectly known.

The Hindus believed that the body contained three elementary substances, microcosmic representatives of the three divine universal forces, which they called spirit (air), phlegm, and bile. These were comparable with the humours of the Greeks. Health depends on the normal balance of these three elementary substances. The spirit has its seat below the navel the phlegm about the heart, and the bile between the heart and the navel. The seven primary constituents of the body-blood, flesh, fat, bone, marrow, chyle, and semen are produced by the action of the elementary substances. Semen was supposed to be produced from all parts of the body and not from any individual part or organ.

Both Charaka and Sushruta state the existence of a large number of diseases (Susruta says 1,120). Rough classifications of diseases are given. In all texts "fever" of which numerous types are described, is regarded as important, phthisis (wasting disease, especially pulmonary tuberculosis) was apparently common, and the Hindu physicians knew the symptoms of cases likely to terminate fatally. Smallpox was common, and it is probable that smallpox inoculation was practised.

HINDU WRITINGS ON DIAGNOSIS AND PROGNOSIS

In diagnosis, the Hindu physicians used all five senses. Hearing was used to distinguish the nature of the breathing, alteration in voice, and the grinding sound produced by the rubbing together of broken ends of bones. They appear to have had a good clinical sense, and their sections on prognosis contain acute references to symptoms that are of grave import. Magical beliefs still persisted, however, until late in the classical period, the prognosis could be affected by such fortuitous factors as the cleanliness of the messenger sent to fetch the physician, the nature of his conveyance, or the types of persons whom the physician met on his journey to the patient.

Indian therapeutics was largely dietetic and medicinal. Dietetic treatment was important and preceded any medicinal treatment. Fats were mostly used internally and externally. The most important methods of active treatment were referred to as the "five procedures"; the administration emetics, purgatives, water enemas, oil enemas, and sneezing powders, inhalations were frequently employed, as were leeching, cupping and bleeding.

The Indian materia medica was extensive and consisted mainly of vegetable drugs, all of which were from indigenous plants. Charaka knew 500 medicinal plants, and Susruta knew 700. But animal remedies (such as the milk of various animals, bones, gallstones) and minerals (sulfur, arsenic, lead, copper sulfate, gold) were also employed. The physicians collected and prepared their own vegetable drugs. Among those that eventually appeared in western pharmacopoeias are cardamom and cinnamon.

As a result of the strict religious beliefs of the Hindus, hygienic measures were important in treatment. Two meals a day were prescribed with indications of the nature of the diet, the amount of water to be drunk before and after the meal, and the use of condiments. Bathing and care of the skin were carefully prescribed, as were cleaning of the teeth with twigs from named trees, anointing of the body with oil, and use of eyewashes.

HINDU SURGERY

In surgery, ancient Hindu medicine reached its zenith. Detailed instructions about the choice of instruments and the different operations are given in the classical texts. It has been said that the Hindus knew all ancient operations except the arrest of haemorrhage by the ligature. Their operations were grouped broadly as follows: excision of tumors; incision of abscesses, punctures of collections of fluid in the abdomen; extraction of foreign bodies; pressing out of the contents of abscesses; probing of fistulas; and stitching of wound.

The surgical instruments used by the Hindus have received special attention in modern times. According to Susruta, the surgeon should be equipped with 20 sharp and 101 blunt instruments. The sharp instruments included knives of various patterns, scissors, trocars (instruments for piercing tissues and draining fluid from them), saws and needles. The blunt instruments included forceps, specula (instruments for inspecting body cavities or passages), tubes, levers, hooks and probes. The SUSHRUTA SAMHITA does not mention the catheter, but it is referred to in later writings. The instruments were largely of steel. Alcohol seems to have been used as a narcotic during operations.

Especially in two types of operations the ancient Hindus were outstanding. Stone in the bladder (vesical calculus) was common in ancient India, and the surgeons frequently carried out the operation of lateral lithotomy for removal of the stones. They also introduced plastic surgery. Amputation of the nose was one of the prescribed punishments for adultery, and repair was carried out by cutting from the patient's cheek a piece of tissue of the required size and shape and applying it to the stump of the nose. The results appear to have been tolerably satisfactory, and the modern operation is certainly derived indirectly from this ancient source. The Hindu surgeons, also performed an operation for the cure of anal fistula and in this they were definitely in advance of the Greeks.

In the past there had been much speculation as to whether the Greek derived any of their medical knowledge from the Hindus. Mid-20th-century opinion held that there was certainly intercommunication between Greece and India before the time of Alexander the Great.

A brief description of chronological events related to development of health and medicine in India is given below:

3000 BC: In the Indus Valley Civilisation, one finds evidence of well developed environmental sanitation programmes such as underground drains public baths, etc. 'AROGY' or 'Health' was given high priority in daily life and this concept of health included physical, mental, social and spiritual well-being.

2000 BC: RIGVEDA marks the beginning of the Indian system of medicine. Medicine was considered part of VEDAS or Scriptures. 'AYURVEDA', a 'Science of life and art of living' said to be founded by Sage 'ATREYA'. Good health implies an ideal balance between tridoshic factors, i.e. wind, bile, phlegm (VATA-PITTA AND KAPHA) according to AYURVEDA. Health promotion and health education were also emphasized by following 'Dinacharya'.

1000 BC: ATHARVAVEDA mentions the twin aims of

medical sciences as health and longevity and curative treatment. Hygiene and dietetics are considered important in treatment. Beneficial effects of milk are described in detail.

800 BC: A codification of medical knowledge scattered through vedas by BHELA called BHELA-SAMHITA.

700 BC: A codification of medical knowledge by AGNIVESA, said to be disciple of ATREYA, called AGNIVESA SAMHITA became the basis of later CHARAKA.

600 BC: A treatise by KASYAPA mainly dealing with paediatrics.

500 BC: 'CHIVARAVASTU', a book written by unknown author is found. It mentions prince Jivika, the court physician of Bimbasara, King of Magadh, as a marvellous physician and surgeon. He is credited with such difficult operations as piercing the skull to operate on the brain, surgery of the eyes, etc. and medical treatment of dropsy, internal tumors and varicose veins.

272 BC-236 BC: King Asoka, a convert to Buddhism, built number of hospitals. More emphasis was laid on the preventive aspects. Doctors, nurses, and midwives were to be trustworthy and skilful. The nurses were usually men and old women. This period saw famous medical schools at Taxila and Nalanda.

237 BC-201 BC: St. Buddha instituted a state medical system, appointed doctors for every 10 villages on the main roads of India. Pharmaceutical gardens were also maintained.

200 BC-100 BC: Patanjali explored the yoga system of philosophy of men and physical discipline–the starting point of yoga therapy later continued

100 BC: CHARAKA SAMHITA, the first classical exposition of Indian system medicine deals with an almost all the branches of medicine, anatomy, physiology, aetiology, prognosis, pathology, treatment procedure, and sequence of medication and an extension MATERIA MEDICA for more than 600 drugs. This treatise formed the basis of the ATREYA School of Medicine in India, in (100) A.D. The qualification of attending nurse, enshrined in the CHARAKA samhita, i.e. knowledge of preparation and compounding of drugs for administration, cleverness, devotedness to patient under care and purity of both mind and body.

200-300 AD: SUSHRUTA SAMHITA appears to have been revised by Nagarjuna, laid main emphasis on surgery. This great treatise described more than 300 operations, 43 different surgical processes and 121 different types of instruments. The MATERIA MEDICA is also extensive covering more than 650 drugs of animals, plant and mineral origin. This treatise forms the basis of DHANWANTARI School (300 AD).

Sushruta defines ideal relations of doctor, patient, nurses and medicine as the four feet upon which a cure must rest.

500-600 AD VAGBHATA wrote ASTANGA HRIDAYA (8 limbs and heart). The eight limbs refer to the eight traditional branches of Ayurvedic knowledge, i.e. therapeutics, surgery, ENT, mental and superstitious diseases, infantile diseases and treatment, toxicology, arresting physical and mental decay, and rejuvenation or regaining lost virility potency and procreative ability.

This book is the most concise and scientific exposition of AYURVEDA. It is in verse form, making it easy to memorise. It incorporates the teachings of the sages ATREYA and DHANWANTARI and the RASAYANA school of medicine. It is distinguished but its knowledge of chemical reactions and laboratory processes. This book has been translated into foreign language.

600-800: A.D. SODHALA (700 AD) two treatises, Gandanighraha, a medical treatise and Sodhala a medical Lexicon.

VRUDUKUNTA (750 AD) writes SIDDAYOGA, the earliest treatise on RASA CHIKITSA now existing intact. The RASA CHIKITSA system considers mercury as the king of all medicines. SIDDAYOGA explain the various preparations of mercury and other metals, alloys, metallic compounds, salts and sulphur. This school of medicine is called SIDDHA school. All of them are made of metals, salts and sulphur. It is supposed to be a continuation of the pre-Aryan medical system in India. It is popular in eastern and southern India.

SIDDHA NAGARJUNA Two treatises on the SIDDHA systems, RASARATHANAKARA and AROGYA MANJARI.

MADHAVACHARYA (700-800 AD) wrote Madhava Nidana. This is a compilation from the earlier works of Agnivesa, Charaka, Sushruta, Vagbhata. It is specially useful as a chemical guide to preparations. It is famous allover India as the best Ayurvedic work on the diagnosis of diseases.

800-1300 AD: A number of treatises were written in India during this period. ARKAPRAKASHA, a book on tincture extraction, SARANGADHARA SAMHITA, Chikitsa, Sangraha and YOGA RATNAKARA are the better known among them.

The period also witnessed a spirit of writing on the RASA CHIKITSA system. RASHA HRIDAYA by Govind Vagbhata, RASARATNAKARA by Siddha Nityananda, RASARATNASAMMUKTA by Vagbhata (another), RASARNAVA by Sambhu, RASENDRACHINTAMANI by Ramachandra, and RASENDRA CHOODAMANI by Somadeva.

1300-1600 AD: BHAVAMISRA wrote BHAVA PRA-KASHA. This is the most renowned Indian treatise during the period. It contains an exhaustive list of diseases and their symptoms and complete list of drugs including many not mentioned in the earlier works. It includes aetiology and treatment of syphilis, a disease brought into India by Portuguese seamen.

Other works of this period are CHIKITSALIYE by Trisata, a

manual on diagnosis; CHINTAMANI by Ballbhendra on aetiology and diagnosis; and VAIDYAMRUTHA by Moreswara on the treatment of diseases.

Another class of works produced during this period are Medical Lexicons by Madanapala, Nagahari, Bimapala, and Rajavallabha.

1600: East India Company established British Rule in India. Western medical and surgery started to be practized and became popular in India.

NURSING IN INDIA

Beginning of Modern Nursing

In the past, the progress of nursing in India has been hindered by many difficulties, such as: the low status of women, the system of purdah among Muslim women, the caste system among Hindus, illiteracy, poverty, political unrest, language differences, and the fact that nursing has been looked upon as servant's work.

Since Independence Day 1947, many changes have taken place and the attitude towards nursing is changing. More women are being educated and many are taking up nursing as their profession.

We have very little information about medicine and nursing in India until the 15th century, when Vasoco de Gama came to India. He set up trading posts on the west coast. Franciscan, Dominican and Jesuit missionaries came to minister to the sick and needy. The Portuguese set up European type of dispensaries at Goa and Madras and physicians from Europe were invited to India. One of these, Garcia da Orta, in 1550 wrote SIMPLES AND DRUGS OF INDIA.

Military Nursing

Military Nursing was the earliest type of nursing. In 1664, the East India Company helped to start a hospital for soldiers at Fort St. George, Madras. Later, a civilian hospital was built and the medical staff, appoined by the East India Company, served in both hospitals. In 1797 a Lying-in-Hospital was built and in 1854 the government sanctioned a Training School for Midwives. In 1861, through the efforts of Miss Nightingale, reforms in military hospitals led to reforms in civil hospitals. Efforts were made to provide health services for the people of India. This laid the foundation for public health nursing.

Nursing in the military hospitals was of poor quality carried on by male orderlies and menial staff. In 1871 the Government General Hospital, Madras undertook a plan to train nurses. Nurses were brought from England to be in-charge and the first six students were those who had previously received their diploma in midwifery. Later this plan was reversed. General training was taken first followed by a course in midwifery.

In Bombay, among the one of the earliest hospitals is the Jamsetjee Jeejeebhoy group, the first of which was opened in 1843. Another hospital which was to play an important part in the development of modern nursing in India was the Pestani Hormusji Cama Hospital for women and children, which was founded in 1883 but not opened until 1886.

Provision for the nursing care of patients in these early hospitals was very limited. In the JJ Group, nursing was done by medical students and menials until 1868 when the government invited the Sisters of the Community of All Saints to come from England and take over the work of nursing. Their work was appreciated and the need for training nurses was felt. At this time, it was difficult to get nurses. There were only a few Anglo-Indian and Indian Christian girls working in mission hospitals. The sisters of all saints took the first steps to establish a training school for nurses in this hospital. In 1891, **Bai Kashibai Ganpat** was the **first Indian nurse** to come for training. Training was at first two years but became three years when the Bombay Presidency Nursing Association was established in 1909.

An outstanding graduate of the JJ Group of hospitals was Miss. TK Adranvala. After her graduation, she worked as a ward sister, then became assistant Matron under the sisters and finally, superintendent of the hospitals. She held this position until she was asked to accept the position of Nursing Superintendent and Nurse adviser to the government of India. She remained in this position until retiring in 1966. She continues active participation in nursing as a WHO representative in Nepal. Miss Adranvala has worked very hard to raise the status of the nursing profession in India. She has given much of her time to the interests of the TNAI having held the office of president for two terms and that of treasurer until she was released at her own request. The nursing profession in India is fortunate to have had such a capable person as Miss Adranvala as its representative on the World Health Organization. She is highly respected by all and many seek her wise counsel.

Mission Hospitals

Mission Hospitals were the first to begin the training of Indians as nurses, very gradually overcoming the prejudices of parents against sending their girls for a training which was felt to be beneath the dignity of decent educated girls. Religion prevented Hindu and Muslim girls from joining at all and so only Christian girls could be trained at first. But for many years, even they felt nursing was an inferior profession.

In the beginning there was no uniformity of courses or educational requirements. About 1907-1910 the North India United Board of Examiners for Mission Hospitals was organized and set up rules for admissions and standards of training and conducted a public examination. On 24th May 1909 the Indian Medical Mission Association granted the Nursing Diploma after examining student by Central Board for Nurses' Training Schools in South India. A few years later the Mid-India and the South India Boards of Nurse examiners were similarly set up.

These are Examining Boards of the Nurses' League of the Christian Medical Association of India. The name of the South India Board was changed to 'The Board of Nursing Education, Nurses' League of Christian Medical Association of India branch in 1975.

The Dufferin Fund

Until the late 19th century there were no women doctors and therefore, no care for women except in mission hospitals. This fact was brought to the attention of Queen Victoria. At this time, Lady Dufferin was coming out to India with her husband who was on government service. Queen Victoria instructed Lady Dufferin about the need for medical care for women and children in India and asked her to take a special interest in this problem. Lady Dufferin wrote to her friends and influential people to get financial aid. Thus, in 1885, Lady Dufferin was responsible for starting the 'National Association for supplying Medical Aid by Women to Women of India'. This is commonly called the Dufferin Fund and continues to provide medical education for women, to train nurses and midwives for hospitals and private work, and to improve medical facilities for women.

Between 1890 and 1900, many schools under either missions or government were started in various parts of India. The directors fo these schools were English or American. Each school sets up its own pattern of training familiar to the director. There was a need for systematic training of nurses like that given in the Nightingale School in England. Thus it was, that in 1886, money from the Dufferin Fund was made available for this purpose. Miss Atkinson, a Nightingale nurse, was brought out from England to Bombay to set up and be the superintendent of the FIRST MODERN TRAINING SCHOOL FOR NURSES IN INDIA. The school was established in the Cama Hospital for Women and Children in 1891. It began with a one year course but by 1995 it had been extended to three years.

The leaders of nursing in India realized that more and better qualified teachers and ward supervisors were needed if standards were to be maintained and nursing was to advance. Hence, courses were set up in several places to give Indian nurses an opportunity to prepare themselves for responsible positions in hospitals and schools of nursing. Post-certificate courses were first offered in nursing administration, supervision and teaching. These originated at the College of Nursing, New Delhi; the College of Nursing, CMC Hospital Vellore and the Government General Hospital, Madras.

The first four-year-basic bachelor degree programmes were established in 1946 at the Colleges of Nursing in Delhi and Vellore. This programme is now offered in a number of other colleges.

In 1963, the School of Nursing in Thiruvananthapuram instituted the first two year post-certificate bachelor degree programme. Other schools have begun this programme since that time.

In recent years, as higher education for nurses has developed around the world, courses in India have developed so that the nurse can specialize in almost any subject and continue education through the level of the Master's degree. The first Master's degree course, a two-year postgraduate programme was begun in 1960 at the College of Nursing in Delhi. (Now Rajkumari Amrit Kaur College of Nursing, New Delhi-110024). In 1970, many colleges of nursing were started and offering PCBSc Nursing and Basic BSc Nursing courses in various parts of India. In Karnataka, Bangalore University instituted Ph D programme for nurses in 1991. The author of this book is the first person to get Doctoral degree in the State of Karnataka.

Auxiliary Nursing

The use of auxiliary nursing personnel to ease the shortage of professional nurses had been common in some countries when it was first put into practice in India. A two-year programme for the Auxiliary Nurse-Midwife was first established in 1951 at St. Mary's Hospital, Tarn Taran in Punjab state. By 1962, there were 263 courses being offered in India. The auxiliary nurse midwife is prepared to practise elementary nursing and full midwifery. She functions primarily in the community rather than the hospital. The practice of the auxiliary nurse-midwife has helped to improve the amount of care given to the patient as well as the health teaching given to the public. In 1977 the ANM course was completely revised by the Indian Nursing Council and expanded to include sociology health education and communication skills and subjects necessary to equip the multipurpose health worker/ANM to serve effectively as a primary health care worker in the community. Such workers are key persons for achievement of the goal of 'Health for all by 2000 AD" to which we in India are committed.

Textbooks

One of the handicaps in the development of nursing schools was the lack of textbooks. In other countries books had been written by doctors and nurses. Some of these were translated into the vernacular for the early schools and colleges. Many English and American textbooks are being used in the schools today. There is a great nccd for textbooks which have been written by Indian nurses. A beginning had been made in this work and the first TEXTBOOK FOR NURSES IN INDIA was printed by the South India Examining Board of the Nurses' League of the Christian Medical Association of India in 1941. The Nurses' League has also directed the publishing of a TEXTBOOK FOR AUXILIARY NURSE-MIDWIVES, first printed in 1967. This book was completely revised and published in two volumes in 1985 as a TEXTBOOK FOR THE HEALTH WORKER (ANM) to meet the needs of the health worker. Several manuals related to the basic sciences and nursing have been published by other professional nursing bodies. Although progress has been made in the publication of textbooks by the nurses of India, there remains a wide area of subjects which have not been touched upon and the general need for more and varied textbooks continues. Since a few nursing educator started writing texts on Nursing, to quote, Late Dr. (Mrs) Kasturi Sunder Rao wrote text on 'Community Health Nursing, and a few Bombay-based Nurses made an effort to write guides and two books on Nursing. In later part of 1990s the author of this book also has written on **'Nursing Research'** (1998), **Community Health Nursing** (1998), **Nursing Administration, Nursing Education** and Fundamentals of Nursing on the basis of present needs in Indian context.

Nursing education in India began with very brief periods of training as mentioned in the first part of this chapter. Orderlies and midwives were often chosen for this and were given a period of two to six months of closely supervised practical experience in general nursing, then called 'sick nursing'. This was training in the hospital, and certificates were given after completion of a training.

The basic programme for combined general nursing and midwifery developed rapidly after 1871. The need for theory as well as practical experience was felt. The training for general nursing was extended to two years and then three years before the student went on for midwifery training. The present basic programme for nursing education throughout India consists of a three-year programme in general nursing and six to seven months in midwifery. Uniformity of training is maintained by recognition of schools which meet the standards and requirements given by the Indian Nursing Council. The basic certificate programme now includes all areas of nursing as integrated community health nursing.

REGISTRATION OF NURSES

As training for nurses, midwives, and health visitors progressed, the need for legislation to provide basic minimum standards in education and training was felt. It was also felt that registration would give greater professional status. For some years, nurses struggled to obtain proper examinations and examiners and registration for nurses. In 1926 Madras State formed the first Registration Council. While most states now have a recognized Registration Council, all do not. It is now possible for the students of all schools in India to be registered in one of the State Registration Councils.

The Indian Nursing Council

The Indian Nursing Council Act was passed by an ordinance on December 31st 1947. The council was constituted in 1949. The purpose of the council is to co-ordinate activities of the various State Registration Councils, to set up standards for nursing education and to make sure these standards are carried out. Before this time, nurses registered in one state were not necessarily recognised for registration in another. The condition to mutual recognition by the State Nurses Registration Council called reciprocity was possible only if uniform standards of nursing education was maintained. Therefore, the INC was given authority to prescribe curricula for nursing education in all of the states. At the same time, it was given authority to recognize programmes of nursing education or refuse recognition. The Indian Nursing Council is not itself a registering body nor examining body but it can enforce its standards by recognizing or refusing to recognize schools.

Community Health Nursing

In India community health nursing had its beginning when the terrible conditions under which children were born were recognized as a cause for the high civilian mortality rate. It was realized that the untrained *dais* who attended women during delivery must be given training. This was not an easy job as the *dais* were unwilling to be trained and the patients were very willing to accept the old customary methods and could see no need to change. The first attempts to train *dais* were carried out by missionaries as early as 1886. In 1900, Lady Curzon brought about the establishment of the Victoria Memorial Scholarship for the purpose of improving safe delivery practices. The need for training a better type of midwife was felt. In this, Madras State led the way when they passed the Madras Registration of Nurses and Midwives Act of 1926.

Slowly the need for trained personnel for maternal and childhealth, as part of community health nursing was felt. To supply this need a Health School for the training of health visitors was started in Delhi in 1918. This has now become the Lady Reading Health School.

A further step forward was taken in 1948, when community health nursing was integrated in the basic programme of the new degree courses which were started at the College of Nursing, Delhi and the School of Nursing, CMC Hospital, Vellore under the University of Delhi and Madras respectively.

Since 1953, a post-certificate course in community health nursing has been given at the All India Institute of Hygiene and Public Health in Calcutta. In 1960, a course was established by the Lady Reading Health School in Delhi. Several other schools now offer this programme.

To prepare more community Health nurses, in 1957 the Government of India selected ten schools of nursing and gave assistance so that they could integrate community health nursing into their basic course. Since that time, recognition of a programme of basic nursing education required that community health nursing be integrated into the basic course. Thus, all professional nurses today can function in the hospital and the community at the level of a staff nurse.

Various international organizations, such as WHO, UNICEF and Colombo Plan have assisted by supplying trained personnel and equipment to help in the training of students in the rural field, maternity work and paediatrics.

THE NURSES' RESPONSIBILITY FOR THE FUTURE OF NURSING

Throughout this study of nursing we have seen nursing advance from the kindly ministrations of a mother or a neighbour to the highly organized service of today. In the beginning individuals were inspired to help one another in distress. This essential care or service still remains but time has brought about changes in our ideas regarding nursing. Today we are not only relieve and give comfort but help our patients to live upto their optimum health. The new emphasis is on health nursing—nursing the mind, the family as a whole and as part of the community with the nurse as the health teacher.

Growing specialisation in medicine is resulting in a trend towards increased specialisation in nursing. The development of new tests and diagnostic procedures, new medicines and new equipment make specialisation even more necessary as the amount of scientific knowledge needed for a certain speciality becomes greater. Developments in other professions also influence trends in the nursing profession. As other members of the health team become more available and more highly specialized, the work of the nurse is changing towards more specific nursing functions. It has also added to the number and kind of professional relationships which must be maintained by the nurse. The power of spiritual factors is becoming of increasing interest as reports of the healing power of spiritual activity such as meditation is receiving more attention. Just as advances in technology tend to take the nurse away from the bedside and a direct relationship with the patient, so these developments are showing the need for a deeper therapeutic relationship between the nurse and the patient. The future will demand a balance of these factors in order to meet the total health needs of the individual and the community. Future trends are likely to show an effort to make this balance.

Many trends leading to professionalism are taking place because of the untiring efforts of nurses dedicated to achieving the aim of becoming a profession. In 1970, WHO recognized *Nursing* as a profession. It has often been a difficult struggle requiring real courage and vision by nursing leaders in the face of serious obstacles. Today nurses enjoy many rights and privileges, though desired standards are still not achieved in all areas, because nursing leaders have struggled to achieve them. Nurses who are going to be the future leaders have to carry on this work of greater achievement through growing amounts of writing and research.

Nursing today provides an ever widening scope of opportunity for service. With present trends leading towards greater opportunities, varieties of services and growing social and professional recognition, it should be exciting and challenging for nurses to know that all nurses members of this profession since they fulfill the criteria of the profession. (for further details please read the authors text on "NURSING ADMINISTRATION".

Nursing Process Application

In the past, nurses have prided themselves on comforting those, who are ill and on executing with precision such tasks as dressing wounds administering medications, and bathing, feeding and ambulating client. Many of these tasks were ordered by doctors and few nurses would have characterized their 'Job' on being independent, scientifically based or creative. Now health care delivery system has changed, and nursing has changed with it. Nurses now work with well and ill clients in all settings. In addition to their role as caregiver, nurses fill specialized roles as care managers—co-ordinators, teachers, counsellors, advocates, nursing administrators, nurse-educators and nurse researchers. Nurses are responsible for a unique dimension of health care "the diagnosis and treatment of human responses to actual or potential health problems" (ANA 1980) and as such are knowledgeable, competent, and independent professionals who work collaboratively with other health care professionals to design and deliver holistic care.

As the practice of nursing became more complex, nurses began to study the process of nursing to both understand and improve the means nurses used to accomplish their aims. It has been assumed that professional nursing practice is interpersonal in nature. Recognizing the importance and effect of the nurse's relationships with the client /patient professional nurses use this knowledge throughout the nursing process. It is also assumed that professional nurses view human being as holistic, thereby acknowledging that mind and body are not separate but function as a whole. People respond as unique whole beings. What happens is one part of mind or body affects the person as a whole. These assumptions give clue that nursing is interpersonal in nature and the professional nurses view human beings as holistic, give guidance and directions to the use of the nursing process.

NATURE OF NURSING PROCESS

As studied earlier, "nursing is the diagnosis and treatment of human responses to actual or potential problems". The fundamental basis of nursing practice is "Process". Every aspect of practice is affected by an understanding and utilization of nursing practice.

Nursing process is an organized approach to problem-solving and decision-making that describes the intellectual activity of the nurse. It is the accepted methodology for nursing practice. The nursing process is the underlying scheme that provides order and direction of nursing care. It is the essence of profession—Nursing practice. It is the 'tool' and methodology of the nursing profession and as such it helps nurses in arriving at decisions and in predicting and evaluating consequences.

The nursing process is a *"deliberate, intellectual activity* by which the practice of nursing is approached in an orderly *systematic* manner. Each of these terms for defining the process can be further delineated as follows:

- 'Deliberate' refers to careful, thoughtful and intentional process.
- 'Intellectual' refers to the process has rational, knowledgeable, reasonable and conceptional.
- 'Activity' refers to state or condition of functioning, *initiating*, changing and behaving.
- 'Orderly' refers to that it is methodological, efficient, and has logical arrangement.
- 'Systematic' means to purposeful and pertaining to classification.

The nursing process is a method of making clinical decisions. It is a way of thinking and acting in relation to the clinical phenomena of concern to nurses. Classifically the nursing process comprises of five phases or dimensions: assessment, nursing diagnosis, planning, implementation and evaluation. The nursing process is a systematic decision-making model that is cyclic not lineal (Fig. 2.1). By virtue of evaluational phase, the nursing process incorporates a feedback loop that maintains quality control of its decision-making outputs.

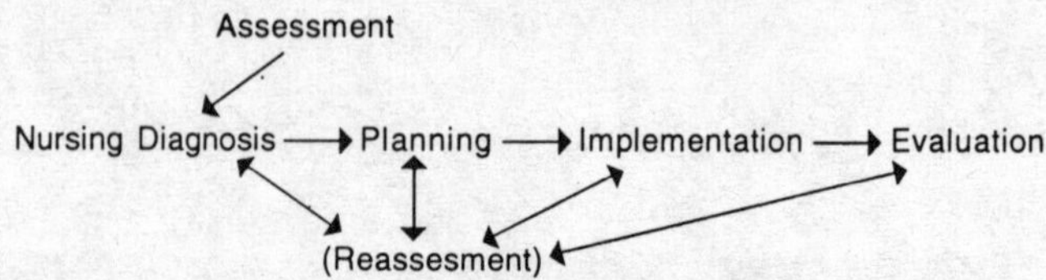

Fig. 2.1: The Nursing Process

The nursing process is indeed a method of solving clinical problems but it is not merely a problem-solving method. Similar to a problem-solving method, the nursing process offers an organized, systematic, approach to clinical problems. Unlike a problem solving method, the nursing process is continuous, not episodic. The five phases constitute a continuous cycle throughout the nurses' moment-to-moment data interpretation and management of patient care. The phases of nursing process being not only continuous, but "interactive" in other words, all phases of the nursing process operate and influence each other and the patient simultaneously. This illustrates interactive nature of the nursing process, wherein each phase represented by a line that intersects with others and converges at point in time to which the nurse attends.

The nursing process was developed as a specific method for applying a scientific approach or a problem-solving approach to nursing practice. Problem-solving approaches are not unique to nursing. For example, health planners have long used a health planning process that is a problem-solving approach aimed at planned social change. Physicians use a specific process for gathering assessment data to make a medical diagnosis. The nursing process deals with problem specific to nurses and their clients/patients. In nursing client/patient may be an individual, family, or community, and the nursing process has been adapted for use with each type of client/patient (Christensen and Kenny 1990).

Students of nursing using the nursing process are learning to behave as professional nurses in practice behave. Since the nursing process is the essence and tool (methodology) of professional nursing practice, student must become familiar with and adopt at using it as their basis of practice. The nursing process also provides, a means for evaluating the quality of nursing care given by nurses and assures their accountability and responsibility to the client/patient.

To use the nursing process effectively, nurses need to understand and apply appropriate concepts and theories from nursing, the theological, physical and behavioural sciences and the humanities. These concepts and theories provide a rationale for decision making, judgements, interpersonal relationships and actions. These concepts provide the framework for nursing care.

DEFINITION OF NURSING PROCESS

The nursing process is often defined as the application of critical thinking to client-care activities. In addition, because nursing is a human-caring discipline, other styles of thinking influence nursing decision. Four ways of thinking which include ritual, random, appreciative and critical thinking. Ritual thinking underlies the development of habits-actions we perform so often or regularly, that we do them automatically, without conscious decisions. Random thinking is the free association of ideas at the unconscious level that can lead to impulsive implementation of the first problem solving solution that comes to mind it can also be creating source of new problem-solving ideas and approaches. Appreciative thinking reflects awareness of human values and respect for client's individual needs. Critical thinking is based on the acientific method, i.e. the deliberate and systematic use of rational informed thought processes in problem finding and problem solving. It is the key stone of sensible decision making using the nursing process and it yields predictable, repeatable results.

The nursing process can be defined in terms of three major dimensions which include purpose, organization and properties.

Purpose

The primary purpose of the nursing process is to help manage each client care scientifically, holistically and creatively. To do this successfully the nurse needs many intellectual, technical and interpersonal and ethical/legal competencies as well as the willingness to use them creatively when working with the clients to promote wellness, to prevent disease, or illness, to restore health and to facilitate coping with altered functioning.

Organization

The nursing process has traditionally defined as a systematic method for assessing health status, diagnosing health care needs, formulating a plan of care, initiating and implementing plan and evaluating the effectiveness of plan of care. The nursing process consists of five sequential steps or inter-related phases, i.e. assessment, nursing diagnosis, planning implementation, and evaluation. These are considered as organized steps or components or nursing process.

Properties

The nursing process has seven properties, that is, systematic dynamic, interpersonal, flexible, theoretically-based, goal-oriented and universally applicable. Here the various words and phrases have been used to describe the nursing process.

1. *Systematic:*

The nursing process is a systematic method that directs the nurse and client as together determine the need for nursing care, plan and implement the care and evaluate the results. The steps in this client-centred, goal-oriented process are interrelated each of the five steps preceding it. The process provides a framework that enables the nurse and client to do the following.

- Collect systematically clients' data (assessing)
- Clearly identify client strengths and problem (diagnosing)
- Develop holistic plan of individualized care that specified the desired client goals and related outcomes and the nursing interventions most likely to assist the client to meet those expected outcomes (planning)
- Execute the plan of care (implementing)
- Evaluate the effectiveness of the plan of care in terms of the client goal and achievement (evaluation).

The nursing process directs each step of nursing care in a sequential order/manner. So it is systematic.

2. *Dynamic:*
The nursing process is dynamic, because it involves continuous change. It is an ongoing process focussed on the changing responses of the client that are identified throughout the nurse-client relationship.

3. *Interpersonal:*
The nursing process is interpersonal. Always at the heart of nursing is the human being. It is interactive because the interactive nature is based on the reciprocal relationship that occurs between the nurse and the client, family and other health professionals.

4. *Flexible:*
The nursing process is flexible, because the flexibility of the process may be demonstrated in two contexts.

- It can be adapted to nursing practice and any setting or area of specialization dealing with individuals, groups or communities.
- Its phrases may be used sequentially and concurrently, i.e. the nursing process is most frequently used in sequence, however, the nurse may use more than one step at a time.

5. *Theoretically based:*
The nursing process is theoretically based because the process is devised from a broad-based knowledge including the sciences and humanities and can be applied to any other theoretical models of nursing.

6. *Goal-oriented:*
The nursing process is goal oriented because it offers a means for nurses and clients to work together to identify specific goal related to wellness promotion, disease and illness prevention, health restoration and coping with altered functioning, which are most important to client, and to match them with appropriate nursing actions. Once these are recorded in the plan of care, each nurse can quickly determine the client's priorities and begins nursing with a clear sense of how to proceed. The client benefits from continuity of care and each nurse can move the client close to good achievement.

7. *Universally applicable:*
The nursing process is universally applicable the one constant in health care is changed. Once nurses have a working knowledge of the nursing process, they find that they can practice nursing with well or ill persons, young or old, in any type of practice setting. Efforts made by the nurses to master nursing process will result in their possession of a valuable tool that can be used with ease in any nursing situation.

STEPS OF NURSING PROCESS

Nursing process involves five steps which include assessment, nursing diagnosis, planning, implementation and evaluation. In earlier writings about the nursing process, many authors agreed that four phases components, steps or stages were necessary; assessment, including nursing diagnosis or problem identification, planning, intervention or implementation and evaluation. Because nursing diagnosis is the considered essential component of the nursing process, majority of them are accepted as one step in the nursing process, Let us examine in brief of each step.

Assessment

Assessment is the first phase in the nursing process and has two subphases which include data collection and data analysis or synthesis. Assessment consists of the systematic and orderly collections and analysis of data about the health status of the client/patient for the purpose of making the nursing diagnosis. If incorrect or insufficient assessment leads to incorrect nursing diagnosis which could mean inappropriate planning, implementation and evaluations. Therefore, the importance of accurate assessment cannot be overemphasized. It is vital to the process and is the basis for all other phases. Although assessment is the first phase, it may also occur as reassessment during any other phase of the process when new data are obtained as shown in Figure 2.1.

The systematic and orderly collection of data is essential for the nurse to know if sufficient data have been collected. It also provides a method of quick retrieval of information about the client/patient for auditing professional practice and for doing research. In addition, it serves as a means of communicating information to their health care providers, assessing involves, a thorough, ongoing, comprehensive collection of subjective and objective data of the patient-family-environment, interactions. Such data are obtained via history-taking, observation, physical examination, laboratory data, X-rays and other diagnostic studies. Use of *functional health* pattern (GORDON. M. 1987) assists in eliciting information concern in nursing. A holistic view during assessment phase ensures that the biological, psychological, social, cultural and spiritual spheres of the client are considered. Any assessment guidelines include the following:

- Biographical data.
- A health history including family members.
- Subjective data and objective data about current health status including physical examination and reason for contact with health care professional, medical diagnosis, if the client/patient has a medical problem, and results of diagnostic studies.
- Social, cultural, and environmental data.
- Behaviours that may place a person at risk for potential disease/problems.

By using these guidelines, the data collected are classified into discrete areas that can be compared, contrasted for relationships and clustered during the analysis of data. The current health status of the client is also ascertained through interviewing the client or the person responsible for the client (subjective data) and thorough examination and observation of the client to obtain data that can be seen or measured objectively (objective data). For example, client's description of pain is considered subjective data, whereas vital signs are an example of objective measurement.

By virtue of nursing's unique orientation and commitment to holism, nurses collect an enormous amount of data about a patient's biopsychosocial health status. And by virtue of an array of techno-physiologic monitoring devices, nurses process an additional layer of data in the form of physiologic parameter measurements. Consequently, assembling this data base, nurses need some place to file the information as it is collected. Ideally, this storage system would contain compartments, which could keep the data separated and organized. Such system is called as *assessment* or *organizational framework*.

Organizational framework can also serve as guides for assessment and their compartments consists of headings corresponding to the attributes the nurse accepts as constituting the nature of human health illness and nursing. In this way, framework helps guide the identification of diagnosis that are within the domain of nursing.

Assessment frameworks are neither new nor unique to nursing. Traditionally nursing used medical assessment framework for the collection and organization of data, but a nursing knowledge base and conceptual orientations become increasingly differentiated and complex, the biologic mechanistic scheme of medicine was found to be insufficiently comprehensive for its use by nurses as a tool for holistic assessment.

- The assessment framework for the generalist medical practice include body systems like cardiovascular, respiratory, neurologic, endocrine metabolic, hematopoietic, integumentory, gastrointestinal, genitourinary, reproductive, and psychiatric.
- The functional health pattern typology developed by *Marjory Gordon* are categories of human biologic, psychologic, developmental, cultural, social and spiritual assessment, has gained wide acceptance in nursing service and education systems as assessing framework which includes:
  - Health perception—health management
  - Nutritional—metabolic
  - Eliminations
  - Activity—exercises
  - Sleep—rest
  - Cognitive—perceptual
  - Self-perception—self-concept
  - Role—relationship
  - Sexuality—reproductive
  - Coping—stress tolerance
  - Value—belief
- And Nine human responses revised by NANDA (1986) named NANDA (North American Nursing Diagnostic Association).

Taxonomy I (system of classification that organizes known phenomena into a hierarchic structure and helps direct the discovery of new phenomena). The specifications of a nomenclature and its successor, a taxonomy, is an important preliminary step in building nursing theory and science. The Nine human responses patterns of taxonomy I revised are as follows:

1. Exchanging: A human response pattern involving mutual giving and receiving.
2. Communicating: A human response pattern involving sending messages.
3. Relating: A human response pattern involving establishing bonds.
4. Valuing: A human response pattern involving the assigning of relative worth.
5. Choosing: A human response pattern involving selection of alternatives.
6. Moving: A human response pattern involving activities.
7. Perceiving: A human response pattern involving reception of informations.
8. Knowing: A human response pattern involving the meaning associated with information.
9. Feeling: A human response pattern involving the subjective awareness of information.

The selection of any one framework over another, as long as it is designed to organize nursing data is an individual choice.

Nursing Diagnosis

Nursing diagnosis, the second phase of the nursing process is recognized in ANA definition of nursing as the diagnosis and treatment of human responses to actual or potential health problems. The concept of nursing diagnosis, a process whereby nurses interpret assessment data and apply standardized labels to health problems they identify and anticipate treating, is rapidly evolving in clinical and educational settings. Critical attention is being focused on aspects of nursing practice and education that either foster or inhibit the establishment of the discipline nursing as a profession. A traditional reliance on the language and therapeutics of other sciences is inhibiting the establishment of nursing as a free-standing profession. Effort to identify and name the conditions that nurses study and treat, on the other hand, foster nursing professional identity by clarifying its distinct services to society and providing a vehicle for the building of its science.

A nursing diagnosis is a clinical judgement about individual, family or community responses to actual or potential health problems/life processes provide the basis for selection of nursing interventions to achieve outcomes for which the nurse is accountable" (NANDA 1990). This diagnostic statement identifies the client's actual or potential health problems deficit or concern, which can be affected by nursing actions. It describes a group of data with interpretation based on the client's ability to meet basic needs. Models for these diagnostic statements have been provided by many authors based on the taxonomy developed by NANDA. For most clients, there will be more than one nursing diagnosis (in medicine also now there will be more than one medical diagnosis).

Nursing diagnostic statements are derived from the nurse's *inferences* which are based on the assessed and validated data coupled with nursing, scientific and humanistic concepts and theories. The term 'inference' is very useful in defining nursing diagnosis, because it emphasizes the tentative and assumptive nature of diagnoses. *Inference* refers to the process of arriving at a conclusion by reasoning from evidence" and warns that "if the evidence is slight the term comes close to surmise". In recognizing that *element* of both judgement and inference are part of nursing diagnosis, one can appreciate the need to limit or control the influence of bias on the part of the nurses and in the act of diagnosing so that the diagnostic conclusion reached is as logical and factually based as possible.

The human response to health and illness situation constitutes the focus of phenomenon, of concern to nurses, and it is the object of nurse's diagnostic activities. As one proceeds through the analysis of data, certain patterns develop and the use of relevant concepts and theories become appropriate. Nursing diagnosis can be considered a client-related behavioural statement that identifies the area for focus of nursing action. A diagnosis may deal with an actual (present-oriented) or a potential (future-oriented) health problem. It is based on conclusions reached in the assessment phase.

Formulating Nursing Diagnosis Statements

Guidelines for use of the taxonomy of approved nursing diagnosis. It is important to recognize that classification of the phenomena to which a profession addresses itself is a sizable and ongoing task. The development and refinement of nursing's nomenclature of health status are in their earliest stages and subject to much revision based on the reserved and clinical reports presented and reviewed at each of NANDA's conferences and by the Diagnosis Review Committee. Work on existing diagnoses also is incomplete. Several have eitiologies and defining characteristics yet to be developed, making clinical use difficult and frustrating. Other diagnosis may be deleted from the approved list from conference to conference. Such changes are both necessary and usual in the process of taxonomy development. One has only to look at the system of names describing health problems treated by physicians not many years ago (for example, chilblain's consumption, dropsy) to appreciate nursing's progress to date.

Guidelines for Diagnostic Labels

Definitions of health problems Nearly all approved diagnoses have accompanying definitions to better explain the health state they represent. These definitions are important for the student of nursing diagnosis to consider, because they clarify more about the health state than is apparent from the label alone. For example, the definition accompanying the disgnose's fear and anxiety draw a particularly useful distinction between the two problems. Fear is an emotion that has an identifiable source or object that the patient validates, whereas anxiety is an emotion whose source is non-specific or unknown to the patient. Other good examples of such definitions accompany the diagnoses social isolation, powerlessness, altered parenting, and caregiver role strain.

Until definitions accompany all approved diagnoses, it is important for nurses collaborating in care to establish consensus about the meaning and scope of the health problems stated.

Making diagnostic labels specific Some nursing diagnoses need accompanying qualifiers or specifiers based on the characteristics of the health problem as it manifests itself in a particular patient. For example, the diagnosis fear needs specification as to the object of the patient's particular fear, such as death, pain, disfigurement, or malignancy. Similarly, the diagnosis knowledge deficit needs specification about the content of the deficit, such as use of incentive spirometer, counting the pulse rate or respiratory muscle strengthening exercise. Following is a list of nursing diagnoses needing specification, each with an example of a particular patient circumstance so specified:

Fear: Postoperative pain.

Knowledge deficit: Self-monitoring of oral anticoagulation therapy.

Altered peripheral: Tissue perfusion.

Altered nutrition: Less than body potassium requirements.

Altered nutrition: More than body *kilocalorie* requirements.

Self-care deficit: Bathing and feeding.

Non-compliance: Prescribed activity restrictions.

Guidelines for Aetiologic/related factors

Making aetiologies specific In many instances, NANDA's aetiologies are broad categories or examples needing to be made specific based on characteristics of the health state and the patient being treated. For example, one of several possible etiologies for the diagnosis fluid volume excess is COMPROMISED REGULATORY MECHANISM. Considering this, the cause of the fluid excess in a particular patient, the nurse needs to specify which regulatory mechanism and in what way compromised (for example, inappropriate ADH secretion by the neurohypophysis) before the diagnosis can be formally stated (disregarding the question of whether the problem is treatable by nurses or needs referoal).

Several aetiologies needing to be made specific follow-up along with examples of such specification in parenthesis;

- Situational crisis (recent diagnosis of terminal illness).
- Psychologic injuring agent (hurtful relationship, verbal abuse).

- Developmental factors (developmental arrest, extremes of age).

Nursing diagnoses as aetiologies Nursing diagnostic labels may rightfully serve as aetiologies for other diagnoses. Examples are anxiety R/T* knowledge deficit, and activity intolerance R/T decreased cardiac output.

Aetiologies as the focus of treatment The treatment plan formulated for a given diagnosis must include interventions aimed at resolution or management of the aetiologic factors, as well as the health state. In fact, in some instances nursing treatment is directed exclusively at the aetiology of a diagnosis, with the logical expectation that, if the causative factors are reduced in influence, the problem should begin to resolve. This is true especially in instances where a nursing diagnosis has as its aetiology another nursing diagnosis, consider treatment approaches to the diagnosis. In effective breathing pattern R/T there is high abdominal incision pain. Predictably, little effectiveness is shown if the interventions are focused solely on reviewing the rationale for slow, deep symmetrical, breathing; demonstrating the technique; and encouraging the patient in its performance without some plan for manipulation of the pain variable.

Medical diagnoses as aetiologies Because, as mentioned, the aetiology of a nursing diagnosis becomes a focus of intervention in the management of the overall health state, citing a medical condition or diagnosis as the aetiology is conceptually inadvisable if the diagnostic statement is to retain its identity as a health problem primarily resolved by nursing therapies. And yet, many health states of concern to critical care nurse and amenable to their treatment are consequent to medical conditions. Examples are the ineffective airway clearance that results from chronic obstructive pulmonary disease (COPD), and sensory-perceptual alterations that result from coronary artery bypass graft surgery. In these instances the nurse should isolate those aspects of the contributing pathologic state that are modifiable by nursing intervention and cite these factors as aetiologic, for instance, ineffective airway clearance R/T thick tracheobronchial secretions, respiratory muscle weakness, and knowledge deficit; effective cough and hydration techniques, and sensory-perceptual alterations R/T sensory overload, sensory depression, and sleep pattern disturbance. These diagnostic statements are more clearly worded and provide a much sharper focus for nursing intervention.

Guidelines for Defining Characteristics

Making defining characteristics specific As with diagnostic labels and statements of aetiology, defining characteristics cited for diagnoses are in non-specific form and often need to be modified to reflect the particular situation presented by the patient being diagnosed. For example, the diagnosis impaired gas exchange has as one of the possible defining characteristics ABNORMAL BLOOD GASES. In the nurses' formulation of this diagnostic statement for clinical use, the specific blood gas value used to diagnose the problem should be cited in the statement (e.g. PO_2 : 54 mm Hg and /or PCO_2 : 50 mm Hg) versus the non-specific sign category, abnormal blood gases.

Several defining characteristics are cited as following non-specific form with accompanying examples of proper specification:

- Respiratory depth changes (hypoventilation)
- Blood pressure changes (hypotension)
- Autonomic responses (dilated pupils, tachycardia)
- Altered electrolytes (hypokalemia)
- Change in mental state (confusion, obtundation, apprehension)

Major or critical defining characteristics Major or critical defining characteristics are designated signs and/or symptoms that must be present for the health problem to be considered present. Major defining characteristics, when applicable, must be present in the nurse's assessment profile to diagnose the corresponding health state with any degree of certainty. For example, the diagnosis unilateral neglect has as its major defining characteristic *Consistent in attention to stimuli on affected side*. It is essential, then, that the characteristic be present in the patient's situation (in addition, perhaps, to several other noncritical signs) for the diagnosis of the problem. The assignment of major or critical status to a defining characteristic is based on research or extensive clinical experience in which the signs and symptoms of a health problem are tested for their ability to meet reliably predict the presence of the diagnosis and can therefore be used with confidence by the nurse diagnostician.

Guidelines for Diagnosing High-Risk States

Determining a risk state for diagnosis Predicting a potential health problem in a given patient involves an estimation of probability. The potential for an event, or pattern of response, to occur can truly be said to exist in almost any situation. Consider the high-risk health problems facing the postoperative patient. This risk state includes high-risk for non-compliance with the rehabilitative regimen, high-risk for body image disturbance, high-risk for sleep pattern, disturbance, high-risk for ineffective airway clearance, high-risk for constipation and high-risk for aspiration, to name only a few. To state each of these diagnoses on a treatment plan without regard for probabilities and develop desired patient outcomes and interventions for each is pointless.

What should occur is an appraisal of the patient's health status and the identification of risk factors that place him or her at higher risk for the health problem than the general population. For example, all persons recovering from abdominal surgery have high-risk for constipation because of the effects of general anaesthesia and narcotic analgesics, manipulation of abdominal viscera, and postoperative immobility. All nurses have a tacit understanding of this risk, and monitoring and intervention are carried out as part of routine nursing care to avert the problem. Hence there is no need to state the problem*.

A patient is at higher risk than the general population of postoperative patient if there is, for example, a history of dependence on laxatives, fluid volume deficit, prolonged immobility, or non-compliance with nursing prescriptions for ambulation. The diagnosis indicating this potential and its risk factors could be stated so that additional and/or more intensified interventions, over those that are routine, can be planned.

Stating high-risk diagnosis Several of the approved diagnoses address potential dysfunctional status and cite risk factors. Examples of such diagnoses are the following.

Altered Nutrition: High-risk for more than body requirements.

High-risk for aspiration
High-risk for disuse syndrome
High-risk for impaired skin integrity
High-risk for infection
High-risk for injury
High-risk for poisoning
High-risk for suffocation
High-risk for trauma
High-risk for violence.

In addition to those diagnoses formally listed as high-risks, any diagnosis from the approved list can be stated as an at risk problem by simply adding the modifier high-risk to the label. For example, self-esteem disturbance can be written high-risk for self esteem disturbance by virtue of the presence of factors but not yet the actual health problem.

High-risk nursing diagnoses have only two parts to the statement: the HEALTH PROBLEM AT RISK and the RISK FACTORS (e.g. high-risk for ineffective individual coping, risk factors, malignant biopsy results, absence of inter personal support system, and history of alcohol abuse).

Guidelines for Stating Wellness Diagnoses

Wellness nursing diagnoses represent clinical judgements regarding an individual, family, or community in transition from a specific level of wellness and functioning to a higher level of wellness and functioning. The terms potential for enhanced (specify) is the designated diagnostic label. Wellness diagnoses are one-part statements, for example, potential for enhanced parenting, potential for enhanced coping.

Diagnostic reasoning Diagnostic reasoning is the critical thinking process through which the nurse moves to arrive at a nursing diagnosis. Like any process, it is often orderly and systematic, However, unlike a process, not all of its factors and operations exist in one's conscious awareness. The challenge of refining one's diagnostic reasoning is to bring into awareness the factors and operations that influence the process and are necessary in arriving at an accurate "answer" or diagnosis. Four key components of diagnostic reasonings are collecting and organizing the data base, identifying cues, making inferences, and validating inferences.

Collecting and organizing the data-base Collecting and organizing a data-base was discussed earlier.

Identifying cues A cue is a piece of information, a raw fact. Nurses notice and seek cues regarding patients' health status and functioning. Sweaty palms, restlessness, and a heart rate of 102 beats/min. are cues. In the process of diagnostic reasoning, cues are the units of information that are collected and recorded for later analysis.

Making inferences An Inference is the assignment of meaning to cues. A nursing diagnosis is an example of an inference. When individual cues are clustered and interpreted collectively, they begin to assume an identity different from what each represents individually. Sweaty palms, restlessness, and a heart rate of 102 beats/min. when interpreted as a cluster could now represent anxiety, shock, fear or pain.

Inferences are created, whereas cues exist. The process of creating inferences from cues, therefore, carries with it the risk of error in logic. If the cues sweaty palms, restlessness, and a heart rate of 102 beats/min were grouped and interpreted in a patient, who also manifested gargling respiratory sounds and a rapid shallow breath in pattern and these additional cues were overlooked or ignored by the person assigning meaning to the cluster—the inference might be erroneous, the more probable inference now might be erroneous, the more probable inference now being ineffective airway clearance. Nursing diagnoses are inferences, and defining characteristics and risk factors are the cues that lead to these inferences.

Validating inferences Once a diagnostic inference is formulated, the nurse will develop and implement a treatment plan designed to resolve or reduce the problem represented by that inference. Erroneous inferences carry, an obvious implication in terms of potential patient harm resulting from treatment of a non-existent health problem or from treatment withheld for a missed diagnostic nursing malpractice. Consequently, it is assential to seek validation of diagnostic interferences before implementing treatments.

Four approaches to the validation of interferences are recommended. First, consult with an authoritative source. This may be a clinical nurse specialist, nurse educator, textbook or published research, for example, Seek confirmation of the logical and scientific integrity of your diagnostic statement. Second, reexam the cues; could the ones in the diagnostic statement support and other diagnosis or only the one chosen? Could the cues from the data base believe not to be a part of the cluster supporting this diagnosis belong to some other cluster, or could several of them, together with cues supporting this diagnosis, suggest an altogether different diagnosis? Third, validate inferences with the patient. Nurses may share with the patient the cluster of cues identified and what is represented.

*(No need to state the problem on an individualised nursing care plan; however, this high risk diagnosis should be on record in a standards of care manual or standardized care plan.)

Patients often have remarkable insight into what underlies their pattern of response and can be a great resource in validating the nurse's conclusions. Additionally, people benefit significantly from having their situations reflected back to them. Indeed, collaborating with the patient in this way may be all the interversion that is necessary. Fourth seek evidence of the reliability of the diagnostic inference from within the appropriate reference group. Do most professional peers conclude the same explanation for the available cues?

These approaches are workable strategies for seeking validation of diagnostic references before the institution of treatment, however the only way to achieve or confirm validation of a diagnosis is to treat the problem and evaluate the outcome. If favourable and predicted outcomes result, strong evidence exists that the problem and its aetiology or risk factors and defining characteristics were accurately inferred.

Source of diagnostic error Much scientific curiosity exists within the nursing profession regarding the diagnostic reasoning process, strategies employed by experts and those used by notices. The following discussion focuses only on the most common type of diagnostic error. THE INFERENTIAL LEAP, and several of the sources. For more in-depth examinations of the skills of clinical problem solving and decision-making, the reader is referred to Gordon, Carneveli, Tanner and Benner.

Inferential leap As the term implies, the inferential leap involves a jump to a conclusion based on premature termination of the data gathering/data analysis phase of the nursing process. Numerous studies show that this jump to an erroneous conclusion is most frequently made because not all of the variables are known or examined at the time the inference is fomulated. Of interest, the novice often closes the SEARCH for cues prematurely, whereas the expert will more often prematurely terminate the ANALYSIS of cues.

The novice may close the search for cues prematurely because of a lack of understanding of the scope of the problem to be diagnosed. Diagnose such as disturbance in self-concept and infective individual coping are reported to be at the highest level of abstraction among nursing diagnoses and are, therefore, more difficult to fully grasp, let along discriminate from other diagnostic possibilities. The expert has an advantage in this regard by virtue of a greater breadth of experience, both with the label and the clinical presentation of patients demonstrating the diagnosis.

Professional advantages of nursing diagnosis Baer assembled from the literature the following statements in advocacy of nursing diagnosis. They are presented here to highlight the advantages nursing diagnosis brings to the profession. Nursing diagnosis does the following:

- Assists in organizing, defining and developing nursing knowledge or scope.
- Aids in identifying and describing the domain and scope of nursing practice.
- Focus as nursing care on the patient's response to problems.
- Prescribes diagnosis-specific nursing interventions that should increase the effectiveness of nursing care.
- Facilitates the evaluation of nursing practice.
- Provides a framework for testing the validity of nursing interventions.
- Provides a standardized vocabulary to enhance intraprofessional and interprofessional communication.
- Prescribes the content of nursing curricula.
- Provides a framework for developing a system to direct third party reimbursements for nursing services.
- Indicates specific rationales for patient care based on nursing assessment.
- Leads to more comprehensive and individualized patient care.

In summary, nursing diagnoses are standardized labels that represent clinical judgements made by professional nurses and describe health states resolved primarily by nursing therapies. Nursing diagnosis focuses on nursing assessment and intervention on the human response to altered health states thus constituting a unique, distinct, and imperative component to critical health care. Nursing diagnosis is mandated as part of competent registered nurse performance criteria by most state nurse practice acts, as well as constituting the core of the ANA's formal definition of nursing.

Diagnosing involves the identification of the patients' actual or potential problem, and the aetiology or cause of the problem that nurses can independently treat. The most essential and distinguishing feature of any nursing diagnosis is to describe a health condition primarily resolved by nursing intervention or therapies. Nursing diagnosis is a pivotal component of nursing process. On the one hand it is the judgement, conclusion or decision determined by the nurses as a result of the assessing and problem-solving process. It reflects the process involved in gathering analyzing and interpreting the assessment data. On the other hand, nursing diagnosis provides the basis from which patient outcomes are derived and a plan of appropriate nursing interventions is developed and implemented. Put another way, nursing diagnosis emerges from the collection, analysis and interpretation of assessment data, and provides the framework from which the patient's plan of nursing care involves.

Nursing, as a diagnosis-based practice, demands the nurses become expert at assessing patient's needs and problems formulating nursing diagnosis based on that assessment, evolving and implementing, a plan of care and documenting this nursing care process in a manner reflective of the professional, skilled nursing care rendered. It is the only documenting nursing activities that professional practice can be validated and financially rewarded. Nursing diagnosis reflects a patient's problems or unhealthful response and the problem or aetiology that nurses can treat independently. It is a definitive statement of an actual or potential problem, alteration or deficit in the life process (i.e., physiologic, psychologic, sociologic, and spiritualism) of an individual. After the nursing diagnosis are identified, they should be ranked in order of priority. This ranking should consider both the clients' and the nurses' opinions. Those areas that have the greatest impact on the client, the family or both should receive particular attention. The nurse should also determine priorities based on past nursing experience and on scientific knowledge of the needs and functions of human beings. Therefore, a continuum of priorities of nursing diagnosis is developed that is based on the degree of threat to the level of wellness of the client.

The nursing diagnosis can be considered a decisive statement concerning the client's nursing needs. It is important to remember that diagnoses are based on the client's concerns as well as an actual or potential problem that may be symptoms of physiological disorder or of behavioural psychosocial or spiritual problem.

Nurses are encouraged to use the nursing diagnostic categories (as listed) in their daily practice when formulating nursing diagnosis. But it should be remembered and noted that nurses need not feel restricted to the use of NANDA's list but rather should be motivated to develop in practice. Other nursing diagnosis which may be submitted included in NANDA's list or to make separate better list of nursing diagnosis. In this way, nurses are able to share their ideas, experiences, logic and creativity. The procreation of nursing language, along with an ever-increasing awareness of the intellectual activity involved in its process and implementation is every nurse's professional responsibility.

Planning

Planning is the third phase of the nursing process. The plan for providing nursing care plan can be described as the determination of what can be described as the determination of what can be done to assist the client. Planning involves the mutual setting of goals and objectives judging priorities and designing methods to resolve actual or potential problems. Two things are accomplished in the planning phase of nursing process, which includes

- Establishing goals and objectives.
- Selection of nursing intervention,

Goals and Objectives

Goals and objectives which are derived from the nursing diagnoses evolve from and are predicted by the problem portion of the nursing diagnoses, and are established for each nursing diagnosis listed. Goals are stated in broad terms to identify effective criteria for evaluating nursing action. These goals pertain to rehabilitation, prevention of complications associated with stressors, the ability of the client to adapt to these stressors, or all three other goals may deal with the achievement of the highest health potential for a client. For example, "Client will have an adquate understanding of basic food groups and their relationship to RDA = Recommeded Daily Allowance requirements within one month".

Objectives are the short statement of desired or expected outcomes of the client/patient. Objectives are determined from the goals and need to be stated in terms of observable behaviour. Objectives should define the conditions under which the expected or desired end behaviours are to occur and should specify the performance level and specific behaviours that will be accepted as evidence that desired outcomes have been met. The behaviour in question refers to psychological, physiological, social, cultural and intellectual activities and other observable responses. The desired behavioural outcomes (objectives) should be stated in a manner that everyone can understand without having to seek clarification. The criteria for stating objectives include the following.

Objectives should:

- Be written as the patient behaviours or goals. Patient's outcomes reflect those human responses (physiologic, psychologic, emotional) that must occur if the patient problems is to be resolved. Patient outcomes do not reflect goals that the nurse will achieve. The nurse's role is to support and assist the patient to identify and use his/her capabilities and coping mechanisms more effectively in dealing with the problem.
- Be written in precise and consise terms using action verbs.
- Provide directions for care.
- Specify appropriate time frame within which the patient is reassessed and the care plan is reevaluated. This serves to determine the effectiveness of the nursing intervention in assisting the patient to achieve the desired outcome(s).
- Be realistic.
- Be measurable. It is crucial that patient outcomes be stated in measurable terms so that nurses caring for the patient can use the same criteria to evaluate the patient's response to therapy.

Nursing Interventions

The second subphase in nursing care planning is the identification of nursing actions. For each nursing diagnosis, i.e. nursing interventions, nursing interventions evolve from the aetiology position of the nursing diagnosis. For learning experiences (learning by doing) each nursing action is based on carefully thought out scientific rationale and specifies what kind of nursing care is to be done to meet the client's problems effectively. Nursing action should be spelled out precisely. These actions are part of the scheme for providing good nursing care. The characteristics of nursing interventions will include the following.

- Determining the nursing intervention requires that the nruses have a strong theoretical and experiential knowledge base. The nurse must be able to establish appropriate rationale for each nursing intervention implemented.

- Nursing interventions need to be specific: Their implementation is directed towards treating the cause and resolving the patient's problems.
- Nursing interventions prescribe nursing treatments, that is, what it is, the nurse must do to treat the aetiology (cause) of the patient's problem. Behaviours described by nursing interventions reflect those of the nurse and not necessarily those of the patient.
- Clear and concise documentation of nursing interventions on the patient care plan is essential to communicate the activities and behaviours of the nurses to colleagues and other health care providers.
- In writing the nursing interventions, the care plan needs to be revised systematically in terms of patient's responses and outcomes. Decisions can then be made as to when specific interventions should be revised, updated, renewed or discontinued. Specific dates and time frames should be documented accordingly (Please note that specific dates and times are not included in the nursing care plan presented in this text because they need to be individualized for the specific patient).
- Each documented nursing intervention should be dated and signed by the nurse. The nurse's signature is particularly important in terms of accountability and in the sharing of information (feedback), including clarification of goals and rationales underlying care.

Interventions are the power of nursing and a distinct strength, also known as nursing orders or nursing prescriptions which constitute the treatment approach to an identified health alterations. Interventions are selected to satisfy the outcome criteria and prevent or resolve the nursing diagnosis or problem. Planned interventions should provide clarity, specificity, and direction to the spectrum of nurses implementing care of the patients, e.g. "Check vital signs", "measure intake and output". "Monitor heart state", etc.

Nursing interventions are said to be hypotheses established for testing if they contribute to the solution of the problem. It is upto the nurse with the client, the family or both to select appropriate action to produce desired results. In selecting nursing action, it is important to analyze the available options and to determine the probability of success in reaching the objective. Sometimes compromises must be made to provide the best care for the client, and the nurse needs to be aware of this when specifying nursing actions.

The nursing care plan deals with actual or potential problems. Nursing interventions are based on scientific principles and theories of nursing and they need to be specific. The plan serves as a means for resolving the problems and for meeting established goals in an orderly fashion. Also it provides a means for organization, giving direction and meaning to the nursing action used in helping the client, the family or both to resolve the health problems. A plan of action is necessary, because it aids in the efficient use of time. It saves both time and energy by providing essential data for those individuals who are responsible for giving care. Since the clients' condition is continuously changing, the written nursing care plan needs to reflect these changes. Therefore, planning becomes a continuous process based on evaluation and reassessment. The written plan is the most efficient way of keeping all individuals involved in the client's care informed of modification in the plan of nursing care.

Documentation of the patient's nursing care plan reflects the culmination of the problem-solving/decision-making activities of the professional nurse. Such documentation demonstrates the ability of the nurse to apply nursing knowledge to clinical situations and to integrate this knowledge in the implementation of the component of the nursing process.

The nursing care plan (NCP) format is used throughout this text to afford the reader the opportunity to examine the interrelatedness of the components of the process and to appreciate how documentation of language of process which includes problem, reason, objectives, nursing intervention (with rationale) and evaluation.

Problem refers actual or potential problems, stated in the form of nursing diagnosis, which is the product of assessment.

Reason refers to an inference in the diagnostic reasoning. Diagnostic reasoning is the critical thinking process through which the nurse moves to arrive at a nursing diagnosis, which includes the key point of subjective data (client complaints) and objective date (please note that examples of NCP 'reasons', are shown in this chapter: but throughout the text it has not (given/shown) included in nursing care plan presented in the text because they need to be individualized for each patient).

Objectives refer to short statement of derived or expected outcomes of the patient, in the subphase of planning component of nursing process.

Nursing Intervention refers to planned interventions which will provide clarity, specificity and direction to the spectrum of nurses implementing care for a patient. Implementation of nursing intervention is the action component of the planning. It is the phase of the nursing process in which the nursing treatment plan is carried out.

Evaluation of the attainment of the exepcted patient outcomes occurs formally at intervals designated in the outcome criteria. Please note that evaluation column is not included in the nursing care plans presented in this text, because they need to be individualized for each patient).

Author used the following 'PRONE' format for nursing care plans when 'P' stands for **problem**, 'R' stands for **reason** and 'O' stands for **objectives**.

Problem	Reason	Objective	Nursing intervention	Evaluation

This is where and 'N' stands for nursing intervention and 'E' stands for evaluation. The sample of nursing care plan with 'PRONE' format are in the end of this chapter.

Implementation

After planning, implementation is the next, or fourth phase of the nursing process. Implementation refers to the actions initiated to accomplish the defined goals and objectives. Implementation is often considered as the actual giving of nursing care. It is putting the plan into action. Other terms used to describe this part of the process are Action or intervention. The words implementation and intervention are not synonymous. Implementation refers to putting a plan into action; intervention speaks to involvement in the affairs of another, a coming between the other and a problematic situation. Therefore, the term implementation seems more appropriate to describe this phase of the process if nursing actions directed towards resolving the problem and meeting the health care needs of the client. It is an ongoing process through which the nurse is reassessing reviewing and modifying the plan of care, and if necessary, seeking assistance in meeting the client's health care needs.

Since the nursing process is interpersonal in nature, it must take place between the nurse and the client. The client may be a person, a group, a family, or even a community. The beliefs that the nurse and the client have about human beings, nurses, and clients and about interactions between nurses and clients will affect the types of actions that both consider appropriate. If human beings are considered unique, then nursing actions should reflect this uniqueness. Therefore, the philosophy of nursing that a nurse develops will affect the nursing actions that he or she uses in meeting the needs of clients. Yura and Walsh (1973) indicated that the implementation phase of the nursing process draws heavily on the intellectual, interpersonal, and technical skills of the nurse. Wilkinson (1992) supports the importance of critical thinking throughout the nursing process. Although the focus is on action, the action is intellectual, interpersonal, and technical in nature.

The implementation phase begins when the nurse considers various alternative actions and selects those most suitable to achieve the planned goals and objectives. Just as goals and objectives have priorities in the plan, actions may also have priorities. Nursing actions may be carried out by the nurse who developed the nursing care plan or by other nurses or nursing assistants. Nursing actions may also be carried out by the client or family. To carry out a nursing action, the nurse refers to the written plan for specific information. Many nursing actions fall into the broad categories of counselling, teaching, providing physical care, carrying out delegated medical therapy, co-ordination of resources, referral to other sources of help, and therapeutic communication (verbal and non-verbal).

According to the goals and objectives for client, as discussed earlier, several nursing actions could be implemented. For example, under objective 1 (identify the basic food groups from a chart), the following actions could be considered.

1. Establish and agreed upon time when client and her family could meet with the nurse in their home during the next week.
2. Establish a baseline knowledge about the client and the family members' understanding of basic food groups.
3. Take chart and booklets containing information about the basic food groups to client home.
4. Teach family about using the basic good groups for good nutrition (base teaching on information gained from baseline knowledge).
5. Focus on the value of the food groups for each family member based on age, height, weight, and activity.
6. Request a return demonstration in which client and other family members will identify foods by planning the food in a food group and will state why each food group is important.

In Campbell's (1980) study of nursing diagnoses and nursing actions, seven categories of nursing actions were developed. These are assertive hygienic, rehabilitative, supporting, preventive, observational, and educative. Wilkinson (1992) speaks to doing, delegating, and recording. Both point out that almost all nursing actions are initiated by nurses without medical direction. Nurses initiate and carry out all activities that fall within the nursing domain. In the hospital setting, nurses are also asked to assist physicians in carrying out medical prescriptions and to follow institutional policies. Therefore, nurses need to be clear about their dependent and independent functions.

For every nursing action, the client responds as a total person, that is, as a whole, the concept of HOLISM, which states that a person is more than the sum of that person's parts, means that the nurse may be treating a person's leg but the person will respond as a whole person (Leddy and Pepper, 1993). The concept is used in thinking about the consequences of any nursing actions. For example, the simple action of turning the patient every two hours will have a variety of consequences. Some of these consequences could or should be (1) increased circulation, (2) improved muscle tone, (3) improved breathing (4) less flatus (gas) in the intestinal track, (5) prevention of pressure sores, (6) increased or decreased pain, (7) opportunity for communication with caregiver, (8) increased ability to socialize with patient in next bed, and (9) increased or decreased ability to reach articles at bedside. There may be other consequences that could not have been predicted, such as an opportunity to express values or beliefs. Therefore, in planning nursing actions, it is important to consider the cluster of consequences of both positive and negative value that can be expected to occur with and following each action (Oermann, 1991). Using this knowledge will help the nurse select the most appropriate actions. Although not all consequences are predictable for a specific client, it is possible to develop a general knowledge of expected consequences. Knowledge of consequences is an important aspect of the implementation phase of the nursing process. The implementation phase is completed when the nursing actions are finished and the results are recorded against each diagnosis.

Evaluation

Evaluation is the fifth and final phase of the nursing process. It may be defined as the appraisal of the client's behavioural changes that are a result of the action of the nurse (Christensen and Kenney, 1990; Leddy and Pepper, 1993; Wilkinson, 1992). Although evaluation is considered to be the final phase, it frequently does not end the process. As mentioned earlier in this chapter, evaluation may lead to reassessment, which in turn may result in the nursing process beginning all over again. The main questions to ask in evaluation are: Were the goals and objectives met? Were there identifiable changes in the client's behaviour? If so, why? If not, why not? Where the consequences of nursing actions predict. These questions help the nurse to determine which problems have been solved and which problems need to be reassessed and replanned. Unsolved problems cannot be assumed to reflect faulty or inadequate data collection; rather, each part of the nursing process may need to be evaluated to determine the cause of ineffective actions.

The key to appropriate evaluation of nurse-client actions lies in the planning phase of the nursing process. When objectives are described in behavioural terms with clearly stated expected outcomes, it is easy to determine whether or not the nurse-client actions were successful. These objectives become the criteria for evaluating nurse client actions. Just as goals should be mutually set with a client whenever possible, it is also important for the nurse and client to mutually establish the objectives (criteria for evaluation).

According to Wilkinson (1992), evaluation consists of the following five steps.

1. Review the goals or predicted outcomes.
2. Collect data about the client's responses to nursing action.
3. Compare actual outcomes to predicted outcomes and decide if goals have been met.
4. Record the conclusion.
5. Relate nursing plans to client outcomes.

The first three steps are specific to client outcomes. Step 1 has been briefly discussed in relation to the planning phase of the process. In addition to stating the desired behaviour change, it is also important for the nurse to decide how the change will be measured (predicted outcome) and when it will be measured.

Step 2 involves the collection of evidence (data). Although data are collected in both assessment and evaluation, the data collected during evaluation are used differently from data collected during assessment. In assessment, data are collected for the purpose of making a nursing diagnosis. In evaluation, data are collected as evidence to determine whether the goals and objectives were met. This is an important difference to note in using the nursing process.

Step 3 in evaluation is the one that is often the most difficult because it is easy to use different measurements in making judgements. For example, if a nurse observed that a client "ate well", would this mean the same thing the client or to another nurse? "Ate well" could be interpreted to mean that the client was able to chew, swallow, and digest the food with no difficulty, or it could refer to the amount and kind of food consumed. Therefore, in evaluation, it is not only important to determine the criteria (objectives) and be specific in predicting outcomes, it is also important to determine the exact way(s) in which evidence is gathered and interpreted to ascertain whether the criteria were met.

When predicted outcomes are not reached, reassessment should occur, and the process begins again. If the evaluation shows that the nurse-client objectives have been met, the nursing process is complete.

Evaluation based on behavioural changes is *outcome evaluation*. There are two other types of evaluation, both of which are reflected in wilkinson's two other types of evaluation, both of which are reflected in Wilkinson's (1992) evaluation steps. *Structure evaluation* relates to such things as appropriate equipment to assess the client or to carry out the plan and to record evaluation conclusions (Step 4). For example, if the scales were inaccurate, then correct data could nto be obtained. Structure evaluation may also relate to the organization within which the nurse works. The nurse may be unable to carry out the nursing process appropriately because of agency limitations on time; this must be considered a part of the evaluation. *Process evaluation* which focuses on the activities of the nurse, can be done during each phase of the nursing process, or it may be carried out at the end of the process (Step 5). The following are examples of process evaluation questions that can be used in evaluating each phase of the process.

Assessment

1. Were historical data that might be related to health problems collected?
2. Was a physical examination carried out and the results recorded?

3. Was the analysis logical? Did it make use of the collected data? Were significant findings mentioned in the analysis?

Diagnosis

1. Was the diagnosis based on the analysis?
2. Is the diagnosis a logical conclusion from the data collected?

Planning

1. Are goals and objectives stated?
2. Does the plan rationally follow from the diagnosis?
3. Were goals and objectives mutually established with the client?

Implementation

1. What activities did the nurse carry out?
2. What activities did the client carry out?
3. Were the activities consistent with the objectives?

Evaluation

1. Were the predicted outcomes achieved?
2. What evaluation methods were used?
3. Were the conclusions recorded?

The nurse and the client are responsible for carrying out outcome evaluation. Structure and process evaluations are typically carried out by the nurse, others in nursing administration, or both within an agency.

HEALTH ASSESSMENT

Health assessment is an integral part of holistic nursing. It provides the basis for nursing process. The nurse works in a variety of settings, seeking information about client's health status. The purposes of the health assessment are to:

- Establish a nurse-client relationship
- Gather data about the client's general health status, integrating physiologic, psychologic, cognitive, socio-cultural, developmental and spiritual dimensions.
- Identify clients' strengths.
- Identify actual and potential health problems.
- Establish a base for the nursing process.

There are two components of health assessment which includes health history and physical assessment.

A. Health History

Health history is a collection of subjective and objective data that provides a detailed profile of the client's health status. The *subjective* data are the symptoms which are indications of illness that are perceived by the patient or client. For example, (pain, nausea, feeling nervous, etc.) *The objective* data are the signs of illness, as perceived by the examiner, i.e. doctor or nurse. For example, rashes, altered vital signs, visible drainage, etc.

The nurse collects information through interview with the client. An interview is a planned communication. During the assessment, the nurse conducts the interview in a relaxed, unhurried manner in a quiet, private, well-lighted settings. To conduct an effective and informative interview, the nurse must develop interviewing skills, gain the patient's trust, and convey feelings of compassion while remaining objective. The patient must feel the information being given is important to the nurse, the nurse must demonstrate an interest in the patient's state of wellness. The nurse initially establishes trust by introducing himself or herself and asking what name the patient wishes to be called by and then using the name during the interview. An accepting posture in which the nurse is sitting in a relaxed manner at eye level with the patient, will foster trust. A pleasant facial expression will help and eye contacts make the patient feel he has the nurse's full attention. The nurse can enhance communication by using non-judgemental language. The tips of maintaining effective communication are as follows:

(i) Promoting Effective Communication

Maintaining silence Silence can help the nurse and patient to organize their thoughts. It also enables the nurse to observe the patient more closely.

Listening attentively Attentive listening allows one to understand an entire message conveyed, verbally and non-verbally. It also facilitates trust.

Conveying acceptance Acceptance means that one is non-judgmental. Acceptance is not synonymous with agreement; rather, it is a willingness to hear the person's message. One conveys acceptance through positive feedback and making sure verbal and non-verbal cues match.

Asking related questions Questioning is a direct method of communicating. Asking related questions allows the patient to give information logically. Open-ended questions are useful for eliciting more information from the patient about a subject.

Paraphrasing Paraphrasing sends feedback to the patient that information has been accurately received.

Clarifying Clarifying helps retain important information. Using examples can clarify abstract ideas. All clarification should be specific.

Focusing When a discussion becomes vague or ill-defined, focussing directs conversation to a specific topic or issue. It limits the area of discussion to which the patient can respond. The nurse seeks meaning in the patient's message.

Stating observations Describing a patient's observed behaviour can provide feedback as to whether an intended message was received. It can clarify conflicts between verbal and non-verbal cues.

Offering information Offering information provides a patient with relevant data and prevents one-sided conversations. It is useful for health teaching and helps in decision making.

Summarizing Summarizing is a concise review of main ideas from a discussion. It sets the tone for further interactions. By reviewing a conversation the participants can focus on key issues and any relevant information previously deleted.

(ii) Inhibiting Effective Communication

Giving an opinion Giving an opinion takes decision making away from the patient. It inhibits spontaneity, stall problem solving, and creates doubt. If offering suggestions, the nurse should stress that they are only options.

Offering false reassurance Offering false reassurance can do more harm than good. False reassurance may allow the nurse to promise something that will not occur or is unrealistic.

Being defensive Defensiveness in the face of criticism implies that the patient has no right to an opinion. The patient's concerns often become ignored. Attentive listening helps the patient open up but does not imply agreement.

Showing approval or disapproval Showing approval or disapproval is judgmental and may halt a conversation. It inhibits the patient's ability to share ideas and make decisions independently. Disapproval can indicate rejection.

Asking why Asking why may imply an accusation. It can cause resentment, insecurity, and mistrust. If additional information is needed, the nurse can phrase a question to avoid use of "why."

Changing the subject inappropriately Changing the subject inappropriately is rude and shows a lack of empathy. It stalls communication. The patient may then give incomplete or inadequate information.

Forming communication barriers Forming communication barriers by saying something inadvertently that blocks a patient's communication can break down communication. By acknowledging the mistake, the nurse can start the communication process anew.

The health assessment interview also provides information about how the client perceives his or her health status or problems. Although you may not agree with the client's perceptions, it is important to understand these perceptions when planning nursing care.

Any uncertainty about the client's perceptions should be clarified during the interview. Communication techniques such as: direct questioning, or reflecting, or restating the client's comments, may enhance understanding. For example, you can say, I am not certain I understand. Did you mean....?

The Interview Process

The health assessment interview may be formal and structured to collect a wide range of information, or informal and focussed on a specific area of concern. In a formal interview, your primary concern is to establish a comprehensive data base. In an informal interview, you may discuss specific questions with the client while givign nursing care. Assessment through interviewing and questioning should be continuous, ongoing process lasting as long as you and the client interact.

The health care setting may influence the choice of interview topics. In well-child clinics, for example, the interview usually focusses on routine health practices, nutrition, and normal growth and development, whereas in the intensive care unit, data collection focuses on physiological or psychological stability and on maintaining vital functions.

Three interrelated phases constitute an effective interview; the introductory phase, the working phase and the termination phase.

A. The Introductory Phase

The introductory phase sets the tone and direction of the interview and establishes a mutual understanding of the purpose of the exchange. The purpose of the introductory phase are as follows:

- To establish rapport
- To ensure a comfortable setting
- To define what both parties expect from the interview.

(i) Establishing rapport Establishing rapport begins with demonstrating respect for the client as a person with problems, rather than regarding the person as a problem to be solved.

You should demonstrate respect at the beginning of the interview by extending a cordial greeting, addressing the client by name and then introducing yourself by name. You should not address an adult client with his or her first name unless invited. Offering to shake hands is one way of demonstrating warmth and acceptance.

Non-verbal behaviours, especially on your part, may also help build rapport. Mutual respect best can be expressed when you and the client face each other and maintain eye contact. If possible you should avoid standing over the person, because this may be intimidating. Of course, such a position may be appropriate if you are informally interviewing the person while providing care. If the interview is conducted at the bedside, you should sit beside the bed with the siderail down, leaning slightly toward the person. Non-vertal behaviours such as: expressions of disgust, boredom, or impatience may interfere with establishing rapport or may imply lack of interest.

Beginning the interview with a brief, casual conversation that focuses on the client may help dispel tension or awkwardness. If your comments are predominantly self-centred, the person may feel neglected or unimportant.

(ii) Ensuring comfort If possible, you should conduct the interview in a private setting, free from interruptions. When privacy is difficult to maintain, such as in acute care settings, you can at elast close the door or wait until other people have left the room before initiating the interview. Pulling the curtains or moving to the corner of the room also helps to promote a sense of privacy, even though these gestures may not necessarily prevent others from hearing what is said.

It is also helpful to demonstrate concern about physical comfort by asking how the client is feeling, whether he or she is comfortable or needs to use the bathroom before proceeding. If the client is in pain or is fatigued, consider postponing the interview.

(iii) Defining expectations It is important to clarify what both you and the client expect from the interview and to establish an agreement about the rules and norms of the interview. This process is known as CONTRACTING. You should explain how discussing the person's health concerns will help in planning nursing care and encourage the person to participate in the interview. The client who answers questions, responds honestly, and shares relevant personal information is most likely to benefit from the health assessment interview.

In addition, you should inform the client aboutother professionals who will see the written account of the interview and the way in which the information will be used. To ensure confidentiality, you should ask if the client does not want certain information recorded.

You may also discuss the length of time the interview will run and the possibility that future sessions may be needed. Finally, you and the client should discuss decision-making. For example, if you intend to make some decisions for the client, the client should be so informed. If you intend to encourage the client to make his or her own decisions, the client should be made aware of the expectation.

B. The Working Phase

During the working phase of the interview, which is the most time-consuming phase, you should collect data that are pertinent to the client's overall health status. Such information will be invaluable in forming an appropriate care plan. Both verbal responses and non-verbal behaviour should be recorded. The purposes of the working phase are:

- To collect biographic data
- To collect data pertinent to the client's health status
- To identify and respond to the client's needs

The Structured interview A structured interview may be used to facilitate data collection during the working phase. Familiarity with the forms before the interview will enable you to concentrate on the client's responses. Formats for structured interviews vary. Traditionally, nurses have followed a medical model in conducting health assessment interviews. However, nursing models are now being used in many settings. The structured interview usually begins with biographic information including name, age and birthddate, sex, address, birth place, marital status, and occupation. Although asking about previously recorded biographic information is unnecessary, you should always review such data, because it is relevant to the person's social identify and self concept.

The next portion of the structured interview concentrates on determining the person's functional status. (subsequent chapters discuss specific interview guidelines for each functional area). You can proceed smoothly from one topic to the next by using transitional phrases such as "Now I'd like to discuss how you feel about your sleep habits," or "Now I'd like to ask some questions about your bowel and bladder functions".

The structural interview should proceed from general to specific. Gather general biographic information and data pertaining to health perceptions before discussing sexuality, personal values, and relationships. You must establish trust and rapport before discussing intimate topics.

If the client is reluctant to discuss specific topics, you should provide an opportunity to talk about what he or she feels is most important. Use broad opening statements, such as, "Why don't you begin by telling me what brings you here," or "what's troubling you today?" Once the client has expressed immediate concerns, he or she is more likely to discuss other subjects.

You should view the structured interview as a guide rather than a rigid series of questions that must be asked in a set order. Excessive questioning may undermine rapport, inhibit responses, and encourage the client to assume a passive role of merely answering questions. Applying principles of therapeutic communication rather than direct questioning may result in a more productive interview, as is discussed in more detail in the next section. Such techniques encourage free expression about the topics raised.

Communication is also enhanced when both you and the client speak the same 'language'. The terminology you use should be simple and appropriate and not based on medical jargon. When necessary, definite terms and structure questions to allow time for the client to respond thoughtfully and meaningfully.

Completing the health assessment interview in one session may not always be possible. If the client shows signs of fatigue or a limited attention span, bring the interview to a close. Trying to continue under these circumstances.

C. The Termination Phase

The termination phase serves to end the interview. Saying how long the interview will last at the beginning will prevent the client experiencing a sense of premature closure at the end of the interview.

Presummary, summary and follow-up techniques may be incorporated into the termination phase. Presummary involves providing cues to indicate that the interview is coming to an end. For example, you could say, "I see that we only have 10 minutes left. Is there anything else you would like to discuss before our time is up?" or "There are three more questions I'd like to ask." Planning additional interview sessions may be necessary if all relevant topics have not been adequately discussed.

Next, a brief summary of the points covered will allow both you and the client a chance to validate perceptions. Specific plans for follow-up or additional interviewing are discussed at this time.

PHYSICAL ASSESSMENT

The Physical Examination is usually conducted in a head-to-toe sequence, but can be adapted to meet the need of the client being examined. It offers objective information about the client. The nurse uses the skills of physical assessment to make clinical judgement. The client's condition and response affects the extent of the examination. The accuracy of Physical assessment influences the choice of therapies a client receives and the determination of the response to those therapies. Continuity in health care improves when the nurse makes ongoing, objective, and comprehensive assessment. An examination should be designed for the client's needs. If a client is acutely ill, the nurse may assess only the involved body system. A more comprehensive examination conducted when the client feels more at ease and the nurse learns about the client's health status.

Preparation for Physical Assessment

It is very important that some preparation needed for client while conducting physical assessment in the physical environment. Physical examination requires privacy. An examination room should be well-equipped for all necessary procedures. Adequate lighting is needed for proper illuminations of body parts. The room should be sound proof, well-ventilated, and should be warm enough to maintain client's comfort. There should be proper examination table or bed with pad or mattress with necessary articles and linen including small pillow and others.

Client or Patient

Preparation of the client, both psychologically and physiologically also is very important. By which nurse explains to client that body structures will be examined, and asks the client to use toilet to void. For emptying the bladder and bowel, if needed, instruct to collect the specimen required. Physical preparation involves being sure that client is dressed and draped properly.

Equipment

The equipment or instrument needed for examination should be readily available and arranged in order for easy use.

Instruments	*Equipment and supplies*
• Blood pressure apparatus or spygmomanometer	• Alcohol swabs.
	• Cotton applicators
	• Disposable pad
• Stethoscope	• Drape or sheet
• Ophthalmoscope	• Gauze dressing (4 and 4)
• Snellen's chart	• Gloves (sterile or non-sterile)
• Otoscope	• Lubricants
• Nasal speculum	• Penlight
• Scale with height measurement	• Flash light and spot light
	• Safetypin
• Vaginal speculum	• Substance for testing smell
• Tuning fork	• Tap measure
• Percussion hammer	• Gown for client
• Thermometer	• Wrist watch with second hand
• Tongue dipressor	• Paper towels
	• Swabs and sponge forceps
	• Specimen container

POSITIONS FOR EXAMINATIONS

A number of positions are used during physical assessment, because during examination, the nurse asks client to assume proper positions so that the body parts are accessible and clients stay comfortable. The positions and their uses during physical assessment are as follows:

Sitting Positions

The client may sit upright in a chair or on the side of the examining table or bed. Sitting upright provides full expansion of lungs and provides better visualization of symmetry of upper body parts and facilitates full-lung expansion. It is used to assess the head and neck, posterior and antherior thorax, and lungs, breasts, axillae, heart and upper extremities, and also to take visual signs. If physically weakened, client may be unable to maintain an upright position, may be supine in the bed with the head elevated.

Supine Positions

In supine position, the client lies flat on the back with legs together but extended and slightly bent at the knees. The head may be supported with a small pillow. This is most normally relaxed position. It prevents contracture of abdominal muscles and provides easy access to pulse sites. This position can be used to assess the head and neck, anterior thorax and lungs, breasts, heart, abdomen extremities and peripheral pulses. In this position client becomes short of breath easily, examiner may need to raise the head of the bed.

Dorsal Recumbent Position

In the dorsal recumbent position, the client lies on the back with legs separated, knee bent, and soles of the feet flat on the bed. In this position clients with painful disorders are more comfortable with knees flexed. This position also is used to assess the head and neck, anterior thorax, and lungs, breasts, heart, extremities and peripheral pulse. It is used for client who have difficulty in maintaining supine position. This position should not be used for abdominal assessment because it promotes contraction of abdominal muscle.

Sims Position

In this, the client lies on either the right or left side. The lower arm behind the body and upper arm is bent at the shoulder and elbow. The knees are both bent, with the uppermost leg more acutely bent. Here the flexion of hip and knee improves exposure of rectal area. This position is used to assess the rectum and vagina. It should not be used for person with joint deformities which may hinder client's ability to bend hip and knee.

Prone Position

In this, the client lies on the abdomen, flat on the bed, with the head turned, to one side. This position is used only to assess extension of hip joint; and can be used to assess the posterior thorax. This position is intolerable for client with respiratory difficulties and difficult in assuming this position for older adults.

Knee-Chest Position

Here, the client kneels, using the knees and chest to bear the weight of the body. The body is at 90° angle to the hips, with the back straight, the arm above the head, and the head turned to one side. This position provides maximal exposure to rectal area, used to assess rectal area. This position is embarassing and uncomfortable. Clients with arthrities or other joint deformities may be unable to assume this position.

Lithotomy Position

In this position, the client is in the dorsal recumbent position with the buttocks at the edge of examining table and the feet supported in stirrup. This position provides maximum exposure of genitalia and facilitates insertion of vaginal speculum, so used to assess rectum and the area of female genitalia and genital tract.

Lithotomy position is also embarrassing and uncomfortable, so examiner minimizes time that the client spends in it. Client is kept well draped. It is uncomfortable for older persons and difficult for clients with severe arthritis or other deformities.

Standing Position

The standing or erect position may be used to assess posture, gait, and balance.

Client's abilities to assume positions will depend on their physical strength and degree of wellness. As stated earlier, some positions may be embarrassing and uncomfortable. Therefore, clients should be kept in these positions no longer than necessary. The examiners explain the positions and assist clients in attaining them. The drapes are adjusted to be sure that the area to be examined is accessible and that no body part is unnecessarily exposed. The nurse chooses the position according to part of body of the client examined on priority wise.

TECHNIQUES OF PHYSICAL EXAMINATIONS

Observation

The basic techniques of physical examination are inspection, palpation, percussion, and auscultation, together referred to as OBSERVATION. These skills enable you to collect data systematically using the senses of sight, touch, hearing and smell. Physical appearance, behaviour, communication patterns, and activity abilities can all be observed, as can a person's environment and events that affect him or her. Observing facial expression for signs of discomfort, detecting odours that indicate infection, listening to chest sounds to determine airway patency, and touching the skin to determine body temperature are all examples of observation.

Inspection

Inspection is systematic and deliberate visual observation to determine health status. Begin the physical examination with a general survey or inspection of the client, including an assessment of age, posture, stature, body weight, grooming and mobility patterns. Next carry out a more thought observation in a head-to-toe fashion. Note the shape and size of the head, hair distribution, general skin condition, and facial expressions. Inspect the face for symmetry of eyes and balance of facial expression. While inspecting the neck note visible pulsations, bulges, or venous distension. Inspect the chest and abdomen, noting symmetry, masses, pulsations, skin condition and visible signs of discomfort, such as holding the abdomen. Inspect the lower extremities, noting especially ankle swelling and skin integrity.

Following the general survey, more detailed observations are made as the physical examination progresses to specific body parts or systems. Inspection always precedes palpation, percussion, or auscultation of a particular area. More specific guidelines on examination skills are provided in subsequent chapters.

Effective inspection is facilitated by good lighting and exposure. Occasionally, instruments such as the ophthalmoscope and the otoscope may be used as well.

PALPATION

With palpation you rely on the sense of touch to make judgments about (1) the size, shape, texture and mobility of structures and masses; (2) the quality of pulses; (3) the condition of bones and joints; (4) the extent of tenderness in injured areas or structures; (5) skin temperature and moisture; (6) fluid accumulations and edema and (7) chest wall vibrations.

Different parts of the hand are used to palpate different types of structures. Breasts, lymph nodes and pulses should be palpated with the fingertips, where nerve endings are most concentrated. The tumb and index fingertips are used to evaluate tissue firmness. Temperature can be quickly assessed with the back of the hand, where temperature sensory nerves are most concentrated and the skin is thin. Vibrations can be felt most strongly with the palm of the hand especially along the metacarpal joints.

Palpitation should be carried out in such a way as to avoid discomfort. Your hands should be warm and the client relaxed to avoid muscle tensing. Palpate painful areas last. The amount of pressure you apply is governed by the type of structure you are examining and the degree to which palpation may cause discomfort. Any expression of distress or pain should prompt you to palpate lightly.

Palpation may be light, deep, or bimanual. *Light Palpation* the safest and least uncomfortable involves exerting gentle pressure with the fingertips of your dominant hand, moving them in a circular motion. Place your hand parallel to the part of the body surface you are examining and extend your fingers to depress the skin surface approximately 0.5 to 0.75 inches (1 to 2 cm). Exert and release fingertip pressure several times over an area. Exerting continuous pressure would tend to dull the tactile discrimination senses.

Deep Palpation, which is done after light palpation, is used to detect abdominal masses. The technique is similar to light palpation except that the fingers are held at a greater angle to the body surface and the skin is depressed about 1.5 to 2 inches (4 to 5 cm). A variation of this technique involves placing the fingertips of one hand over the fingertips of the palpating hand. The top hand should press and guide the bottom hand to detect underlying masses.

Bimanual Palpation involves using both hands to trap a structure between them. This technique can be used to evaluate the spleen, kidneys, breasts, uterus and ovaries.

PERCUSSION

Percussion involves tapping the body lightly but sharply to determine the position, size, and density of underlying structures, as well as to detect fluid or air in a cavity. Tapping the body creates a soundwave that travels 2 to 3 inches (5 to 7 cm) towards underlying areas. Sound reverberations assume different characteristics depending on the features of the underlying structures. Percussing the right upper abdominal quadrant, for example will usually elicit dull sounds, indicating the presence of the liver, tapping over the lungs should reveal resonant sounds associated with airfilled spaces. Percussion should usually be performed after an area has been palpated.

Three percussion methods can be used: mediate or indirect, immediate, and fist percussion. The method chosen depends on the area to be percussed. *Mediate or indirect percussion* should be used to percuss the abdomen and thorax, and can be performed by using the finger of one hand as a plexor (striking finger) and the middle finger of the other hand as a pleximeter (the finger being struck). *Immediate percussion*, used mainly to evaluate the sinuses or an infant's thorax, involves striking the surface directly with the fingers of the hand only. *Fist percussion*, used to evaluate the back and kidneys for tenderness, involves placing one hand flat against the body surface and striking the back of the hand with a clenched fist of the other hand.

Procedure

Mediate or indirect percussion is the basic technique of percussion and is performed in the following manner.

1. Place the pad of the middle finger of your non-dominant hand firmly against the surface being percussed. The other fingers as well as the heel of this hand, should be raised to avoid contact with the body surface. Hold the finger firmly against the body surface throughout percussion, even when it is not being tapped by the other hand.
2. Use the middle finger of your dominant hand as the plexor. Hold the forearm horizontal to the surface being percussed. Keep the forearm stationary and use wrist motion to make striking movements.
3. Quickly strike the distal phalanx of the finger that is positioned on the body surface with the tips of the finger of the other hand. Use only the wrist to generate motion, and quickly remove the striking hand after percussing to avoid muffling the percussion sound. You may percuss a single area two or three times before moving to the next area. Light tapping is more effective than heavy tapping.
4. Identify the percussion sound. Skillful percussion reveals one of the five percussion sounds, depending on the density of underlying structures, flatness, dullness, resonance, hyperresonance, and tympany. (Table 2.1) *A Flat sound* is elicited by percussing over solid masses such as bone or muscle. *A Dull sound* which has a lower pitch than a flat sound, is elicited when high density structures, such as the liver, are percussed. *Resonance* is a hollow sound heard, for example, by percussing the lung. *Hyperresonance* is an abnormal sound with a pitch between resonance and tympany, and may indicate an emphysematous lung or pneumothorax. *Tympany* is a drum-like sound heard over airfilled body parts such as the bowel or stomach.

Table 2.1: Percussion sounds

Sound	*Pitch*	*Intensity*	*Quality*	*Location*
Flatness	High	Soft	Extreme dullness	Normal: Sternum, thigh Abnormal: Atelectatic lung
Dullness	Medium	Medium	Thudlike	Normal: Liver, diaphragm Abnormal: pleural effusion
Resonance	Low	Loud	Hollow	Normal: lung
Hyper-sonance	Lower than reso-nance	Very Loud	Booming	Abnormal: emphysematous lung, pneumothorax
Tympany	High	Loud	Musical, drum-like	Normal: gastric air bubble; puffed-out cheek Abnormal: air-distended abdomen

5. Proceed to the next percussion area. Move from more resonant to less resonant areas, because detecting a change from resonance to dullness is easier than detecting a change from dullness to resonance.

Common Errors in Percussion

The most common errors in performing mediate percussion are as follows:

- *Moving the forearm of the dominant hand* Remember, all motion should be generated from the wrist.
- *Pressing, the striking finger into the positioned finger* Remove the striking finger immediately after tapping.
- *Causing injury to oneself or the client* by inadvertently striking the client or your own hand with a long fingernail. The fingernail of the plexor finger should be kept short.
- *Falling to hear the percussion note* Eliminate environmental noise including noise caused by bracelets or loose-fitting watches. If the note is still difficult to hear, check your technique.

AUSCULTATION

Auscultation is the skill of listening to body sounds created in the lungs, heart, blood vessels, and abdominal viscera. Auscultation is usually the last technique used during the examination. The sequence usually progresses from inspection to palpation, percussion, and auscultation, except during the abdominal examination, when auscultation is the second step (following inspection).

Immediate auscultation involves placing one's ear directly on the skin, such as over the lung. This method is rarely used because environmental noise frequently interferes with hearing. The usual method is *Mediate auscultation*, for using a stethoscope to detect sounds. The best results are gained using a good quality stethoscope. You should eliminate extraneous poise such as televisions, voices, and equipment sounds before performing auscultation. Do not create noise by moving the stethoscope over the body hair or clothing or by touching the stethoscope tubing.

Auscultated sounds are described in terms of pitch, intensity, duration and quality. *Pitch* is determined by the frequency of sound vibrations and should be classified as high or low. *Intensity* refers to the loudness of the sound. *Duration* refers to how long the sound lasts or how long it takes to occur in relation to a physiological event such as systole. Quality of sound must be described using subjective terms such as tinkling, harsh or blowing. Specific auscultatory guidelines are discussed throughout the test.

SYMPTOM ANALYSIS

Symptoms are detected during the physical examination or identified during the interview. Symptoms that indicate a possible change in physical status include pain, nausea, dizziness, dysphagia, and dyspnea. Such symptoms are systematically evaluated to aid in diagnosing physiological alterations. Evaluate each reported physical symptom according to the following criteria (elicited by questioning the client).

- *Onset* When did you first notice the symptom (time and date) was the onset sudden or gradual? Has this symptom occurred at other times in the past? What circumstances precipitated the symptom?
- *Location* (*may be relevant only when the symptom is pain*): Where did the pain occur? (ask the client to point to the exact location.) Does the pain radiate?
- *Quality* How did you feel when it occurred? How would you describe it?
- *Quantity* How intense was the symptom (mild or severe, or rated on a scale of 1 to 10)? Did the symptom interfere with your usual activities, such as: walking, sleeping or talking?
- *Frequency and duration* How frequently did the symptom occur and how long did it last?
- *Aggravating or alleviating factors* What makes the symptom worse or better?
- *Associated factors* Did you notice any other changes when you noticed this symptom? (ask about factors normally associated with the symptom, such as nausea with chest pain).
- *Course* How has the symptom changed or progressed over time?

PHYSICAL EXAMINATION INSTRUMENTS

The physical examination is conducted with the aid of several instruments. Some are simple, such as safetypins and cotton wisps used to evaluate sensory function. Others are complex, such as stethoscopes, which are used to evaluate heart tones. Some of the more complex, commonly used physical examination instruments are discussed in this chapter as well as in other chapters. During a complete physical examination, the instruments and equipment listed in display may be used.

Stethoscope

A stethoscope is used to evaluate sounds that are difficult to hear with the human ear, such as: heart, bowel, vascular and lung sounds. The stethoscope transmits sound to the ears while blocking out environmental noise.

The chestpiece of the stethoscope is designed to detect high or low-frequency sounds and consists of two main parts: the diaphragm and the bell. The flat, closed diaphragm filters out low-pitched sounds and is used to detect high-pitched sounds such as lung sounds. Best results are obtained by placing the diaphragm evenly and firmly over the person's exposed skin. Because the diaphragm has a relatively large surface, it transmits acute sounds over a wide area. The diaphragm should be at least 1.5 inches in diameter. Smaller diaphragm pieces are available for examining children.

The open bell portion of the chestpiece is used to detect low-frequency sounds such as diastolic heart murmurs. The bell should be at least 1 inch in diameter. The bell is placed gently on the person's skin. If too much pressure is applied, the bell will function as a diaphragm. Fain sounds may be difficult to detect with the bell because of its relatively small size.

The stethoscope tubing is made of flexible rubber or plastic that is thick enough to block environmental sounds. Double tubes that are less than 12 inches long further enhance sound transmission.

The binaurals are placed in the ears and are positioned to project sound towards the tympanic membrane. The tips of the earpieces approximate the angle of the ear canal, and should fit snugly and comfortably. Manufacturers usually supply several earpieces so that a comfortable pair can be selected.

Doppler Probe

The Doppler probe is used to evaluate blood flow, especially when traditional methods such as pulse palpation or auscultation are inappropriate or ineffective. Common clinical applications include evaluating fetal heart sounds and peripheral pulses such as brachial, radial, femoral, popliteal, dorsalis pedis, and posterior tibial pulses. The Doppler probe or transducer is placed on the skin in order to send a low-energy, high-energy sound beam (ultrasound beam) towards underlying red blood cells. Ultrasound waves are reflected off moving objects, in this case, the red blood cells, and return to the Doppler transducer, which also functions as a receiver. The Doppler probe detects the change in sound frequency as sound is returned and converts the sound into an audible signal. When blood is flowing through the vessel that is being evaluated, a pulsatile sound can be heard.

Doppler probes are available as pencil-shaped probes, flat disks, or stethoscope-like units. Each device usually has an on/off switch and a volume control dial. A small amount of gel can be applied between the end of the Doppler transducer and the client's skin to eliminate air interference. The probe is then placed gently on the skin over the vessel at approximately a 60° angle to the flow within the vessel. Excessive pressure applied to the skin may occlude the vessel.

Ophthalmoscope

An ophthalmoscope is used to inspect internal eye structures. The head of the ophthalmoscope is placed on a battery base, and may be exchanged for an otoscope head. To understand the effective use of this instrument, it is important to become familiar with the structures of the ophthalmoscope head.

Internal eye structures can be viewed by directing a light source toward the person's pupil and looking through the viewing aperture. Light is directed away from the headpiece by a front mirror window. The viewing aperture may be adjusted by turning the aperture selection dial. To see the different apertures available on the ophthalmoscope model, shine the light towards a piece of paper and adjust the aperture selection dial. Usually, the large aperture is selected if pupils are dilated and the small aperture chosen if pupils are constricted. The slit aperture may be used to examine the anterior portion of the eye and evaluate fundal lesion levels. The grid aperture may be used to characterize, locate and measure fundal lesions. The red-free filter or green beam may be used to evaluate the retina and disc, especially for any haemorrhaging, which appears black with this filter, while melanin pigments usually appear gray.

The ophthalmoscope lens can be adjusted to bring the internal eye structures into sharp focus, compensating for nearsightedness or farsightedness of the client or examiner. If necessary, you may wear contact lenses or glasses during the examination if the lens adjustment does not provide sufficient compensation. The lens can be adjusted by rotating the lens selection dial with the index finger while looking through the viewing aperture. At the zero diopter setting on the lens indicator, the lens neither converges or diverges light. The black numbers, obtained by moving the lens selection dial clockwise, have positive values (+1 to +40) and improve visualization if the client is farsighted. The red numbers obtained by counterclockwise rotation, have negative values (–1 to –20) and improve visualization if the client is nearsighted.

Otoscope

An otoscope is used to inspect the structures of the internal ear. The head of the otoscope should be placed on a battery base and may be exchanged for an ophthalmoscope head.

Internal ear strctures should be viewed by looking through the illuminated magnifying lens and speculum. The lens may be displaced to the side so that instruments can be inserted or foreign bodies removed. The size of the speculum should allow maximal visualization with minimal discomfort to the client.

Some otoscopes are equipped with pneumonic devices to introduce a small amount of air against the tympanic membrane, and may be used to evaluate the flexibility of the tympanic membrane.

GUIDELINE FOR HEAD-TO-TOE APPROACH TO PHYSICAL EXAMINATION

General Approach

The physical examination is performed in a systematic manner, such as in a head-to-toe fashion. The guidelines presented here apply to the comprehensive examination of an ambulatory adult. The examination sequence may be modified depending on your preference and the client's condition. Variations are usually recommended when examining persons who are seriously ill or injured, or when examining infants, children, and frail elderly patients.

Preliminary Evaluation

At the beginning of the examination, while the person is ambulatory and before he or she changes into an examining gown, you may evaluate the following:

- Height and weight
- Posture and gait
- Snellen visual acuity
- Cerebellar function.

Sensory Testing

Sensory testing may be performed throughout the examination.

Examination Guidelines
Head-to-Toe Examination

Procedure	*What to observe and record*
1. INITIATE THE GENERAL SURVEY	• General state of health
a. The general survey begins when you first meet the client, in the waiting room or examination room, or while delivering bedside care.	• Signs of distress such as breathing difficulty, pain • Awareness, behaviour, facial expression, mood
b. Survey mobility and gait as the person walks into the room	• Height, weight, nutritional status.
c. Continue the general survey as you examine each body region.	• Hygiene, grooming, clothes. • Skin condition • Odours • Posture, motor activity, physical deformities. • Speech pattern • Apparent age vs. actual age.
With the client seated on the examination table, bed, or chair,	
2. MEASURE VITAL SIGNS	• Blood pressure • Pulse • Respiratory rate Body temperature
3. EXAMINE THE HEAD	
a. Inspect and palpate the cranium	• Hair • Size, shape, and symmetry • Tenderness • Scalp smoothness
b. Palpate and auscultate the temporal arteries	• Thickening • Tenderness • Bruits
c. Inspect and palpate the face.	• Symmetry • Movements • Tenderness • Nodules • Sinus tenderness
d. Test cranial nerves V and VII	• Motor and sensory response
e. Inspect the nose and test cranial nerve I	• Patency • Septum • Mucosa • Sense of smell
4. EXAMINE THE EYES AND TEST VISION	
a. Inspect and palpate to evaluate external eye structures.	• Shape and symmetry • Eyelids and eyelashes • Lacrimal glands, puncta, and lacrimal functions. • Upper and lower conjunctiva • Lens, cornea, iris, and pupil.
b. Evaluate visual acuity. Perform near vision new or SnellerJaeger chart testing of chart testing of far vision at the beginning of the examination.	• Eye chart readings. • Peripheral vision.

Procedure	*What to observe and record*
c. Test extraocular muscle function (cranial nerves III, IV and VI).	• Extraocular eye movements • Eye movement during cover-uncover test. • Eye alignment and symmetry.
d. Test pupillary reflexes	• Reaction to light
e. Inspect internal eye structure with the ophthalmoscope; darken the room if possible	• Accommodation • Retina • Retinal vessels • Optic disc • Mascula.
5. EXAMINE THE EARS AND TEST HEARING.	
a. Inspect and palpate the external ear	• Skin integrity. Structure, alignment and symmetry • Tenderness.
b. Evaluate hearing	• Ability to distinguish sounds varying in pitch and intensity • Sound laterelization. • Perception of air conduction of sound vs. bone conduction.
c. Inspect the ear canal and tympanic membrane with the otoscope	• Skin integrity. • Obstructions, foreign bodies • Colour, light reflection, landmarks, and configuration of the tympanic membrane
6. EXAMINE THE ORAL CAVITY	
a. Inspect and palpate the outer structures of the oral cavity.	• Lips • Jaw • Temporomandibular joint. • Parotid glands
b. Inspect and palpate the inner structures of the oral cavity.	• Oral mucosa • Tongue • Inner cheek • Hard and soft palates • Oropharynx • Uvula
c. Test cranial nerves V, IX and XII.	• Motor responses
7. EXAMINE THE NECK	
a. Inspect musculoskeletal structures	• Alignment • Symmetry
b. Palpate the lymph nodes	• Consistency • Enlargement • Nodules • Tenderness
c. Inspect and palpate the thyroid gland	• Consistency • Enlargement • Nodules • Tenderness
d. Test neck musculoskeletal function and cranial nerve XI.	• Muscle strength and tone • Range of motion.
e. Palpate and auscultate the carotid arteries	• Pulsations • Vascular sounds
f. Test neck musculoskeletal function and cranial nerve XI.	• Muscle strength and tone • Range of motion.

Contd...

Contd...

Procedure	*What to observe and record*
g. Palpate and auscultate the carotid arteries	• Pulsations • Vascular sounds
8. EXAMINE THE UPPER EXTREMITIES	
a. Inspect the masculoskeletal structure, skin and nails	• Skin integrity • Muscle mass • Alignment and symmetry
b. Test musculoskeletal function	• Muscle strength and tone • Range of motion.
c. Palpate branchial and radial arteries	• Pulsations
d. Test deep tendon reflexes	• Motor response
9. EXAMINE THE ANTERIOR CHEST	
a. Inspect and palpate the breasts and axillae	• Skin integrity • Size, shape, and symmetry • Consistency
b. Inspect, palpate, percuss, and auscultate the thorax	• Skin integrity • Ventilatory pattern • Shape and symmetry • Chest excursion • Vibrations • Percussion tones • Breath sounds
c. Inspect, palpate, and auscultate the precordium.	• Pulsations • Vibrations • Heart sounds
10. EXAMINE THE BACK.	
a. Inspect and test musculo-skeletal structures	• Spinal alignment • Muscle tone • Range of motion
b. Perform fist percussion over the spine and kidneys.	• Tenderness
c. Inspect, palpate, percuss and auscultate the posterior thorax	• Same as anterior thorax

Position client supine on the examining table or bed. Elevate the head 30 degrees to inspect the neck veins.

Procedure	*What to observe and record*
11. INSPECT THE NECK VEINS	• Jugular venous pulsations • Central venous pressure
12. EXAMINE THE ANTERIOR CHEST (as above, adding palpation of glandular breast tissue and precordial auscultation in the left lateral position)	
13. EXAMINE THE ABDOMEN	
a. Inspect, auscultate, palpate and percuss the four abdominal quadrants	• Contour and symemtry • Skin integrity • Bulges • Bowel sounds • Vascular stands • Muscle tone • Masses • Organ characteristics • Percussion tones • Tenderness

Contd...

Procedure	*What to observe and record*
b. Palpate and percuss specific organs (liver, spleen, kidneys)	• Size • Consistency • Tenderness
14. EXAMINE THE LOWER EXTREMITIES	
a. Inspect musculoskeletal structures, skin, and toenails	• Skin integrity • Muscle mass • Alignment and symmetry
b. Test musculoskeletal function	• Muscle strength and tone • Range of motion
c. Palpate politieal, posterior tibial, and pedal arteries	• Pulsations
d. Test deep tendon reflexes and plantar reflex	• Motor response

Position the female client in the lithotomy position with stirrups.

Procedure	*What to observe and record*
15. EXAMINE THE GENITALS AND PELVIS	
a. Inspect the external genitals	• Skin integrity • Contour and symmetry • Discharge
b. Inspect the vagina and cervix	• Skin integrity • Masses • Discharge
c. Palpate the vagina, uterus, and cervix	• Muscle tone • Position • Size Consistency and masses
16. EXAMINE THE RECTUM-	• Muscle tone • Stool • Tenderness • Masses • Bleeding, discharge

Assist the male client to a standing position.

Procedure	*What to observe and record*
17. EXAMINE THE EXTERNAL GENITALS	
a. Inspect and palpate the peins	• Skin integrity • Masses Discharge
b. Inspect and palpate the scrotum	• Skin integrity • Size and shape • Testicular descent and mobility • Masses • Tenderness
c. Inspect and palpate for hernias	• Bulges
18. EXAMINE THE RECTUM (for male patients, different positions may be used and special attention is given to prostate palpation)	

After examination, documentation is necessary; this should be specific, descriptive and objective. The following descriptive terminology suggested for documentation.

OVERALL APPEARANCE INSPECTION

SEX: male/female
GENERAL GROOMING: Clean? hair combed? make-up?
POSITION/POSTURING: Supine? prone? rigid? opisthotonos? erect? slumped?
BODY SIZE: Thin? fat? obese? emasciated? flabby? weight proportionate to height? mesomorph? endomorph? ectomorph?
FACIAL EXPRESSIONS: Smiling? frowning? blank? apathetic?
BODY LANGUAGE: Eye contact? no eye contact? arms folded over chest?
OTHER OBSERVATIONS: Restless? fidgeting? lying quietly? listless? trembling? tense?

SKIN INSPECTION AND PALPATION

COLOUR AND VASCULARITY: Pink? tan? brown? dark brown? grayish? pasty? yellowish? flushed? jaundiced?
TURGOR AND MOBILITY: Elastic? non-elastic? tenting? wrinkles? oedematous tight?
TEMPERATURE AND MOISTURE: Cold? cool? warm? hot? feverish? moist? dry? clammy? oily? sweating? diaphoresis?
TEXTURE: Smooth? rough? fine? thick? coarse? scaly? puffy?
NAILS: Clean, manicured? smooth? rough? dry? hard? brittle? splitting? cracking? angle of nail bed? clubbing? curved? flat? thick? yellowing? paronychia? NAIL BEDS AND LUNULE: pale? pink? cyanotic? red? shape of lunule? blanching? spooning?
BODY HAIR GROWTH: Colour? thick? thin? coarse? fine? location and distribution on body? hirsutism?
SKIN INTEGRITY: Intact? not intact? LESIONS, BIRTHMARKS, MOLES, SCARS AND RASHES: (describe shape, size and location) nevi? fissures? maculas? papules? pustules? nodules? vullae? cysts? carbuncle? wheals? erythema? excoriation? desquamation? abrations? cherry angiomas? senile lentigines? senile purpura? senile keratoses? seborrheic keratoses? bruises? insect bites? crusts? warts? pimples? blackheads? bleeding? drainage? lacerations? scaly? ulcers? lichenification?

HEAD INSPECTION AND PALPATION

SHAPE: Round? Oval? square? pointed? normocephalic?
FACE: Oval? heart-shaped? pear? long square? round? thin? high cheekbones? symmetrical?
SENSATION (TRIGEMINAL CN V): Sensation on three branches? clenched teeth?
FACIAL CN VII: Facial expressions, smiles?
HAIR: Color and growth coarse? fine? thick? thin? sparse? alopecia? long? short? curly? straight? permed? glossy? shiny? greasy? dry? brittle? stringy? frizzy?
CONDITIONS OF SCALP: Clean? scaly? dandruff? rashes? sores? drainage?
MASSES AND LUMPS: (describe location and shape, measure size.)

EYES INSPECTION AND PALPATION

EYEBROWS: Colour and shape: alignment? straight? curved? thick? thin, sparse? plucked? scaly?
EYELASHES: Long? short? curved? none? artificial?
EYELIDS: Dark? swollen? inflamed? red? stye? infected? open and close simultaneously? ptosis? entropion? ectropion? lid lag? xanthomas?
SHAPE AND APPEARANCE OF EYES: Almond? rounded? squinty? prominent? exophthalmic? sunken? symmetrical? bright? clear? dull? tearing? discharge? (serous? purulent?) exotropia? esotropia? nystigmus? strabismus?
SCLERA: White? cream? yellowish? jaundiced? injected? pterygium?
CONJUNCTIVA: Pale pink? pink? red? inflamed? nodules? swelling?
IRIS: Colour and shape: round? not round? coloboma? arcus senilis?
CORNEA: Clear? mulky? opaque? cloudy?
PUPILS (OCULOMOTOR-CN III) (PERRLA): SIZE AND SHAPE: (measure in mm) round? not round? (describe EQUALITY: symmetrical? anisocoria? right larger than left? left larger than right? convergence? Reaction to light and accommodation? consensual reaction? EXTRAOCULAR MOVEMENTS (OCULOMOTOR), TROCHLEAR, ABDUCENS, CN III, IV, VI): intact?
LACRIMAL GLANDS: Tender? non-tender? inflamed? swollen? tearing?
AIDS: Glasses? contact lenses? prosthesis?
VISUAL FIELDS (OPTIC-CNII): Intact?
VISION (OPTIC-CNII): Reads newsprint? reports objects across room?

EARS INSPECTION AND PALPATION

PINNAE: Size and shape: large? small? in proportion to face? protruding oval? large lobes? small lobes? symmetrical? right larger than left? left larger than right? pinnae irregular? colour? skin intact? redness? swelling? tophi? cauliflower ear? furuncles? Darwin's tuburcle?
LEVEL IN RELATION TO EYES: Top of pinnae level with outer canthus of eyes? top of pinnae lower than outer canthus of eyes? top of pinnae higher than outer canthus of eyes?
CANAL: Clean? discharge? (serous? bloody? purulent?) nodules? inflammation? redness? foreign object? CILIA: Present/absent? CERUMEN: Present/absent? colour? consistency?
TYMPANIC MEMBRANE: Colour? pearly white? injected? red? inflamed? discharge? cone of light? landmarks? scarring? bubbles? fluid level?
HEARING (AUDITORY-CN VII): Right-present/absent? left-present/absent? hears watch tick? hears whisper? responds readily when spoken to? WEBER: Laterlizes equally? to left? right side? RINNE: Air conduction: bone conduction 2:1? Hearing aid: right/left.

NOSE AND SINUSES INSPECTION AND PALPATION

SIZE AND SHAPE: Long? short? large? small? in proportion to face? flat? broad? broad based? thick? thin? enlarged? nares symmetrical/ asymmetrical? pointed? swollen? bulbous? flaring of nostrils?
SEPTUM: Midline? deviated right? left? perforated?
NASAL MUCOSA AND TURBINATES: Pink? pale? bluish? red? dry? moist? discharge? (purulent? clear? watery? mucus?) cilia present/absent? rhinitis? epistaxis? polyps?
PATENCY OF NARES: (close each side and ask client to breathe) right - patent/partial obstruction/obstructed? left? patent/partial obstruction and obstructed?
OLFACTORY (CN I) Correctly identifies odors?
SINUSES: Tender? non-tender? transillumination?

MOUTH AND PHARYNX INSPECTION

LIPS: COLOR: Pink? red? tam? pale? cyanotic? SHAPE: Thin? thick? enlarged? swollen? symmetrical? asymmetrical? drooping left side? drooping right side? CONDITION: Soft? smooth? dry? cracked? fissured? blisters? lesions? (describe)
TEETH: Color and condition: white? yellow? grayish? spotted? stained? darkened? pitting? notched? straight? crooked, protruding? separated? crowded? irregular? broken? notching? peglike? loose? dull? bright? dentulous? malocclusion? CARIES AND FILLINGS: Number and location? DENTAL HYGIENE: Clean? not clean?
BREATH ODOR: Sweet? odorless? halitosis? musty? acetone? foul? fetid? odor of drugs or food? hot? sour? alcohol?
GUMS: Pink? firm? swollen? bleeding? sensitive? gingivitis? hypertrophy nodules? irritated? receding? moist? ulcerated? dry? shrunken? blistered? spongy?
FACIAL AND GLOSSOPHARYNGEAL (CN VII and IX): Identifies taste? or note?
TONGUE: Macroglossia? microglossia? glossitis? geographic? red? pink? pale? bluish? brownish? swollen? clean? thin? thick? fissured? raw? coated? moist? dry? cracked? glistening? papillae?
HYPOGLOSSAL (CN XII) TONGUE MOVEMENT: Symmetry? lateral? fasciculation?
MUCOSA: Colour? leukoplakia? dry? most? intact? not intact? masses? (describe size, shape and location) chancre?
PALATE: Moist? dry? colour? intact? not intact?
UVULA: Colour? midline? remains at midline when saying "ah"? gag reflex present?
PHARYNX: Colour? petechia? injected? beefy? dysphagia?
TONSILS: Present/absent? cryptic? beefy? size 1 + to 4 + ?
TEMPOROMANDIBULAR JOINT: Fully mobile symmetrical? tenderness? crepitus?

NECK INSPECTION AND PALPATION

APPEARANCE: Long? short? thick? thin? masses? (describe size and shape) symmetrical? not symmetrical?
THYROID: Palpable? nodules? tender?
TRACHEA: Midline? deviated to right/left?
LYMPH NODES: (Occipital- preauricular, postauricular, submental, sub-maxillary, tonsilar, anterior cervical, posterion cervical, superficial cervical, deep cervical, supraclavicular) non-palpable? tender? lymphadenopathy? shotty? hard? firm?

THORAX AND LUNGS INSPECTION, PALPATION, PERCUSSION AND AUSCULTATION

RESPIRATIONS: Rate? tachypnea, eupnea, bradypnea? apnea? orthopnea? laboured? stertorous? RHYTHM: Regular/irregular? inspiration time greater than expiration time? expiration time greater than inspiration time? spasmodic? gasping? orthopnic? gasping? deep? eupnic? shallow? flaring of nostrils with respirations? symmetrical asymmetrical? right thorax greater than left? left throax greater than right? ratio of AP diameter to lateral diameter between 1:2 and 5:7? ribs sloped downward at 45° angle? well? defined costal space? accessory muscles used? pigeon chest? funnel chest? barrel chest? abdominal or chest breather? skin intact? lesions? colour? thin? muscular? flabby?
POSTERIOR THORAX: Tenderness? masses? RESPIRATORY EXCURSION: Symmetrical? asymmetrical? no respiratory movements on right/left? subcutaneous emphysema? crepitus? fremitus? estimation of level of diaphragm? spine alignment? tenderness? CVA tenderness? resonance? dull? hyperresonance? diaphragmatic excursion 3-5 cm? comparison of one side to the other? suprasternal north located? costochondral junctions tender? chest wall stable? vocal fremitus?
LUNG AUSCULTATION: Vesicular? bronchovesicular? bronchial? whispered pectroliloquy? adventitious sounds? rales? rhonchi? wheezes? crackles? rub? bronchophony? egophony?

BREASTS AND AXILLAE INSPECTION AND PALPATION

BREASTS: Male? female? present/absent? colour? large? small? well developed? firm? pendulous? flat? flabby? symmetrical? asymmetrical? dimpling? thickening? smooth? retraction? peau d'orange? venous pattern? tenderness? masses? (describe) gynecomastia?
NIPPLES: Present? absent? circular? symmetrical? asymmetrical? inverted? everted? pale? brown? rose? extranipples? discharge? deviation? supernumerary?
AXILLA: Shaved/unshaved/odor? masses or lumps? (describe size and shape)
LYMPH NODES: (Lateral, central, subscapular, pectoral, epitrochlear) Palpable? tender? shotty?

HEART AND PERIPHERAL VASCULAR INSPECTION, PERCUSSION, AUSCULTATIONS AND PALPATION

HEART: Precordial bulge? abnormal palpations? PMI? thrills?

heave or lift with pulsation? S_1, loudest at apex? S_2 loudest at base? S_3? S_4? splits? clicks? snap? rub? gallop? MURMURS: systolic? diastolic? holosystolic? harsh? soft? blowing? rumbling? grading 1 through 6? high pitch? medium pitch? low pitch? radiating?
CAROTID PULSE: Note: Do not check both right and left cartoid pulses simultaneously. VOLUME: Bounding? forceful? strong? full? weak? feeble? thready? symmetrical? right less than left? left less than right? RHYTHM: Regular? irregular? symmetrical? asymmetrical? bruits present? absent?
APICAL PULSE: Record rate; tachycardia? bradycardia? pounding? forceful, weak? moderate? regular? irregular?
PERIPHERAL PULSES: (Do not count rate of these pulses except radial) Record character, volume, rhythm, and symmetry of brachial, radial femoral, popliteal, dorsalis pedis, and posterior tibial pulses. VOLUME: Full? strong? forceful? bounding? perceptible? imperceptible? weak? thready? symmetrical? asymmetrical? right greater than left? left greater than right? RHYTHM: Regular? irregular? symmetrical? asymmetrical? SYMMETRY: Record as symmetrical? right greater than left or left greater than right? pulse deficit, pulse pressure, BP in both arms, BP lying, sitting and standing if applicable. Jugular venous distention? (record cm above level of sternal angle).

ABDOMEN INSPECTION, AUSCULTATION, PERCUSSION, PALPATION

CONTOUR: Irregular? protruding? enlarged? distended? scaphoid? concave? sunken? flabby? firm? flat? flaccid?
SKIN: Colour; intact? not intact? shiny? smooth? scars? lesions? (describe size, shape, and type of lesion) striae? umbilicus?
BOWEL SOUNDS: Present? absent? hyperactive? high-pitched tickling? gurgles? borborygmus?
PERCUSSION: Tympanic? dull? flat? (describe where) liver size 6-12 cm? splenic dullness 6-10th rib? ascites?
PALPATION: Splenomegaly? hepatomegaly? organomegaly? masses? aotic pulse? diastasis recti? tenderness? bulges? lower pole of kidneys palpable? inguinal or femoral hernia? inguinal nodes? (describe).

MUSCULOSKELETAL INSPECTION AND PALPATION

BACK: Shoulders level? right shoulder higher than left? left shoulder higher than right? alignment? lordosis? scoliosis? kyphosis? ankylosis?
VERTEBRAL COLUMN ALIGNMENT: Straight? lordosis? scoliosis? kyphosis?
JOINTS: Redness? swelling? deformity? (describe) crepitation? size? symmetry? subluxation? separation? bogginess? tenderness? pain? thickening? nudules? fluid? bulging?
RANGE OF MOTION: Describe as full, limited or fixed, estimate degree of limitation, assess range of motion of neck, shoulders, elbows wrists, fingers, back, hips, knees, ankles, toes.
EXTREMITIES: Compare extremities with each other; describe colour and symmetry; temperature; hot, warm, cool, cold, moist, clammy, dry; muscle tone descriptors are firm, muscular, flabby, flaccid, atrophy? fasciculation? tremor?
LOWER EXTREMITIES: Symmetry? (describe any variations from normal abrasions? bruises? swollen? edema? rashes? lesions? (describe) prosthesis? varicose veins?

GENITOURINARY AND RECTUM INSPECTION

RECTUM: Haemorrhoids? inflammation? lesions? skin tags? fissures? excoriation? swelling? mucosal bulging? retrocele?
FEMALE GENITALIA: Pubic hair distribution and colour? nits? pediculosis? lesions? nodules? inflammation? swelling? pigmentation? dry? moist? shrivelled, atrophy or full labia? discharge? (describe) odor? asymmetry? varicosites? uterine prolapse? smegma? rash?
MALE GENITALIA: Pubic hair distribution and colour? nits? pediculosis? circumcised? uncircumcised? phimosis? epispadius? hypospadius? smegma? priapism? varicocele? cryptorchism? hydrocele? swelling? redness? chancre? crusing? rash? discharge? (describe) edema? scrotal sack rugated? atrophy?

NEUROLOGIC

Describe tics, twitches, paresthesia, paralysis, co-ordination.
GAIT: Balanced? shuffling? unsteady? ataxic? parkinsonian? swaying? scissor? spastic? waddling? staggering? faltering? swaying? slow? difficult? tottering? propulsive?
ACCESSORY- CN XI: Shrugs shoulder? symmetry?
REFLEXES: Report as present or absent
CO-ORDINATION: Report as to test done.
CRANIAL NERVES: May be reported here.

MENTAL STATUS

LEVEL OF ALERTNESS: Alert? stuporous? semicomatose? comatose?
ORIENTATION: Oriented to time, place and person? confused? disoriented?

If confused, check orientation as follows:

TIME: Ask client year, month, day, date.

PLACE: Ask client's residence address, where she/he is now.

PERSON: Ask client's name, birthday.

MEMORY: RECENT MEMORY: Give client short series of numbers and ask client to repeat those numbers later. LONG-TERM: Ask client to recall some event, that happened several years ago.
LANGUAGE AND SPEECH: Language spoken? SPEECH: Slurred? slow? rapid? difficulty forming words? aphasis?
RESPONSIVENESS: Responds appropriately to verbal stimuli? responds readily? slow to respond?

It is probable that all of the questions in each system will not be included every time you take a history. Nevertheless, some questions regarding each system should be included in every history. These essential races are listed in bold type in the outline that follows. More comprehensive and detailed areas for questions relating to each system are listed afterward and should be included whenever the patient gives positive responses to the first group of questions for that system. Keep in mind that these lists do not represent an exhaustive enumertion of questions that might be appropriate within an organ system. Even more detailed questions may be required, depending on the patient's problem.

General Constitutional Symptoms

Fever, chills, malaise, fatigability, night sweats; weight (average, preferred, present, change, appetite).

Skin

Rash or eruption, pruritus, pigmentation or texture change; excessive sweating, abnormal nail or hair growth.

Skeletal

Joint stiffness, pain, restriction of motion, edema, erythema, heat, bony deformity.

Head

1. General: frequent or unusual headaches, dizziness, syncope, severe injuries.
2. Eyes: visual acuity, blurring, diplopia (double vision), photophobia (abnormal sensitivity to light), pain, recent change in appearance or vision; glaucoma, use of eyedrops or other eye medications, history of trauma or familial eye disease.
3. Ears: hearing loss, pain, discharge, tinnitus, vertigo.
4. Nose: sense of smell, frequency of colds, obstruction, epistaxis, postnasal discharge, sinus pain.
5. Throat and mouth: hoarseness or change in voice; frequent sore throats, bleeding or edema of gums; recent tooth abscesses or extractions; soreness of tongue or buccal mucosa, ulcers; disturbance of taste.

Endocrine

Thyroid enlargement or tenderness, heat or cold intolerance, unexplained weight change, diabetes, polydipsia (excessive thirst), polyuria, changes in facial or body hair, increased fat and glove size, skin striac.

1. Males: onset of puberty, erections, emissions, testicular pain, libido, infertility.
2. Females:
   a. Menses: onset, regularity, duration of flow, dysmenorrhea, last period, intermenstrual discharge or bleeding, pruritus date of last pap smear, age at menopause, libido, frequency of intercourse, sexual difficulties.
   b. Pregnancies: number of miscarriages, abortions, duration of pregnancy or postpartum period; use of oral or other contraceptives.
   c. Breasts: pain, tenderness, discharge, lumps, mammograms.

Respiratory

Pain relating to respiration, dyspnea, cyanosis, wheezing, cough, sputum (character and quantity), hemoptysis (expectorating blood from respiratory tract, night sweats, exposure to TB; date and result of last chest X-ray examination.

Cardiac

Chest pain or distress, recipitating causes, timing and duration, relieving factors, palpitations, dyspnea, orthopnea (number of pillos needed), edema, claudication (weakness of legs accompanied by cramp-like pain), hypertension, previous myocardial infarction, estimate of excerise tolerance, past ECG or other cardiac tests.

Haematological

Anemia, tendency to bruise or bleed easily, thromboses, thrombophlebitis, any known abnormality of blood cells, transfusions.

Lymph Nodes

Enlargement, tenderness, suppuration to produce purulent (*pus*) material.

Gastrointestinal

Appetite, digestion, intolerance for any class of foods, dysphagia, heartburn, nausea, vomiting, haematemesis, regularity of bowels, constipation, diarrhea, change in stool colour or contents (clay-coloured, tarry, fresh blood, mucus, undigested food), flatulence, haemorrhoids, hepatitis, jaundice, dark urine; history of ulcer, gallstones, polyps, tumor; previous X-ray examinations (where, when, findings).

Genitourinary

Dysuria, flank or suprapubic pain, urgency, frequency, nocturia, hematuria, polyuria, hesitancy, dribbling, loss in force of stream, passage of stone; edema of face, stress incontinence, hernias, sexually transmitted disease inquire what kind and symptoms, and list results of serological test for syphilis (STS), if known.

Neurological

Syncope (brief lapse in consciousness caused by transient cerebral hyposiz), seizures, weakness or paralysis, abnormalities of sensation or co-ordination, tremors, loss of memory unusual frequency, distribution, or severity of headaches, serious head injury in past.

Psychiatric

Depression, mood changes, difficulty concentrating, nervousness, tension, suicidal thoughts, irritability, sleep disturbances.

GUIDE TO TREATMENTS: An advice to public by nurses

Introduction

Taking charge of your own health care, deciding when to see a doctor, when an alternative practitioner might be more appropriate, and what you can handle yourself, is an intelligent, perhaps even necessary approach these days. Unfortunately, there are no easy guidelines—many physicians with years of training and experience often find such decisions difficult. Still, the more you know about how diseases can be treated, the more likely you are to make appropriate choices in managing your own and your family's medical care.

When to Call a Doctor

Thousands of people will die needlessly each year because of denial and delay. Among them are heart attack victims who wait an average of six hours to call a doctor, and other people who ignore for months the common warning signs of a major disease such as cancer.

By contract, those who run to a medical specialist for every ache, pain, and sniffle not only drive up medical costs, but also increase their risk of adverse reactions from overtreatment. The ideal is to find a middle ground based on common sense and knowledge.

Whom to See

Everyone should have a primary-care physician to oversee and co-ordinate medical care. This might be a family practitioner, an internist, an osteopath, a pediatrician (for children), or a gynecologist (for women). The doctor may have his or her own practice or be part of a group practice or a clinic. The important thing is that your practitioners know your medical history and have a stake in maintaining your health.

When you are injured or acute illness strikes, always turn first to a conventionally trained medical doctor. These practitioners are the best qualified to treat trauma and other emergencies, infections, diabetes, heart disease, cancer, and other serious illnesses.

If you suffer from a chronic pain syndrome or some other conditions for which conventional medicine can do little, you might be better off seeing an alternative practitioner. And in many cases, you may be the best person to manage your illness, often under the guidance of a medical professional.

In the box to the right and on the next two pages is a listing of medical signs and symptoms and their possible causes.

PROBLEMS THAT DEMAND PROMPT MEDICAL ATTENTION

Call your local emergency service or get to the nearest emergency room if any of the following develop:

Possible Heart Attack

- Severe pain, light-headedness, fainting, sweating, nausea, or shortness fo breath
- Feeling of pain, pressure, fullness, or squeezing in the center chest that lasts more than two minutes
- Pain spreading from the center chest to the shoulders, neck, or arms.

Possible Stroke or mini-stroke

- Sudden weakness or numbness on one side of the body, usually affecting the face, an arm, or leg
- Sudden loss of speech, or difficulty speaking or understanding speech
- Loss of vision or dimness, usually in one eye or half of both eyes
- Unexplained dizziness, unsteady gait, lack of co-ordination, or falling
- Sudden severe headache unlike any experienced in the past
- Abrupt loss of memory or altered mental abilities.

Possible Shock

- Cold, clammy, and pale skin
- Weakness and light headedness
- Rapid, weak pulse
- Rapid, shallow, and irregular breathing
- Agitation and feeling of apprehension.

Possible Anaphylactic Reaction

- Severe swelling, especially around the eyes, mouth, and face
- Weak, rapid pulse
- Difficulty breathing
- Possible nausea, vomiting, and abdominal cramps
- Bluish tinge to skin and nails
- Confusion, dizziness, possible loss of consciousness.

Possible Internal Bleeding

- Coughing or vomiting up blood, which may look like coffee grounds
- Blood in the stool or urine
- Bleeding from a body opening, such as the ears, nose, or mouth
- Abdominal swelling and tenderness
- Excessive thirst.

Fevers

See a doctor as soon as possible if:
- Body temperature rises to 100.5° F (38° C) in a baby younger than 3 months
- Body temperature rises to 103° F (39.4° C) in a child or adult of any age
- Body temperature rises to 101° F (38.3° C) and stays there for three days
- Low-grade fever recurs or persists for two or more weeks
- Fever of any degree is accompanied by severe headache, stiff neck, swelling of the throat, or mental confusion.

SIGNS AND SYMPTOMS

In medical terms, a sign is any visible indication of disease—bleeding, a rash, or swelling, for example. A symptom is something you can feel, such as pain, fever, or nausea, and it may or may not be accompanied by a physical change. Below are common signs and symptoms and their possible causes.

COMMON SIGNS AND SYMPTOMS

Signs or symptoms	*Possible causes*
Anxiety	Alcoholism, panic attack, premenstrual syndrome, stress, a thyroid disorder
Belching	Gallbladder disease, indigestion, a malabsorption syndrome
Bleeding and bruises	
Gums	Periodontal disease, leukemia, vitamin deficiency
Eye	Diabetes, high blood pressure
Nose	A clotting disorder, high blood pressure, injury, nasal polyps or tumors
Rectal	Anal fissure, colon cancer or polyps, diverticulitis or other intestinal disorder, haemorrhoids, ulcers
Skin	Allergic reaction, anemia, a blood or clotting disorder, Cushing's syndrome, drug reaction, haemophilia, injury, leukemia
Sputum	Bronchitis, lung cancer, pneumonia, pulmonary embolism, throat infection, tubeculosis
Urine	Bladder infection, urinary tract cancer, kidney stone, prostate disorder
Vagina	Abortion or miscarriage, cancer, a hormonal disorder, infection, menstrual abnormalities, injury, polyps
Vomit	Cirrhosis of the liver, esophageal tear, ulcers
Breathlessness	Anemia, anxiety, asthma, heart disease, hyperventilation, a lung disorder
Confusion	Addiction, alcoholism, Alzheimer's disease or other dementia, drug reaction, head injury, stroke
Constipation	Appendicitis, colon cancer or other bowel disorder, diabetes, diet, drug side effects, inactivity, pregnancy, a thyroid disorder
Coughing	Asthma, bronchitis, common cold, croup, cystic fibrosis, flu, pneumonia
Cyanosis (bluish skin)	A circulatory disorder, congenital heart defect, cystic fibrosis, heart failure, respiratory failure, Raynaud's disease
Delirium	Alcohol or drug abuse, brain tumor or abscess, encephalitis, head injury, heat stroke, meningitis, mountain sickness, poisoning, psychosis, Reye's syndrome
Diarrhea	AIDS, allergies, celiac disease, food poisoning, inflammatory bowel disease, irritable bowel syndrome or other colon disorder, infection, a malabsorption syndrome, traveler's diarrhea
Dizziness	Alcohol or drug abuse, anemia, a brain disorder, cardiac arrhythmia, drug reaction, ear infection, Menière's disease, stroke or mini-stroke, tumor
Fatigue	Anaemia, cancer, chronic fatigue syndrome, depression, flu or other infectious disorders, heart disease, hepatitis, mononucleosis, premenstrual syndrome, respiratory disorders

Signs or symptoms	*Possible causes*
Fever	Abscess, AIDS, appendicitis, cancer, infection (bacterial or viral), medication side effects, rheumatoid arthritis or other autoimmune diseases
Fainting	Anxiety, blood loss, cardiac arrhythmias, heart attack or other heart condition, hyperventilation, hypoglycemia, stroke
Gait changes	Arthritis, a back disorder, multiple sclerosis or other neuromuscular disorder, Parkinson's disease, stroke
Hallucinations	Alcoholism, drug reaction, fever, schizophrenia or other psychotic disorder
Hirsutism	Cancer, Cushing's syndrome, drug side effects, hormonal imbalances, polycystic ovaries or other ovarian disorder
Hoarseness	Anxiety, asthma, bronchitis, cancer, common cold, croup, polyps, smoking, thyroid deficiency
Impotence	Alcoholism, depression, diabetes, drug reaction, multiple sclerosis, hormonal abnormalities, a nerve disorder, surgery for prostate tumors or disease, a thyroid disorder
Insomnia	Alcohol and caffeine use, anxiety or depression, drug side effects, a thyroid disorder
Intestinal gas	Colic, colon cancer or other bowel disorder, diet, indigestion, a malabsorption syndrome
Itching	Allergies, chickenpox or other rash, dry skin, eczema, fungal or other infection, liver disease, stress, vaginitis
Jaundice	Anaemia, blocked bile duct, cirrhosis, hepatitis or other liver disorder, gallbladder disease, a pancreatic disorder, infant prematurity
Loss of appetite	AIDS, anemia, cancer, depression, a digestive disorder, drug reaction, an eating disorder, infection, loss of taste
Mood changes	Alcohol or drug abuse, depression or other psychological disorder, drug reaction, a hormonal disorder, menopause, premenstrual syndrome, psychological stress
Nausea and vomiting	Alcohol abuse, appendicitis, brain injury, drug reaction, ear infection, gallbladder disease, food poisoning, gastritis, glaucoma, heart attack, hepatitis, indigestion, infection, intestinal obstruction, Mènière's disease, morning sickness, motion sickness, ulcers, vertigo
Nightmares	Alcohol or drug abuse, anxiety, depression, fever, posttraumatic stress syndrome
Numbness or tingling	Bell's palsy, carpal tunnel syndrome, a circulatory disorder, neuropathy, Raynaud's disease, shingles
Pain	
Abdomen	Appendicitis, a digestive disorder, gallstones, hepatitis, intestinal disorders

Contd...

Contd...

Signs or symptoms	*Possible causes*
	menstrual cramps, pelvic inflammatory disease, tubal pregnancy
Back	Arthritis, muscle spasms or strain, osteoporosis, ruptured disk
Chest	Angina, an esophageal disorder, heart attack, heartburn, pleurisy, pneumonia, pneumothorax
Ear	Infection, foreign body
Eye	Conjunctivitis, glaucoma, foreign body, iritis, sinus infection, injury, sty, tumours
Face	Bell's palsy, dental disease, headache, shingles, sinus infection, temporomandibular joint disorder
Foot	Arthritis, bunions, corns or calluses, gout, neuromas, warts
Generalized aches	Flu, lupus, mononucleosis, rheumatoid arthritis, shingles
Head	Brain tumor, migraine or other type of headache, muscle tension, sinusitis, stroke
Knee	Arthritis, chondromalacia patella, infection, Lyme disease, strain or other injury
Leg	A circulatory disorder, fracture, muscle injury, phlebitis, shin splints
Mouth	Canker sores, cold sores, dental cavities, gum disease, infection
Neck	Arthritis, meningitis, muscle injury slipped disk, stress
Joint/muscle	Arthritis, lupus, strain or sprain, tendinitis
Throat	cold, flu, laryngitis, strep infection, tonsillitis, quinsy
Painful intercourse	
In males	Penile warts, prostatic or urethral infection
In females	Menopausal dryness, vaginitis, premenstrual syndrome
Palpitations	Anemia, anxiety, caffeine, heart disease, hypoglycemia, menopause, medications, premenstrual syndrome, a thyroid disorder
Rashes	Allergies, drug reactions, eczema, an infectious disease, lupus, rosacea, toxic shock syndrome
Runny nose	Allergies, common cold, sinus infection
Seizures	Brain tumor, drug side effect, cerebral palsy, epilepsy, fever, head injury, hypoglycemia, toxemia of pregnancy, meningitis, poisoning
Speech problems	Alcohol abuse, Alzheimer's disease, Bell's palsy, multiple sclerosis, stroke, Parkinson's disease
Swallowing problems	Anxiety, diphtheria, an esophageal disorder, pharyngitis, strep throat, throat cancer, tonsillitis, quinsy
Sweating	Anxiety, drug reaction, fever, heart attack, infection, menopause, stress, a thyroid disorder

Signs or symptoms	*Possible causes*
Swelling and lumps	
Abdominal	Cancer, heart failure, hernias, internal bleeding, intestinal gas, kidney failure liver disease, pregnancy, uterine tumor
Breast	Cancer, fibrocystic condition, mastitis
Generalized	Anaphylactic reaction, drug reaction, heart failure, kidney disease, phlebitis, a liver disorder, thyroid disease
Joints	Arthritis, sprains
Skin or body surface	Abscess, cysts or other benign growths, cancer, edema, enlarged or obstructed lymph glands, ganglion, hives, infection, moles, warts
Taste changes	Bell's palsy, cancer, drug reaction, gum or dental disease, liver disease, loss of smell, pregnancy, a salivary disorder
Thirst	Diabetes, fever, heat exhaustion
Tinnitus (ringing in the ears)	Brain injury or tumor, cold or flu, drug side effects, ear infection, exposure to loud noise, Mènière's disease, earwax build-up, otosclerosis, vertigo
Tremor	Alcoholism, anxiety, Parkinson's disease, a thyroid disorder
Urinary problems	
Discoloured urine	Bladder or kidney infection, kidney stones, liver or gallbladder disease, urinary tract cancer
Incontinence	Aging, Alzheimer's disease, a bladder disorder, nerve deterioration, spinal injury, stroke
Urgency	Bladder infection, bladder tumor, diabetes, interstitial cystitis, drug reaction, pregnancy
Painful urination	Bladder infection, gonorrhea or other sexually transmitted disease, kidney infection, kidney or bladder stones, prostatitis, urethritis, vaginitis
Vaginal discharge	Cancer, cervicitis, gonorrhea, vaginitis, pregnancy, premenstrual syndrome
Vision problems	Cataracts, detached retina, glaucoma, iritis, macular degeneration, mini-stroke, retinopathy
Weakness	Anaemia, cancer, Guillain-Barré syndrome, heart disease, infection, liver disease, multiple sclerosis, muscular dystrophy, myasthenia gravis, rheumatoid arthritis
Weight changes	
Unexplained gain	Heart failure, kidney disease, liver disease, medications, toxemia of pregnancy, underactive thyroid
Unexplained loss	AIDS, anaemia, cancer, diabetes, an eating disorder, infection, an intestinal disorder, malabsorption syndrome, ulcers
Wheezing	Allergies, asthma, bronchitis, emphysema, heart failure, lung disorders

NURSING CARE PLAN OF FEVER

Fever is a term used to refer to an evaluation of body temperature above the normal (37.8°C or 38.2°C). Fever may be related to an altered set points of the hypothalaemia thermostat mechanism due to excessive heat production (as in hyperthyroidium salicylate poisoning, malignant hyperthermias) or due to reduced heat loss (heat stroke, Datura poisoning ectodermal dysplasia). Fever due to infectious diseases is usually to the first mechanism.

Infective agents also called exogenous pyrogens are engulfed by phagocytic leukocytes in the tissues. The inflammatory response triggered by the exogenous agents, agent lead to the production of compounds grouped together as leukotrienes that help the leukocytes, monocytes and macrophages to engulf the infective agent. Activated phagocytic cells produce several polypeptide compounds, such as interleukin-1, cachectin, (also called tumor necrosis factor), interleukin-6 and interseron-a. These compounds are examples of 'endogenous pyrogens' interleukin-1 acts on the arachidonic acid path-way, stimulating the production of prostaglandins by the vascular endothelial cells of the hypothalamus. Increased levels of prostaglandins E_2 within the hypothalamus accelerate the "firing rate" of the "cold sensitive" cells in the preoptic anterior hypothalamia nuclei and reduce the activity of the "warm sensitive" cells. This results in the shifting of the set point of the hypothalaemia thermostat towards a higher temperature setting. The vasomotor centre responds by increasing peripheral vascular tone; cutaneous vasoconstriction decreases heat loss. Shivering thermogenesis may also be initiated. These mechanisms continue until the temperature of blood bathing and the hypothalamic neurons reache the new set point.

AETIOLOGY OF FEVER

Pyrexia of unknown origin (PUO) has been arbitrarily defined as a temperature in excess of 38.3°C (101°F) for a duration of at least three weeks, which remains undiagnosed after a week of investigation in the hospital. The causes of PUO are as follows:

1. Infections
   - Pyogenic infections: Pyogenic abscess, cholangitis, pelvic abscess, liver and subphrenic abscess, diverticular abcess, thrombophlebitis.
   - Vascular infection: Infective endocarditis, infected vascular access devices.
   - Chronic glomerulomatus infection: Tuberculosis, atypical mycobacterial infections, fungal infections.
   - Other prolonged bacterial, reckettisial, and viral illnesses, brucellosis, chronic meningococcemia.
2. Immune inflammatory diseases: Systemic lupus erythematosus, juvenile rheumatoid arthritis (skin disease), vasculitis including giant cell arteritis.
3. Neoplasms: Primary (renal, pancreas, hepatic, lung, colon), secondary (hepatid secondaries) lymphoid neoplasms.
4. Granulomatous conditions (non-infections) Sarcoidosis.
5. Metabolic and familial conditions: Familial metaranian fever. Fabry's disease.
6. Drug-induced fever.
7. Pacititious fever.
8. Undiagnosed fever.

Table 2.2: Nursing care plan of patient with fever

Problem	*Reason*	*Objective*	*Nursing intervention (rationale)*	*Evaluation*
1. Altered comfort R/T increased body temperature (infection)	Due to infection • Temperature↑ • Malaise+ • Heart rate↑ • ↑Respiratory rate • ↑WBC count	Have body temperature below 100° F (37.8°C)	• Assess the patient, temperature 4th hourly (to monitor temperature) • Administer antipyretic drugs 4th hourly if ordered (to reduce temperature) • Keep environmental temperature at 70°F (21.1°C) • Avoid heavy layers of clothing or bed covers (to aid in lowering body temperature) • Give tepid sponge bath, after antipyretic therapy (to reduce temperature through evaporation rapidly) • Use skin lotions (to prevent drying) • Change the linen frequently if patient is diaphoretic (to prevent chilling and subsequent rise in body temperature from muscular activity) • Implement appropriate measure (to treat causes of fever)	(Pl response to be written in the column)
2. Risk for fluid volume deficit	• Metabolic rate • Diaphoresis • Decreased oral intake	Have no signs of dehydration	• Assess for rapid respiration and pulse • Assess damp skin, clothing and bed clothing • Assess unwillingness or inability to ingest fluids • Assess signs of dehydration. (to determine risk for fluid deficit) • Encourage fluid intake to 3-4 2/day (to replace fluids loss due to fever) • Monitor TPR and BP 4th hourly. (to know any indication of hypovolemia) • Administer IV fluids if necessary. • Monitor intake and output accurately • Give careful estimate of insensible losses (to evaluate need for replacement)	
3. Risk for altered nutrition: less than body requirement R/T increased. caloric need.	• Metabolic rate↓ • Oral intake↓	Have no weight loss	• Assess intake and monitor weight daily (to know the risk) • Give high caloric, high proteins, easily digested food and fluidity (to maximise intake and minimize energy expanse) • Help patient balance activity and rest to conserve energy (to ensure preferred activity) • Monitor alternate method of nutritional intake, i.e. enteral, parenteral.	

↑ = Increased ↓ = Decreased + = Present

Table 2.3: Nursing care plan of MI

Problem	*Reason*	*Objective*	*Nursing intervention (rationale)*	*Evaluation*
1. Pain	Imbalance of O_2 supply and demand (write subjective and objective data of pain)	Reducing pain	• Position the patient in bed in Semi Fowler's position	Pain in resting is semi Fowler's position
			• Handle the patient while providing care, while IV. giving taking vital signs, ECG, etc.	
			• Administer oxygen by nasal cannula at 4 L/min. • Offer support and reassurance. • Administer sublingual nitroglycerin as directed. • Monitor NP. heart rate, respiration rate, frequently every five minutes. • Administer narcotics as prescribed. • Obtain basal vital signs.	Colour improved and patient verbalizes decreased pain BP remains stable. HR within limits
			• Give IV nitroglycerin as prescribed. • Review with patient frequently the importance of the reporting any chest pain, discomfort, without delay	No signs of bleeding
2. Anxiety	Chest pain (other subjective and objective data)	Allebiating anxiety	• Explain equipment, procedure and need for frequent assessment to patient and family. • Explain the visiting hours and importance of limiting number of visitors. • Offer family members preferred times and phone unit to check on patient status.	Patient and family verbalize understanding.
			• Observe autonomic signs of anxiety such as increased HR, BP, RR tremulousness. • Administer anti-anxiety agents as prescribed, e.g. diazepam. • Observe adverse effects of sedation such as lethargy, confusion, etc.	No autonomic signs of anxiety
			• Offer touch and massage (may promote relaxation).	Verbalizes decrease of anxiety
			• Maintain continuity of care (consistency of routine and staff, promote trust and confidence.	Co-operation with care and talkative with staff
3. Decreased Cardiac output	(write subjective and objective data)	Cardiac output will improve or maintaining hemodynamic stability	• Monitor BP Every 2 hours or as directed. • Monitor respiration and lung fields every 2 to 4 hours by auscultating and observing. • Evaluate heart rate and heart sounds every 2 to 4 hours or as directed. • Administer IV fluids as ordered. • Note presence of JVD and liver engorgement. • Evaluate major arterial pulses. • Take body temperature every 4 hours or as directed. • Observe presence of oedema. • Monitor skin colour and temperature. • Be alert to change in mental status. • Evaluate urine output (30 ml/hr). • Monitor life-threatening dysrhythmias. • Correct dysrhythmias immediately as directed.	

Contd...

Contd...

Problem	Reason	Objective	Nursing intervention (rationale)	Evaluation
4. Activity intolerance	Insufficient oxygenation and deconditioning effect on bedrest. (+ add subjective and objective data)	Increasing activity tolerance	• Promote rest with following measures: – Minimise environmental noise. – Provide confortable environment temperature. – Avoid unnecessary procedures and interruptions. – Structure routine care measures including rest. – Discuss the patient and family about visiting hours and limiting visitors. – Promote restful diversional activities (e.g. reading, listening to music, etc.) – Encorage frequent changes of position gently. – Assist the patient with prescribed activities, e.g. change of position ROM exercises, etc.	
5. Risk for injury	"	Prevent bleeding	• Take vital signs every 15 minutes during infusion fo thrombolytic agents. • Observe the presence of hematomas or skin breakdown in pressure areas sacrum, back, elbows ankles • Be alert verbal complaints of backpain • Observe all punctured sites every 15 minutes. • Apply manual pressure to arterial or venous sites of bleeding occurs or use pressure dressings. • Observe for blood in stool, emesis, urine and sputum. • Minimize venipuncture and arterial punctures • Avoid IM injection • Caution about vigorous tooth brushing. • Avoid trauma to patient by gentle handling. • Monitor CT, BT, HR% PTT, HCT. • Check current blood type and cross match • Administer antacids as directed • Administer IV fluid and transfusion as directed • Monitor changes in mental status • Avoid vigorous oral suctioning (if)	
6. Altered tissue perfusion	"	Maintaining tissue perfusions	• Observe for persistent and/or recurrence of signs and symptoms of MI. • Report immediately. • Administer oxygen/as directed • Record a 12-load ECG • Prepare patient for possible emergency procedure (catheterization or surgery.)	
7. Ineffective individual coping	"	Strengthening coping abilities	• Listen carefully to patient and family to ascertain their clarification. • Assist the patient to establish positive attitude towards illness and progress • Manipulate environment to promote restful sleep. • Be alert to signs and symptoms of sleep deprivation • Minimize possible emotional response to transfer for ICU	

Contd...

Contd...

Problem	*Reason*	*Objective*	*Nursing intervention (rationale)*	*Evaluation*
8. Knowledge deficit R/T care of MI patient		Educate the patient and family for health maintenance and management	• Inform the patient and family members about what has happened to heart. • Instruct patient on how to judge the body's response to activity (oxygen requirement, importance of rest, taking pulse, review signs and symptoms). • Design an individual activity progression program for patient as directed. – Walk daily gradually increasing distance and time as directed. – Avoid activities that tense muscles – Avoid working with arms overhead – Gradually return to work – Avoid extremes in temperature – Do not rush, avoid tension • Tell the patient that sexual relations may be resumed on the advice of health care provider. Usually after exercise tolerance is assessed. – If the patient can walk briskly or climb two flights of stairs, can usually resume sexual activity with familial partner. – Sexual activity should be avoided after heavy meals, after alcohol or when tired. • Advise getting at least 7 hours sleep at each night and take 20-30 minutes rest period in day. • Advise limiting visitors • Advise eating 3 to 4 small meals per day • Advise limiting caffeine and alcohol intake • Driving car must be on advice of physician • Teach patient to notify when following symptoms occur: – Chest pain or pressure – Shortening of breath – Unusual fatigue – Swelling of feet and ankles – Fainting and dizziness – Very slow or rapid heart beat • Assist patient to reduce risk for another MI by risk factors modification avoid smoking, reducing high blood cholesterol levels – Reducing high BP, obesity, diabetes, stress, etc. – Control of the condition can be achieved through appropriate measures against obesity, control of serum cholesterol and hypertension and active exercise and physical fitness high dose of vitamin C can effectively reduce the serum cholesterol level in hypercholestremia. – Long-term use of beta-adrenoceptor blocking drugs can reduce cardiovascular mortality.	(Patients response to nursing measures, treatment and progress to be written in this column)

Table 2.4: Nursing care plan of patient in hypovolemic shock

Problem	*Reason*	*Objectives*	*Nursing intervention (rationale)*	*Evaluation*
1. Hypovolemic shock R/T blood loss	Subjective and objective data, e.g. one of the following • Massive trauma • GI bleeding • Ruptured aortic aneurysm • Surgery • Erosion of vessel from lesion, tubes or other devices. • DIC (diminished intravascular coagulation)	• Treat shock • bring patient to normal level	• Stop external bleeding with direct pressure, pressure dressing tourniquet • Reduce intra-abdominal or retro-peritoneal bleeding by applying MT or prepare for emergency surgery • Administer lactated Ringer's solution or normal saline • Transfuse with fresh whole blood, packed cells, fresh frozen plasma or platelets if no significant improvement with crystalloids • Use non-blood plasma expanders (albumen, dextran) until blood is available • Autotransfusion if appropriate	
2. Shock R/T plasma loss	• Burns • Accumulation of intra-abdominal fluid. • Malnutrition • Severe dermatitis.	"	• Administer low dose cardiotonics (dopamines) • Administer Ringer's lactate solutions or NS • Administer albumin. Fresh frozen plasma or dextran if CO is still low	
3. Shock R/T crystalloid loss.	• Dehydration • Protracted vomiting or diarrhea • Nasogastric suction	"	Administer isotonic or hypotonic solution	

Note: When crystallized or colloid solution is administered, proper precautions to be followed and every significant information documented.

Table 2.5: Nursing care plan for cardiogenic shock

Problem	*Reason*	*Objective*	*Nursing intervention (rationale)*	*Evaluation*
1. Cardiogenic shock R/T Myocardial disease or injury.	(Subjective and objective data of one of the following.) • Acute MI • Myocardial contusion • Cardiomyopathies	– To rule out hypovolaemia – To maintain ventricular filling pressure	• Fluid challenge with upto 300 ml of NS or RL solution to rule out hypovolaemia unless CCF or pulmonary oedema pressure • Insert CVP (central venous pressure) or pulmonary artery catheter; – monitor cardiac output, pulmonary pressure – monitor PCWP (pulmonary capillary wedge pressure) • Administer IV fluids to maintain ventricular filling pressure of 15-20 mm Hg. • Administer inotropics (e.g. dopamines or dobutamine) • Administer vasodilators (e.g. sodium nitroprusside) • Administer diuretics (e.g. mannitol or furasemide) • Use cardiotonics (digitalis) beta blockers (propanol) • Use crycosteroids	
2. Shock R/T valvular disease or injury	• Ruptured aortic cusp • Ruptured papillary muscles • Ball thrombosis		Same as above (hypovolaemia shock)	

Table 2.6: Sample nursing care plan for the patient with a carotid artery aneurysm and middle cerebral artery syndrome

Problems	*R*	*Objective*	*Nursing interventions*	*Rationales*
Nursing Diagnosis #1 Alteration in cerebral perfusion, related to: 1. Cerebral infarction with consequent cerebral edema. 2. Vasospasm associated with subarachnoid bleeding		Patient will: 1. Maintain cerebral perfusion pressure more than 60 mm Hg; ICP less than 15 mm Hg; mean arterial blood pressure ~ 80 mm Hg	• Monitor for signs/symptoms of increasing ICP:	• Initial treatment is focused on stabilizing and supporting intracranial dynamics, and reducing and/or preventing rebleeding.
			◆ Establish baseline parameters for level of consciousness, mentation, respiratory rate and pattern, pupillary reactions, and sensorimotor function.	◆ Baseline measurements are used to compare subsequent responses
		2. Remain without cardiac dysrhythmias. 3. Exhibit intact level of consciousness and mentation:	• Maintain the integrity of the ICP monitoring system:	• ICP monitoring is a highly invasive technique, which places the patient at considerable risk of infection.
		• Oriented to person/ place	◆ Check for leaks, air; stopcocks in appropriate positions. - Perform insertion site care as per protocol.	◆ Inadvertent loss of CSF in the presence of increased ICP can alter intracranial haemodynamics and precipitate herniation
		• Memory intact	• Obtain and record accurate pressure measurements:	
			◆ Confirm accurate placement of transducer at level of foramen of Monro.	◆ Venting port of transducer should always be at pressure source (i.e., the foramen of Monro). For every inch above or below the pressure source, the pressure reading may be as much as 2 mmHg off
			◆ Analyze waveforms and pressure readings and identify trends. ◆ Calculate and record cerebral perfusion pressure hourly.	◆ Trends are more significant in determining status of ICP and intracranial compliance
			• Implement measures to prevent and/or reduce ICP:	
			◆ Maintain proper positioning and body alignment; elevate head of bed; avoid head rotation or flexion on chest.	◆ Allows for optimal venous drainage from cranium via gravity. Prevents jugular vein compression or obstruction
			• Prevent increase in cerebral blood flow: ◆ Initiate and maintain hyperventilation via mechanical ventilation to maintain $PaCO_2$ at 25-35 mmHg; PaO_2 more than 80 mmHg.	• Hypercapnia and hypoxemia predispose to cerebral vasodilation and increased cerebral blood flow.
Nursing Diagnosis # 2 Alteration in comfort: Headache, related to: 1. Meningeal irritation 2. Surgical incision		Patient will: 1. Verbalize feeling relieved of pain. 2. Demonstrate a relaxed demeanor.	• Assess for signs/symptoms of meningeal irritation: ◆ Nuchal rigidity, photophobia, headache, positive Kernig's and Brud-zinski's signs	• Intracranial bleeding is highly irritating to meningeal and brain tissues
			• Implement nursing measures to reduce headache and prevent bleeding	
			◆ Move patient carefully, minimizing head movement or sudden jarrign of patient or bed; turn q2h.	◆ Turning helps to mobilize tracheobronchial secretions and redistribute pressure points to maximize circulation.

Contd...

Problems	*R*	*Objective*	*Nursing interventions*	*Rationales*
			◆ Dim the patient's bedside light, and maintain a quiet environment with minimal stimuli. - Handle patient gently when providing care. - Caution patient not to cough, sneeze, or strain.	◆ Dimming the lights helps reduce the discomfort of photophobia ◆ These activities cause an increase in ICP
			• Administer analgesics as prescribed, and monitor effectiveness of medication in relieving pain and relaxing the patient.	• Headache can be excruciating.
Nursing Diagnosis #3 Potential for injury: Seizures, related to: 1. Cranial cerebral insult (cerebral infarction and edema; intracranial bleeding).		Patient will: 1. Remain seizure free. 2. Maintain serum levels of phenytoin within the acceptable therapeutic range.	• Assess/monitor for seizure activity, documenting characteristics: onset, location, type of movement, associated changes in body function. • Maintain seizure precautions as per protocol. • Administer prescribed anticonvulsants. ◆ Monitor serum elvels of phenytoin (dilantin), (serial)	• Craniocerebral insults place the patient at risk of having seizures; anticonvulsant medications are usually prescribed prophylactically.
Nursing Diagnosis # 4 Nutrition, alteration in, less than body requirements, related to: 1. Altered state of consciousness 2. Compromised protective reflexes 3. Ineffective chewing or swallowing 4. Fatigue 5. Depression		1. Patient will maintain an anabolic state: • Body weight within 5% of baseline. • Total serum proteins within the acceptable range: albumin 3.5-5.0 g/ 100 ml. 2. Patient will verbalize having an appetite	• Consult with nutritionist to determine caloric and nutritional needs. • Initiate prescribed nutritional regimen: ◆ Hyperalimentation; fluid restriction • Monitor response to hyperalimentation: ◆ Intake and output ◆ Laboratory parameters; BUN, creatinine, total protein, and albumin ◆ Daily weight when patient's condition permits • Maintain the integrity of the hyperalimentation system as per unit protocol.	• Critical illness increases nutritional needs; these patients can rapidly experience a catabolic state when maintained on intravenous fluid replacement therapy. (one liter of dextrose and water contains 600 calories.)
Nursing diagnosis #5 Airway clearance, ineffective, related to: 1. Compromised cough 2. Need for minimizing activity of any kind during the acute phase 3. Limited mobility.		Patient's airway will remain patent; breath sounds will be normal, without adventitious sounds (e.g., crackles, wheezes, rhonchi).	• Assess breath sounds/adventitious sounds. • Suction patient only when absolutely necessary, using meticulous technique. ◆ Limit each pass to 10 seconds ◆ Prevent accumulation of secretions. • Maintain ventilation and oxygenation as prescribed.	• Abnormal breath sounds or the presence of adventitious sounds suggests accumulation and pooling of secretions. • Suctioning may increase interacranial pressure. ◆ Pneumonia is a frequent complication and usually develops on the paralyzed side (in this case, the right upper and lower lobes). A decrease in thoracic excursion and altered pulmonary haemodynamics are contributory factors.
Nursing Diagnosis #6 Communication impaired, related to: 1. Dysphasia and dysarthria		Patient will: • Demonstrate use of alternative means of communication (e.g., nodding the head, pointing the finger, writing on a tablet, slate board).	• Assess the patient's communication status: ◆ Ask simple questions and determine patient's ability to answer. ◆ Evaluate appropriateness of the answer, and the use of words, grammar, and syntax.	• Assessment identifies the skills that remain intact. • Lesions of the left cerebral hemisphere frequently disturb Broca's area, resulting in an expressive aphasia.

Contd...

Contd...

Problems	*R*	*Objective*	*Nursing interventions*	*Rationales*
			◆ Evaluate the patient's understanding of the spoken word by asking the patient to follow simple instructions.	
		• Demonstrate ease and comfort when groping for words.	• Loss of the ability to communicate can be devastating. A calm, reassuring approach and supportive manner are essential. • Encourage and reassure patient; anticipate needs; verbalize fears, frustrations for patient. ◆ Convey acceptance of the patient's behaviour • Approach to the patient: ◆ Encourage verbalization. ◆ Spend time with patient. ◆ Assure patient that speech will improve overtime and with rehabilitation.	• Develop a system of communication that facilitates understanding, taking into consideration the patient's deficits. ◆ Feeling unhurried may be reassuring as the patient searches for words to express herself.
Nursing Diagnosis # 7 Anxiety, related to: 1. Fear of dying. 2. Potential sequelae related to neurologic deficits.		1. Patient will write out needs and concerns on a slate board or tablet. 2. Demonstrate relaxed demeanor and perform relaxation techniques as condition permits.	• Assess for signs/symptoms of anxiety: ◆ Wide-eyed look, clenched fists, increased heart rate. ◆ Identify cause, if possible, and treat. • Initiate interventions to reduce anxiety: stay with patient to reassure; verbalize fears/frustrations the patient may be experiencing; indicate acceptance of the patient.	• Severe anxiety can aggravate the patient's overall condition. Because Mrs M. is unable to communicate verbally, her anxiety level may be especially high.

Table 2.7: Sample nursing care plan for the patient with spinal cord injury

Problems	*R*	*Objective*	*Nursing interventions*	*Rationales*
Nursing Diagnosis #1 Ineffective breathing pattern: alveolar hypoventilation, related to: 1. Altered ventilatory mechanics: hypoventilation associated with paralysis of intercostal and abdominal muscles		Patient will: 1. Demonstrate effective minute ventilation with trend of improving: • Tidal volume >7 – 10 ml/kg	• Perform a comprehensive respiratory assessment: ◆ Airway potency; rate, rhythm, depth of breathing; chest and diaphragmatic excursion; use of accessory muscles; breath sounds and presence of adventitious sounds.	• Major goal of airway management is to establish/maintain adequate alveolar ventilation. ◆ Increased rapid, shallow respirations may signal deterioration of respiratory function.
		• Respiratory rate <25/min. 2. Achieve a vital capacity of >15 – 25 ml/kg.	• Assess neurologic status: mental status, level of consciousness, status of protective reflexes (cough, gag, swallowing).	• Hypoxia may be reflected by changes in mental status or behaviour (restlessness, irritability).
		3. Verbalize ease of breathing.	• Monitor serial pulmonary function tests: tidal volume, vital capacity.	• Serial monitoring enables trends to be identified in pulmonary function.
Nursing Diagnosis #2 Ineffective airway clearance, related to: 1. Ineffective cough associated with paralysis of intercostal and abdominal muscles. 2. Immobility.			• Assess ability to cough and handle secretions.	• Loss of intercostal and abdominal muscles compromises the patient's ability to cough effectively.
		Patient will: 1. Demonstrate a secretion-clearing cough. 2. Maintain arterial blood gas values: • PaO_2 >80 mmHg • $PaCO_2$~35 – 45 mmHg • pH 7.35 – 7.45	◆ Monitor quality, quantity, colour, and consistency of sputum; obtain specimen for culture/sensitivity • Implement measures to ensure adequate respiratory function:	◆ Loss of protective reflexes places patient at increased risk of developing aspiration pneumonia. • Airway obstruction frequently occurs with spinal cord injury or injuries involving head and neck.

Contd...

Contd...

Problems	*R*	*Objective*	*Nursing interventions*	*Rationales*
			• Establish and maintain patent airway. • Monitor serial arterial blood gases; establish baseline function. • Initiate oxygen therapy to maintain arterial blood gases within acceptable range.	• Hypoxemia in the spinal cord injured patient is most commonly associated with retained secretions.
			• Initiate measures to handle secretions; provide humidified oxygen; maintain hydration; nasotracheal suctioning only when necessary.	• Suctioning increases risk of infection; suctioning-associated vagal stimulation may precipitate bradycardia in the spinal cord injured patient who may already be bradycardiac.
			• Initiate chest physiotherapy when overall condition is stabilized: postural drainage; percussion and vibration; deep breathing and coughing exercises.	• Loosens and dislodges secretions and enhances movement of secretions toward trachea where they may be accessible to removal by coughing/suctioning.
			• Instruct in use of incentive spirometry.	• Use of incentive spirometry encourages deep breathing, reducing risk of atelectasis.
			• Use a calm, reassuring approach: anticipate needs, offer explanations, be accessible to patient/family.	• Anxiety is a major problem in the spinal cord injured patient.
Nursing Diagnosis # 3 Cardiac output, alteration in: descreased, related to: 1. Loss of systemic vasomotor tone (neurogenic shock).		Patient's vital signs will stabilize: • BP > 90 mm Hg systolic (or within 10 mmHg of baseline) • Heart rate ~ 60/min. • Body temperature 98.6°F.	• Assess cardiovascular function and presence of neurogenic (spinal) shock: • Blood pressure, pulse, body temperature: skin temperature. • Cardiac monitoring for dysrhythmias. • Hydration status.	• Spinal cord injury (T_{4-6} and above) precipitates spinal shock with loss of sympathetic autonomic reflexes: loss of systemic tone leads to hypotension; unopposed parasympathetic tone predisposes to bradycardia; interruption of sympathetic innervation underlies hypothermia with impaired temperature regulation.
			• Implement measures to stabilize cardiopulmonary function: • Initiate prescribed intravenous therapy ~75 - 100 ml/hr. • Monitor intake and output.	
			• Initiate measures to minimize orthostatic hypotension: apply antiembolic stockings: abdominal binder. • Elevate lower extremities at regular intervals.	• Orthostatic hypotension results from venous stasis associated with impaired vasomotor tone and skeletal muscle paralysis.
Nursing Diagnosis # 4 Urinary climination, alternation in, related to: 1. Loss of voluntary control of micturition. 2. Compromised micturition reflex.		Patient will maintain: • Urine output > 30 ml/hr. • Weight within 5% of baseline. • Balanced intake and output. • Stable serum electrolytes, BUN, and creatinine. • Infection-free urinary tract.	• Monitor renal and hydration status: • Specific parameters to assess include body weight (daily), intake/output, serum electrolytes, BUN and creatinine, hematology profile (Hct, Hgb).	• Urinary retention predisposes to complications, such as urinary tract infection, and autonomic dysreflexia. • Accurate intake/output and daily weight assist in determining adequacy of renal/urinary function, and fluid balance. • Adequate hydration functions to prevent urinary infection and urinary calculi.

Contd...

Contd...

Problems	*R*	*Objective*	*Nursing interventions*	*Rationales*
			• Implement straight catheterization protocol using aseptic technique noting amount, colour, clarity, and specific gravity of urine. • Assess for bladder distention at regular intervals and straight catheterize PRN.	• Adequate renal perfusion maintains filtration and renal function: haemoconcentration may predispose toelectrolyte imbalance; increased blood viscosity may cause thromboembolic complications.
Nursing Diagnosis #5 Skin integrity, impairment of, related to: 1. Immobility. 2. Sensory loss.		Patient will maintain: • Intact skin with good turgor. • Body weight within 5% of baseline.	• Maintain skin integrity. • Assess skin carefully q 2h for signs of compromised circulation especially at pressure points.	• Pressure ulcer develops when there is lack of movement and distribution of weight; pressure is most concentrated between bone and skin surfaces that support body weight.
			• Initiate therapeutic regimen: • Turn/position q 2h; document rotation of positions.	• Implementation of therapeutic regimen maximizes tissue perfusion, prevents venostasis and tissue ischemia.
			• Maintain proper body alignment.	• Maintenance of proper body alignment prevents further neurologic damage.
			• Passive ROM exercises. • use of footboard, splints, sheepskin or air mattress, elbow/heel pads. • Administer lotion to pressure points. • Monitor and evaluate response to therapy.	• Passive ROM exercises help to maintain muscle tone and to improve circulation.
			• Consult with nutritionist to initiate necessary nutritional regimen.	• Breakdown of body proteins (gluconeogenesis) impairs tissue healing and places the patient at increased risk of pressure ulcer development and infection.

Table 2.8: Sample nursing care plan for the patient with acute head injury

Problems	*R*	*Objectives*	*Nursing interventions*	*Rationales*
Nursing Diagnosis # 1 Alteration in cerebral perfusion pressure, related to: 1. Large, right sided acute subdural hematoma. 2. Potential cerebral edema formation.		Patient will: 1. Maintain: • Cerebral perfusion pressure > 60 mmHg. • Intracranial pressure <15 mm Hg. • Arterial blood pressure ~ 80 mm Hg (mean). 2. Exhibit intact level of consciousness and mentation: • Oriented to person, place. • Memory intact. 3. Demonstrate intact sensorimotor function: • Distinguish pinprick from crude pressure. • Purposeful motor response to painful stimulus.	• Assess: level of consciousness, mentation, respiratory rate and pattern, pupillary size and reactivity, sensorimotor function (muscle tone, deep tendon reflexes, posturing). • Assess vital signs: BP, pulse, body temperature.	• Patient responses to increases in ICP can change rapidly from moment to moment; a sustained increase in ICP (>25-30 mmHg for greater than 15-20 minutes) can compromise cerebral perfusion pressure: • A rise in BP, widening pulse pressure, and slow-bounding pulse are late occurring signs of increasing ICP.
			• Maintain integrity of intracranial monitoring system: scrupulous hand-washing and aseptic technique; monitor system for leaks, avoid drainage of CSF. • Obtain/record pressure readings using appropriate procedure/protocol: • Venting port of transducer at level of foramen of Monro.	• ICP monitoring is a highly invasive system with a high risk of infection. • Maintaining a closed system reduces risk of infection; ensures valid readings. • For every inch that the measurement is off, approximately 2 mm Hg is added or subtracted from the digital readout.

Contd...

Contd...

Problems	*R*	*Objective*	*Nursing interventions*	*Rationales*
			◆ Monitor waveform configuration/digital readouts.	◆ Monitoring trends provides essential information regarding status of ICP and intracranial compliance.
			• Implement measures to prevent and/or reduce ICP: ◆ Maintain proper positioning; elevate head of bed; body in proper alignment.	◆ Elevation of head facilitates drainage from cranium via gravity.
			◆ Maintain controlled hyperventilation and oxygenation; prevent accumulation of tracheobronchial secretions; use meticulous suctioning technique.	◆ Hypercapnia causes cerebral vasodilation, increasing intracerebral blood flow. ◆ Proper suctioning technique reduces hypoxemia.
			• Monitor response to prescribed therapy to reduce cerebral edema: ◆ Diuretic therapy/hyperosmolar therapy. ◆ Corticosteroid therapy. ◆ Strict intake and output.	◆ Fluid restriction coupled with pharmacologic therapy helps to reduce extracellular fluid volume; a mildly dehydrated state is maintained.
			◆ Monitor laboratory data: BUN, creatinine, electrolytes, serum osmolality, urine specific gravity.	◆ Craniocerebral insults frequently predispose to diabetes insipidus. – Increased serum osmolality helps draw fluid from brain interstitium and reduce cerebral edema.
Nursing Diagnosis # 2 Ineffective breathing pattern, related to: 1. Expanding right-sided acute subdural hematoma with consequent brainstem compression.		Patient will: 1. Demonstrate effective breathing pattern: • Respiratory rate < 25/min. • Rhythm and depth eupnelc. 2. Maintain adequate pulmonary function: • Tidal volume >7-10 ml/kg. • Vital capacity >12-15 ml/kg.	• Assess respiratory function hourly: ◆ Spontaneous breathing: rate/rhythm/depth. ◆ Monitor arterial blood gases (serially).	• Maintenance of adequate ventilation/oxygenation is imperative because hypercapnia and hypoxemia cause cerebral vasodilation.
			• Implement measures to improve breathing pattern: ◆ Maintain semi-Fowler's position.	◆ Allows maximal chest excursion; facilitates drainage of blood and CSF from cranium.
			◆ Maintain nasogastric decompression.	◆ Prevents abdominal distention, which can compromise diaphragmatic excursion.
			◆ Maintain mechanical ventilation and oxygenation: assess tidal volume and vital capacity at bedside.	◆ See Chapter 32.
Nursing Diagnosis # 3 Ineffective airway clearance, related to: 1. Compromised protective reflexes (eg., gag, cough, epiglottal closure). 2. Altered state of consciousness.		Patient will: 1. Maintain patent airway: • Normal breath sounds. • Absence of adventitious breath sounds (e.g., crackles, wheezes). 2. Demonstrate secretion-clearing cough (unless contraindicated by intracranial hypertension).	• Assess airway patency hourly:	• Hypercapnia and hypoxemia increase cerebral blood flow.
			◆ Status of protective reflexes (gag, cough).	◆ Compromised protective reflexes place patient at risk of aspiration.
			◆ Auscultate breath sounds. ◆ Assess characteristics of sputum: – Colour, tenaciousness, amount, odor.	◆ Presence of crackles, wheezes, and rhonchi suggests increased pulmonary secretions; or inability to mobilize or clear secretions.
			◆ Assess hydration status. ◆ Maintain hydration as prescribed. – Humidity oxygen administered.	◆ Dehydration causes tracheobronchial secretions to become thick, tenacious, and difficult to clear.

Contd...

Contd...

Problems	*R*	*Objective*	*Nursing interventions*	*Rationales*
Nursing Diagnosis # 4 Impaired gas exchange, related to: 1. Widespread atelectasis. 2. Potential neurogenic pulmonary edema.		Patient will: 1. Be alert, oriented to person/place. 2. Demonstrate appropriate behaviour. 3. Maintain optimal arterial blood gases: • $PaCO_2$ ~ 30 mm Hg • PaO_2 > 80 mm Hg • pH ~ 7.35-7.45	• Assess cardiopulmonary function: ◆ Heart rate, skin colour. ◆ Haemodynamic parameters: systemic arterial BP, PCWP, cardiac output. ◆ Presence of cardiac dysrhythmias. • Monitor laboratory data: ◆ Arterial blood gases: – pH. – PaO_2, $PaCO_2$ • Calculate $AaDO_2$ • Implement oxygen therapy as prescribed. • Implement positive end-expiratory pressure (PEEP) therapy as prescribed. Monitor: ◆ ABGs, mixed venous oxygen tension (SVO_2). ◆ Lung compliance. ◆ Haemodynamic parameters (PCWP, PAP, CO). • Monitor for complications of PEEP therapy: ◆ Reduction in venous return to the heart and cardiac output; reduction in cerebral perfusion; barotrauma.	• Haemodynamic parameters reflect tissue perfusion. Evidence of cyanosis is a late sign of altered perfusion:>5 g haemoglobin are unsaturated. ◆ Hypoxemia is associated with myocardial irritability. – Metabolic acidemia is associated with decreased tissue perfusion as the lack of oxygen predisposes to anaerobic metabolism with lactate production. – Metabolic acidemia may depress myocardial function predisposing to dysrhythmias. ◆ Most closely reflect effectiveness of gas exchange. • Alveolar-arterial gradient < 250 to 300 mmHg with an FIO_2 ~ 60% in the presence of deteriorating pulmonary function is highly suggestive of ARDS: ◆ O_2 concentration should maintain PaO_2 > 60 mm Hg. • PEEP therapy maintains airway opening pressure at end-expiration above the atmospheric pre-ssure,thus increasing the FRC (functional residual capacity), preventing airway collapse, and enhancing gas exchange and oxygen transport. ◆ Lung compliance is determined by dividing the peak inspiratory pressure (PIP) into the tidal volume. (See Chap. 34) ◆ Positive intrathoracic pressures generated reduce venous return via the great veins. – Overdistention and rupture of alveoli are major complications of PEEP therapy.
Nursing Diagnosis#5 Potential for injury: Seizures, related to: 1. Cerebral hypoxia associated with an increase in ICP with consequent decrease in CPP. 2. Cerebral irritation associated with cerebral trauma with bleeding.		Patient will: 1. Remain seizure-free. 2. Maintain effective serum levels of phenytoin. • Usual serum levels: ~10-20 mg/ml.	• Assess characteristics of seizure activity: ◆ Onset, influencing factors, duration. ◆ Type of movement: tonic-clonic. ◆ Associated changes in level of consciousness, pupillary size/reactivity. ◆ Vomiting, urinary/bowel incontinence. • Implement measures to prevent seizure activity:	• Seizure activity can precipitate a significant increase in ICP; it increases cellular metabolism and the oxygen demand; it raises body temperature.

Contd...

Contd...

Problems	*R*	*Objective*	*Nursing interventions*	*Rationales*
3. Surgical manipulation of fragile brain tissue and meninges.			◆ Avoid activities that cause a substantial sustained increase in ICP (>25-30 mm Hg/15 to 20 minutes). ◆ Monitor for signs/symptoms of meningeal irritation: nuchal rigidity, photophobia, persistent headache, positive Kernig's and/or Brudzinski's signs. • Initiate and maintain seizure precautions: ◆ Oral airway; padded side rails and headboard, side rails in up position, bed in low position. ◆ Administer prescribed anticonvulsant therapy. ◆ Evaluate patient's response to anticonvulsant therapy (obtain serial blood levels of phenytoin).	
Nursing Diagnosis#6 Alteration in fluid and electrolyte balance (potential), related to: 1. Aggressive diuretic therapy and corticosteroid therapy. 2. Diabetes insipidus.		Patient will: 1. Maintain hemodynamic function: • Mean systolic BP ~80 to 100 mmHg. • Heart rate at patient's baseline. • Regular rhythm without dysrhythmias.	• Assess hydration status: ◆ Daily weight if not contraindicated by the presence of a labile ICP. ◆ Intake and output. ◆ Status of skin/mucous membranes; edema. • Implement fluid replacement regimen as prescribed.	• Patients at risk of developing cerebral edema, or an increase in ICP, are maintained in a slightly dehydrated state.
		2. Maintain balanced intake/output. • Stable weight (unless contraindicated). • Urine output: > 30 ml, < 200 ml/hr. • Urine specific gravity: 1.010 to 1.025.	• Monitor for signs/symptoms of diabetes insipidus: ◆ Presence of polyuria, polydipsia. ◆ Urine specific gravity ~ 1.005. ◆ Presence of dehydration: poor skin turgor, sunken eyeballs. • Monitor laboratory parameters: serum electrolytes, osmolality, BUN, creatinine, hematology profile.	• Diabetes insipidus may occur secondary to craniocerebral trauma, infection.

Table 2.9: Nursing care plan for the patient receiving thrombolytic therapy: Streptokinase and tissue plasminogen activator

Problems	*R*	*Objectives*	*Nursing interventions*	*Rationales*
Nursing Diagnosis#1 Potential for physiologic injury: Bleeding, related to manipulation of clotting cascade.		1. Patient will not have active bleeding as evidenced by: • Stable hematocrit, haemoglobin levels. • Guaiac-free stools, Secretions. • Absence fo haematoma, bruising, ecchymosis. • Stable blood pressure. • Stable mentation.	• Perform complete assessment of patient at least every 4 hrs including: ◆ Neurologic assessment. ◆ Inspection of skin for areas of discolouration. ◆ Quality of peripheral pulses. ◆ Guaiac results of secretions, excretions. ◆ Evaluation of current laboratory values (haemoglobin, haematocrit, PTT, fibrinogen levels).	• Complete assessment will allow for rapid detection of any possible bleeding complications. ◆ Haemoglobin and haematocrit will determine the volume and oxygen-carrying capacity of red blood cells in the circulation. PTT will estimate the blood's ability to clot. Fibrinogen will estimate the amount of coagulation proteins available to make clots.

Contd...

Contd...

Problems	*R*	*Objective*	*Nursing interventions*	*Rationales*
			• Monitor vital signs and clinical status every 15-30 minutes until stable, then every 24 hrs.	• Frequent clinical assessment will allow for rapid detection of bleeding.
			• Inspect insertion sites for bleeding when taking vital signs	• Previous sites of clotting frequently are dissolved during administration of thrombolytic agent.
			• Observe for retroperitoneal ecchymosis and severe lower back pain when taking vital signs.	• Catheterization via the femoral artery predisposes patient to iliac or femoral dissection.
			• Observe for retroperitoneal ecchymosis and severe lower back pain when taking vital signs.	
			• Avoid patient care activities that would predispose patient to bleeding or bruising: ◆ Shaving. ◆ Venipuncture. ◆ Vigorous toothbrushing. ◆ Aggressive patient manipulation. ◆ Use of non-invasive blood pressure cuffs.	• Haemostatic mechanisms are impaired after thrombolytic therapy, preventing rapid resolution of bleeding.
			• Maintain alignment of extremity involved in the procedure and place 5-10-lb sandbag over site.	• Movement of extremity may dislodge newly formed clots. Direct pressure promotes haemostasis.
			• Co-ordinate blood work if venipuncture is required, or maintain large-bore IV with saline lock for blood sampling.	• Maintenance of vascular-integrity is critical in preventing uncontrolled bleeding.
			• Monitor patient's laboratory work: ◆ Thrombin time. ◆ Prothrombin time. ◆ Partial thromboplastin time. ◆ Fibrinogen split products. ◆ Fibrinogen levels. ◆ Haematocrit. Haemoglobin.	• All indicators of clotting will be prolonged for 6-12 hrs after administration of streptokinase. ◆ Indicators of bleeding should not decrease during post-procedure period.
			• Alert all personnel that patient is anticoagulated by placing a sign at bedside.	• Increased communication among health care team minimizes risk of complications.
			• If invasive procedures are required avoid noncompressible vessels. ◆ Subclavian vein. ◆ Internal jugular vein.	• Predisposes patient to uncontrolled bleeding.
Nursing Diagnosis # 2 Potential of physiologic injury: Bleeding, related to thrombolytic therapy (diminished clotting ability).	1.	Patient will remain haemodynamically stable and bleeding will be controlled with minimal blood loss as evidenced by: • No change in blood pressure. • No change in haemoglobin, haematocrit levels.	• Hold pressure to site for at least 1/2-3/4 hr. • Notify physician immediately of any bleeding.	• Haemostasis is prolonged due to manipulation of clotting cycle.
			• Monitor vital signs and document.	• Blood pressure will drop and heart rate increase if significant volume loss has occurred.
			• Be prepared to administer blood products containing clotting factors (FFP, packed RBC, cryoprecipitate).	• Supplementing clotting cycle is effective in maintaining haemostasis.
			• Administer aminocaproic acid as prescribed, and monitor response to therapy.	• Aminocaproic acid is a haemostatic agent used to prevent excessive formation of plasmin. This helps to control bleeding caused by thrombolytic agents.

Contd...

Contd...

Problems	*R*	*Objective*	*Nursing interventions*	*Rationales*
			• Administer fluid and plasma expanders.	• May require volume to maintain adequate cardiac output.
Nursing Diagnosis #3 Potential alteration in comfort, related to allergic response (specific to streptokinase only).		Patient will not demonstrate discomfort related to manifestations of an allergic response (i.e. itching, musculoskeletal pain, respiratory distress, fever, anaphylaxis).	• Monitor temperature every 4 hrs. ◆ Inspect skin every 30 minutes - 1 h for 6 h, then every 4 h. ◆ If febrile, administer medication that does not affect haemostasis (i.e., acetaminophen).	• Manifestations of allergic response will occur soon after administration of streptokinase as antigen is encountered. ◆ Aspirin may contribute to patient's inability to clot.
			• Monitor patient closely if signs/symptoms of reaction occur and document.	• Patient who has recently had exposure to beta-haemolytic streptococcal proteins will develop a severe response to the therapy.
			• Be prepared to administer-corticosteroids, Benadryl or life support measures if reaction is severe.	
Nursing Diagnosis #4 Potential alteration in cardiac output, related to dysrhythmias		Patient will remain haemodynamically stable as evidenced by: • Maintenance of MAP greater than 70 mmHg. • Lack of signs and symptoms of decreased cardiac output: dizziness, nausea, shortness of breath.	• Monitor patient's rhythm continuously, noting and documenting any change from baselines. • Treat all dysrhythmias with standard protocols, noting patient's response. • Reassure patient that this is not unexpected and signals success of the procedure.	• Reperfusion dysrhythmias occur frequently after successful thrombolysis. • Patients often fear that dysrhythmias mean the procedure has been unsuccessful.
Nursing Diagnosis #5 Potential alteration in tissue perfusion, related to reocclusion of coronary arteries.		Patient will remain pain-free or chest pain will be alleviated, with resolution of ECG changes indicative of ischemia, infarction.	• Instruct patient to notify nurse immediately at onset of chest pain; reinforce significance of time. • Observe patient for nonverbal signs of discomfort. • Obtain a 12-lead ECG with any patient discomfort and observe for ischemic changes. ◆ Notify physician immediately. ◆ Administer standard medications for myocardial ischemia.	• Patients may not understand the importance of communicating chest pain or are afraid to admit that the problem has not resolved. • Electrocardiographic indicators of ischemia differentiate true angina from other kinds of discomfort.
			• Prepare patient for possibility of repeat procedure, emergent IABP, or open-heart surgery.	• It may be necessary to revascularize the myocardium by more conventional methods if reocclusion occurs. ◆ Counterpulsation will help with coronary artery perfusion and minimize myocardial demands.

Table 2.10: Sample care plan for the patient with pulmonary embolism

Problems R	*Objectives*	*Nursing interventions*	*Rationales*
Nursing Diagnosis #1 Impaired gas exchange, related to: 1. Altered pulmonary blood flow. 2. Ventilation/perfusion mismatching. 3. Right-to-left shunting.	Patient will maintain optimal arterial blood gas parameters: • pH 7.35 - 7.45. • PaO_2 > 80 mm Hg. • $PaCO_2$ 35-45 mm Hg. • HCO_3 22-26 mEq/liter.	• Assess for signs/symptoms of hypoxia, anxiety, tachypnea, dyspnea, dyspnea, air hunger, tachycardia, hypertension, or hypotension.	• A classic sign of a pulmonary embolism is a subtle, mild dyspnea. In the presence of pulmonary infarction associated with an embolism, sudden and severe dyspnea may reflect an underlying total or partial obstruction of pulmonary blood flow.
		• Assess level of fatigue	• The increased work of breathing may predispose to fatigue; fatigue may result in alveolar hypoventilation with worsening hypoxemia; and it predisposes to hypercapnia.
		• Monitor arterial blood gas parameters.	• A metabolic acidemia is often associated with decreased tissue perfusion; the consequent anaerobic metablolism causes a rise in serum lactate levels. Arterial blood gas parameters most closely reflect effectiveness of gas exchange and pH.
		• Administer prescribed humidified oxygen therapy.	• Oxygenation is effective in the treatment of ventilation/perfusion mismatch.
		• Prepare for intubation.	• Compromised ventilatory effort, ventilation/perfusion mismatch, and right-to-left shunting may compromise gas exchange sufficiently to require mechanical ventilation.
Nursing Diagnosis #2 Cardiac output, alteration in: Decreased, related to: 1. Pulmonary hypertension. 2. Right sided heart failure. 3. Decrease in left ventricular end diastolic pressure.	Patient will maintain stable haemodynamics: • Heart rate < 100 beats/min. • CVP 0-8 mmHg. • PCWP < 25 mmHg. • Cardiac output 4-8 liters/min.	• Assess for signs/symptoms of right sided heart failure: Weight gain, imbalance in intake and output; haemodynamic changes—neck vein distention, tachycardia, extra heart sounds (S_3 and S_4); edematous lower extremities.	• Pulmonary hypertension is the major haemodynamic disturbance of pulmonary embolism. Hypoxemia, acidemia, and a reduced cross-sectional area of the pulmonary capillary bed contribute to the development of pulmonary hypertension.
		• Administer prescribed medication regimen to treat right heart failure: • Vasopressor therapy, cardiac glycosides, morphine, diuretics, and sedatives. • Monitor response to drug therapy.	• Therapies are directed towards decreasing myocardial oxygen consumption and demand. • Morphine increases systemic venous capacitance; the reduced venous return decreases the work of the heart.
Nursing Diagnosis #3 Tissue perfusion, alteration in, related to: 1. .....disorder 2. Deep venous thrombosis.	Patient will remain without recurrent pulmonary embolism as • Absence of pain • Stable vital signs (for patient). • Stable arterial blood gases.	• Assess for signs/symptoms of venous thrombosis: Tenderness, warmth, pain, and peripheral .... • Measure circumference of each extremity at designated point daily.	• Predominantly, pulmonary emboli arise from deep venus thrombosis: Edema in a characteristic manifestation in the presence of disruption in venous blood flow.

Contd...

Contd...

Problems	*R*	*Objectives*	*Nursing interventions*	*Rationales*
3. Pulmonary embolism.			◆ Assess for Homans' sign each shift.	◆ A positive Homans' sign occurs when pain in the calf is experienced upon dorsiflexion of the foot. It is highly suggestive of venous thrombosis.
			• Apply antiembolic hose to both lower extremities; remove for 20 min/shift.	◆ Periodic removal allows filling of superficial capillaries.
			• Assist patient to perform active range of motion exercises each shift unless otherwise contraindicated.	• Exercise enhances "skeletal-muscular pump," which functions to prevent pooling of blood in the lower extremities (venostasis) and maintains venous return to the heart.
			• Instruct patient to avoid positions that compromise blood flow in the extremities.	• Positions that compromise blood flow can cause circulatory stasis.
			• Encourage deep breathing hourly.	• Expands lungs and minimizes atelectasis.
			• Caution to avoid straining, breath-holding, or other Valsalva's maneuver.	• Such activities increase risk of dislodging thrombi.
Nursing Diagnosis #4 Potential for physiologic injury, bleeding, related to anticoagulant therapy.		Patient will experience an absence of bleeding: • Stable hematocrit/haemoglobin (for patient).	• Assess closely for signs/symptoms of bleeding.	• Anticoagulant therapy is major treatment in patients with deep venous thrombosis. Major adverse effect of heparin is the risk of bleeding.
		• Stable vital signs. • Absence of petechiae, ecchymosis, hematuria, occult blood in stools, or bleeding at invasive sites.	• Teach patient to examine self for signs of bleeding: Petechiae, easy bruising, changes in colour of urine or stools.	• An average patient may afford early recognition of subtle bleeding.
			• Obtain daily serum coagulation parameters (prothrombin and partial thromboplastin times); monitor closely for desired range.	• Usual PT/PTT is maintained 1½–2 times the control.
			• Monitor all invasive sites every shift. • Limit puncture sites and blood drawing to only when necessary. ◆ Use only small gauge needles when drawing blood. • Teach patient to use an electric razor and to avoid vigorous toothbrushing.	• Puncture sites and invasive lines will not be able to clot as quickly during anticoagulant therapy. Large haematomas may occur without appropriate application of pressure post-injection and at puncture sites. It may be necessary to apply direct pressure to these sites for as long as 10 min, followed by application of pressure dressing.
			• Maintain access to protamine sulphate for patients receiving heparin therapy.	• Protamine sulphate is the antidote for heparin and should be readily available for administration if necessary.

Table 2.11: Sample care plan for the patient with myocardial infarction

Problems	*R*	*Objectives*	*Nursing interventions*	*Rationales*
Nursing Diagnosis #1 Alteration in comfort, related to: 1. Myocardial ischemia		Patient will verbalize feeling free of pain.	• Assess for presence of chest discomfort.	• Continuous assessment of patient to determine verbal and nonverbal cues of pain episodes is essential as patient may be experiencing denial of his condition.

Contd...

Contd...

Problems	*R*	*Objectives*	*Nursing interventions*	*Rationales*
			◆ Have patient rate discomfort on a scale of 1-10, with 10 being most severe.	◆ Patient may not appear to be in distress, but because he may mask signs of pain as a result of such factors as stoicism and cultural differences, pain may be severe. A scaling system is a more objective tool.
			◆ Notify physician of any episodes of chest pain and take appropriate actions: Obtain vital signs, get a 12-lead ECG.	◆ Enhanced sympathoadrenal response associated with pain and anxiety may increase heart rate and oxygen demand, and may provoke myocardial ischemia.
			• Minimize discrepancy between O_2 supply and demand. ◆ Provide periods of rest. ◆ Regulate activities. ◆ Maintain a quiet environment.	• Goal in treatment is to maximizse O_2 supply and minimize O_2 demand.
Nursing Diagnosis #2 Potential for anxiety, related to: 1. CCU environment. 2. Newly diagnosed disease.		Patient will: 1. Verbalize anxiety and/or fears. 2. Demonstrate behaviour suggesting decreased anxiety: Relaxed facies and demeanor. 3. Heart rate 60-80 beats/minute. 4. Blood pressure within 10 mmHg of baseline.	• Assess for verbal and nonverbal cues of anxiety.	• Patient may verbalize he is not feeling anxious but may be demonstrating anxious behaviour.
			◆ Provide patient/family with information regarding diagnosis, diagnostic procedures.	◆ Family members can be helpful in relaxing patient but must be included when giving information regarding care.
			• Orient patient and family to CCU environment: Staff, equipment, visiting hours, when and whom to call for information about the patient's condition.	• Knowing what to expect assists in coping; family may feel reassured knowing when they can visit or whom to call to get progress reports on the patient's condition.
			• Sedate as necessary, and monitor response.	• Quiet rest and relaxation are essential especially during acute phase when oxygen demands need to be reduced.
Nursing Diagnosis #3 Alteration in cardiac output: Decreased, related to: 1. Dysrhythmias. 2. Left ventricular dysfunction.		Patient will: 1. Maintain electrophysiologic stability: • Heart rate 60-80 beats/minute. • Rhythm: regular. 2. Maintain haemodynamic stability: • Blood pressure within 10 mmHg of baseline. • Mental status: Alert, oriented to person, time, and place. 3. Skin warm, usual colour. 4. Urine output greater than 30 ml/hr.	• Initiate continuous cardiac monitoring. ◆ Monitor rate, rhythm.	• Early detection of serious dysrhythmias allows early treatment and prevention of complications.
			• Treat serious or "warning" dysrhythmias as per unit protocol.	• "Warning dysrhythmias" may precipitate episodes of ventricular tachycardia and/or fibrillation.
			• Initiate haemodynamic pressure monitoring as prescribed/indicated: Arterial pressure, central venous pressure; PAP, PCWP, CO should the patient's condition become complicated.	• Rhythm and conduction disturbances may be associated with haemodynamic compromise, particularly in the patient with marginal left ventricular function.
			• Monitor for signs and symptoms of left ventricular dysfunction: Sinus tachycardia, dyspnea, orthopnea, crackles, S_3 gallop, jugular venous distention; hypotension, elevated pulmonary pressures, and decreased cardiac output.	• Myocardial ischemia and/or infarction predisposes patient to left ventricular dysfunction.

Contd...

Contd...

Problems	*R*	*Objectives*	*Nursing interventions*	*Rationales*
			• Initiate treatment protocol should left ventricular dysfunction occur: ◆ Administer vasopressors as prescribed and monitor response to therapy. ◆ Administer antidysrhythmics as prescribed and monitor response to therapy. ◆ Administer vasodilator therapy and monitor resposne to therapy.	• Prompt treatment to reduce ischemia and decrease oxygen demand may prevent myocardial injury and necrosis and preserve left ventricular function. ◆ Dysrhythmias may reduce cardiac output and compromise coronary artery perfusion. ◆ Should left ventricular function become compromised, therapy to reduce preload and afterload may be initiated to reduce the work of the left ventricle and, thus, oxygen demand.
Nursing Diagnosis #4 Coping, potentially ineffective (individual), related to: 1. Diagnosis, and fear of dying. 2. Necessary changes in lifestyle, occupation.		Patient will: 1. Verbalize feelings of depression, fears about heart disease.	• Assess for signs and symptoms of depression: Withdrawal, insomnia, listlessness, crying, lack of self-esteem, feelings of hopelessness, anorexia. • Encourage verbalization of feelings.	• Depression may interfere with patient's ability to deal realistically with situation, and may compromise recovery.
		2. Use denial as a mechanism to help control fear and anxiety, but not to interfere with ultimate acceptance of diagnosis and rehabilitation.	• Assess use of denial as a defense mechanism. ◆ Support appropriate use of denial by the patient.	• Denial is commonly used by patients who have myocardial infarctions; this mechanism can reduce overwhelming anxiety and enable the patient to progress through the acute phase without further physiologic compromise.
			• Monitor physiologic parameters (heart rate, blood pressure, pulse) closely during conversations that involve potentially stressful topics.	• Potentially distressful topics include pain, fear of dying, and consequences of death for family members, as well as changes in lifestyle and occupation as may be necessitated by the myocardial infarction. ◆ Such topics can cause changes in physiologic parameters and may reflect the patient's coping ability.
Nursing Diagnosis #5 Knowledge deficit regarding: 1. Coronary artery disease.		Patient will have knowledge of disease: • Risk factors. • Medications. • Rest/exercise. • Changes in lifestyle. • Follow-up care.	• Assess knowledge base and learning needs of patient and family. ◆ Utilize resources in patient teaching (pamphlets, video tapes, as appropriate).	• Patient has a cardiac history and may have received teaching previously. Assessment of learning needs is essential at this time. ◆ Patient may not be ready for teaching while in the CCU, but the foundation for learning can begin.
			• Document knowledge base, teaching, and patient's response to teaching in progress notes.	• This facilitates continuity of care.

Table 2.12: Nursing care plan for the patient with neoplastic-related surgery of the head and neck

Problems	*R*	*Objectives*	*Nursing interventions*	*Rationales*
Nursing Diagnosis #1 Alteration in breathing pattern, related to: 1. Postoperative tracheostomy.		Patient will: 1. Maintain adequate respiratory function: A. Respiratory < 25/ minutes. B. Tidal volume 5-7 ml/ kg. C. Arterial blood gases: • pH 7.35-7.45. • $PaCO_2$ 35-45 mm Hg. • PaO_2>60 mm Hg. 2. Maintain intact neurological function: • Mental status alert and oriented to person, place, and date.	• Note preoperative respiratory status and history from records. • Assess respiratory status q 4 hr include auscultution of anterior and posterior chest, respirations, and arterial blood gases (as indicated). • Tracheostomy care q 4 hr (as per institutional guidelines). • Encourage coughing, turning, and deep breathing q 2 hr. • Encourage use of incentive spirometer. • Administer humidified air/oxygen. • Keep head of bed elevated 30°. • Assess neurological status q 4 hr and PRN.	• May already be compromised. • To mobilize secretions. • To moisten secretions. • Note physician recommendations. • Changes in level of consciousness may result from decreased oxygen.
Nursing Diagnosis #2 Potential for alteration in haemodynamics and tissue perfusion, related to: 1. Manipulation of major vessels in neck intraoperatively.		Patient will: 1. Maintain presurgical circulatory status. • Heart rate 60-80/ minute. • Rhythm: Regular sinus. • Blood pressure within 10 mmHg of baseline. • Haemodynamic parameters within acceptable range (arterial pressure, pulmonary artery and pulmonary capillary wedge pressures). • Usual skin colour, skin warm to touch. • Brisk capillary refill.	• Note preoperative circulatory status and history from records. • Assess pulse and blood pressure q 4 hr. • Encourage range of motion to unaffected extremities q 2 hr with assistance. • Note colour and temperature of extremities PRN and record. • Observe for signs and symptoms of phlebitis every shift. • Encourage early ambulation. • Keep tracheostomy ties loosely applied. • Avoid use of excessive dressings on neck and chest as per physician recommendations.	• May have history of circulatory problem (e.g. carotid arterial insufficiency, risk of cerebral vascular accident). • Will prevent venous stasis. • Will prevent decreased circulation to flaps. • Improves visibility of area and facilitates assessment.
Nursing Diagnosis #3 Alteration in fluid balance, related to: 1. Surgical procedure. Patient will:		Patient will: 1. Maintain balanced intake and output, and body weight within 5% of baseline. 2. Maintain stable laboratory values: • Serum osmolality 285-295 mOsm/kg. • Serum electrolytes within acceptable range. • Urine specific gravity: 1.010-1.025.	• Assess present fluid balance. • Record accurate intakes and outputs and report imbalances. • Administer intravenous fluids/blood products as prescribed. • Note and record colour and type of drainage from drains, EG and NG tubes. • Begin tube feedings when indicated.	• Note estimated blood loss, insensible losses, urine output, intravenous infusions bllood products, gastric and wound drainage. Clear fluid from drains may indicate improper placement into lymph channels.

Contd...

Contd...

Problems	*R*	*Objectives*	*Nursing interventions*	*Rationales*
Nursing Diagnosis #4 Impaired skin integrity, related to: 1. Surgical incision. 2. Poor wound healing.		Patient will: 1. Not experience an infection at surgical sites. 2. Have skin become/remain intact.	• Note preoperative skin integrity from history. • Assess skin integrity q 4 hr. • Assess unaffected areas in neck and chest area for swelling and discolouration. • Cleanse incisions as per institutional protocol.	• May already be compromised.
Nursing Diagnosis #5 Alteration in body image, related to: 1. Surgical procedure.		Patient will: 1. Verbalize feelings about body image changes. 2. State ways to adapt to body alterations.	• Discuss potential changes in body image preoperatively. • Encourage patient to voice feelings, comments, and questions about surgery. • Answer questions and reinforce information given by physician. • Encourage support from family or significant others. • Offer realistic hope whenever possible. • Refer patient for additional professional help, when indicated.	• Important to assess previous problems, adjustment difficulties, or coping mechanisms.

Common Problems of Adult Patient

(1) STRESS AND ITS MANAGEMENT

Stress is a state produced by a change in the environment that is perceived as challenging, threatening or damaging to the persons dynamic balance or equilibrium. There is an actual or perceived imbalance in the person's ability to meet the demands of the new situation. The change or stimulus that evokes this state is the 'Stressor'. The nature of the stressor is variable, an event or change that will produce stress in one person will be neutral for another, and event that may produce at one time and place for one person may not do so for the same person at another time and place. A person appraises and copes with changing situations. The desired goal is *adaptation* or adjustment to the energy and ability to meet new demands. This is stress-coping process, a compensatory process with physiologic and psychologic components.

Adaptation is a constant, ongoing process that requires a change in structure, function, or behaviour so that the person is better suited to the environment. The process involves an interaction between the person and the environment. The outcome depends upon the degree of fit between the skills and capacities of the person and his or her sources of social support, on the one hand and the types of challenges or stressors being confronted on the other. As such adaptation is an individual process with each individual having different levels of ability to cope and/or respond. As new challenges are met, this ability to cope and adapt can change, thereby providing the individual with a wide range of adaptation ability from which to draw. Adaptation goes on throughout the lifespan and during that process many developmental and situational challenges will be encountered, especially in situations of health and illness. The goal of these encounters is to promote adaptation. In situations of health and illness, this goal is realized by optional wellness.

Theories/Approach to Stress

There were three different theoretical approaches which have been used to define stress in nursing.

1. Stress as response
2. Stress as stimulus
3. Stress as transaction

The first theory conceptionalizes *stress as a response* to an environmental stressor. This theory was first proposed by Hans Selye (1956, 1976) who identified/defined "stress as a non-specific response of the bod·· to any demand made upon it, regardless of its nature" Selye referred to these stress-inducing demands as 'stressor'. Stressors can be physical (e.g. noise, burns, running a marathon, infectious disease, pain, etc.) or emotional (e.g. diagnosis of cancer, promotion at work, watching a loved one die, failing an examination, financial loss, winning a beauty contest) and pleasant or unpleasant, as long as they require the individual to adopt. In response to either physical or psychologic stressors, a series of physiologic changes occur. Selye called/labelled this pattern of responses as General Adaptation Syndrome (GAS) (the detailed discussion included in this chapter).

A second stress theory, views *stress as a stimulus* that causes a response. This theory originated with Holmes TH, (1967), Rahe RH and Masuda (1967, 1975) who developed a tool to assess the effects of life changes on health. Life changes are defined as conditions ranging from minor violation of law to death of a loved one. They define stress as a stimulus, or the cause of the response. In this context, stress is viewed as external to the individual. In this psychosomal model, life events are measured as predictors of illness. Stress is considered as a predisposing or precipitating factor increasing the individual vulnerability to illness. The life events that make people more vulnerable to illness and their mean values are as follows: (Holmes, Rahe 1967).

Sl.No.	*Life event stressors*	*Mean value*
1.	Death of spouse ..	100
2.	Divorce ..	73
3.	Marital separation from male ..	65
4.	Detention	
5.	Death of a close family member ..	63
6.	Major personal injury or illness ..	53
7.	Marriage ..	50
8.	Being fired at work ..	45
9.	Marital reconciliation with mate ..	45
10.	Retirement from work ..	45
11.	Major changes in health of a family member ..	44

Contd...

Contd...

Sl.No.	*Life event stressors*	*Mean value*
12.	Pregnancy	40
13.	Sexual difficulties	39
14.	Gaining a new family member (through birth, adoption, etc.)	39
15.	Major business readjustment (merger, reorganization, bankruptcy)	39
16.	Major changes in financial state (worse or better than early)	38
17.	Death of a close friend	37
18.	Changing to different line of work	36
19.	Major change in number of arguments with spouse	35
20.	Taking out a mortgage or loan for a major purchase	31
21.	Foreclosure on a mortgage or loan	30
22.	Major changes in responsibilities at work (promotions demotions, transfers)	29
23.	Son or a daughter leaving from home	29
24.	Trouble with in-laws	29
25.	Outstanding personal achievement	28
26.	Spouse beginning or ceasing work outside home	26
27.	Beginning or ceasing normal schooling	26
28.	Major change in living conditions (building new house, deterioration of house or neighbourhood)	25
29.	Revision of personal habits (dress, manners, association)	24
30.	Trouble with boss	23
31.	Major change in working hours or conditions	20
32.	Change in residence or changing to a new school	20
33.	Major change in usual type and amount of recreation	19
34.	Major change in social activities	17
35.	Taking out a mortgage or loan for a lesser purchase	17
36.	Major changes in sleeping habit	16
37.	Major changes in number of family get together & eating habits	15
38.	Vacation	13
39.	Christmas or any major festival	12
40.	Minor violation of law (traffic tickets, disturbing peace, etc).	11

The factors that affect are individual response to life events indicating the importance of using a holistic approach when assessing the patient/client.

A third stress theory focuses on person-environment-transactions and is referred to as the "transaction or interaction" theory. In this, stress is defined as *transaction*. In the transactive model, there is an exchange or transaction between the person and the environment, which provides feedback to the person-environment-relationship. A proponent of this theory is Richard Lazarus, who emphasized the role of *Cognitive Appraisal* in assessing stressful situations and selecting coping options. Lazarus and Folkman (1984) defined "Psychologic stress" as a particular relationship between the person and the environment that is appraised by the person as taxing his or her resources and endangering his or her well-being.

Lazarus theory focuses on the person-environment-transactions and cognitive appraisal of demands and coping options. Appraisal is a judgement process that includes recognizing the degree of demands or stressors, placed on the individual. The appraisal process also involves the recognition of available resources or options that help when dealing with potential or actual demands.

During primary appraisal, demands are according to the possible impact on the individual well-being. Demands can be judged as irrelevant, benign-positive, or stressful. If demands are appraised stressful, they can be classified as representing harm or loss, threat or challenge. Harm or loss demands involve actual damage and threat demand, involve anticipated harm or loss, challenge demand differes from threat and harm or loss because they are viewed as a potential for personal gain or growth.

Secondary appraisal refers to the process of recognizing the coping resources and options that are available. Primary and secondary appraisal often occur simultaneously and interact with each other in determining stress. *Cognitive reappraisal* is the process of continually relabelling cognitive appraisals. Certain factors influence tne labelling of appraisals. Situational factors include the intensity of the external demands, the immediacy of the expected impact, and ambiguity. Person-related factors include motivational characteristics, belief systems and intellectual resources and skills.

Appraisal and coping are affected by the internal characteristics of the person. These include health and energy, as well as the person's belief system including existential belief (faith, religious beliefs, commitments or life goals (motivational properties), and the persons own sense of self including self-esteem, control and mastery. They also include knowledge, problem-solving skills and social skills which include ability to communicate and interact with others.

Physiologic Response to Stress

An understanding of the physiological changes associated with stress provide the foundation for the assessment of the client experiencing stress and the implications for health outcomes. The physiologic response to a stressor is a protective and adaptive mechanism to maintain the haemostatic balance of the body.

Stressors or demands may be physical; psychologic or social. The body will respond physiologically to both actual or symbolic stressors. The complex processes by which an event is perceived as a stressor and by which the body responds is not fully understood. However, there are three interrelated systems viz. nervous system, endocrine system, immune system.

Nervous System

Neural and hormonal actions to maintain haemostatic balance are integrated by the hypothalamus. Hypothalamus is located in the center of the brain, surrounded by the limbic system and the cerebral hemispheres. It integrates autonomic nervous system mechanism, that maintains the chemical constancy of the internal environment of the body. Hypothalamus participates in both emotional and physiologic response to stressors. This control is significant because most stressors precipitate an emotional reaction. In addition to the hypothalamus, other parts of the CNS including cerebral cortex, limbic system and reticular formations are involved in the neural control of emotions and the physiologic responses to stress. The functions of these structures are closely interrelated.

- *Cerebral cortex*: After an external event has occurred, afferent input is sent to the cerebral cortex via sensory impulses from the peripheral nervous system including the eyes and ears. In stress response, afferent impulses are carried from sensory organs (eyes, ear, nose, skin) and internal sensors (baroreceptors, chemoreceptors) to nerve centers to the brain. Afferent impulses that travel to the cortex from the periphery via the spinal cord (spinopthalmic pathway) also activate the reticular formation in the area of the brainstem. The reticular formation then relays input to the thalamus and from the thalamus to the cerebral cortex. The cerebral hemispheres are concerned with cognitive functions, through processes, learning and memory. (the limbic system has connection with the both cerebral hemispheres and the brainstem). The network of neurons which is involved with arousal and consciousness is called reticular activating system (RAS). The RAS functions to maintain wakefulness and alertness. The somatic, auditory and visual associative areas and the cerebral cortex receive input from the peripheral sensory fibres and then interpret it. The prefrontal area serves to reduce the speed of the associative functions so that the person has time to evaluate the information in light of the past experiences and future consequences and to plan a course of action. All these functions are involved in the perception of a stressor.

Limbic System:

The limbic system, which lies in the inner mid-portion of the brain, near the base includes the septum, cingulate gyrus, amygelula, hippocampus, and anterior muscle of the thalamus. The function of the limbic system is thought to be involved with emotions and behaviour. When these structures are stimulated, emotions, feelings, and behaviours can occur that ensure survival and self-preservation such as feeding, sociability and sexuality. (drinking, eating, temperature control, reproduction defense and aggression).

The cerebral cortex and limbic system instruct to serve the experiential and executive functions of emotions. Endorphins are found in this system and around, reduce the perception of painful stimuli.

- *Reticular Formation* is also located in between the lower end of the brainstem and the thalamus. It contains the RAS, which sends impulses contributing to the limbic system and to the cerebral cortex and thalamus. In addition to receiving input, from thr periphery, the RAS also receives impulses from the hypothalamus, when the RAS stimulates it increases its output of impulses leading to wakefulness. Both physiologic stresses, usually increase the degree of wakefulness.
- *Hypothalamus* which lies just above the pituitary gland has many functions as given below:

i. Co-ordinates impules:
   - Autonomic nervous system
   - Body temperature regulation
   - Food intake
   - Water balance
   - Urine formation
   - Cardiovascular function.

ii. Secretes releasing factors —regulation of anterior and posterior pituitary hormone.

iii. Affects behaviour:
   - Emotion and alertness.

The hypothalamus receives information regarding traumatic stimli via the spinopthalmic pathway, pressure - sensitive input from the baroreceptors via brainstem, and emotional stimuli via limbic system. Because the hypothalamus secretes peptide hormones and factors that regulate the release of hormones by the anterior pituitary, it is central to the connection between the nervous and endocrine system responding to stress. In addition, the hypothalamus regulates the function of both sympathetic and parasympathetic branches of the autonomic nervous system.

Endocrine System

Once the hypothalamus activated in response to stress, the endoctrine system becomes involved. The sympathetic nervous system stimulates the adrenal medulla to release the hormones epinephrines and the sympathetic nervous system including adrenal-medulla, is referred to as sympathoadrenal response. These hormones prepare the body for the "Fight or flight response" response. This response activated by physical stressors such as hypovelemia and hypoxia, and emotional status, particularly anger, excitement and fear.

The hypothalamas released corticocotrophin releasing hormones(CRH) which stimulates the anterior pituitary to release preopiomelanocortin (POMC). Both adrenocorticotrophic hormones (ACTH) and endorphin are derived from POMC. ACTH, in turn stimulates adrenal cortex to synthesize and secretes glucocorticoids, and to a lesser degree aldosterone and androgen. Glucocorticoids in particular, cortisol, are essential for the stress response. Cortisol produces a number of physiologic effects that include increasing the glucose level, potentiatory action of catecholamines on blood vessels and inhibiting inflammatory response. Aldosterone acts to increase sodium reabsorption in the kidney tubules, and as a result increases ECF. During stress, neural stimulation of the posterior pituitory results inthe secretion of ADH which also promotes water reabsorption by the distal and collecting tubules of the kidney.

Stimulation of both the adrenal medulla and cortex results in an increased blood glucose levels. This elevation provides the additional fuel for the increased metabolism needed for fighting or fleeing. The increased cardiac output, due to increased (HR & ECF) increased blood glucose level, and increased metabolic rate make the physical response possible. In addition dilatation of the skeletal muscle blood vessels and the brain provide quick movement and increased alertness.

Immune System

Negative stressors lead to alterations in immune functions in humans through processes involving the hypothalamic-pituitary adrenal axis and the autonomic nervous system that affect immune function. In return, the immune system also affects endocrine and CNS responses. Both corticostrenoids and catedholomines are known to suppress immune function. Interluccin-I (which is released by activated macrophages), one type of cytokine, may directly stimulate the release of ACTH and thus initiate the stress response. glucocorticoids depress the immune system, when there are present in high concentrations, there is a reduction in the inflammatory response to injury or infection. The steps of inflammation process is inhibited, lymphocytes are destroyed in lymphoid tissues and antibody production is decreased. As a result, the ability of the persons to resist infections is reduced.

Selye's Theory of Stress

In 1936, Selye, experimenting with animals, first described a syndrome consisting of the enlargement of the adrenal cortex, shrinkages, and thymus, spleen, lymph nodes and other lymphatic structures and the appearance of deep, bleeding ulcers in the stomach and duodenum. He identified this as a non-specific response to diverse, noxious stimuli. From this, he developed a theory of adaptation to biologic stress, which he titled The General Adaptation Syndrome (GAS).

The General Adaptation Syndrome (GAS) has three phases: Alarm, resistance, and exhaustion. Once the stressor or stimulus is integrated, into CNS, multiple responses occur because of activation of the hypothalamic pituitary adrenal axis and autonomic nervous system. The nature of these responses, in which the stimulus and its effects successively cause changes in nervous, endocrine and immune systems is fundamental to understanding the physiologic and behavioural changes that occur in an individual experiencing stress.

Stage of Alarm Reaction

The first stage of the stress response is the alarm reaction of the GAS, in which the individual perceives a stressor physically or mentally and the 'Fight or Flight' response is initiated. When the stressor is of sufficient intensity to threaten the steady of state of the individual, it requires a reallocation of energy so that adaptation can occur. In this stage, the sympathetic fight or flight response is activated with release of adrenal medullary hormones and the ACTH-adrenal cortical response begins. The alarm reaction is defensive and anti-inflammatric but self-limited. This temporarily decreases the individual's resistance and may even result in disease or death, if the stress is prolonged and severe, (because it is impossible to live in a continuous state of alarm).

The physical signs and symptoms of the alarm reactions are generally those of sympathetic nervous system stimulation. These signs include increased blood pressure, increased heart and respiratory rate, decreased gastrointestinal motility, pupil dilatation, and increased perspiration. The patient may complain of such symptoms as increased anxiety, nausea and anorexia.

Stage of Resistance

Since it is impossible to live in a continuous state of alarm, the person moves into the second stage, resistance. Ideally, the individual quickly moves from the alarm reaction to the stage of resistance, in which physiologic forces are mobilized to increase the resistance to stress. During this stage, adaptation to noxious stressors occurs. At this time, adaptation may occur, involving modification of the external and internal environment. Resistance is high at this time as compared with the normal state due to increased cortisol activity. The amount of resistance varies among individuals, depending on the level of physical functioning, coping abilities, and total number and intensity of stressors experienced. Although few overt physical symptoms and signs occur in this state as compared with the alarm stage, the person is expending energy in an attempt to adapt. This adaptive energy is limited by the resources of the individual.

Stage of Exhaustion

The stage of exhaustion occurs when all the energy for adaptation has expended. Exhaustion sets in and endocrine activity increases, producing deleterious effects on the body systems (especially circulatory, digestive and immune) that can lead to death. The physical symptoms of alarm reaction may briefly reappear in a final effort by the body to survive. This is exemplified by a terminally ill person who becomes alert and has stronger vital signs shortly, before death. The individual in this stage of exhaustion usually becomes ill and may die if assistance from outside sources is not available. This stage can often be reversed by external sources of adaptive energy such as medications, blood transfusion or psychotherapy. According to Selys, there is also a local adaptation syndrome (LAS). This syndrome includes inflammatory response and repair process that occur at the local site of tissue injury. The LAS occurs in small, topical injuries such as in contact dermatitis. If the local injury were severe enough, the GAS would be activated also.

Nursing Management

The client faces an array of potential stressors, or demands that can have health consequences. The nurse needs to be aware of the situations, that are likely to result in stress and also must assess the client's appraisal of the situations. The major areas that provide the nurse with useful guide in the assessment process include demands, human response to stressors and coping. It is always better to observe the following indices of stress, in which some are psychologic, some are physiologic, some behavioural, and some reflect social behaviour and thought process. Some of these reactions may be coping behaviours.

- General irritability, hyperexcitation or depression.
- Dryness of the throat and mouth.
- Overpowering urge to cry or run and hide.
- Easily fatigued, loss of interest.
- Floating anxiety "- do not know what or why.
- Easily startled.
- Stuttering or other speech difficulties.
- Hypermobility, pacing, moving about, cannot sit still.
- GI symptoms—butterflies in the stomach, diarrhea, vomiting.
- Change in menstrual cycle.
- Loss or excessive appetite.
- Increased use of legally prescribed drugs, e.g. tranquilizers.
- Accident proneness.
- Disturbed behaviour.
- Pounding of the heart.
- Impulsive behaviour, emotional instability.
- Inability to concentrate
- Feelings of unreality, weakness or dizziness.
- Tension, alertness,
- Nervous laughter.
- Grinding of teeth.
- Insomnia.
- Perspiring
- Increased frequency of urination.
- Muscle tension and migraine, headache.
- Pain in the neck and lower back.
- Increased smoking.
- Alcohol and drug addiction.
- Nightmares.

The probable nursing diagnosis in coping-tolerance pattern will be

- Impaired adjustment.
- Caregiver role strain.
- Ineffective individual coping: defensive coping/Ineffective denial.
- Ineffective family coping; compromised.
- Ineffective family coping; disabled.
- Family coping: potential for growth.
- Post-trauma response.
- Relocation stress syndrome.
- Risk for self-harm
- Risk for violence

And plan the nursing interventions accordingly to the situation or event and stress.

Nursing Interventions in Stress Management

The first step in managing stress is to become aware of its presence. This includes identifying and expressing stressful feelings (as stated above). The role of the nurse is to facilitate and enhance the coping and adaptation. Nursing interventions depend on the severity of the stress experience and demand. The nurse's efforts are directed to life-supporting interventions and to the inclusion of approaches aimed at the reduction of additional stressors to the client. The importance of cognitive appraisal in the stress experience should prompt the nurse to assess if changes in the way the client perceives and labels particular events or situations (cognitive reappraisal) are possible. So the nurse should also consider the positive effects that result from successfully meeting stressful demands. Greater emphasis should also be placed on the part of cultural values and beliefs enhancing or constraining various coping options.

An individual personal resource that aids in coping include health and energy. A health promoting lifestyle provides these resources and buffers or cushions the impact of stressors. Lifestyle or habits that contributed to the risk of developing illness can be reduced or eliminated. Health risk appraisal is an assessment method designed to promote health by examining the individual personal habits and recommending change where health risk is identified. For example, smoking, causes lung cancer and can be prevented by reducing or leaving the habit of smoking.

Coping Enhancement

It is a nursing intervention (and defined as "assisting a patient to adapt to perceived stressors, changes, or threats which interfere with meeting life demands and roles" (McCloskey,

Bulechek 1992). After completing a health-risk approach, the nurse could use "Coping enhancement to assist the patient in an analysis of the appraisal and to explore methods to improve the person's coping abilities including appraisal of his or her own personal resources.

The activities of coping enhancement are as follows:

- Appraise the patient's adjustment to change in body image as indicated.
- Appraise the impact of the patient's life situations on roles and relationships.
- Encourage the patient to identify a realistic description of change in role.
- Approve the patient's understanding of the disease process.
- Approve and discuss alternative responsis to situation.
- Use a calm reassuring approach.
- Provide an atmosphere of acceptance.
- Assist patient in developing an objective appraisal of an event.
- Help the client to identify the information he/she made ineterested in obtaining.
- Provide factual information concerning diagnosis, treatment and processis.
- Provide the patient with realistic choices about certain aspects of care.
- Encourage an attitude to realistic hope as a way of dealing with feelings of helplessness.
- Evaluate patients decision-making ability.
- Seek to understand the patient's perspective of a stressful situation.
- Discourage decision-making when patient is under severe stress.
- Encourage gradual mastery of the situation.
- Encourage patience in developing relationships.
- Encourage relationships with persons who have common interests and goals.
- Encourage social and community activities.
- Encourage the acceptance of limitation of others.
- Acknowledge the patient's spiritual/cultural background.
- Encourage the use of spiritual resources if desired.
- Explore the patient's previous achievements of success.
- Explore patient's reason for self-criticism.
- Confront patient's ambivalent (anger or depression) feelings.
- Foster constructive outlets of anger and hostility.
- Arrange situations that encourage patient's autonomy.
- Assist patient in identifying positive responses from others.
- Encourage the identification of specific life values.
- Explore with the patient previous methods of dealing with life problems.
- Introduce the patient to persons (or group) who have successfully undergone the same experience.
- Support the use of appropriate defence mechanisms.
- Encourage verbalization of feelings, perceptions and fears.
- Discuss consequences not dealing with guilt and shame.
- Encourage the patient to identify own strength and abilities.
- Assist patient in identifying appropriate short and long-term goals.
- Assist the patient in breaking down complex goals into manageable steps.
- Assist the patient in examining available resources to meet the goal.
- Reduce stimuli in the environment that could be misinterpreted as threatening.
- Appraise patient's needs/desires for social support.
- Assist the patient to identify available support systems.
- Determine the risk of the patient's inflicting self-harm.
- Encourage family involvement as appropriate.
- Encourage the family verbalize feelings about ill family member.
- Provide appropriate social skills training.
- Assist the patient in problem-sloving in a constructive manner.
- Instruct the patient on the use of relaxation techniques as needed.
- Assist the patient to grieve, and work through the losses of chronic illness and/or disability if appropriate.
- Assist the patient to clarify misconceptions.
- Encourage the patient to evaluate his/her own behaviour.

Relaxation Techniques

Synder (1993) and Egan (1993) identified relaxation technique as the major method used to relieve stress, included in nursing interventions. Commonly used techniques cited were progressive muscle relaxation, relaxation with guided imagery, and Benson's relaxation response. The goal of relaxation training is to produce response that counters the stress response.

- *Progressive Muscle Relaxation* involves tensing and releasing the muscles of the body in sequence and sensing the difference in feeling. It is best if the person lies on a soft cushion on the floor, in a quiet room, where he can breath easily. Self-taught or instructor-directed exercise that can involve learning to contract and relax muscles in a systematic way beginning with face and ending with feet. This exercise may be combined with breathing exercises that focus on inner-self.
- *Relaxation with Guided Imagery* is the 'purposeful use of imagination to achieve relaxation and/or direct attention away from undesirable sensations. The nurse helps the person to select a pleasant scene or experience from his or her past. This image serves as the mental device in this technique. As the person sits comfortably and quietly the nurse guides him to review the scene trying to feel and

relieve the imagery with all of the senses. A tape recording can be made for description of science or experience the pleasant one.

Benson's Relaxation Response

Benson and Proctor (1984) describe the following steps for this response which include:

Step 1. Pick a brief phrase or word that reflects your basic belief systems.
Step 2. Choose a comfortable position.
Step 3. Close your eyes.
Step 4. Relax your muscle.
Step 5. Become aware of your breathing and start using your selected focus word.
Step 6. Maintain a passive attitude.
Step 7. Continue for a set period of time.
Step 8. Practise the technique twice a day.

The response combines meditation with relaxation.

The other techniques of stress management will also include the following.

- *Thought stopping*: It is a self-directed behavioural approach used to gain control of self-defeating thoughts. When these thoughts occur the individual stops the thought process and focuses on conscious relaxation.
- *Exercises*: Regular exercise, especially, aerobic movement, results in improved circulation, increased release of endorphins on an enhanced sense of well-being.
- *Humour* in the form of laughter, cartoons, funny movies, riddles, audiocassettes, comic books and joke books can be used for both the nurse and patient.
- *Assertive behaviour*: Open honest, sharing feelings, desires and opinions in a controlled way. The individual who has control over one's own life is less subject to stress.
- *Social support*. This may take the form of organised support and self-help groups, relationships with family and friends and professional help.

In addition, meditation, breathing techniques, therapeutic touch, music therapy, biofeedback can be used as stress management technique.

(2) PAIN AND ITS MANAGEMENT

INTRODUCTION

Pain is a complex, multidimensional phenomenon. Everyone has experienced some types or degrees of pain. Pain prompts people to seek health care more often than any other problem. Pain is one of the most common problems faced by nurses when they are dealing with the patients. And also nurses are in an excellent position to work with the client in pain and to help that client overcome the pain. For which nurse has to earn more knowledge about pain and its management. The nurse has a responsibility to understand the experience of pain and to initiate measures that provide relief or help the client learn to cope. Because, the nurse spends more time with the patient in pain than any other health care professionals and has the opportunity to help relieve pain and its harmful effects. Some of the definitions enhance the nurse's ability to assess the client who is in pain by focusing on specific aspects of the pain experience.

DEFINITIONS OF PAIN

1. Pain is defined by McCaffery as "whatever the person experiencing the pain says it is, existing whenever the person says it does". It is subjective experience with no objective measurement.
2. The International Association for the Study of Pain (IASP) defined, "pain is an unpleasant sensory and emotional experience associated with actual or potential tissue damage or it is described in terms of such damage". Pain can be a major factor inhibiting the ability and willingness to recover from illness.
3. Mount Castle defined pain as "that sensory experiences evoked by stimuli that injure or threaten to destroy tissue, defined introspectively by every man as that which hurts".
4. Sternbach defined pain as (i) an abstract concept which refers to a personal, private-sensation of hurt, (ii) a harmful stimules that signals current or inpending tissue damage, and (iii) a pattern of responses to protect the organism from harm".

The nursing definition of pain is "whatever bodily hurt, he says it does". The cardinal rule in the care of patients with pain is that all pain is real, even if its cause is unknown.

NATURE OF PAIN

As stated earlier pain is whatever the experiencing person says it is and existing whenever the person says or does. This statement/definition makes the client the expert about his or her own pain. Because clinical pain is subjective and no objective measures of it exists, the only people who can accurately define their own pain are experiencing that pain. Although it is subjective in nature, the nurse charged with accurately assessing and helping to relieve the client's pain. To help a client gain relief, that nurse must believe that the pain exists.

Pain is a protective physiological mechanism. A person with a sprained ankle avoids bearing full weight on the foot to prevent further injury. Pain is a warning that tissue damage has occurred. The client who is unable to feel sensation, such as one with spinal cord tumor, is unaware of pain-inducing injuries. Pain is a leading cause of disability. As the average lifespan increases more people have chronic diseases in which pain is a common symptom. In additional medical advance have resulted in diagnostic and therapeutic measures that are uncomfortable. Nurses care daily for clients in pain.

DIMENSIONS/COMPONENTS OF PAIN

Pain consists of five components, i.e. affective, behavioural, cognitive, sensory, and physiologic. Affective component includes the emotions related to the pain. Behavioural components include the behavioural responses to the pain. Cognitive components include the beliefs, attitudes, evaluation and goals about the pain, and sensory components include the control how pain is perceived by altering transmission of nociceptive stimuli to the brain, that is, physiologic components of pain. These components are also called as dimensions of pain which help in assessment and management of pain. Pain results from complex interactions among these dimensions and can be understood by considering first the physiologic and thereafter the sensory, affective, behavioural and cognitive dimensions.

PHYSIOLOGY OF PAIN/PAIN PROCESS

Pain is a complex phenomenon. It is a mixture of physical, emotional and behavioural reactions. One way to gain the understanding the pain experience is to conceptualize pain as a process made-up of three physiological steps, i.e. reception, perception and reaction. Examining these steps of the process helps the nurse better understand the pain experience and better treat the client in pain.

Reception of Pain

Reception components involves three major steps: Transduction, transmission and modulation.

Pain Transduction

The strain of events that leads to pain begins where primary afferent nociceptors (PAN) fibres are excited by a variety of stimuli. The stimuli consist of mechanical events such as stretching of organs or pressures, extremes of temperature, i.e. heat or cold, and chemical changes such as ischemia. Specific fibres that react to these stimuli are classified as mechanical, thermal or chemical nociceptors. Fast pain is usually elicited by mechanical and thermal type of receptors (A-delta fibers) whereas slow pain can be elicited by all receptors (C-fibers). Together these fibres referred to as primary afferent nociceptors-primary afferent nociceptors fibers.

Fast pain It is the pain that occurs in about 0.1 second when painful stimuli are applied. It is often referred to as sharp, prickling, acute or electric pain. It is transmitted through a A-delta fibers. Fast pain is mostly caused by a more superficial stimulus.

Slow pain It is pain that begins one second or more after stimulation and increases slowly over seconds or minutes. This pain is also known as burning, aching, throbbing or chronic pain. It is often associated with tissue distraction and is felt in both superficial and deep tissues. It is transmitted through the more primitive type of fibers. A wide variety of chemical substances, including bradykinin, serotinin, histamine, substances of potassium, iron, acids, proteolytic enzymes, prostaglandins, and acetylcholine are significants in slow pain that often follows tissue injury.

Pain Transmission

Once the PAN (primary afferent nociceptors) are stimulated, the impulse they discharge travel as electrical activity to the spinal cord and on to the brain. This electrical activity becomes the experience of pain when it reached the brain. There will be no experience of pain, when/if the neural pathway for these impulses is blocked by surgical cutting or medications which inhibit the activity of pathways fibers or natural methods (endogenous) that block portion/the pain pathways.

Nerve fibers that carry somatosensory information from the body periphery to the spinal cord include A-beta, A-delta, and C fibers. A-type fibers have a myelin sheath that speeds up information transmission. A-delta fibers, transmit pain stimuli, A-beta fibers are larger and carry other sensory information such as touch. C-fibers transmit pain stimuli more slowly because they have no myelin sheath. C-fibers also conduct thermal, chemical and strong mechanical impulses. Pain sensation following stimulation of A-delta fibers differ from that following C-fiber stimulation. A-delta fiber activity is felt more slowly after painful stimulation but the sensation is more constant and continuous. It is persistent, dull and acting and is difficult to localize. These different fibers enter the dorsal root of the spinal cord, which transmits the pain impulses. The fibers separate as they enter the cord and then reform in the dorsal horn. This area receives, transmits and processes sensory impulses. The afferent nociceptors end at the level of the first, second and fifth laminae. The substation gelatinosa is found in the second laminae hypothized to be gating mechanism (Gate control theory).

Gate control theory A pain proposed by Melzack and Wall (1965) suggests that pain impulse can be regulated or even blocked by gating mechanisms along with central nervous system. The proposed location of the gates is in the dorsal horn of the spinal cord. Further findings suggested other gates exist (Melzact, denis 1978). When gates are open, pain impulses flow freely. When gates are closed, pain impulses become blocked. Partial opening of the gates may also occur. Small fibres carry most potentially painful impulses. Excitation of C-fibres inhibits gating mechanisms so that pain stimuli flow easily to cortical controls of brain. Large A-fibres pass through the same gating mechanisms. Whether the gates remain open or closed depend on whether competing passages from larger nerve fibres stimulate the gating mechanism. A bombardment of a large fibre sensory impulses such as those from the pressure of the back sub or heat of a warm compress closes the gates to PAN stimuli. Transmission of pain impulses from the spinal cord to the cerebral cortex can be inhibited or facilitated thus altering perception. This gate control theory gives the nurse a conceptual basis for pain relief measures to some extent.

Pain Modulation

There is a great deal of variations in the way clients perceive similarly painful stimuli. The pain modulation system is one reason, thus occurrence of variance. There are variety of mechanisms that contribute modulation are as follows.

Modulation via the dorsal horn The dorsal horn was once considered a simple relay for impulses, but is now known to contain extremely complex circulatory and multiple biochemical agents that both transmit and modulate nociceptive input. The dorsal horn is now thought to modulate the nociceptive impulses rather than simply receive and transmit these impulses. A high degree of processing of the sensory impulses occurs at this level.

Modulation via descending pathways The descending serotoninergic inhibitory fibres originate in the peraquaductual gray matter (PAG) of the midbrain and descend downward into the nuclear raphe magnus. Neurons from the PAG project downward into the dorsal horn at the first and fifty lamae levels. The neurotransmitters serotonin and substance P are released into these areas, contributing modulation of pain.

Modulation via endogenous chemicals Some chemical compounds release by injury or inflammation stimulate nociceptors, for example, histamine, bradykinin, serotonin, substance P and prostaglandin E. Pain may be reduced by medication that block these agents such as steroids, aspirin and other non-steroidal anti-inflammatory drugs (NSAIDs) that reduce inflammation and block prostaglandins. There is also a naturally occurring system within the nervous system called the "analgesia systems".

This analgesia system described by Guyton and Hall has three parts: (i) neurons from the periadaductal gray area of the mesencephalon and upper pons surrounding the adequate of sylvius send their signals to (ii) the raphe magnus nucleus, a thin midline nucleous located in the lower pons and upper medulla. Where the signals are sent down the dorsolateral columns in the spinal cord to (iii) a pain inhibitory complex located in the dorsal horns of the spinal cord. At this point in the system, pain can be blocked.

Perception of Pain

Pain perception refers to interpretation of the next phasé of the pain process. Once the nociceptive input has been received and transmitted, it must be perceived or interpreted. Because every individual perceives and interprets pain based on his or her individual experience, this one point at which pain becomes different for each person. Pain modulation occurs as it is being transmitted. For example other sensory input will help reduce, the amount of nociceptive information that is transmitting supraspinally.

Pain perception does not depend solely on the degree of physical damage. It is generally agreed both physical stimuli and psychosocial factors influence a person's experience of pain. Although there is little consensus on the specific effects of these factors, it is known that anxiety, experience, attention, expectation and measuring of the situation in which injury occurs affect pain perception. Brain activities such as distraction or anxiety may also affect the severity and quality of the pain experience.

In the past, pain was viewed as a primary sensation and motivational and cognitive processes were believed to influence only our reaction to pain, it now seems apparent that there are mechanisms within the body that can modify pain-related neural impulses even before they are transmitted to the brain. Thus, pain is likely to be determined by a relative balance between the sensory peripheral input and mechanisms of central control (brain) input to gating mechanisms in the spinal cord.

The first point the nurse needs to consider is the client's pain threshold. This is defined as the lowest intensity of a painful stimulus that is perceived by the client as pain. The pain threshold may vary based on physiologic factors such as inflammation or injury near pain receptors, but essentially it is similar for all people if the central and peripheral nervous system are intact. The second part of pain pertains to the individuals tolerance of pain. Tolerance is different for each person who experiences pain. This may vary within each person based on many subjective factors, such as meaning of pain and the setting. It really refers to the amount of pain the client willing to endure. Some individuals have high tolerance, that is, they can tolerate a lot of pain without distress, whereas others have a very low tolerance. This tolerance will also vary for a given individual depending on a variety of factors that influence pain such as nausea, fatigue and other sensory input. Only the client, not the health care team, can tell the tolerance level. The nurse must remember that pain tolerance can vary from situation to situation or from event to event.

Another aspect that will alter a person's perception of pain is his or her experience with pain. This may be the reason that people incorrectly assume that infants do not have pain. When infants feel pain, it is simply that the infant has no experience with pain and therefore, is unable to interpret it, and cannot communicate what is being felt. The reverse is also true. When a person has a bad experience with pain, the anticipation that future pain may be bad can make any work. There is also a physiologic reason if the pain is in the same area, that is persons with recurrent low back pain actually have a lower pain threshold and that area than persons who have not had low back pain.

Reaction to Pain

The reaction to pain is the physiological and behavioural responses that occur after pain is perceived. In physiological responses; as pain impulses ascend the spinal cord towards the brain system and thalamus, the automatic nervous system becomes stimulated as part of the stress response. Pain of low to moderate intensity and superficial pain elicits the flight or flight reaction of the general adaptation syndrome. Stimulation of the sympathetic branch of the autonomic nervous system results in physiological responses. If the pain is unrelenting, reverse or deep, typically originating from involvement of the visceral organs (such as with myocardial infarction, and colic from gallbladder or renal stones). The parasympathetic nervous system goes into action. Sustained physiological responses to pain could cause serious harm to an individual. Except in case of severe traumatic pain, which may send a person into shock, most people reach a level of adaptation in which physical signs return to normal. Thus, a client in pain will not always exhibit physical signs.

The behavioural responses of pain may be described in three phases of a pain experience which include anticipation, sensation and aftermath (Mein Hart and McCaffery 1983). Usually anticipation phases occur before pain received except some unforseen painful situations. Anticipation of pain often allows a person to learn about pain and its relief. With adequate instruction and support, client learn to understand pain and control anxiety before it occurs. Nurses play an important role in helping clients during the anticipatory phases with proper guidance, which help clients make aware of unknown and they cope with their discomfort. Sensation of pain occur when pain is felt. The ways that people choose to react to discomfort vary widely. A person's tolerance of pain is the point at which there is an unwillingness to accept pain of greater severity, or duration. The extent to which a person tolerates pain depends on attitudes, motivation and value. Pain threatens physical and psychological well-being. Typical body movements and facial expressions that indicate pain include holding the painful part, bent posture and grimaces. A client may cry moan. Often the client expresses discomfort through restlessness and frequent requests to the nurse. The nurse soon learns to recognize patterns of behaviour that reflect pain. Aftermath phase of pain occurs when it is reduced or stopped. Even though the source of discomfort is controlled, a client may still require the nurse's attention. Pain is a crisis. After painful experience client may experience physical symptoms such as chills, nausea, vomiting, anger or depression. If there are repeat episodes of pain, aftermath responses can become serious health problems. The nurse helps clients gain control and self-esteem to minimise fear over potential pain experience.

The individual reaction to pain adds even more variation to the pain process. There are many variable factors in this part of the process, including situation, culture, age, sex, cause of pain, tolerance, value and meaning of pain and various psychological factors such as fear, anxiety and depression.

FACTORS INFLUENCING PAIN

Situation

The situation associated with the pain influence the person's response to it. A person's responses to pain experienced in a formal crowded situations may differ greately from the responses were he or she alone or in a hospital.

Culture

Culture influences how people learn to react to express pain. People respond to pain in different ways. The nurse must neve assume to know how clients will respond. However, an understanding of cultural background, socio-economic status, and personal attitudes help the nurse more accurately assess pain and its meaning for clients. A young girl in a stoic culture may be allowed to cry because of pain whereas boys are not allowed to cry in some culture.

Age

Age is an importatn variable that influences pain, particularly in children and older adults. Age may release a client from culturally imposed norms in relation to pain expression. Developmental differences found among these age groups can influence how children and older react to the pain experience. Young children have difficulty in understanding pain and the procedures nurses administer that may cause pain. Young children who have not developed vacabularies also have difficulty verbally describing an expressing pain to parents/caregivers. Cognitively toddlers are unable to recall explanations about pain or associate pain as experiences that can occur in various situation. Older people may assign different meanings to that pain. Pain is often thought by the elderly as natural manifestation of aging.

Sex

Gender may be an important influence in pain. In most cultures boys are expected to show less expression of pain than girls. As they grow older men are also expected to express pain less than that of women.

Meaning of Pain

The meaning of a person's pain is a factor that influences his or her responses to pain. A person will perceive pain differently if it suggests a threat, loss, punishment, or challenges. For example a woman in labour perceives pain differently from a woman expressing pain from a recent back injury or pain caused by childbirth. If the cause is unknown, more negative psychological factors use such as fear, anxiety, etc. Come into play and the pain may be misinterpreted resulting in an inappropriate response. A client copes differently with pain, depending on its meaning.

Anxiety

The degree of anxiety the client is experiencing also may influence the client's response to pain. It is not possible to separate the mind from the body, so pain is always has both physiologic and psychological components. When anxiety is high, pain is felt greater. Emotionally healthy persons are usually able to tolerate moderate or even severe pain than those whose emotions are less stable.

Fatigue

Fatigue heightens perceptions of pain. This intensifies pain and decreases coping abilities. Pain is often experienced less after a restful sleep than at the end of a long day.

Attention

The degree to which a client focuses on pain can influence pain perception. Increased attention has been associated with increased pain, whereas distraction has been associated with a diminished pain response. This concept is one that nurses apply in various pain relief measures such as relaxation, guided emergency and massage.

Previous Experience

Each person learns from painful experiences. Previous experience does not necessarily mean that a person will accept pain more easily in the future. If a person has had frequent episodes of pain without relief or bouts of severe pain, anxiety or even fear may occur. In contrast if a person had repeated experience of pain, may be better prepared to tolerate or take necessary actions to relieve pain to some extent.

Coping Style

The experience of pain can be lonely, when client experiences pain in health care setting such as hospitals, the loneliness can be unbearable. Frequently, client feels a loss of central pain and an inability to control their environments or the outcome of event's coping style thus influences the ability to deal with pain.

Family and Social Support

Parents and attitudes of significant others also affect pain response. People in pain often depend on family members for support, assistance or protection. An absence of family members or friends can often make the pain more stressful. For children, presence of parents is very essential.

TYPES OF PAIN

There are different ways to define types of pain, which include according to onset, duration, severity, modes of transmission, location, causation and causative force. The examples of which are as follows:

- Onset or time of occurrence, e.g. postoperative pain
- Duration, e.g. chronic pain or acute pain
- Severity or intensity, e.g. severe, mild or scored (0 to 10 on a scale)
- Location or source, e.g. superficial, deep or central pain
- Causation, e.g. pain due to receptor stimulation or nerve damage, or psychophysiologic pain.
- Causative force or agent, e.g. spontaneous, self-inflicted or other pain.

The common terms used to classify pain are as follows.

Acute Pain

Acute pain is usually of recent onset and is most commonly associated with a specific injury. It is time limited and generally has a defined cause and purpose. It may be mild, moderate or severe in nature and is usually sudden in onset. It occurs abruptly after an injury or disease, persists until healing occurs, and often intensified by anxiety or fear. Acute pain consistently, increasing during wound care, ambulation, coughing and deep breathing. It is described in sensory terms such as sharp, stabbing and shooting. Acute pain indicates that damage or injury has occurred. It draws the attention to the fact that it is occurring and teaches us to avoid similar potentially painful situation. So acute pain is seen as a useful and limiting pain in that indicates injury and motivates the person to get relief by treatment of the pain and usually the cause. Acute pain is usually reversible or controllable with adequate treatment. If no lasting damage occurs or systematic disease exists, acute pain usually decreases as healing occurs; this generally occurs in less than six months and usually less than one month. Acute pain can be described as lasting from a few second to six months, e.g. prick of finger in a second and fracture for six months.

Usually the acute pain leads to discomfort, uncomfortable and disturbs the individual in many aspects according to the nature and extent of pain. An unrelieved acute pain can affect the pulmonary, cardiovascular, gastrointestinal, endocrine and immunologic system. It leads to autonomic response that is considered with sympathetic stress response. The significant negative effects are increased heart rate, increased stroke volume, increased blood pressure, increased pupillary dilation, increased muscle tension, decreased gastrointenstinal motility, decreased salivary flow (dry mouth). The stress response may increase the patient risk for physiologic disorder (MI, pulmonary infection, thromboembolism, prolonged paralytic ileus) and the psychologic disorders which include anxiety and persists. If acute pain is not effectively managed, it may progress to a chronic pain.

Chronic Pain

Chronic pain is a complex physiological and psychological phenomenon that causes varying degrees of disability in a large portion of the population. Chronic pain is constant or intermittant in nature that persists over a period of time. It lasts beyond the expected time and often cannot be attributed to a specific cause or injury. Chronic pain is often defined as pain that lasts for six months or more. It may begin as acute pain but it persists over an extended period of time. The pain may be mild, moderate or severe and may be intermittant or continuous.

Chronic pain is classified as malignant or non-malignant.

Non-malignant Pain

Chronic pain is usually considered pain that lasts more than six months or one month beyond the normal end of the condition causing pain and has no forceable and except very slow healing, as with burns, or death. It is continuous or persistent and recurrent. Chronic pain may have an identifiable cause although the cause may be difficult to determine; and is often described using effective terms, such as 'hateful' or 'sickening', and is often much more difficult to treat than acute pain. It is considered useless pain because it is not usually a manifestation of impending damage. For example, severe rheumatic arthritic chronic pain is often frustrating and difficult for a person to live with. It gives no clues about how to lessen it. Clients experiencing continuous and continually recurring chronic pain often become increasingly ingrossed by their illness. They may seem fearful, tense, fatigued and depressed. Many persons with an unending chronic pain become withdrawn and isolated. Their pain often exhausts them and their families, physically and emotionally.

Malignant Pain

Malignant pain is considered to have qualities of both acute and chronic pain. It can be of different types. An individual's mental response to pain depends on the duration and possibility and the intensity of the pain. Pain that is constant, continuous and moderate is often described by the client (patient as far more difficult to bear that pain than paraxysmal and intense). The duration of chronic pain includes months and years of pain, not minutes or hours. It is associated withdrawal and despaire. Anxiety may give way to depression. Some chronic pain patients/clients learn to adapt and cope with the pain, adjusting their lives.

The sympathetic arousal that may be associated with acute pain diminishes over weeks or months even though the pain itself persists. Sympathetic adaptation occurs over time. The nurse must remember, however, that the absence of expected expression of severe pain does not mean, that the pain is gone. The nurse must depend on the client's description, the manifestations are not expected to find in the clients. Most clients have major effective and behavioural changes when experiencing pain for prolonged period. Such changes may be compounded and chronic pain syndrome can develop. The following are the characteristics of chronic pain syndrome:

- Depressed mood
- Increased or decreased appetite and weight, decreased libido capacity, poor physical tone and increased depression
- Social withdrawal—withdrawal from outside interests and relationship
- Preoccupation with physical manifestation
- Poor sleep and chronic fatigue, leads to inactivity, analgesics, depression.

For example, in cases of cancer pain, arthritis, trigeminal neuralgia, etc. Some clients with chronic pain may not exhibit any of the above mentioned manifestations or they may exhibit only a few. However, once these changes take place, they may become more significant to treatment than the pain's original physical source. Unfortunately psychosocial implications about pain sometimes reinforce the idea that clients may make too much fuse over that pain.

Superficial Pain

Superficial pain occurs when the receptors in surface tissues are stimulated. Superficial or cutaneous pain is classified into two types:

i. Pain with an abrupt onset and a sharp or stinging quality, and
ii. Pain with a slower onset and burning quality.

Superficial pain may be delineated by having the client point to the painful area. It may occur along each segment representing a portion of the body surface innervated by one dorsal root, a dermatome or skin segment in an area of skin supplied by one dorsal root. Each spinal nerve has dorsal and sensory root. The boundaries of dermatome may appear to be distinct in anatomic drawings, but nerve distribution actually overlaps. Irritation of one posterior root produces pain in adjacent dermatomes. A spinal nerve attaches the spinal cord with two roots anterior and posterior. The anterior root contains efferent nerve fibers that carry impulses from the CNS to the periphery of the body. The posterior root contains afferent nerve fibers that carry impulses from the body's periphery towards CNS. Cutaneous pain is relatively uncomplicated because it is readily localized, that is, which client can indicate exactly where it hurts.

Deep Pain

Deep pain arises from deeper tissues. Deep pain is divided automatically into splanchnic which refers to pain in the viscera and deep somatic refering to pain in deep structures other than the viscera, such as-muscle, tendons, joints and periosteum.

Splanchnic Pain

Viscera refers to abdominal viscera. Actually, a viscus (plural viscera) in any of the large interior body organs occupies any body cavity such as the cranial, thoracic, abdominal or pelvic cavities. Visceral pain tends to be diffuse, poorly localized, vague, dull pain. Nerve fibers innervating body organs follows the sympathetic nerves to the spinal cord. This may be the reason why autonomic manifestations (e.g. diarrhhea, cramps, sweating, hypertension) frequently accompany visceral pain. Typical visceral pain includes acute appendicitis, cholecystitis, inflammation of the biliary and pancreatic tract, gastroduodenal disease, cardiovascular disease, pleurisy and renal and ureteral colic. Visceral pain is transmitted through the sympathetic and parasympathetic fibers of autonomous nervous system, with the pain being referred to the body surface, often in sites at a distance. Visceral pain also may be sent through the nerve fibers in the parietal pleura, pericardium, or peritoneum and is called parietal pain. Parietal pain is transmitted directly to the spinal nerves, with the pain being felt directly over the painful area. Parietal tissue is well supplied with spinal nerve instead of sympathetic nerves. Pain starting in the parietal tissue is often very sharp.

Deep Somatic Pain

Somatic structures are those of the body wall, such as muscles and bones. Pain in the somatic structures is complicated phenomenon. The main difference between superficial pain and deep pain is difference between cutaneous and deep sensitivity (i.e. the capacity to receive stimulus and respond to them is the difference in nature) of the pain evoked by noxious or harmful stimuli. For example, unlike cutaneous pain, deep pain is poorly localised, may produce nausea, and is frequently associated with sweating and changes in the blood pressure. Deep somatic pain is generally diffuse, less localizable than cutaneous pain. This is because the area supplied by one posterior nerve root (sclerotome) is less well defined than in dermatome and does not correspond with a dermal segment. Also pain from deep structures frequently radiates/spreads from primary site, e.g. pain from lumbar disc is felt along the sciatic nerve.

Somatic structures vary in their sensitivity to pain. Highly sensitive structures include tendons, deep fascia, ligaments, joints, bone periosteum, blood vessels and nerve. Skeletal muscle is sensitive only in stretching and ischemia. Bone and cartilage respond to extreme pressure and chemical stimulation, for example, Rh arthritis, osteomyelitis.

Localized Pain

Localized pain arises directly from the site of the disturbance.

Referred Pain

Referred pain is one which is felt in a part of the body which is remote from the actual point of stimulation. The impulses usually arise in an organ, but the pain is projected to a surface area of the body. Both visceral and somatic pains are usually referred to as segment of skin because visceral fibrosynapse at the level of the spinal cord close to fibers innervating some subcutaneous tissue. A classifical example of referred pain is that associated with 'angina pectoris', the pain originates in the heart muscle as a result of ischemia, but it may be experienced in the midsternal region, the base of the neck and down the left arm. Similarly, in myocardial infarction, pain is not felt in the heart, but it is felt at left arm shoulder or jaw pain. It may be due to the fibers innervating these areas are close to those innervating the myocardium resulting in the referred pain. Similarity in pain of appendicitis is often reported by the patient as being in the midline of the abdomen, above the umbilicus whilst the appendix is usually located deep in the abdomen, close by the appendix, on the right side.

Identification of the segment of the spinal cord that is involved, is transmitting referred pain is diagnostically helpful. Pain arising from a deep structure, whether a deep somatic structure or a viscus has a referred segmental distribution or a pattern of pain, determined according to the spinal cord segment supplying to this structure.

Intractable Pain

Persistent, severe pain that cannot be effectively controlled by the usual medication is referred to as "intractable pain". Intractable chronic pain states, producing prolonged and intense bombardment of the central nervous system are very difficult to bear. The client may become suicidal or at least take no steps to prolong life.

Headache

Headache is the most common type of pain, frequently discomfort experienced by many people, and applies to the pain sensation that is perceived as being in the cranial vault (excluding facial pain, toothache and earache). There are many causes of headache involving both intracranial and extracranial structures. The brain itself is almost insensitive to pain, although the venous sinuses, tentorium, dura, some of the cranial nerves and associated vasculature are pain sensitive. One of the most sensitive areas in the brain is middle meningeal artery. Changes in intracranial pressure, either decrease or increase, may lead to headache, because the pressure changes cause the pain sensitive structures in the head to shift.

There are many types of headache of intracranial origin. Vascular headache is common type of intracranial headache. This headache can be caused by a variety of problems such as: hypertension, sepsis, hypoxia, and various medications. Other causes of intracranial headache include infection, haemorrhage, and changes in intracranial structures. Migraine is also a type of headache of intracranial origin but cause is unknown.

There are many types of headaches of extracranial original which are common and have many causes. Many extracranial structures are sensitive to nociceptive stimuli. These structures include the skin, subcutaneous tissues, muscles, arteries and periosteum of the skull. Problem in the eyes, sinuses, ears, teeth, nose, and jaws also may lead to headache. The mechanisms of these headaches are similar to headaches of intracranial origin. Stimuli such as: traction, distention, dilation and spasms of vessels, irritation of nerves and inflammation of various structures can cause them. The common types of extracranial headache are muscle tension, temporomandibular joint syndrome, ocular sinus, dental and otic.

Headaches can be best treated by first identifying the cause.

Psychogenic Pain

Psychogenic pain is that experience when there is no detectable organic lesion. However, pathology may still be present. Psychogenic pain refers to pain that believed primarily due to emotional factor rather than physiologic dysfunctions. Clients experiencing psychogenic pain have a real pain experience. Psychogenic pain is different from pretended pain. Although psychogenic pain starts without a physical basis, repeated severe stress probably alters the complex physiology of pain transmission, modulation, and perception. The pain the client feels is real to that client and the tension and/or stress the client is feeling may lead to pronounced physiologic changes. When the psychogenic effect of stress, anxiety, fear and anger produces painful alteration in physiology, these can be called "psychophysiologic pain". Psychogenic pain requires that the cause may be found and treated.

NURSING MANAGEMENT OF PAIN

In the management of pain, nursing has an important role in anticipating and preventing pain, and in supporting clients who have been thorough physically painful experience. Appropriate information effectively communicated can do much to help provide a sense of control and minimizing anxiety. Advance knowledge of the physiological and psychological dimensions of plan provides a challenge for the nurse critically to examine nursing practices in pain assessment and management.

Assessment

Assessment is essential for diagnosis and for planning of pain control measures. Pain is difficult to measure because pain is a subjective experience or phenomena. One of the priorities for adequate treatment of pain is an accurate assessment. The goal of pain assessment is to identify the aetiology of the pain; to understand the patient's sensory, affective, behavioural and cognitive pain experience for the purpose of implementing pain management techniques; and to identify the patient's goal for therapy and resources for self-management of the pain. It is the nurse often who is responsible for gathering and documenting assessment data.

Assessment, however, is highly influenced by the client's ability to delineate aspects of the pain experience accurately. If the client cannot communicate clearly (e.g. child, unconscious patient) then this aspects of the pain assessment is altered. Without the subjective information, it is difficult to intervene effectively except by trial and error. Ongoing assessment of pain is useful. This ongoing assessment should include subjective and objective assessment, that is, the individuals' verbal description of the pain and observation of person's behaviour.

Each person has a basic human need to be free to pain and discomfort. Humans are motivated to avoid pain. Pain can occur as a result of inadequate satisfaction of other basic human needs. For example, need to eliminate urine not met because urinary stones block the bladder outlet and pain occurs. Part of the nursing assessment is to identify any unmet needs that may contribute to person's pain.

Each person experiences and expresses uniquely and attaches personal meaning or explanations to pain experiences. The personal meanings nurses attach to pain may interfere with the assessment. The personal meanings attached to pain result from personal pain experience throughout life and may arise from a person's individual experience and sociocultural experiences. The cultural and familial role modeling one supposes to teach a child is as the following:

- What pains are appropriate or inappropriate to talk about
- Behaviour that is a appropriate or inappropriate when one experiences pain
- Circumstances likely to produce pain, which should therefore be avoided
- Various methods to avoid pain
- Reasons, why one may experience pain such as punishment, testing by supernatural or devine powers, or bad thoughts
- Possible consequence of pain, such as attention or lack of attention from others, imminent death.

A pain experience is also affected by personal factors:

- Pain expectancy (the anticipation of pain)
- Pain experience (willingness to experience pain)
- Pain apprehension (generalized desire to avoid pain)
- Pain anxiety (the anxiety of pain provokes because of its associated mystery, loneliness, helplessness, threat).

Since the pain evokes emotional responses, observation of behaviour of the client/patient provides a nurse with understanding of a person's feelings and of what pain means to a particular person. By accepting behaviours and trying to understand their origins, nurses can help individuals experiencing pain. To do this well, nurses must:

- Accurately observe client's behaviour
- Listen to all that clients say
- Never judge clients or jump to conclusions.

The perception, pain, is influenced by number of factors, which include integrity of the nervous system, state of consciousness, age, physical states (fatigue, debility, lack of sleep, and prolonged suffering all reduce a client's ability to tolerate pain) and emotional states (worry, fear, and anxiety reduce a person's ability to tolerate pain).

Assessment Process

The assessment process should provide the nurse with understanding of the patient's/client's pain, as well as establishing the nurse as a partner in the patient's search for pain relief. Patient teaching is an integral part of assessment, as information is provided clarifying the nurse's questions or responding to the patient's concern. As the patient discomfort is a source of stress to the family, it is important to involve the family and other members of the patient's network in the pain assessment. If the patient's ability to speak for himself or herself is limited, it is imperative to involve the family.

An accurate history is essential to assess a client's/patient's experience of pain. A detailed system analysis is performed using the following guidelines, to find out various aspects of pain.

Location The location should be identified as specifically as possible. To determine the location of the patient's pain ask the following questions:

- Where is pain in the body?
- Is the pain internal or on the surface (external)?
- Is the pain always in these areas?
- If the pain is in more than one spot, are the pains equal, or does one trigger the others?
- Is the pain on both sides of your body? If so, is it the same on each side?

The site may be well-defined or diffused or the pain may radiate, involving wider area. To determine the extension and radiation of patient's pain ask the following questions:

- Does the pain extend from where it started? Does it cover a wider area, or can you point to where it is?
- Is there a pattern in which the pain spreads?
- Is the pain on the surface or deep inside?

Observing the pain locations on the patient's body will help localize the sites of pain as well as identify any physical changes at the site such as swelling/or discolouration.

Onset and duration When the pain first began and how the pain has changed over time should be determined. To determine the onset and pattern of the patient's pain ask the following questions:

- When did the pain begin? Is it a regular pain or does it vary? Does it occur in cycles, e.g. sometimes, every day; every month or every spring
- What triggers the pain? Are there specific things that always trigger it? Can you identify particular patterns?
- Does the pain begin suddenly or gradually over time? Is it continuous, or does it vary? Are there separate episodes of pain? If, so, does the pain go away completely between episodes or does it just get better?
- Has the pain pattern changed at all since it began?
- Has your lifestyle changed since the pain began?

To determine the duration of the patient's pain, ask the following questions:

- How long does the pain last? Are you free of pain between episodes?
- Is the pain constant, intermittent or rhythmic?

Character or quality A description of the pain, using patient's own words is helpful in determining the origin of pain and possible pain relief measures. To determine the character or quality of the patient's pain, ask the client the following question to describe it.

- Is the pain, dull, sharp, throbbing, burning, electric or shooting?

If the patient is unable to provide such descriptions the descriptors used in the McGill-Melzack pain questionnaire can be used.

Exacerbating factors Often patients may be comfortable at rest, but have difficulty in morning due to pain. Activities which exacerbate the pain should be identified. To determine the factors, that precipitate, aggravate and alleviate the patient's pain ask the following questions:

- What seems to trigger pain? Can you identify a specific cause or event that always or sometime precedes the pain?
- Does anything alter the pain? Does anything make it worse, such as smoking, drinking alcohol, eating, heat or tension? Is there anything that makes the pain better, such as rest, activity–heat or cold or medications.

Associated manifestations The impact of pain on the person's physical functioning should be explored. To determine whether there are any manifestations associated with client's pain, ask the following questions:

- Are there any other problems caused by your pain
- Do you have any nausea/vomiting, restlessness, insomnia, excessive sleeping, or loss of appetite.

Associated manifestations also include profuse perspiration, fainting, inability to perform usual functions, dulling of senses, apathy, clouding of consciousness, disorientation and inability to rest and sleep.

Effect on activities of daily living To determine how the client's pain affects activities of daily living, ask the following questions:

- Does the pain interfere with work, sleep, driving, eating, school work, sexual relations, housework, social activity or other activity
- Has the pain caused any changes in your lifestyle
- When did you last have a good night's sleep.

Intensity A new pathogenic condition must be ruled out when there is sudden increase in pain intensity, the intensity of the pain can be measured in several ways which are summarised as follows:

- *Visual analogue scale (VAS)* – consists of a 10 cm line vertical or horizontal with one end marked 'no pain' and other 'worst possible pain' (Fig. 3.1).

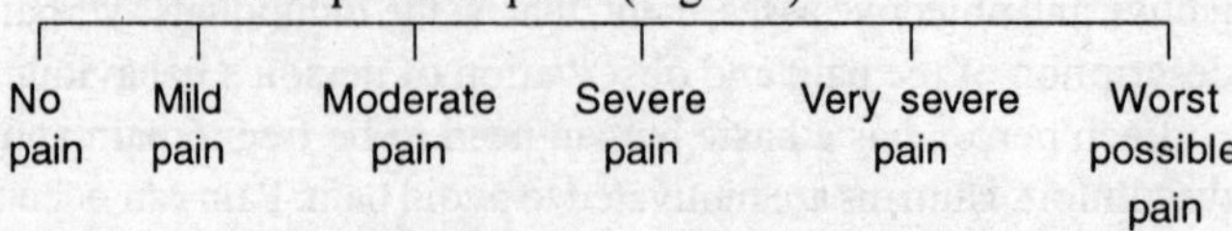

Fig. 3.1: Visual analogue scale

The patient marks the line to show where the pain lies. This approach works well for acute pain. It is not useful in chronic pain. Some patients have difficulty in understanding the basic concept involved in it, and may not be able to use the scale at all.

- *Numerical rating scale (NRS)* – typically runs from 0 (no pain) to 10 (unbearable) although 0-5 or 0-7 may be used. Here the patient simply gives a score to indicate that pain level (Fig. 3.2).

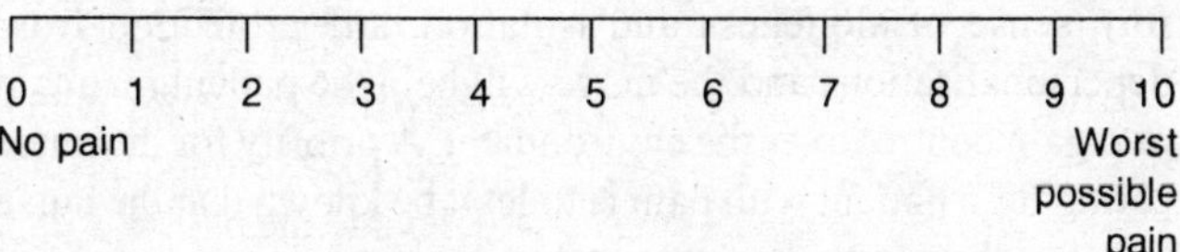

Fig. 3.2: Numerical rating scale

- *Verbal descriptor scale (VDS)* – here, a range of words are used to describe the potential spectrum of pain and the patient states which word most accurately reflects how they feel.
- *McGill pain questionnaire* – is complex but reliable and sensitive tool which involves multidimensional measurements of pain with time, the effect it has on the patient, location and intensity of pain.

To determine the intensity of patient's pain the following should be done:

- Ask, on a scale of 0-10 with '0' being 'no pain' and '10' being 'the worst pain you can imagine' how would you rate your pain now? How would you rate it worst? How would you rate it with activity?
- Note what non-verbal manifestation of pain the client exhibits—grimacing, crying, moaning, sleeping, appearing exhausted, or remaining immobile.

Relief measures The efficacy of measures used by the patient to relieve pain should be identified. To determine how the patient obtains pain relief, ask the following questions:

- What do you do to relieve the pain (ask about both invasive and non-invasive pain relief measures)
- What has not worked to relieve your pain?

This includes both those activities suggested by the medical and nursing staff such as the use of analgesic, as well as measures employed by the patient himself, such as distraction, visualization, rubbing, etc. All drugs used by the patients and their dose.

Physical examination Start the examination by having the patient show where the pain is and describe how it feels. Pain is subjective and the patient himself is an expert about his/her pain, but objective manifestations that observed by nurse and other health care providers give clue to its cause. Objective manifestations of pain can be divided into three categories which include sympathetic responses, parasympathetic responses and behavioural responses.

Sympathetic responses are often associated with minimal to moderate pain intensity or superficial pain. They signify the other body defenses are mobilized and that the fight-or-flight response has begun. Objective manifestations include pallor, increased pulse, increased blood pressure, increased respiration, skeletal muscle tension, dilated pupils and diaphoresis.

Parasympathetic responses are often associated with pain of severe intensity or with deep pain. In this, body defenses may collapse in an attempt to lesson the effects of external threat. Manifestations of parasympathetic response include decreased blood pressure, decreased pulse, nausea and vomiting, weakness, prostration, pallor and loss of consciousness.

The patient may exhibit the behavioural responses in the acute pain as follows (Table 3.1).

Table 3.1: Behavioural indications of effects of pain

• *Vocalization*	: Moaning, crying, screaming, gasping, grunting.
• *Facial expression*	: Grimace, clenched teeth, wrinkled forehead, tightly closed or widely opened eyes or mouth, lip biting, tightened jaw
• *Body movement*	: Restlessness, immobilization, muscle tension, increased hand and finger movements, pacing activities, rhythmic or rubbing motions, protective movement of body parts
• *Social interaction*	: Avoidance of conversation, focus only on activities for pain relief, avoidance of social contact, reduced attention span.

- Assume a posture that minimizes pain such as lying rigidly, guarding drawing up the legs, or assuming the fetal position
- Moan, sign, grimace, clench the jaws or fist, become quiet, or withdraw from others
- Blink rapidly
- Cry, appear frightened, exhibit restlessness
- Have a drawn facial expression
- Have twitching muscles
- Withdraw when touched
- Hold or protect the painful area or remain motionless.

Although it is unreasonable to think that the nurse would be performing the detailed assessment constantly with a patient, portions of it are important and should be done at regular intervals.

Nursing Diagnosis

An accurate diagnosis made only after a complete assessment clusters of defining characteristics reveal the nursing diagnosis best fitted to the client/patient condition and needs. The nursing diagnosis should focus on the specific nature of these pains to help the nurse identify the most useful types of interventions for alleviating pain and minimizing its effect on the client's lifestyle and function.

The nursing diagnoses are directly associated with care of patients with pain, i.e. chronic pain. The other nursing diagnoses that may be appropriate because of the effects of pain on other aspects of a patient's life include the following (Table 3.2):

- Anxiety
- Knowledge deficit (specify)
- Body image disturbance
- Altered nutrition
- Colonic constipation
- Impaired physical mobility
- Ineffective family coping, disabling
- Ineffective individual coping
- Powerlessness
- Altered family processes
- Altered role performance
- Fatigue
- Selfcare deficit (specify)
- Fear
- Sexual dysfunction
- Anticipatory grieving
- Sleep pattern disturbance
- Social isolation
- Altered thought process.

Following are the examples of nursing diagnoses for pain:

1. Anxiety related to (R/T) unrelieved pain.
2. Pain R/T physical injury/reduced blood supply to tissue/natural childbirth process.
3. Chronic pain R/T chronic physical disability/psychosocial disability/inadequate pain control.
4. Hopelessness R/T chronic malignant pain.
5. Ineffective individual coping R/T chronic pain.
6. Impaired physical mobility R/T musculoskeletal pain/incisional pain.
7. Risk for injury, R/T reduced pain reception.
8. Self-care deficit (specify) R/T musculoskeletal pain.
9. Sexual dysfunction R/T arthritic hip pain.
10. Sleep pattern disturbance R/T low back pain.

Planning

For each nursing diagnosis identified, the nurse develops a care plan for the client/patient needs. Together the nurse and patient discuss realistic expectation for pain-relief measures and the degree of pain relief to expect. Objectives of the care are selected on the basis of the nursing diagnosis and client condition. Appropriate measures and therapies are chosen on the basis of the related factor contributing to the patient's pain or health problem.

A critical element in the management of a patient with a pain syndrome is the establishment of a trusting relationship and good rapport with the patient and the family. The patient and the family need to know that the nurse considers the pain significant and understands that pain may totally disrupt a person's life. The nurse's goal is to help the patient cope with the pain by using medications and techniques to help with relaxation, comfort, sense of aloneness and isolation, and protection from depersonalisations and the nurse will help the patient maintain or regain control over the environment. A priority for the nurse caring for a patient with pain is to let it be known that the nurse believes the person has pain and to explain some of the physiologic mechanism of pain.

Nursing actions that promote the establishment of an effective relationship with the person who is experiencing pain and with the family should include the following.

Believe the patient The patient needs to be able to trust the nurse to believe in the pain's existence. This message can be conveyed verbally to the patient by saying "I know you are in pain". The nurse may need to help the family believe the patient.

Clarify responsibilities in pain relief Discuss what the nurse is going to do, and what the patient and the family are expected to do.

Respect the patient's response to pain The nurse should accept the right of the patient to respond to the pain in the necessary manner. The family also needs help in this area. The patient may need help to accept the reasons to pain; the behaviour may be less than is expected by the patient and the family.

Collaborate with the patient The patient should be encouraged to use coping techniques that have been effective in the past. The patient and the family should be helped to participate actively in setting goals for pain relief.

Explore the pain with the patient The nurse needs to find out the meaning of the pain to the person enduring the pain and to the family.

Be with the patient often The nurse should act as buffer for the patient and the family during difficult times. The nurse's physical presence may reassure or distract the patient or it may offer variety, thus relieving the pain.

Guidelines for Individualising Pain Therapy

When providing pain relief measures, the nurse chooses therapies suited to the client's unique pain experience, McCaffery (1979) suggests nine useful guidelines for pain therapy. The following guidelines are eleven which include nine.

Establish a relationship of mutual trust Always believe the client and try to convey concern. An adversial relationship between nurse and client lessens the effectiveness of pain therapies.

Table 3.2: Nursing care plan for pain relief

Problems	*Reasons*	*Objectives*	*Nursing interventions*	*Evaluation*
Pain related to abdominal incision movement	c/o sharp, localized pain over lower abdominal incisions worsening during coughing and movement. Guards abdomen rigidly while turning and breathing deeply.	1. Client will achieve control of pain within 24 hours after surgery. 2. Patient will initiate movement in bed without painful behavioural cues. 3. Client will express relief during PCA infusion	1. Position client anatomically on side with knee flexed and small pillow below legs. 2. Have colleagues available to lift client in bed for repositioning. Encourage cient to ask for assistance. 3. Explain the purpose of PCA device, method for initiating device and expected response. 4. Demonstrate and coach client through relaxation exercise.	
Impaired physical mobility R/T musculoskeletal pain	c/o pain, edema manifested by painful movement, decreased range of motions. Loss of muscle strength.	Patient will demonstrate increase in mobility of joints.	Place the patient in position of comfort, suggests joints anatomically with pillow or pads and change position every hour: • Assist in ROM exercise • Avoid restrictive clothing • Assist to ambulate as tolerated • Maintain save environment	
Self-care deficit R/T pain	Not dressed Not groomed	Patient's independence in self-care activities will increase within the parameters of disability	• Teach self-care activities • Establish and teach routine plan of ADLs • Set goals with patient, encourage short-term easily accomplished goal • Discuss the use of snaps on clothing and slip-on shoes	
Chronic low-self-esteem R/T inability to work	Preoccupation with body changes and verbalization fo powerlessness.	Patient will verbalize understanding of changes in body image caused by disease process and will begin to exhibit increased confidence in dealing with self-esteem.	• Encourage verbalization about fears and anxiety of disease process • Deal with behavioural change denial, powerlessness, etc. • Be supportive and kind in setting goals • Encourage independence • Modify environment	
Knowledge deficit R/T home care management	Having misconception about medication regimen, exercise programme and diet.			

Use different types of pain relief measures Using more than one therapy has an additive effect in reducing pain. In addition, the character of pain may change throughout the day, requiring several different therapies.

Provide pain relief measures before pain becomes severe It is easier to prevent severe pain than to relieve it after it exists. Giving analgesics half an hour before, client must walk or perform an activity is an example of controlling pain early.

Consider the client's ability or willingness to participate in pain relief measures Some client cannot actively assist with pain therapy because of fatigue, sedation or altered level of consciousness. However, there are variations of pain-relief measures that require little effort, such as relaxation exercises in bed or listening to music as a distraction. The nurse will not relieve pain by forcing an unwilling patient to participate in therapy.

Choose pain-relief measures on the basis of the clients behaviour reflecting the severity of pain It would be poor judgement to administer a patient narcotic if a client has only mild pain. The nurse carefully assesses the client's comments and behaviour before choosing pain therapy. Some clients acquire relief from severe pain after using only mild analgesics. Only the client can determine the potency of an effective therapy.

Use measures that the client believes are effective The client is the expert of pain. The client may have ideas about measures to use (e.g. rubbing lotion on a swollen finger) and times to use them will make pain therapy successful.

If a therapy is ineffective at first, encourage client to try again before abandoning it Often, anxiety or doubt prevents a therapy from relieving pain, or the measure may require adjustment or practice to become effective. The nurse should be patient and understanding in helping the client learn to use measures that do not afford immemdiate relief.

Keep an open mind about what may relieve pain New ways are often found to control pain. There is still much to be learned about the pain experience. Rejecting non-conventional therapies leads to mistrust. The nurse should be sure all therapies are safe.

Keep trying The nurse can easily become frustrated when efforts at pain relief fail. The nurse should not abandon the client when pain persists but reassess the situation and consider alternative therapies.

Protect the client A pain therapy should not cause more distress than the pain itself. The nurse always observes the client's response to therapy. The nurse's aim is to relieve pain without disabling the client mentally, emotionally or physically.

Educate the client about the pain When possible, the nurse should explain the cause of the pain, time of occurrence, duration and quality and ways to gain relief. Education promotes the prevention of pain.

The basic nursing responsibility is protecting the client from harm. One simple way to promote comfort is by removing or preventing painful stimuli. The following measures can be performed by the nurse to assist in pain control:

- Tighten and smooth wrinkled bed linen
- Reposition drainage tubes/other objects on which patient is lying
- Place warm bath blankets for coolness
- Loosen constricting bandages (unless specifically applied as a pressure dressing)
- Change wet dressings
- Position the client in an anatomical alignment
- Check temperature of hot or cold applications including bath water
- Lift client on bed—do not pull. Patient up in bed; handle gently.
- Position patient correctly on bed pan.
- Avoid exposing skin or mucous membrane to irritants (e.g. diarrheal stool, wound drainage)
- Prevent urinary retention by keeping Foley's catheters' patent and free flowing
- Prevent constipation with fluids, diet and exercises.

Nursing Intervention

Nursing interventions for pain relief can be grouped and discussed in two broad categories:

1. Non-invasive or non-pharmocological intervention/pain relief strategy.
2. Invasive interventions/pain relief strategies.

Nonivasive Interventions

The noninvasive techniques which may be offered by the nurses often used as adjuncts to the analgesic regimen, not alternatives.

Trusting relationship Develop good trusting relationship as already explained.

Alleviate anxiety To Alleviating anxiety, stay with the client for a while. Allow the client to talk and express feelings and fears. Communicate empathy and willingness to listen. Take measures to relieve anxiety in positive direction according to experience of nurses. With patient with pain, for example, self-directed pain prevention/reduction techniques such as meditation, using therapeutic touch, backrub, applying cool cloth, etc.

Distraction or diversion It is one of the measures used to pain relief. Distraction helps to focus attention away from the pain and to some extent, any contact the nurse with the patient which is not focused on pain per se. Distraction which reduces the conscious awareness of pain usually works with mild pain than severe pain. Distraction may take many forms, viz. occupational therapy, conversation, reading, watching television, listening to radio, meditation, self-hypnosis, biofeedback, and autosuggestion, etc. Distractions serve to increase pain tolerance, that is, it makes the pain more bearable.

Combating anticipatory fears Anticipatory fears are those fears that occur prior to an experience of pain-producing stimuli. These help prepare clients to meet pain realistically by talking with them about the pain they fear.

Providing physical care Effective physical nursing care for clients experiencing pain is directed at reducing mechanical, chemical and thermal stressors that lower pain tolerance. This includes protecting patient from local irritations or inflammation such as infection or thrombosis, muscle spasm or muscle strain, interference with local blood supply and venous and lymphatic drainage, distention of hollow visceral organs such as the bowel and bladder and further damage to traumatised tissue.

There are several important principles of physical nursing care as follows:

- Identify the source of pain and eliminate or reduce the pain
- Handle sensitive or injured tissue carefully
- Always perform painful procedures when pain-relieving medications are producing their maximal effect
- Check drainage tubes frequently to ensure that they are not caught, stretched, pulled, kinked, or looped and that they are positioned correctly
- Protect the client from fatigue and helping the client to get a good night's sleep
- Be alert to inflammation and ischemia caused by immobilization—take suitable measure to reduce it
- Change the position to relieve muscle spasms, maintain good body alignment of the client
- Use gentle massage and application of heat or cold if needed.
- Use dormal stimulation, i.e. application of pressure, acupressure, massage. TENS (transcutaneous electric nerve stimulation), ice massage (massaging area with ice).

Invasive Intervention

The drugs used to relieve pain work by altering pain sensation, depressing pain perception or modifying the patient's response to pain as the nurse has considerable control over and responsibility for the effective use of medicines to reduce pain, knowledge of the drugs used in pain control, their routes of administration and side effects is needed. Examples of analgesic are of four types as follows:

1. Non-narcotic analgesics
   - Acetaminophen (tylenol, datnol)
   - Acetyl salycyclic acid (aspirin)
   - Choline magnesium trisalycylate (tritisate)
2. NSAIDs
   - Ibuprofen (brufen)
   - Naproxen (naprosyn)
   - Indomethacin
   - Tolmetin
   - Piroxicam
3. Narcotic analgesics
   - Meperidine
   - Methylmorphine (codiene)
   - Morphine sulphate (morphine)
   - Fentany (sublimzae)
   - Butorphanol (butarin)
   - Hydormorphene HCl
4. Adjuvants
   - Amitriptyline
   - Dydroxyzine
   - Caffeine
   - Chloropromozine
   - Diazepam

There are four types of analgesic as mentioned below which include (i) non-narcotic analgesics (ii) NSAIDs (iii) opioids and (iv) adjuvants or coanalgesics. Non-narcotic and NSAIDs provide relief for mild and moderate pain, such as the pain.

(3) MANAGEMENT OF FLUID, ELECTROLYTE AND ACID-BASE IMBALANCES

The cells that make-up body tissues exist in a chemically constant but physiologically dynamic internal environment. Physiologic processes function to regulate this environment so that responses to stimuli minmally affect the body. The chemical consistency achieved through fluid, electrolyte and acid-base balance. Physiologic homeostasis and life itself depends on normal fluid and electrolyte balance and acid-base balance. It is essential to maintain bomeostasis. Homeostasis is the term used to describe the ability to maintain internal balance in the presence of external stressors.

The homeostatic mechanisms that regulate fluid and electrolyte balance represent interaction between chemical and physiologic processes. Promoting balance in either a wellness or an illness state can prevent fluid and electrolyte imbalances that may be life-threatening. Nurses have primary professional contact with most clients. In any setting, it is natural for them to play an action role in the prevention, early detection and treatment of fluid and electrolyte imbalances. Now nurses not only have the opportunity, but they have broad base of knowledge of normal physiology and pathology, to assist in the identification of clients at risk and recognizing early manifestations of imbalance and taking measures to correct imbalance through nursing process.

Water Content of the Body/Fluids

Water is the primary component of all body fluids. It is the solvent used to transport nutrients to cells and to remove waste products produced by the cellular metabolism. Temperature regulation is assisted by evaporation of water on the body surface. Approxiately 60% of weight in a typical adult is composed of fluids, i.e. water and electrolytes. Factors that influence the amount of body fluids are age, gender, and body content. As a general rule, younger people have a higher percentage of body fluid than that of older people and men have proportionately more body fluid than that of women. Obese people have less fluid than thin people because fat cells contain little water. Adipose tissues contain less water than an equivalent amount of muscle tissue. In an older adult, body water content averages 45 to 55% of the body weight. In the infant, water content averages 70 to 80% of body weight. Therefore, the young are at risk because they have less fluid reserve. Both the very young and very old have a decreased ability to compensate for fluid loss.

Body fluid is located in the two compartments viz., intracellular space (fluid in the cells) and the extracellular space (fluids outside the cells). Intracellular fluid (ICF) is located (primarily in the skeletal muscle mass) and constitutes 40% of body weight or 70% or two thirds of the total body fluids/water. Extracellular fluid (ECF) constitutes about 20% of the body weight or 30% or one-third of total body fluids/water. Extracellular fluid (ECF) constitutes about 20% of the body weight or 30% or one-third of total body water. ECF consists of interstitial (between cells and lymph) intravascular (fluid within the cells is plasma), cerebrospinal, and intraocular fluid, as well as secretions of the gastrointestinal (GI) tract. Sometimes, the term 'transcellular' i.e., a product of secretion and diffusion from cells is used to refer to cerebrospinal, pericardial, synovial, intraocular and pleural fluids, sweat and diagestive secretions.

ECF transports nutrients, electrolytes and oxygen to cells; carries waste products for excretion; regulates heat; lubricates and cushions, joints and membranes; hydrolizes food for digestive processes, and maintains vascular volume by passing easily through the capillary walls. ICF provides the cell with the internal aqueous medium necessary for its chemical functions. Normally, the fluid volume inside and outside of the cells maintains a steady state due to compensatory responses. 'Fluid spacing' is a term used to classify the distribution of body water. The term 'fluid' is used because more than water is found in these ICF and ECF compartments such as glucose, sodium and potassium. *First spacing* is a normal distribution of fluid in both the ECF and ICF components. *Second spacing* refers to an excess accumulation of interstitial fluid (oedema). *Third spacing* occurs when fluids accumulate in areas that normally have no fluid or only a minimum amount of fluid. (For example, of third spacing are, ascitis, sequestration of fluid in the bowel in peritonitis and oedema associated with burns).

Water is not only responsible for the body's structure and functions but it is also necessary for the maintenance of equilibrium (homeostasis) and of life itself. Body fluids normally shift between the two major compartments or spaces in an effort to maintain the equilibrium between the spaces. Loss of fluid from the body can disrupt the equilibrium. Sometimes, fluid is not lost from the body, but it is unavailable for use by either ICF or ECF space. Loss of ECF into a space that does not contribute to equilibrium between ICF and ECF is referred to as *third space fluid shift*. Third spacing is a concern because it takes fluid away from the normal fluid compartments and may produce hypovolemia. An early clue of a third space fluid shift is a decrease in urinary output, despite adequate fluid therapy. Urine output decreases because fluid shift out of the intravascular space; the kidneys that receive less blood flow and at-tempt to compensate by decreasing urine output. Other signs and symptoms of 'third spacing' that indicates an intravascular fluid volume deficit, include increased heart rate, decreased blood pressure, decreased central venous pressure, oedema, increased body weight and imbalance in fluid intake and output. For example, third space occurs in ascitis, burns, massive bleeding into a joint or body cavity.

Physiology

As the primary body fluid, water is the most important nutrient of life, whereas life can be sustained for only a few days without water. The following are the primary functions of water in the body.

- Provide a medium for transporting nutrients to cells and wastes from cells and transporting nutrients to cells and wastes from the cells, and transporting such substances as hormones, enzymes, blood platelets, and red and white blood cells.
- Facilitate cellular metabolism and proper cellular chemical functioning.
- Act as a solvent for electrolytes and non-electrolytes.
- Helps maintain normal body temperature.
- Facilitates digestion and promotes elimination.
- Act as a tissue lubricant.

Regulation of Body Flow

As water moves through all parts of the body it is constantly being lost. Fluid leaves the body through the kidneys, lungs, skin, and GI tract. To maintain homeostasis, the normal daily loss must be met by the normal daily intake. Haemostasis is a relatively constancy in the internal environments of the body, naturally maintained by adaptive responses and that promote healthy survival. An approximate daily water intake and output of an adult eating 2500 calories per day are as follows:

Intake		*Output*	
Route	*Gain(ml)*	*Route*	*Amount of loss (ml)*
Water in food	1,000	Skin	500
Water from oxidation	300	Lungs	350
Water as liquid	1,200	Faeces	150
		Kidney	1,500
Total	2,500	Total	2,500

Mechanisms Controlling Fluid and Electrolyte Movement

There are many different processes which control the movement of fluid and electrolytes between the ICF and ECF spaces. These processes include simple diffusion, facilitated diffusion, active transport, osmosis, fluid presence (hydrostatic pressure and oncotic pressure).

Simple Diffusion

Diffusion is defined as the natural tendency of a substance or solutes to move from an area of higher concentration to one of lower concentration. It occurs through the random movement of ions and molecules. It occurs in liquids, gases, and solids. For example, exchange of oxygen and carbon dioxide between pulmonary capillaries and alveoli. Net movement of the molecules stops when the concentrations are equal in both areas. The membrane separating the two areas must be permeable to the diffusing substance for the process to occur. These molecules move without external energy. Diffusion is an efficient mechanism for the movement of molecules in and out of cells. Diffusion does not require energy.

Facilitated Diffusion

Some molecules diffuse slowly into the cell because of the composition of cellular membrane. However, when they are combined with a specific carrier molecule, the rate of diffusion accelerates. Like simple diffusion, facilitated diffusion moves molecules from an area of high concentration to one of low concentration. Glucose transport into the cell is an example of facilitated diffusion. The hormone insulin increases the rate of facilitated diffusion of glucose in most tissues.

Active Transport

Active transport is a process in which molecules move in the absence of a favourable diffusion gradient. In which, the physiologic pump (Naik) that moves fluid from an area of lower concentration to one of higher concentration. External energy is required for this process because molecules are being moved against a concentration gradient. Active transport requires adenosine triphosphate (ATP) for energy. The energy production of energy depends on oxygen and glucose availability. The concentration of sodium and potassium differs greatly intracellularly and extracellularly. By active transport, sodium moves out of the cell and potassium moves into the cell. The energy source for the sodium-potassium pump is ATP which is produced in the mitochondria. By definition, active transport implies that entry expenditure must take place for the movement to occur against a concentration of gradient.

Osmosis

Osmosis, a special type of diffusion, is the flow of water between two compartments separated by a membrane permeable to water but not to solute. Here the movement of fluid across a semipermeable membrane from an area of low solute concentration to an area of high solute concentration. This process stops when the solute concentrations are equal on both sides of the membrane. In this, water moves from the compartments that is more dilute (has more water) to the side that is more concentrated (has less water). The semipermeable membrane prevents movement of solute particles. Osmosis requires no outside energy sources and stops when concentration differences disappear. In addition to diffusion, osmosis is very important for maintaining the chemical stability of body cells.

Osmotic pressure or force is a term used to describe the movement of water by the process of osmosis. It can be described as a pulling of water. Osmotic pressure is an important factor in the movement of water between fluid compartment, 'Osmolarity' and 'Osmolality' both measurement of osmotic pressure.

Osmolality measures to osmotic force of solute per unit of weight of solvent. It reflects the concentration of fluid that affects the movement of water between fluid compartments by osmosis, osmolality measures the solute concentration per kilogram in blood and urine. It is measured inmiliosmoles per kg of water (mOsm/kg). The normal osmolality of body fluids between 275 and 295 mmol/kg or mOsm/kg. The major determinants of osmolality are sodium, glucose, and urea with sodium. Increase in the concentration of these substances in the plasma causes fluid movement into plasma because of its increased osmotic pressure.

Osmalality measures the total miliosmols of solutes per unit of a total volume of solution. The number of osmoles, the standard unit of osmotic pressure per liter of solution. It is expressed as miliosmols per liter (mOsm/L) used to describe the concentration of solutes or dissolved particles.

In clinical practice, osmolality is used most oftenly. Serum osmolality may be measured directly through laboratory tests or estimated at the bad side by doubling the serum sodium level or by utilizing the following formula.

$$Na^{+} \times 2 + \frac{\text{glucose}}{18} + \frac{\text{BUN (blood urea nitrogen)}}{3} = \text{Approximate value of serum osmolality.}$$

In *osmotic movement of fluid* cells are affected by the osmolality of the fluid that surrounds them. Where fluids are added to the body those that have same osmolality as cell interior are *"isotonic"*. solutions that contain more water than the cell are *hypotonic* (hypoosmolar), those with less water than the cell are hypertonic (hyperosmolar).

Fluid Pressure

As a result of pressure, body fluids shift between the interstitial space and the vascular space within the capillary. The pressure in the body fluids are either hydrostatic or oncotic.

Hydrostatic pressure is the force exerted by a fluid against the walls of its container. The heart is a main component in generating pressure in blood vessels. Hydrostatic pressure in the vascular system gradually decreases as the blood moves through the arteries until it is about 40 mm Hg at the arterial end of a capillary. Because of the size of the capillary bed and fluid movement into the interstitium, the pressure decreases to about 10 mm Hg at the venous end of the vessel. Hydrostatic pressure in the capillaries tends to filer fluid out of the vascular compartment into the interstitial fluid.

Oncotic pressure (colloidal osmotic pressure) is an osto-motic pressure exerted by colloidal, in solution. In plasma, proteins molecules attract water and contribute to the total osmotic pressure in the vascular system. Unlike electrolytes, the large molecular size prevents proteins from leaving the vascular space through pores in capillary walls. Plasma oncotic pressure is approximately 25 mm Hg. Some proteins are found in the interstitial space, and they exert an oncotic pressure of approximately 1 mm Hg.

The movement of the fluid through a capillary via the above stated two pressures (hydrostatic and oncotic) is called 'filtration'. An example of filtration is the passage of water and electrolytes from the arterial capillary bed to the interstitial fluid. In this instance, the hydrostatic pressure is furnished by the pumping action of the heart. Through filtration absorption or reabsorption resorption will take place. *Absorption* usually refers to the initial movement of substances such as end products of digestion or medications from organ such as GI tract or tissues such as the muscle, subcutaneous or dermal tissue, buccal or pharyngeal tissues, into the vascular system. *Reabsorption* refers to movement of water, electrolytes, vitamins, amino acids, glucose, lactate or other essential substances from one compartment, such as the interstitial or renal tubules, back into vascular capillaries. *Resorption* refers to the process of calcium salts leaving the bone and moving into the blood in an ionized form.

REGULATION OF FLUIDS AND ELECTROLYTES OR HOMEOSTATIC MECHANISM

The body is equipped with remarkable homeostatic mechanisms to keep the composition and volume of body fluid within narrow limits or normal. Organs involved in the homeostatic mechanism or regulation of fluid and electrolytes include hypothalamus, pituitory gland, adrenal gland, kidney, GI tract, parathyroid gland, heart, blood vessels and lungs, etc.

Hypothalamus

Water ingestion in the conscious client is regulated by the thirst receptors located in the hypothalamus. The thirst mechanism is stimulated by the hypotension and increased serum osmalality. In addition, thirst may result from polyuria, fluid volume depletion as small as 0.5% excess sodium intake, hypertonic feedings, and hypertonic IV fluids. Although thirst can be reported and is an important clinical manifestation of fluid imbalances, it is not a true indicator of fluid balance in all persons. The thirst mechanism depressed in the elderly. The desire to consume fluids is also affected by social and psychologic factors not related to fluid balance. A dry mouth will cause the client to drink, even when there is no measurable body water deficit. Water ingestion will equal water excretion in the individual who has free access to water, a normal thirst and ADH mechanism and normally functioning kidneys.

Pituitary Gland

The hypothalamus manufactures a substance known as anti-diuretic hormone(ADH) which is stored in vesicle in the posterior pituitary gland and released as needed. ADH which regulates water retention by kidneys. The distal tubules and collecting ducts in the kidneys respond to the ADH by becoming more permeable in water so that water is absorbed into the blood and not excreted. When there is a normal plasma osmolality and normal circulating plasma volume, continued ADH secretion is called "Syndrome inappropriate anti-diuretic hormone (SIADH). ADH is released in response to many conditions an increase in plams osmolality, ECF volume depletion, pain, stress, and use of certain medications such as narcotics, barbiturates, and anaesthetics. Stress may be physiologic or psychologic. The factors which suppressing ADH include hypo-osmolality of the ECF, increased blood volume, exposure to cold, acute alcohol ingestion, carbon dioxide inhalation, administration of some diuretics, lithium and some anti-psychotic medications. ADH prevents urine production and promotes water reabsorption from the renal tubules. Stimulation of the thirst mechanism and ADH release usually occurs concurrently in response to a body fluid deficit.

Adrenal Gland

ECF volume is maintained by a combinations of hormonal influences. ADH affects only water reabsorption. Hormones released by the adrenal cortex help regulate both water and electrolytes. Two groups of hormones secreted by the adrenal cortex include glucocorticoids and mineralocorticoids. The glucocorticoids primarily have an anti-inflammatory effect and increase serum glucose, whereas mineralocorticoids (e.g. aldesteron) enhances sodium retention and potassium excretion. When sodium is reabsorbed, water follows as a result of osmotic changes. *Cortisol* is most common 'hormone which are the properties of gluco and minerlocorticoids properties. Adrenocorticotrophic hormone (ACTH) from the anterior pituitary is necessary for aldosterone secretions. Hypovolemic is a common clinical condition in which aldesterone is secreted to maintain homeostasis.

Kidneys

The kidneys maintain fluid volume and concentration of urine by filtering the ECF through the glomeruli. Reabsorption and excretion of ECF occurs in the renal tubules in response to ADH, aldesterone and ANP (atrial natriuretic peptides). ANP released from the atria in response to atrial distention, vasoconstriction, or direct cardiac damage. These factors increase the excretion of sodium and water and results in vasodilation. Renal prostaglandins and renal rennin-kinin system also increases sodium excretion. The major function of kidneys in maintaining normal fluid balance include the following.

- Regulation of ECF volume and osmolality by selective retention and excretion of body fluids.
- Regulation of electrolytes level in the ECF by selective retention of needed substances and excretion of unneeded substances.
- Regulation of pH of ECF by retention of hydrogen ions.
- Excretion of metabolic wastes and toxic substances.

Parathyroid Gland

The parathyroid glands embedded in the corners of thyroid gland, regulate calcium and phosphate balance by means of parathyroid hormone (PTH). PTH influences bone resorption, calcium absorption from the intestine and calcium reabsorption from the renal tubules.

GI Tract

Daily water intake and output are between 2000 to 3000 ml. The gastrointestinal tract accounts for the most of the water intake, water intake includes fluids, water from food metabolism and water present in solid foods. Lean meal is approximately 70% water whereas the water content of many fruits and vegetables is about 100%. Most of the body water is excreted by kidneys. A small amount of water eliminated by GI tract is faeces.

Lungs

The lungs are also vital in maintaining homeostasis. Insensible water loss, which is unavoidable vaporization from the lungs and skin assists in regulating body temperature. Normally, about 900 ml per day is lost. The amount of water loss is increased by accelerated body metabolism, which occurs with increased body temperature and exercise. Through exhalation, the lungs remove approximately 300 ml of water daily in the normal adult.

Heart and Blood Vessels

The pumping action of the heart circulates blood through the kidneys under sufficient pressure for urine to form. Failure of the pumping action interferes with renal perfusion and thus with water and electrolytic regulation.

In addition, neural mechanisms also contribute to the balance of water and sodium. Mechano-receptors and baroreceptors are nerve receptors involved in neural mechanism.

ORGANS THAT MAINTAIN HOMEOSTASIS

Kidneys

- Regulate ECF volume and osmolality by selective retention and excretion of body fluids.
- Regulate electrolytic levels in the ECF by selective retention of needed substances and excretion of unneeded substances.
- Regulate pH of ECF by excretion or retention of hydrogen ions
- Excrete metabolic wastes (primarily acids) and toxic substances.

Heart and Blood Vessels

- Circulate blood through the kidneys under sufficient pressure of urine to form (puping action of the heart).
- React to hypovolemia by stimulating fluid retention (stretch receptors in the atria and blood vessels).

Lungs

- Eliminate about 13, 000 mEq of hydrogen ions (H^+) daily, as opposed to only 40 to 80 mEq excreted daily by kidneys.
- Act promptly to correct metabolic acid-base disturbance, regulate H^+ concentration (pH) by controlling the level of CO_2 in the ECF as follows.
  - Metabolic alkalosis causes compensatory hypoventilation resulting in CO_2 excretions (increased acidity of the ECF).
  - Metabolic acidosis causes compensatory hyperventilation, resulting in CO_2 excretion (decreased acidity of the ECF).
- Remove approximately 300 ml of water daily through exhalation (insensible water loss) in the normal adult.

Adrenal Glands

- Regulate blood volume and sodium and potassium balance by secreting aldosterone; a mineralocorticoid secreted by the adrenal cortex.
  - The primary regulator of aldosterone appears to be angiotensin II which is produced by the reninangiotensin system. A decrease in blood volume triggers this system and increases aldosterone secretion, which causes sodium retention (and thus water retention) and potassium loss.
  - Decreased secretion of aldosterone causes sodium and water loss and potassium retention.
- Cortisol, another ACTH, has only a fraction of the potency of aldosterone.
- However, secretion of cortisol in large quantities can produce sodium and water retention and potassium deficit.

Pituitary Gland

- Stores and releases ADH, which makes the body retain water. Functions of ADH include:

- Maintains osmotic pressure of the cells by controlling renal water retention or excretion.
- When osmotic pressure of the ECF is greater than that of the cells (as in hypernatremia or hyperglycemia), ADH secretions is increased causing renal retention of water.
- When osmotic pressure of the ECF is less than that of the cells, (as in hyponatremia) ADH secretion is decreased, causing renal excretion of water.

– Controls blood volume (less influential than aldosterone)
- When blood volume is decreased, an increased secretions of ADH results in water conservation.
- When blood volume is increased, a decreased secretion ADH results in water loss.

Parathyroid Glands

– Regulate calcium (Ca^{2+}) and Phosphate (HP_4^{2-}) balance by means of PTH; PTH influences bone reabsorption, calcium absorption from the intestines and calcium reabsorption from renal tubules.
- Increased secretion of PTH causes:
  i. Elevated serum calcium concentration
  ii. Lowered serum phosphate concentration
- Conversely, decreased secretion of PTH causes:
  i. Lowered serum calcium concentrate.
  ii. Elevated serum phosphate concentrate.

FLUID IMBALANCES

Fluid imbalances occur when the body's compensating mechanisms are unable to maintain homeostatic state. Fluid imbalances may relate to either volume or distribution of water or electrolytes.

Fluid Volume Deficit (FVD)

Fluid volume deficit can be caused by a deficiency in the amount of both water and electrolytes in ECF, but the water and electrolytes proportions remain near normal. The state is commonly known as 'hypovolemia'. Both osmotic and hydrostatic pressure changes for the interstitial fluid into intravascular space. As the interstitial space is depleted, its fluid becomes hypertonic, and cellular fluid is then drawn into the interstitial space, leaving cells without adequate fluid to function properly.

Fluid volume deficit results from the loss of body fluids expecially if fluid intake is simultaneously decreased. The related factors of FVD are:

i. Loss of water and electrolytes, as in:
- Vomiting
- Polyuria
- Diarrhoea
- Fever
- Excessive laxative use
- Excessive sweating
- Fistulas
- Third-space fluid shifts
- Gastrointestinal suction.

ii. Decreased intake, as in:
- Anorexia
- Inability to gain access to fluids
- Nausea
- Inability to swallow fluids.
- Depression

The main characteristics of fluid volume deficits are:

- Weight loss over short period (except in third-space losses).
- Decreased skin and tongue turger.
- Dry mucus membranes.
- Urine output less than 30 ml. per hour in adult.
- Postural hypotension (systolic pressure drops by more than 15 mmHg when client moves from lying to standing or sitting position).
- Weak, rapid pulse.
- Slow-filling peripheral veins.
- Decreased body temperature, such as 95° to 98°F (35°C to 36.7°C) unless infection is present.
- CVP less than 4 cm H_2O.
- BUN elevated out of proportion to serum creatinine.
- Specific gravity (urine) high.
- Haematocrit elevated.
- Flat neck veins in supine position.
- Marked oliguria, late.
- Altered sensorium.

Nursing Intervention for FVD

1. Assess for presence or worsening of FVD
2. Administer oral fluids if indicated.
   - Consider the client's likes and dislikes when offering fluids.
   - If the client is reluctant to drink because of oral discomfort select fluids that are non-irritating to the mucosa, and provide frequent mouth care (offer saline gargle and apply lubricant to lips).
   - Offer fluids at frequent intervals.
   - Explain the need for fluid replacement to the client.
   - Administer medications if nausea is present, to provide relief before fluids are offered.
3. Consider the following interventions for clients with impaired swallowing.
   - Assess gag reflex and ability to swallow water before offering solid foods; have a suction apparatus on hand.
   - Position the client in an upright position with a head and neck flexed slightly forward during feeding (tilting the head backward during swallowing predisposes to aspiration because this position opens the airway).
   - Provide thick fluids or semisolid foods (such as pudding or gelatine). These are more easily swallowed because of their consistency and weight than are thin liquids.

4. If the client is unable to eat and drink, discuss possibility of tube feeding or TPN with the physician.
5. Monitor response to fluid intake, either orally or parenterally.
6. Monitor clients with tendency for abnormal fluid retention (such as renal or cardiac problems) for signs of overload during aggressive fluid replacement.
7. Turn client frequently, apply moisturising agents to skin.

Sometimes dehydration used as synonym for hypovolemia; technically it is wrong. Dehydration refers only to a decreased volume of water; but water is not decreased without electrolyte charges also. Hydration is the union of a substance with water and is often used to indicate that there is normal water volume in the body.

Fluid Volume Excess

Excessive retention of water and sodium in ECF in near normal proportions results in a condition termed as FLUID VOLUME EXCESS. It is also called "HYPERVOLEMIA". Overhydration refers only to above-normal amounts of water in extracellular spaces. Malfunction of the kidneys causing an inability to excrete the excesses and failure of the heart to function as a pump resulting in accumulation of fluid in the lungs and dependant parts of the body, are common causes. When water is retained in excessive amount, so as sodium.

Due to increased extracellular osmotic pressure from the retained sodium, fluid is pulled from the cells to equalize the tonicity. By the time intrcellular and extracellular spaces are isotonic to each other, an excess of both water and sodium are in ECF, while the cells are nearly depleted The excessive ECF may accumulate in tissue spaces, thus is known as "Oedema". Oedema can be observed around eyes, fingers ankles and sacral space and also accumulate in or around body organs. It may result in a weight gain in excess of 5 per cent. When the excess fluid remains in the intravascular space, the concentration of solids in the blood is decreased.

Interstitial to plasma shift is the movement of fluid from the space surrounding the cells to the blood. This shift, also called hypervolemia is a compensatory response to volume or osmotic pressure changes of the intravascular fluid. Although the body attempts to mainfain normal balance in all fluid spaces, the intravascular fluid is usually protected at the expense of interstitial fluid and ICF.

The common related factors which lead to fluid volume excess (FVE) are as follows:

- Compromised regulatory mechanisms such as
  - Renal failure
  - Congestive heart failure.
  - Cirrhosis of liver
  - Cushing's syndrome.
- Overzealous administration of sodium containing IV fluids
- Excessive ingestion of sodium containing substances in diet or sodium containing medication.

The characteristics of fluid volume excess will include:

- Weight gain over short period.
- Peripheral oedema excess of fluid in interstitial space)
- Distended neck veins
- Distended peripheral veins
- Slow-emptying peripher veins
- CVP over 11 cm H_2O
- Crackles and wheezers in lungs
- Polyuria (if renal function normal)
- Ascitis, pleural effusion (when FVE is severe, fluid transudes into body cavities)
- Decreased BUN (due to plasma dilution)
- Decreased hemalocrit (due to plasma dilution)
- Bounding, full-pulse
- Pulmonary oedema, if severe.

Nursing Intervention

- Assess the presence or worsening of FVE
- Encourage adherence to sodium restricted diet if prescribed
- Teach client requiring sodium restricitions to avoid over-the-counter drugs without first checking with the health care adviser/nurse
- When fluid retention persists despite adherence to dietary sodium intake, consider hidden sources of sodium, such as water supply or use of water softener
- When indicated, encourage rest period, lying down favours diuresis of oedema fluid
- Monitor the client's response to diuretics. Discuss significant findings with physician
- Monitor the rate of parenteral fluids and the client response. Discuss significant finding with physician
- Teach self-monitoring of weight and intake and output measurements to clients with chronic fluid retention (such as those of CCF, renal failure, cirrhosis of liver).
- If dyspnea or orthopnea are present, position the client in semi-Fowler's position to facilitate lung expansion
- Turn and position the client frequently, be aware that oedematous tissue is more prone to skin breakdown than in normal tissue.

ELECTROLYTES

Electrolytes are substances whose molecules dissociate or split into ions when placed in water. These substances are found in ECF and ICF that dissociate into electrically charged particles known as ions. Cations are positively charged ions. For example, Sodium (Na^+), Potassium (K^+), Calcium (Ca^{2+}) and Magnesium (Mg^+), Hydrogen (H^+) ions. Anions are negative charged ions. For example, Bicarbonates (HCO_3^-) Chloride (Cl^-) and phosphate (PO_4^3) ions and proteins. The ionic charge is termed valence. Cations and anions combine according to their valency.

The concentration of electrolytes can be expressed in milligrams per deci-litre (md/dl), millimeter per liter (mmo/L) or milli equivalent per liter (mEq/L). See the normal level of electrolytes in appendix. The role of electrolytes in cellular functions includes the following.

1. Regulation of water distribution, and osmolality
2. Regulation of acid-base balance
3. Transmission of nerve impulses, i.e. neuromuscular activity
4. Contraction of muscles
5. Clotting of blood
6. Enzyme reaction.

ELECTROLYTES

Regulation of Electrolytes

Electrolytes regulate water distributiion regulate acid-base balance and maintain a balanced degree of neuromuscular excitability. There are many different kinds of electrolytes in the body. These include Sodium (Na^+) Potassium (K^+), Calcium (Ca^{++}) Magnesium (Mg^{2+}), Chloride (Cl^-) Bicarbonate (HCO_3^-), Phosphate (PO_4^-), etc.

Sodium

Sodium is the chief electrolyte of ECF. It moves easily between intravascular and interstitial spaces and moves across cell membrane by active transport. Many chemical reactions in the body are influenced by sodium, particularly in nervous tissue cells and muscle tissue cells.

The functions of sodium are as follows:

- It controls and regulates the volume of body fluids
- It maintains waterbalance throughout the body
- It is the primary regulator of ECF volume
- It influences ICF volume
- It participates in the generation and transmission of nerve impulses
- It is an essential electrolyte in the sodium-potassium pump.

The sources and losses of sodium are:

- An average daily intake is not known; but the average adult intake is eliminated to be between 6 and 15 g. and the RDA for sodium for adults is approximately 500 mg for 0.5 g.
- Sodium is found in many foods. Particularly, bacon, ham, sausage, catsup, mustard, relish, processed cheese, canned vegetables, bread, cereal, and salted snack food. It is found in table Sal (NaCl) which is about 46% sodium.
- Sodium excess are eliminated primarily by the kidneys. Small amounts are lost in faeces and perspiration.

Regulation of Sodium

- Sodium normally is maintained in the body within a relatively narrow range, and deviations quickly result in a serious health problem.
- Salt intake regulates sodium concentrations.
- Sodium is conserved through reabsorption in the kidneys, a process of stimulated by aldosterone.
- The normal extracellular concentrations of sodium is 135 to 145 mEq/L (mmol/L).

Potassium

Potassium is the major cation of ICF. Potassium and sodium work reciprocally. For example, an excessive intake of sodium results in an excretion of potassium and vice versa. The functions of potassium are as follows:-

- It is the chief regulator of cellular enzyme activity and cellular water content.
- It plays a vital role in such process as the transmission of electric impulses, particularly in nerve, heart, skeletal, intestinal, and lung tissue; protein and carbohydrate metabolism and cellular building.
- It assists in regulation of acid-base balance by cellular exchange with H^+.

The sources and losses are:

- An average daily requirement of K^+ is not known; but an intake of 50 to 100 m Eq. daily maintains potassium balance.
- A well-balanced diet contains adequate quantities of potassium. Major sources include bananas, peaches, kiwi, figs, dates, appricots, oranges prunes, melons, raising, broccoli, and potatoes. Meat and dairy products also provide adequate amounts of potassium.
- Potassium excreted primarily by the kidneys. The kidneys have no effective method of conserving potassium. Therefore, deficits develop readily if excreted in excess without being replaced simultaneously.
- Gastrointestinal secretions contain potassium in large quantities. Some is also found in perspiration and saliva.

Regulation of K^+

- Cellular potassium is conserved by the sodium pump when sodium is excluded.
- The kidneys conserve potassium when cellular K^+ is decreased.
- Aldosterone secretions trigger potassium excretion in urine.
- The normal range for serum potassium is 3.5 to 5 mEq/L.

Calcium

Calcium is the most abundant electrolyte in the body. Upto 99 per cent of the total amount of calcium in the body is found in bones and teeth in ionized form. There is close link between concentration of calcium and phosphorus. The functions of calcium are:

- It is necessary for nerve impulse transmissions and blood clotting.
- It is catalyst for muscle contraction. Strength of contractions (especially cardiac muscle contraction) is directly related to the serum concentration of calcium ions.
- It is needed for vitamin B_{12} absorption and for its use by body cells. "It acts as a catalyst for many cell chemical activities.

- It is necessary for strong bones and teeth.
- It establishes thickness and strength of cell membrane.

The sources and losses of calcium

- The average daily requirements for calcium is about 1 g for adults. Higher amounts are required according to body weight, for children, for pregnant and lactating women, and postmenopausal women.
- Calcium found in milk, cheese and dried beans. Some calcium is present in meats and vegetables.
- Use of calcium is stimulated by vitamin D. The most active form of vitamin D (calcitriol) promotes calcium absorption and limits calcium excretion when levels are inadequate.
- It leaves bones and teeth to maintain normal blood calcium levels if necessary.
- It is excreted in urine, faeces, bile, digestive secretion and perspiration.

Regulation of calcium

- When ECF calcium levels decrease, the parathyroid glands increase the secretions of PTH, which acts on bones to increase the release of calcium into the blood and acts on the kidney tubules and the intestinal mucosa to increase the absorption of calcium from the kidneys and the intestine.
- A high serum phosphate concentration increases serum calcium; a low serum phosphate concentration decreases serum calcium.
- Calcitonin, a hormone secreted by the thyroid gland has an opposite effect of calcium than PTH. Increases in calcitonin reduce the serum calcium concentration primarily by opposing osteoclast bone resporption.

Magenesium

Most of the cation magnesium is found within body cells. It is present in heart, bone, nerve, and muscle tissues. Magnesium is the second most important cation of ICF. The functions of magnesium are as follows:

- It is important for the metabolism of carbohydrates and proteins.
- It is important for many vital reactions related to the body's enzymes
- It is necessary for protein and DNA synthesis, DNA and RNA transcription, and translation of RNA-
- It maintains normal intracellular levels of potassium.
- It serves to help maintain electric activity in nervous membranes and muscle membranes.

The sources and losses of magnesium are:

- The average daily adult requirement for magnesium is about 18 to 30 mEq. Children required larger amount.
- Magnesium found in most foods but especially in vegetables, nuts, fish, wholegrains, peas and beans.

Regulation

- Magenesium is absorbed by the intestines and secreted by the kidneys.
- Plasma concentration of magnesium range from 1.3 to 2.1 mEq/L with about one-third of that amount bound to plasma proteins.

Chloride

Chloride, the chief extracellular anion, is found in blood, interstitial fluid, and lymph and in minute amounts in intracellular fluid. The functions of chlorides are as follows:-

- It acts with sodium to maintain the osmotic pressure of the blood.
- It plays a role in the body's acid-base balance.
- It is important in buffering action when O_2 and CO_2 exchange in RBCs.
- It is essential for the production of HCl in gastric juices.
- The average daily requirement of chlorides are unknown. It is found in foods high in sodium, in dairy products and meat.

Regulation of Cl^-

- It is normally paired with sodium and excreted and conserved with sodium by the kidneys.
- Chloride deficits lead to potassium deficit and vice versa.
- Normal serum chloride levels range from 95 to 105 mEq/L.

Bicarbonate

The bicarbonate molecule is an anion. It is the major chemical base buffer within the body and is found in both ECF and ICF. The bicarbonate is essential for acid-base balance. Bicarbonate and carbonic acid constitute the body's primary buffer systems.

Phosphate

The phosphate ion is the major anion in body cells. It is a buffer anion in both ICF and ECF. The functions of phosphate are:

- It helps maintain acid-base balance.
- It is involved in important chemical reactions in the body; For example it is necessary for many B. Vitamins to be effective; helps promote nerve and muscle action, and plays role as carbohydrate metabolism.
- It is important for cell division and for the transmission of heredity traits.

An average daily requirement for phosphorous are similar to those for calcium. It is found in most foods especially in beef, pork, and dried peas and beans. It is metabolised in the same manner as calcium.

Phosphate is regulated by PTH and by activated vitamin D. Calcium and phosphates are inversely proportional and increase in one results in a decrease in the another. The normal range of phosphate is 2.5 to 4.5 mEq/L (mmol/L).

ELECTROLYTE IMBALANCES

Human body contains quite large volume of water as ICF and ECF and the fluid contains several inorganic ions such as sodium, potassium, chloride, bicarbonate, sulphate, phosphate, calcium and magnesium. The complex mechanism of human life maintains the concentration and volume of the body fluids at a constant level and in general, it is not influenced by dietary intake and metabolism, while kidneys play a vital role in maintaining the balance. When clients present with deficit or excesses of sodium, potassium, calcium, magnesium or phosphate, special nursing care is required. A brief description of the common electrolyte imbalances are as follows:

Hyponatraemia

Hyponatraemia refers to a sodium deficit in ECF caused by loss of sodium or a gain of water. It is a condition on lowered level of plasma volume. In this condition, osmotic pressure changes results in ECF, moving into the cells. When this occurs, an examiner's fingerprints tend to remain on the client's skin over the sternum where pressure is applied with the fingers.

The related factors leading to hyponatraemia are:

- Loss of sodium as in: loss of GI fluids, use of diuretics; adrenal insufficiency.
- Gains of water as in: excessive administration of D_5W, diseases associated with SIADH; pharmoscologic agents that impair renal water excretion.
- Hyponatraemia or sodium depletion occurs from loss of body fluids through sweating, vomiting, diarrhoea, intestinal fistula, dialysis and from aspiration of gastric contents.
- Chronic pyelonephritis, chrome uremia, diutretic phase of acute renal failure, diabetic ketoacidosis, cystic diseases of the kidney, and excessive or prolonged use of diuretics results excessive loss of sodium through urine.
- Endocrine diseases show as myroedema, Addison's disease, hyperaldosteronism, and uncontrolled diabetes mellitus also leads to sodium depletion.
- Excessive loss of sodium can also occur through the skin as in extensive burns, generalized dermatitis, etc. in children, cystic fibrosis.

Sodium is mainly an extracellular ion, and its depletion causes migration of water in the intracellular compartments, making the extracellular fluid hypotonic. Consequently plasma becomes hypo-osmolar and plasma volume falls.

The main characteristics of hyponatraemia are:

- Anorexia
- Nausea and vomiting
- Lethargy
- Confusion
- Muscle cramps
- Fingerprint overstrenum
- Muscular twitching
- Seizures
- Coma
- Serum sodium below 135 mEq/L

This condition presents with tiredness, lethargy, muscular weakness, mental confusion, and in severe cases, convulsions and coma. The skin appears cold, pale and inelastic. Tongue is dry. Reduction in plasma volume causes reduction in cardiac output and results tachycardia fall of blood pressure and raising pulse rate. The eyeballs become soft due to reduced intraocular pressure, urine output is reduced and soon oliguria supervenes and finally leads to uraemia. When the plasma serum concentration falls exaggeratedly to 120 mmol/litre; litre of blood or less, muscle cramps occur. It can produce acidosis and circulatory failure as complication.

Treatment

Mild cases are treated with frequent drink of water with added sodium chloride or with isotonic (0.9%) Saline solution by IV injection. In other cases, 2-4 litres of isonoic saline solution is given IV infusion over 6-12-hours. More severe cases are treated with 2-3-litre of IV isotonic solution in first 2-3-hours, followed by further 2-5 litres within 24-48 hours. If there is associated water intoxication water intake is restricted to 500-1000 ml in 24 hours. In addition, the client is given treatment for the underlying condition.

Nursing Intervention

- Identify clients at risk for hyponatraemia.
- Monitor fluid losses and gains. Look for loss of sodium containing fluids, particularly in conjunction with low-sodium-intake.
- Monitor presence of gastrointestinal symptoms, such as: anorexia, nausea, vomiting, and abdominal cramping.
- Monitor laboratory date for serum sodium levels less than normal.
- Check specific gravity of urine.
- With clients able to consume a general diet, encourage foods and fluids with high sodium content.
- Be familiar with the sodium content of commonly used parenteral fluids. Monitor client with cardiovascular disease receiving sodium-containing fluids closely for sign of circulatory overload such as moist rales in the lungs.
- Use extreme caution when administering hypertonic saline solution (3 to 5% NaCl) Be aware that these fluids can be lethal if infused carelessly.
- Avoid giving large water supplements to clients receiving isotonic tube feedings, particularly if routes of abnormal sodium loss are present or water is being retained abnormally.

HYPERNATRAEMIA

Hypernatraemia or sodium excess refers to surplus of sodium in ECF that can result from excess water loss or overall excess of sodium. Because of the increased extracellular osmotic pressure, fluids move from the cells, leaving them without sufficient fluid. It is a condition which excess of sodium occurs in the ECF, giving rise to cellular dehydration.

The related factors which lead to hypernatraemia are:

- Deprivation of water, most common in those unable to perceive or respond to thirst.
- Hypertonic tube feeding with inadequate water supplement.
- Increased insensible water loss (as in hyperventilation)
- Ingestion of salt in unusual amounts.
- Excessive parenteral administration of sodium-containing solution-
  - Hypertonic saline (3% or 5% NaCl.)
  - 7.5% sodium bicarbonate
  - Isotonic saline.
- Profuse sweating.
- Diabetes insipidus.
- Heat stroke
  Drowning in sea water.
- Hypernatraemia also occurs when water losses of the body exceed sodium loss as that is seen in diabetes insipidus, marked glycosuria, hypercalcaemia, hypokalaemia, chronic renal failure, and recovery phase of acute renal failure.
- Sodium excess may occur along with water excess when due to inadequate clearance of the kidneys both sodium and water accumulate in the extracellular space, leading to oedema, for example, nephrotic syndrome, cardiac failure, nutritional or thiamine deficiency, cirrhosis of liver and in cases of usage of drugs such as corticosteroids, androgens, phenylbutazone, oral contraceptive and carbenoxelone.

It causes retention of sodium, increased volume of ECF and oedema in the interstitial compartment.

The main characteristics of hypernatraema are:

- Thirst.
- Elevated body temperature.
- Tongue dry and swollen, sticky mucus membranes.
- In severe hypernatremia
  - Disorientation
  - Hallucinations
  - Lethargy when disturbed
  - Irritable and hyperreactive when stimulated
  - Focal or grand mal seizures, coma, low blood pressure, tachycardia.
- Serum sodium above 145 mEq/L.
- Urinary specific gravity.015 provided water loss from nonrenal route.

It may produce hyponatraemia, hyperglycaemia and shock as complication.

Treatment

Management of the condition calls for an immediate attention and treatment instituted within 24-48 hours can avoid occurrence of cerebral oedema.

Mild cases are given IV influsion 5% dextrose solution. Other cases need restriction of water and salt by mouth. Management of the condition depends upon the underlying condition. Diuretics and other measures are taken on the advice of the physician according to condition of patient.

Nursing Intervention

- Identify clients at risk of hypernatraemia.
- Monitor fluid losses and gains. Look for abnormal losses of water or low water intake, and for large gains of sodium as might occur with ingestion of proprietory drugs with high sodium content. And also consider that prescription drugs may have high sodium content. Of coruse, one should look for excessive intake of high sodium foods.
- Monitor changes in behaviour such as restlessnes, disorientation and lethargy.
- Look for excessive thirst, and elevated body temperature. If present, evaluate in relation to other signs.
- Monitor serum sodium level.
- Prevent hyponatraemia in debilitated clients unable to perceive or respond to thirst by offering them fluids at regular intervals. If fluids intake remains inadequate, consult the physician to plan an alternate route for intake, either by tube feedings or by the parenteral route.
- If tube feedings are used, give sufficient water to keep the serum sodium and the BUN level within normal limits. Beware that the higher the osmolality of the feeding, the greater the need for water supplements.

HYPOKALAEMIA

Hypokalaemia refers to a potassium deficit in ECF. When the extracellular potassium level falls, potassium moves from the cell, creating an intracellular potassium deficiency. Sodium and hydrogen ions are then retained by the cells to maintain isononic fluids. These electrolyte shifts influence normal cellular functioning, the pH of ECF, and function of most of the body systems. Skeletal muscles are generally the first to demonstrate a potassium deficiency. It is a condition associated with depletion of potassium characterized by muscular weakness, leg cramps, apathy, mental confusion and paralysis.

The related factors leading to hypokalemia are:

- It develops from excessive loss of potassium in the urine and stool and from severe water depletion.
- Potassium-losing diuretics, i.e. frusemide, thiazide, etc.
- Steroid administration.
- Use of carbenicillin, sodium penicillin, amphotorecin B.
- Hyperaldosteronism
- Hyperalimentations
- Poor intake as in anorexia nervosa, alcoholism, potassium free parenteral fluids.
- Osmotic diuresis (as occurs in uncontrolled diabetes mellitus or mannitol administration).

The main characteristics of hypokalaemia are:

- Fatigue
- Anorexia, nausea and vomiting.
- Muscle weakness
- Decreased bowel motility (intestinal ileus)-Paralytic ileus.
- Cardiac arrhythmia
- Increased, i.e. sensitivity to digitalis.
- Polyuria, nocturia, dilute urine (if hypokalaemia prolonged). Mild hyperglycaemia
- Serum K below 3.5 mEq/L
- Paresthesias or tender muscles.
- ECG Changes- Fattened T waves, ST segment depressions
- Respiratory. hyperventilation.

Treatment

Management of the condition requires adequate management of the underlying conditions.

Nursing Intervention

- Beware of clients at risk for hypokalaemia and monitor for its occurrence.
- Assess digitalized clients at risk for hypokalaemia especially closely for symptoms of digitalis toxicity.
- Take measures to prevent hypokalemia when possible
  - Prevention may take the form of encouraging extra potassium intake for at-risk patient (when the diet allows).
  - When hypokalaemia due to abuse of laxatives or diuretics education of the client may help alleviate the problems.
- Administer oral potassium supplement when prescribed.
- Be aware that clients may not need potassium supplements if they are using salt substitutes because these substances usually contains viable amounts of potassium.
- Be thoroughly familiar with the critical facts related to administering potassium intravenously.

HYPERKALAEMIA

Hyperkalaemia refers to an excess of potassium in ECF. It is a condition with excess of potassium, characterized by conduction defect in the heart and myoneural junction of the muscle.

The related factors which lead to hyperkalaemia are:

- Decreased potassium excretions as in
  - Oliguric renal failure.
  - Potassium-conserving diuretic usage
  - Hypoaldosteronism.
- High potassium intake, especially in presence of renal insufficiency:-
  - Improper use of oral potassium supplements.
  - Rapid excessive administration of IV potassium.
  - High-dose potassium penicillin.
  - Foods high in potassium (such as dried apricots)
- Shift of potassium out of cells due to acidosis, tissue trauma, and malignant cell lysis.
- Potassium excess also occurs in acute renal failure, severe crush injuries and burns. Severe haemorrhages and adrenal insufficiency.
- It is also seen in diabetic keto acidosis.

The main characteristics of hyperkalaemia are:

- Vague muscular weakness is usually first sign.
- Cardiac arrhythmias, bradycardia and heart block can occur.
- Paresthesias of face, tongue, feet and hands.
- Flaccid muscle paralysis (spreads from legs to trunk and arms, respiratory muscle may be affected).
- Gastrointestinal symptoms such as nausea, intermittent intestinal colic, or diarrhoea may occur.
- ECG changes tall, peaked T waves, absent P waves widened QRS complex.
- Serum K, above 5.0 mEq/L (mmol/L).

It can produce cardiac arrest, metabolic acidosis and respiratory acidosis as complications.

Treatment

Management of the condition is done by replacement of water loss and correction of electrolyte imbalance. The client is given diet with restricted protein but with as much as fat and carbohydrate and also managing the underlying condition.

Nursing Intervention

- Beware of clients at risk for hyperkalaemia and monitor for its occurrence. Hyperkalaemia is life-threatening; it is imperative to detect it easily.
- Take measures to prevent hyperkalaemia when possible by following guidelines for administering potassium safely both intravenously or orally.
  - Follow rules for safe administration of potassium-
  - Avoid administration of potassium conserving diuretics, potassium supplements or salt substitutes to client with renal insufficiency.
  - Caution client to use salt substitute sparingly if they are taking other supplementary form of potassium or taking potassium-conserving diuretics. (example, spironolactone, triamaterine, and amiloride).
  - Caution hyperkalaemic clients to avoid foods high in potassium content. Some of these are coffee, cocoa, tea, dried fruits, dried beans, wholegrain breads.

HYPOCALCAEMIA

Hypocalcaemia refers to a calcium deficit in ECF. If the condition is prolonged calcium is taken from bones. This results in osteomalacia, which is characterized by soft and pliable bones. Common signs and symptoms for hypocalcaemia include numbness and tingling of fingers, muscle, cramps and tetany.

The related factors leading to hypocalcaemia are:

- Surgical hypoparathyroidism (may follow thyroid surgery or radical neck surgery for cancer)
- Malabsorption
- Vitamin D deficiency
- Acute pancreatitis
- Excessive administration of citrated blood
- Primary hypothyroidism
- Alkalotia states (decreased ionized calcium) Hyperphosphataemia
- Medullary carcinoma of thyroid
- Hypoalbuminaemia (as in cirrhosis, nephrotic syndrome and starvation)
- Hypomagnesaemia
- Decreased ultraviolet exposure.

The main characteristics of hypocalcaemia will include:

- Numbness-tingling fingers, circumoral region and toes
- Cramps in the muscle of extremities
- Hyperactive deep tendon reflexes (such as patellar and triceps)
- Trousseau's sign
- Chvostek's sign
- Mental changes such as confusion and alteration in mood and memory
- Convulsions, usually generalized but may be focal
- Spasm of laryngeal muscles
- EGK shows prolonged QT interval
- Spasms of muscles in abdomen (can stimulate acute abdo-emergency)
- Total calcium level below 8.5 mg/dL or ionized level below normal (below 50%)
- Hypocalcemic state occurs when calcium loss occurs causing a fall in serum calcium level. This may eventuallycause tetany and death.
- It is usually asymptomatic and the neurological manifestation develop slowly.
- It then gives rise to diffuse encephalopathy, depression and psychosis
- In severe cases there may be laryngiospasm and gen convulsion
- It may also give rise to papilloedema and cataract.

Treatment

Most cases respond well to adequate or supplemented calcium and phosphorus. The patient may be given calcium carbonate, 2.52 to 3.78 g daily orally or calcium gluconate 0.5 - 1.5 g along with calciferol 15.45 μg daily orally. Otherwise, 10 ml of 10% calcium gluconate is given by slow IV. Adequate management and control of predisposing causes can prevent the occurrence of the condition.

Nursing Interventions

- Beware of clients at risk for hypocalcemia and monitor its occurrence.
- Be prepared to take seizure-precautions.
- Monitor condition of airway closely because laryngeal stridor can occur.
- Take safety precautions if confusion is present.
- Be aware of factors related to the safe administration of calcium replacement salts.
- Educate people in high-risk groups for osteoporosis (especially postmenopausal women not on oestrogen therapy). If adequate amounts are not consumed in the diet (as is often the case), calcium supplements should be considered.
- Educate people at risk for osteoporosis about the value of regular physical exercise in decreasing bone loss.
- To prevent osteoporosis in later years, educate young women about the need for a normal diet to ensure adequate calcium intake. Also discuss the calcium-losing aspects of alcohol and nicotine use.

HYPERCALCAEMIA

Hypercalcaemia refers to an excess of calcium in ECF. It presents an emergency situation because this condition often leads to cardiac arrest. It is a condition of excess of calcium and is characterized by polyuria, polydipsia, skeletal muscle weakness and hypertension.

The related factors that lead to hypercalcaemia are:

- Hyperparathyroidism
- Malignant neoplastic disease
- Prolonged immobilization
- Large doses of vitamin D or viv d. intoxication
- Overuse of calcium containing antacids or calcium supplements thiazide diuretics
- Milk-alkali syndrome
- Sarcoidosis
- It is also seen in person with Paget's disease, myxoedema, Addison's disease and osteoporosis in aged persons.

The common features of hypercalcaemia are:

- Muscle weakness
- Tiredness, listlessness, lethargy
- Constipation
- Anorexia, nausea, and vomiting
- Decreased memory span, decreased attention span, and confusion
- Polyuria, and polydipsia
- Renal stones
- Neurobic behaviour progressing to frank psychosis may occur (reversible with correction of hypercalcaemia)
- Cardiac arrest may occur in hypercalcaemic crisis
- ECG shows shortened QT interval

- Serum calcium over 10.5 mg/dl
- It may produce renal failure, shock and death in complication.

Treatment

In mild cases, adequate rehydration is often effective. Management of the condition also includes management of the underlying conditions. In other cases, intravenous infusion of isotonic saline is given to promote calciuria. Calcium is also eliminated or maintained in the lower level by giving sodium phosphate 1-2 g orally daily and client is encouraged to take more fluids.

Nursing Intervention

- Be aware of clients at risk for hypercalcaemia and monitor its occurrence.
- Increase client mobilization when feasible.
- Encourage the oral intake of sufficient fluids to keep the client well hydrated.
- Discourage excessive consumption of milk products and other high calcium foods.
- Encourage adequate bulk in the diet to offset the tendency for constipation.
- Take safety precautions if confusion or other mental symptoms by hypercalcaemia are present.
- Be aware that cardiac arrest can occur in clients with severe hypercalcaemia be prepared to deal with this emergency.
- Be aware that bones may fracture more easily in clients with chronic hypercalcaemia because bone resorption has been excessive, weakening the bony structure. Transfer clients cautiously.
- Educate home-bound oncology clients with a predisposition for hypercalcaemia and their families, to be alert for symptoms that occur with this condition and to report them to the health care providers before they become severe.
- Be alert for signs of digitalis toxicity when hypercalcaemia occurs in digitalized clients.
- Help prevent formation of calcium renal stones in clients with long-standing hypercalcaemia or immobilization by:
  - Forcing fluids to maintain a dilute urine, thus avoiding supersaturation of precipitates.
  - Encouraging fluids that yield an acid ash (prune or crannberrymilk) because a urinary pH less than 6.5 favours calcium deposits.
- Preventing urinary stasis by turning the immobilized client, elevating head of the bed and having the client sit up if this can be tolerated.

HYPOMAGNESEMIA

Magnesium is an important and plentiful cation and is essential for many enzymatic system associated with protein, carbohydrate and lipid metabolism.

Hypomagnesemia refers to magnesium deficit. It is condition of low plasma concentration of magnesium, characterized by neuromuscular and CNS hyperirritability.

The related factors which lead to hypomagnesemia are:

- Chronic alcoholism.
- Intestinal malabsorption syndrome.
- Diarrhoea.
- Nasogastric suction—prolonged
- Aggressive refeeding after starvation (as in TPN)
- Prolonged administration of magnesium-free IV fluids
- Uncontrolled diabetes mellitus—diabetic ketoacidosis
- Hyper aldosteronism.
- Drugs–prolonged use of
  - Diuretics, aminoglycoside, antibiotics (e.g. gentamycin), cisplatin
  - Excessive dose of vitamin-D or calcium supplements
  - Citrate preservative in blood products.
- Pancreatitis, thyrotoxicosis, hyperparathyroides
- Severe osteotis fibrosa, PEM.

The common characteristics of hypomagnesemia are:

- It presents with multiple metabolic and nutritional deficiency
- It gives rise to anorexia, lethargy, vomiting, weakness, and tetany
- Neuromuscular irritability
  - Increased reflex
  - Course tremors
  - Positive chvostek's and Trousseau's signs.
  - Convulsions.
- Cardiac manifestations will include
  - Trachyarrhythmias
  - Increased susceptibility to digitalis toxicity
  - ECG changes in severe cases. PR and QT interval prolongation, Widened QRS complex, ST segment depression and T-wave inversion.
- Mental changes
  - Disorientation in memory
  - Mood changes
  - Intense confusion
  - Hallucination
- Serum magnesium level below 1.3 mEq/L.

Treatment

Repletion of the cases are done through magnesium sulphate and chloride. It is customary to give double the amount required because half of magnesium given excreted by the kidneys. The repletion is done gradually and is given orally or intravenously. In severe cases, IV only.

Nursing Intervention

- Be aware client at risk for hypomagnesaemia, especially closely for symptoms of digitalis toxicity because a deficit of magnesium predisposes to toxicity.

- Be prepared to take seizure precautions when hypomagnesaemia, especially closely for symptoms of digitalis toxicity, because a deficit of magnesium predisposes to toxicity.
- Monitor condition of airway, because laryngeal stridor can occur.
- Take safety precautions if confusion presents.
- Be familiar with magnesium replacement salts and factors related to these safe administration.
- Be aware that magnesium-depleted clients may experience difficulty in swallowing.
- When magnesium deficit is due to abuse of diuretics in laxatives, educating the client may help alleviate problem.
- Be aware that most commonly used IV fluids have either no magnesium or relatively small amount. When indicated, discuss the need for magnesium replacement with physicians.
- For clients experiencing abnormal losses, but able to consume a general diet, encourage intake of magnesium, rich foods (such as green-leafy vegetables, nuts, legumes and fruits such as bananas, oranges, and grape fruits).

HYPERMAGNESAEMIA

Hypermagnesaemia refers to a magnesium excess. It can occur especially in end stage renal failure. When kidneys fail to excrete magnesium and excessive amounts are administered therapeutically. It is a condition associated with excess of magnesium and is characterized by muscular weakness and ECG changes.

The related factors which lead to hypermagnesaemia are:

- Renal failure (particularly when magnesium containing medication is administered).
- Adrenal insufficiency.
- Excessive magnesium administration during treatment of eclampsia.
- Hemodialysis with excessively hard water or with dialysate inadvertantly high in magnesium content.

Magenesium has a direct action on the myoneural junction. Its excess creates blockage causing impairment of neuromuscular transmission and that results in diminished excitability of the muscle cells.

The main characteristics of hypermagnesaemia are:

- Early signs (serum level of mg of 3 to 5 mEq/L)
  - Flushing and a sense of skin warmth (due to peripheral vasodilation)
  - Hypotension (due to blockage of sympathetic ganglia as well as to direct effect on smooth muscle)
- Depressed respiration
- Drowsiness, hyoactive reflexes and muscular weakness
- Cardiac abnormalities-cardiac arrest may develop
- Weak or absent cry in newborn
- ECG shows prolonged PR interval, widened QRUS Complex and elevated T-wave amplitude
- Elevated serum magnesium level.

Treatment

In severe cases and also in other cases cardiac and respiratory support are given by IV injection of 10-20 ml of 10% calcium gluconate maintenance of adequate hydration is essential. The client is also given frusemide by IV injection to promote excretion of magnesium. In more severe cases haemodialysis is done.

Nursing Intervention

- Be aware of client at risk for hypermagnesaemia and assess for its presence. When it is suspected assess the following parameters:
  - Vital signs: look for low blood pressure and shallow respirations with periods of apnea
  - level of consciousness: Look for drowsiness, lethargy and coma.
- Do not give magnesium containing medication to clients with renal failure or compromised renal function.
- Be particularly careful in following 'standing order' for bowel preparation for X-ray because some of these include the use of magnesium citrate.
- Caution clients with renal disease to check with their health care providers before taking over the counter-medication.
- Be aware of factors related to safe parenteral administration of magnesium salts.

HYPOPHOSPHATAEMIA

Hypophosphataemia refers to a below-normal serum concentration of inorganic phosphorous. It is a clinical manifestation of phosphate depletion, characterized by progressive encephalopathy and osteomalacia.

The related factors which lead to hypophosphataemia are:

- Inadequate intake or absorption of phsophorous - malabsorption
- It is associated with vomiting and diarrhea
- Prolonged injestion of alluminium hydroxide or bicarbonate
- It is also seen in:
  - Prolonged use of glucose insulin, fructose, administrations
  - Refeeding after starvation
  - Hyperalimentation
  - Alcohol withdrawal
  - Diabetic ketoacidosis
  - Respiratory alkalosis
  - Phosphate-binding antacids use
  - Recovery phase after severe burns
  - Use of anabolic steroids
  - Chronic haemodialysis.

The main characteristics of hypophosphataemia are:

- Progressive encephalopathy
- Paresthesias
- Muscle weakness

- Muscle pain and tenderness
- Mental changes, such as apprehension, confusion, delirium coma
- Cardiomyopathy
- Acute respiratory failure
- Seizures
- Decreased tissue oxygenation
- Joint stiffness
- Serum phosphate below 2.5 mg/dL
- Phosphate compounds are present in all normal foods and are essential for metabolism of carbohydrate, protein and fat. They are also responsible for changes, transfer, or depletion occurs from prolonged negative phosphate balance and form chronic malnutrition.

Treatments

Management of the condition includes treatment of the underlying cause, repletion of phosphate, and maintenance of body fluids.

Nursing Intervention

- Identify clients at risk for hypophosphataemia;
  - severely malnourished clients
  - alcoholic clients
  - clients with diabetic ketoacidosis.
- Monitor clients at risk for the presence of hypophosphataemia.
- Be aware that severely hypophosphatemic clients are thought to be greater risk for infection because of changes in WBCs.
- Administer IV phosphate products cautiously.
- Be aware that in adults the usual maintenance dose of phosphorous is 10 to 15 mmol/L of TPN solution.
- Be aware of the need to introduce hyperalimentation gradually in clients who are malnourished.
- Because it is possible to give too much phosphorous when administering phosphate solutions, moniter for signs of hyperphosphatemia and of the salt in which it is administered.
- Monitor for diarrhea in clients taking oral phosphorus supplements; consult physician if it persists or is severe.
- Mispowdered oral phosphorus supplements with chilled or ice water to make them more palatable.

HYPERPHOSPHATAEMIA

Hyperphosphataemia refers to above-normal serum concentrations of inorganic phosphorous. It is a condition associated with increased level of phosphate and is characterized by hypocalcemia.

The related factors which lead to hyperphosphatemia are:

- Excessive intake of phosphataemia
- Excessive intake of phosphate
- Hypervitomınosia D.-Large vitamin D intake
- Acute renal failure
- Chronic renal insufficiency
- Chemotherapy: particularly for acute lymphoblastricluekamia and lymphoma
- Large intake of milk
- Use of cow's milk in infants
- Excessive intake of phosphate containing laxatives
- Overzealous administration of phosphorous-supplements (oral or IV)
- Excessive use of Fleets Phosphosoda as enema solution particularly in children and people with slow bowel elimination
- Hypoparathyroidism
- Hyperthyroidism.

The main characteristics of hyperphosphatemia are:
This condition by itself does not give rise to any symptoms but manifested with that of hypocalcaemia which includes:

- Short-term consequences: Symptoms of tetany, such as tingling of fingertips and around mouth, numbness and muscle spasms.
- Long-term consequences: precipitation of calcium phosphate in non-osseous sites; such as kidneys joints, arteries, skin or cornea.
- Serum phosphate above 4.5 mg/dl.

Treatment

Management of the condition requires correction of underlying condition.

Nursing Intervention

- Identify clients at risk for hyperphosphatemia.
- Monitor signs of tetanus and other features of hypocalcemia.
- Be aware that soft-tissue calcification can be long-term complication of a chemically-elevated serum phosphate level. Calcification may occur in site such as kidney, arteries, joints.
- Administer prescribed oral or IV phosphate supplements cautiously and monitor serum phosphorous levels periodically during their use.
- When appropriate, instruct clients that use of phosphate, containing laxatives may result in acute phosphate poisoning.
- Beware that phosphate containing enema can result in hyperphosphataemia if used injudiciously, particularly in children and those with slow bowel emptying, instruct clints accordingly.
- When low-phosphorus diet is prescribed, instruct clients to avoid foods high in phosphorous content. Such foods include hard cheese or cream, nuts and nut products; whole grain cereals (e.g. bran and oatmeal) dried fruits, dried vegetables; special meats such as kidneys, sardines, and sweet breads and desserts made with milk.

ACID-BASE IMBALANCES

Arterial blood gases (ABGs) are most commonly used to assess and treat acid-base imbalances. Results from venous, blood are only specific for particular extremity or area where the blood was sampled and do not provide information on how well the lungs oxygenating the blood. The pH of plasma indicates balance or impending acidosis or alklosis. In addition however, a study of the blood oxygen and carbon dioxide gases is important. The partial pressure (indicated by 'p') of these gases, or their tensions are determined by the use of a nomogram, which reflects the chemical and physical activities of two gases. The partial pressure of carbon dioxide $PaCO_2$; for oxygen, it is PaO_2. The "a" indicates an arterial specimen. When the PaO_2 is low, haemoglobin carries less than normal amounts of oxygen, when the PaO_2 is high, the haemoglobin carries more oxygen, oxygen saturation readings (SaO_2) reveal the percentage of O_2 in the blood that combines with haemoglobin. The $PaCO_2$ is influenced almost entirely by respiratory activity. When $PaCO_2$ is low, carbonic acid leaves the body in excessive amounts; When the $PaCO_2$ is high, there are excessive amounts of carbonic acid in the body.

Acid-base imbalance occurs when the carbonic acid or bicarbonate levels become disproportionate. When there is a single primary cause, these disturbances are known as respiratory acidosis or alkalosis and metabolic acidosis or alkalosis. These disturbances are a result of an upset in acid-base balance, as follows:

- Respiratory disturbance alters carbonic acid portion:
  - Respiratory acidosis and alkalosis are the results of respiratory disturbances
  - Compensation occurs to resolve balance in the kidneys by either conserving or excreting more bicarbonate.
- A metabolic disturbance alters the bicarbonate portion.
  - Metabolic acidosis and alkalosis are almost entirely the result of metabolic processes
  - The primary organs for compensation to restore balance are lungs, which either try to conserve or excrete more CO_2 which is available in weakly ionized carbonic acid.

The brief description of management of acid-base imbalances are as follows:

Respiratory Acidosis (Carbonic Acid Excess)

Respiratory acidosis is primary excess of carbonic acid in ECF. Any decrease in alveolar ventilations that result in retention of CO_2 can cause respiratory acidosis. Because the lungs are the source of the problem, they are unable to participate in compensation. As the carbonic acid content increases, the kidney attempts to retain more bicarbonate and increase their hydrogen excretion. It is a clinical state of altered hydrogen excretion. It is a clinical state of altered hydrogen ion concentration characterized by hypoventilation.

RA = high $PaCO_2$ because of alveolar hypoventilations.

The related factors for respiratory acidosis (RA) are:

- Acute respiratory acidosis:
  - Acute pulmonary oedema
  - Aspiration of a foreign body
  - Atelectasis
  - Pneumothorax, hemothorax
  - Overdose of sedatives or anaesthetic
  - Position on operative room table that interferes with respiration
  - Cardiac arrest
  - Severe pneumonia
  - Laryngospasm
  - Mechanical ventilation improperly regulated
  - Chronic respiratory acidosis
  - Emphysema
  - Cystic fibrosis
  - Advanced multiple sclerosis
  - Bronchiactasis
  - Bronchal asthma.
- Factors favouring hypoventilation.
  - Obesity
  - Tight abdominal binders and dressings
  - Postoperative pain (as in high abdominal or chest incisions)
  - Abdominal distention from cirrhosis or bowel obstruction.

The main characteristics of respiratory acidosis are:

i. Acute respiratory acidosis:
   - Mental cloudiness
   - Dizziness
   - Palpitations
   - Muscular twitching
   - Convulsions
   - Warm flushed skin
   - Unconsciousness

   Ventricular fibrillation may be first sign in anaesthetized patient (related to hypokalemia)

   - Arterial blood gases (ABGs)
     - PH below 7.35
     - $PACO_2$ over 45 mm Hg (primary)
     - HCO_3^- normal or only slightly elevated.

ii. Chronic respiratory acidosis:
   - Weakness
   - Dull headache
   - Symptoms underlying disease process
   - ABGs – pH below 7.35 or within lower limits of normal.
     - $PaCO_2$ over 4.5 mm Hg (primary)
     - HCO_3^- over 26 mEq/L (compensatory).

Treatment

Administer respiratory stimulants, i.e. Nikethamide 2-4 ml of 25% solution by IV repeated every one or two hour and treating the underlying condition.

Nursing Intervention

- Treatment is directed at improving ventilation; exact measures vary with the cause of inadequate ventilation.
- Pharmocological agents are used as indicated. For example, bronchodilators help reduce bronchial spasm; antigiotic for infection.
- Pulmonary hygienic measures are used when necessary to rid the respiratory tract of mucus and purulent drainage.
- Adequate hydration (2 to 3 L/day) is indicated to keep mucous membranes moist and thereby facilitate removal of secretions. Supplemental oxygen is used as necessary.
- A mechanical respirator, used cautiously, may improve the pulmonary ventilation. One must remember that overzealous use of a mechanical respirator may cause rapid excretion of CO_2 that the kidneys will be unable to eliminate excess bicarbonate with sufficient rapidity to prevent alkalosis and convulsion. For this reason the elevated $PaCO_2$ must be decreased slowly.

Respiratory Alkalosis (Carbonic Acid Deficit)

Respiratory alkalosis is a primary deficit of carbonic acid in ECF. It is the result of the increased alveolar ventilation and therefore, a decrease in CO_2. An increase in respiratory rate and depth causes the CO_2 loss because the CO_2 is excreted faster than normal. Because of the deficit of the CO_2, which is a respiratory stimulant sensed in the medulla of the brain. Depression of cessation of respiration eventually can occur. Because the lungs are the source of the problem, they are unable to participate in compensation. Therefore, kidneys attempt to alleviate the imbalance by increasing bicarbonate excretion and by retaining more hydrogen. Respiratory alkalosis = Low $PaCO_2$ because of alveolar hyperventilation.

It is a clinical disorder of altered hydrogen's ion concentration that is developing from hyperventilation.

The related factors which lead to respiratory alkalosis are:

- Extreme anxiety (most common cause)
- Hypoxemia
- High fever
- Early salicylate intoxication (stimulates respiratory center)
- Gram-negative bacteremia.
- CNS lesions involving respiratory center, meningitis, encephalitis.
- Pulmonary emboli, pneumonea
- Thyrotoxicosis
- Excessive ventilation by mechanical ventilators
- Pregnancy (high progesterone level sensitizes the respiratory centre to CO_2 : Physiologic).

The main characteristics of respiratory alkalosis are:

- The condition presents with anxiety
- Light-headedness (a low $PaCO_2$ causes cerebral vasoconstrictions and thus decreased cerebral blood flow)
- Respiratory symptoms—frequent, deep-sighing, or rapid and deep breathing.
- Hyperventilation syndrome, i.e. tinnitus, palpitations, sweating, dry mouth, tremulousness, precordial pain (tightness) nausea and vomiting, epigastric pain, blurred vision, convulsions and loss of consciousness.
- ABGs – pH over 7.45
  - $PaCO_2$ below 35 mm Hg (primary)
  - HCO_3^- under 22 mEq/L (compensatory)

Treatment

Treatment is given by correction of underlying causes.

Nursing Intervention

- If the cause of respiratory alkalosis is anxiety, the client should be made aware that the abnormal breathing practice is responsible for the symptoms accompanying this condition.
- Instruct the client to breathe more slowly (to cause accumulation of CO_2) or to breathe in closed system (such as paper bag).
- Usually sedative is required to relieve ventilation in very anxious patients (If alkalosis severe enough to cause fainting, the increased ventilation ceases and respiration reverts to normal).
- Treatment for other causes of respiratory alkalosis is directed at correcting for the underlying problem.

METABOLIC ACIDOSIS (Base Bicarbonate Deficit)

Metabolic acidosis is a proportionate deficit of bicarbonate in ECF. The deficit can occur as the remit of an increase in acid components or an excessive loss of bicarbonate. The lungs attempt to increase the CO_2 excretion by increasing the rate and depth of respirations. The kidneys attempt to compensate by retaining bicarbonate and by excreting more hydrogen. If the body is unable to achieve normal balance, the person may lose consciousness as metabolic acidosis increases and death eventually results. Thus

Metabolic acidosis = Low bicarbonate, non-volatile acid present use up HCO_3^- in disproportionate amounts

It is a condition of hydrogen ion concentration characterized by rise of hydrogen ion and reduction in plasma bicarbonate level.

The related factors which lead to metabolic acidosis are:

- Normal anion gap related to
  - Diarrhea
  - Intestinal fistulas
  - Ureter sigmoidostomy

- Hyperalimentation-vomiting excessively
- Acidifying drugs (such as ammonium chloride)
- Renal tubular acidosis (RTA).

- High anion gap related to
  - Diabetic ketoacidosis
  - Starvational ketoacidosis
  - Lactic acidosis
  - Renal failure
  - Ingestion of toxins (such as salicylates, ethylene glycol, and methanol)
  - acute alcoholic

The main characteristics of metabolic acidosis are:

- Headache, confusion, drowsiness
- Increased respiratory rate and depth (may not become clinically evident until HCO_3^- is quite low)
- Nausea and vomiting
- Peripheral vasodilation (may be present, causing warm flushed skin)
- Decreased cardiac output when pH below 7. Bradycardia may +
- ABGs – Fall in pH below 7.35
  - HCO_3^- under 22 mEq/L (primary)
  - $PaCO_2$ under 35 mm Hg (compensatory by lungs)
  - Base excess always negative.
- Hypokalaemia frequently present
- Hyperapnoea - Kussmauls respiration
- It eventually produces circulatory shock in complication.

Treatment

Salt and water repletion, and treating underlying conditions Treatment is directed towards correcting the metabolic defect. If the cause of the problem is excessive intake of chloride, treatment obviously focusses on eliminating the source, when necessary, bicarbonate is administered.

Control of the condition requires avoidance of and adequate management of the conditions which gives rise to the condition.

Nursing Intervention

Metabolic alkalosis (base bicarbonate excess)

Metabolic alkalosis is a primary excess of bicarbonate in ECF. This may be the result of excessive acid losses or increased base ingestion or retention. The body attemtps to compensate by retaining CO_2. The respirations become slow and shallow, amid periods of breathing may occur. The kidneys attempt to excrete potassium and sodium with the excessive bicarbonate, and retain hydrogen in carbonic acid. Thus,

Metabolic alkalosis = High bicarbonate - non-volatile acid is lost and it is not using up HCO_3^- or HCO_3^- gained is disproportionate amount.

It is a disorder of hydrogen ion concentration disturbance characterized by hypocalaemia and hypokalaemia.

The related factors which lead to metabolic alkalosis are:

- Vomiting or gastric suction
- Hypokalaemia
- Hyper aldosternonism
- Cushing's syndrome
- Potassium losing duretics '(e.g. thiazide, frusemide, ethacrynic acid)
- Alkali ingestion (bicarbonate containing antacids)
- Parenteral $NaHCO_3$ administration for cardio-pulmonary resuscitation
- Abrupt relief of chronic respiratory acidosis.

The main characteristics of metabolic alkaloids are:

- Irritation and neuromuscular excitation
- Those related to decreased calcium ionization are:
  - Dizziness, tingling of fingers and toes, circumoral paresthesia, carpopedal spasm, hypertonic muscles.
- Depressed respiration (compensatory action by lungs)
- ABGs – pH above 7.45, bicarbonate over 26 mEq/L,
  - $PaCO_2$ over 45 mm Hg (compensatory)
  - Base excess always possible.
- Hypokalemia often present
- Serum Cl. relatively lower than Na.

Treatment

Correction of the underlying cause is essential for proper management of condition. Treatment is aimed at reversal of the underlying disorder. Sufficient chloride must be supplied to the kidney to absorb sodium with chloride (allowing the excretion of excessive bicarbonate).

Treatment also includes restoration of normal fluid volume by administration of sodium chloride fluids because continued volume depletion serves to maintain the alkalosis.

Nurses wishing to be a role model of self-care behaviours that promote fluid, electrolyte, and acid-base balance should meet the following goals:

The nurse will:

- Daily ingest the quantity and type of fluids (to include six to eight glasses of water) that promote healthy hydration and urinary functioning.
- Evaluate use of food diets, diuretics, laxatives, and alcohol, identifying potential risks to health.
- Identify situations of high risk for fluid and electrolyte imbalance and intervene appropriately.

Perioperative Nursing

Surgery long back became a medical speciality, because often the treatment of a wide variety of illness and injuries includes some type of surgical intervention. Surgery is an invasive method of treatment that may be planned or unplanned, major or minor, and that may involve any body part or system. Care for the client during all phases of the surgical experience needs to be continuous and integrated surgical procedures require physical and psychosocial adaptations and are stressors for both the client and the family. The client's recovery from a surgical procedure requires skillful and knowledgeable nursing care whether the surgery is one on outpatient bases or in the hospital setting. Nurses working in both settings must understand the principles of caring for surgical clients.

As stated earlier, a client faces variety of stressors when confronting surgery. Anticipatory surgery leads to fear and anxiety for client who associate surgery with pain, possible disfigurement, dependence, and perhaps even loss of life. Family members often fear a disruption in lifestyle and experience a sense of powerlessness as the surgery approaches. The trauma sustained during surgery creates physical needs requiring close supervision and skilled intervention by the nurse and surgeon. Nurses use all phases of nursing process used in perioperatively to make assessment and provide interventions necessary to promote the recovery of health, prevent further injury or illness, and facilitate coping with alterations in physical structure and function.

DEFINITION OF PERIOPERATIVE NURSING AND NURSE

Perioperative nursing refers to the role of the nurse during the preoperative, intraoperative and postoperative phases of a client's surgical experience. The concept of perioperative nursing stresses the importance of providing continuity of care.

- A perioperative nurse is defined as the registered nurse, who, using the nursing process, designs, co-ordinates and delivers care to meet the identified needs of the clients whose protective reflexes or self-care abilities are potentially compromising because they are under the influence of anaesthesia during operative or other invasive procedures.
- Perioperative nurse, possesses and applies knowledge of the procedure and the client's intraoperative experience throughout the client care continuum. And also they assess, diagnose, plan, intervene and evaluate the outcome of interventions based on criteria and support of a standard care targeted towards the population.
- The perioperative nurse addresses the changing physiologic, pathophysiological, sociocultural and spiritual responses of the client that have been initiated by the prospect of performance of the invasive procedure.

SCOPE OF THE PERIOPERATIVE NURSING

The scope of perioperative nursing practice consists of three phases:

- Preoperative
- Intraoperative, and
- Postoperative.

Preoperative Phase

Begins where the decision for surgical intervention is made and ends with transference of the client to the operative suite. Nursing activities range from a baseline assessment of the client during the preoperative interview and continues with assessment in the pre-admission unit, client room, holding area, or induction room on the day of surgery. Before surgery, the nurse prepares the client and family for the surgery, performs diagnostic tests, and assesses the client in preparation for the operation.

Intraoperative Phase

Intraoperative phase begins where the client is transferred to the operating room bed and ends when the client is transferred to an area of recovery from anaesthesia. In this phase, nursing interventions range from communicating the client's plan of care, identifying nursing activities, necessary for expected outcome and establishing priorities for nursing actions. During surgery, the nurse assists surgeons and other operating room nurses to ensure that the client receives optimal care. The nurse also co-ordinates client needs with team members and personnel from other disciplines, co-ordinates the use of supplies and equipment, controls the environment, prepares for potential emergencies, and communciates and documents the client's plan of care.

Postoperative Phase

Postoperative phase begins with the client's transfer to an area for recovery and ends with client's recovery from surgery. Nursing activities range from communicating pertinent information about the client's surgery. To assist the client to physical stability and wakefulness and institute measures to help the client achieve maximum recovery.

CLASSIFICATION OF SURGICAL PROCEDURE

Surgery can be defined as the art and science of treating disease, injuries and deformities by operation and instrumentation. The surgical procedure involves the interaction with the patient, the surgeon, and the nurse. Surgical procedures usually are classified on the basis of urgency, degree of risk, and purposes.

Based on Urgency

Surgery may be classified as elective surgery, urgent surgery and emergency surgery.

Elective Surgery
It is preplanned and performed on the basis of client's choice. It is not essential and may not be necessary for health and delay in surgery has no ill effects, can be scheduled in advance based on the choice of client.

The purpose of elective surgery is:

- to remove or repair a body part
- to restore function
- to improve health
- to improve self-concept.

For example, tonsillectomy, hernia repair, cataract extraction and lens implant, hip prosthesis, haemorrhoid ectomy.

Urgent Surgery
In which the surgery is the necessity for the client's health, but not an emergency. This is performed for the purposes as in elective surgery and to prevent further tissue damage. For example, removal of gallbladder, coronary artery bypass, surgical removal of tumour, etc.

Emergency Surgery
When surgery must be done immediately to preserve the client's life, remove or repair body part, restore function, improve health and self-concept. For example, control of haemorrhage, repair of trauma, perforated ulcer, intestinal obstruction, tracheostomy and caesarean section.

Based on Degree of Risk or Seriousness

Surgery has been classified as major or minor on the basis of risk for the client.

Major Surgery
Involves extensive reconstruction or alteration in body parts, poses great risks to well-being. It requires hospitalization usually prolonged to well-being; has a high degree of risk; involves major body organs, life-threatening situations and potential postoperative complications. Major surgery may be elective, urgent, or emergency. For example, nephrectomy, cholecystectomy, colostomy, hysterectomy.

Minor Surgery
Is primarily elective; it is usually a brief, carries low risk and results in few complications. It can be performed in clinics, outpatient clinic and minor operation theatres. For example, teeth extraction, removal of warts, skin biopsy, laparoscopy, dilatations and curettage.

Based on Purpose

- *Surgical procedures* based on purpose will include diagnostic, ablative palliative, reconstructive, transplant, constructive.
- *Diagnostic* is surgical exploration that allows physician to make or to confirm diagnosis, may involve removal of tissue for further diagnostic testing. For example, breast biopsy, laparoscopy, bronchoscopy, exploratory laparotomy (incision in peritoneal cavity to inspect abdominal organs).
- Ablative is excision or removal of diseased body part. Example: Appendicectomy, sub-total thyroidectomy, partial gastrectomy, colon resection, amputation, cholecystectomy, etc.
- *Palliative:* surgery performed to relieve or reduce intensity of an illness or disease symptoms will not produce cure. For example, colostomy, nerve root resection (rhizotomy) debridement of necrotic tissue, balloon angioplasty, arthroscopy, etc.
- *Reconstructive* surgery is performed to restore function to traumatise or malfunctioning tissues and to improve self-concept. For example, scar revision, plastic surgery, skin graft, internal fixation of fractures, breast reconstruction.
- *Transplant* is performed to replace organs or structures that are diseased or malfunctioning. For example, kidney, cornea, liver, heart, joints, total hip replacement.
- *Constructive* surgery is performed to restore function lost or reduced as a result of congenital anomalies. For example, repair of cleft palate, closure of atrial defect in heart.

Sometimes combination of several surgery explained above also are performed as and when needed.

The common prefixes and suffixes used to explain the type of surgical procedure are as follows (see on next page):

ROLE OF NURSE IN PERIOPERATIVE CARE

General Care

Each surgical client, responds differently in surgery, when he enters the health care setting in different stages of health. Many variables influence a person's physiologic and psychological responses to the surgical experience. These include physical and mental status, extent of disease, magnitude of the surgery, social and financial resources and psychological and physiologic preparation for surgery. When consideres effectively, these variables reveal the degree of risk for a client undergoing surgery.

Common Prefixes and Suffixes in Surgery

Prefixes		*Suffixes*	
Term	*Definition*	*Term*	*Definition*
Supra-	Above, beyond	-oma	Tumour, swelling
Artho-	joint	-ectomy	Removal of organ
Chole-	Bile or gall	-rrhapy	The suturing or stitching of part of an organ
Cysto-	Bladder		
Encephalo-	Brain	-scopy	Looking into
Hysten-	Uterus	-ostomy	Making an opening or stoma.
Mast-	Breast	-otomy	cutting into
Meningo-	Membrane	-plasty	To repair or restore
Myo-	Muscle	-cele	Tumour, Hernia, Swelling
Nephro-	Kidney	-itis	Inflammation of
Oophor-	Ovary		
Pneumo-	Lung		
Pyelo-	Pelvis, Kidney pelves		
Salpingo-	Fallopian tube		
Thoraco-	Chest		
Viscero-	Organ Especially Abdomen.		

While making physiologic assessment before surgery, nurse elicits information about age; presence of pain; and nutritional status; fluid and electrolyte balance; presence of infections; physical mobility, skin integrity, cardiovascular; pulmonary, renal, gastrointestinal, liver, endocrine, neurologic and haematologic function; sensory medication history, abnormalities, injuries and previous surgeries, health habits, and socio-cultural history (see health assessment) and note any abnormalities and report to the concerned and take suitable measures to correct and sending the client to operating room.

The possible preoperative tests include the followign and reasons for those tests and normal ranges stated are as given below:

- Complete blood count and picture should be tested.
- Serum potassium (normal 3.5-5 mEq/L to identify hyperkalaemia or hypokalaemia.
- Serum sodium (normal 136 to 145 mEq/L) to identify hypernatraemia, dehydration or overhydration.
- Serum chloride (normal 96-100 mEq/L) to identify hypercholeraemia, hypocholoraemia, or metabolic disorder.
- Glucose (normal: 60-100 mg/dl to identify hypoglycomia or hyperglycomia.
- Creatinine (normal: 0.7-1.4 mg/dl) to identify acute or chronic renal disease.
- Blood urea nitrogen (BUN) - (10-20 mg/dl) to identify impaired liver or kidney function or excessive protein or tissue catabolism.
- Haemoglobin (Hgb) - (Female-12 to 15 gm/dl; Male 13-17 gm/dl)—to identify the presence and extent of anaemia.
- Haematocrit (Hct)—Female 36 to 46%, Male 39-51%) to identify the presence and extent of anaemia.
- Prothrombin time (PT) or clotting time (CT)-(11-18 seconds)—to identify dysfunction of blood clotting (Prothrombin level).
- Partial thromboplastin time (PTT)—to identify deficiencies of coagulation factors.
- Chest X-ray - (no abnormal heart or lung lesion) to determine size and contour of heart, lungs, and major vessels.
- Electrocardiogram (ECG) - normal rate and rythm)—to determine the electrical activity of the heart.
- Urin analysis—to identify abnormalities.

Any deviations from the normal, should be noted and reported to take precautions during surgery. And the common medical conditions that increase the high risk in surgery will include bleeding disorders, diabetes mellitus, heart diseases, upper respiratory infection, liver diseases, fever, chronic respiratory diseases, and immunological disorders. (leukaemia ......). A special precaution should be taken on these cases before, during and after surgery.

Preoperative Nursing Care

Persons who require surgical intervention and nursing care enter the health care settings in a variety of situations, ranging from essentially healthy people who have planned elective procedure to emergency admissions for treatment of trauma. Surgical client may be of any age group and at any point on the health-illness continuum. It is the nurse's responsibility to identify factors that affect risk from a surgical procedure, assess physical and psychosocial needs of the client and family and establish a plan of care, based on appropriate nursing diagnoses, that include interventions to meet needs and facilitate recovery as the client progresses through the perioperative period.

Preoperative Assessment Teaching

The nurses make preoperative assessment by taking history, conducting physical examination, performing diagnostic tests as required preoperatively according to clients' status/requirements, and takes informed consent in preoperative phase. Informed consent is very essential for anyone who is undergoing any invasive procedure like surgery. A consent form is the legal document which signifies the client's informed consent for the procedure. The consent form guards the client against unwanted invasive procedure. It also protects the health care facility and health care professional (see consent form in appendix).

In addition, preoperative teaching is an important component in the client's operative experience. Teaching about postoperative activities is implemented in the preoperative phase and is the nurse's responsibility. Clients and families need to know about surgical events, and sensations, how to manage pain, and how to perform physical activities necessary to decrease postoperative complications and facilitate recovery. The teaching-learning process is individualised to meet both specific and common client needs. Preoperative teaching allays anxiety and encourages clients to participate actively in their own care. The basic areas that must be covered in preoperative teaching are the following:

Deep-Breathing Exercises and Coughing Exercises
To help expand collapsed lung and prevent postoperative pneumonia and atelectasis, coughing exercises help to guard the suture.

Turning Exercises
Which help to prevent venuos stasis, thrombophlebitis, decubitus ulcer, formation, and respiratory complications.

Extremity Exercises
Help to prevent circulatory problems, such as thrombophlebitis, by facilitating venous return to the heart.

Ambulation
Early ambulation when appropriate, helps prevent postoperative complications.

Pain Control
Regarding medication (IV or IM) or NPO (nothing per oral), Relaxation technique are advisable. In addition TENS and PCA are taught for pain control measure.

Postoperative Equipments
Clients may be instructed about equipments that may be used postoperatively. Depending upon the surgery, various tubes, drained and IV lines are used.

Physical Preparation
The physical preparation of the client for surgery may vary, depending on the client's physical status and special needs, type of surgery to be done and surgeon's order. Certain nursing interventions are appropriate for all surgical clients in the areas of hygiene and skin preparation, elimination, nutrition, and fluids, and rest and sleep. The nurse is responsible for the preparation and safety of the client on the day of surgery.

Skin preparation The skin is cleaned by scrubbing the operative site one or more times with an antiseptic soap or solution to remove bacteria. This can be done by the client while taking a bath or shower. Ideally, a shower is taken in the evening before or the morning of surgery. Shampooing the hair and the cleaning of the fingernails also help to reduce number of organism present. The incisional area usually is shaved before surgery because hair serves as a reservoir of bacteria. Usually the operative area is treated at the night before surgery with an antiseptic such as povidone-iodine (betadine) to clean and disinfect the skin.

Elimination The gastrointestinal tract needs special preparation on the evening before surgery to

- reduce the possibility of vomiting and aspiration during anaesthesia.
- reduce the possibility of a bowel obstruction, and
- prevent contamination from faecal material during intestinal tract or bowel surgery.

Emptying the bowel of faeces is no longer routine procedure before surgery, but the nurse should use preoperative assessment to determine the need for an order of bowel elimination. If the client is scheduled for surgery of the GI tract, cleansing enema usually ordered.

Insertion of an indwelling urinary catheter may be ordered before surgery, especially in clients having pelvic surgery, to prevent bladder distension or accidental injury. If an indwelling catheter is not in place, the client should void immediately before receiving premedication to ensure an empty bladder during surgery.

Nutrition and fluids Preparation involves restricting food and fluid. If a client undergoing surgery is to receive a general anaesthesia, foods and fluids are restricted 8 to 10 hours before the operation. This restriction significantly reduces the possibility of aspirations of gastric contents, which can cause aspiration pneumonia. Most clients have an NPO status after midnight.

Rest and sleep Rest and sleep are important components in reducing stress before surgery and in healing and recovery after surgery. The nurse can facilitate rest and sleep in the immediate preoperative period by meeting psychological needs, carrying out teaching, providing a quiet environment, and administering prescribed bed time sedative medication.

Preoperative Care on the Day of Surgery

Immediate preoperative preparations begin at least 1 to 2 hours before surgery in the hospital. The nurses' responsibility on the day of surgery will include

- Note allergies according to institutional policy.
- Take and record the vital signs, assess and report any abnormalities for elevated temperature.
- Check the identification band to make sure it is legible, accurate and securely fastened to the client.
- Be sure that informed consent has been obtained and is clearly documented.
- If a skin preparation has been ordered, check that it has been completed accurately and thoroughly.
- Check for and carry out any special orders, such as administering enema or starting an IV line, secured previous records, inserting nasogastric tube, giving medications.
- Verify that the client has not eaten for the last eight hours. Check that fluids have been restricted although sometimes the physician will order clients to take their usual oral medication with a small sip of water.
- Ask the client to void, measure and record the amount of urine (if indicated).
- Assist the client with oral hygiene if necessary.

- Have the client to remove jewellery to prevent loss or injury from swelling, during or after surgery. Many facilities allow the client to keep wedding band or Mangal Sutra (Tali) on as long as they are taped securely. If jewellery is removed, it should be stored according to policy or given to authorised member of their family.
- Remove all hairpins or hairpieces. This prevents injury to the client during surgery as well as possible loss or hairpieces or wigs.
- Remove coloured nail polish from at least one nail for the pulse oximeter to allow intraoperative and postoperative assessment of skin and nail beds for circulation and oxygenation of tissues.
- If the client is wearing hearing aid, notify the operating room nurse. Leave it in place so that operating room personnel know it is there and can communicate with the client.
- Remove all prosthesis, such as dentures, or partial plates, eye glasses, contact lenses and artificial limbs and keep them safely (dentures may cause respiratory distress).
- Give the preoperative medications that are prescribed, either at a scheduled time or "on call". The commonly ordered medication are:
  - Sedatives and tranquilisers to alleviate anxiety and facilitate anaesthesia, induction. For example nembutol, chloro-promozen, or diazapam.
  - Anticholenergic to decrease pulmonary and oral secretions to prevent laryngospasm, e.g. atrophine.
  - Narcotic analgesics to facilitate client's sedation and relxation and to decrease the amount of anaesthetic agent need, for example morphine.
  - Neurolephanalgesics agents to cause a general state of calmness and sleepiness.

To prevent omissions and preoperative nursing intervention, most facilities supply nurses with a preoperative checklist. As each intervention on the list is completed, the nurse initiats it. Documents through checklists and narrative charting, the nursing intervention carried out.

- Assist in moving client from the bed to the operating room stretcher when it is time to transport the client to surgery, ensuring accurate identification.

INTRAOPERATIVE NURSING

Intraoperative phase begins when the client enters the surgical suite and ends with admission to the recovery area. Nursing care during this phase focuses on the client's emotional wellbeing, as well as on physical factors such as safety positioning, maintaining asepsis and controlling the surgical environment. The nurses are the client's advocates upon induction of anaesthesia.

In the surgical holding area, the nurse is responsible for reviewing the record for completeness, ensuring proper identification of the client, client's safety and providing emotional support. It is important to deal with the fears and concerns of a frightened or agitated client. A relaxed client undergoes anaesthetic induction easier than who is anxious. If the client still seems anxious despite sedation and reassurance, notify the surgeon or anaesthesia personnel. Here the anaesthetologist sees the client., IV fluids starts time him or her or nurse-anaesthetist. Nurse-anaesthetist also can administer medication needed during surgery. The procedures vary among institutions of health care.

Introduction to Anaesthesia

Anaesthesia means the absence of pain (Greek: an=without + aisthesis = feeling). Anaesthesia is an artificially-induced state of partial or total loss of sensation, with or without loss of consciousness. Anaesthesia produces muscle relaxation, blocks transmission of nerve impulses and suppresses reflexes.

There are two types of anaesthesia i.e., general anaesthesia and regional anaesthesia.

General anaesthesia Is a drug-induced depression of the central nervous system (CNS) that is reverted either by metabolic elimination in the body or by pharmocologic means. General anaesthetic agents produces analgesia, amnesia and unconsciousness, characterized by loss of reflexes and muscle tone.

There are four stages of anaesthesia. Brief explanation and nursing intervention in these stages are as follows:

Onset Starts from anaesthetic administration to loss of consciousness. In this stage, client may be drowsy or dizzy and may experience auditory or visual hallucinations. Nursing action in this stage will include, close operating room doors, keeping room quiet, and standby to assist client.

Excitement Starts from loss of consciousness to loss of eyelid reflexes. Here there will be increase in automatic activity, irregular breathing, client may struggle. In this stage, nurse has to remain, quitely at client's side, assist anaesthetists if needed.

Surgical anaesthesia This stage starts with loss of eyelid reflexes, to lose of motor reflexes and depression of vital function. Here client is unconscious, muscles are relaxed and no blink or gag reflexes. In this stage, begin preparation (if indicated) only when anaesthetists indicate stage III has been reached and client is under good control.

Danger (death) Stage experiences. Vital functions too depressed may lead to respiratory and circulatory failure. In this stage, client is not breathing and he may or may not have a heartbeat. If arrest occurs, nurse responds immediately to assist establishing airway, provide cardiac arrest tray, drugs, syringes, long needles, assist surgeon with closed or open cardiac massage.

General anaesthesia can be administered by inhalation or intravenously. An inhalation agent will include nitrous oxide, halothene (fluothene) enflurane (ethrane) and isofluorane (porane) and the intravenous drugs are thiopental sodium (penthathol), fentanyl citratedroperidol (innovar) and ketamine hydrochloride. The selections of anaesthetic agents are according to decision of the anaesthesiologist. But continuous monitoring of side effects of the drugs, vital signs are essential.

Regional Anaesthesia

Regional anaesthesia blocks the pain stimulus at the origin and along afferent neurons of along the spinal cord. Regional anaesthesia produces a loss of painful sensation in only one region of the body and does not result in unconsciousness. The client may receive sedative that produces drowsiness. The Regional anaesthetic agents block the conduction of impulses in nerve fiber without depolarizing the cell membrane are: Local agents and topical agents. An example of local agents are Bupivacaine HCl (Marcaine HCl) (xylocane) and examples of topical agents will include benzocaine, ethylchloride spray, tetracain HCl. All these agents have their own side effects. Contraindication for children, test dose can be given prior to use of these agents to know any allergies to these agents.

The types of regional anaesthesia are:

- Topical anaesthesia
- Local infiltration anaesthesia
- Field block anaesthesia
- Peripheral nerve block anaesthesia
- Spinal anaesthesia
- Epidural anaesthesia
- Caudal anaesthesia.

The other types of anaesthesia are used in modern drugs acupuncture, cryothermia and hypnoanaesthesia. The type of anaesthesia chosen depends on the surgery performed and level of unconscious desired.

NURSING CARE DURING SURGERY

Nursing care during surgery will include providing emotional care, assessing the client with positioning (as required for type of surgery) maintaining safety, maintaining surgical asepsis, prevent client heat loss, monitoring malignant hyperthermia, assisting with surgeon to perform surgery by providing proper equipments and supplies, assisting with wound closure, assessing drainage, and transferring client to recovery room.

Postoperative Nursing

The postoperative phase of surgery is final phase of the surgical experience. Nursing plays a critical role in returning the client to an optimal level of functioning. The postoperative period can be divided into two phases, i.e. immediate postanaesthesia and postoperative period, and later in postoperative phase.

Immediate Postoperative Phase

Immediate postoperative phase is the first few hours after surgery when the client is recovering from the effect of anaesthesia. Here the nurse has to keep all emergency equipment and drugs, etc. for use for patient's recovery from anaesthesia and on admission to postoperative unit, the nurse performs the following:

- Assess airway patency and support as needed, and assess for the presence of hoarseness, cramp, strider, wheezes or decreased breath sounds.
- Applies humidified oxygen via nasal cannula or facemask (unless otherwise ordered).
- Records vital signs (blood pressure, heart rate, strength and regularity, respiratory rate and depth, oxygen saturation, skin colour, and temperature).
- Assess the client's level of consciousness, muscle strength and ability to follow commands.
- Observe the client's IV infusions, dressings, drains and special equipment.
- Remain at the client's bedside, continuing close observations of the client's conditions.

After the client has been positioned safely and the baseline vital signs status has been ascertained, the nurse receives verbal report regarding surgery in detail, i.e. type of surgery, time of incision, patient's condition during surgery, type of anaesthesia, sedative, all untoward incident happened and everything about surgery and documents the reliable and retainable information for further care that follow surgeon's and anaesthetist's instructions for patient's recovery.

It is very important, that nursing intervention associated with immediate recovery (ABCs) are as follows:

A. Airway:
- Maintain patency, keep head tilted up and back may position one side with the face down and neck slightly extended.
- Note presence or absence of gag/swallowing reflex
- Suction until awake and alert
- Provide oxygen if necessary.

B. Breathing:
- Evaluate depth, rate, sounds, rhythm and chest movement.
- Assess colour of mucous membrane
- Place hand above nose to detect respirations if shallow
- Initiate coughing and deep breathing as soon as able to respond
- Chart time oxygen is discontinued.

C. Consciousness:
- Able to extubate airway
- Responds to command
- Verbalizes responses
- Reacts to stimuli.

C—Circulation:
- Monitor TPR every 15 minutes; take axillary or rectal temperature if necessary
- Assess rate, rythm, quality of pulse
- Evaluate colour and warmth of skin and nailbeds

- – Check peripheral pulse if indicated
- – Monitor IVs solution, rate, site.

S—System review:
- – Assess neurological functions
- – Monitor drains, tubes, colour and amount of output
- – Evaluate pain response, may need to give analgesics
- – Observe for allergic reactions
- – Assess urinary output if Foley catheter is in place.

For remaining postoperative period, nurse has to take following measures to:

- Continuous assessment of respiratory and circulatory assessment
- Ensure optimal respiratory function—deep breath and coughing exercises
- Relieving postoperative discomforts—relieving pain, restlessness nausea and vomiting, abdominal distension, hiccups, etc.
- Maintaining normal body temperature
- Avoid injury—by providing proper positioning in bed
- Maintaining normal nutrional status—by IV fluids, total parenteral nutrition
- Promoting normal urinary functions
- Promoting bowel eliminations—preventing paralytic ileus, and constipation
- Restoring Mobility—by positioning in proper
- Early ambulation—bed exercises
- Prevent and treatment of complication like shock, hemorrhage, deep venous thrombosis (DVT), pulmonary embolism, *respiratory* complication like undetected hypoxemia, atelectasis, bronchitis, bronchopneumonia and lobar pneumonia, hypostatic pulmonary congestion, pleuracy, etc. and gastric complication like nutritional anaemia, intestinal obstruction and postoperative psychosis.
- Wound healing.

COMMON TRAYS USED IN PREOPERATIVE NURSING

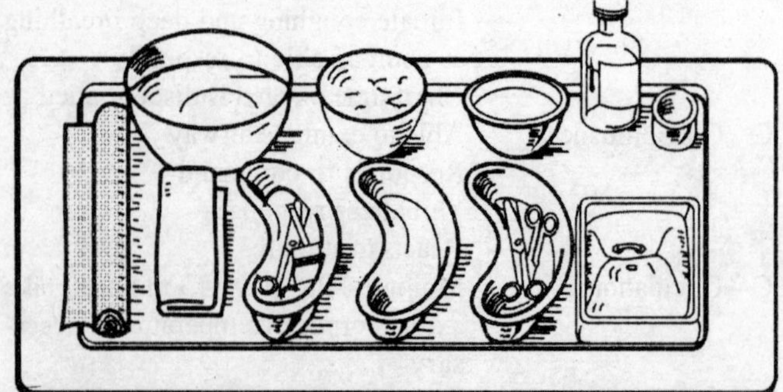

Fig. 4.1: Tray for preoperative skin preparation

1. A bowl of hot water.
2. A bowl with cotton wool and gauze swabs.
3. A receiver with a razor and a pair of scissors.
4. A small bowl with warm ether soap.
5. A receiver or disposal bag for soiled swabs.
6. A protection for the bed.
7. A disposable drape.

When a skin disinfectant and sterile dressing is to be applied add:

a. A bottle with the ordered disinfectant, e.g., hibitane.
b. A gallipot for the lotion.
c. A receiver or suitable container with set of dressing forceps.
d. A small packet containing the necessary sterile dressings and towels.

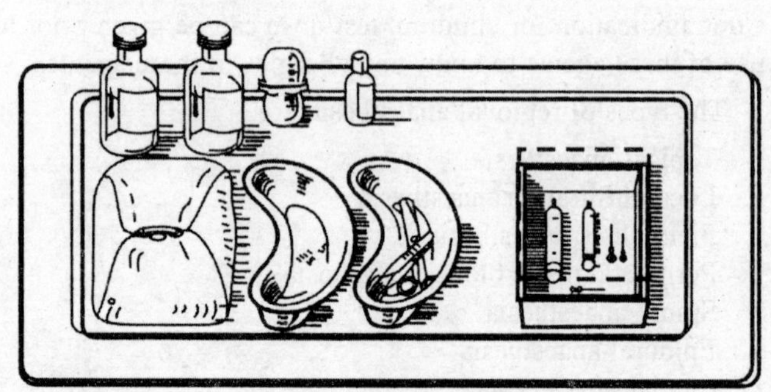

Fig. 4.2: Tray for local anaesthetic by injection

1. Small packet containing sterile towel and swabs.
2. A bottle with cetavlon (1%).
3. A bottle of methylated spirit.
4. Two sterile gallipots.
5. Bottle containing the local anaesthetic, e.g., xylocaine (0.5%).
6. Packet or box with 5 and 2 ml dry sterile syringes and assorted suitable-sized needles.
7. A receiver or suitable container with three pairs of sterile dressing forceps.
8. A receiver or disposal bag for soiled swabs.
   (local anaesthesia may also be produced using, e.g., a spray or drops.)

1. A bowl of gauze swabs.
2. A jar with dressed wooden probes.
3. A bottle with the local anaesthetic, e.g. cocaine (10 %).
4. A suitable measure for the anaesthetic.
5. De Vilbiss spray.
6. A small tray with laryngoscope(s).

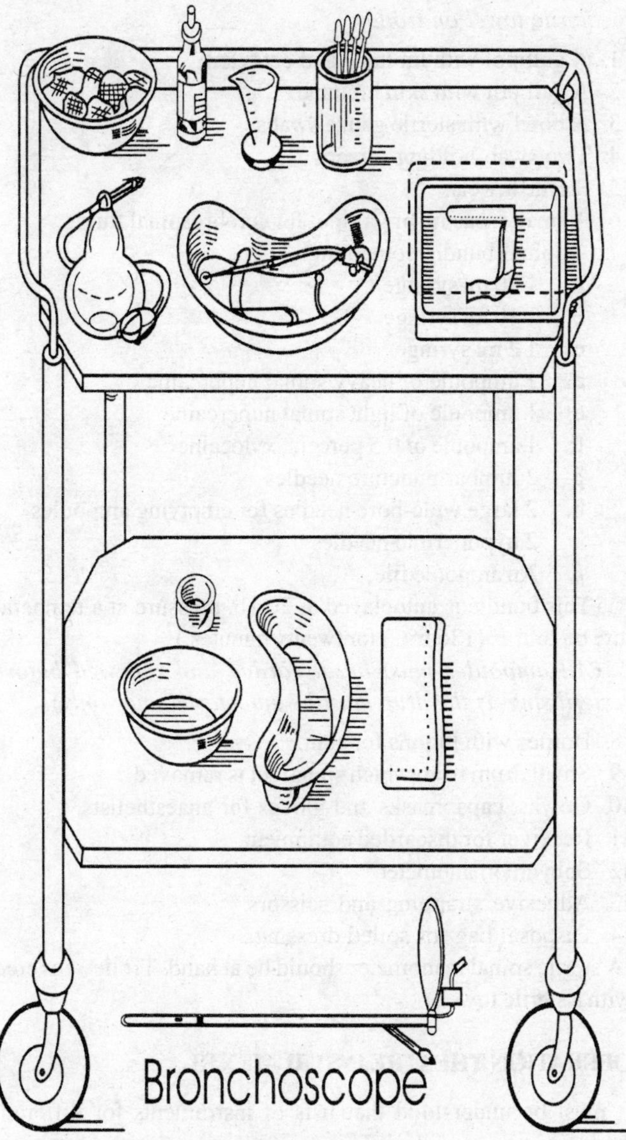

Fig. 4.3: Trolley for direct laryngoscopy

7. A receiver with angled tongue depressor and grasping forceps.
8. Sickness basin.
9. Denture jar.
10. A receiver or disposal bag for soiled swabs.
11. A disposable drape.

(*N.B.*—Patient premedicated. Several sizes of laryngoscope available. Extra-electric bulbs at hand. Suction apparatus in readiness.)

(It may be necessary to have tracheotomy instruments also in readiness.)

For bronchoscopy.—Requirements are similar with the addition of a bronchoscope.

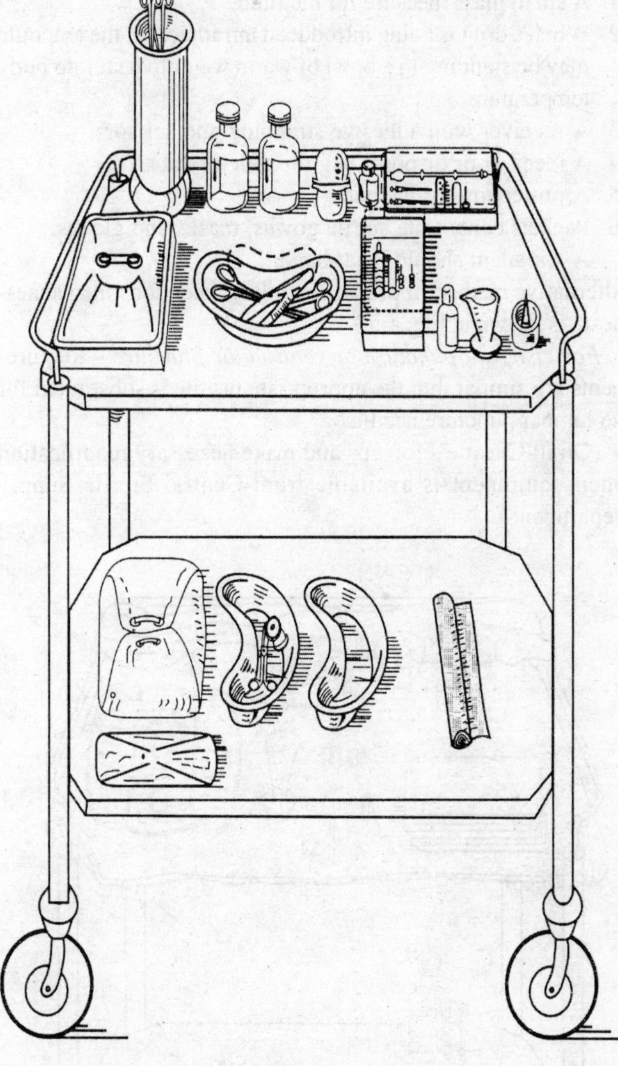

Fig. 4.4: Trolley for lumbar puncture

1. A jar with Cheatle's forceps.
2. A small tray with a packet containing sterile towels and dressings.
3. A bottle of cetavlon (1%).
4. A bottle of methylated spirit.
5. Two sterile gallipots.
6. A covered receiver or suitable container with three pairs of sterile dressing forceps.
7. Hypodermic syringe and needles in syringe box or packet.
8. A bottle with local anaesthetic, e.g. novocaine (2%) or xylocaine (0.5%).
9. Two lumbar puncture needles, a spinal manometer, 10 or 20 ml syringe and cannula; these may be autoclaved in a packet or a special covered tray. A tenotomy knife may also be required.
10. A sterile specimen bottle.

11. A small glass measure for the fluid.
12. When a drug is being introduced intrathecally, the ampoule may be standing in a bowl of warm water to heat it to body temperature.
13. A receiver with adhesive strapping and scissors.
14. A receiver or disposal bag for soiled swabs.
15. A protection for the bed.
16. Packets containing sterile gowns, masks and gloves.
17. A stimulant should be at hand.

(alternative method of preparing trolley when for spinal anaesthesia is shown in Fig. 4.5.)

For cisternal puncture or ventricular puncture—Requirements are similar, but the appropriate needle is substituted for the lumbar puncture needle.

(Omit: Cheatle's forceps and make necessary modification when equipment is available from Central Sterile Supply Department.)

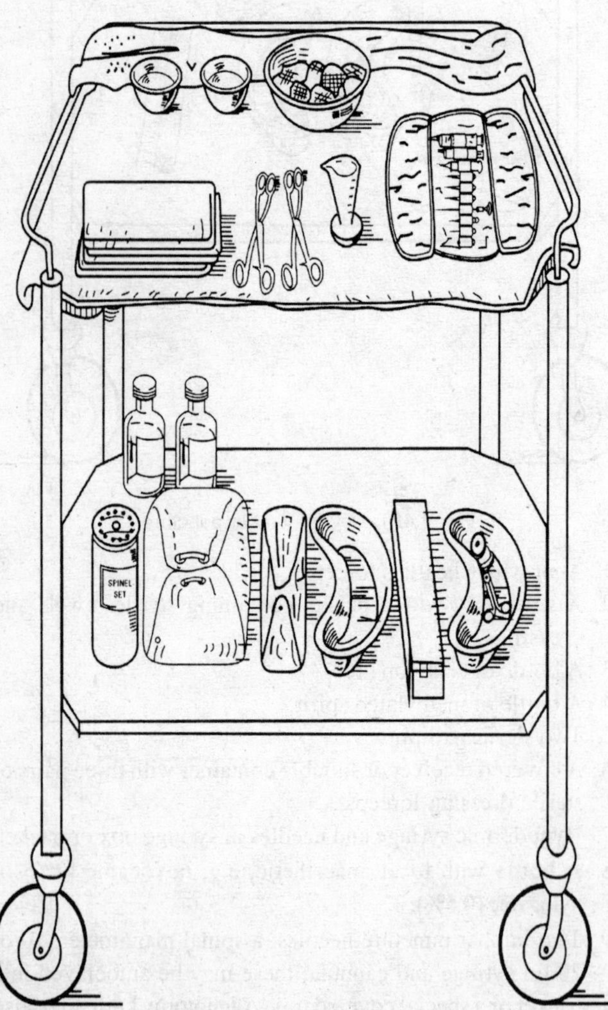

Fig.4.5: Trolley for spinal anaesthesia

Sterile towel on trolley—

1. A gallipot with hibitane and cetavlon.
2. A gallipot with skin hibitane.
3. A bowl with sterile gauze swabs.
4. Two swab-holding forceps.
5. Sterile towels.
6. A small measure or gallipot for cerebrospinal fluid.
7. A spinal bundle containing:
   a. 1 20 ml syringe
   b. 1 10 ml syringe
   c. 1 2 ml syringe
   d. 1 ampoule of heavy spinal nupercaine
   e. 1 ampoule of light spinal nupercaine
   f. 1 ampoule of 0.5 percent, xylocaine
   g. 2 lumbar puncture needles
   h. 2 large wide-bore needles for emptying ampoules
   i. 2 hypodermic needles
   j. An ampoule file.

(This bundle is autoclaved at 20 1b. pressure at a temperature of 260° F. (126.6°C) for twenty minutes.)

(*All ampoules must be discarded and renewed before resterilising as the drug must be autoclaved once only*).

8. Bottles with lotions for skin.
9. Small drum from which spinal set is removed.
10. Gowns, caps, masks and gloves for anaesthetists.
11. Receiver for discarded equipment.
12. Sphygmomanometer.
13. Adhesive strapping and scissors.
14. Disposal bag for soiled dressings.

(A sterile spinal manometer should be at hand. Trolley covered with a sterile towel.)

OPERATION THEATRE INSTRUMENTS

It must be understood that lists of instruments for different operations vary with different surgeons and circumstances, but the following have been found generally satisfactory:

General Set (Plate I)

15 Lane's tissue forceps (I, 1).
9 Spencer Wells' artery forceps (I, 2).
9 Mayo Ochsner's forceps (I, 3).
4 Toothed dissecting forceps (I, 4).
2 Non-toothed dissecting forceps (I, 5).
2 Retractors (I, 6).
2 Sponge-holding forceps (I, 7).
4 Towel clips (I, 8).
1 Small probe (I, 9).
1 Long probe (I, 9).
1 Grooved director (I, 10).
1 Blunt dissector (I, 11).
1 Raspatory (I, 12).

(the last five items bracketed: 9 extras)

1 Sharp spoon (I, 13).
1 Aneurysm needle (I, 14).
1 Needle holder (I, 15).
1 Suture holder (I, 16).
(9 extras)
1 Pair curved scissors (I, 17).
2 Pairs straight scissors (I, 18).
2 Scalpels (I, 19).

Plate I

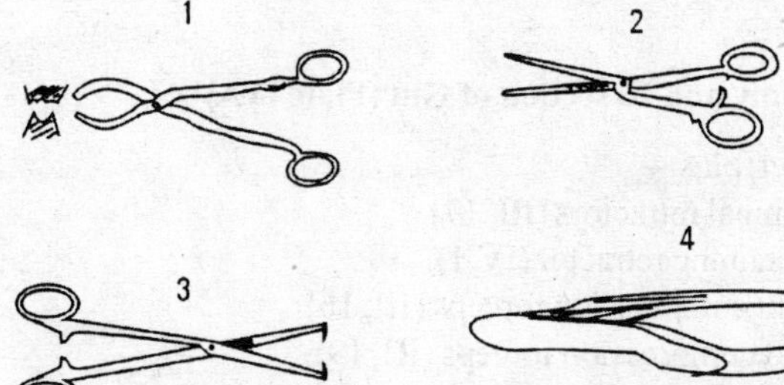

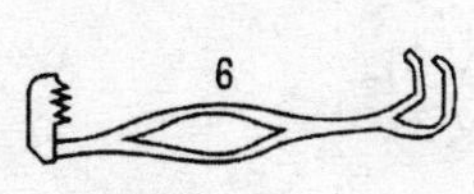

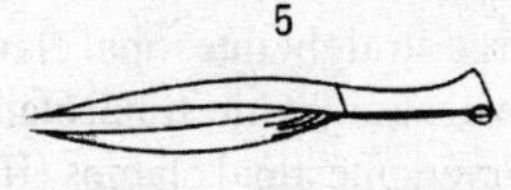

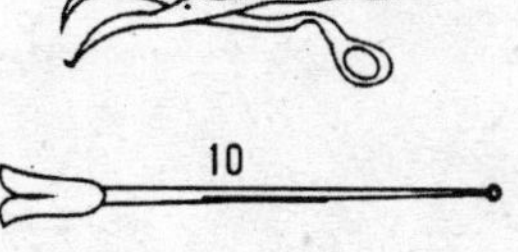

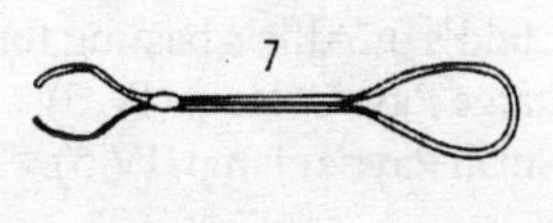

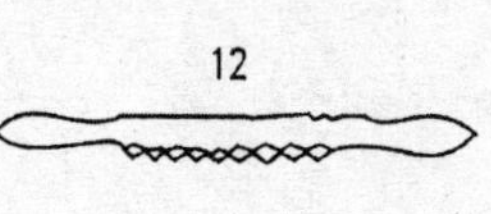

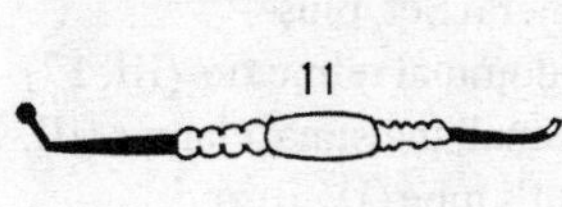

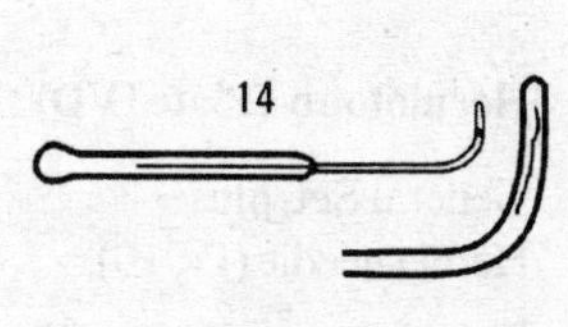

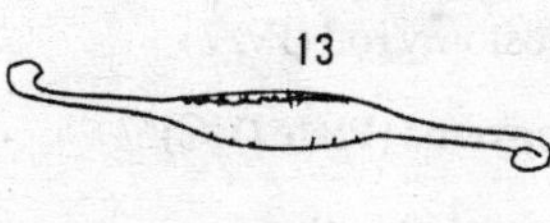

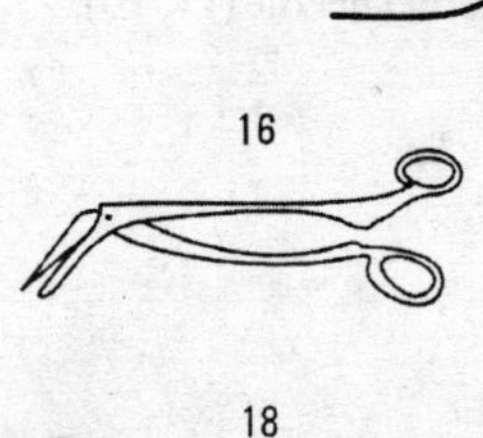

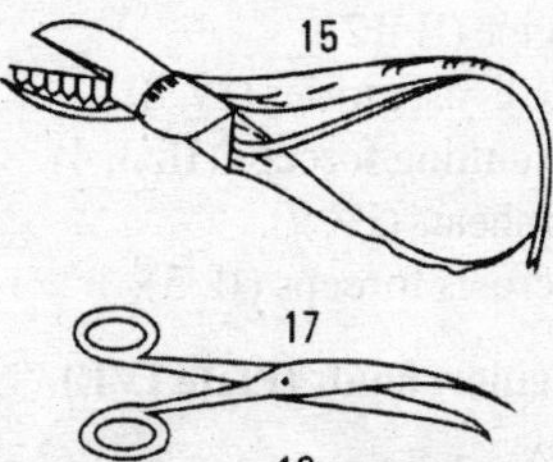

Bone Set (Plate II)

9 Skin clips (II, 1).
2 Lion bone-holding forceps (II, 2).
2 Small lion-holding forceps (II, 2).
1 Large straight bone cutting forceps (II, 3).
1 Large curved bone cutting forceps (II, 4).
1 Small straight bone cutting forceps (II, 4).
1 Small curved bone cutting forceps (II, 4).
2 Pairs necrosis forceps (II, 5).
1 Pair sequestrum forceps (II, 6).
1 Awl (II, 7).
1 Grooved awl (II, 8).
1 Mallet (II, 9).
Langenbeck retractors (II, 10).
1 Pair sinus forceps (II, 11).
2 Rugines (II, 12)
1 Pair large bone levers or spikes (II, 13).
1 Pair medium bone levers (grooved) (II, 14).
1 Pair small bone levers (or more according to operation)
1 File (II, 15).
1 Mechanical drill and drill points (II, 16).

Plate II

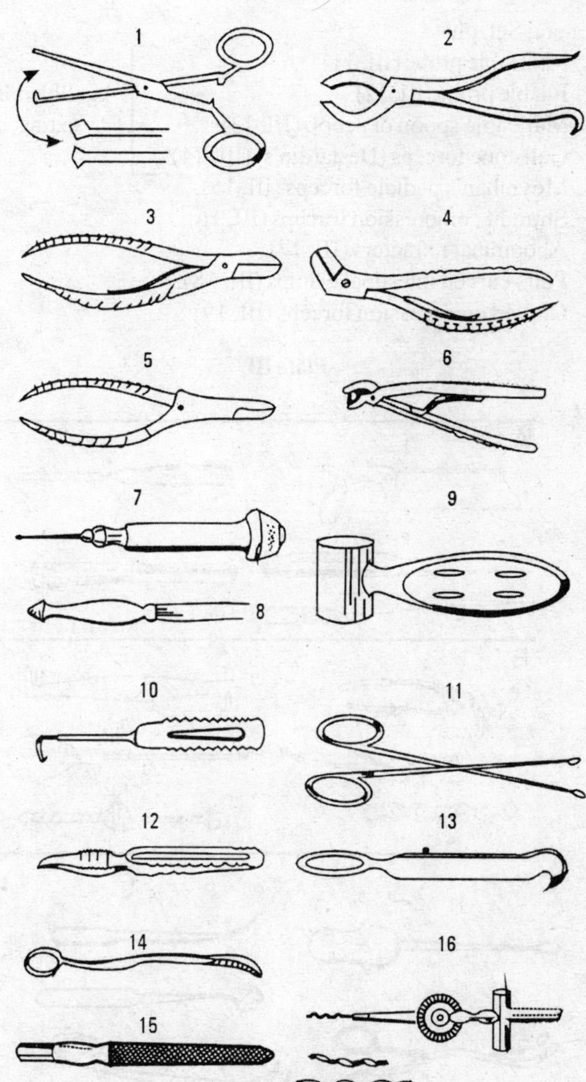

Bone Sharps (Plate IIIA).

1 Large saw (III, 1).
1 Small saw.
Chisels of varying sizes (III, 2).
Osteotomes varying sizes (III, 3).
Gouges varying sizes (III, 4).
Drill points varying sizes (II, 16).

Bone Plating Set (Plate IIIB).

General Set and Bone Set, plus—
2 Plate-holding forceps (III, 5).
2 Plate benders (III, 6).
2 Screw-holding forceps (III, 7).
2 Screwdrivers (III, 8).
Plates (III, 9) and screws (III, 10).

Extra Laparotomy Instruments (Plate IIIC).

General Set, plus.—
1 Malleable probe (III, 11). ⎤
1 Pliable probe (III, 12). ⎥ 4 gallbladder
1 Malleable spoon or scoop (III, 13). ⎥ extras
1 Gallstone forceps (Desjardin's) (III, 14). ⎦
2 Moynihan's pedicle forceps (III, 15).
2 Straight compression forceps (III, 16).
2 Abdominal retractors (III, 17).
2 Pairs curved intestinal clamps (III, 18).
2 Curved compression forceps (III, 19).

Plate III

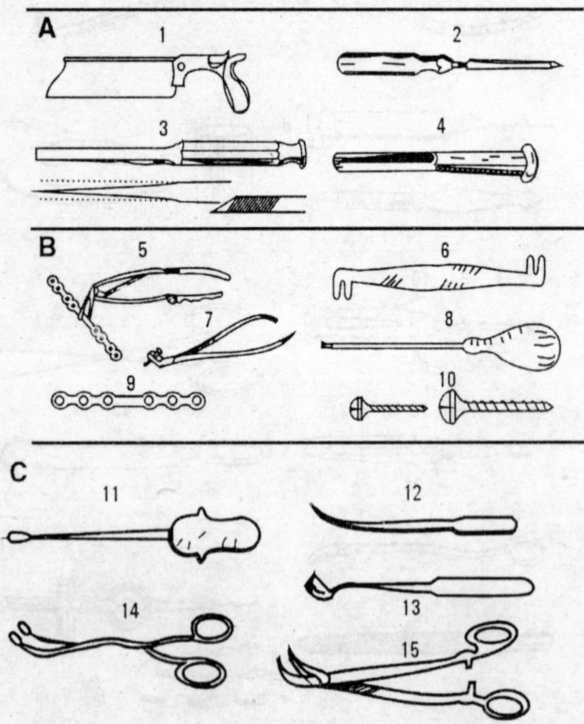

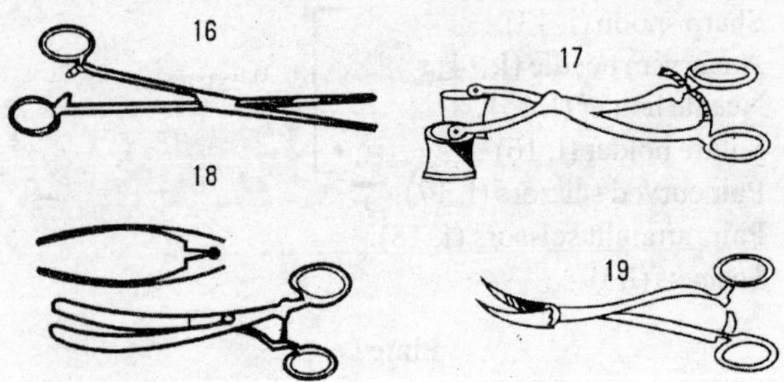

Gastrectomy and Resection of Gut (Plate IVA)

General Set, plus.—
2 Abdominal retractors (III, 17).
1 Self-retaining retractor (IV, 1).
2 Straight compression forceps (III, 16).
2 Curved compression forceps (III, 19).
2 Moynihan's pedicle forceps (III, 15).
1 Double intestinal clamp (IV, 2).
2 Large straight intestinal clamps (IV, 3).
2 Small straight intestinal clamps (IV, 3).
2 Curved intestinal clamps (III, 18).
4 Ludd's or Allis's basting forceps (IV, 4).
1 Large Payr's clamp (IV, 5).
1 Small Payr's clamp (IV, 5).

Colostomy (Plate IVB)

General Set, plus—
Abdominal retractors (III, 17).
2 Small intestinal clamps (III, 18).
Paul's tube (IV, 6) and
colostomy rod (IV, 7).

Empyema (Plate IVC)

General Set, plus-
Rugine (II, 12).
2 Rib raspatories (IV, 8).
Rib cutting forceps (II, 3, 4).
Rib shears (IV, 9).
Necrosis forceps (II, 5).

Herniotomy (Plate IVD)

General Set, plus•-
Hernia needle (IV, 10).

Haemorrhoids (Plate IVE)

General Set, plus—
Proctoscope (IV, 11).
4 Haemorrhoid clamps (IV, 12).

Amputation (Plate IVF)

General Set, plus—
Extra artery forceps (I, 2).
Bone set (II).
Bone sharps (IIIA).
Flat retractor (IV, 13).
Amputation knife (IV, 14).

Plate IV

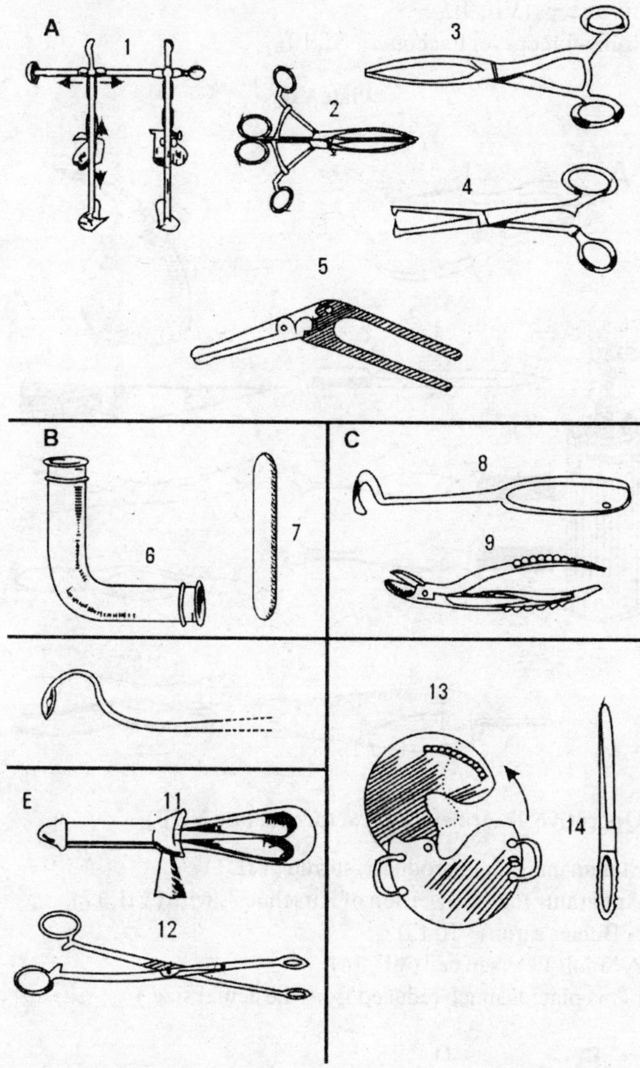

Tonsillectomy (Plate V)

1 Towel clip (I, 8).
4 Tongue depressors (V, 1).
1 Davis gag (V, 1).
Suspension apparatus for gag (V, 2).
2 Tonsil guillotines (V, 3).
2 Doyen's gags (V, 4).
2 Mayo Ochsner's artery forceps (I, 3).
1 Tracheotomy dilator (V, 5).
2 Tonsil snares (V, 6).
1 Tonsil dissector (V, 7).
2 Adenoid curettes (V, 8).
2 Pairs toothed dissecting forceps (I, 4).
2 Curved tonsil forceps (V, 9).
1 Toothed tonsil forceps (V, 10).

4 Straight artery forceps (I, 2).
4 Curved artery forceps (I, 2).

Plate V

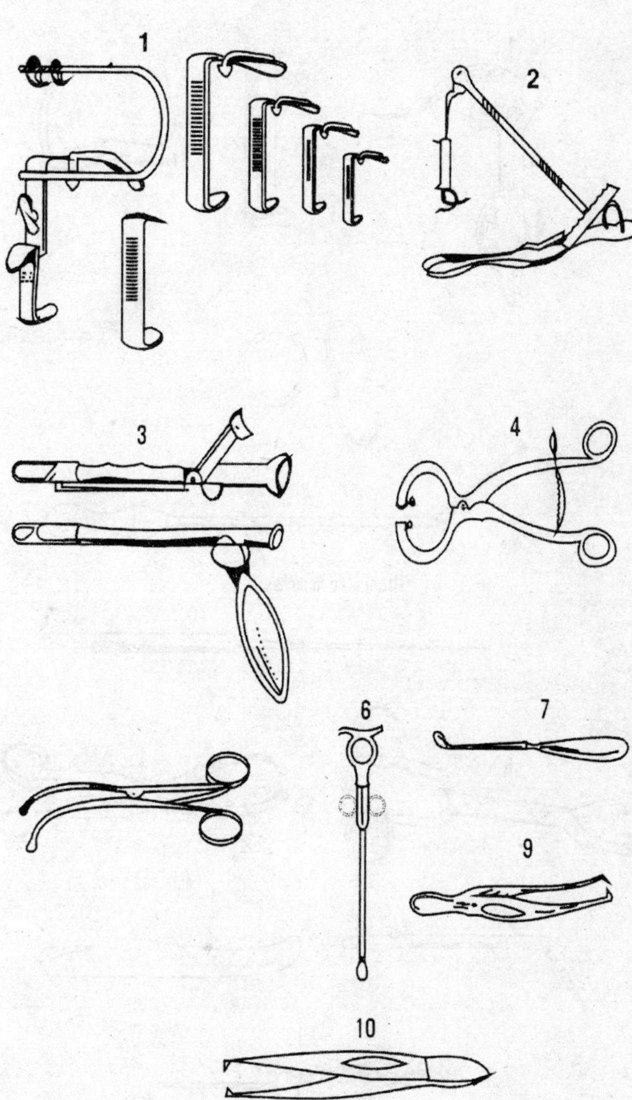

Some Special Instruments for Gynaecological Work Plate VI

Vaginal speculae, Auvard's (VI, 1).
Vaginal speculae, Sims' (VI, 2).
Vaginal speculae, Fergusson's (VI, 3).
Pessaries (VI, 5).
Uterine sound (VI, 6).
Playfair's probe (VI, 7).
Ovum forceps (VI, 8).
Vulsellum forceps (VI, 9).
Intrauterine douche nozzle (VI, 10).

Dilators for cervix (VI, 11).
Intrauterine flushing curette (VI, 12).

Plate VI

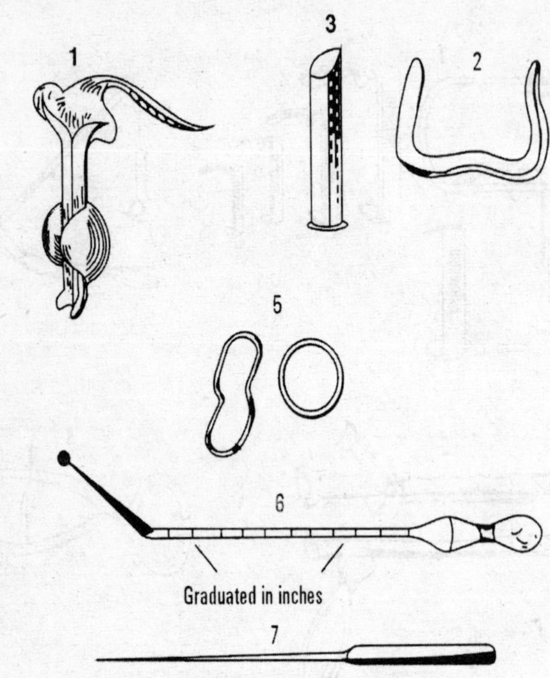

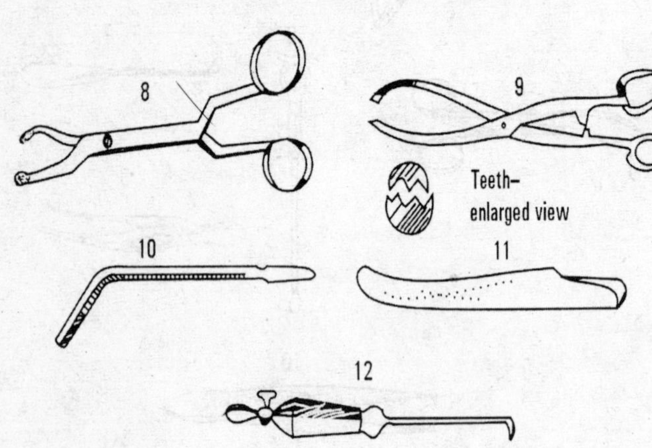

Some Special Instruments for Ophthalmic Work (Plate VIIA)

Retractor (VII, 1).
Undine (VII, 2).
Ophthalmoscope (VII, 3).
Graefe's knife (VII, 4).
Keratome (VII, 5).
Beer's knife (VII, 6).
Iris scissors (VII, 7).
Elliott's trephine (VII, 8).
Iris forceps (VII, 9).
Roller forceps for trachoma (VII, 10).

Plate VII

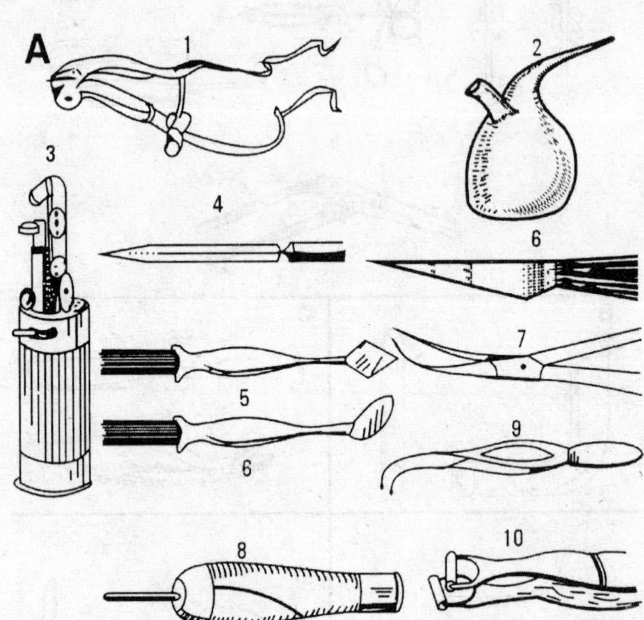

Operative Treatment of Fractures (Plate VIIB)

Steinmann's pin, introducer, stirrup (VII, 11).
Apparatus for the insertion of Kirschner's wire (VII, 12).
A Bohler's iron (VII, 13).
A Smith-Petersen nail (VII, 14).
(This plate is much reduced from the actual size.)

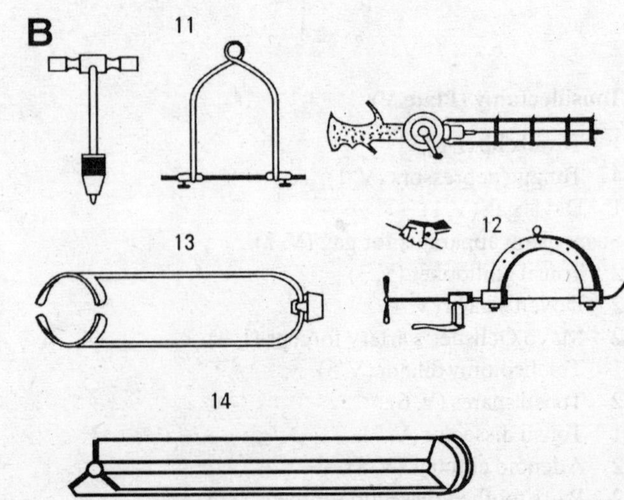

Cancer Nursing/ Oncological Nursing

Cancer was recognized in ancient times by skilled observers who gave it the name "Cancer" (Latin word Canceri-crab) because it stretched out in many directions like the legs of a crab. The term cancer is an "umbrella" word used to describe a group of more than 270 diseases in which cells multiply without restraint, destroy healthy tissue endangering life. The psychological and physiological impact on cancer patients and their families results in profound changes in their lifestyles. Cancer may result in death for some and mutilation for others. The legends, surroundings, malignant diseases often focussing on its incurability help foster feelings of hopelessness and dread. Yet, much progress has been made in prevention, early detection and treatment of cancer and research continue in these areas.

Oncology nurses must have a broad base of knowledge in both pathophysiology and psycholosocial arena. They care for patients of all ages, both gender and in a variety of settings. The oncology nurse feels and fills the role of care provider, manager, researcher, teacher and consultant. To provide comprehensive care, the nurse must have accurate knowledge about prevention, control and treatment of cancer. Nurse has to teach about cancer in all settings. In addition to teaching, the nurse has an active role in treatment and control programs of cancer. To be effective as a helping person, the nurse must be aware of the emotional impact that the diagnosis of cancer has on the patient and family, because this emotional response affects every aspect of nursing care. Cancer nursing challenges the creativity, skill and commitment of the nurses.

CANCER

The word Cancer, often abbreviated Ca, is a term that frightens most people. Cancer is synonymous with the term "malignant neoplasma". Other terms suggest malignant neoplasm includes tumour, malignancy, carcinoma and aberrect cell growth. Strictly speaking, these words are not interchangeable.

Cancer is a disease of the cell in which the normal mechanisms of control of growth and proliferation are disturbed. This results in distinctive morphological alteration of the cells and aberration in tissue pattern. Cancer is a collective term describing a large group of diseases characterized by uncontrolled growth and spread of abnormal cells. This group of diseases:

- arise from any tissue or organ,
- differ greatly from one another in appearance and growth
- may follow very different courses of developments in their host.
- respond differently to the variety of therapies applied to them.

The word 'neoplasm' is derived from Greek words neos: new, and plasis: molding. Thus, neoplasm is defined as an abnormal new growth or formation of tissue that serves no useful purpose and may harm the host organism.

A neoplasm may be either benign or malignant.

- Benign is defined as a usually harmless growth that does not spread or invade other tissues.
- Malignant is defined as a harmful tumour, capable of spread and invasion of other tissues far removed from the site of origin.

In addition, some other important terms used in cancer are:

- Anaplastic refers to those tumour cells that are completely undifferentiated and bear no resemblance to cells of tissues of their origin.
- Hyperplasia refers to an increase in the number of normal cells in a normal arrangement in a tissue or organ, usually leads to an increase in the size or part and an increase in functional activity.
- Metaplasia refers to the replacement of one type of fully differentiated cell by another fully differentiated cell in another part of the body where the second cell type does not normally occur.
- Dysplasia refers to an alteration in the size, shape, and organization of differentiated cells; cells lose their regularity and show variability in size and shape, usually in response to an irritant; cells may revert to normal when the irritant is removed, but may transform to neoplasia.
- Metastasis refers to the ability of neoplastic cells to spread from the original site of the tumour to distant organs, spreading as the same cell type as the original neoplastic tissue.
- Carcinoma-refers to a form of cancer that is composed of epithelial cells that tend to infiltrate surrounding tissues and may eventually spread to distant sites.
- Oncogenes refer to cancer genes that are altered versions of normal genes.

- Proto-oncogenes refer to repressed oncogenes existing in normal which can be activated by many different factors and cause the host cell to become malignant.
- Tumour refers to usually synonymous with neoplasm.

Pathophysiology of Cancer

The exact cause and method of the development of cancer are unknown. Cancer is a group of many diseases of multiple causes that can arise in any cell of the body capable of evading regulatory control over proliferations and differentiation. The two major dysfunctions present in the process of cancer of "defective cellular proliferation (growth)" and "defective cellular differentiation".

Defective Cellular Proliferation
Cancer cells usually proliferate in the manner and at the same rate of the normal cells of the tissue from which they arise. However, cancer cells respond differently than normal cells to the intracellular signals that regulate the state of dynamic equilibrium. Cancer cells divide indiscriminately and haphazardly. Sometime, they produce more than two cells at the time of mitosis. The loss of intracellular control of proliferations may be result of a mutation of the stem cells. The stem cells are viewed as the target or the origin of cancer developed. The DNA of the stem cell is substituted or permanently rearranged. When this happens the stem cell is mutuated and has the potential to become malignant. It will usually proliferate at the rate of the tissue origin, and some subpopulation can promote tumour progression to generate malignant cells. The malignant cells can differentiate to form normal tissue cells.

Defective Cellular Differentiation
Cellular differentiation is normally and orderly a process that progresses from a state of immaturity to a state of maturity. Because all body cells are derived from the fertilized ova, all cells have the potential to perform all body functions. As cell differentiates, this potential is repressed and the mature cell is capable of performing only specific functions. Genes that are important regulators of these normal cellular processes are the "cellular oncogenes or proto-oncogenes. Mutations that alter the expression of genes or their products can activate proto-oncogenes to function as 'oncogenes' (tumour-inducing genes) by inducing mitosis but inhibiting differentiation of the cell.

The proto-oncogene has been described as the genetic lock that keeps the cell in its mature functioning state. When this lock is 'unlocked' it may occur through exposure to carcinogens or oncogenic viruses, genetic alterations and mutations occur. The abilities and properties that the cell had in fetal development are again expressed. Although oncogens and oncogenic products, contribute to normal cell function, oncogens intefere with normal cell expression under some conditions, causing cell to become malignant. The comparison of the characteristics of normal and malignant cells (Table 5.1) are as follows:

Table 5.1: Characteristics of normal and malignant cells

Normal cells	*Malignant cells*
A. *Mitotic cell division*	
Mitotic cell division leads to two daughter cells	Mitosis leads to multiple cell that may or may not resemble the parent, multiple mitotic spindles
B. *Appearance*	
• Cells of same type homogeneous in size, shape and growth	• Cells larger and grow more rapidly than normal, pleomorphic, i.e. heterogeneous in size and shape
• Cells cohesive, form regular pattern of expansion	• Cells not as cohesive, irregular pattern or expansion
• Uniform size to nucleus	• Larger, more prominent nucleus
• Have characteristics pattern of organization	• Lack of characteristic pattern of organization of host cell
• Mixture of stem cells (Precursors) and well-differentiated cells	• Anaplastic, lack of differentiated cell characteristic, specific functions
C. *Growth pattern*	
• Do not invade adjacent tissue	• Invade adjacent tissues
• Proliferate in response to specific stimuli	• Proliferate in response to abnormal stimuli
• Growth in ideal conditions (e.g. nutrients, oxygen, space, correct biochemical environments)	• Growth in adverse conditions such as lack of nutrients
• Exhibit contact inhibition	• Do not exhibit contact inhibition
• Cell birth equals or in less than cell death	• Cell birth exceeds cell death
• Stable cell membrane	• Loss of cell control as a result of cell membrane charges
• Constant and predictable cell growth rate	• Erratic cell growth rate
• Cannot grow outside specific environment, e.g. breast-cell growth and only in breast	• Able to break off cells than migrate through blood stream or lymphatics or seed to distant sites and grow in other sites
D. *Function*	
• Have specific and designated purpose	• Serve no useful purpose
• Contribute to the overall well-being of the host	• Do not contribute to the well-being of the host, parasitic
• Cells function in specific pre-determined manner (e.g. cells in thyroid secrete thyroxine)	• If cells function at all, do not function normally or they may actually cause damage. (e.g. malignant lung cancer cells secrete ACTH, causing excessive stimulated...cortex)

Contd...

Contd...

Normal cells	Malignant cells
E. *Others*	
• Develop specific antigens, characteristic of particular cell formed	• Develop antigens completely different from normal cell
• Chromosomes remain constant throughout cell division	• Chromosomal aberrations occur as cell matures
• Complex metabolic and enzyme pattern	• Have more primitive and simplified metabolic and enzyme pattern
• Cannot invade, erode or spread	• Invade, erode and spread
• Cannot grow in the presence of necrosis or inflammation	• Grow in presence of necrosis and inflammatory cells such as lymphocytes and macrophages
	• Exhibit periods of latency that vary from tumour to tumour.
	• Have own blood supply and supporting stroma

The cause and development of each type of cancer are likely to be multifactorial. It is not known how many tumours have chemical, environmental, genetic, immunologic, or viral origin. It is common belief that the development of cancer is rapid, haphazard event. Although scientists have learned a great deal about the causes of cancer, the exact mechanism by which these agents transform healthy cells into neoplastic cells remains obscure. One accepted perception is that cancer developes as a result of genetic alteration from one or more causes, resulting in uncontrolled cellular reproduction and growth. When a defective cell divides, the new cells contain defective genetic code within the DNA. Overtime defective cells divide and multiply and the malignancy grows.

Carcinogens are substances that when introduced into the cell cause changes in the structure and function of the cells that lead to cancer. It is not a simple cause and effect mechanism. However, the natural history of cancer is an orderly process causing several stages and occurring over a period of time. There are three identified stages of carcinogenesis, i.e. initiation, promotion and progression.

i. *Initiation* The first stage, initiation, is an irreversible alteration in the cells' genetic structure resulting from the action of a chemical, physical or biologic agent. This altered cell has the potential for developing into a clone of neoplastic cells. Most carcinogens (*pl. see etiology*) are detoxified by protective a enzymes and are harmlessly excreted. If this protective mechanism fails, carcinogens enter the cells' nucleus and may irreversibly bind to DNA. DNA repair is possible. However, if repair does not occur before all divisions, the cell will replicate into daughter cells, each with the same genetic alterations. After this damage of DNA cells are more susceptible to progression into malignancies. Irreversibly initiated cells do not display their changes and are not detectable until exposed to a promoting agent.

ii. *Promotion.* Promotion is usually the result of a second factor acting on the initiated cell. A single alteration of the genetic structure of the cell is not sufficient to result in cancer. At least one or more mutation must occur in cells in which a mutation already occurred. The chances of this occurring, given the billions of cells in the human body, seem highly unlikely. However the odds of cancer development are increased with the presence of promoting agents.

Promotion—the second stage in the development of cancer is characterized by the reversible proliferation of the altered initiated cells and consequently, with an increase in the initiated cell population likelihood of second cell mutation is increased. Some agents are called complete carcinogens because they produce both initiation and promotion. However, promotion may occur after very long periods of latency, which varies with the type of agent, dose, and characteristics of the target cell. Promoting agents work by changing the expression of genetic information within the cell, increasing DNA synthesis, increasing the number of copies of a particular gene, and altering cellular communication. Often exposure to the promoting agent is under the control of the client as with the tobacco, alcohol and dietary.

An important distinction between initiation and promotion is that the activity of promoters is reversible. This is a key concept in cancer prevention. Promoting factors include such agent as dietary fat, obesity, cigarette smoking, and alcohol consumption. Prolonged stress may also be a promoter. The withdrawal of these factors can reduce the risk of neoplastic formation.

iii. *Progression* Progression is the final stage in the nature/history of a cancer; it involves the morphologic and phenotypic changes in cells, which are associated with increasingly malignant behaviour leading to invasion of surrounding tissue and metastasis to distant body parts. In other words, this stage is characterized by increased growth rate of the tumour, as well as by increased invasiveness and metastasis.

Metastasis can occur via the vascular system, lymphatic system and the process of implantations. Metastasis via the *Vascular system* occurs in a variety of ways, which includes:

- Proliferating cancer cells in draining lymph nodes may enter a large collecting lymph vessel, such as thoracic duct, that empties into the larger veins leading to the heart.
- Surrounding tissue may be invaded from the primary site of the cancer cells. The cancer cells penetrate the blood vessels and are released into blood stream.
- Cancer cells aggregates are trapped in the small capillaries of the tissues and organs.
- Through the segregation of proteolytic enzymes, cancer cells penetrate the walls of the capillary and enter the adjacent tissue where they begin to proliferate.

The *lymphatic spread* occurs in a manner similar to vascular spaces in the body, conducting particles and fluid into lymph nodes. Cancer cells that break free from tissue or invade a lymph vessel almost always become trapped in the meshwork in the draining lymph node. If these cancer cells proliferate, the result is lymphadenopathy. Continued proliferation may result in the release of cancer cells into the lymph vessels leading from the lymph node to the next lymph node up the chain.

Implantation may occur when cancer cells become embedded along the serosal surfaces of body organs, such as the peritoneal cavity or the pleural cavity. During the surgical procedure, implantations may also occur in the primary organ or in the regional area if the environment is suitable.

METASTASIS

Implantation	Lymphatic system	Vascular system
• Serosal seeding.	↓	↓
• Surgical manipulation	Lymph nodes	Emboliformation
↓	↓	
Body cavities	Distant site	

Aetiology of Cancer

There are approximately 150 types of cancers found in human beings and there are probably at least 500 different cancer-causing agents. Some of the causes on the basis of several studies are as follows:

Viruses

The study of viruses in tumours has lead investigators to discover oncogenes. Oncogenes are small segments of genetic DNA that can transform normal cells into malignant cells, independently or incorporated into a virus. Viruses probably do not, as a single agent cause cancer. However, viruses may be one of multiple agents acting to initiate carcinogenesis. Certain DNA and RNA viruses termed 'CONCOGENIC' can transform the cells they infect and induce malignant transformations. It has been found that viruses have been associated with hepatocellular carcinoma (hepatinus G. Virus) T-cell lymphoma, T-cell leukaemia, Burkitt's lymphoma (Epstein-Barr virus), nasopharyingieal carcinoma, and cervical cancer.

Chemical Carcinogens

The chemical carcinogens thought to cause cancer in human beings due to close and prolonged contact and persons who are affected usually are workers in industries where these chemicals are used as by-products. The chemical carcinogens and associated neoplasm are as follows:

Carcinogen	*Affecting organ*
• Cigarette smoking	Lungs, upper respiratory tract, bladder, cervix, etc.
• Asbestos	Mesothelioma, lung
Acrylonitrile	Lung, colon, prostate.
• Arsenic	Skin, lung, liver
• Benzene	Luekaemia
• Cadmium	Prostate, kidney
• Chromium compound	Lung
• Nickel	Lung, nasal sinuses.
• Uranium	Lung
• Aflatoxin	Liver
• Nitrates	Stomach
Chloromethyl ethers	Lung
• Isopropyl oil	Nasal sinuses
• Benzidene	Bladder
• Vinyl chloride	Angiosarcoma of liver
• Radiation	Numerous locations
• Polycyclic hydrocarbons	Lung, skin
• Mustard gas	Lung

Physical Carcinogens

Physical carcinogens cause cellular damage just as chemical carcinogens. The classification of physical carcinogen exists:

- Ionizing radiation.
- Ultraviolet radiation, and
- Foreign bodies.

Excessive exposure to *ionizing radiation* can cause permanent DNA mutation and transformation into a malignant growth. Most radiation from natural resources (radon, cosmic, terrestrial and internal radiation). Certain malignants have been correlated with radiation as carcinogenic agents are leukaemia, lymphonce, thyroid cancer, childhood cancer (if exposed) bone cancer (exposed persons include radiologists, radiation chemises, uranium miners).

Ultraviolet radiation from the sun can cause changes in DNA structure that can lead to malignant transformation if it is not repaired. Basal and squamous cell carcinomas of the skin as well as melanoma are linked to ultraviolet exposure.

Foreign bodies that are not biodegradable, such as asbestos fibers and bekelite disc and cellophane implants can induce the development of cancer by stimulating reactions to constant tissue damage such as scar formations, thus increasing the probability of neoplastic formations.

Drugs and Hormones

Certain drugs and hormones have also been identified as carcinogens. Drugs that are capable of interacting with DNA (e.g. alkylating agents) as immunosuppressive agents, have the potential cause neoplasm in human beings. And certain hormones administered to women has also been linked to the development of cancer. Certain cancers related to drug and hormone exposure in human beings are as follows:

Carcinogen	*Associated cancer*
a. Radioisotopes	
• Phosphorus (32 p)	Acute leukaemia
• Radium, mesothorium	Osteosacroma, sinus carcinoma
• Thorotrast	Hemangioendothelioma of liver
b. Immunosuppressive agent.	
• Antilymphocyte serum	Reticulum-cell sarcoma, epithelial
• Antimetabolites	cancer of skin and viscera, acute
• Alkylating agents	myelogenous leukaemia
• Corticosteroids	
c. Cytotoxic drugs	
• Phenylalanine mustard	Bladder cancer
• Cyclophosphomide	Acute melogenous leukaemia
d. Hormones	
• Synthetic ostrogen-prenatal	Vaginal and cervical
• Synthetic ostrogen-postnatal	Endometrial carcinoma (adenosquamous type)
• Androgenic-anabolic steroids	Hepatocellular carcinoma
• Diethylstilbestrol (DES)	Vaginal cancer
e. Others	
• Arsenic	Skin, liver cancer
• Phenacetin containing drug	Renal pelvis carcinoma
• Coal Tar ointments	Skin cancer
• Diphenyl hydantoin	Skin cancer
• Chloromphenical	Leukaemia
• Amphetamine	Hodgkin's disease

In addition to the carcinogen described above, there are also certain predisposing factors that influence the host susceptibility to various aetiologic agents.

i. *Age:* There is an increasing incidence of cancer in the young and in persons more than 55 years of age. Many cancers such as prostate, and colon cancer and some chronic leukaemia occur in older people. Testicular cancer is found in men between 20 to 40 years of age. Ovarian cancer is most common in women over 55 years of age. Many cancers occur mainly in childhood, e.g. Ewing's sarcoma, certain acute leukaemias, Wilms' tumour and retinoblastoma.

ii. *Sex:* Women are most susceptible to certain types of cancer than men, i.e. cancer cervix, cancer breast, etc.

iii. *Occupation:* People in certain occupations are more susceptible to certain cancers because of their greater contact with specific carcinogens. For example, industrial workers, who expose to certain physical and chemical carcinogens,.

iv. *Heredity:* Actually, none of the specific types of cancer are considered heredity. But there are a number of cancers that provide evidence of inheritable predisposed... to cancer. Fanconi anaemia, atelangiectasia, and xeroderma pigmentosum are examples of autosomal recessive conditions that predisposes persons to a variety of malignancies. Fasmilial polyposis, coli retinoblastoma, Wilms' tumour, and neurofibromatosis are examples of autosomal dominant disorders that follow classic mendelian patterns of inheritance. Breast, overian and colon cancers may also show a familial pattern.

v. *Diet and nutrition:* A diet high in fat may be a factor in the development of breast, colon and prostate cancer. Excessive alcohol, especially when accompanied by cigarette smoking, increases the risk of cancers of mouth larynx, throat, oesophagus and stomach has been noted as area of world where salt-cured smoked, and nitrate cured goods are eaten frequently. People who have more weight have an increased risk of colon breas prostate, gallbladder, ovary and uterine cancer.
Studies have shown that daily consumptions of vegetables and fresh fruits is associated with decreased risk of lung, prostate bladder, oesophagus, colorectal, and stomach cancers. High fiber diet may reduce the risk of colon cancer.

vi. *Stress:* Studies suggest that stress may increase the risk of cancer. Chronic physical and emotional stress preys on the hypothalamus, the portion of the pituitary gland that regulates hormone and immune systems. Increased stress causes hormonal and immunologic changes or both, which may in turn may spur the growth and proliferation of cancer cells.

vii. *Precancerous lesions:* Common precancerous lesions include pigmented moles, burn scars, senile keratoses, leukoplakia, and benign adenomas or polyps of the colon or stomach. These lesions need to be periodically assessed for malignant changes.

Classification of Cancer

Neoplastic tumours classified according to behaviour of tumour (benign or malignant) anatomic site, histologic analysis (grading) and extent of disease (staging). This classification systems are intended to provide a standardised way:

- To communicate the status of cancer to all members of health team.
- To assist in determining the most effective treatment plan.
- To serve as a factor in determining the prognosis, and
- To compare like groups for statistical purposes.

Benign and Malignant

Tumours can be classified on the basis of behaviour as benign or malignant.In general, benign neoplasm, are well differentiated and malignant neoplasms range from well-differentiated to undifferentiated. The difference between benign and malignant tumours are as follows; on the basis of their characteristics:

Benign tumour	*Malignant tumour*
a. Speed of growth:	
• They grow slowly usually continue to grow throughout life unless surgically removed; may have periods of remission.	• They usually grow rapidly, tend to grow relentlessly through life, rarely, neoplasm regress spontaneously
b. Mode of growth:	
• Growth by enlarging and expanding, always remaining localized, never infiltrates surrounding tissues.	• Grows by infiltrating surrounding tissues; may remain localized (*in situ*) but usually infiltrates other tissues
c. Cell characteristics:	
• Usually well-differentiated; mitotic figure absent or scanty mature cells; anaplastic cells absent, cell function poorer in comparison with normal cells from which they arise, if neoplasm arises in glandular tissue, cell may secrete hormones	• Usually poorly differentiated large number of normal and abnormal mitotic figures present, cells tend to be anaplastic, i.e. young embryonic type; cells too abnormal to perform any physiologic functions; occasionally a malignant tumour arising in glandular tissue secretes hormones
d. Recurrence:	
• Recurrence extremely unusual when surgically removed	• Recurrence common following surgery because tumour cells spread into surrounding tissues.
e. Metastasis:	
• Metastasis never occurs	• Metastasis very common
f. Effect of neoplasm:	
• Not harmful to host unless located in area where it causes compression of tissues or obstruction of vital organs, does not produce cachexia (weight loss, dabilitation, anaemia, weakness, wasting).	• Always harmful to host. Results in death unless removed surgically or destroyed by radiation or chemotherapy, causes disfigurement, disrupted organ function, nutritional imbalance may result in ulceration, sepsis, perforations, haemorrhage, tissue slough, almost always produces cachexia which leaves person prone to pneumonia anaemia, etc.
g. Prognosis:	
• Prognosis is very good tumour generally removed surgically	• Depends on cell type and speed of diagnosis, poor prognosis indicated if cells are poorly differentiated and evidence of metastatic spread exists; good prognosis indicated when cells still resemble normal cells and there is no evidence of metastasis.

Anatomic Site Classification

In the anatomic classifications of tumours, the tumour is identified by the tissue origin, the anatomic site and the behaviour of the tumour, i.e. benign or malignant. Carcinoma originates from embryonical ectoderm (skin and glands) and endoderm (mucous membrane linings of the respiratory tract, GI tract and genitourinary tract). Sarcoma originates from embryonal mesoderm (connective tissue, muscle, bone and fat). Symphomas and leukaemias originate from the hematopoietic system. The classification of tumour by tissue origin is as given below.

Tissue origin	*Benign*	*Malignant*
a. *Connective tissue*	...	Sarcoma
• Embryonic fibrous tissue	Myxoma	Myxosarcoma
• Fibrous tissue	Fibroma	Fibrosarcoma
• Adipose tissue	Lipoma	Liposarcoma
• Cartilage	Chandroma	Chondrosarcoma
• Bone	Oesteoma	Osteogenic sarcoma
b. *Epithelium tissue*	...	Carcinoma
• Skin and mucous membrane	Papilloma	Squamous cell carcinoma
• Glands	...	Basal cell carcinoma.
	...	Transitional cell carcinoma
	Adenoma	Adenocarcinoma
	Cystadenoma	Cystadenocarcinoma
• Pigmented cells (malanocytes)	Nevus	Malignant melanoma
c. *Endothelium*		Endothelioma
• Blood vessels	Hemangioma	Hemangioendothelioma Hemangiosarcoma Kaposi's sarcoma
• Lymph vessels	Lymphangioma	Lymphangiosarcoma Lymphangioendothelioma
• Bone marrow	...	Multiple myeloma Ewing's sarcoma Leukaemia
• Lymphoid tissue		Malignant lymphoma Lymphosarcoma Reticulum cell sarcoma
d. *Muscles tissue*		
• Smooth muscles	Leiomyoma	Leiomyosarcoma
• Straited muscle	Rhabdomyoma	Rhabdomyosarcoma
e. *Nerve tissue*		
• Nerve fibres and sheaths	Neuroma	Neurogenic sarcoma
	Neurinoma	
	Neurofibroma	Neurofibrosarcoma
• Ganglion cells	Ganglioneuroma	Neuroblastoma
• Glial cells	Glioma	Glioblastoma
• Menenges	Meningioma	Malignant meningioma
f. *Gonads*	Dermoid cyst	Embryonal carcinoma Embryonal sarcoma Terato carcinoma

Histologic Analytic Classification

The histologic grading of tumours, the appearance of the cells and the degree of differentiation are evaluated. For many tumours, four grades are used.

Grade I	Cells differ slightly from normal cells (mils displasia) and are well differentiated.
Grade II	Cells are more abnormal (moderate displasia) and moderately differentiated.
Grade III	Cells are very abnormal (severe dysplasia) and poorly differentiated.
Grade IV	Cells are immature and primitive (anaplaxia) and undifferentiated, cell of origin difficult to determine.

Extent of Disease Classification

The extent of disease classification is often called 'staging'. The clinical staging classification determines the extent of the disease process of cancer by stages:

Stage '0' :	Cancer *in situ*. It is defined as a neoplasm of epithelial tissue that remains confined to the site of origin.
Stage I :	Tumor linked to the tissue of origin, localized tumour growth.
Stage II :	Limited local spread.
Stage III :	Extensive local and regional spread.
Stage IV :	Metastasis.

This type of classification is used as a basis for staging in cancer of cervix and Hodgkin's disease.

The TNM classificatiaon system represents the standardization of the clinical staging of cancer. It is used to determine the extent of disease process of cancer according to three parameters. Tumour size (T), degree of regional spread to the lymph nodes (N) and absence of metastasis (M). TNM system has been used in cancer of breast.

Table 5.2: TNM Staging classificatiaon system

Tumour	
T_0	No evidence of primary tumour
T_S	Carsinoma *in situ*
T_1, T_2, T_3, T_4	Ascending degrees of tumour size and involvement.
Nodes	
N_0	No evidence of disease in lymph node
N_{1a}, N_{2a}	Disease found in regional lymph nodes, metastasis not suspected.
N_X	Regional lymph nodes cannot be assessed clinically.
Metastasis	
M_0	No evidence of distant metastasis.
M_1, M_2, M_3	Assending degrees of metastatic involvement of the host, including distant nodes.

Prevention of Cancer

The nurse plays a prominent role in all the levels of prevention of cancer. Cancer nursing is directed towards the prevention and early detection of neoplasm as well as the care of the patient in treatment, recovery or advanced stage of cancer. At present, it is not possible to prevent all types of cancer, but some cancers can be prevented by avoidance of recognized carcinogens and by altering health behaviours.

Primary Prevention

Primary prevention of cancer is activity taken to prevent the occurrence or reduce the risk of cancer in healthy persons. Activities in this area of health promotion include identifying risk factors, reduction and cancer prevention programmes. For example the dietary changes to reduce cancer which include:

a. Increased intake of high-fiber foods such as fruits and vegetables and whole grain cereals. Dark green and deep yellow fruits and vegetable rish in vitamin A and C (cabbage, broccoli cauliflower, brussels sprouts and kohlrabi).
b. Reduced intake of salt-cured, smoked and nitrite-cured foods, fats and oils especially from animal sources; alcoholic beverages and excess calories leading to obesity.

So, one important aspect of the nurse and other health care provider is to educate the public to do the following:

- Reduce or avoid exposure to known or suspected carcinogens and cancer-promoting agents.
- Eat balanced diet that includes vegetabels (green, yellow and orange), fresh fruits, wholegrains, adequate amount of fiber, and low level of facts and preservatives.
- Participate in regular exercise regimens.
- Obtain adequate, consistent, periods of rest (at least 6 to 8 hours per night).
- Have a health examination on consistent basis that includes health history physical examination and specific diagnostic tests for common cancers, i.e., lung cancer, colon and rectal cancer, prostate cancer, cervical cancer and breast cancer, etc.
- Eliminate, reduce or change the perceptions of stressors and enhance the ability to positively cope with stressors.
- Enjoy consistent periods of relaxation and leisure.
- Know the seven warning signals of cancer- which include "CAUTION" as follows.
  1. Change in bowel or bladder habits.
  2. A sore that does not heal.
  3. Unusual bleeding or discharge.
  4. Thickening or lump in the breast or elsewhere.
  5. Indigestion or difficulty in swallowing.
  6. Obvious change in a wart or more.
  7. Nagging cough or hoarseness.
- Learn and practice self-examination of breast and testicles.
- Seek immediate medical care if cancer is suspected.

In some occupations, the employees may have contact with carcinogenic substances such as asbestos, chromium, ether, vinyl-chloride and benzyprene, etc. In such industries, proper regulation and protective measures can be taken accordingly to reduce the risk of cancer.

The nurses can have a definite im1pact in convincing people that a change in the lifestyle pattern will have a positive influence on health.

Secondary Prevention

Secondary prevention of cancer is focussed on the early diagnosis of which early detection and screening are the major components. Screening and detection programmes are concentrated on some of the most common cancers including cancers of the breast, cervix, colon/rectum, prostate, skin and oropharynx.

The screening for specific cancer sites which have high risk profile are as follows:

Lung The risk of lung cancer can occur with a person of

- History of 20/ pack-years of smoking (1 pack a day for 20 years).
- Exposure to air-borne carcinogens especially asbestos, uranium, hydrocarbon.
- Age range 40-80 years.
- Chronic lung disease.

The method of screening any such case will be observation by patient for change in respiratory status, increased frequency of infections and change in cough, sputum, breathing, and voice. Some doctors advise annual chest X-rays.

Colon and rectum The risk of colon and rectal cancer occurs with a person's

- History of familial polyposis, ulcerative colitis, Crohn's disease
- Personal or family history of colon or rectal cancer.
- Taking diet high in fat and low in fiber.
- Age range 40-75 years.

The method of screening will be

- Blood test on stools every year after age of 50 years.
- Digital rectal examination annually after age of 40 years.
- Sigmoidoscopic examination (preferably flexible) every 3-5 years after 50 years.
- Observations by patients for change in bowel pattern, i.e., diarrhoea, constipation, pain, flatus, black tarry stools, bleeding.

Prostate The risk of prostatic cancer occurs with presence of prostatic hyperplasia and presence of prostatic infection. The methods of screening of such case will be;

- Digital rectal examination of age 40 years and annually thereafter.
- Prostate specific antigens blood test every year.
- Observation on men aged 50 and older, for dysuria, blood in urine, difficulty in producing stream of urine.

Cervix The risk of cervical cancer occurs with a person

- Who has a history of early intercourse (before the age of 20 years) with multiple partners.
- Who maintains poor personal hygiene including poor menstrual hygiene.
- Who has history of herpes virus type II infections and cervical dysplasia.

For such cases screening measures will include:

- Pap test and pelvic examination every year for those who are or have been sexually active or who have attained the age of 18 years.
- Calposcopy if suspicious area is noted.
- Observation by patient for abnormal vaginal bleeding or discharge, pain, or bleeding with sexual intercourse.

Endometrium The risk of endometrial cancer occurs with a person's having infertility, ovarian dysfunction, obesity, uterine bleeding, estrogen therapy over long period of time, diabetes and age range 30-80 years.

By such cases, screening measures will include

- Pap test every year.
- Pelvic examination every year.
- Endometrial biopsy every year for women of menopause and
- Observation by patient for abnormal uterine bleeding, pain, change in menstrual pattern.

Skin The risk of skin cancer occurs with person, having prolonged exposure to sun, and previous radiation exposure; fair, thin skin, and positive family history of dysplasia *nevus* syndrome.

For such cases, screening measures include, self examination monthly with suspicious lesions evaluated promptly, physical examination every year, and observation by patient for sore that does not heal, change in wart or mole.

Breast The risk of breast cancer occurs with persons who are caucasian, who has early menarche, late menopause, fibrocystic disease, and infertility, more than age of 30 years for first pregnancy, and who has a personal history of breast cancer mother or sister with history of breast cancer, obesity, and whose age range is 35-65 years.

The screening measure will be

- Monthly breast self-examination.
- Breast examination by health professional every 3 years for women aged 20-40 and every year after the age of 40.
- Baseline mammogram of age 40 and every 1-2-years between ages 40-49 and every year after the age of 50.
- Observation by patient for lungs or thickening discharge from nipple, pain in the breast.

In order to assume the expected role in cancer prevention and early detection programmes, the nurse must keep informed about the trends in the incidence of cancer and advances being made. If the nurse is to have a significant impact, the challenge needs to be recognized and strategies must be developed to teach cancer control effectively.

To sum up, the early detection of cancer in asymptomatic population according to American Society Guidelines (1995) are as follows:

1. *Chest X-ray*: It is no longer recommended for smokers to screen for lung cancer, but can be done.
2. *Sputum cytology*: -do-
3. *Physical examination*: For both male and females, after the age of 40 years, yearly including examination of skin, lymph nodes, mouth, thyroid, breast, testes, rectum and prostate.
4. *Health teaching*: For both male and females, who attained the age of 20 years. It has to be done every 3 years to teach about proper diet, exercise, health habits, breast and testicular self-examinations, avoidance of sunlight, and smoking cessation.
5. *Breast self examination*: For females who have attained menarchy or 20 years and above, every month after menses before menopause; after menopause, monthly on any specified day such as the first or last of the month.
6. *Mammography*: For women who are between 35-40 years of age, baseline mammogram; between 40-49 years mammogram should be done every 1-2 years and yearly after 50 years; high risk women should check with their physicians.
7. *Pap smear*: For females who are above 18 years of age, and sexually active women should have pap smears regardless of age, should be performed yearly until there are three negative examinations in a row; at this point, they can be performed yearly or as physician advises.
8. *Pelvic examination*: For females who are between 20-40 and 40 and above, every 3 years, earlier if sexually active, yearly after 40 years.
9. *Endometrial tissue sample*: For female at menepause, high risk women (obese, abnormal uterine bleeding, estrogen therapy, history of infertility, diabetes, hypertension, failure to ovulate) should have this test performed at menopause.
10. *Testicular self-examination*: For males, monthly, on a set date such as the first of the month following a shower.
11. *Breast physical examination*: For females every 3 years for those who are between 20-39 years and annually for those who are above 40.
12. *Digital rectal examination*: For both male and females who are above 40, annually rectal cancer and prostate in men.
13. *Fecal occult blood*: For both males and females those who are above 20 years, done on advice of physician.
14. *Proctoscopy, flexible sigmoidoscopy*: For both men and women who are above 50 years every 3-5-years.

Diagnosis of Cancer

A diagnostic plan for the person in whom cancer is suspected, includes health history, identification of risk factors, physical examination and specific diagnostic studies.

Health History

The health history includes particular emphasis on risk factors, such as family history of cancer, exposure to or use of known carcinogen (e.g. cigarette smoking and exposure to occupational pollutants or chemicals, disease characterised by chronic inflammation (e.g. ulceration colities) and drug ingestions (e.g. hormone therapy). Other important information related to dietary habits, ingestion of alcohol, lifestyle and patterns and degree of coping with perceived stressors.

Physical Examination

The physical examination should be thorough and particular attention should be given to the respiratory system, the gastrointestinal systems, including colon, rectum, and liver), the lymphatic system (including spleen), the breast, the skin, the reproductive system of the male (testicles, prostate) and of the female (cervix, uterus, ovary and the muscule-skeletal and neuologic systems.

When a malignant tumour is in the early stages, there are often few manifestations. Clinical manifestations usually appear once the tumour has grown to a sufficiently large size to cause one or more of the following problems:

- Pressure on surrounding organs or nerves
- Distortion of surrounding tissue
- Obstruction of lumen of tubes
- Interference with the blood supply of surrounding tissues
- Interference with the organ function
- Disturbance of body metabolism
- Parasitic use of the body's nutritional supplies
- Mobilization of the body's defensive responses, resulting in inflammatory changes.

Common clinical manifestations that may arise secondary to cancer include weight loss, weakness or fatigue, CNS alterations, pain and haematologic and metabolic alterations. Close assessment of such manifestations may reveal that they are directly or indirectly related to the tumour growth.

Anorexia, weight loss, weakness and fatigue are related to the body's inability to consume and use nutrients appropriately. Mechanical interference by tumours, malabsorption, paraneoplastic endocrine secretions (such as excessive secretions of thyroid hormone) and tumour, use of nutrient, may all contribute to a cycle that must be interrupted to avoid general physical debilitation.

Pain may occur as a result of obstruction or destruction of a vital organ, pressure on sensitive tissues or bone, or involvement of nerves. If it occurs and is not adequately treated, it may become constraint and progressively severe.

The client who has difficulty with vision, speech, co-ordination or memory may be experiencing primary or metastatic CNS disease. Increased intracranial pressure caused by tumour growth may cause headache, lethargy, nausea, and vomiting.

Unexplained anaemia often indicates a malignancy. Haematologic changes also include leukopenia, leukocytosis, and bleeding disorders. Which in some diseases may occur before local manifestations. Metabolic manifestations also signify the possibility of malignant disease.

A localized tumour usually produces manifestations related to increased pressure or obstruction in a single region. Metastatic disease and extensive tumours of major organs may display a variety of local and systemic manifestations.

Diagnostic studies Diagnostic studies to be performed will depend on the suspected primary or metastatic site (s) of the cancer. The common diagnostic studies that may be included in the process of diagnosing cancer include the following:

- Cystologic examination, e.g. pap smear
- Basic X-ray studies for identifying the destructive tumours of the GI, respiratory and renal tracts
- Complete blood count
- Proctoscopic examination
- Liver function studies
- Radiographic studies, e.g. mammogram, (in breast cancer)
- Radioisotopic scans (for liver, brain, bone, lung cancer)
- Computed tomography (CT) scan
- Magnetic resonance imaging (MRI)
- Antigen skin testing (to know the presence of oncofetal antigens)
- Bone marrow examination
- Lymphangiography
- Biopsy (surgical excision of a small piece of tissue for microscopic examination, i.e. needle biopsy, incisional biopsy, excisional biopsy).

Treatment of Cancer

When caring for the patient with cancer, the nurse should know the goals of the treatment plan to appropriately communicate with and support the patient. The goal of cancer treatment is 'cure', 'control' or palliation.

The Major objective of cancer therapy is to treat the client effectively with appropriate therapy for sufficient duration so that cure results with minimal functional and structural impairment. When *cure* is the goal, it is expected that after treatment the patient will be free of disease and will have a normal life. Many kinds of cancer have the potential to go into permanent remission with an initial course of treatment or with treatment extending for several weeks, months or years. (e.g. Basal cell carcinoma of skin is usually cured by surgical removal of lesion or radiation therapy).

When cure is not possible, important alternative goals are:

i. to prevent metastasis
ii. to relieve manifestations, and
iii. to maintain a high quality of life for as long as possible.

Here, the *control* is the goal of the treatment plan for many cancers considered to be chronic. The patient undergoes the initial course of therapy and is contineud on maintenance therapy for a period of time or is followed closely so that early signs and symptoms of recurrence can be detected. These cancers are usually, not cured., but they are controlled by therapy for long periods of time (e.g. chronic lymphocytic leukaemia).

Palliation can also be a goal of the cancer treatment plan. With this treatment, goal, relief of symptoms and the maintenance of a satisfactory quality of life are the primary objective rather than cure or control of the disease process. For example, radiatioan therapy given to relieve the pain of bone metastasis.

The goals of cure, control and palliation are achieved through the use of four treatment modalities for cancer, which includes;

1. Surgery
2. Radiation therapy
3. Chemotherapy
4. Biologic response modifiers.

Surgery

Surgery is the oldest form of cancer treatment and for many years it was the only effective method of cancer diagnosis and treatment. It is also an integral part of the rehabilitation and palliation of patients with cancer. The types of surgical procedures used in surgical management of cancer are as follows.

i. *Biopsy* is the surgical removal of a piece of tissue from the questionable area, and the tissue sample is sent to the pathology laboratory for diagnostic verification. The sample of tissues can be obtained through the needle biopsy or incisional biopsy or excisional biopsy.

ii. *Reconstruction/Rehabilitative surgery* Advances in reconstructive surgery offer a different perspective on rehabilitation to the patient who has experienced curative surgery. Here, performing the repair of defects from previous radical surgical resection. It can be performed early (as in head and neck surgery). Restoration of form and function is possible in varying degrees depending on the site and extent of surgery. Reconstructive surgery may be performed concurrently with the radical procedure or delayed for optimal outcome. The major goal of reconstructive surgery is to improve the patient's quality of life by restoring maximal function and appearance.

iii. *Palliative surgery* refers to a surgery that attempts to relieve the complications of cancer. Because of surgical procedures carry an inherent potential for morbidity, use of surgery in palliative care is carefully considered and used only if the risk-benefit ratio is favourable. Palliative surgery can benefit the clients with cancer and improve quality of life include the procedure than reduce pain; relieve airway obstruction, relieve obstructions in the GI and GU tract; relieve pressures on the brain and spinal cord; prevent haemorrhage remove infected and ulcerating tumours and drain abscess. Example of palliative surgical procedure are cordotomy, colossomy, laminectomy, etc.

iv. *Adjuvant surgery* refers to the use of various surgical techniques to facilitate the overall management. These procedures are used to provide supportive care throughout the disease process of cancer. These procedures include.

- Insertion of feeding tubes in the esophagus or stomach
- Creation of a colostomy to allow a rectal abscess to heal
- Suprapubic cystotomy for the patient with advnced prostatic cancer
- Vascular access devices
- Radiotherapy implants
- Peritoneal access
  Ventricular access
- Drainage of peritoneal or pleural effusions.

v. *Surgery for primary lesions* is the removal of the primary site of malignancy. The goal of therapy is cure. This depends on the biology of that particular cancer. For example basal cell carcinoma of skin, early tumour of the rectum or colon.\

vi. *Surgery for metastatic lesion* or resection of metastatis is used in selected case where a cure can be obtained or reasonable prolongation of survival is possible. The primary cancer must be under control. The decision to proceed is influenced by the type of histology, number of lesions, their locations and whether they are bilateral, solitary metastatic lesions that appear in the lungs, liver or brain can be removed to effect a surgical cure.

vii. *Preventive/prophylactic surgery* is the removal of lesion, that if left in the body are apt to develop into cancer. Certain conditions or diseases increase the risk of cancer occurrence so significantly that removal of the target organ is justified to prevent cancer development. For example, polyps in the rectum. Clients with high risk factors may consider prophylactic surgery (e.g. prophylactic mastectomy, or oophorectomy).

viii. *Curative surgery* is the removal of the primary site of malignancy and any lymph nodes to which the neoplasm has extended. Such surgery may be all that is required. For example, radical neck dissection, lumpectomy, mastectomy, Pneumonectomy, orchiectomy, thyroidectomy and bowel resection.

ix. *Debulking surgery* is the removal of bulk of the tumour; should be performed before the start of chemotherapy whenever possible. This procedure may be used if the tumour cannot be completely removed (e.g. attached to a vital organ). This type of procedure makes the adjuvant therapy more effective.

Radiation Therapy

Radiation therapy (RT) is a local treatment modality for cancer. RT is the use of high energy ionizing rays to treat a variety of cancer. Ionizing radiation destroys the cell's ability to reproduce by damaging the cells DNA. Rapidly dividing cells, such as some cancer cells are more vulnerable to radiation than more slowly dividing cells. Furthermore, normal cells have greater ability than cancer cells to repair the DNA damage from radiation. In addition to the DNA effects, a complex chain of chemical reactions occurs in the extracellular fluid resulting in the formation of free radicals. Well oxygenated tumour show a much greater reaponse to radiation than poorly oxygenated tumors. Oxygen free radicals formed during ionization interact readily with nearby molecules causing cellular damage including genetic material.

Radiation is the emission and distribution of energy through space or a material medium. The energy produced by radiation, when absorbed into tissue, produces ionization and excitation. This local energy is sufficient to break chemical bonds in DNA, which leads to biologic effect. The major target of radiation effect is DNA. The ionization that occurs eventually causes damage to DNA, which renders cells incapable of surviving mitosis. Loss of proliferative capacity yields cellular death at the time of division. Cellular death is dependent on the cell going through its mitotic cycle. Thus death occurs at different rates for different cell types. This is true for both normal cells and cancer cells. However, cancer cells are more likely to be dividing because of the loss of control of cellular divisions. Furthermore, these cells are unable to repair the radiation damage to DNA. Therefore, cancer cells are more likely to be permanently damaged by the cumulative doses of radiation. Normal tissues are usually able to recover from radiation damage of therapeutic doses are kept within certain ranges.

Goals of radiation therapy The goals of radiation therapy are cure, control and palliation. To accomplish these treatment goals, radiation therapy can be used alone or as an adjuvant treatment modality in combination with surgery chemotherapy and biologic response modifiers.

- *Cure* is the goal when radiation therapy is used alone as a curative modalityfor treating patients with basal cell carcinoma of the skin, tumours confined to the vocal cord, and Stage I or II A Hodgkin's disease. Radiation therapy can be combined with surgery and chemotherapy to cure certain cancers such as Stage II B, III A and III B, Hodgkin's disease, Ewing's sarcoma, head and neck cancer and Stage I and II breast cancer.

- Control of the disease process of cancer for a period of time is considered to be a reasonable goal in some situations. Initial treatment is offered at the time of diagnosis, and additional treatment is given each time symptoms of disease recur. Most of the patients enjoy a satisfactory quality of life during symptom-free period. It can be combined with surgery to further enhance the local control of cancer. It can be given preoperatively, intraoperatively and also postoperatively as assessed accordingly.
- *Palliation* is often the goal of RT. The patient can be treated to control the distressing symptoms that are occurring as a result of disease process. Tumours can be reduced in size to relieve symptoms more as pain and obstruction. Example of the use of RT for palliatives include the relief of:
  - pain associated with bone metastasis
  - pain and neurologic symptoms associated with brain metastasis
  - Spinal cord compression
  - Intestinal obstruction
  - Superior vena cava obstruction
  - Bronchial or tracheal obstruction
  - Bleeding (e.g. bladder and intrabronchial).

Types of radiation therapy Radiation therapy can be administered from a variety of sources. Sources can be classified into those used outside (i.e. external RT) and those used close to the surface of the body or inside the body (Internal RT).

External radiation Radiation treatment can be given by external beam radiation delivered from a source placed at some distance from the target site. It is usually administered by high energy X-ray machine (e.g. the betatron and linear accelerator) or machine containing a radioisotope (cobalt 60).

The main advantage of high-energy radiations is its skin-sparing effect. This means that the maximum effect of radiation occurs within the tumour deep in the body and not on the skin surface. Neutron beam therapy is delivered from a cyclotron particle accelerator is currently used to treat many types of cancer (tumour in salivary gland, prostate, lung).

Internal radiation Internal RT involves the placement of specially prepared radioisotopes directly enter near the tumour itself. This is known as brachy therapy in which the implantation or insertion or radioactive materials directly into the tumour or in close proximity of the tumour. An implant may be temporary with the source placed into a catheter or tube inserted into the tumour area and left in place for several days. This method is commonly used for tumours of the head and neck, and gynecologic malignancies.

There are two types of internal RT.

i. *Sealed-source* in which the radioactive material is enclosed in a sealed container. Sealed source RT includes intracavity and interstitial therapy. In *intracavity* therapy, the radioistopes, usually cesium 137 or radium 226, is placed into an applicator, then placed in body cavity for a carefully calculated time usually 24 to 72 hours (e.g. used to treat cancer of uterus or cervix).

   In interstitial therapy, the radioisotope of choice (iridium 192, iodine 125, cesium 137, gold 198 or radon 222) is placed in needles, beads, seeds, ribbons or catheters and then implanted directly into the tumours (e.g. as used in prostate cancer).

ii. *Unsealed-sources RT* are used in systemic therapy. Radioisotopes may be administered intravenously into a body cavity or orally. For example, sodium phosphate P32 is administered intravenously to treat polycythemia vera, Iodine 131 is given orally in very low doses to treat Graves' disease.

Measurement of radiation There are different units which are used to measure radiation as follows:

i. *Curie* (ci) - A measure of the number of atoms of a particular radioisotope that disintegrate in one second.
ii. *Rontgen* (R) - A measure of the radiation required to produce a standard number of ions in air; a unit of exposure to radiation.
iii. *Rad* - Measurement of radiatiaon dosage absorbed by the tissue.
iv. *Rem* - Measurement of the biologic effectiveness of various forms of radiation on the human cell (1 Rem = 1 Rad).
v. *Gray* (Gy) - 100 rads - 1 Gy.

The grays and centigrays are the units currently used in clinical practice.

Safety precautions in radiation therapy There are three key principles to follow to protect nurses and others from excessive radiation exposure, viz., distance, time and shielding.

i. *Distance* The greater distance from the radiation source, the less exposure dose of ionizing rays. The intensity of radiation decreases inversely to the square of the distance from the source. For example, if a person stands 4 ft from a source of radiation, the person is exposed to approximately 1/4 the amount of radiation the person would receive at 2 ft.
ii. *Time* Minimal exposure time should be promoted, although patient care needs must still be met. A nurses exposure is generally limited to 30 minutes of direct care per 8 hours shift.
iii. *Shielding* The dose of X-rays and gamma rays is reduced as the thickness of the lead shield is increased. In practice, nurses have found that leadshielding can be cumbersome to work with. So it is better to maintain maximum distance

from the radioactive source and limiting duration of exposure as safety measure.

The following guidelines will help protecting staff and others from radiation.

1. Place the client in a private room–It prevents undue exposure to other clients and to nurses caring for these clients.
2. Plan care well so that minimal time is spent in direct contact with the client. Do not spend more than 30 minutes per shift with the client.
3. Stand at the client's shoulder (for cervical implants) or at the foot of the bed (for head and neck implants) avoiding close contact with unshielded areas.
4. In case, if you must have prolonged contact with the client or if you will be exposed to an unshielded area, use a lead shield.
5. Do not care for more than one client with a radiation implant at one time.
6. All health care personnel should wear appropriate monitoring devices.
7. The room should be marked with appropriate signs stating the presence of radiation, do not allow children under 18 or pregnant women to visit; limit visitors' time to 30 minutes at a distance of at least 6 feet from the radioactive source; do not care for these patients if you (female nurse) are pregnant.
8. Carefully check all linens or other materials from the bed for the presence of implants.
9. Keep long handled forceps and lead-lined container available on the nursing unit or in the client's room while the implant is in place.

Chemotherapy

Chemotherapy is the systemic treatment of cancer with chemicals, i.e. drugs. Here the use of antineoplastic drugs to promote tumour cell destructions by interfering with cellular function and reproduction. It includes the use of various therapeutic agents and hormones.

The goal of chemotherapy is to destroy as many tumour cells as possible with minimal effect on healthy cells. It can be used for cure, control, and palliation. The objective of chemotherapy is to reduce the number of cancer cells present in the primary tumour site(s) and metastatic tumour site(s). Several ractors will determine the response of cancer cells to chemotherapy as given below:

i. *Mitotrio rate of the tissue* from which the tumour arises. The more rapid the mitotic rate, the greater response to chemotherapy. Chemotherapy is the treatment of choice for acute leukaemia, choriocarcinoma of the placenta, Wilms' tumour (used in conjunction with surgery) and neuroblastoma. These cancer cells have a rapid rate of cellular proliferation.
ii. *Size of the tumour* The smaller the number of cancer cells, the greater the response to chemotherapy.
iii. *Age of the tumour* The younger tumour, the greater the response to chemotherapy. Younger tumours have a greater percentage of proliferating cells.
iv. *Location of the tumour* Certain anatomic sites provide a protected environments from the effects of chemotherapy. For example, only few drugs cross the blood-brain barrier (nitrosourceus and bleomycin).
v. *Presence of resistant tumour cells* Mutation of cancer cells within the tumour mass can result in varient cells that are resistant to chemotherapy. Resistance can also occur because of the biochemical inability of some cancer cells to convert the drug to its active form.
vi. *Physiologic and psychologic status of the host* A state of optimum health and positive attitude will allow better withstand aggressive chemotherapy.

Classification of chemotherapy Chemotherapeutic agents generally are classified according to their pharmacologic action and effect on the cell generation cycles. However, the method by which cancer cells are inhibited or destroyed is not always unknown.

The two major categories of chemotherapeutic drugs are cell cycle-nonspecific and cell cycle-specifier. The cell cycle nonspecifiers have their effect on the cells that are in the process of cellular replication and proliferation, as well as on the cells that are in the resting phase (Go). The *cell cycle-specific* have their effect on cells that are in the process of cellular replication or proliferation (G_1, S_1, or M). These drugs are effective at only one specific phase of cell cycle.

The common drugs used as chemotherapeutic agents are as follows:

1. *Alklating agent*
   - Nitrogen musturd (Mechlorethemine)
   - Cyclophosphamide (Cytoxan)
   - Chlorambucil (Leukeran)
   - Busulfan (Myleran)
   - Melphalan (Alkeran)
   - Thiotepa (Thiotepa)
   - Ifosfamide (Ifex).
2. *Antimetabolites*
   - Methotrexate
   - 6 Mercaptopurine (6 MP)
   - 6 Thioguanine (6 TG)
   - 5 Fluorouracil (5 Fu)
   - Cystosine arabinoside ((A-RA-C) Cytosar-4)
   - Fludarabine phosphate
   - Deoxycoformycin (Pentastatin).

3. *Antitumour antibiotics*
   - Deunorubicin (Cerubidins)
   - Doxorubicin (Adriamycin)
   - Dactinomycin (Cosmegen)
   - Bleomycin (Blenoxane)
   - Mitomycin (Mutamycin)
   - Picamycin (Mittracin, mitramycin)
   - Idarubiun (Idamycin)
   - Mitoxantrone (Novamtrone).
4. *Hormonal agents*
   i. *Androgens*
      - Testosterone propionate
      - Fluoxymesterone (Halotestin)
      - Dromostanolone (Drolban)
      - Testosactone (Teslac)
      - Methyltestosterone.

   ii. *Corticosteroids*
      - Cortisone acetate
      - Prednisone (Meticorten)
      - Dexamethosone (Dedadron)
      - Methyl prednisolone sodium (Solu-Medrol)
      - Hydrocartison sodium succinate (Solu-cortef).

   iii. *Oestrogen*
      - Diethyl stilbestrol (DES)
      - Ethinyl estradiol (Estriny).

   iv. *Progesterones*
      - Hydroxy progesterone caporate (Prodrox)
      - Megestrol (Megace)
      - Metroxyprogesterone (Provera)
      - Estramustine (Emcut).

   v. *Oestrogen antagonists*
      - Tamoxifen (Norvadex)
      - Leuprolide (Lupron).

   vi. *Antiadrenal*
      - Amino gluthimide.
5. *Vinca alkaloids*
   - Vincristine (Oncovin)
   - Vinblastine (Velban)
   - Vindesine sulfate.
6. *Epipodophyllotoxins*
   Etoposide (VP-16).

Nursing Intervention in Chemotherapy

1. *Alkalating* agents are cell cycle nón-specific and act against already formed nucliec acid by cross-linking DNA strands, thereby preventing DNA replication and trancription of RNA. The major toxin of alkalatings are dependent upon drugs given which include hematopoietic anaemia, leukopenia, thrombocytopenia, GI-nausea and vomiting, dirrhoea, reproductive-infertility, change in libido, Gu-cystitis and renal toxicity.

The nursing intervention for these toxicities are

i. Haematopoietic toxicity:
   - Monitor WBC, RBC, platest count biweekly for pancytopenia
   - Observe for signs and symptoms of infections, bleeding, anaemia
   - Provide rest periods and 8 hours sleep per night
   - Teach benefits of good personal hygiene
   - Provide comfort and suggestion measures.

ii. Gastrointestinal toxicity:
   - Document nausea and vomiting times and amount
   - Administer antiemetic drug PRN
   - Hydrate to 2000 ml/24 hour if not contradicted
   - Record intake and output
   - Avoid noxious odors
   - Use relaxation techniques or distractions
   - Provide small frequent meals.

iii. Reproductive toxicity:
   - Inform of possibility of temporary or permanent infertility and danger to growing foetus.
   - Provide reproductive counselling as needed.

iv. Genitourinary toxicity:
   - Inform that haemorrhagic cystitis can occur with cytoxan and ifosfamide therapy.
   - Administer mesna (urothelial protection agent) to help to prevent cystitis.
   - Encourage hydration and complete and frequent emptying of bladder.

2. *Antimetabolites* act by interfering with synthesis of chromosomal nucleic acid, antimetabolites are analogs of normal metabolites and block the enzyme necessary for synthesis of essential factors or are incorporated into the DNA or RNA and thus prevent replication are cycle-specific.

The major toxicities of antimetabolites are dependant on drugs given which are as follows:

- Haematopoietic – Bone marrow suppression
  – Anaemia.
  – Leukopenia.
  – Thrombocytopenia
- Gastrointestinal – Mucositis/stomatitis.
  – Diarrhea.
  – Nausea and vomiting.

The nursing intervention of these toxicities are as stated in alkalating agents and in addition to the above, the following has to be performed.

For Mucosites and Stomatitis

- Inspect oral cavity daily for presence of sores, change in taste and sensation.

- Teach oral care and encourage immediately after meals and at bed time, soft toothbrush and prescribed mouthwash. (Peroxide, oral saline, baking soda and water or provide anaesthetic agent for mouth sores (e.g. Stomatitic cocktail).
- Report signs and symptoms of oral infection.
- Soft diet with non-irritating foods high in protein, calories, offer high caloric liquid supplements.

For Diarrhoea

- Low residue diet, high protein and calories maintain hydration
- Monitor and document number and frequency stools
- Administer antidiarrhoeal medication as needed
- Provide meticulus skin care in perirectal area
- Promote good hygiene habits.

3. *Antitumour antibiotics* interfere with synthesis and function of nucleic acids and inhibit RNA and DNA synthesis. These are cycle-specific. The major toxicities of antitumour antibiotics include:
   - Hematopoietic - Bone marrow suppression
   - GI - Mucositis/Stomatitis, anorexia, nausea and vomiting
   - Integumentary-alopecia, tissue necrosis (if extravasate)
   - Cardiac and pulmonary toxicity.

In addition to above stated nursing interventions, for other chemotherapeutics, the added nursing interventions for;

i. Integumentary - For alope a, warn of potential for hair loss and ways of minimizing loss.

For Extravasation

- Monitor IV infusion to prevent infiltration. When infiltrated stop immediately and institute agency protocol to prevent tissue necrosis-notify doctor immediately and keep extravasation kit available at all times.

ii. Cardiac toxicity may occur with bleomycin (Pneumonitis and progressive pulmonary fibrosis), should not exceed a lifetime dose of 400 iu. Assess respiratory status and document changes.

4. *Hormonal agents*
   - Androgens alter pituitary function and directly affects the malignant cell. Toxicitis of androgens include fluid retention and masculinization.
   - *Corticosteroids* lyse lymphoid malignancies and have indirect effects on malignant cells. The major toxicitis include fluid retention, hypertension, diabetes, and increased susceptibility to infection.
   - *Oestrogen* and progestrone suppress testosterone production in males and alter the response of breast cancer to prolectin and promote differentiation of malignant cells. The major toxicities include fluid retention, feminization and uterine bleeding.
   - *Oestrogen anagonists* compete with oestrogens for binding with oestrogen receptor sites on malignant cells. Toxicites are minimal with occasional headache and hotflash.
   - *Antiadrenals*. Produce the equivalent of a medical adrenalectomy, thereby inhibiting the formations of oestrogen and androgenesis and function of nucleic acids and inhibit RNA and DNA synthesis. These agents are cycle non-specific toxicity in adrenal insufficiency.

The nursing interventions during chemotherapy with harmful agent are:

- For fluid retention
  - Warn of potential weight gain
  - Weight biweekly
  - Maintain intake and output if needed.
- For feminization in males
  - Inform about chance of gynaecomastia—change in voice, distribution of body fat and hair and cardiovascular problem.
- Assess fears and concerns and provide psychological support as needed.
- For virisization in females.
  - Discuss the risk for facial hair, lowered voice, clitorial enlargement - fluid retention.
  - Assess fears and concerns and provide psychological support.
- For uterine bleeding
  - Prepare postmenopausal woman for occurrence
  - Provide support and reassurance.
- For diabetes
  - Inform patient of potential occurrence
  - Monitor blood sugar changes.
  - Observe signs and symptoms of diabetes.
- For adrenal insufficiency
  - Instruct on need to comply with replacement therapy while on medication.
  - Reassure that need for therapy will cease when drug is discontinued.

5. *Vinca alkaloid* bind to proteins within the cells causing metaphase arrest thus inhibiting RNA and protein synthesis. Major toxicites are bone marrow suppression and alopecia- (See nursing intervention as stated above).
6. *Epiplodophyllotoxins* cause breaks in DNA and RNA protein cross links. The major toxicities are neurological, i.e. neurotoxicity, muscle weakness, peripheral neurities, paralytic ileus, loss of deep tenden reflexes.

The nursing intervention for neurological toxicities will include:

- GI – Check for peristalsis frequently.

   - determine usual pattern of bowel elimination
   - facilitate elimination with laxative regimens.
- Peripheral – Observe for numbness, tingling in extremities
   - Institute safety measure (e.g. wearing shoes, using cane or walker for ambulation)
   - Seek assistance for ambulation as needed
   - Teach signs and symptoms to report to concerned doctor
   - Provide supportive care and reassurance.

Guidelines for Care of Client with Chemotherapy

1. *Teach the patient and significant others*
   - Signs and symptoms of infection, thrombocytopenia
   - How to read thermometer and when to notify the doctor
   - Good hygienic practices—cleansing the perinium from front to back, change underwear daily and handwashing
   - Information about prescribed drugs—name, dose, side effects, importance of taking as prescribed
   - Use of antiemetics
   - Importance of medical follow-up and blood studies
   - Available support group for chemotherapy patients.
2. *Prevent infection*
   - Good hygiene especially handwashing—patient, family, health personnel.
   - Prevent exposure to people with known infection (other staff, family, etc.)
   - Meticulous septic technique during IV infusion and dressing changes
   - Avoid use of aspirin or acetaminophen to prevent masking fever
   - Maintain intact skin and mucous membrane
     - Avoid bumping and breaking the skin
     - No injections
     - Keep finger nails short, to prevent small skin breaks. (nurses, patients other care givers)
     - Avoid anal intercourse
     - Avoid enemas, rectal medications, rectal thermometers
     - Avoid excessive friction and provide vaginal lubrication during sexual intercourse (use water soluble jelly...).
   - Maintain meticulous oral hygiene
     - Maintain teeth and gums in good condition
     - Use mouthwash or oral irrigations with normal saline... baking soda or sodium bicarbonate solution
     - Use mycostatin tablets or suspension as necessary
     - Relieve drynes, drink water and other fluids
     - Use artificial saliva as needed in form of spray
     - Stimulate saliva with gum, candies, buttermilk, yoghurt
     - Brush teeth with soft toothbrush (small soft bristle) or use foam stick or swab
     - Brush teeth in short horizontal strokes at least for 3 to 4 minutes, at least 3 times a day
     - Use flouridated toothpaste or rinse to prevent caries
     - Use water pik under low pressure or irrigation, if platelet count is low
   - Maintain optimal respiratory functions, encourage, turn, cough and deep breathe (if confined to bed).
3. *Maintain optimal gastrointestinal function*
   - Give antidiarrheal medication as needed.
   - Plan daily bowel regimen for constipation, give stool softener as prescribed.
   - Treat stomatitis oral nystatin, or other prescribes
   - Oral irrigations every 2 hours.
   - Soft, bland foods, cold liquids, tolerated by some persons.
   - Treat nausea and vomiting.
     - Give antiemetics 30 to 45 minutes before chemotherapy, use large doses
     - Use auditory or diversional stimulation (music slides, phonograph)
     - Give anti-emetics around the clock for severe nausea and vomiting.
     - Use texation techniques were hypnosis, therapeutic touch.
     - Eat foods which can minimise nausea and vomiting.
4. *Minimising or preventing alopecia*
   - Encourage use of wigs, scarves, eyebrow pencils, false eyelashes
   - Avoid frequent shampooing, combing, or brushing
   - Use soft-bristle hair brush
   - Advise against permanent and hair colouring. (increase rate of hair loss).
5. *Minimising or preventing urinary effects*
   - Hemorrhage, cystitis, renal toxicity.
   - Force fluids when take cyclophosphamide
   - Take cyclophosphamide early in the day
   - Check serum creatinine or 24 hour urine for creatinine clearance before giving cisplatin and streptolorecin.
6. *Minimising reproductive effects*
   - Provide birth control information and reproductive counselling
   - Provide informatioan about sperm banking before initiation of therapy for male patients.

Administration of Chemotherapy

Chemotherapy can be administered by several routes.

- Oral Ex. Cyclophosphomide
- Intramuscular Ex. Bleomycin

• Intravenous	Ex. Doxorubicin, vincristine
• Intracavitary (pleural, peritoneal)	Ex. Radioisotopes, alkalating agents
• Intrathecal	Ex. Methotrexate, cytosine, arbinoside
• Intraarterial	Ex. DTIC, 5-Fu, Methotrexate, fluxuridine
• Perfusion	Ex. Alkalysing, alkalating agents
• Continuous infusion	Ex. 5-Fu, Methostreate, cytosine, arbinoside
• Subcutaneous	Ex. Cytosine arabinoside
• Topical	Ex. 5-Fu cream
• Intraperitoneal	Ex. Methotrexate, 5-Fu

Mostly used common routes are IV and oral. One of the major concerns with the IV administration of antineoplastic drugs is possible irritation of vessel wall by the drugs, or even worse, extravasation (infiltration of drugs into tissues surrounding the infusion site), causing local tissue damage. Many chemotherapeutic drugs are vesicants agents that when accidentally infiltrated into the skin cause severe local tissue breakdown and necrosis. Some guidelines to promote safe use of chemotherapeutic drugs by IV administration follows:

1. Know specifics about the safe administration of chemotherapy.
2. Start an IV infusion and normal saline solution or 5% dextrose in water or saline solution with a small-lumens short needle or catheter. Ensure that recent venipunctures have not been performed to the proximal to the IVSa. Avoid using on arm that has poor lymphatic drainage or that has previously received radiation therapy.
3. Select a vein that is larger enough to promote infusion without irritating the intima of the vein. When a vesicant is administered, avoid the veins in the hand, wrist, and antecutital area.
4. Instruct the patient to immediately report any changes in sensation especially burning or stinging pain.
5. Check for blood return before infusing the chemotherapeutic drug. However, a blood return does not always indicate an intact vein.
6. If more than one drug is to be used, give the vesicant agents. First, when the vein is at its optimum integrity. (note this metod is controversial, so confirm with the concerned).
7. Slowly push those drugs that are to be given by the push or bolus method. Give in small increments (0.5 to 1.0 ml). Pause 30 to 60 seconds after each increment and allow the IV infusion to flush the vein, check blood returns, and again gently push 0.5 to 1.0 ml of the medication. Repeat until the medication has been given and allow the IV infusion to flush the vein for several minutes.
8. Avoid continuous peripheral IV infusion of vesicant agents. If given peripherally, the administration of vesicant agents must be motivated directly at all times.
9. Stop the IV infusion immediately if the patient complains of a burning or stinging pain or if an infiltration is suspected. If the drug is an irritant, check for blood return and if present continue to administer the drugs. If it is vesicant, stop the infusion and begin appropriate extravasation procedure.
10. If extravasation occurs:
    - Stop the IV infusion immediately; notify the doctor or use the standing written orders for the treatment related to the specific vesicant agent.
    - Remove the IV infusion tubing and aspirate any remaining drug with a new syringe.
    - Inject the prescribed antidote (if one is available) in the infusion needle or in a 'pincushion' fashion in the skin surrounding the needle site.
    - Apply a topical corticosteroid cream, if prescribed.
    - Elevate the site.
    - Apply cold compresses for the first 24 to 48 hours unless a vinca alkaloid has been infiltrated; heat is applied following extravasation of vinca alkaloids.
    - Document the extravasation.
    - Observe site at designated intervals
    - A plastic surgeon may be consulted, depending on the extent of anticipated damage.

Principles of Chemotherapy Administration

1. Combination chemotherapy is far superior to single agent chemotherapy.
2. Complete remission is the minimum requisite for cure and even increased survival.
3. The first round chemotherapy offers the best chance for significant benefit, therefore, the initial therapy should be the type with maximum effectiveness.
4. Maximum doses of drugs are used to attain maximum tumour cell kill; Dose reduction to minimised toxicity has been called "killing patients with kindness".
5. Neoadjuvant or induction chemotherapy is always recommended for some specific cancer (e.g. breast cancer).
6. Chemoprevention shows promise in prevention of some second-primary cancers (head and neck).

Side effects of radiation therapy and chemotherapy The common side effects of radiation therapy and chemotherapy classified according to systemwise are as follows:

1. *Gastrointestinal system*
    i. *Dryness of the mucous membranes of the mouth* When salivary glands are located in the radiation treatment

field, they are frequently damaged. This may be a permanent side effect of the radiation therapy and it can be quite disturbing because it is difficult to eat, swallow, and talk when the mucous membranes are dry. Artificial saliva is available.

ii. *Stomatitis and mucositis* This problem occurs when epithelial cells of the oral mucosa and intraoral soft tissue structures are destroyed by chemotherapy or radiation therapy. These cells are extremely sensitive because of their normal high cell turnover rate. Mucositis can precipitate complications of infection and haemorrhage.

iii. *Oesophagitis* Inflammation and ulceration of mucous membranes or esophagus as a result of rapid cell destructions occur as a side effect of chemotherapy and radioactive therapy to the area of the neck, chest and back.

iv. *Nausea and vomiting* The vomiting center in the brain is stimulated by products of cellular breakdown that occurs in response to chemotherapy and radiation therapy. The drugs used in chemotherapy also stimulate the vomiting center. Destruction of the epithelial lining of the GI tracts occurs in response to both these therapies to chest, abdomen and back. A strong psychologic impacts is associated with nausea and vomiting and the high stress level associated with concern cancer and cancer treatment.

v. *Anorexia* It is site specific side effect of radiation therapy dry mouth, mucositis, esophagitis, nausea, vomiting, and diarrhea occur. Side effects of chemotherapy include nausea, vomiting, stomatitis, esophagitis, and diarrhea. Fatigue, pain and infection are present. Alteration in the sensation of taste occurs when tumours release waste products into the blood stream. Psychological and social impact of cancer and cancer therapy result in an increased level of stress and changes in the usual lifestyle pattern.

vi. *Altered taste sensations* Due to destruction of the taste buds in the treatment field occurs in radiation therapy. The amount of taste alterations or loss depends on the radiation dosage and the extent field. Complete loss of taste often occurs. Taste changes may be a permanent outcome of therapy. Waste products occur in response to cellular destructions from radiation therapy and chemotherapy. These waste products are thought to be responsible for alteration in task sensations. Reduction in the amount of saliva occurs because of the locatioan of the salivary glands in the treatment field. Food must be in solution to be tasted.

vii. *Diarrhea* Due to denuding of the epithelial lining of the small intestine occurs as a side effect of both the therapies to the abdomen or the lower back.

viii. *Constipation* Due to dysfunction of the antonomic nervous system from neurotoxic effects of plant alkaloids (Vincristine, Vinblastine) occurs.

ix. *Hepatotoxicity* Toxic effects of certain chemotherapy drugs such as methotrexate, mitomycin, 6-MP and cytosine arabinoside are product.

2. *Haematopoietic system*

i. *Anaemia* These therapies result in depressant effect on bone marrow function. Malignant infiltration of bone marrow by cancer occurs. Ulceration, necrosis and bleeding of neoplastic growth occurs.

ii. *Leukopenia* As stated earlier, these therapies result in depressant effect on bone marrow. The effect is especially significant because of the short span of white blood cells. Infection is the most frequent cause of morbidity and death in the patient with cancer. Usual sites of infection are the respiratory and genitourinary system.

iii. *Thrombocytopenia* Depressant effect on bone marrow functions may lead to malignant infiltrations of the bone marrow. Abnormal destruction of circulating platelets is present. When platelet count decreases spontaneous bleeding can occur.

3. *Integumentary system*

i. *Alopecia* Alopecia occurs as a side effect of some chemotherapy agents and radiation therapy to the skull. Hair loss that occurs in response to radiation therapy is usually permanent. The hair begins to fall out during the first week of therapy, and this may progress to complete hair loss.

ii. *Skin reaction* Extravasation of vesicant chemotherapeutic drugs (e.g. doxorubicin) gives intravenously causes severe necrosis of tissues exposed to the drug.

4. *Genitourinary tract*

i. *Cystitis* This problem occurs when the epithelial cells of the lining of the bladder are destroyed as a side effect of chemotherapy (e.g. cyclophosphomide) and as a side effect of radiation therapy when the bladder located in the treatment field. Clinical manifestation of urgency, frequency, and haematuria are present.

ii. *Reproductive dysfunction* This problem occurs as a result of the effect of chemotherapy on the cells of the testes or ova or as a result of the effect of radiation therapy when the cells of the testes or ova are located in the treatment field. Symptoms of cancer and cancer therapy include fatigue, diarrhea nausea, vomiting, anxiety, fear and pain.

iii. *Nephrotoxicity* Necrosis of proximal renal tubules present as a result of an accumulation of drugs (e.g. cisplatin) in the kidney.

5. *Nervous system*
   i. *Increased intracranial pressure* This problem may result from radiation oedema in the CNS. This phenomenon is not well understood but is easily controlled with steroids and pain medication.
   ii. *Peripheral neuropathy* Paresthesia, areflexia, skeletal muscle weakness and smooth muscle dysfunction (e.g. paralytic ileus, constipation) can occur as a side effect of plant alkaloids (e.g. vimblastine, vincristine) and cisplatin.
6. *Respiratory system*
   i. *Pneumonitis* When the lungs are located in the treatment field, radiation pneumonitis may develop 2-3 months after start of treatment. It is characterised by a dry, hacking cough, fever and exertional dyspnea. After 6-12 months, fibrosis will occur and will be persistently evident on X-ray. The patient with fibrosis is more susceptible to respiratory infection. This problem can also occur as a result of chemotherapy (e.g. bloomycin, busulfin).
7. *Cardiovascular system*
   i. *Pericarditis and myocarditis* This problem is an infrequent complication when the chest wall is radiated. It may occur upto one year after treatment.

PROCEDURE GUIDELINES—ADMINISTERING IV CHEMOTHERAPY

a. Examine the site for erythema or selling. Over a period of days to weeks, the site can become mottled and lead to necrosis.
b. Stop the infusion of the chemotherapeutic agent.
c. Aspirate all residual chemotherapeutic agent in the IV needle/catheter.
d. Administer antidote (see accompanying table) inject intradermally in circular motion around the extravasation site to prevent leakage of drug to surrounding tissues (if appropriate or inject via the IV catheter)
e. Antidote may prevent tissue necrosis. If unable to aspirate from IV catheter, catheter may be blocked and antidote will not reach extravasation.

MANAGEMENT OF AN EXTRAVASATION

Chemotherapeutic agent	*Local antidote*	*Method of administration*
Decarbazine (DTIC) Dactinomycin (actinomycin D) Mitomycin C (mutamycin) Mechlorethamine (nitrogen mustard)	Isotonic sodium thiosulfate 10% Mixing 4.0 ml of sodium thiosulfate 10% with 6.0 ml sterile water for injection	1. Inject 5-6 ml mixture through the existing line and so in divided doses into the extravasated site with multiple injections. Repeat SQ dosing over several hours. 2. Apply cold compresses 6-12 hr after the extravasation.
Vinblastine (velban) Vincristine (oncovin)	Hyaluronidase (Wydase) 150 units/ml	1. Inject 1-6 ml (150-900 units) Sq into extravasated site with multiple injections.
Temposide (Vm 26)	Add 1 ml USP NaCl	2. Apply warm compresses.
Etoposide (vepesid)- Streptozocin (zanosar) Mithramycin (mithracin)		
Dauno rubicin (cerubidine) Doxorubicin (adriamycin) Mitaxantrone (navantrone) AMSA	Hydrocartisone 50-100 mg/ml	1. Inject 1/2ml (50-100 mg) IV through the existing line and SQ into the extravasated site with multiple injections. Total dose not to exceed 100 mg. 2. Apply cold compresses for 15 minute 4 times in a 24-hour period.
BCNU (carmustine)	Sodium bicarbonate (0.5 mEq/ml) prefilled syringe	1. Inject 2-6 ml of mixture (1.0–3.0 mEq) I.V. through the existing IV line and into the extravasated site with multiple injections. 2. Total dose not to exceed 10 ml of solution (5.0 mEq). 3. Apply cold compresses. Do not apply pressure.
Pachtaxel (taxol)	None	1. Apply warm compresses to the extravasation site for 24 hours.

1. Nursing care plan of cancer client

Problem	*Reason*	*Objective*	*Nursing intervention*	*Evaluation*
1. Pain related to effects of disease or its treatment	• As manifested by facial mask, complains of pain pain, guarding.	• Reduction of pain to a tolerable and manageable level.	• Assess the pain to provide a baseline treatment. • Confront and correct fears of addiction to reduce the possibility of understanding the patient's pain. • Use an analgesic ladder (1. non-opioid 2. weak opioid 3. strong opioid). • Teach patient complementary pain management techniques (imagery, relaxation, biofeedback, etc. to augment pain management strategies.	
2. Altered nutrition, body requirement R/T anorexia and other symptoms.	• Anorexia nausea, vomiting as manifested by fatigue. • Inadequate food intake requirement with or without weight loss.	• Maintenance of body weight and adequate energy of AOL. • Decreased episodes of nausea and vomiting.	• Avoid punitive or judgemental statements about food intake or weight loss. • Administer antiemetic medication as prescribed to minimise GI effects. • Maintain pleasant, quiet, restful environment to avoid triggering nausea and vomiting and to allow maximum rest. • Modify diet to include bland, lukewarm, high calorie, high protein foods to prevent triggering vomiting and provide additional calories. • Try small frequent feedings every few hours rather than fewer larger meals to facilitate gastric emptying and prevent early satiety. • Teach patient to eat and drink slowly to allow patient to enjoy taste and to prevent bloating. • Ensure adequate fluid hydration with chemotherapy to dilute drug level and reduce stimulation of vomiting receptor. • Provide a well-balanced diet that includes all food groups with increased protein-caloric intake to promote positive nitrogen balance. • Gently encourage patient to eat but avoid nagging to prevent establishing a negative meal environment. • Avoid foods that are gas forming, such as salads, cabbage, broccoli, fruits and bear, because they can promote nausea and a sense of fullness. • Serve all foods attractively and in a pleasant environment to stimulate appetite. • Teach the patient to sip the nutritional supplement slowly between meals to avoid bloating. • Teach the patient what to eat rather than stressing the fact that more food should be eaten (advise home prepared items.)	
3 Ineffective management of therapeutic regimen R/T Lack of knowledge of long-term management of cancer.	• As manifested by frequent questions by patients and care given regarding – Self care	• Patient and nurses express confidence in management of cancer patient.	• Determine the knowledge and technical skills needed by patient and nurses to plan needed instruction. • Assess current level of knowledge and skill to determine the abilities and of patient and caregivers to perform tasks correctly.	

Contd...

Contd...

Problem	*Reason*	*Objective*	*Nursing intervention (rationale)*	*Evaluation*
	– treatment – Side effects – Observed inability, etc.	• Adequate knowledge base to provide care	• Teach required skills and provide information to patient and caregiver to increase their knowledge level. • Provide opportunity for follow-up evaluation and teaching to increase patient/caregiver confidence and ensure correct performance task.	
4. Altered oral muscous membrane R/T chemotherapy or radiation therapy	• As manifested by verbalization or signs of pain or discomfort in mouth-coated tongue, xerestomia, halitosis, swollon membranes, oral lesions, haemorrhagic gingivitis, leukoplakin, stomatitis.	• No oral pain • No infection in oral mucosa. • No break in integrity of oral mucosa.	• Assess oral mucosa daily. • Teach patient to inspect oral cavity because stomatitis occurs 4 to 14 days after treatment begins • Remove dentures at night to avoid further irritation. • Observe for dryness, redness and white or yellow membrane and the presence of any breaks in integrity of tissues. • Distinguish stomatitis from candidiasis and other oral problems, such as xerostomia, and herpes for appropriate treatment. • Use mouthwashes of baking soda, baking soda and lime, or normal saline solution every 2 hours to provide comfort. • Use soft-bristle-toothbrushes, sponge-tipped applicators, or an irrigation syringe as cleansing agents to prevent trauma. • Avoid the use of lemon and glycerine swabs for mouth care because they increase dryness and irritation. • Apply topical anaesthetics such as viscous xylocaine as ordered to provide pain relief. • Modify diet to avoid hot, spicy acidic foods to avoid irritation. • Discourage use of irritants such as tobacco and alcohol. • Encourage drinking of water or other liquids at frequent intervals to keep moist the mucous membrane. • Apply small amount of petroleum jelly lip gloss or moisturises to lips to promote comfort and prevent dryness.	
5. Fatigue R/T the effects of cancer or its treatment	As manifested by verbal report of lack of energy and inability to maintain usual routine	Satisfactory activity level relative to phase of disease or environment.	• Inform the patient that fatigue is an expected side effects of therapy and that it usually begins during the first week of therapy, reaches its peak in 2 weeks, continues and then gradually disappears 2 to 4 weeks after treatment has been ended. • Encourage patient to rest when fatigued, to maintain usual lifestyle pattern as closely as possible and to pace activities in accordance with energy level because rest periods are essential to conserve energy.	
6. Ineffective individual coping R/T depression secondary to diagnosis and treatment	– Uncertain outcome of treatment, – disruption in lifestyle, or – financial burden as manifested by verbalised or observed inability to manage	• Appropriate response to problems. • Able to seek and/or accept support and assistance	• Have paient direct own care when possible to encourage patient independence. – Provide information to allow patient to make informed choices regarding treatment regimen and plan of care. – Facilitate communication between patient and family to foster a supportive network. – Assess and mobilize patient's support systems. – Refer patient to social services for financial assistance if appropriate to provide additional resources. – Assess need for further counselling.	

Contd...

Contd...

Problem	*Reason*	*Objective*	*Nursing intervention*	*Evaluation*
	effective components of diagnosis and resulting symptoms, threats or attempts ot commit suicide, concern ove over financial implications of disease.			
7. Body-image disturbance R/T hairloss, disfiguring surgery, and weight loss	As menifested by expressions of concern with changes in body; refusal to interact with visitors, isolation, frequent crying, refusal to care of self or to look in mirror	Able to verbalize acceptance of changes in body appearance and function	• Provide psychologic support and prepare patient for expected hairloss to lessen shock of event when it occurs. • Encourage patients to select a wig and begin to wear it before hairloss begins and to wear a scarf or turban to conceal hairloss. • Use a mild, motion-based shampoo, cream rinse, and hair conditioner every 4 to 7 days to avoid drying remaining hair. • Avoid excessive shampooing, brushing an combing of hair to reduce hair loss. • Avoid use of electric hair dryers, curlers, curling rods, and hair spray to minimise scalp irritations and decrease hairloss. • Help patient select clothing and colours that minimise weightloss or effects of disfiguring surgery. • Assure patient that value as a person is not associated with external appearance. • Discuss expected physical changes with family members and advise them of ways to assist patient with acceptance to prepare the family and to foster family relationships.	
8. Altered family process R/T cancer diagnosis of family member.	As manifested by observed communication problem among family members, lack of family support related to physical, emotional and for spiritual needs of the patient.	• Family members communicate about patient and cooperate in care of the patient • Family will seek outside help when needed.	• Assess family structure and support system to determine amount and quality of support available to patient. • Teach needed skills to family members. • Provide opportunities for discussion of caregiving and emotional implications of role changes to promote verbalization of feelings and shared understanding of problems • Assist family members to set realistic expectations for patient and themselves. • Provide guidance on course of disease and anticipated outcome so planning can be accomplished.	
9. Risk for infection R/T Lukopenia, depressed immune system and multiple exposure to microscope	(Please see concerned chapters for NCP)			
10. Potential for bleeding related to thrombocytopen.				

Contd...

Contd...

Problem	*Reason*	*Objective*	*Nursing intervention*	*Evaluation*
11. Potential for hyperuricemia R/T chemotherapy		• Monitor signs of hyperuricemia • Report deviations from acceptable parameters. • Carry out medical and nursing interventions	• Monitor for high level uric acid excretion in urine, high serum uric acid excretion in urine, high serum uric acid, obstructed uropathy, decreased urine output, nausea vomiting, lethargy. • Record intake and output to determine fluid balance. • Encoruage fluids to prevent uric acid crystals from causing obstruction. • Evaluate blood urea nitrogen (BUN) and scruro-creatinum levels to identify early changes in renal functions. • Administer allopurinol (Zyloprim) as ordered to reduce endogenous uric acid production.	

NURSING ALERT

DO NOT INJECT AN ANTIDOTE VIA THE IV CATHETER IF UNABLE TO ASPIRATE THE CHEMOTHERAPEUTIC AGENT.
Remove the needle.
Apply ice or heat to the site, depending on the chemotherapeutic agent which has extravasated.

FOLLOW-UP PHASE

1. Document drug dosage, site and any occurrence of extravasation including estimated amount of drug extravasated, management. Photograph if possible.
2. Observe regularly after administration for pain, erythema, induration, and necrosis.

2. If only a small amount of drug extravasated and frank necrosis does not occur, phlebitis may still result, causing pain for several days or induration at the site that may last for weeks or months.

3. Monitor for other side effects of infusion.
   a. Patient may describe sensations of pain, stretching, or pressure within the vessel, originating near the venipuncture site or extending 7.5-12.5 cm (3-5 inches) along the vein.
   b. Discoloration-red streak following the line of the vein (called a flare reaction) or darkening of the vein.
   c. Itching, urticaria, muscle cramps, or pressure in the arm.

3.
   a. Caused by irritation to the vein.
   b. Flare reaction common with doxorubicin (andriamycin). Darkening of vein may occur with 5-fluorouracil (5-FU)
   c. Caused by irritation of surrounding subcutaenous tissue.

Respiratory Nursing

The act of breathing involves two inter-related processes, ventilation and respiration–ventilation is the movement of air into and out of lungs. Respiration refers to the exchange of oxygen and carbon dioxide across cell membrane. The primary purpose of the respiratory system is gas exchange, which involves the transfer of oxygen and carbon dioxide between the atmosphere and blood. The respiratory system is divided into two parts, i.e. the upper respiratory tract and lower respiratory tract. The upper respiratory tract includes the nose, pharynx, adenoids, tonsils, epiglottis, larynx and trachea. The lower respiratory tract consists of bronchioles, alveolar ducts and alveoli. With the exception of the right and left main stem bronchi, all lower airway structures are contained in the lungs. The right lung is divided into three lobes—upper, middle and lower and the left lung into two lobes (upper and lower). The structure of the chest walls (ribs, pleura, muscle of respiration) are also essential to respiration.

ASSESSMENT OF RESPIRATORY SYSTEM

Respiratory assessment should be tailored to the individual's health status. The most common symptoms or reason, a person seeks health care include dyspnoea, cough, sputum production, haemoptysis, wheezing or chest pain. Upper airways symptoms may include obstruction of noses, nasal discharge, sinus pain, sore throat or hoarseness.

Dyspnoea

Dyspnoea means breathlessness, but the terms used to describe difficult or laboured breathing observable by others. It may cause other problems such as constipation or poor nutrition, as well as psychosocial problem related to poor self-esteem or changes in lifestyle. Individual experiencing pulmonary dysfunctions, such as breathlessness, tend to perceive their illness in terms of its impact on their ability to carry out activities of daily living. Which includes

- Bathe, dress and groom
- Perform chores or hobbies
- Walk or exercise
- Get to the bathroom
- Prepare meals and rest
- Maintain family and social relationships
- Getting into home or Client's stairs
- Maintain employment
- Sleep
- Perform scanality
- Attend activities away from home

Analysis of dyspnoea according to its time and characteristics.

i. *Timing*: Chronic or acute, episodic or paroxysmal, onset, duration and frequency.
ii. *Characteristics*:
   - Perceived severity
   - Phases of respiratory cycle–Inspiratory, expiratory, throughout cycle.
iii. *Other symptoms related to dyspnoea:*
iv. *Associated factors*:
   - Time of day
   - Seasonal or weather changes
   - Environmental irritants.
   - Anxiety
   - Body position – paroxysmal nocturnal dyspnoea (PND). Sudden onset while sleeping in recumbent position.
     – Orthopnoea: breathlessness on assuming recumbent position.
   - Activity.

Cough

Coughing has two main functions. It protects the lungs from aspiration and it helps propel foreign matter and excess mucus up through the airways. The individual can describe the cough in terms of timing and characteristics as follows:

i. *Timing*:
   Chronic, acute paroxysmal (periodic forceful episode difficult to control) onset (graded or sudden).
ii. *Characteristics*:
   - Perceived severity.
   - Pattern, occasional, upon rising, with activity (talking exercising, eating).
iii. *Quality*:
   - Productive - non-productive
   - Dry progression to productive
   - Barking

- Hoarse
- Hacking

iv. *Other symptoms*:

- Chest tightness
- Fever, coryza
- Choking.

Sputum Production

The mucous blanket lines the epithelial layer of the trachobronchial tree and cleanses it of inhaled particles and debris. Mucus is produced by the globet cells and submucosal glands. The cilia propel the mucous (which contains foreign particles, pus, blood and debris) upward toward the pharynx where it is coughed up, suctioned or swallowed. Normal sputum is clear and thin and average 100 ml/day. However, individuals with pulmonary disease often have sputum associated with these conditions making it important to assess the baseline super characteristics, describes as thick, viscous (gelatanious) tenacious (sticky), frothy, mucoid (colourless, clear, non-infectious watery, mucopurulent, and casts (from bronchioles, rubbery).

The mucopurulent sputum may be:

- Creamy yellow: Staphylococcal pneumoniae.
- Green: Pseudomonas pneumoniae
- Current jelly: Klebsiella pneumoniae.
- Rusty: Pneumococcal pneumonia.
- Pink frothy: Pulmonary oedema

The quantity of amount of sputum may be teaspoon, tablespoon or cups used as a measurement.

Haemoptysis

Haemoptysis is the coughing up of blood or blood-tinged sputum. It may contain air bubbles. The source of bleeding may be from any where in the upper or lower airways or from the lung parenchyma. Blood that originates in the GI tract and is coughed up as dark brown or resembling coffee grains in appearance termed as 'haematemesis'. It is usually never frothy, may be mixed with food particles, pH acidic dark-red or coffee coloured. Bleeding from the nares (epistaxis) should be assessed as a cause for coughing up blood or vomiting of blood.

In haemoptysis, blood is usually frothy, pH alkaline, bright red. The coughing up of 400-1600 ml of blood in 24 hours period is considered massive and severe, needs immediate medical attention.

Wheezing

Wheezing is a continuous high-pitched, whistling sound produced when air passes through narrowed or obstructed airways. It is generally occurring during expiration, however, wheezing can be heard throughout respiratory cycle. Wheezing is usually heard with a stethoscope; however, wheezing may be audible to the person or heard by others in close proximity to the person. An analysis of this symptom should include factors that can cause bronchospasm and produce wheezing such as asthma, exposure to physiological irritants, stress, anxiety. Snoring or stridor cloud snoring may be experienced.

Chest Pain

Chest pain can result from several conditions. Chest pain may be cardiac origin. The chest pain of pulmonary origin can originate from the chest wall. Parietal pleura or lung parenchyma. The characteristics of pulmonary chest pain are:

- Pain from the *chest wall* is well-localised, constant ache increasing with movement. It may be due to trauma, cough and herpes zoster.
- Pain is parietal pleura is a sharp, abrupt onset, increasing with inspiration or with sudden ventilatory effort (cough, sneeze) unilateral.
- Pain from lung parenchyma is dull, constant poorly localised in benign pulmonary tumours and carcinoma; well-localised sharp, sudden onset in pneumothorax; sudden onset, increasing stabbing pain on inspiration, may radiate in cases of pulmonary embolus and infarction.

In addition to review of symptom or reason the person is seeking health care, the person should be interviewed about risk factors associated with respiratory dysfunction, including smoking, past pulmonary illnesses or exposure to respiratory infections, predisposition to genetic disorders, exposure to environmental irritants (dust, fume gases, etc.) and the psychosocial effects of respiration disorders.

The emotional responses include anxiety, depression, hostility, fear or panic, etc. and ask the person's problems with swallowing and ambulating as well as neuromuscular diseases.

The common abnormalities of the thorax and lungs found by physical examinations are as follows:

Inspection

- *Pursed-lip breathing* Is an exhalation through mouth with lips pursed together to slow exhalation. As seen in COPD, asthma suggests increasing breathlessness. Strategy taught is slow expiration, decrease dyspnoea.
- *Tripod position* Inability to be flat, i.e. leaning forward, with arms and elbows supported on overbed table. Seen in COPD, asthma in exacerbations, pulmonary oedema, indicates moderate to severe respiratory distress.
- *Accessory muscle use* In intercostal retractions neck and shoulder muscles are used to assist breathing. Muscles between ribs pull in during respiration. Due to COPD, asthma in exacerbation-secretion retention, indicate severe respiratory distress, hypoxaemia.
- *Splinting* A voluntary decrease in tidal volume to decreased pain on chest expansion. It is due to thoracic or abdominal incisions, chest trauma, plurasy.

- *Increased AP diameter* AP chest diameter equal to the lateral, slope of ribs more horizontal (90°) or spine. One to COPD, asthma, cystic fibrosis, lung hyperinflation, advanced age.
- *Tachypnoea* Increased rate of 20 breaths/minute, > 25 breath/minute in elderly. Due to fever, anxiety, hypoxaemia, restrictive lung disease. Magnitude of increasing above normal rate reflects increased work of breathing.
- *Kussmaul's respiration* Regular rapid and deep respirations are due to metabolic acidosis. Increase in rate aids body in CO_2 excretion.
- *Cyanoses* Refer to a bluish colour of skin best seen in earlobes, under eyelids or nailbeds. It is due to decreased oxygen transfer of lungs, decreased cardiac output, non-specific unreliable indicator.
- *Clubbing of fingers* Refer to increased depth, bulk, sponginess, of distal digit finger. It is due to chronic hypoxaemia, cystic fibrosis, lung cancer, bronchiectasis.
- *Abdominal paradox* An inward (rather than normal outward) movement of abdomen during inspiration. It is due to insufficient and ineffective breathing pattern–non-specific indicator of severe respiratory distress.

Palpation

- *Tracheal deviation* is a leftward or rightward movement of trachea from normal midline position. It is non-specific indicator of change in position of mediasternoid structure, medical emergency if caused by tension pneumothorax.
- *Altered tactile fremitus* is increase or decrease in vibrations. It is due to increased in pneumonia, pulmonary edema; decreased in pleural effusion, atelectic area, lung hyperinflation, absent in pneumothorax, large atelectasis.
- *Altered chest movements* i.e. unequal or equal but diminished movement of two sides of chest with inspiration. Usually unequal movement caused by atelectasis, pneumothorax, pleural effusion, splinting, equal but diminished movement caused by barrel chest, restrictive disease and neuromuscular disease.

Percussion

- *Hyper resonance* is loud, laver-pitched sound over areas that normally produce a resonance sound. It is due to lung hyper inflation (COPD), lung collapse (pneumothorax) air trapping (asthma).
- *Dullness* is medium-pitched sound over areas that normally produce a resonant sound. It is due to increased density (pneumonia, large atelectasis). Increased fluid pleural space (pleural effusion).

Auscultation

- *Fine crackles* are series of short explosive, high-pitched sounds heard just before the end of inspiration: result of rapid equalisation of gas pressure when collapsed alveoli or terminal bronchioles suddenly snap open similar sound to that made by rolling hair between fingers just behind ear. Can be heard in fibrosis (asbestos interstitial oedema, early pulmonary oedema), alveolar filling (pneumonia) loss of lung volume (atelectasis), early phase of congestive heart failure.
- *Coarse crackles* are series of short, low-pitched sounds caused by air passing through airway intermittently occluded by mucus unstable bronchial wall, of fold of mucosa, evident on inspiration and at times, expiration; similar sound to bowling quality with more fluid. These can be heard in congestive heart failure, pulmonary oedema, pneumonia with severe congestion, COPD.
- *Ronchi* are continuous rumbling, snoring, or rattling sounds from obstructions of a large airways with secretions most prominent on expiration; change often evident after coughing or suctioning. These are heard in COPD, cystic fibrosis, pneumonia, bronchietasis.
- Wheezing are continuous musical sound of constant pitch: result of partial obstruction of larynx or trachea. It is due to epiglottis, vocal cord oedema after extubation, foreign body.
- *Absent breath sounds* no sound evident over entire lung or area of lung. It is due to pleural effusion, main stem bronchi, obstruction, large atelectasis, pneumonectomy, lobectomy.
- *Pleural friction rub* is cracking or grating sound from roughened inflamed surfaces of the pleura rubbing together, evident during inspiration. It is due to pleurasy, pneumonia, pulmonary infarction.
- *Bronchophony, whispered pectoriloguy* a spoken or whispered syllable more distinct than normal on auscultation as in pneumonia.
- Egophony is a spoken "e" similar to "a" on auscultation because of altered transmission of voice sounds seen in pneumonia, pleural effusion.

DIAGNOSTIC STUDIES OF RESPIRATORY SYSTEM

Blood Studies

i. *Haemoglobin* test reflects amount of haemoglobin available for combination with oxygen. Venous blood is used. The normal level of adult man is 135-180g/dl (13.5-18 g/l) = Normal level of adult woman is 12-16 g/dl (120-160 g/l). The nursing responsibilities during the procedure is to explain the procedure and its purpose. No special care is required.
ii. *Haematocrit* test reflects ratio of red blood cells to plasma increased haematocrit (polycythaemia) found in chronic hypoxaemia. Venous blood is used. Normal for adult man is 40-54 per cent and woman is 38-47 per cent. The nursing responsibility is as in HB%.

iii. *Antitrypsin assay* is valuable in the identification of individuals with the genetic abnormality that leads to emphysema. This is a globulin that inhibits certain enzymes. The normal values of a_1-antitrypsin assay.

MM genotype: 2.1-3.8 u/ml
M2 phenotype: 1.05-2.1 u/ml
22 phenotype:0.5-0.7 u/ml

The nursing care includes as in haemoglobin. No food or fluid restrictions are necessary.

iv. *Complete blood count* The normal counts of RBCs in male 4.6-6.2 million/D. 4.2-5.4 million/L in females. The normal level of WBC 4.0-11.0 × 10^3/L.

v. *Arterial blood gases (ABG)*: Arterial blood is obtained through puncture of radial or femoral artery or through arterial catheter. ABGs are performed to assess acid-base-balance, ventilation status, need for oxygen therapy, change in oxygen therapy, or change in ventilation settings. Continuous ABG monitoring is also possible via a sensor or electrode inserted into the arterial catheter.

Nursing responsibility in this test, thus includes.

Explain the purposes of the test and its procedure to the patient in using oxygen (percentage, L/min). Avoid change it for 20 minutes before obtaining sample. Assist with positioning (e.g. palm up, wrist slightly hyperextended if radial artery is used). Collect blood into heparanised syringe. To ensure accurate results, expel all air bubbles, and place sample in ice, unless it will be analysed in less than 1 minute. Apply pressure to artery for 5 minutes after specimen is obtained to prevent haematoma at the arterial puncture site.

The normal values, parameters of ABGs are

- *Acid-base-balance* measured as pH (hydrogen ion concentration. Normal 7.35-7.45. Alkalaemia increased 7.45. Acedemia decreased 7.35.
- *Oxygenation* PaO_2 (partial pressure of dissolved O_2 in blood. Normal 80–100 mm Hg. Hyperoxaemia ↑ 100 mm Hg, hypoxaemia ↓ 80 mm Hg.
- *Ventilation* SaO_2 percentage of O_2 bound haemoglobin. $PaCO_2$ partial pressure of CO_2 dissolved in blood. The normal SaO_2 is 95–98 per cent. The normal $PaCO_2$: 35–45 mm Hg hypercapnia ↑ 45 mm Hg. Hypocapnia ↓ 35 mm Hg.

vi. *Oximetry*: Test monitors arterial or venous oxygen saturation device attached to the ear lobe, finger or nose for SPO_2 monitoring or is contained in a pulmonary artery catheter for SVO_2 monitoring. Oximetry is used for continuous monitoring in ICUs, inpatient and outpatient sortings and exercise testing.

The nursing responsibilities include, applying probe to finger, forehead, earlobe or bridge of nose. When interpreting SPO_2 and SVO_2 values, first assess patient status and presence of factors that can alter accuracy of pulse oximeter reading. For SPO_2, these include motion, low perfusion, bright lights, use of intravascular dyes, acryling nails, dark skin colour. For SVO_2 these include change in O_2 delivery or O_2 consumptions. For SPO_2 notify physician of ± 4 per cent change from baseline or decrease to less than 90 per cent. For SVO_2 notify physician of ± 10 per cent change from baseline or decrease to less than 60 per cent.

Sputum Analysis

The nursing responsibilities include explain purposes. Some tests require specimens, collected in consecutive days usually 4 ml of sputum is sufficient. Coughing upon awakening is more likely to result in collecting sputum and not saliva. Instruct individual to rinse the mouth with water, demonstrate effective deep breathing and coughing, have individual practice deep breathing and coughing, instruct individual to notify staff as the specimen is collected. Following are different test and nursing care.

i. Culture and Sensitivity

Single sputum specimen is collected in a sterile container. For diagnosing bacterial infection, select antibiotic and evaluate treatment. Here instruct patients on how to produce of good specimen for Gram stain test as given below if patients cannot produce specimen bronchoscopy may be used.

ii. Gram Stain

Staining of sputum permits classification of bacteria into Gram-negative and Gram-positive types. Results guide therapy until culture and sensitivity results are obtained. Here nurse instructs patient to expectorate sputum into the container after coughing deeply. Obtain sputum in early morning because secretions collect during night. If unsuccessful try increasing oral fluids, intake unless fluids are restricted. Collect sputum in sterile container (sputum trap) during suctioning or by aspirating secretions from the trachea. Send specimen to laboratory promptly.

iii. Acid-fast Smear Culture

Test is performed to collect sputum for acid-fast bacili (AFB). A series of 3 early morning specimen is used. Nursing responsibility as in Gram stain and cover specimen and send to laboratory for analysis.

iv. Cytology

In this single sputum specimen is collected in special container with fixative solution. Purpose is to determine presence of abnormal cells that may indicate malignant condition. The nurse should send specimens to laboratory promptly and take measure in other tests.

Radiological Studies

i. Chest X-ray

Test is used to screen, diagnose, and evaluate change. Most common views are postero-anterior and lateral. In this nurse instructs patient to undress to waist, put on gown, and remove any metal between neck and waist.

ii. Computed Tomography (CT)

Test is performed for diagnostic of lesions difficult to assess by conventional X-ray studies, such as those in the hilum, mediastenum, and pleura. Images show structures in cross section. Nursing care is same as for chest X-ray.

iii. Magnetic Resonance Imaging (MRI)

Test is used for diagnosis of lesions difficult to assess by CT scan (e.g. lung apex near the spine). Here, nurse explains purpose, takes measures as in chest X-ray and instructs the patient to remove all metal (e.g. jewellery, watch) before test. It takes about an hour.

iv. Ventilation/Perfusion (V/P) Lung Scan

Test is used to identify areas of the lung not receiving air flow (ventilator) or blood flow (perfusion). It involves injection of radioisotope and inhalation of small amount of radioactive gas (Xenon). A gamma detecting device is used to record radioactivity. Ventilation without perfusion suggests pulmonary embolus. The nursing measures are as for chest X-ray. Also check for dye allergy. Obtain an accurate weight so that the dosage of radioactive agent can be calculated. No special care or precaution is needed afterwards (post test) because the gas and isotope transmit radioactivity for only brief interval.

v. Pulmonary Angiogram

Study is used to visualize pulmonary vasculature and locate obstructions or pathologic conditions such as pulmonary embolus. A radio-opaque dye is injected, usually through a catheter into the pulmonary artery or right side of the heart. Nursing measures same as chest X-ray. Know that dye injection may cause flushing, warm sensation, and coughing. Check pressure dressing site after procedure. Monitor blood pressure, pulse rate and circulation distal to injection site. Report and record significant changes.

vi. Positron Emission Tomography (PET)

Test is used to distinguish benign and malignant lung nodules. It involves IV injection of a radioisotope with short-half life. Nursing measures same as V/P.

Endoscopic Examination

Bronchoscopy

This study is typically performed in outpatient procedure room. Flexible fiberoptic scope is used for diagnosis, biopsy, specimen collection, or assessment of changes. It may also be done to suction mucous plugs or to remove foreign objects. In this examination, the nurse instructs patient to be on NPO status for 6-12 hours. Obtain signed permit (consent). Give diazepam if ordered by physician before procedure to aid relaxation. After procedure, keep patient NPO until gag-reflex returns and monitor for laryngeal oedema. If biopsy was done, monitor for haemorrhage and pneumothorax.

Mediastinoscopy

Test is used for inspection and biopsy of lymph nodes in mediastinal area. Nurse prepares patient for surgical intervention, obtains signed permit. Afterwards monitor as for bronchoscopy.

Biopsy

In lung biopsy specimen may be obtained by transbronchial or open-lung biopsy. This test is used to obtain specimens for laboratory analysis. Nursing measures same as bronchoscopy.

Others

Thoracentesis

Test is used to obtain specimen of pleural fluid for diagnosis, to remove pleural fluid or to instill medication. The physician inserts a large bore needle through chest wall into pleural space. Chest X-ray is always obtained after procedures to check pneumothorax. Nursing responsibility includes explaining procedures to patient and obtain signed permit prior to procedure. Position patient upright, instruct not to talk or cough, and assist during procedure. If large volume of fluid is removed, monitor for decrease in shortness of breath, send labelled specimen to laboratory.

Pulmonary Function Test

It is used to valuate lung function. It involves use of a spirometer to diagram air movement as patient performs prescribed respiratory manoeuvres. Nurse has to avoid scheduling immediately after meals times. Avoid administration of inhaled bronchiodilator for 6 hours before procedure.

Explain procedure to patient. Provide rest after procedure.

DISORDERS OF NOSE AND SINUSES

Deviated Septum

Deviated septum is deflection of the normally nasal septum. It is most commonly caused by trauma to the nose or congenital disproportion, a condition in which the size of the septum is not proportioned to the size of the nose.

On inspection, septum is to one side, altering the air passage symptoms are variable. The patient may experience obstruction to nasal breathing, nasaloedema, or dryness of the nasal mucosa with crusting and bleeding (epistaxis). A severely deviated septum may block drainage of mucus from the sinus cavities, resulting in infection (sinusitis). Nasal breathing is subjective and only the patient can gauge the degree of 1obstruction and amount of discomfort it causes.

Health promotion is aimed at prevention of precipitating factors such as accidental falls in childhood. Medical management of deviated septum includes the use of decongestants or a nasal corticosteroid only to reduce nasal oedema. Before using the inhaler, ask the person to gently blow their nose, making sure that their nostrils are clear. Then follow these steps.

- Remove the cap from the nasal inhaler.
- Shake the container well.
- Hold the inhaler between the thumb and forefinger.
- Tilt the head back, slightly and insert the end of the inhaler into the nostril, painting it slightly towards the outside nostril wall. Hold the nostril closed with one finger.
- Press down the container to release one dose and at the same time inhale gently.
- Ask patient to hold the breath for a few seconds then breathe out slowly through the mouth.
- Withdraw the inhaler from the nostril and repeat the process for the other nostril if more than one puff is prescribed for nostril repetition.
- Replace the protective cap on the inhaler.

Surgery is an option for patient with severe symptoms. A nasal septoplasty is performed to reconstruct and properly align the deviated septum. Nasal septoplasty can be performed alone or with a rhinoplasty.

Nasal Fracture

Nasal fracture is most often caused by trauma of substantial force to the middle of the face. Complications of the fracture include airway obstruction, epistaxis and cosmetic deformity. Nasal fractures are classified unilateral, bilateral or complex. A unilateral fracture typically produces little or no displacement. Bilateral fractures, the most common fractures, give the nose a flattened look. Powerful frontal blows cause complex fractures, which may also shatter frontal bones. Diagnosis is based on the health history, direct observation and X-ray finding.

On inspection, nurse should assess the patient's ability to breathe through each side of the nose and note the presence of oedema, bleeding, or haematoma. There may be ecchymosis under one or both eyes. The nose is inspected internally for evidence of septal deviation, haemorrhage or clear drainage, which suggest leakage of CSF. If clear drainage is observed, a specimen may be sent for determining CSF. Injury of sufficient force to fracture nasal bones results in considerable swelling of soft tissues. With extensive swelling, it may be difficult to verify the extent of deformity or the repair the fracture until several days later when oedema is subsiding.

The goals of nursing management are to reduce oedema, prevent complications, educate the patient and provide emotional support. Ice may be applied to the face and nose to reduce oedema and bleeding. When a fracture is confirmed, the goal of management is realignment of the fracture using closed or open reduction (septoplasty, or rhinoplasty). These procedures re-establish cosmetic appearance and proper function of the nose and provide an adequate airway.

Nursing management of nasal surgery (Rhinoplasty, septoplasty, or nasal fracture reductions) includes the following.

- Before surgery, the patient should be instructed to avoid taking aspirin-containing drugs for 2 weeks to reduce bleeding.
- In postoperative period, include assessment of respiratory status, pain management, and observation of the surgical site for haemorrhage and oedema.
- Health teaching is important, because, these procedures involve a short hospital stay and the patient must be able to detect early and late complications.

The problem of patient undergoing surgery may have certain problems needing nursing care.

- *Altered health maintenance* R/T Lack of knowledge of the procedure, for which nurse has to explain the procedure, expected postoperative course, and required self care to decrease anxiety and increase patient cooperation. Answer questions as needed and assess the patient perception about body image and expectation of surgery to obtain information to use in patient care.
- *Ineffective breathing pattern related to presence of packaging*, nasal oedema, intranasal splints, as manifested by complaints of shortness of breath, alterations in respiration rate, rhythm or depth. Here, the nurse has to assess for respiratory distress, elevate head of bed, provide supplemental oxygen (if prescribed).

Instruct the patient to blow nose, open mouth when sneezing, and coughing to maintain correct position of packing. Apply cold compress to incisional area to promote vasoconstriction and reduce oedema. Instruct the patient to call nurse for any untoward effects.

- *Pain related to oedema* from surgical procedure, for which nurse should teach patient correct analgesic schedule, describe to patient the amount of pain expected, and teach patients non-pharmacological measures (elevation of head, cold compress) and avoid using aspirin on NSAIDs. Teach patient gentle cleaning techniques such as use of cotton swabs, with hydrogen peroxide to clean crusting and application of water-soluble jelly to lubricate when packing has been removed to promote cleanliness and prevent infection and promote use of bedside humidifier to decrease drying of mucosa and promote comfort and management of nasal haemorrhage or epistaxis.

Simple first aid measures should be used first to control epistaxis. The nurse should keep the patient quiet, position the patient in a sitting stature, leaning forward, or if not possible, in a reclining position with head and shoulders elevated; apply direct pressure by pinching the entire soft laven portion of the nose for 10 to 15 minutes; apply ice compresses to the nose, and have the patient suck on ice; partially insert a small guaze pad into the bleeding nostril and apply digital pressure if bleeding continues and obtain medical assistance, if bleeding does not stop. When first aid measure is not effective, management involves localisation of the bleeding site and application of a vasoconstrictive agent cauterization or anterior packing indicated. Anterior packing may consist of ribbon guaze impregnated with antiseptic ointments that is wedged firmly in the desired location and remain in place for 48 to 72 hours. If posterior packing is required, the patient should be hospitalised. Inflatable balloons may be used as the nasal pack on gauze rolls may be inserted. Stringes attached to the packaging are brought to the outside and taped to check for ease of removal. A nasal sling (folded 2 × 2 in gauze pad) should be taped over the nares to absorb drainage. Since packing is painful, mild narcotic analgesic is administered.

Failure of posterior packing indicates surgical correction.

Rhinitis

Rhinitis refers to inflammation of the mucous membrane of the nose. It may be acute or chronic or allergic rhinitis. All forms of rhinitis cause sneezing, nasal discharge with nasal obstruction and headache. Aetiology, pathophysiology and diverse manifestations are according to this type as follows:

Acute Rhinitis

Aetiology: Acute rhinitis (coryza, common cold) is caused by viruses that invade the upper respiratory tract. It is an inflammatory, condition of the mucous membrane of the nose and accessory sinuses caused by a filterable virus. It affects almost everyone at some time and occurs most often in winter with additional high incidences in early rain fall and spring. Some of the known causes of the common cold are 100 serotypes of rhinoviruses, coronoviruses, adenoviruses, echoviruses, influenza and parainfluenza viruses and coxsackieviruses.

It is the most prevalent infectious disease and is spread by airborne droplet sprays emitted by the infected person while breathing talking, sneezing or coughing or by direct hand contact. Frequency increases in winter months, when people stay indoors and overcrowding is more common. Other factors such as chilling, fatigue, physical and emotional stress and the patient compromised immune status, may increase susceptibility.

Clinical manifestations: The patient with acute viral rhinitis typically first experiences tickling, irritation, sneezing or dryness of the nose or nasopharynx followed by copious nasal secretions, some nasal obstruction, watery eyes, elevated temperature, general malaise, and headache. After the early profuse secretions, the nose becomes more obstructed and the discharge is thicker, within few days, the general symptoms improve, nasal passages reopen, and normal breathing is established. Secondary invasion by bacteria may cause pneumonia, acute bronchitis sinusitis and otitis media.

Management: No specific treatment exists for the common cold. The goals of treatment are to:

- Relieve symptoms
- Inhibit spread of infections, and
- Reduce the risk of bacterial complications.

Rest, fluids, proper diet, antipyretics and analgesics are helpful. Complications of acute rhinitis include pharyngitis, sinusitis, otitis media, tonsilitis, and chest infection. Treat with proper antibiotic therapy. Antibiotics have no effect on virus if taken unjudiciously, may produce resistance organisms.

Allergic Rhinitis

Aetiology: Allergic rhinitis (hayfever) is a type I-hypersensitive reaction. It is the reaction of the nasal mucosa to a specific antigen (allergen). Attacks of seasonal rhinitis usually occur in spring and fall and are caused by allergy to pollens from trees, flowers or grasses or weeds. Inhaled allergens are classified as outdoor (seasonal) also called acute or indoor (perennial), also called chronic. The outdoor allergens are pollen of trees, grasses or weeds. Inhaled allergens are classified as outdoor (seasonal) also called acute or indoor (perennial), also called chronic. The outdoor allergens are pollen of trees, grasses or weeds. The indoor allergens are spores of molds, dustmites, and animal danders.

Clinical manifestation: Manifestations of allergic rhinitis are nasal congestion, sneezing, watery, itchy eyes and nose, altered sense of smell and thin watery nasal discharge. The nasal turbinates appear pale, boggy and swollen. The turbinates may fill the air space and press against the nasal septum. The posterior ends of the turbinates can become so enlarged that they obstruct sinus aeration or drainage and result in sinusitis. With chronic exposure to allergens the patient responses include, headache, congestion, pressure and postnasal drip. The patient may complain of cough, hoarseness, or the recurrent need to clear throat. Congestion may be sufficient to cause snoring. Nasal polyps may be present if the allergy has persisted for a long time.

Management: There are several measures used in management of allergic rhinitis. The measures to reduce symptoms of allergic rhinitis are:

- Avoidance is the best treatment.
- *Avoid house dust* Use the approach "less is best". Focus on the bedroom. Remove carpeting. Limit furniture. Enclose the pillows, mattresses and springs in airtight, zipper-sealed, vinyl cloth bags, install an airfilter if possible. Close the airconditioning vent into the room.
- *Avoid house dust-mites* Wash building in hot water (130°F) weekly. Wear a mask when vacuuming. Double bag the vacuum cleaner. Install a filter on the outlet post of the

vacuum cleaner. Avoid sleeping or lying on upholstered furniture. Remove carpets that are laid down on concrete. If possible, have someone else for cleaning the house.

- *Avoid mold spores* The three 'D's that promote growth of mold spores are darkness, dampness, and drafts. Avoid places where humidity is high (e.g. basements, camps on the lake, clothe hampers, greenhouses, stables, barns). Dehumidifiers are rarely helpful. Ventilate closed rooms, open doors and install fans. Consider adding windows to dark room. Consider keeping lights on in closets. A basement light with a timer that provides light several hours a day decreases mold growth.
- *Avoid pollens* Stay inside with closed doors and windows during high-pollen season. Avoid the use of fans. Install an airconditioner with a good airfilter. Wash filter weekly during high pollen season. Put the car air-conditioner on "recirculate" when driving.
- *Avoid pet allergens* Remove pets from the interior of the home. Clean the living area thoroughly. Do not expect instant relief. Symptoms usually do not improve significantly for 2 months following pet removal.
- *Avoid smoke* The presence of a smoker will sabotage the best of all possible symptom reduction programme.

The drug therapy involves the use of antihistamines, decongestants and nasal sprays. An oral antihistamine or oral decongestant is typically used first. If therapy is not effective, a nasal corticosteroid spray may be used to decrease inflammation. Corticosteroid administered by a nasal spray are purely absorbed in the system in circulation.

i. *Antihistamines* bind with H_1 receptors on target cells, block of histamine binding. Relieve acute symptoms of allergic response (itching, sneezing, excessive secretions, mild congestions) may cause sedation (diminished alertness, slow reaction time, somnolence) and stimulation (restlessness, nervous insomnia) and may cause palpitation tachycardia, urinary retention or frequency. So, the nurse warns the patient regarding side effects and teaches the patient to report palpitations, change in heart rate, change in bowel, bladder habits and instruct the patient not to use alcohol with antihistamines because of additive depressive effects.

An example of antihistamine includes first generation agents such as ethanalamines (e.g. benzedrine) ethylenediamines, alkylamins (chloropheniramine) piperazines, piperidine, phenothazine (phenergan), etc. The second generation agents such as Astemizole, Loratadine, Cetrizone, etc.

ii. *Decongestants* stimulate adrenergic receptors on blood vessels promote vasoconstriction and reduce nasal oedema and rhinorrhoea. Example oral pseudoephedrin (sudafed), topical-nasal-spray: e.g. oxymetazoline, phenylephrine. The side effects include CNS stimulation causing insomnia, excitation, headache, irritability, increased blood and ocular pressure, dysuria, palpitations, tachycardia. Here the nurse advises patient of adverse reactions. Advise some preparations are contraindicated for patients with cardiovascular diseases, hypertension, diabetes, glaucoma, prostate hyperplasia, hepatic and renal disease. Teach patient that these drugs should not be used for more than 3 days or more than 3-4 times a day. Longer use increases risk of rhinitis medicamentosa.

iii. *Corticosteroids* nasal spray inhibits inflammatory response. At recommended dose, systemic side effects are unlikely because of low systemic absorption. If used greater than prescribed dose, mild transient nasal burning and stringing occurs. Here nurse should teach patient correct use instruct patient to use on regular basis and not p r n reinforce that spray acts to decrease inflammation, and discontinue the use of nasal infection develop.

iv. *Mast cell stabilizer* i.e. nasal spray (cromolyn spray, nidocromia spray) inhibits degranulation of sensitized mast cells which occurs after exposure to specific antigen. Has minimal side effects. Teach patient correct use, explain occurrence of nasal irritation or burning.

v. *Anticholenergic* nasal spray (ipratropium bromide), blocks hypersecretory effects by competing in binding sites on the cell. Reduces rhinorrhea and common cold, allergic and non-allergic rhinitis. The side effects include dryness of mouth and nose. Does not cause systemic side effects.

Chronic rhinitis is a chronic inflammation of the mucous membrane with increased nasal mucosa caused by repeated acute infections, by an allergy or by vasomotor rhinitis. The cause of vasomotor rhinitis is unclear but this condition may result from an instability of the autonomic nervous system caused by stress, tension or some endocrine disorders. Rhinitis may also be caused by the overuse of nose drops.

In addition to measures of management of rhinitis suggestion is made in acute allergic rhinitis, that the patient should be taught to *self-administration of nose drops* as given below.

- Wash hands
- Assume a position that will facilitate flow of medication:
  - Sit on chair and tip head well backward, or
  - Lie down with head extended over the edge of bed, or
  - Lie down with pillow under shoulders and head tipped backwards.
- Turn head to side that will receive the drops.
- Place no more than 3 drops of solution into each nostril at one time (unless otherwise prescribed).
- Remaining position with head tilted backward for 3 to 5 minutes to permit solution to reach posterior nares.
- If marked congestion is still present 10 minutes after nose drop insertion, another drop or two of solutions may be administered (nasal constriction from first insertion may facilitate additional drops reaching posterior nares).

And advise the person with rhinitis regarding

- Obtain additional rest.

- Drink at least 2 to 3 litres of fluid daily
- Medications: Use nasal spray or nose drops two or three times per day as ordered.
- Prevention of further infection.
  - Blow nose with both nostrils open to prevent infected matter from being forced into eustachian tube.
  - Cover mouth with disposable tissues when coughing and sneezing to prevent droplet nuclei from contaminating the air.
  - Dispose of used tissues carefully.
  - Avoid exposure when possible (i.e. avoid crowds, people with cold specific allergens). Elderly persons and those with chronic lung diseases are particularly vulnerable and should have a flu shot yearly.
  - Wash hands frequently and especially after coughing, blowing the nose, sneezing, and so on. Evidences suggest that several types of colds are transmitted from person to person by hand contact and from touching objects handled by persons with a cold.
  - Seek medical attention if the following are present.
- High fever, severe chest pain, earache
- Symptoms lasting longer than 2 weeks
- Recurrent cold.

Sinusitis

The sinuses are airfilled cavities lined with nucleus membranes. Any inflammation of the mucous membrane of the sinuses is termed as "Sinusitis".

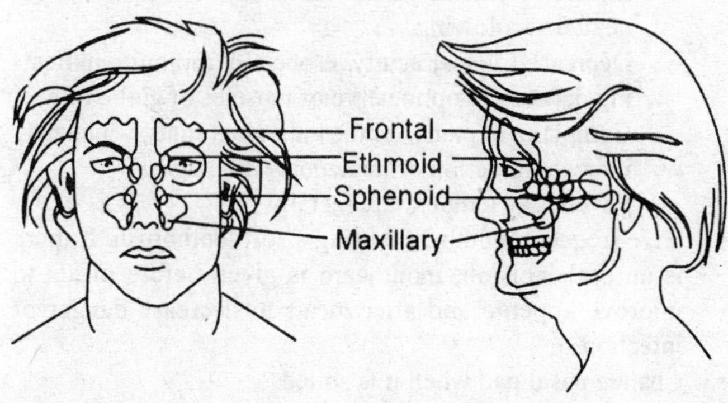

Fig. 6.1: Paranasal sinuses

Aetiology

Sinusitis develops when the ostia (exit) from the sinuses is narrowed or blocked by inflammation or hypertrophy (swelling) of the mucosa. The secretions that accumulate behind the obstruction provide a rich medium for growth of bacteria, viruses and fungi all of which cause infections.

- Bacterial sinusitis is most commonly caused by streptococcus pneumoniae, *Haemophilus influenzae*, or moraxella catarrhalis, betahaemolytic streptococcus, Klebsiellapneumoniae, anareobic organism.
- Viral sinusitis follows an upper respiratory infection in which the virus penetrates the mucous membrane and decreases ciliary transports, e.g. rhinovirus, parainfluenza, adenovirus.
- Fungal sinusitis is uncommon and is usually found in patients who are debilated or immunocompromised.

Acute sinusitis usually results from an URI, allergic rhinitis, swimming or dental manipulations all of which cause inflammatory changes and retention of secretions. Chronic sinusitis generally results from repeated episodes of a acute sinusitis that result in irreversible loss of the normal ciliated epithelium lining the sinus cavity.

Pathophysiology

The first symptom of acute bacterial sinusitis is usually a stuffy nose followed by slowly developing pressure over the involved sinus. Other signs and symptoms include general malaise and toxicity, persistent cough, postnasal drip, headache slightly elevated or normal temperature and mild leukopnoea. Symptoms worsen over 48 to 72 hours culminating in severe localised pain and tenderness over the involved sinus. The patient often believes that the pain is due to an infected tooth.

In acute frontal and maxillary sinusitis pain usually does not appear until 1 to 2 hours after awakening. It increases for 3 to 4 hours after awakening and then becomes less severe in the afternoon and evening. There may be bloody or blood-tinged discharge from the nose in the first 24 to 48 hours. The discharge rapidly becomes thick, green and copious, blocking the nose. The throat may become inflamed and sore on one side, because of the purulent discharge.

Clinical Manifestation

Acute sinusitis causes significant pain over the affected sinus purulent nasal drainage, nasal obstruction, congestion, fever and malaise. The patient looks and feels sick. Assessment involves inspection of the nasal mucosa and palpation of the sinus points for pain. Findings that indicate acute sinusitis include a hyperemic and edematous mucosa, enlarged turbinates and tenderness over the involved sinuses. Pain is caused by the accumulation of pus and absorption of air behind a blocked ostium. The patient also experiences recurrent headaches that change in intensity with position or when secretions drain.

Management

For most patients, diagnosis is made without any studies. Certain cases of radiographic studies are indicated particularly chronic sinuses, conventional sinus X-rays, computed tomography (CT) and MRI. Fibrocystic examination of the nose (Rhinoscopy) may also be used. Management of acute bacterial sinusitis centers on relief of pain and shrinkage of the nasal mucosa. Ibuprofen and oral decongestant such as pseudoephedrine are commonly prescribed. In some patients, codeine may be required for pain relief. The antibiotic of choice is limited for 10 days. If patient does not improve after 5 days of amoxicilline a changes of antibiotics may be necessary, which includes Loracarbef amoxicillin clavulanate potassium (Augmentin), cefacler, doxycycline, trimethoprim, and sulfamethoxazole, clarithromycin, azithromycin (5 days).

Patient may obtain relief from saline nasal sprays steam, from a shower, or a humidifier. Hot wet packs applied to the face over the infected sinus (es) either continuously or for 1 to 2 hours at a time for four times a day may provide symptomatic relief. A washcloth wrung out in hot water is convenient way to provide wet pack.

Acute frontal sinusitis with pain, terness and edema of the frontal or sphenoid sinus may require hospitalization because of the risk of intracranial complications and osteomyelitis. High dose of intravenous antibiotic and nasal congestants orally or spray may be ordered.

Fungal sinusitis can range from mild infections resembling chronic sinusitis to severe life-threatening invasive infections, needs prolonged and necessary antibiotics or surgical drainage of sinuses.

Invasive fungal sinusitis is most likely to occur in transplant patients, patients on chemotherapy, patients with AIDS, or persons with controlled diabetes. Aspergillus and Mucor are two types of fungi most prone to cause invasive disease. Symptoms include facial fullness, cranial neuropathies, and pain. Proptosis of the eye, facial swelling and blood-stinged discharge may be present. These patients need hospitalization. Treatment includes IV amphoterun B, aggressive surgical management are required.

The types of sinus surgery are:

- Functional endoscopic sinus surgery (FESS): Here sinus endoscope enters sinus and removes diseased mucosa and opens ostia. It is used for chronic sinusitis and removal of polyps.
- Caldwell-Luc (Radical Antrum perforation): Here clearing out of maxillary sinus through incision under upper lip, It is used as chronic maxillary sinusitis.
- *Transnasal external or trânsantral ethimoidectomy* Various approaches used to excise inject ethmoid and sphenoid cells. It is used in chronic ethimoid and sphenoid sinusitis.
- *Erontal sinusectomy* A complete removal of diseased mucosa of both frontal sinus, space packed with subcutaneous fat from abdomen. Performed in chronic frontal sinusitis.
- *Epheroid sinus surgery* Ethmoid sinus removed and anterior wall of sphenoid sinus opened. Performed in chronic sphenoid sinusitis.

The nurse has to perform preoperative teaching for the person undergoing sinus surgery, which includes.

– Determine patients' understanding about the surgical procedure. Clarify misconceptions and answer patients' and family questions. Explain that the patient will:

- Have nothing to eat or drink for 6 to 8 hours preoperatively.
- Receive a sedative before surgery.
- Feel pressure, not pain during surgery.
- Have a nasal pack for 24 to 48 hours postoperatively and may feel like he or she has a "head cold".
- Have a "black eyes" and swelling around the nose and eyes for 1 to 2 weeks postoperatively.
- Have prescription for pain medication as needed.

Postoperative care of the person undergoing sinus surgery will include:

- After general anaesthesia, position patient well into the side to prevent swelling of aspiration of blood drainage.
- Administer cool mist via face tent or collar, or provide humidifier.
- When the patient is awake, remind him or her to expectorate secretions and not swallow them.
- Encourage mid-Fowler's position when fully awake to promoted drainage and decrease oedema.
- Apply ice compresses over nose (or ice bag over nose, (or ice bag over maxillary and frontal sinuses) in the early postoperative period.
- Monitor patient for
  - Excessive bleeding from nose (may be evidence of repeated swallowing.
  - Decreased visual acuity, especially diplopia, indicating damage to optic nerve or muscles of globe of eye.
  - Complaint of pain over the individual sinus, which may indicate infection or inadequate drainage.
  - Fever–take temperature rectally.
- Give frequent mouth care using a soft toothbrush. If there is an oral incision, mouthcare is given before meals to improve appetite and after meals to decrease danger of infection.
- Change nasal pad when it is soiled
- Apply ice compresses to ecchymosis areas to constrict blood vessels, decrease oozing and oedema, and help relieve pain.
- Encourage liberal fluid intake. Patient may be very thirsty because of dry mouth from mouth breathing.
- Teach patient to:
  a. Avoid blowing nose for at least 48 hours after packing is removed to prevent bleeding.
  b. Avoid sneezing: If the patient must sneeze he or she should keep mouth open.

c. Avoid lifting heavy objects.
d. Report signs of infection–fever, purulent discharge to surgeon.
e. Expect tarry stools from swallowed blood for a few days.
f. Avoid constipation (Valsalvas manoeuvre–i.e. straining can cause bleeding).
g. Expect that ecchymosis of nose and eyes will begin to change colour over next 1 to 2 weeks.
h. Take prophylactic antibiotics as prescribed. Do not stop until all medication is taken.

In addition, patients are advised to take more rest to heal; precaution to be given blowing and sneezing. Keep head ele-vated for proper breathing, small dressing pad → around dressing to absorb drainage, and instruct the patient not to take aspirin or any product containing aspirin, which can cause bleeding and caution with oral hygiene to avoid injury to the incisions.

Acute Pharyngitis

Acute pharyngitis is an acute inflammation of the pharyngeal walls. It may include the tonsils, palate, and uvula.

Aetiology

It may be caused by haemolytic streptococci, staphylococci, other bacteria, filterable virus or fungi. Acute follicular pharyngitis (strep throat) results from beta haemolytic streptococcal invasion. Neisseria gonorrhoea and corynebacterium diphtheria and other bacteria causing pharyngitis. Fungal pharyngitis caused by candidiasis can develop prolonged use of antibiotics or inhaled corticosteroids as in immunosuppressed patient (e.g. AIDS).

Pathophysiology

Dryness of the throat is common complaint. The throat appears red, and soreness may range from slight scratchiness to severe pain with difficulty in swallowing. A. hacking cough may be present. Children often develop a very high fever, whereas adults may have only a mild elevation of temperature, symptoms usually precede or occur simultaneously with the onset of acute rhinitis or acute sinusitis.

Clinical Manifestation

In follicular pharyngitis uniform infection of pharyngeal walls, purulent exudate, oedema of lymphoid tissue of palate, tonsils uvula, occur and show sore throat, slightly elevated temperature, and malaise.

In gonococcal or viral pharyngitis, vesicles may be present on pharyngeal walls and tonsils occurs. There will be minimal discomfort, fever, diffuse sore throat.

In infectious mononucleosis (Epstein-Barr virus), exudate on pharyngeal walls and tonsils, spleen may be enlarged. There will be a sore throat, cervical lymphadenopathy, and fever.

Fungal pharyngitis (e.g. especially cardidiases-Thrush) develop in patient who is immune suppressed and in prolong antibiotics. There will be pus, dysphagia, white plaque, in mouth or on pharyngeal walls.

Management

Acute pharyngitis is usually relieved by hot saline throat gargles. An ice collar may make the person feel more comfortable. For adults acetylsalicylic acid administered orally Aspergum may be prescribed. Lozenges containing a mild anaesthetic may help relieve local soreness. Moist inhalations may help relieve local soreness. A liquid diet usually is better tolerated than solid food and fluids to at least 2.5 litre per day is encouraged.

Oral hygiene may prevent drying and cracking of the lips and usually refreshes the mouth. If the temperature is elevated, the person should remain in bed and even if ambulatory and a febrile, should have extra rest.

A throat culture is necessary to identify the offending organism. For follicular pharyngitis, the choice of antibiotic is penicillin. If person is allergic to penicillin, erythromycin or other antibiotic is prescribed. Candida infections are treated with nystatin and antifungal, antibiotic.

The goals of nursing management are infection control, symptomatic relief and prevention of secondary complications. The patient should be encouraged to increase fluid intake, cool, bland liquids and gelatin will not irritate pharynx. Citrus fruits juice should be avoided because they irritate the mucous membrane. And make the patient understand the need to take prescribed antibiotic until the course is completed.

Acute Follicular Tonsillitis

Acute follicular tonsillitis is an acute inflammation of the tonsils and their crypts. It is usually caused by the streptococcus organism. It is more likely to occur when the persons's resistance is low, and it is common in children.

Pathophysiology and Clinical Manifestation

The onset is almost always sudden, and symptoms include sore throat, pain on swallowing, fever, chills, general muscle aching and malaise. These systems often last for 2 to 3 days. The pharynx and tonsils appear red, and the peritonsillar tissues are swollen. Sometimes a yellowish exudate drains from crypts in the tonsils. A throat culture usually is taken to identify the offending organism.

Complications of untreated tonsillitis include heart and kidney damage, chorea and pneumonia. Incidence of these complications is decreasing with early diagnosis and widespread use of penicillin. Recurrent attacks of tonsillitis need to undergo tonsillectomy. This procedure is usually performed from 4 to 6 weeks after an acute attack is subsided.

Peritonsillar abscess typically occurs as a complication of acute pharyngitis and acute tonsillitis if bacterial invasion of one or both tonsils. The tonsils may enlarge sufficiently to threaten airway patency. Infections extend from the tonsils to form an access in the surrounding tissues. The presence of pus behind the tonsils causes difficulty in swallowing, talking and opening the mouth, the difficulty in swallowing may be so great that the person is unable to swallow. Pain is severe and may extend to the ear on the affected side. The patient will experience high fever, leukocytosis and chills.

Management

The patient with acute tonsillitis is encouraged to rest and take generous amounts of fluid orally. Warm saline throat gargle (irrigation) may be ordered, and antibiotics are given for streptococcal pharyngitis, acetaminophen (tyclerol) and codeine sulfate may be ordered for pain and discomfort. An ice collar applied to the neck may relieve discomfort.

Early detection and treatment with IV antibiotic therapy may clear the infection and prevent abscess development. If antibiotics to which the offending organism is sensitive are administered early, infection subsides. If the peritonsillar abscess caused by anaerobic organisms hydrogen peroxide (an oxidizing agent) in the form of mouthwash may help to relieve symptoms. If an abscess develops incision and drainage are required. An emergency tonsillectomy may be performed, or an elective tonsillectomy may be scheduled after the infection subsided.

Chronic Enlargement of Adenoids and Tonsils

Tonsils and adenoids are lymphoid structures located in the oropharynx and nasopharynx. They reach full size in childhood and then begin to atrophy during puberty. When adenoids enlarge, usually results of chronic infections but sometimes for no known reason they cause nasal obstructions. The person breathes through mouth, snores loudly, may have a dull facial expression and may have reduced appetite, because the blocked nasopharynx can interfere with swallowing. Hypertrophy of the tonsils does not usually block the oropharynx but may affect speech and swallowing and cause mouth breathing.

Pathophysiology

The tonsils are red and swollen with yellow or white exudate found mainly in the crypts of the tonsils. Signs and symptoms include fever, dry throat, malaise, dysphagia, otalgia, and a feeling of fullness in the throat. Lymph nodes in upper part of the neck is swollen and palpable.

Management

The tonsils and adenoids are removed when they become enlarged and cause symptoms of obstruction, when they are chronically infected. When the person has repeated attacks of tonsillitis or after repeated peritonsillar abscess. Chronic infections of these structures usually do not respond to antibiotics and may become foci of infections by spreading organisms to other parts of the body such as heart and kidney.

Tonsillectomy is performed with either general or local anaesthesia. After tonsils are removed, pressure is applied to stop superficial bleeding. Bleeding vessels are tied off with sutures or by electrocoagulation. The person is monitored carefully for haemorrhage, especially when sleeping, because a large amount of blood may be lost without any external evidence of bleeding. The person who is bleeding excessively often is returned to the operating room for surgical treatment to stop the haemorrhage. If sutures are used, the person will have more pain and discomfort than that occurring after simple tonsillectomy and may be unable to take solid food for several days.

The tough, yellow, fibrous membrane that forms over the operative site begins to break away between the fourth and eight postoperative days and haemorrhage may occur. The separation of the membranes accounts for throat being more painful at this time.

Pink granulation tissue soon becomes apparent and by the end of the third postoperative week, the area is covered with normal mucous membrane.

The following points to be kept in mind while taking care of a person after tonsillectomy:

- Position patient on side until fully awake after general anaesthesia of in mid-Fowler's position when awake.
- Monitor for haemorrhage
  - Frequent swallowing (inspect throat)
  - Bright red vomitus
  - Rapid pulse
  - Restlessness.
- Comfort
  - Give 30 per cent cool mist via collar
  - Apply ice collar to neck (will also reduce bleeding by vasoconstriction)
  - Use acetamonephin in place of aspirin (in tendency on bleeding)
- Food and fluids
  - Give ice-cold fluids and bland foods during initial period (e.g. ice chips, popsicles, jella)
  - Milk is usually not given, because it may increase mucus and cause the patient to clear the throat.
  - Advance to normal diet as soon as possible.
- Patient and family teaching
  - Avoid attempting to clear throat immediately after surgery (may initiate bleeding)
  - Avoid coughing, sneezing, vigorous nose blowing and vigorous exercise for 1 to 2 weeks
  - Drink fluids (2 to 3 L/day) until mouth odour disappears
  - Avoid hard, scratchy foods such as pretzels, popcorn or toast, until throat is healed

- Report signs of bleeding to physician immediately
- Expect more throat discomfort between 4th and 8th postoperative days because of membrane separation
- Expect stool to be black or dark for a few days because of swallowed blood
- Resume normal activity immediately as long as it is not stressful and does not require straining.

Acute Laryngitis

Acute laryngitis is an inflammation of the mucous membrane lining of the larynx accompanied by oedema of the vocal cords. It may be caused by cold, by sudden changes in temperature or by irritating fumes.

Pathophysiology/Clinical Manifestation

Symptoms vary from a slight huskiness to complete loss of voice. The throat may be painful and feel scratching, and a cough may be present.

Management

Laryngitis management requires only symptomatic treatment. The person is advised to remain indoors in an even temperature and to avoid talking for several days or weeks, depending on the severity of the inflammation. Steam inhalation may be soothing and cough syrups or home remedies for cough to provide relief to some patients. Smoking should be avoided. Additional fluids by mouth help prevent dehydration and drying of throat.

The nursing role is mainly patient teaching, which could include the following.

- Need to take antibiotics as prescribed (Full course as prescribed)
- Need to increase fluid intake
- Need to stop smoking for smokers
- Need to avoid smoky environment
- Refferral to a support group of persons wanting to stop smoking
- Precautions to be observed in using steam inhalations.

Chronic laryngitis may occur in persons who use their voices excessively, who smoke a great deal or who work continuously where there are irritating fumes. Hoarseness usually is worse in early morning and evening. There may be dry, harsh cough. Treatment of chronic laryngitis includes removal of irritants, voice test, correction of faulty voice habits, steam inhalation. Additional fluid by mouth care are encouraged.

Laryngeal Paralysis

Laryngeal paralysis may result from disease or injury of either the laryngeal nerves or the vagus nerve.

Aetiology

Laryngeal paralysis may be caused by

- Aortic aneurysm
- Mitral stenosis
- Laryngeal cancer
- Subglottic or cervical esophageal tumours
- Bronchial carcinoma
- Neck injury
- Severing or stretching of the recurrent laryngeal nerve during thyroidectomy
- Prolonged intubation of patients in intensive care units.

Pathophysiology

Either one or both vocal cords may be paralyzed. If only one cord is affected, the airway is adequate and now the voice may be affected. Efforts to improve the voice in persons with unilateral cord paralysis have been accomplished by injecting a small quantity of Gelfoam or Teflan into paralyzed cord. This swells the cord and pushes it towards the midline where the other cord can approximate it better during phonation.

Bilateral paralysis causes a poor airway that results in incapacitating dyspnoea, stridor on exertion and a weak voice. A sudden bilateral vocal cord paralysis is not common and usually a result of massive cerebrovascular accident or blunt trauma both of which are incompatible with life.

Management

Diagnostic tests performed include:

- Indirect laryngoscopy to diagnose vocal cord abnormality
- Videostroboscopy (observe vocal cords vibration during phonation). Here fibreoptic laryngoscope is attached to videotape to record actual cord motion. This is to diagnose abnormal vibrations of cord.
- Electromyography to determine innervation and thus movement of vocal cords.
- CT scan to determine cause of vocal cord paresis or paralysis such as tumour or aneurysm along course of recurrent laryngeal nerve.

Treatment of laryngeal paralysis is symptomatic.

- Antacids are used if patient experiencing gastroesophageal reflux which neutralize gastric acid.
- H_2 inhibitor, used to reduce the amount of gastric acid produced.
- Antibiotics are used for infection.
- Tracheostomy may be necessary to maintain airway
- Other procedures are followed according to causes.

Laryngeal Oedema

Acute laryngeal oedema may be caused by anaphylaxis, urticaria, acute laryngitis, scream inflammatory diseases to the throat or oedema after intubation. It causes the airway to narrow or close and required immediate restoration of the airway.

Treatment of acute laryngeal oedema consists of administration of an adrenocorticosteroid or epinephrine. Intubation or tracheostomy may be necessary.

Airway Obstruction

Airway may be complete or partial. Complete airway obstruction is medical emergency. Partial airway obstructions may occur as a result of aspiration of food as foreign body. In addition, partial airway obstruction may result from laryngeal oedema following extubation laryngeal or tracheal stenosis, and neurologic depression.

Symptoms include stridor, use of accessory muscles, suprasternal and intercoastal retractions, wheezing, restlessness, tachycardia and cyanosis.

Management

Prompt assessment and treatment are essential because partial obstructions may quickly progress to complete destruction. Interventions to maintain a patient airway include use of obstructed airway (Heimlich) manoeuvre, endotracheal intubation and tracheostomy.

An endotracheal tube is usually chosen initially as a means of providing airway, tracheostomy is performed only if airway maintenance is necessary for longer than 10 to 14 days or if trauma to the airway prevents the use of an endotracheal tube.

In endotracheal intubation, a tube is passed through either the nose or mouth into the trachea, whereas in a tracheostomy, an artificial opening is made in the trachea into which a tracheostomy tube is inserted. The procedures are used to:

- Establish and maintain patent airway
- Prevent aspiration by sealing off the trachea from digestive tract in the unconscious or paralysed person
- Permit removal of tracheobronchial secretions in the person who cannot cough adequately, and
- Treat the patient who requires positive pressure mechanical ventilation that cannot be given effectively by masks.

The endotracheal tubes is made of plastic with an inflatable cuff so that a closed system with the ventilator may be maintained. The tube is inserted via the mouth or nose through the larynx into the trachea. If an oral endotracheal tube is used, a rubber airway or bite block is often necessary to prevent the patient from biting down on the tube and obstructing the airway.

Tracheostomy

A tracheostomy is a surgical incision into the trachea for the purpose of establishing an airway. It is the stoma (an opening) that results from the tracheostomy. Indications for a tracheostomy are to:

- Bypass an upper airway obstruction,
- Facilitate removal of secretions,
- Permit long-term mechanical ventilation, and
- Permit oral intake and speech in the patient who requires long-term mechanical ventilation.

Nursing Care

Before the procedure the nurse should explain to the patient and the family the purpose of the procedure and inform them that the patient will not be able to speak if an inflated cuff is used.

The patient and family should be informed the normal speech will be possible as soon as the cuff can be deflated.

A variety of tubes are available to meet individual patient needs, which includes:

i. Tracheostomy tube with cuff and inflated balloons: When properly inflated, lower pressure, high-volume cuff distributes cuff pressure over large areas, minimizing pressure on tracheal wall.
ii. Fenestrated tracheostomy tube with cuff and inner cannula and decannulation plug: when inner cannula is removed, cuff deflated, and decannulation plug inserted, air flows around the tube through fenestration in outer cannula and up over vocal cords. Patient can then speak.
iii. Speaking tracheostomy tube (Portex, National) with cuff, two external tubings; It has two tubings, one leading to cuff and second to opening above the cuff. When port is connected to air source, air flows out of opening and up over the vocal cords, allowing speech in the cuff inflated.
iv. Tracheostomy tube (Bivona Fome-cuff) foam filled cuff: This cuff is filled with plastic foam. Before insertion, cuff is deflated. After insertion, cuff is allowed to fill passively with air. Pilot tubing is not capped and no cuff pressure monitoring is required.

All tracheostomy tubes contain a face plate or flange, which rests on the neck between the clavicles and outer cannula. In addition, all tubes have an obturator, which is used when inserting the tube. During insertion of the tube, the obturator is placed inside the outer cannula with its rounded tip protruding from air end of the tube to ease insertion. After insertion, the obturator must be immediately removed so that air can flow through the tube. The obturator should be kept in an easily accessible place at the bedside (e.g. taped to the wall) so that it can be used quickly in case of accidental decannulation.

Nursing Management of Endotracheal or Tracheostomy Tube

An endotracheal or tracheostomy tube provides a direct route for introduction of pathogen, into the lower airway, increasing the risk of infection. It is essential that the following preventive nursing intervention be consistently implemented.

1. Minimize infection risk
    - Endotracheal airways irritate the trachea resulting in increased mucus production. Assess the patient regularly for excess secretions and suction as often as necessary to maintain a patent airway.

- Provide constant airway humidifications. Endotracheal airways bypass the upper airway which normally humidifies and warms inspired air. An external source of cool, humidified air must be provided to avoid thickening and crusting of bronchial secretions.
- All respiratory therapy equipment should be changed every 6 hours. In addition:
  – Replace any equipment that touches the floor,
  – Remove water that condenses in equipment tubing. Do not pour condensed water back into humidifier reservoir, because it may contain pathogens.
- Provide frequent mouth care. Secretions tend to pool in the mouth and in the pharynx, particularly if the cuff of the tube is inflated. An endotracheal tube or oral airway increases the risk of ulceration or abrasion of the lips and oropharynx.
  – Gently suction oropharynx as needed
  – Inspect the lips, tongue and oral cavity regularly
  – Clean the oral cavity with swab soaked in saline
  – Apply moisturising agent to cracked lips.
- Maintain adequate nutrition levels.

a. The person with endotracheal tube is allowed nothing by mouth. Nourishment will be given parenterally or gastrointestinal feedings. Gastrointestinal supplemental feedings are preferred because they maintain the function of the gut, proposeless infection risk, and more economical than IV fluids. While administering GI feeding to the intubated patient, nurse will:
   – Assess for bowel sounds and tube placement,
   – Elevate head of the bed at least 45 degrees, and
   – Inflate the tracheostomy tube cuff.
     - If using a Salem sump nasogastric tube, check the amount of residual feeding. If the half volume of the feeding to be given remains, the tube feeding is withheld.
     - Administer the tube feeding over 20-30 minutes.
     - Keep head of bed elevated for 45-60 minutes after feeding.
     - Assess at regular intervals for aspiration.
     - Regularly assess for tube placement and residual stomach contents.

b. The patient with a tracheostomy tube is usually able to swallow and have a normal oral intake. Some experts prefer that the cuff on the tracheostomy tube be inflated while the patient is eating to prevent aspiration. Others believe that cuff bulges into oesophagus and make swallowing more difficult, and they therefore prefer that cuff be deflated. Nursing assessment will determine which technique to be used. Methyline blue dye can be swallowed before each feeding or mixed with tube feeding. If the dye does not appear in tracheal secretions, it is safe to proceed with the meal.

2. Ensure adequate ventilation and oxygenation
   - Assess lung sounds regularly. Unless the individual's underlying pathology alters lung ventilations, sounds should be heard bilaterally, and chest expansion should be symmetrical. If an endotracheal tube is inserted too far it will slip into one of the mainstems of bronchi (usually the night) and occlude the opposite bronchus and lung resulting in atelectasis on the obstructed side. Even if the endotracheal tube is still in the trachea, airway obstruction will result if the end of the tube is located on the carina. This will result in dry secretions that obstruct both bronchi. So the tube is pulled back until it is positioned below the larynx and above the carina. The tube is then fastened securely in place.
   - Turn and reposition the patient every 2 hours for maximum ventilation and lung perfusion.
   - Assess respiratory frequency, tidal volume and viral capacity
   - Perform postural drainage, percussion and vibration as appropriate

3. Provide safety and comfort.
   - Most endotracheal and tracheostomy tubes have cuffs for the following reasons
     – To provide a sealed airway for positive pressure mechanical ventilation, and
     – To prevent aspirations in the unconscious person during tube feedings
   - Assess tube placement in regular intervals.
     – The tube is secured around neck with tape or specially designed ties, and
     – The endotracheal tube is marked to establish a landmark for position comparison and to measure and document the length of the tube that extends beyond the patient lips.
   - Change tapes or ties whenever soiled to decreased skin irritation.
   - Always keep a spare tube at the bedside.
   - Minimize sensory deprivations. Because patients with these tubes with cuff-inflated cannot talk. Therefore, an acceptable communication mode must be established as follows:
     – Organise questions so that patient can use a simple 'Yes' or 'No' response (nodding head, using hand signals, or squeezing the nurse's hand),
     – The patient may be able to use an erasable board or note pad to communicate,
     – Always talk to the patient and explain all procedures,

- Reorient the patient frequently,
- Encourage family and friends to talk to patient and offer encouragement,
- Keep call light (or tap bell) within the patient's reach
- Reinforce that the ability to speak will return when the tube is removed.

4. Observe special precautions during the immediate extubation period
   - Monitor for signs such as increased respiratory distress, increased restlessness, hoarseness and laryngeal stridor indicating upper airway obstruction secondary to laryngeal oedema.
   - Assess for adequacy of cough and gag reflex
   - After removal of a tracheostomy tube there is a temporary air leak at the incision site. To speak, the patient will have to occlude the opening with a finger.
   - The tracheal stoma can be suctioned. However, frequent use of the stoma for suctioning can delay closure and healing of tracheostomy incisions.

Procedure for Suctioning a Tracheostomy Tube

1. Assess the need for suctioning 4th hourly. Indications include coarse crackles or rhonchi over large airways, moist cough, increase in peak inspiratory pressure and mechanical ventilator and restlessness or agitation if accompanied by decrease in SPO_2 or PaO_2. Do not suction routinely or if patient is able to clear secretion with cough.
2. If suctioning indicated, explain the procedure to the patient.
3. Collect necessary equipment; suction catheters no larger than half the lumen of the tracheostomy tube), gloves, water, cup, and drape. If a closed tracheal suction is used, the catheter is enclosed in a plastic sleeves and reused for 24 hours. No, additional equipment is needed.
4. Check suction source and regulator. Adjust suction pressure until the dial reads-120 to 150 mm Hg pressure with tubing occluded.
5. Wash hands,. put on goggles and gloves.
6. Use sterile technique to open package, fill cup with water, put on gloves, and connect catheter to suction. Designate on hand as contaminated for disconnecting, bagging and operating the suction control. Suction water through the catheter to test the system.
7. Assess SPO_2 heart rate and rhythm to provide baseline for detecting change during suctioning.
8. Provide preoxygenation by (i) adjusting ventilator to deliver 100 per cent O_2, (ii) using reservoir-equipped manual resuscitate bag (MRB) connected to 100 per cent O_2; or (iii) asking patient to take 3-4-deep breaths. While administering oxygen, the method chosen will depend on the patient's underlying disease and ability or illness. The patient who has tracheostomy for an extended period of time and is not acutely ill, may be able to tolerate suctioning without use of an MRB or the ventilator.
9. Gently insert the catheter without suction to minimize the amount of oxygen removed from the lungs. Insert the catheter approximately 5-6 inches. Stop if any obstruction is met.
10. Withdraw the catheter 1-2 cm and apply suction intermittently, while withdrawing catheter in a rotating manner. If secretion volume is large, apply suction continuously.
11. If the patient develops mucous plugs or thick secretions a 3-5 ml bolus of normal saline may be instilled into the airway to loosen secretions sufficiently to clear the airway either through coughing or suctioning.
12. Limit suction time to 10 seconds. Discontinue suctioning if heart rate decreases from baseline by 20 beats, increases from baseline by 40 beats per minute, an arrhythmias or SPO_2 decreases to less than 90 per cent.
13. After each suction-pass, oxygenate with 3-4 breaths by ventilator, MRB or deep breaths with oxygen.
14. Rinse catheter with sterile water.
15. Repeat procedure until airway is clear. Limit insertions of suction catheter to three passes.
16. Return oxygen concentration to prior setting.
17. Rinse catheter and suction the oropharynx or use mouth suction.
18. Dispose of catheter by wrapping it around fingers of gloved hand and pulling glove over catheter. Discard equipment in proper waste container.
19. Auscultate to assess changes in lung sounds. Record time, amount, and character of secretions and response to suctioning.

Tracheostomy Care

Although nursing care of persons with either endotracheal or tracheostomy tube is similar, patients with tracheostomies have additional nursing care needs. Nursing care includes maintaining air humidification, providing nourishment, and weaning for the tracheostomy tube. The care of the tracheostomy tube. The care of the tracheostomy is as follows:

1. Explain procedure to the patient.
2. Collect necessary sterile equipment (e.g. suction catheter, gloves, water, basin, drape, tracheostomy-ties, tube brush or pipe cleaners, 4x4s, hydrogen peroxide 3 per cent, sterile water and tracheostomy dressing (optional)

   Note: Clean rather than sterile technique is used at home.
3. Position patient in semi-Fowler's position.
4. Assemble needed materials on bedside table next to patient.
5. Wash hands, put on goggles and gloves.
6. Auscultate chest sounds. If rhonchi or coarse crackles are

present suction the patient if unable to cough up secretions.

7. Unlock and remove inner cannula, if present. Many tracheostomy tubes do not have inner cannula. Care for these tubes includes all steps except for inner cannula care.
8. If disposable inner cannula is used, replace with new cannula. If non-disposable cannula is used:
   - immerse inner cannula in 3 per cent hydrogen peroxide and clean inside and outside of cannula using tube brush or pipe cleaner,
   - Drain hydrogen peroxide from cannula. Immerse cannula in sterile water and shake to dry.
   - Insert inner cannula into outer cannula with the curved part downward and lock in place.
9. Remove dried secretions from stoma using 4 × 4 soaked in sterile water. Gently pat area around the stoma dry. Be sure to clean under the tracheostomy face plate, using cotton swabs to reach this area.
10. Maintain position of tracheal retention sutures if present, by taping above and below the stoma.
11. Change tracheostomy ties. Tie tracheostomy ties securely with room for one finger between ties and skin. To prevent accidental tube removal, secure the tracheostomy tube by gently applying pressure to flange of the tube during the tie changes. Do not change tracheostomy ties for 24 hours after the tracheostomy procedure.
12. As an alternative some patients prefer tracheostomy ties made of velero, which are easier to adjust, other patients use plastic IV tubing because it is easily cleaned and dries without need to replace the ties.
13. Unless excessive amounts of exudate are present avoid using a tracheostomy dressing since this keeps the site moist and may predispose to infection.
14. If drainage is excessive, place dressing around tube. A tracheostomy dressing or unlined gauze should be used. Do not cut the guaze because threads may be inhaled or wrope around the tracheostomy tube. Change the dressing frequently. Wet dressings promote infection and stoma irritation.
15. Repeat care three times a day and as needed and also follow manufacturers' instructions.

ACUTE BRONCHITIS

Bronchitis is an inflammation of the lower respiratory tract that is usually due to infection and occurs most frequently in patients with chronic respiratory disease. Bronchitis can be acute or chronic bronchitis.

Acute bronchitis is an inflammation of the bronchi and usually the trachea (tracheobronchitis).

Aetiology

Acute bronchitis occurs most often in persons with chronic lung disease. It also occurs as an extension of the URI in persons without underlying any lung disease, and is therefore communicable. It may be caused by physical and chemical agents such as dust, smoke, or volatile fumes. As air pollution increases, the incidence of acute bronchitis increases.

Acute bronchitis is typically viral, but bacterial pathogens such as *Streptococcus pneumoniae* and *Haemophilus influenzae* may also cause bronchitis, either primary or secondary infections which includes:

- Viruses: Rhinovirus, adenovirus, influenza A and B, parainfluenza virus and respiratory syncytial virus (RSV).
- Bacteria: Streptococcus pneumonia, Haemophilus influenza Moraxella catarrhalis, Bordetella pertussis, Mycoplasma pneumonia, Chlamidia pneumonia.

Pathophysiology

As a part of the inflammatory process, there is increased blood flow to the affected area, causing an increased in pulmonary secretions. A painful cough with sputum productions, low-grade fever, and malaise are common symptoms. The patient may have pain beneath the sternum caused by inflammation of the tracheal wall. Bronchitis without tracheitis never seen, and tracheobronchitis is more appropriate term for this condition. Symptoms usually last 1 for 1 to 2 weeks but may continue for 3 to 4 weeks. Rhonchi and wheezes heard on chest examination. If symptoms worsen and there is a high fever, shortness of breath, pleuritic chest pain (pain on inspiration) rapid respirations and rales or sign if consolidation on physical examination of the chest, pneumonia suspected.

Management

Treatment of acute bronchitis is mainly supportive and includes the following.

- Codeine or dextromethorphan is prescribed for nocturnal cough
- Bronchodilator therapy is prescribed for patients who are wheezing and for those whose peak expiratory rate prolonged, e.g. albuterol, or ipoatropium.
- Decongestants and antihistamines are used sparingly, if at all, because they tend to dry secretions and make them more difficult to remove.
- Oral fluids intake of 2 to 3 litre per day is encouraged if there is no contraindications to it.
- Aspirin helps to reduce fever and alleviate some of the symptoms and inflammation
- Patients who are smokers are urged to quit.
- Antibiotics are usually not prescribed unless there is evidence of bacterial infections.
- Rest is encouraged to give the body a chance to heal.

Nursing care is supportive and is directed towards helping the patient with prescribed therapy and avoiding future infections. Emphasis on assisting the patient to cough effectively, assisting with comfort, assisting with activities of daily living and teaching the patient and family.

To produce an effective cough, a deep inspiration must be followed by maximal expiratory effort against a closed glottis. This results in a tremendous increase in intrathoracic pressure. As glottis opens, mucus and inhaled particles are forced out of the airways at a high velocity. Persistent coughing can be annoying and tiring to the patient and those around him or her. Complications of persistent coughing includes, insomnia, exhaustion vomiting, urinary incontinence, rib or muscle trauma, pneumothorax, and fainting. If cough persists, give cough medication as prescribed. A semi-Fowler's position or high-Fowler's position usually facilitates breathing. Provide for good drainage of trachobronchial secretions and give antibiotics as ordered and assist in ADL.

PNEUMONIA

Pneumonia or pneumonitis is an acute inflammation of the lung tissue (lung parenchyma).

Aetiology

Pneumonia is resulting from inhalation or transport via the bloodstream of infectious agents or noxious fumes or from radiation treatment. Pneumonia is classified according to whether infection was acquired in the community or in the hospital. Thus pneumonia is classified as "community acquired pneumonia (CAP) or hospital acquired pneumonia (HAP). HAP is also called nosocomial pneumonia. The causes of pneumonia are as follows.

i. Community-acquired pneumonia caused by:
   - *Streptococcus pneumoniae*
   - *Haemophilus influenzae*
   - *Mycoplasm pneumoniae*
   - Respiratory viruses
   - *Chlamydia pneumoniae*
   - Legionella pneumophila
   - Oral anaerobes
   - Moraxella catarrhalis
   - *Staphylococcus aureus*
   - Nocardia
   - Enteric aerobic Gram-negative bacteria (e.g. Klebsiella)
   - Fungi
   - *Mycobacterium tuberculosis.*

ii. Hospital acquired pneumonia caused by:
   a. Pseudomonasaeru inosa
   b. Enterobacter
   c. *Escherichia coli*
   d. Proteus
   e. *Klebsiella*
   f. *Staphylococcus aureus*
   g. *Streptococcus pneumoniae*
   h. Oral anaerobes.

The risk factors which predispose to pneumonia are:
- Smoking
- Air pollution
- Altered consciousness: Alcoholism, head injury, seizures, anaesthesia, drug overdose
- Tracheal intubation (endotracheal intubations, tracheostomy)
- Upper respiratory tract infection
- Chronic diseases: Chronic lung diseases, diabetes mellitus, heart disease, uremia, cancer
- Immunosuppression
  - Drugs (carciosteroids, cancer chemotherapy, immunosuppressive therapy after organ transplant)
  - HIV
- Malnutrition
- Inhalation of aspiration of noxious substances
- Debilitating illness
- Bedrest and prolonged immobility
- Altered oropharyngeal flora.

The risk factors for hospital acquired pneumonia are:
- Residence in an ICU
- Mechanical ventilation (those who required 48 hours or more ventilation)
- Endotracheal intubation or tracheostomy
- Recent surgery
- Debilitation, i.e. malnutrition
- Invasive devices
- Neuromuscular disease
- Depressed level of alertness
- Aspiration
- Antacid use
- Age 60 or older
- Prolonged hospital stay
- Any serious underlying disease.

Pathophysiology

Normally, the airway distal to the larynx is sterile because of protective defence mechanisms. These mechanisms include:
- Filtration of air
- Warming and humidification of inspired air
- Epiglottis closure over the trachea
- Cough reflex
- Mucociliary escalator mechanism
- Secretion of immunoglobulin A
- Alveolar macrophages.

Pneumonia results in inflammation of lung tissue. Depending on the particular pathogen and the hosts' physical status, the inflammatory process may involve different anatomical areas of the lung parenchyma and the pleurae. The normal function of respiratory system and primary pathophysiology and clinical manifestation are as follows:

i. Normally 'mucociliary system' cleanses inhaled air by trapping particles. In pneumonia, hypertrophy of mucous membrane lining lung, resulting in hypersecretions leads to increased sputum production and cough:
   - Anaerobic - Foul-smelling, sputum
   - Klebsiella - Current Jelly colour
   - Staphylococcus - Creamy yellow
   - Pseudomonas–Green
   - Viral/mucopurulent

And bronchospasms from increased secretions, leads to localised or diffuse wheezing dyspnea.

ii. Generally 'alveolocapillary membrane' exchanges oxygen-carbon dioxide. In pneumonia, there is increased permeability resulting in excess fluid in interstitial space, shows consolidation (in chest X-ray films) localised/bacterial; diffuse/viral, and also there is decreased surface area for gas exchange leads to hypoxaemia.
iii. Normally pleura maintains close approximation of lungs and chest wall; minimizes friction during lung expansion and contraction. In pneumonia there is inflammation of the pleura which shows, chest pain, especially on inspiration, pleural effusion, dullness on percussion, decreased breath sounds and decreased vocal fremitus.
iv. Normally respiratory muscle expands and contracts chest wall and thus pleura and lungs. In pneumonia there is hypoventilation and respiratory acidosis (in presence of underlying disease) leads to decreased chest expansion and hypercapnoea and low arterial blood pH.
v. The lung defense system protects normally sterile lung from invasion. In pneumonia there is bacteremia, shows elevated blood cell counting; leukocytes (15,000 to 25000/mm), neutrophilia and tachypnoea and fever.

In pneumococcal pneumonia there is congestion, red hepatisation and gray hepatisation.

Clinical Manifestation

CAP has been traditionally thought to present any two syndromes; typical and atypical, although the distinctions are not clear.

Typical pneumonic syndrome is characterised by sudden onset of fever, chills, cough productive of purulent sputum, and pleuritic chest pain (in some cases). On physical examination signs of pulmonary consolidations such as dullness, percussion, increased fermitus, bronchial breath sounds, and crackles may be found. In elderly or debilitated patient, confusion or stupor may be predominant. Usually two types of pneumonia caused by *S. pneumoniae* and *H. influenzae*.

The atypical syndrome is characterised by a more gradual onset dry cough, and extrapulmonary manifestation such as headache, myalgia, fatigue, sore throat, nausea, vomiting and diarrhoea. On physical examination, crackles are often heard. This type of classically produced by mycoplasm, pneumonia and legonell chlamydia pneumonia. Viral pneumoniae are characterised by an atypical presentation with chills, fever, dry non-productive cough and extrapulmonary symptoms. Most of the pneumoniae run uncomplicated. If occurs, the complications are pneumonia including pleurisy, pleural effusion, atelectasis, delayed resolution, lung abscess, empyema, pericarditis, arthritis, meningitis and endocarditis.

Management

History, physical examination and chest X-ray often provide enough information to take management decisions without costly laboratory tests. Diagnostic tests include:

- Chest X-ray film to conform consolidation and distribution and pleural effusions.
- Sputum studies for culture and sensitivity if unable to obtain specimen by usual means, may use,
  – Transtracheal aspiration,
  – Bronchoscopy with aspiration, biopsy or bronchial brushings.
- Arterial blood gas studies or pulse oximetry.
- Haematology: WBC count, cole agglutinin and compliment fixation for viral studies.
- Thoracentesis to obtain pleural fluid specimen if pleural effusion is present.

The possible nursing diagnosis on the basis and assessment will be:

- Airway clearance, ineffective R/T decreased energy, fatigue, tracheobronchial inflammation.
- Impaired gas exchange R/T alveolar capillary membrane changes altered oxygen delivery.
- Pain R/T pleural inflammation, coughing paroxysms.
- Rest for infection R/T compromised lung defense system.
- Knowledge deficient R/T condition, treatment.
- Anorexia R/T infection process-sputum production.
- Altered nutrition/body requirement R/T increased metabolic needs.

Prompt treatment with the appropriate antibiotic almost always cures bacterial and mycoplasmal pneumonia. In uncomplicated cases, the patient responds to drug therapy within 48 to 72 hours. Indications for improvement including decreased temperature, improved breathing, and reduced chest pain. Abnormal physical finding lasts for more than 7 days. The nursing intervention includes.

i. Maintaining effective airway clearance
   - Monitor for increased respiratory distress
   - Assist patient to cough effectively
   - If unable to clear down airway, suction airway using sterile technique

- Assist with nebuliser therapy
- Administer bronchiodilator as ordered. Monitor for side effects and response to therapy
- Change position frequently to assist in mobilising secretions
- Ensure fluid intake adequate to thin secretions.

ii. Facilitate breathing

Help the patient breathe deeply and expand the chest to increase ventilation.

- Place the patient in position to facilitate breathing, usually upright or semiupright position.
- A pillow may be placed lengthwise at the patient's back to provide support and thrust thorax slightly towards allowing free use of the diaphragm.
- The patient who must be upright to breathe may find it restful to place head and arms on a pillow placed on an overbed table.
- For the patient with severe hypoxaemia, side rails should be in place. The patient can use them to assisting about in bed.
- Some patients who breathe best when sitting up in a large armchair while leaning on a smaller chair. Placed in front of that. This chair is blocked to prevent it from slipping.
- Assist with ADL pacing activities to prevent fatigue and respiratory distress.

iii. Administration of medication and treatment

- Before starting prescribed antibiotic, collect sputum for culture and blood for culture if ordered
- Maintain antibiotic blood levels by giving antibiotic at scheduled time
- Give medication prescribed to relieve pain. Codeine may be ordered because it is less likely to inhibit cough reflex than more potent narcotics.
- Begin oxygen therapy.

iv. Administering oxygen therapy

v. Promoting comfort

- Place in position of comfort. Preferably head of bed elevated 45 to 90 degrees.
- Assess character and location of chest pain.
- Administer analgesic for chest pain e.g. acetylsalicylic acid, acetominophen and codeine.
- Splint chest with hands when patient coughs.
- Administer frequent mouth care. Protect lips and nares with lubricants.
- Keep patient warm and dry and avoid chilling.

vi. Preventing spread of infection.

- Standard precautions are used.

vii. Facilitating learning.

The major teaching emphasis is on prevention.

- Assess patient's understanding of pneumonia with questions concerning such information on how pneumonia is transmitted and risk factor.
- Teach proper handling of secretions. Cover nose and mouth with tissue when coughing or sneezing. Discard tissues in paper or plastic bag for disposal. Expectorate into specimen container provided.
- Stress importance of handwashing after coughing, sneezing and expectorating.
- Reinforce importance and follow-up care
- Reinforce the need for immunization, i.e., inlfuenza vaccine and pneumococcal vaccine. (Pneumonia Polysaccaride vaccine is given only every 3 to 5 years.

viii. Promoting adequate hydration and nutrition

- Encourage oral fluids. If patient is receiving IV fluids, monitor rate. Observe for signs of fluid volume deficit or excess.
- Ask patient what foods he or she would like to eat.
- Offer small, frequent feedings.
- Encourage high-carbohydrate and high-protein foods.

TUBERCULOSIS

Tuberculosis is an infectious disease caused by mycobacterium tuberculosis. It usually involves the lungs, but it also occurs in the kidneys, bones, adrenal glands, lymph nodes and meninges and can be disseminated throughout the body.

Aetiology

Mycobacterium tuberculosis, a gram-positive, acid-fast bacillary, is usually spread via air-borne droplets, which are produced when the infected individual coughs, sneezes or speaks. Once released into a room, the organisms are dispersed and can be inhaled. Brief exposure to a tubercle bacilli rarely causes an infection. Rather it is more commonly spread to the individual who has had repeated close contact with an infected person. It is not highly infective and transmitted. It usually requires close, frequent or prolonged exposure. The disease cannot be spread by hands, books, glasses, dishes or other fomites.

Pathophysiology

When an individual with no previous exposure to TB (negative tuberculin reactor) inhales a sufficient number of tubercle bacilli into the alveoli, tuberculosis infection occurs. The body's reaction to the TB bacilli depends on the susceptibility of the individual, the size of the dose and the virulence of the organisms. Inflammation occurs within the alveoli (parenchyma) of the lungs, and natural body defenses attempt to counteract the infection.

When the bacilli is inhaled, they pass down the bronchial system and implant themselves on the respiratory bronchioles or alveoli. The lower part of the lungs are usually the site of initial bacterial implantation. After implantation, the bacilli multiply with no initial resistance from the host. The organisms are engulfed by phagocytosis (initially neutrophils and later macrophages) and may continue to multiply within the phagocytes.

Macrophages ingest the organism and present the microbacterial antigens to the T cells. CD4 cells secrete lymphothine than enhance the capacity of the macrophages to ingest and kill bacteria. Lymph nodes in the hilar region of the lung become enlarged on their filter drainage from the infected site. The inflammatory process and the cellular reaction produce a small, firm, white nodules called the 'primary tubercle'. The centre of the nodules contain tubercle bacilli cells gather around the centre and usually the outer portion becomes fibrosed. Thus, blood vessels are compressed, nutrition of tubercle is impaired, and necrosis occurs at the centre. The area becomes walled off by fibritic tissue, and the centre gradually becomes soft and cheesy in consistency. This later process is known as "Caseation necrosis". This material may become calcified (calcium deposits) or it may liquify (liquification necrosis). The liquified material may be coughed up, leaving a cavity or hole in the parenchyma of the lung. This cavity or cavities are visible on chest X-ray films and results in the diagnosis of cavitary disease. The only X-ray evidence of TB infection is a calcified nodule known as "Ghon's tubercle". Ghon's tubercle is referred to as the "primary complex". When a tuberculosis lesion regresses and heals, the infection enters a latent period in which it may persist without producing a clinical illness. The infection may develop into clinical disease if the persisting organism begins to multiply rapidly, or it may remain dormant. If the initial immune response is not adequate, control of the organisms is not maintained and clinical disease results. Certain individuals are at a higher-risk for clinical disease including those who are immunosuppressed, e.g. HIV, cancer, person who received chemotherapy or corticosteroid therapy) or have diabetes mellitus. Dormant but viable organism persists for years. Reactivation of TB can occur if the host defense mechanisms become impaired.

Clinical Manifestation

In the early stages of TB, the person is usually free of symptoms. Many cases, if it is found that incidentally when routine chest X-rays are taken, especially in older adults. Systemic manifestation may initially consist of fatigue, malaise, anorexia, weight loss, low grade fever (especially in late afternoons) and night sweats. The weight loss may not be excessive until late in the disease and is often attributed to overwork or other factors. Irregular menses may also be present in premenopausal women.

A characteristic pulmonary manifestation is 'cough that becomes frequent and produce mucoid or macopurulent's sputum. Chest pain characterised as dull or tight may also be present. Hemoptysis is not a common finding and is usually associated with more advanced cases. Sometimes TB has more acute, sudden manifestation, the patient has high fever, chills, generalised of the like symptoms, pleuritic pain and a production of cough.

The complication of TB are miliary tuberculosis, pleural effusion, TB pneumonia, involvement of other organs, e.g. bone, kidney, brain, etc.

Management

This will be diagnosed by taking prompt health history and physical examination. The diagnostic studies of TB include

- Tubercular skin testing, montoux test
- Chest X-rays
- Bacteriological studies–sputum smear, sputum
- WBC. Serologic test by ELISA (enzyme-linked immunosorbent assay).
- CSF.

The common drugs used for management of tuberculosis are:

i. *Isoniazid (INH)*: Interferes with DNA metabolism and tubercle bacilli. It is bactericidal, penetrates all body tissues and fluids, including CSF. The side effects include peripheral nueritis, hepatotoxicity, hypersensitivity (skin rash, arthralgin, fever). Optic neuritis, vitB_6 neuritis. INH metabolizes primarily by liver and excretion by kidneys, pyridoxine (Vit B6) administration during high-dose therapy as prophylactive measure, use as single prophylactic agent. For active TB in individuals whose PPD converts to positive, ability to cross blood-brain barrier. Avoid alcohol and antacids during therapy. Daily alcohol intake interferes with metabolism of isoniazed and increases risk of hepatitis, antacids containing alluminium hydroxide also interferes with absorption of INH.

ii. *Rifampin* has broad spectrum effects, inhibits RNA polymerase of tubercle bacillus. It is bactericidal, penetrates all body tissues, including CSF. It is most commonly used with INH, low incidence of side effects, suppression of effects of birth control pills, possible orange urine. The other side effects may develop are hepatitis, febrile reactions, thrombocytopenia (Rare) GI disturbance, peripheral neuropathy, hypersensitivity, hepatotoxicity increases when given with INH. During its therapy, urine, sweat, tears may turn orange temporarily decrease effectiveness of oral contraceptives, anticoagulants, corticosteroids, barbiturates, hypoglycemics and digitalis.

iii. *Ethambutal* inhibits RNA synthesis and a bacteriostatic for the TB bacilli and does not penetrate all body fluids except CSF. The common side effects are skin rash, GI disturbance, malaise, peripheral neuritis, and optic neuritis. It has no significant reaction with other drugs. Should be given with food. Periodic checking of vision needed. It is most commonly used as substitute drug when toxicity occurs with Refampicin and INH.

iv. *Streptomycin* inhibits protein synthesis and is bacteriocidal. Poor penetration into body tissues and CSF. The side effects of.................... and INH include (eighth cranial nerve damage streptomycin vestibular or occular) damage often irreversible, nephrotoxicity and hypersensitivity. It should be used cautiously in older adults those with renal disease and pregnant women; must be given parenterally. During its use patient should be monitored monthly for kidney function, vestibular function with caloric stimulation test, and hearing with audiogram.

v. *Pyrazinamide* is bacteriostatic or bacteriocidal depending on susceptibility of mycobacterium (exact mechanism not known). Usual side effects of fever, skin rash, hyperuricemia, jaundice (rare) hepatitis, arthrolgia, GI irritation. High rate of effectiveness when used with streptomycin or capreomycin.

In addition, ethionamide, capromycine, kanamycin and paraamino salicylic acid (PAS) cycloserine (seromycin) and used as second line of drugs for TB treatment.

A problem with antituberculosis therapy is the length of time medication must be taken. In the past, 18 to 26 months was the usual period of time required for individuals to adhere to the medical regiment. Shorter courses of therapy (6 to 9 months) have been shown to be effective. Now three options for treatment are available. Regimen option for the initial treatment of tuberculosis include:

Option 1. Four drug regimen consisting of isoniazid, rifampin, pyrazinamide and either ethambutl or streptomycine. Therapy may be given daily or 2-3 times weekly if DOT (directly observed therapy). Ethambutol or streptomycin may be discontinued if susceptibility to isoniazed or rifampin is documented. Pyrazinamide should be discontinued after 8 weeks. The total duration of the therapy should be at least 6 months and at least 3 months after sputum culture converts to negative. Fixed dose combination of all these drugs are available to simplify therapy.

Option 2. Daily isoniazed, rifampin, pyrazinamide and streptomycin or ethambutol for 2 weeks followed by DOT twice weekly administration of the same drugs for 6 weeks followed by rifampin for 16 weeks.

Option 3. DOT 3 times/weekly administration of isoniazed, rifampin, pyrazinamide, and ethambutol or streptomycin for 6 months.

For TB with HIV infection cases, option 1, 2, 3 can be used, but treatment regimens should continue for a total of 9 months and at least 6 months beyond culture conversion.

Medical therapy is the primary treatment of tuberculosis, but surgery may be used to remove residual pulmonary lesions and patients. The surgical procedures then are used include wedge resection, segmental resection, lobestomy, etc.

A well-balanced diet containing the essential food groups with a vitamin supplement is recommended. Those who are poorly nourished or underweight may benefit from six small feedings of high-calorie, high protein foods daily rather than three meals.

The major nursing responsibility is to teach the patient about TB and how it is transmitted. Preventing contamination of air with tubercle bacilli is accomplished by treating the patient antituberculosis drugs and teaching the patient to cover the nose and mouth with tissues when sneezing and coughing. Advise the patient, he must take antituberculosis drugs as prescribed and drugs are always taken as combination of at least four drugs initially and drugs must be taken uninterruptedly.

To improve airway clearance, the patient is taught to sit upright in a chair or bed. If the patient is confined to bed at home, he or she may find it helpful to sit on the side of the bed with the feet on a chair. The patient may be taught to take two or three deep breaths cover the mouth with tissues and then cough. Using this method when coughing decreases, fatigue because it requires less expenditure of energy than does repeated ineffective coughs. Many patients can cough most effectively when the mouth is moist and sips of water or a warm beverage such as tea or coffee can be encouraged before coughing.

For patients with thick tenacious sputum, fluid intake is encouraged to thin the secretions and make them easier to expectorate. Water is considered by many experts to be the most effective sputum liquifying agent.

To reduce fear about the disease and what lifestyle changes it will require, patients are encouraged to ask questions about anything they do not understand or anything that concerns them. The nurse who sits while talking with the patients signals them he or she will take the time to listen to the patient. All questions should be answered as completely as possible, supplying information appropriate to the patients' educational level and ability to comprehend what is being taught. Written materials with diagram and drawings that reinforce what is being taught are helpful. The materials are given to the patient for use later on.

Nurses and other health care workers need to know the protective measures they can use when caring for patients who have a positive TB smear or culture.

BRONCHIECTASIS

Bronchiectasis is a disorder characterised by permanent, abnormal or irreversible dilation of the bronchial tree or one or more large bronchi.

Pathophysiology

When infection attacks the bronchial lining, inflammation occurs, and an exudate forms. The progressive accumulation of secretions obstructs the bronchioles. The obstructed bronchioles then breakdown, and ciliated columnar epithelium is replaced by non-ciliated cuboidal epithelium and sometimes fibroitic tissue, resulting in localised areas of dilations or saccules. The pathologic changes that result in dilation and destruction of the elastic and muscular structures of the bronchial wall.

There are two pathological types of bronchiectasis, i.e. saccular and cylindrical. Saccular bronchiectasis occurs mainly in large bronchi and is characterised by cavity-like dilations. The affected bronchi end in large sacs. Cylindrical bronchiectasis involve medium-sized bronchi that are mildly to moderately dilated. Fusiform bronchiectasis occurs mainly in large bronchi and is characterized by cavity-like dilations. The affected bronchi end in large sacs cylindrical bronchiectasis involves medium sized bronchi that are mildly to moderately dilated. Fusiform bronchiectasis a subtype of cylindrical tends to involve more 'pouching' of the bronchi. The explosive force of the bronchioles is diminished and they may remain filled with exudate. Only forceful coughing and postural drainage will empty them. Almost all forms of bronchiectasis are associated with bacterial infections and viral infections (adenovir, influenza).

Clinical Manifestations

The condition may develop so gradually that the person is unable to tell when the symptoms first began. Signs and symptoms of bronchiectasis vary with the severity of the conditions and may include the following.

Signs

- Cyanosis
- Clubbing of fingers
- Find crackles and coarse Rhonchi
- Dull or flat sound over the areas of mucus plugs
- Increased vocal and tactile fermitus over the middle and lower lobes
- Decreased diaphragmatic excursion, and
- Paroxysms of coughing on rising in morning and when lying down.

Symptoms

- Severe coughing productive of copious amounts of purulent sputum
- Haemoptysis
- Dyspnoea
- Fatigue and weakness
- Loss of appetite and weight loss.

The diagnostic studies used to diagnose bronchiectasis are chest X-ray, bronchography, sputum examination and CT scanning.

Management

Treatment of bronchiectasis includes:

- Administration of antibiotics on the basis of sputum culture results.
- Administering of bronchodilator, mucolytic agents and expectorants.
- Postural drainage to assist in mobilizing secretions to larger airways where they can be coughed up.

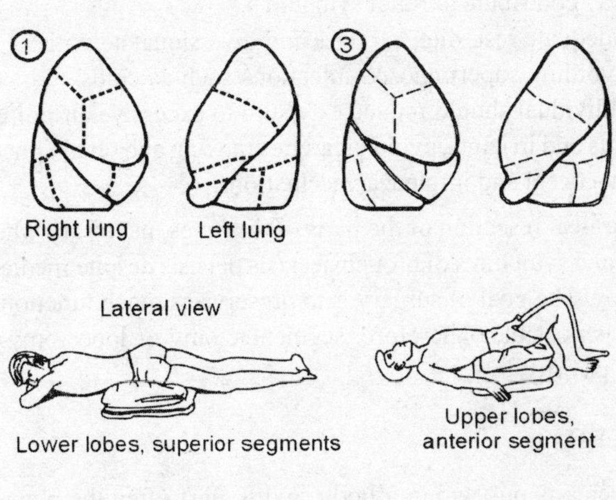

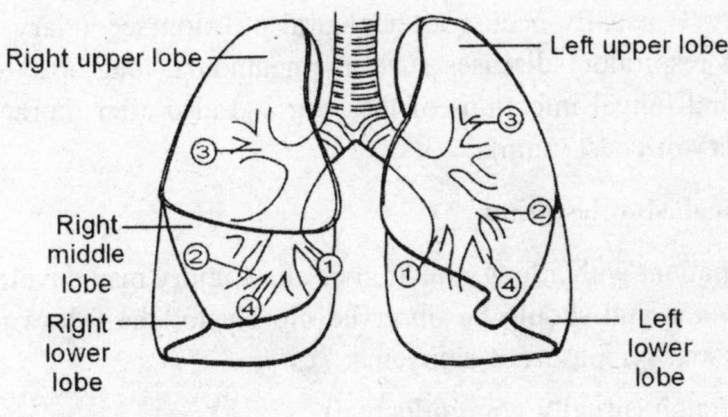

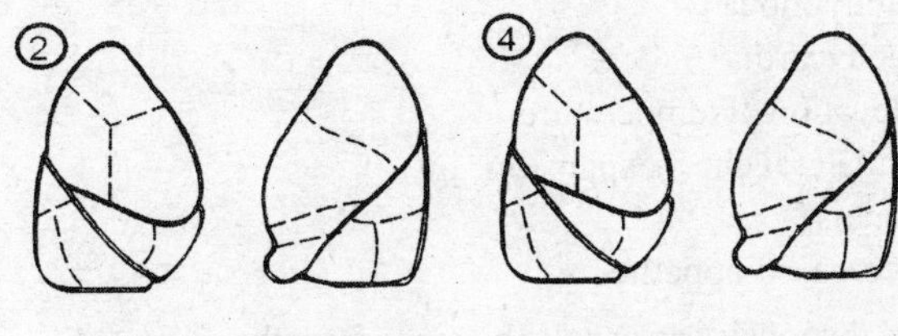

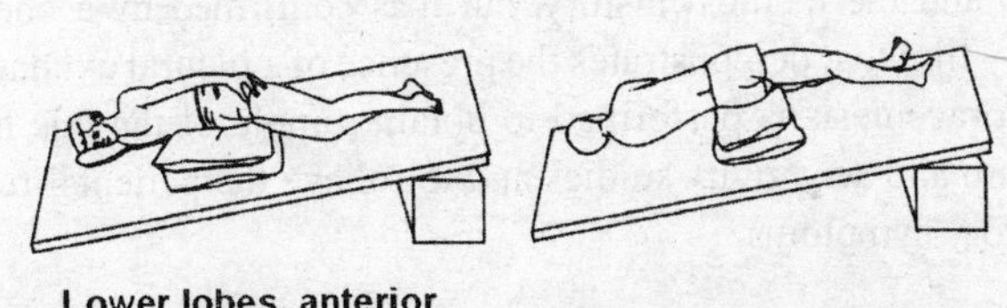

Lower lobes, anterior basal segment
Lower lobes, lateral basal segment

Fig. 6.2: Postural drainage positions. Anatomic segments of the lung with four postural drainage positions. The numbers relate the position to the corresponding anatomic segment of the lung

- Bronchoscopy to remove thicker secretions
- Maintaining good hydration to liquify secretion
- Maintaining good general hygiene including oral hygiene may contribute to relief symptoms.
- Adequate rest, diet, exercise and diversional activities
- Avoiding superimposed infections such as colds
- Individual should reduce exposure to excessive air pollutants and irritants, avoid cigarette smoking and obtain pneumococcal and influenza vaccinations.

Surgical resection of the parts of the lungs, necessary when signs and symptoms of bronchiaectasis persists despite medical therapy. The goal of surgery is to preserve as much functional lung as possible. Therefore, segmentectomy or lobectomy is given priority.

EMPYEMA

Empyema is pus within a body cavity most often the pleural cavity. It usually occurs after pleural effusion secondary to other respiratory diseases such as pneumonia, lung abscess, TB and fungal infections of the lung and also after thoracic surgery or chest trauma.

Clinical Manifestation

The patient with a lung infection or chest injury may develop empyema and should be observed closely for the following signs and symptoms of empyema:

- Cough (usually nonproductive)
- Dyspnoea
- Tachypnoea
- Tachycardia
- Elevation of temperature
- Unilateral chest expansion
- Malaise
- Decreased appetite.

The diagnosis can usually be made from the signs and symptoms and the medical history, but it is confirmed by a chest X-ray film that demonstrates the presence of a pleural exudate. A thoracentesis is performed to obtain sample of the pus for culture and sensitivity studies and to relieve the patients' respiratory symptoms.

Management

The aim of treatment of empyema is to obliterate the pleural space by draining the empyema cavity completely. The cavity can be drained in the following ways.

- Initial treatment is often daily thoracentesis with aspiration of the cavity and instillation of antibiotics into the pleural space. Oral or IV antibiotics may also be given.
- If the cavity cannot be evacuated within a few days and if the lung fails to re-expand to obliterate then space surgery is necessary. The types of surgery depends on the situation and may include:
  - Closed chest drainage
  - Rib resection
  - Decortication and
  - Thoracoplasty.

Nursing depends on the type and effectiveness of the procedure and the patient's symptoms. Some patients require oxygen therapy. Bedrest and couching and deep breathing exercises may be indicated to improve ventilations. In some cases, the patient will go through several treatments before the empyema in space is closed. This can be frustrating, and the patient can become very discouraged. A major nursing role is to support the patient and family during the various procedure.

LUNG ABSCESS

Lung abscess is a pus-containing lesion of the lung parenchyma that gives rise to a cavity. The cavity is formed by necrosis of the lung tissue.

Aetiology

In many cases, the causes and pathogenesis of lung abscess are similar to those of pneumonia. The more common contributing factor to a lung abscess is aspiration of material into the lungs. Risk factors for aspiration include alcoholism, seizure disorder, drug overdose, general anaesthesia, and cerebrovascular accidents. Most of the lung abscesses are caused by infectious agents, i.e., Klebsiella, S. aureus, anaerobic bacilli. Lung abscess also can result from haematogenously spread lung infarct secondary to pulmonary embolus, malignant growth, TB and various fungus and parasitic diseases of the lung.

Pathophysiology

The areas of the lung most commonly affected are the atypical segments of the lower lobes and the posterior segments of the upper lobes. Fibrous tissues usually form around the abscess in an attempt to wall it off. The abscess may erode into the bronchial system, causing the production of foul-smelling sputum. It may grow towards the pleura and cause pleuritic pain. Multiple small abscesses can occur within the lung.

Clinical Manifestation

The onset of a lung abscess is usually insidious, especially if anaerobic organisms are the primary cause. A more acute onset occurs with aerobic organisms. The most common manifestation is cough-producing, purulent (often dark brown) that is foul-smelling and foul tasting. Haemoptysis is common especially at the time that an abscess ruptures into a bronchus. Other common manifestations are fever, chills, prostration, pleuritic pain, dyspnoea, cough and weight loss. History may reveal a predisposing condition such as alcoholism, pneumonia or oral infections.

Physical examination of the lungs indicate the dullness to percussion and decreases breath sounds on auscultation over the segment of lung involved. There may be transmission of breath sounds to the periphery if the communicating bronchus becomes patent and drainage of the segment begins. Crackle may also be present. Oral examination often reveals dental caries, gingivitis and peridontal infection.

Complication can occur include chronic pulmonary abscess, haemorrhage from abscess erosion into blood vessels, brain abscess, bronchopleural fistula, and empyema.

Management

Diagnosis is made on the basis of physical examination, chest X-ray, sputum culture and sensitivity. Prolonged administration of antibiotics (6 to 8 weeks). Penicillin is the choice antibiotics. Recently, clindamycin or metronidazole in combination with penicillin are used.

The patient should be taught how to cough effectively. Chest physiotherapy and postural drainages are helpful. Frequent mouth care (every 2 to 3 hours) is needed to relieve the foul-smelling odour and taste from the sputum. Diluted hydrogen peroxide and mouthwash are often effective. Rest, good nutrition, adequate fluid intake are all supportive measures to facilitate recovery. If dentition is poor and dental hygiene is not adequate and the patient should be encouraged to obtain dental care.

Surgery is indicated but occasionally may be necessary if reinfection of a large cavity lesion occurs.

OCCUPATIONAL LUNG DISEASES

Occupational or environmental lung diseases result from inhaled dust or chemicals. The duration of exposure and the amount of inhalant have a major influence on whether the exposed individual will have lung damage. Another factor is the susceptibility of the host.

Aetiology

Many pulmonary diseases are believed to be caused by substances inhaled in the work place. Occupational lung disease are more common in:

- Blue-collar workers than white collar workers
- Industrial areas than in rural areas, and
- Small and medium-sized business than in larger industrial plants.

In some instances it is debatable whether a person's lung disease is clearly occupation specific. This is true in cases of bronchitis, asthma, emphysema, or cancer, because all of these conditions can be caused or aggravated by several factors found in many different occupations and by non-occupational factors such as smoking and air pollution.

Types

Occupational lung disease can be divided into several categories. The major ones are:

- The pneumoconiosis (black lung disease)
- Asbestos-related lung diseases
- Hypersensitivity diseases including occupational asthma allergic alveolitis and
- Byssinosis (brown lung disease).

Pathophysiology

The pathophysiology, clinical manifestation and prevention of some common occupational diseases are as follows:

i. *Pneumoconiosis* also known as 'dust in the lungs' is called by inhalation and retention of dust particles. Examples of this condition are: silicosis, asbestosis and Byssinosis.
   - *Silicosis* caused if inhaled silica dust, most common form seen in miners, foundry workers, and others who inhaled relatively low concentration of dust for 10-20 years.

In this dust accumulation is tissue or tissue reaction with whorl-shaped nodules throughout lungs. In complicated silicosis there is progressive massive fibrosis throughout lungs decreased lung function and cor pulmonale. In acute silicosis, there is inflammatory reaction within alveoli, diffuse fibrosis. Rapid progression to respiratory failure. The clinical manifestation will include, breathlessness, weakness, chest pain, productive cough with sputum, dies of cor pulmonale and respiratory failure. The preventive measures include dust control and improved ventilation can reduce dust levels. Sand blasters in enclosed spaces can use special suits and breathing apparatus. The complicated progressive massive fibrosis shortens lifespan.

ii. *Asbestos-related lung disease*: Asbestos caused lung cancer, malignant mesothelioma of pleura and periosteum, cancer of the larynx, and certain gastrointestinal cancer, also cause asbestosis of fibrotic lung disease.

Fibrosis caused by asbestos called asbestosis, asbestos fibers, accumulated around terminal bronchioles, surrounds fibers with iron rich tissue, forming asbestos body with characteristic picture on X-ray, more asbestos bodies as more fibers are inhaled, after 20-30 years of exposure fibrosis begins in lungs, interstitial fibrosis develops. Pleural plaques, which are calcified lesions develop on pleura. Dyspnoea, basal crackles, and decreased vital capacity, are early manifestation. The complications include diffused interstitial pulmonary fibrosis. Lung cancer especially in cigarette smokers, mesothelioma (cancer affecting pleura and peritonial membrane).

Treatment with radical pleurectomy and pneumonectomy survival only for 1-2 years. Preventive measures include enforcement for regulations governing mining milling and use of asbestos. Protective masks must be used when working with asbestos.

iii. *Hypersensitivity diseases* fall into occupational category when can occur in bronchi, bronchioles or alveoli, coarse dust causes bronchial reactions, fine dust previous small airway and alveolar reactions.
   - In occupational asthma, hypersensitivity reaction mediated by histamine bronchoconstriction and increased mucus production repeated attacks if cause unrecog-nised and asthma is untreated, may lead to permanent obstructive lung disease; asthmatic response that is well established can be provoked by other factors (i.e. house dust, cigarette smoke) and by fatigue, breathing cold air and coughing where wheezing is major symptom. It can be prevented by total elimination of antigen, desensitization not successful.
   - In farmer's lung (hypersensitivity pneumothitis or allergic alveolitis), alveoli are inflamed, inundated by WBCs, sometimes filled with fluid, if exposure infrequent or level of dust low, symptoms are mild, and treatment not sought, chronic form develops over a period of time eventually fibrosis occurs, and fibrosis may be so well established that it cannot be arrested.

Symptoms begin some hours after exposure to offending dust and include fatigue, shortness of breath, dry cough, fever, and chills. Symptoms may be severe enough to require emergency treatment and hospitalization; acute attacks treated with steroids, recovery may take 6 weeks and patient may have residual lung damage, real cure is permanent separation of patient and antigen.

Preventive measures include properly dried and stored farm products (hay, straw, sugar cane) do not cause allergic alveolitis presumably fungi only grow in moist condition.

iv. *Byssinosis* (Brown lung disease) is occupational disease. Occurs in textile workers; mainly in cotton workers but also afflict workers in flax and hemp industries; cause is found in bales of raw cotton.

In this, chronic bronchitis and emphysema develop in time. Constriction of bronchioles in response to something in crude cotton. Symptoms of asthma and allergy persists long there is exposure to cotton antigen.

Clinical manifestation that develops are tightness in chest on returning to work after a weekend away (Monday fever), strong relationship between amount of dust inhaled and symptoms. Persistent of symptom increases tightness of chest with chronic bronchitis and emphysema, person leaves industry as respiratory cripple.

The preventive measures include–dust control measures, pretreating bales of cotton by washing with steam and other agents may inactivate causative agent, try to detect persons who are likely to become sensitized to cotton dust and keep them out of high risk areas.

Management

Medical therapy of these patients depend on the patient's signs, symptoms and complications. The major role of nurses is to be knowledgeable about the cause and prevention of occupational lung diseases, so that appropriate information and teaching can be presented to community. The best approach to management is, to try to prevent or decrease environmental and occupational risks. Well-designed effective ventilation system can reduce exposure to irritants, wearing mask is appropriate in some occupations. Cigarette smoking must be avoided.

Early diagnosis is essential if the disease process is to be halted. The best treatment is to decrease or stop exposure to the harmful agents. Some places of employment at which there is a known risk of lung disease may require periodic chest X-rays and pulmonary function studies for exposed employees. There is no specific treatment for most environmental lung diseases. Treatment is directed towards symptomatic relief. If there is coexisted problem such as pneumonia, chronic bronchitis, emphysema, or asthma they are treated on providing nursing care accordingly.

LUNG CANCER

Cancer of the lung may be either metastatic or primary. Metastatic tumours may follow malignancy anywhere in the body. Metastasis forms the colon and kidney are common. Metastasis to the lung may be discovered before the primary lesion is known, and sometime locations of the primary lesion may be found only at autopsy.

Aetiology

Cigarette smoking as a chronic respiratory irritant is by far the major risk factor in the development of lung cancer. Heredity may play a role in both the tendency to smoke and the predisposition to develop lung cancer. Another possible risk factor is preexisting pulmonary disease such as TB, pulmonary fibrosis, bronchiectasis and COPD.

Pathophysiology

The pathogenesis of primary lung cancer is not well understood. Usually cancers originate from the epithelium of the bronchus (bronchogenic). They grow slowly and it takes 8 to 10 years for a tumour to reach 1 cm in size, which is smallest detectable lesion on an X-ray. Lung cancer occurs primarily in the segmental bronchi or beyond and have a preference for the upperlobes of the lungs. Pathologic changes in the bronchial system show non-specific inflammatory changes with hypersecretions of mucus, desquamation of cells, reactive hyperplasia of the basal cells, and metaplasia of normal respiratory epithelium to stratified squamous cells. Lung cancers metastasize primarily by direct extension and via. the blood circulation and the lymph system. The common sites for metastatic growth are the liver, brain, bones, scalene lymph nodes and adrenal glands.

Certain lung cancers cause the paraneoplastic syndrome, which is characterised by various manifestations caused by certain substance (e.g. hormones, enzymes and antigens) produced by the tumour cells. Small cell lung cancer most commonly is associated with it.

Clinical Manifestation

Lung cancer is clinically silent for most individuals for the majority of its course. The clinical manifestations of lung cancer are usually non-specific and appear late in the disease process. A patient's signs and symptoms depend on several factors including location of the lesion. Signs and symptoms of lesion in the bronchus and lung include:

- Approximately 10 per cent of patients are asymptomatic and cancer is identified on routine chest X-ray film.
- Approximately 75 per cent have a cough
- Approximately 50 per cent have a haemoptysis
- Shortness of breath and a unilateral wheeze are common. Peripheral lesions that perforate into pleural space shows extrapulmonary intrathoracic signs and symptoms. These include:
- Pain on inspiration
- Friction rub
- Pleural effusion
- Oedema of face and neck when superior vena cava is involved
- Fatigue and
- Clubbing fingers.

Later manifestations include non-specific system and symptoms such as anorexia, fatigue, weight loss, nausea and vomiting. Hoarseness may be present as a result of involvement of the recurrent laryngeal nerve. Unilateral paralysis of the diaphragm, dysphagia and superior vena cava obstruction may occur because of the intrathoracic spread of the malignancy.

Management

Diagnosis may be confirmed by taking accurately the

- Health history and physical examination
- Chest X-ray to depict tumour
- Sputum in cytologic study—for examining bacteria and cancer cells
- Bronchioscopy
- CT scan
- MRI
- Positron emission tomography (PET)
- Spirometry (preoperative)
- Mediastinoscopy
- Pulmonary angiography
- Lung scan

Fine-Needle Aspiration

Surgical resection is usually the only hope for cure in lung cancer. The types of thoracic surgery and indications for their use are as follows:

- Exploratory thoracotomy is performed to confirm suspected diagnosis of lung or chest disease, especially carcinoma; to obtain a biopsy; being replaced by non-invasive procedure (Thoracoscopy).
- Pneumonectomy is removal of a lung, bronchogenic carcinoma when lobectomy will not remove all of lesion, tuberculosis when other surgery will not remove all of diseased lung.
- Pneumonectomy is lung reduction surgery to reduce lung volume and decrease tension on respiratory muscle in persons with emphysema.
- Lobectomy is removal of one lobe of lung, bronchogenic carcinoma confined to a lobe, bronchiectasis, emphysematous blebs or bullae, lung abscess; fungal infections, benign tumours, and tuberculosis.
- Bilobectomy in removal of two lobes from right lungs, bronchogenic carcinoma when lobectomy will not remove all of disease.
- Sleeve lobectomy in the resection of main bronchus or distal trachea with reanastomosis to a distal uninvolved bronchus, bronchogenic carcinoma to preserve functional parenchyma.
- Segmental resection is known as segmentectomy, that is removal of one or more lung segments; bronchiectasis, lung abscess or cyst; metastatic carcinoma and tuberculosis.
- Wedge resection is a removal of pie-shaped section from surface of lung, well-circumscribed benign tumours, metastatic tumours or localised inflammatory disease, including TB.
- Decortication is removal of fibrinous peel from visceral pleura; chronic empyema.
- Thoracoplasty is removal of ribs, residual airspace after resectional surgery; chronic empyema space.

Radiation therapy is used as curative approach in the individual who has resectable tumour but who is considered a poor surgical risk. It is also used as palliative procedure to reduce distressing symptoms such as cough, hemoptysis, bronchial obstruction, and superior vena cava syndrome.

Chemotherapy may be used in the treatment of non-resectable tumours or as adjuvant therapy to surgery in non-small cell lung carcinoma.

Biologic therapy used as adjuvant therapy.

Phototherapy i.e. laser surgery with use of the Nd:YAG also useful in some cases.

The best way to prevent lung cancer is to abstain from smoking. When it is confirmed, nurse has to assist in supporting the patient in all above stated procedures and take suitable nursing measures accordingly.

NURSING MANAGEMENT IN THORACIC SURGERY

Preoperative Care

Preoperative teaching is essential for patients who are undergoing thoracic surgery. The goal of teaching is to prepare the patient for what he or she is expected to do postoperatively. The nurse who is caring for the patient is responsible for determining what the patient understands about the impending surgery and to be sure that preoperative teaching is completed. The points to be discussed in teaching include:

- Patient's knowledge of procedure
- Explanation of procedure is necessary, including intubation for anaesthesia, site of incision and chest tube(s) and drainage system.
- Oxygen
- Blood administration and IV
- Pain medication, including PCA if used
- What the patient will be asked to do
  - Coughing and deep breathing
  - Arm exercise and
  - Ambulation.
- Where patient will be taken after surgery.
  - to recovery–how long
  - to ICU–for how long.
- Where family can wait during surgery.

The other routines of preoperative care of any surgery has to be followed.

Postoperative Care

The care of the patient after thoracic surgery centres on promoting ventilation, and reexpansion of the lung by maintaining a clear airway, maintaining the closed drainage system, promoting nutrition, monitoring the incision for bleeding and subcutaneous emphysema.

In most of the hospitals, the patient is taken from the recovery room to the ICU. The immediate postoperative nursing cares are as follows.

Oxygen Therapy

Oxygen is attached to the endotracheal tube in the immediate postoperative period. After extubation, humidified oxygen is given by cannula, usually at 6L/minute. Oxygen mask should not be used to avoid cough and to rouse secretion.

Haemodynamic Monitoring

The patient is usually attached to a cardiac monitor. A Swan-Ganz catheter and central venous pressure line are used for haemodynamic monitoring.

Position of the Patient in Bed

The patient is kept flat in bed or with head elevated slightly (20 degrees) until blood pressure is stabilised to preoperative levels. Once blood pressure is stabilised, the patient can usually breathe best in semi-Fowler's position with a pillow under the head and neck but not under the shoulders and back, because of the subscapular incision.

Monitoring Vital Sign

Vital signs are taken every 15 minutes until the patient is well recoverd from anaesthesia, every hour until condition has stabilised, and then every 2 to 4 hour. Any deviation should be reported immediately to take suitable measures.

Initiating Coughing and Deep Breathing Exercises

The patient should be assisted to cough as soon as conscious and extubated. If blood pressure is stable, the patient is assisted to sitting position, and the incision is supported anteriorly and posteriorly by the nurse's hands. Firm, even pressure over the incisions with the open palm of the hands is most effective method. The nurse's head should be behind the patient when the patient is coughing. The patient is encouraged to breathe deeply, exhale and then cough. Sips of fluid especially warm ones such as tea or coffee often facilitate coughing. Deep breathing or coughing keep the airway patent, prevent atelectasis and facilitate reexpansion of the lung. Patient is assisted every 2 to 4 hours around the clock. When a patient is unable to cough effectively tracheobronchial suctioning is performed.

Promoting Abdominal Breathing

Abdominal breathing exercises are a valuable adjunct to the care of the patient with chest surgery, because it improves ventilation without increasing pain assist in coughing more effectively.

Promoting Comfort by Pain Relief

Medication for pain should be given as needed and may be required as often as every 3 to 4 hours during the first 48 to 72 hours. PCA and epidural catheters are widely used for pain medication management. Usually morphine is ordered for pain. If medication for pain fails intercostal nerve block may be performed.

Promoting Arm Exercises

Passive arm exercises are usually started in the evening of surgery. The purpose of pulling the patient's arm through range of motion is to prevent restriction of function.

Promoting Nutrition

The patient is encouraged to take fluids postoperatively and to progress to general diet as soon as it is tolerated. Fluid helps liquify secretions and make them easier to expectorate. A diet adequate in protein and vitamins (especially Vit C) facilitates wound healing.

Monitoring the Incision for Bleeding or Subcutaneous Emphysema

The dressing is checked periodically for bleeding. Blood on the dressing is unusual and should be reported to the surgeon at once. The time and amount of blood are recorded in the patient's record. Air leak from the pleural space through the thoracotomy incision or around the chest tubes into the soft tissues indicates subcutaneous emphysema. The presence of air under the skin is readily detected and has been described as feeling like 'tissue paper' "rice krispies" under the skin.

Maintaining Chest Tube(s) and Drainage

All patients who have resectional surgery of the lung, except those having a pneumonectomy will require drainage of the pleural space by one or two chest tubes connected to closed drainage. Precautions to be observed with any type of closed drainage system are as follows:

- Monitor drainage system for tidaling (fluctuating) in one waterseal chamber:
  - Be sure the patient is not lying on the tubes
  - Check connections to be sure the chest tube system is intact
  - Ask patient to cough or change position to see if tidaling is resorted
  - Tidaling will stop when the lung is re-expanded
- Never lift the closed drainage system above the level of the patient's chest, because this allows fluid to be pulled into the pleural space.
- Never clamp chest tubes without a written order from the surgeon because air (positive pressure) will be trapped in the pleural space, further collapsing the lung.
- A liter bottle of sterile water is kept at the bedside at all times. If the patient's chest drainage system cracks or breaks.
  - Insert patiently chest tube into the bottle of sterile water
  - Remove the cracked or broken system and
  - Obtain new system and connect it to patient's chest tube as soon as possible.
- If the patient's tube is accidentally pulled out of the chest (rarely occurs)
  - Apply gloves in accordance with body substance isolation policy
  - Pinch skin opening together with fingers
  - Apply occlusive dressing
  - Cover dressing with overlapping pieces of 2-inch tape
  - Call surgeon immediately.

Chest tubes are removed when there is no tidaling of fluid in the water-sealed chamber and when X-ray films confirm the full re-expansion of the lung.

CHEST TRAUMA AND THORACIC INJURIES

Chest trauma is a major problem often seen in the casualty. Injury to the chest may affect the bony chest cage, pleura and lungs, diaphragm, or mediastinal contents.

Aetiology

Injury to the chest are broadly classified into two groups, blunt and penetrating.

i. *Blunt* trauma or non-penetrating injuries damage the structures within the chest cavity without disrupting chest wall integrity. Blunt injury occurs when the body is struck by a blunt object, such as steering wheel. The external injury may appear minor but the impact may cause severe, life-threatening internal injuries such as ruptured spleen.
   - Blunt steering wheel injury to chest may lead to rib fracture, flail chest, pneumothorax, haemopneumothorax, cardiac contusion, pulmonary contusion, cardiac tamponade, great vessel tears.
   - Shoulder harness seat belt injury may lead to fractured clavicle, dislocated shoulder, rib fractures, pulmonary contusion, pericardial contusion, cardiae temponade.
   - Crush injury (e.g. heavy equipment, crushing thorax) leads to pneumothorax and haemopneumothorax, flail chest, great vessel tears and rupture, decreased blood returned with decreased cardiac output.
   - Countrecoup trauma—a type of blunt trauma, is caused by the impact of parts of the body against other objects. Examples are many head injuries caused by countrecoup trauma.

The causes of blunt injuries are, motor vehicle accident, pedestrian accident, fall, assault with blunt object, crush injury, and explosion.

ii. *Penetrating trauma* or injuries disrupt chest wall integrity and result in alteration in intrathoracic pressures. It occurs when a foreign body impales or passes through the body tissue, e.g. gunshot wound, stabbing, with knife, gunshot, stick, arrow and other missiles. Gunshot or stab wound to chest may lead to open pneumothorax, tension pneumothorax, haemopneumothorax, cardiac tamponade, esophageal damage, tracheal tear, great vessel tears.

Emergency care of the patient with chest trauma requires an accurate assessment of respiratory, cardiovascular and surface finding which include

- Respiratory– Dyspnoea, respiratory distress
  - Cough with or without haemoptysis
  - Cyanosis of the mouth, face, nail beds, mucous membrane
  - Tracheal deviation
  - Audible air escaping from the chest wound
  - Decreased breath sounds on side of injury
  - Decreased oxygen saturation, and
  - Frothy secretions.

- Cardiovascular
  - Rapid, thready pulse
  - Decreased blood pressure
  - Narrowed pulse pressure
  - Asymmetric blood pressure value in arms
  - Distended neck veins
  - Muffled heart sounds
  - Chest pain
  - Crunching sounds synchronous with heart sounds
  - Arrhythmias.
- Surface findings
  - Bruising
  - Abrasions
  - Open chest wounds
  - Asymmetric chest movement
  - Subcutaneous emphysema.

Nursing Intervention

The emergency care are:

- Ensure patient airway
- Administer high-flow O_2 with non-rebreather mask
- Establish IV access with two large-bore catheters. Begin fluid resuscitation as appropriate
- Remove clothing to assess injury
- Cover sucking chest wound with non-porous dressing taped on three sides
- Stabilize impaled objects with bulky dressings. Do not remove
- Assess for other significant injuries and treat appropriately
- Stabilise flail rib segment with hand followed by application of large pieces of tape horizontal across the flail segment
- Place patient in a semi-Fowler's position or position the patient on injured side if breathing is easier after carvical spine injury has been ruled out.

An ongoing monitoring will include:

- Monitor vital signs, level of consciousness, oxygen saturation, cardiac rhythm, respiratory status and urinary output
- Anticipate intubation for respiratory distress
- Release dressing if tension pneumothorax develops after sucking chest wound is covered.

Thorax injuries range from single rib fracture to the life-threatening tears of aorta, vena cava, and other major vessels. The most coronary thoracic emergencies are as follows:

RIB FRACTURES

Rib fractures are the most common type of chest injury (Blunt injury), resulting from trauma ribs (4-9) 3rd to 10th are most commonly fractured because they are least protected by chest muscles. If the fractured rib is splintered or displaced, it may damage the pleura and lungs.

Ribs usually function at the point of maximum impact, but they may fracture at a site distant from impact. Rib fractures are caused by blows, crushing injuries, or strain caused by severe coughing or sneezing spells. When the rib is splintered or the fracture displaced, sharp fragments may penetrate the pleura and lungs, resulting in a haemothorax (blood in the pleural space) or pneumothorax (air in the pleural space) which are penetrating injuries.

Clinical manifestation of fractured ribs include:

- Pain at the site of injury, especially increasing on inspiration
- Localised tenderness and crepitus on palpation
- Splinting of chest and shallow breathing.

Fractures are confirmed by chest X-ray.

The main goal in treatment is to decrease pain so that patient can breathe adequately to promote good chest expansion. Intercostal nerve blocks with local anaesthesia (1% procaine) may be used to provide pain relief and analgesics is given to relieve pain so that the patient can be encouraged to breathe more rapidly.

The patient is observed for splinting of the chest and shallow breathing to which could lead to atelectasis. To improve breathing, the patient is placed in a position of comfort. Most of the patients are able to breathe best in Fowler's or Semi-Fowler's positions.

The patient and family should be educated regarding:

- The patient should rest and do nothing strenuous for several days.
- The patient should take deep breath every hour.
- Narcotic drug therapy must be individualised and used with caution because these drugs can depress respiration.
- The pain is not relieved if analgesic call physician.
- If shortness of breath, sudden sharp chest pain, coughing up blood occurs, rush to casualty part of hospital.

FLAIL CHEST

Flail chest results from multiple rib fractures and thereby causing instability of the chest wall.

When multiple ribs or the sternum is fractured in more than one places, a portion of the chest wall becomes separated from the chest cage, resulting in a flail chest. The chest wall cannot provide the bony structures necessary to maintain bellows action and ventilation. The affected (flail) area will move paradoxically the intact portions of the chest during respiration. During inspiration the affected portion is sucked in, and during expiration it bulges out. This paradoxical chest movement prevents adequate ventilation of the lung in the injured area.

The underlying lung may or may not have a serious injury. Associated pain and any lung injury give rise to loss of compliance, will contribute to an alteration in breathing pattern and lead to hypoxaemia. And may also develop hypercapnia and respiratory acidosis due to increased work of breathing.

Clinical Manifestations

- Severe chest pain
- Paradoxical breathing (asymmetrical chest movement)
- Oscillation of mediastinum
- Increasing dyspnoea
- Rapid shallow respiration
- Accessory muscle breathing
- Restlessness
- Decreased breath sounds on auscultation
- Cyanosis
- Anxiety related to difficult breathing.

Management

- Stabilising the flail segment position end-expiratory pressure (PEEP) used with mechanical ventilation to improve oxygenation will maintain pressure in the lungs throughout the respiratory cycle.
- Provide supplemental oxygen: Monitor with pulse oximetry.
- Correct acid-base balance by mechanical ventilation
- Provide analgesic for pain control
- For severe pain, epidural anaesthesia may be used
- Avoid fluid overload
- Patient should be confined to bed as he or she is on a ventilator.

PNEUMOTHORAX

A pneumothorax is a complete or partial collapse of a lung as a result of an accumulation of air in the pleural space. Pneumothorax may be closed or open.

Closed Pneumothorax

The common form is:

- Spontaneous pneumothorax, which is caused by rupture of small blebs on the visceral pleural space. The cause of the bleb is unknown. This condition occurs most commonly in male cigarette smokers between 20-40 years of age. The other causes include:
- Injury to the lungs from mechanical ventilation
- Injury to the lungs from insertion of a subclavian catheter
- Perforation of esophagus
- Injury to the lungs from broken ribs
- Receptive blebs or bullae in a patient with COPD (e.g. asthma).

Clinical Manifestation

Small or slowly developing pneumothorax may produce no symptoms, but in large or rapidly developing pneumothorax results in:

- Sharp pain on respiration
- Increasing dyspnoea
- Increasing restlessness
- Diaphoresis
- Hypotension
- Tachycardia
- Absence of chest movement in affected side
- Hyper resonance on affected side (topercussion).

Management of closed pneumothorax will include

- Observation on outpatient basis
- Giving supplemental oxygen
- Needle aspiration of air from pleural space, if present, insertion of chest catheter connected to a flutter valve or closed drainage system (suction or vented drainage).
- If frequent recurrences, doxycycline or talc instilled into pleural space to cause adhesion between pleurae, if the procedure fails lung portion with defect resected and parietal pleura abraded.

Open Pneumothorax

Open pneumothorax occurs when air enters the pleural space through an opening in the chest wall. For example, gunshot or stab wound to chest in surgical thoracotomies. A penetrating chest wound is often referred to as a "sucking chest wound, because each time the person inspires, air is sucked into pleural space. In which, sucking sounds at wound site with respiration and tracheal deviation (trachea moves towards unaffected area during inspiration and returns towards midline inspiration are the clinical manifestations.

This will be managed by occlusion of open wound and use other measures as in closed pneumothorax.

Tension Pneumothorax

Tension pneumothorax may result from either in open or a closed pneumothorax. It occurs when air enters the pleural space on inspiration but cannot leave it on expiration. Although usually a result of a closed pneumothorax, a tension pneumothorax can be caused by a penetrating chest injury. The accumulated air builds up positive pressure in the chest cavity resulting in the following:

- Lung collapse on the affected side.
- Mediastinal shift towards the unaffected side.
- Compression of mediastinal contents (heart, great vessels) resulting in decreased cardiac output and decreased venous return.

The clinical manifestation, 'tension pneumothorax will include:

- Severe dyspnoea
- Agitation
- Trachea deviated from midline toward unaffected lung mediastinal shift
- Jugular venous distention
- Absence of chest movement on affected side
- Hypotension, tachycardia
- Breath sounds absent on affected side
- Hyper resonance on affected side
- Diminished heart sounds
- Shock
- Subcutaneous emphysema
- Ineffective ventilation.

Tension pneumothorax is a medical emergency because both the respiratory and circulatory systems are affected. If the tension of the pleural space is not relieved, the patient is likely to die from inadequate cardiac output or marked hypoxaemia. Nurses are now being trained to insert large bore needle and chest tube into the chest walls to release the trapped air. Tension of pneumothorax usually occurs during mechanical ventilation or resuscitative efforts. Since it is the emergency defect in chest wall, covered with a sterile dressing, and insertion of chest tube connected to a flutter valve or closed drainage system.

Haemothorax

Haemothorax is an accumulation of blood in the intrapleural space. It is frequently found in association with open pneumothorax. It may be due to chest trauma, lung malignancy, complication of anticoagulative therapy, pulmonary embolus, and tearing of pléural adhesions.

The clinical manifestations are:

If it is small mild tachycardia, and dyspnoea, air present. If it is large, respiratory distress may be present, which include shallow, rapid, respiration, dyspnoea and air hunger. Chest pain or cough with or without haemoptysis. No breath sounds heard on auscultation.

If tension pneumothorax develops, feature of these also develop as a clinical manifestation.

Treatment of haemopneumothorax depends on air severity of the pneumothorax and the nature of the underlying disease. An emergency management will include chest insertion, autotransfusion of collected blood, treatment of hypovolaemia as necessary. Repeated spontaneous pneumothorax may need to be treated surgically by a partial pleurectomy, stapling or laser pleurodosis to promote adherence of the pleurae to one another. The injection of doxycycline (dry) an irritating agent can be used for pleurodesis.

Nursing intervention for closed, tension and open pneumothorax are as follows:

- Closed pneumothorax patient if he or she admitted performing the following.
  - Place the patient in semi-Fowler's position
  - Administer oxygen
  - Obtain thoracentesis tray and closed drainage equipment.

  For outpatients or for patients after chest tube removal, instruct the patient to:
  - Report any increased dyspnoea to physician
  - Avoid strenous exercises or activity that increases rate and depth of breathing
  - Avoid holding breath
  - Follow physician's instructions about resuming normal activity.
- Tension pneumothorax–is life-threatening event; imperative that intervention be carried immediately to relieve increased intrapleural pressure; intervention same as those listed CP and performed the following.
  - Monitor vital signs frequently
  - Observe for cardiac dysrhythmias
  - Palpate for subcutaneous emphysema in upper chest and neck
  - Use same discharge instruction as in CP (above).
- Open pneumothorax-performed the following.
  - Occlude wound on the non-porous covering
  - Same intervention as CP (closed pneumothorax), and
  - Same discharge instruction as CP.

PULMONARY CONTUSION

A penetrating injury may cause contusion of the lung or pleura. Pulmonary contusion usually results from sudden compression followed by rapid compression of the thoracic cavity, causing blood to extravasate into pulmonary tissue.

The contusion is usually self-limiting because the pulmonary vasculature is a low-pressure system. However, extensive contusion can precipitate pulmonary oedema with resultant hypoxaemia, hypercapnoea, and respiratory acidosis.

Clinical Manifestation

Pulmonary contusion may vary from total absence of symptoms to the full spectrum of symptoms associated with non-cardiogenic pulmonary oedema. Signs and symptoms (some of which may be delayed) include the following.

- Increasing dyspnoea
- Tachypnoea
- Increasing restlessness
- Crackles notes on auscultations, and
- Haemoptysis.

Management

Medical treatment of pulmonary contusion depends on the severity of the injury. Treatment may vary from outpatient monitoring to intubation and mechanical ventilating support when pulmonary oedema present. The nursing care includes the following:

- Administer analgesic as ordered every 3 hours
- Monitor for fluid overload
  - Keep accurate records of all intake and output
  - Monitor vital signs every 30 minutes. Report increased pulse and respiration, and
  - Monitor breath sound every 30 minutes.
- Monitor ventilating status
  - Check for signs of respiratory distress–dyspnoea, increased inspiration, changes in breath sound, and
  - Check ABG results.
- Monitor for sign of symptom of flail chest
- Support patient to stay in bed until physical status is stabilised
  - Stay with patient, listen to patients concerned–explain what is planned, and
  - Assist with ADL
- Teach patient/family how to support pulmonary contusion.

OBSTRUCTIVE LUNG DISEASES

Chronic obstructive pulmonary disease (COPD) is defined as a disease state characterised by airflow obstruction resulting from chronic bronchitis or emphysema. The airflow obstruction is generally progressive, may be accompanied by airway hyperactivity and may be partially reversible.

CHRONIC BRONCHITIS

Chronic bronchitis is defined by the presence of chronic productive cough for minimum of 3 months per year for at least 2 consecutive years in patients in whom other causes have been excluded, it is characterised by physiologically by hypertrophy and hypersecretion of the bronchial mucous glands and structural alterations of the bronchi and bronchioles.

Aetiology

Chronic bronchitis is caused by the inhalation of physical or chemical irritants or by viral or bacterial infections. The most common inhaled irritant is cigarette smoke–heavy cigarette smoking.

Pathophysiology

In chronic bronchitis, there is pathologic changes in the lung consisting of:

- Hyperplasia of mucus secreting glands in the trachea and bronchi,
- Increase in globlet cells
- Disappearance of cilia
- Chronic inflammatory charges and narrowing of small airways, and
- Altered functions of alveolar macrophages, leading to increased bronchial infections.

Frequently airways are colonised with microorganisms. Infection occurs when the organisms increase. Most common infecting agents are *S. pneumoniae* and *H. influenzae*. Excess amounts of mucus are found in the airways and sometimes may occlude small bronchioles and scarring the bronchiole wall may occur chronic inflammation in the primary pathologic mechanism involved in causing the changes characteristics of chronic bronchitis.

Clinically Manifestation

The earliest symptom in chronic bronchitis is usually a frequent, productive cough during most winter months. It is often exacerbated by respiratory irritants and cold, damp air. Bronchospasm can occur at the end of paroxysms of coughing. Frequent respiratory infections are other common manifestation. Somewhat later, dyspnoea on exertion may develop. Unfortunately a patient often attributes chronic cough to smoking rather than lung disease, thus delaying initiation of treatment. In addition, the patient may not be aware of the cough because he/she becomes accustomed to it.

Hypoxaemia and hypercapnoea result from hypoventilation caused by increased airway resistance. The bluish red colour of the skin results from polycythaemia and cyanosis. Polycythaemia develops as a result of increased production of red blood cells secondary to the body's attempt to compensate for chronic hypoxaemia. Haemoglobin concentration may reach 200 g/L. Cyanosis develops when there is at least 5 g/dl or more of circulating unoxygenated haemoglobin.

The complication of chronic bronchitis are cor pulmonale, acute exacerbation of chronic bronchitis, and acute respiratory failure, peptic ulcer, and GERD, and pneumonia.

Management

Diagnostic studies of COPD include

- Chest X-ray film, typical finding in chronic bronchitis and increased bronchovascular markings.
- Sputum studies for culture and sensitivity. Neutrophils and bronchial epithelial cells usually occurs in chronic bronchitis.
- ABG
- ECG
- Exercise testing with oximetry (if indicated)
- EEG or cardia nuclear scan (if indicated).

The primary goal of care for COPD patients are to:

- Improve ventilation.
- Promote secretion–removal.
- Prevent complication and progression of symptoms.
- Promote patient comfort and participation in care and
- Improve quality of life as much as possible.

Medical therapy of chronic bronchitis are depends on symptoms. Pulmonary function tests results in ABG findings. Therapy may include all or some of the modalities outlined here are as follows:

i. Supportive measures:
Education of patient and family about the following:
  - Avoidance of cigarette smoke
  - Avoidance of other inhaled irritants
  - Avoidance of persons with upper respiratory infections
  - Control of environmental temperature and humidity
  - Proper nutrition, and
  - Adequate hydration.

ii. Specific therapy: Medication such as
  - Bronchiodilator–α antitrypsin replacement for those with ↓ levels
  - Antimicrobials–ampicillium or another broad-spectrum antibiotic
  - Corticosteroids—to alleviate acute symptoms: e.g., prednisone
  - Digitalis—to treat LVF if present.

iii. Respiratory therapy in aerosol therapy used to deliver bronchiodilator, through metered cartridge device with spacer at rest.
  - Oxygen therapy for patients who are unable to maintain PaO_2.

iv. Relaxation exercises
  - Meditation for relax

v. Breathing retraining

vi. Rehabilitation.

EMPHYSEMA

Emphysema is defined pathologically by destructive changes in alveolar walls and enlargement of air spaces distal to the terminal non-respiratory bronchioles. It is characterised physiologically by increased lung compliance, decreased diffusing, capacity and increased airway resistance.

Aetiology

The cause of emphysema is not known. However, evidence suggests that proteases released by polymorph nuclear leukocytes or alveolar macrophages are involved in the destruction of the connective tissue of the lungs. Cigarette smoking, infections, ambient air pollution and heredity (AAT–α, antitrypsin) are the other causes of emphysema.

Pathophysiology

Emphysema is a condition of the lungs characterised by abnormal permanent enlargement of the airspaces distal to the terminal bronchioles, accompanied by destruction of these walls and without obvious fibrosis. Structural changes include

- Hyperinflation of alveoli
- Destruction of alveolar walls
- Destruction of alveolar capillary walls
- Narrowed tortuous, small airways, and
- Loss of lung elasticity.

There are two types of emphysema centrilobular and panlobular. In centrilobular emphysema the primary area involvement is the central part of the lobula. Respiratory bronchioles enlarge, the walls are destroyed, and the bronchioles become confluent, chronic bronchioles associate with centrilobular types.

Panlobular emphysema, involves distentions and destruction of the whole lobule. Respiratory bronchioles, alveolar ducts and sacs and alveoli are all affected. There is a progressive loss of lung tissue and decreased alveolar-capillary surface area. Severe panlobular emphysema/usually found in persons with AAT (alpha-antitrypsin) deficiency.

Clinical Manifestation

An early symptom of emphysema is dyspnoea, which becomes progressively more severe. The patient will first complain of dyspnoea on exertion that progresses to interfering with ADL to dyspnoea at rest. Minimal coughing is present, with no sputum or smell amounts of mucoid sputum. As more alveoli becomes over distended increasing amount of air are trapped. This causes flattened diaphragm and an increased anteroposterior diameter of the chest, forming the typical barrel chest. Effective abdominal breathing decreased. The person becomes more of chest breather, relying on the intercostal and accessory muscles. Hypoxaemia may be present. The person is characteristically thin and underweight. The person may suffer from protein-caloric malnutrition. Later clubbing finger may develop. The complications as in chronic bronchitis.

Management of emphysema same as in chronic bronchitis. Nursing intervention for persons with chronic bronchitis and pulmonary emphysema are also the same, which include administration of medication such as digitalis and diuretics as prescribed, improving gas exchange, oxygen therapy, improving efficiency for breathing pattern (pursed lip-breathing, forward-leaving position, abdominal breathing and exercise, pulmonary physiotherapy, segmental postural drainage), improving airway clearance, improving nutrition, preventing infection, preventing fluid volume excess, assisting with breathing in rest, assisting with central of environment, and mounting temperature and humidity, etc.

And teach the following:

i. Progressive relaxation exercise.
  - Contract each muscle to a count of 10 and then relax it.
  - Do exercises in quiet room while sitting or lying in a comfortable position.
  - Do exercises for relaxing muscle, if desired.

- Have another person serve as a "coach" by giving command to contract specific muscles, count to 10 and relax muscle.
- The following are the examples of exercises helpful to some person with (COPD)
  - Raise shoulders, shrug them, and relax for 5 seconds, then relax them completely.
  - Make a first of both hands. Squeeze them lightly for 5 seconds and relax them completely.

ii. Meditation exercises:

1. Sit or lie quietly with eyes closed and attempt to relax all muscles beginning with feet and moving upward.
2. Breathe in through the nose slowly (may help to count slowly to 4 on inhalation) and exhale slowly through pursed lips (mentally count to 6) with a natural rhythm, relaxed and peaceful (this can be coached or performed without assistance).
3. Survey the body points of tension, consciously relax the tense areas. The body is peaceful and relaxed.
4. Continue breathing as above. Aware of the feeling of well-being throughout your body. This can be used for 10 to 20 minutes or after 5 minutes go to step 5.
5. Listen for (or visualize) a special relaxation sound (or image). Listen to it closely (or visualise) all the while breathing as above.
6. At this point, positive suggestion can be used, for example, I am in control of my body. When I find myself getting tense, I can take moment to stop and breathe in all the air that I need and let the tension flow away".
7. After mental suggestion, continue breathing easily and slowly come back to normal alert to mental state.
8. Meditation can be used at any time to induce relaxed state of mind (e.g. to promote sleep).

While taking care of the person with COPD, nurse has to take the following areas should be addressed in a typical teaching programme for persons with chronic bronchitis or emphysema.

i. Patients should be able to explain in lay terms, the basic functions and pathology of their lungs.

ii. Avoidance of respirative irritants and maintenance of a proper environment should be emphasised to people with COPD. Inhaled irritants (especially cigarette smoke) pose a serious threat to these persons. Steps the patient can take to reduce or avoid exposure to these irritants.

- Stop smoking. The nurse should be familiar with community programmes and give a list of them to the patient, to involve in it.
- Ask other persons not to smoke in the patient's room. Inhalation of secondary smoke can exacerbate symptoms.
- Pay heed to announcement on radio and TV warning of pollution alert. Do not go outside during an alert.
- Use an air-conditioner or HEPA filter or electrostatic filter to remove particular matter from air.
  - Keep filters clean and follow manufacturers' directions for use.
  - Use an activated charcoal filter if offending odours or gas pollutants are a problem.
- Avoid abrupt environmental temperature or humidity changes, because they can increase sputum production and cause bronchospasms.
  - Use an airconditioner in hot weather
  - Use a face mask when going out in cold weather
  - Use a dehumidifier or humidifier as appropriate to maintain a humidity of 30 per cent to 50 per cent.
- If air travel is required, check with physician about need for suplemental oxygen.
- Avoid large growds, especially during known influenza.
  - Avoid contact with people who have an upper respiratory infection
  - Receive influenza and pneumonia immunisation.

iii. The patient should be able to explain the following aspects of the home medication or treatment regimen.

- State name, dose, action and side effects of each infection.
- Explain how and where to use medication ordered on an as needed basis (e.g. bronchodilators, antibiotics, steroids, antacids).
- Describe how to obtain and maintain any needed equipment or supplies (e.g. oxygen, nebulizers, humidifiers, aerosols IPPB machines and syringes medications).

iv. The patient should demonstrate how to carry out the specific home exercise programme:

- Specific exercises to be completed
- Frequency of exercise
- Monitor physical response to exercises, such as heart rate increase, increase respiratory rate, or perceived fatigue.

v. The patient should be able to list the names and telephone numbers of the appropriate support services.

ASTHMA

Asthma is an inflammatory disease characterised by hyperresponsiveness of the airways and periods of bronchospasm, resulting in intermittent airway obstruction. The onset of asthma is sudden, contrary to the slow, insidious progression of symptoms seen in chronic bronchitis and emphysema.

Aetiology

Asthma is caused by increased responsiveness of the trachea and bronchi to various stimuli that cause narrowing of the airways and difficulty in breathing. The common factors triggering an asthma attack include:

- Environmental factors
  - change in temperature especially cold air and
  - change in humidity; dry air.
- Atmospheric pollutants
  - Cigarette and industrial smoke, ozone, sulphur dioxide, formaldehyde.
  - Exhaust fumes, oxidants, aerosol sprays.
- Strong odours, perfumes.
- Allergen inhalation.
  - Feathers, animal danders, dust mites molds allergens
  - Foods treated with sulfites, beer, wine fruit juices, snack foods salads, potatoes, shellfish, fresh and dried fruits) and metabisulfites, bisulfites, tartrazines.
- Exercise and cold, dry air
- Stress or emotional upset
- Infection: Vital upper respiratory infection, sinusitis
- Medications: Aspirin and NSAIDs B-blockers (including eyedrops of glaucoma)
- Enzymes: Including those in laundry detergents
- Occupational exposure: Metal salts, wood and vegetable dust, industrial chemicals and plastics
- Chemicals, toluene and others used in solvents, paints, rubber and plastics
- Hormones, menses
- Gastro-esophageal reflex. (GER)

Pathophysiology

The mechanism that induces asthma remains unknown. There are two types of asthma. Extrinsic (atopic) and intrinsic (non-atopic).

Extrinsic asthma results from an inflammatory response of the airway caused by mast cell activation, eosinophil infiltration, and epithelial slughing. An attack is triggered by environmental allergen (dust, pollen, molos, animal dander and foods). An initial encounter with an allergen stimulates plasma cells to produce antigen-specific IgE, antibodies that bind mast cells in airways. When exposed to the allergen IgE antigen binding causes mast cell deregulation and release of inflammatory mediators. The result is an intense inflammatory response in the airways.

Intrinsic asthma occurs in adults 35 years of age in older, the asthma attack is often severe. Factors that precipitate attacks include respiratoy tract infections, drugs (aspirin, B-adrenergic antogonism), environmental irritants, (occupational chemicals) air pollutions, cold, dry, air, exercise and emotional stress. Chemical mediator, interacts with the autonomic nervous systems causing inflammation and bronchoconstriction.

An asthmatic attack results from several physiological alterations, include altered immunological response increased airway resistance, increased lung compliance, impaired mucociliary function, and altered carbon dioxide exchange.

Clinical Manifestation

Asthma is characterised by an unpredictable and variable course. It causes recurrent episodes of wheezing, breathlessness, chest tightness, and cough, particularly at night and in the early morning. An attack of asthma may have an abrupt onset or it may be more gradual. Attacks often occur at night may last for a few minutes to several hours. In between, the patient may be asymptomatic with normal and abnormal pulmonary function. However, in some persons, compromised pulmonary functions may result in a state of continuous asthma and chronic debilitation characterised by irreversible airway disease.

The characteristic clinical manifestation of asthma are wheezing cough, dyspnoea, and chest tightness after exposed to a precipitating factor or trigger. Expiration may be prolonged. Instead of normal inspiratory-expiratory ratio of 1:2 it will be prolonged to 1:3 or 1:4. Normally the bronchioles constrict during expiration. However, as a result of bronchospasm, oedema and mucus in the bronchioles, the airways become narrower than usual. This takes longer for the air to move out of the bronchioles. This produce the characteristic wheezing, air trapping and hyperinflation.

The signs and symptoms associated with asthma are correlated with normal lung functions and underlying pathophysiological origins (see aetiology). The character of asthmatic attacks can vary on a continuum from chronic or acute mild intermittent attacks to life-threatening *status asthmaticus*. Severe acute asthma can result in complication such as rib fractures, pneumothorax, pneumomediastinum, atelectasis, pneumonia and status asthmaticus.

Status asthmaticus is a severe, life-threatening asthma attack that is refractory to usual treatment and places the patient at risk for developing respiratory failure. The causes of which include viral illnesses, ingestion of aspirin or other NSAIDs, emotional stress, increase in environmental pollutants or other allergen exposure, abrupt discontinuation of aerosal medication and ingestion of beta adrenergic blocking agent. In this exhaustion, diminished breath sounds, intubation and mechanical ventilation, complications of status asthmaticus include pneumothorax, pneumomediastenum, acute cor pulmonale with RVF and severe respiratory muscle fatigue leading to respiratory arrest. Death from status asthmaticus is usually the result of respiratory arrest or cardiac failure.

Management

The objective of medical management of asthma are to promote normal functioning of the individual, prevent recurrent symptoms, prevent severe attacks and prevent side effects of medication. The chief aim of various medication is to afford the patient immediate, progressive ongoing bronchial relaxation.

One approach to treat an acute asthmatic attack is as follows:

i. Inhalation of beta-agonist such as albuterol sulphate (proventil, ventalin), salmeterol (Serolvent), or metaproterenol sulphate in normal saline. Which stimulates beta2-receptors in bronchial smooth muscle resulting in smooth muscle relaxation. It starts to act in 10 minutes, effects last 4-6 hours. Here, the nurse has to monitor vital signs, lung sounds, and peak expiratory flow rate (PEFR) before and after treatment. If this is not successful: Go for the following.
ii. Methylprednisoline IV loading dose 2 mg/kg or about 125 mg 6th hrs/then 60-125 mg 6th hourly for 48 hours total or until patient is stable, which reduces inflammation and oedema of airway and decreases hyperactivity of airway. The benefits seen within 6 hours full effect in 6-8 hours.

    When patient is stabilised, change IV to 60 mg oral prednisoline by mouth daily or every other day. The oral prednisoline should be tapered off by 7-10 days, Taper 60 mg over 2 days, 40 mg over 2 days, 30 mg over 2 days and 10 mg over 2 days.
iii. Nebulized atrophine sulphate may be tried, or aminophylline may be given IV a pump is used for better control of infusion... which relax bronchial smooth muscle.

Loading dose of aminophyllin 4 to 6 mg/kg over 15 to 30 minutes and then continuous infusion of 0.45 to 0.70 mg/kg/hour. Patients who have been taking aminophyllin at home will be placed on continuous IV therapy. Rate of infusion is 10-20 mg/ml. Too rapid an infusion may cause severe hypotension, premature ventricular contractions, and cardiac arrest.

Here, the nurse has to monitor heart rate and rhythm closely, and report any change immediately to the concerned. Theophylline metabolised by the liver. For persons with liver disease, small doses are used. Patient taking Cemitidene, erythromycin or ciprofloxacin require smaller doses. Smokers and those taking phenytoin require larger doses to maintain blood level.

Other common medications for asthma are as follows:

- NSAIDs such as cromolym, nedocromil, administered through metered dose inhaler (MDI) or nebulizer, decreases airway inflammation and irritation, headache, bad taste in mouth.
- Corticosteroids (dexamethosone, triamcinolene acetonide, Flunisolid, fluticasone) administered through MDI has an anti-inflammatory action. Side effects are sore throat, hoarseness, cough, oral thrush.
- Leukotriene inhibitors/receptor antagonists such as zafirlukast, zilenton, are anti-inflammatory used orally. Adverse efforts include headache, nausea, diarrhoea, dizziness, myalgia, fever, dyspepsia, elevated glanine aminotransferase level.
- Theophylline can be administered orally or parenterally. It is long acting, bronchiodilator. Side effects are nausea, vomiting, stomach cramps, diarrhea, headache, muscle cramps, tachycardia, irritability, restlessness, serum blood levels should be checked for therapeutic range.
- Anticholenergics (spray) administered through MDI or nebulizer, or nasal spray. It is short-acting bronchiodilator. Side effects are nervousness, dizziness, headache, palpations, blurred vision, nausea, GI distress and dry mouth.
- Beta2-agonist such as salmeterol administered through MDI. It is long-acting bronchiodilator; may lead to adverse effects—headache, tremor, tachycardia, palpations, nasopharyngitis, stomachache, cough, rash.

When administering the above drugs, nurse has to monitor the responses and side effects of the medication and act accordingly. And when using a metered–Dose inhaler (MDI) the nurse has to teach the patient as follows:

- Inhale through nose, then slowly exhale
- Place inhaler 1 to 2 inches off the mouth
- Press down inhaler while simultaneously inhaling one puff deeply. Breath in air from around the mouth piece while inhaling.
- Hold breath for 5 to 10 seconds to allow medication to reach lung.
- Repeat second puff if one is ordered.
- If any untoward effects, stop administering of MDI.

CYSTIC FIBROSIS

Cystic fibrosis is an autosomal recessive, multisystem disease characterised by altered function of the exocrine glands involving primarily the lungs, pancreas, and sweat glands. Abnormally thick, abundant secretions from mucus glands can lead to a chronic, diffuse, obstructive pulmonary disorder in almost all patients.

Aetiology

Cystic fibrosis is an autosomal recessive disease resulting from mutations in a gene located on chromosome 7. The most common mutations in the CF gene is known as the CF transmembrane regulator (CFTR). The primary defect in the CF is abnormally regulated chloride channel activity. This defect alters ionic transport of sodium and chloride across epithelial surfaces. The high concentration of NaCl in the sweat of the patients with CF results from decreased chloride reabsorption in the sweat duct. The basic pathophysiologic mechanism is obstruction of exocrine gland duct with thick viscous secretions that adhere to the lumen of the ducts. The glands distal to the duct eventually undergo fibrosis.

Pathophysiology

Cystic fibrosis is an exocrine gland disease involving various systems, i.e., pulmonary, pancreatic/hepatic, GI, reproductive obstruction of the exocrine glands duct or passage ways occurs in nearly all adult patients with CF. Exocrine gland secretions are known to have a decreased water content, altered electrolyte concentration and abnormal organic constituents (especially no mucus glycoproteins), however, the specific biochemical or physiological defect that leads to obstruction is not known.

The following physiological alterations are found in adults with CF include:

- Pulmonary damage
- Gastrointestinal and pancreatic involvement
- Glucose intolerance.

Clinical Manifestations

The specific clinical manifestation by symptoms are:

- Pulmonary signs and symptoms of CF includes
  - Chronic productive cough and/or recurrent bronchitis or pneumonia
  - Crackles and rhonchi decreased pulmonary compliance, digital clubbing, and
  - Shortness of breath and dyspnoea on exertion, wheezing, and weight loss occurs with respiratory complication and usually indicate need for vigorous therapy.
- Gastrointestinal signs and symptoms include the following:
  - Frequent, bulky, greasy stools
  - Weight loss
  - Cramps and abdominal pain should arouse suspicion of obstruction
- Glucose intolerance signs and symptoms include:
  - Polyuria, polydipsia, polyphagia and
  - Absence of ketoacidosis even with above signs.

Normally mucus production by goblet cells lubricate airways and entraps foreign particles. In CF, excessive amounts of mucus production leads to increased cough and mucus production, inflammation of small airways causing hyperinflation of alveoli give rise to fatigue, shortness of breath, chronic bacterial infections leading to fever, fatigue, shortness of breath, and eroding of a major blood vessel and secondary infection may lead to haemoptysis.

Management

The goals of medical management of CF are to minimize bronchial plugging and to inhibit bacterial colonisation. Measures to minimize bronchial plugging include:

- Chest physiotherapy with chest percussion and postural drainage are performed for 20 minutes two or three times daily and some time much more frequently.
- Administer dornase-alfa 2.5 mg ampule in compressed air-driven nebulizer for reducing visco-elasticity of CF secretion.
- Mucolytic agents may be ordered to thin secretions.
- Humidification of air, according to some physicians
- Antibiotics for infection.

Nursing measures include preventing pulmonary infections, care of haemoptysis, care of pneumothorax and care of cor pulmonale diet, activity and regimen.

- Prevention of pulmonary infection can be made best by:
  - Vigorous postural drainage and percussing
  - Room humidification if ordered
  - Aerosols with a bronchodilator, and
  - Monitoring for infection–and take suitable measure accordingly.
- Nursing care and medical care during haemoptysis include:
  - Elevate head of bed 45 to 90 degrees
  - Turn patient's head to left side to facilitate expectoration of blood
  - Provide clean basin frequently so that patient is not made more anxious by amount of blood
  - Measure amount of hemoptysis and record time and amounts
  - Postural drainage and percussion are contraindicated if haemoptysis present
  - Vitamin K as ordered by mouth or subcutaneously to check bleeding
  - Stay with the patient until bleeding has subsided and made comfortable to less fearful, and
  - Bronchioscopy with endobronchial tamponade may be successful.
- Care of pneumothorax includes proper care for chest tube connected to closed drainage system and other measure used in pneumothorax
- Care of cor pulmonale includes supplement oxygen, long-term diuretic therapy. Digoxin if or as ordered by the physician
- Promoting adequate nutrition–supplemental fat soluble vitamins and multivitamins and vitamin E. Pancreatin enzyme supplemented
- Patient should be encouraged to be upright position as a tolerated
- Patient and family educated about taking care of CF cases.

RESPIRATORY FAILURE

Acute respiratory failure (ARF) is used to describe any rapid change in respiration resulting in hypoxaemia, hypercarnea, or both. ARF can be classified as hypoxaemia or hypercapnia.

Hypoxaemic respiratory failure is also related to an oxygenation failure, because the primary problem is inadequate O_2 transfer. This can be defined as a PaO_2 of 60 mm Hg or less when the patient is receiving an inspired O_2 concentration of 60 per cent or greater.

Hypercapnic respiratory failure is also referred to as ventilatory failure because the primary problem is insufficient CO_2 removal. It is defined as a $PaCO_2$ above normal (> 45 mm Hg) in combination with acedemea (pH < 7.35).

Aetiology

Many disorders can lead to or associated with respiratory failure which can be divided into pulmonary and nonpulmonary diseases.

i. Pulmonary disorders
   - Severe infection
   - Pulmonary oedema
   - Pulmonary embolus
   - COPD - Chronic obstructive pnl. disease
   - CF - Cystic fibrosis
   - ARDS - Acute respiratory distress syndrome
   - Cancer
   - Chest trauma (flail chest)
   - Severe atelectasis, and
   - Airway compromise, secondary to trauma, infection or surgery.

ii. Non-pulmonary disorders
   - CNS disturbance secondary to drug overdose, anaesthesia, head injury
   - Neuromuscular disorders, i.e. Guillain-Barré syndrome. Myasthenia gravis, multiple sclerosis, poliomyelitis, muscular disatrophy, spinal cord injury.
   - Postoperative reduction in ventilation following thoracic and abdominal surgery.
   - Prolonged mechanical ventilation.

Pathophysiology

The respiratory system is made up of two basic parts, the gas exchange organ (Lung) and the pump (the respiratory muscles and the respiratory control mechanism). Any alteration in the function of gas exchange unit or pump can result in respiratory insufficiency or respiratory failure. Regardless of the underlying condition, the resultant events or processes that occur in respiratory failure are the same. With inadequate ventilation, the arterial oxygen falls and tissue cells become hypoxic. Carbon dioxide accumulates, leading to a fall in pH and respiratory acidosis.

Lung or gas exchange unit respiratory failure is usually seen in person with underlying primary pulmonary disease such as COPD. In this situation respiratory failure as a result of pathology directly affects the respiratory unit.

Pump failure is associated with extra-pulmonary disorders that may precipitate respiratory failure. In this situation the underlying disorder decreases the ability of lungs to move oxygen and carbon dioxide into and out of the lungs by altering either the central ventilatory control mechanism (e.g. drug overdose) neuromuscular function (e.g. Gullain-Barré syndrome) or chest wall movement (flail chest).

Acute respiratory failure is defined by predetermined physiological criteria, i.e. sudden onset of the following.

- PaO_2 50 mm Hg or less (measured in room air),
- $PaCO_2$ 50 mm Hg or more, and
- pH 7.35 or less.

Clinical Manifestations

The sign and symptoms associated with hypercapnia, hypoxaemia and respiratory acidosis are

- Headache
- Irritability
- Increasing somnolence coma
- Asterixis (flapping tremor)
- Cardiac dysrhythmias
- Tachycardia
- Hypotension
- Cyanosis.

Management

The management of respiratory failure includes the following.

1. Medical therapy is based on degree of severity.
   - Severe acute respiratory failure, focus on immediate oxygenation and ventilation.
   - Less severe acute respiratory failure: underlying cause determined and treated concurrently while treating hypoxaemia and hypercapnia
2. Clinical evaluation
   a. Diagnosis studies include—ABGs, chest X-ray film, bedside pulmonary spirometry, sputum for culture and sensitivity
   b. Treatment includes
      – Oxygen therapy
      – Ventilation: may require intubation and mechanical ventilatory supports
      – Treatment of underlying causes.

Nursing care includes improving gas exchange, ventilatory support, mechanical ventilation, improving airway clearance, improving breathing pattern, improving cardiac output, maintaining adequate nutrition, health promotion and prevention.

Table 6.1: Nursing care plan for the patient with chronic obstructive pulmonary disease in acute respiratory failure

Problem	*R*	*Objective*	*Nursing interventions*	*Railonales*
Nursing Diagnosis # 1				
Airway clearance, ineffective, related to copious, thick, tenacious secretions.		Patient will: 1. Be alert and oriented to person, place, time. 2. Demonstrate deep breathing techniques and effective secretion-clearing cough. 3. Minimize risk of aspiration. Arterial blood gases will stabilise: • pH > 7.35 < 7.45. • PaO_2 > 60 mmHg. • $PaCO_2$ at level to maintain pH within acceptable range	• Perform a comprehensive respiratory assessment including: ♦ Airway patency; rate, rhythm, and depth of breathing; chest and diaphragmatic excursion.	• Major goal of airway management is to establish and/or maintain adequate alveolar ventilation. ♦ Baseline data are essential to evaluate effectiveness of therapeutic interventions.
			♦ Use of accessory muscles; presence of intercostal retraction.	♦ Increased work of breathing may be caused by small airway obstruction.
			♦ Auscultation of breath sounds.	♦ May detect evidence of secretion accumulation, airway obstruction, atelectasis.
			• Monitor quality, quantity, colour, and consistency of sputum ♦ Obtain sputum for culture and sensitivity on admission, and thereafter as dictated by patient's conditon	• Baseline data enable changes in sputum production and characteristics to be identified. Infection or other pulmonary insult may increase quantity of sputum production.
			♦ Assess secretions for state of hydration or need for mucolytic therapy	♦ Thinning of secretions facilitates mobilisation and clearance.
			♦ Monitor body temperature and white blood count profile.	♦ Early detection of an infectious or inflammatory process affords prompt intervention to minimize the effect of the insult on pulmonary and other body processes.
			• Institute prescribed bronchodilator therapy. ♦ Assess pulmonary function prior to and after bronchodilator therapy	♦ Assists in determining effectiveness of therapy.
			♦ Assist into semi-Fowler's position	♦ Allows for best possible lung expansion.
			♦ Monitor for signs/symptoms of bronchodilator therapy toxicity (especially when theophylline or theophylline salts are used) – Monitor theophylline level.	♦ Theophylline and derivatives have a narrow therapeutic index.
			• Initiate chest physiotherapy techniques: ♦ Postural drainage; percussion and vibration; deep breathing and coughing	• Loosens and dislodges secretions and enhances movement towards trachea from where they are accessible to removal by cough and/or suctioning.
			• Teach appropriate method of coughing	• Achieve most effective cough with least amount of effort.
			♦ Avoid unnecessary or ineffective coughing	♦ May cause irritation of tracheobronchial tree
			• Institute pharyngeal and tracheobronchial suctioning as needed.	• Suctioning is not without risks (hypoxaemia, atelectasis, infection); it should be performed only as indicated.
			♦ Follow appropriate procedure for endotracheal suctioning.	♦ Aseptic technique is essential to minimize risk of infection; oxygenation reduces risk of hypoxaemia.

Contd...

Contd...

Problem	*R*	*Objective*	*Nursing interventions*	*Rationales*
			• Instruct patient in use of incentive spirometry.	• Increases vital capacity and helps to more evenly match ventilation with perfusion.
			• Provide opportunity for rest periods. ◆ Schedule activities to avoid fatigue.	• Reduces oxygen demand; reduces fatigue.
			• Assure hydration state. ◆ Monitor intake and output; daily weight.	• Adequate hydration moistens, loosens, and liquefies secretions.
			• Use a calm, reassuring approach. ◆ Anticipate needs for emotional support.	• Assists to reduce anxiety.
			◆ Be accessible and offer explanations.	◆ An informed patient is usually a cooperative patient.
			◆ Involve in decision-making regarding care when possible.	◆ Allows patient to retain some control over his/her life.
Nursing Diagnosis # 2 Breathing pattern, ineffective, related to reduced maximum expiratory airflow. (See Nursing Diagnosis # 11 below.)		Patient will: 1. Demonstrate effective minute ventilation: Tidal volume (V_T) $>$5-7 ml/kg. Respiratory rate $<$35/min (adult). 2. Achieve a vital capacity (V_C) $>$ 12-15 ml/kg. 3. Verbalise ease of breathing. 4. Demonstrate pursedlip and diaphragmatic breathing. 5. Exhibit breath sounds: • Audible throughout anterior/posterior chest. Reduced to absent adventitious sounds.	• Assess respiratory function: ◆ Rate, rhythm, depth, and pattern of breathing	◆ Reflect work of breathing: Increased work of breathing increases oxygen consumption and results in hypercapnia and physical fatigue/exhaustion.
			◆ Symmetry of chest wall and diaphragmatic excursion.	◆ Effective ventilation requires synchronous movement of chest wall, diaphragm, and abdominal wall. ◆ Rapid, shallow respirations (tachypnoea hyperventilation) move deadspace air, significantly reducing alveolar ventilation. ◆ Asymmetry of respiratory excursion may reflect underlying pathology (e.g., atelectasis, pneumothorax).
			◆ Co-ordination of contraction of inspiratory and expiratory muscles. ◆ Use of accessory muscles. ◆ Auscultation of breath sounds.	◆ Ventilatory dyscoordination (a disordered sequence of the contraction of muscles of inspiration and expiration) may be an early but subtle clue as to the development of ARF.
			◆ Pulmonary lung volumes: Total minute ventilation (V_E), tidal volume (V_T), respiratory rate (f), vital capacity (V_C).	◆ A minimal volume of ventilation is necessary to ensure adequate alveolar ventilation. ◆ Assessment of respiratory volumes allow close evaluation of effectiveness and efficiency of respiratory effort.
			• Assist patient into position of comfort and to allow for best lung expansion.	• Expansion of lungs facilitates more even distribution of ventilation; improves ventilation/perfusion matching.
			◆ Low to semi-Fowler's position; unaffected side down in side-lying position. ◆ Provide table with pillow for patient to lean on.	◆ Reduces ventilation/perfusion mismatch.

Contd...

Contd...

Problem	*R*	*Objective*	*Nursing interventions*	*Rationales*
			• Teach breathing techniques: ◆ Pursed-lip breathing.	◆ Increases expiratory airway resistance which functions to keep airways open longer to allow airflow and to reduce a trapping.
			◆ Diaphragmatic breathing.	◆ Lifting of abdominal wall upward and on ward allows for easier excursion of diaphragm by decreasing pressure within the abdomen.
			◆ Avoid lying flat (supine).	◆ Causes abdominal contents to shift toward chest cavity, limiting diaphragmatic excursion; may predispose to atelectasis.
			◆ Avoid hyperventilation.	◆ May predispose to metabolic alkalosis and patient with chronic lung disease.
			◆ Controlled breathing: Slower, of increased depth; use abdominal muscles.	◆ Conscious control of breathing increased effectiveness of respiratory effort.
			◆ Encourage hourly deep breathing in conjunction with chest physiotherapy techniques and bronchodilator therapy.	◆ Minimises atelectasis; mobilizes section; improves ventilation.
Nursing Diagnosis # 3 Gas exchange, impaired, related to: 1. Alveolar hypoventilation. 2. Ventilation/perfusion mismatch. 3. Diffusion impaired. 4. Right-to-left shunting.		Patient will: 1. Be alert and oriented to person, place, time. 2. Demonstrate appropriate behaviour. 3. Maintain effective cardiovascular function: • Blood pressure within 10 mmHg of baseline. • Cardiac output ~5 liters/min. • Without cyanosis if baseline "pink." • Lab values: Haematocrit Male: 45-52 % Female: 37-48% Haemoglobin > 10-12 g/100 ml. 4. Maintain optimal arterial blood gases: • pH 7.35–7.45. • PaO_2 > 60 mmHg. • $PaCO_2$ at level to preserve normal pH. 5. Maintain alveolar-arterial gradient ($AaDO_2$): Within acceptable range based on FIO_2.	• Perform neurologic examination including:	• Hypercapnia may predispose to carbon dioxide narcosis with depression of central respiratory centers.
			◆ Mental status; level of consciousness; appropriateness of behaviour.	◆ Hypoxaemia may predispose to cerebral tissue hypoxia.
			◆ Deep tendon reflexes.	
			◆ Complaints of headache, dizziness, nervousness, restlessness.	
			• Avoid sedatives, narcotics, hypnotics, tranquilizers.	• Depress central respiratory centers predisposing to alveolar hypoventilation with hypercapnia; may mask signs of significant carbon dioxide retention.
			• Monitor vital signs including: ◆ Blood pressure, heart rate.	• Circulatory impairment will interfere with adequate gas exchange within lungs and at tissue levels:
			◆ Respiratory rate; work of breathing. ◆ Evidence of distress; undue fatigue; secretion build-up.	◆ Increased work of breathing increases oxygen consumption and demand; predisposes to tissue hypoxia.
			• Monitor laboratory data: ◆ Arterial blood gases:	◆ Most closely reflect effectiveness of gas exchange.
			◆ Calculate alveolar-arterial gradient ($AaDO_2$).	◆ Limitation of $AaDO_2$ is that it does not look at cardiopulmonary function as a whole.
			◆ Observe for decreasing PaO_2 and pH, and increasing $PaCO_2$; bicarbonate (HCO_3^-) is elevated.	◆ Patients with COPD will have a different range of normal than healthy individuals.

Contd...

Contd...

Problem	*Objective*	*Nursing interventions*	*Rationales*
			• Increased HCO_3^- reflects renal compensation (i.e., reabsorption of HCO_3^-) in response to decreased blood pH caused by hypercapnia.
		• Haematology profile: Haematocrit (Hct). • Haemoglobin (Hgb).	• Sufficient red blood cells and haemoglobin are required for gas exchange to occur. In patients with long standing COPD, haematology should be monitored for polycythaemia vera.
		• Administer prescribed oxygen concentration:	• Alveolar hypoventilation and V/Q mismatch respond favourably to low-flow supplemental oxygen therapy.
		• Use low-flow supplemental oxygen therapy. • 24-28% by Venturi mask. • 2-3 liters/min by nasal cannula.	• Overzealous oxygen therapy can wipe out hypoxic drive in patients with COPD.
		• Monitor arterial blood gases at regular intervals.	• Reflect effectiveness of lungs in gas exchange.
		• Prevent complications related to precipitous decrease in $PaCO_2$.	• When ventilation has been interrupted (e.g., suctioning) or the FIO_2 has changed, blood sample for analysis should not be obtained for at least 20 minutes after therapy.
		• Monitor criteria for acute respiratory failure. • Additional considerations: Evidence of respiratory distress, "air hunger," secretion build up, undue fatigue	• Patients with COPD may experience difficult weaning from mechanical ventilatory therapy. Timely and aggressive implementation of respiratory support therapies (O_2 therapy, chest physiotherapy, treatment of underlying causes) may successfully prevent need for intubation and mechanical ventilation.
		• Intubate and initiate mechanial ventilation therapy when criteria for acute respiratory failure have been identified.	
Nursing Diagnosis # 4 Cardiac output, alteration in: Decreased (diminished venous return). *Nursing Diagnosis #5* Tissue perfusion, alteration in: Cardiopulmonary.	Patient will: 1. Maintain stable haemodynamics: • Blood pressure within 10 mmHg baseline. • Heart rate < 100 beats/min. • Cardiac output ~5 liters/min. • Central venous pressure (CVP) 0–8 mmHg. • Pulmonary capillary wedge pressure (PCWP) 8-12 mm Hg.	• Perform ongoing cardiovascular assessment: • Continuous cardiac monitoring (establish baseline rate, rhythm, ectopy). • Continuous haemodynamic monitoring (establish baseline): CVP, PCWP,	• Cardiac tissue hypoxia may predispose to dysrhythmias. • Offers significant data regarding cardiopulmonary function. • Positive-pressure mechanical ventilation increases pressure within the thorax, which impedes venous return to the heart; decrease in venous return (preload) reduces cardiac output.

Contd...

Contd...

Problem	*R*	*Objective*	*Nursing interventions*	*Rationales*
		2. Remain without: • Extreme weakness or fatigue. • Peripheral (pedal) oedema. • Neck vein distention. • Chest pain. • Cardiac dysrhythmias. 3. Maintain fluid and electrolyte balance: • Stable body weight. • Balanced intake and output. • Hourly urine output > 30 ml/hr.	◆ Heart sounds—Loudness or intensity, splitting, extra heart sounds (S_3–S_4)? ◆ Breath sounds—Evidence of rales (crackles); altered pulmonary mechanics? ◆ Fatigue, exhaustion? ◆ Neck vein distention? Pedal oedema? ◆ Serial arterial blood gases. • Implement fluid replacement therapy as prescribed. ◆ Monitor hydration status: Daily weight, intake and output, urine specific gravity. ◆ Avoid fluid volume overload.	◆ Loud pulmonic sound or splitting is commonly seen in cor pulmonale; it is related to pulmonary hypertension due to long-standing hypoxaemic state. ◆ In the patient with COPD, diminished breath sounds in a heretofore "noisy" chest may warn of hypoventilation with impending acute respiratory failure • Adequate fluid replacement therapy is essential to maintain blood volume and keep pulmonary secretions moist and easily mobilised. ◆ Long-standing pulmonary disease with pulmonary hypertension predisposes to right heart failure (corpulmonale).
Nursing Diagnosis # 6 Tissue perfusion, alteration in: Cerebral. Patient will:		1. Demonstrate appropriate behaviour: • Oriented to person, place, time.	• Assess ongoing neurologic function. ◆ Mental status, level of consciousness; behaviour appropriate? • Assess fluid and electrolyte status. ◆ Body weight. ◆ Intake and output (hourly urine output). ◆ Serum electrolytes, BUN, creatinine. • Maintain a quiet, relaxed milieu. ◆ Use a calm, reassuring approach. ◆ Provide explanations of care. ◆ Provide frequent periods of rest and relaxation. • Monitor for effects of drugs (e.g., theophylline) on cardiopulmonary function.	• Compromised haemodynamics and hypoxaemia predispose to cerebral hypoxia with altered cerebral function. • Reduced blood volume will further compromise venous return and cardiac output; blood volume may need to be expanded to minimise this effect. ◆ Reduced cardiac output may diminish renal perfusion, placing patient at risk of developing acute renal failure. • Minimise fear and anxiety, which increases oxygen consumption and demand. ◆ The work of breathing is often taxing; it is important to conserve patient's energy. • Drug toxicity may further compromise cardiopulmonary function.
Nursing Diagnosis # 7 Fluid and electrolyte, alterations in		Patient will: 1. Maintain baseline body weight. 2. Balance fluid intake with output. 3. Have: • Good skin turgor. • Absence of peripheral oedema. • Absence of rales (crackles) on auscultation. • Stable vital signs.	• Monitor hydration status: ◆ Daily weight, intake and output, vital signs. ◆ Examine skin for signs of dehydration: Poor skin turgor; sunken eyeballs; dry, parched mucous membranes. ◆ Monitor mental status changes; lethargy; severe weakness; reduced urine output.	• Patients receiving mechanical ventilation with humidified gas therapy are at risk to increase total body water. ◆ Stress increases secretion of antidiuretic hormone (ADH) by posterior pitulitary gland, increasing water retention.

Contd...

Contd...

Problem	*R*	*Objective*	*Nursing interventions*	*Rationales*
		4. Stabilise in terms of serum electrolyte, BUN, creatinine, total protein within acceptable physiologic range.	• Examine for signs of overhydration: peripheral oedema; hypertension; tachycardia; neck vein distention; elevated pulmonary haemodynamics; shortness of breath, dyspnoea. • Monitor serum electrolytes, BUN, creatinine, total protein.	• Stress increases aldosterone secretion by adrenal cortex, which stimulates sodium reabsorption within the kidneys.
Nursing Diagnosis # 8 Acid-base balance, alteration in, related to overzealous oxygen therapy in the patient with long standing COPD.		The patient's arterial blood gases will stabilize as follows: • pH 7.35–7.45. • PaO_2 > 60 mmHg • $PaCO_2$, sufficiently reduced to maintain pH within acceptable range for the patient.	• Administer oxygen therapy cautiously at prescribed concentration (FIO_2).	• In patients with long-standing COPD with chronic hypercapnia and consequent acidemia, the kidneys respond (compensate) by reabsorbing bicarbonate (HCO_3^-). This buffers the excess hydrogen ions associated with the hypercapnia and stabilizes the pH.
			• Closely monitor arterial blood gas values. – $PaCO_2$ must only be reduced to the level that "normalizes" pH	• Overzealous administration of oxygen can cause a precipitous fall in the $PaCO_2$, reducing hydrogenion concentration while leaving excess bicarbonate. The result is metabolic alkalaemia, which, if sufficiently severe, can lead to serious cardiac dysrhythmias and seizures.
Nursing Diagnosis # 9 Nutrition, alteration in: Less than body requirements.		Patient will: 1. Maintain body weight with 5% of baseline weight. 2. Maintain total serum proteins ~6.0–8.4 g/100 ml. 3. Maintain laboratory data within acceptable range: BUN, serum creatinine, electrolytes, fasting blood sugar, serum albumin, haematology profile. 4. Verbalize essentials of adequate diet.	• Arrange consultation with nutritionist and collaborate to perform nutrition assessment: General state of health; baseline body weight; nutritional history: Likes, dislikes, meal preparation, eating habits, cultural, religious considerations. • Lifestyle influences. • Physiologic factors: Height, weight, triceps skinfold, mid-upper arm circumference. • Laboratory studies: Urinary/serum creatinine, BUN, fasting blood sugar, serum electrolytes, total protein (serum albumin), haematology profile.	• Adequate nutritional intake is necessary to meet metabolic requirements to reverse acute respiratory failure. • Nutritional deficiencies (especially in elderly) are often associated with chronic disease.
			• Maintain adequate nutrition with prescribed enteral and/or parenteral feedings. • Special considerations.	• Clinical semi-starvation leads to depression of the hypoxic ventilatory drive. • Patients receiving mechanical ventilation therapy are highly stressed and require nutritional supplements to meet hypermetabolic needs.
			• Avoid large glucose loads to meet caloric needs.	• There is an obligate increase in carbon dioxide with increased glucose intake. Fat emulsions may be used to provide calories. • In patients who are mechanically ventilated or who have reduced respiratory reserve, the increased carbon dioxide can lead to hypercapnia and

Contd...

Contd...

Problem	*Objective*	*Nursing interventions*	*Rationales*
			may precipitate acute respiratory failure in the high risk patient.
		♦ Avoid hypophosphatemia.	♦ Reduced phosphate levels are associated with decreased energy levels, respiratory muscle weakness, and increased risk of infection.
		♦ Avoid high amino acid loads.	♦ Increase O_2 consumption.
		• Place patient in optimal position during feedings (usually semi-Fowler's position).	• Proper positioning and intact protective reflexes reduce risk of aspiration.
		• Confirm placement of nasogastric tube in stomach before initiating feedings. ♦ Assess for protective reflexes (gag, cough, swallowing).	• Proper placement of nasogastric tube helps to prevent aspiration.
		• Provide frequent mouth care and other comfort measures.	• May be aesthetically pleasing to patient/family. ♦ Keep mucus membranes moist and intact.
		• Monitor daily weight; fluid and intake. • Assess bowel function: ♦ Assess bowel sounds. ♦ Initiate bowel regimen, if indicated.	♦ Maintains gastrointestinal smooth muscle tone; prevents constipation or impaction.
Nursing Diagnosis #10 Essential for	Patient will: 1. Maintain normal body temperature ~98.6°F (37°C). 2. Maintain white blood count at acceptable baseline level. 3. Remain without evidence of acute infection: Redness, swelling, pain.	• Identify patients at high-risk of developing an infection: Debilitated or elderly, chronic lung disease, multiple invasive lines, semistarvation state, immunosuppressed.	• Patients with COPD are especially at high risk due to: ♦ Alteration in surfactant activity. ♦ Alterations in respiratory epithelium replication.
		• Obtain baseline cultures: Sputum, urine, blood.	• Upon intubation, a baseline sputum specimen should be obtained. ♦ Use of artificial airway (endotracheal tube or tracheostomy) contaminates the tracheobronchial tree, which is usually considered to be sterile distal to the larynx.
		• Monitor the following parameters: ♦ Body temperature. ♦ Haematology profile—Evidence of leukocytosis; eosinophilia. ♦ Sputum for changes in colour, quantity, consistency, odour; and ability of patient to handle secretions. ♦ Chest X-ray for pulmonary infiltrates.	• Early diagnosis with institution of timely and vigorous therapy (antibiotic) may help to minimise the impact of the infectious process on total body function.
		• Institute vigorous chest physiotherapy and bronchial hygiene.	• Secretion removal improves ventilation and reduces pooling of secretions, which may act as foci of infection.
		• Use aseptic technique for patient care: Tracheobronchial suctioning, care of invasive lines. • Administer prescribed antibiotic therapy. ♦ Monitor culture and sensitivity studies to assess response to therapy. • Maintain nutrition	• Reduces risks of infection.

Contd...

Contd...

Problem	*R*	*Objective*	*Nursing interventions*	*Rationales*
Nursing Diagnosis#11 Pulmonary mechanics, alteration in, related to respiratory muscle atrophy (immobility, mechanical ventilation; see Nursing Diagnosis #2 above).		Patient will: 1. Perform deep breathing exercises. 2. Achieve maximum pulmonary function: • Tidal volume > 7 ml/kg. • Vital capacity > 15 ml/kg. • Maximal expiratory flow.	• Teach deep breathing exercises.	• Use of positive-pressure ventilation predisposes of atrophy of the respiratory musculature, which can present problems for weaning.
			♦ Instruct regarding the importance of deep-breathing exercises.	♦ Improves pulmonary ventilation, mobilises secretions, stimulates circulation. ♦ Teaching regarding pulmonary mechanics forms the foundation of patient's self-care after hospitalization.
			♦ Allow patient to demonstrate pulmonary exercises. ♦ Combine deep-breathing therapy with other chest physiotherapy manoeuvres.	♦ Patient should be allowed to learn one task before proceeding to the next. Always establish readiness to learn on the part of patient and family.
			♦ Involve patient/family in decision-making (e.g., scheduling of exercise activities).	♦ The nature of chronic illness requires cooperation of all family members if exacerbations are to be prevented.
			♦ Encourage early ambulation (e.g., sitting up in chair).	♦ Involvement in planning and decision-making enables patient/family to begin to assume responsibility for their own lives.
			• Assess pulmonary volumes to determine effectiveness of therapy: Tidal volume, vital capacity.	
Nursing Diagnosis#12 Skin integrity, impairment of, related to immobility, and altered nutritional status.		Patient's skin will remain intact.	• Establish routine for turning and repositioning.	• Exercise maintains muscle tone and prevents muscle atrophy.
			• Assist with range-of-motion exercises to extremities. ♦ Provide support stockings to lower extremities. ♦ Assess extremities for calf tenderness. ♦ Measure circumference of thighs and calves daily.	• Exercise stimulates circulation and prevents stasis. ♦ Immobility predisposes to thrombophlebitis.
			• Provide special skin care to back and joints, and all pressure points.	• Maintains circulation to all areas; these patients frequently have a compromised body defense system and are at high risk of infection.
			♦ Establish regimen for: Skin inspection, skin care, decubitus care if necessary. ♦ Provide "egg-crate" or air mattress; sheep-skin; heel and ankle protectors. ♦ Apply local skin care.	♦ It is essential to prevent skin breakdown. ♦ Pressure relief devices.
Nursing Diagnosis#13 Fear. Nursing Diagnosis#14 Knowledge deficit regarding chronic obstructive pulmonary disease.		Patient/family will: 1. He ....verbalize fears and concerns. 2. Identity strengths and coping capabilities. 3. Verbalize knowledge regarding COPD.	• Assess knowledge regarding COPD and ex-............	• Chronic lung disease is a "family disease" impacting every member to some degree.
			• Verbulize fears and concerns for patient and family.	• If the patient/family are to realize optimal function within the limitations of the disease, all family members should be involved in the educating and caring processes.[7]

Contd...

Contd...

Problem	*R*	*Objective*	*Nursing interventions*	*Rationales*
		4. Verbalize intentions to make necessary adjustments in life-style. 5. Demonstrate ability to carry out necessary interventions. 6. Demonstrate self-confidence in their capabilities.	• Help them to recognise and to express their feelings regarding disruption in their life-style. o Encourage them to express fears regarding chronicity of disease: Necessity of oxygen therapy in the home setting; specific medication/other therapies. • Assess readiness to learn (see Chap. 4). o Have patient/family assist in identifying needs and learning objectives. • Assist family in problem-solving techniques. ◆ Help them identify family strengths and resources. ◆ Initiate referral to social services for necessary support: emotional, psychologic, financial, other.	• Assists family in coping; increases self-confidence in their own capabilities. ◆ It is reassuring to have specific resources available to lend assistance and support.

Table 6.2: Nursing care plan for the patient with adult respiratory distress syndrome in hypoxaemic acute respiratory failure

Problem	*R*	*Objective*	*Nursing interventions*	*Rationales*
Nursing Diagnosis #1 Gas exchange, impaired, related to: 1. Right-to-left shunting. 2. Ventilation/perfusion mismatch		Patient will: 1. Be alert and oriented to person, place, time. 2. Demonstrate appropriate behaviour. 3. Maintain effective cardiovascular function: • Blood pressure within 10 mmHg of baseline. • Cardiac output ~5 liters/min. • Without cyanosis if pre-existing pulmonary function normal. • Lab values: Haematocrit Male: 45-52% Female: 37-48% Haemoglobin Male: 13-18 g/100 ml Female: 12-16 g/100 ml. 4. Maintain optimal arterial blood gases: pH 7.35–7.45. PaO_2 > 60 mmHg. $PaCO_2$ ~ 35-45 mmHg. 5. Alveolar-arterial oxygen gradient ($AaDO_2$):<15 mm-Hg on room air.	• Perform neurologic assessment: ◆ Mental status, level of consciousness. ◆ Appropriate behaviour. ◆ Protective and deep tendon reflexes. • Monitor respiratory function: ◆ Respiratory rate and pattern. ◆ Use of accessory muscles. ◆ Status of weakness and fatigue. ◆ Degree of chest wall excursion. ◆ Increase in fremitus? ◆ Presence of dullness on percussion? ◆ Breath sounds: – Abnormal breath sounds. – Adventitious breath sounds. • Assess cardiovascular function: ◆ Heart rate. ◆ Haemodynamic parameters: – Systemic arterial pressure. – Pulmonary capillary wedge pressure. – Cardiac output.	• Hypoxaemia may predispose to cerebral tissue hypoxia. ◆ Increased work of breathing fatigues the patient and predisposes to alveolar hypoventilation with hypercapnia and respiratory acidemia. ◆ Consolidated lung tissue transmits vibrations better than airfilled lung spaces. ◆ Percussion over consolidated lung produces a "dull" sound. ◆ Bronchial breath sounds are often heard in areas of the lung that normally would reflect vesicular sounds; rales (crackles) may also be heard. • Haemodynamic parameters reflect tissue perfusion.

Contd...

Contd...

Problem	*R*	*Objective*	*Nursing interventions*	*Rationales*
			• Evidence of cyanosis.	• Late sign reflecting the desaturation of at least 5 g of haemoglobin; evidence of ventilation/perfusion mismatch and right-to-left shunt.
			• Cardiac dysrhythmias.	• Hypoxaemia is commonly associated with myocardial irritability.
			• Arterial blood gas values: pH.	• A metabolic acidaemia is often associated with decreased tissue perfusion; the consequent anaerobic metabolism causes in rise in serum lactate levels with a progressive metabolic acidosis. • Metabolic acidosis may depress myocardial function and predispose to dysrhythmias.
			• Monitor laboratory data: • Arterial blood gases. pH PaO_2 significantly reduced <60 mmHg. $PaCO_2$ reduced early <35 mmHg. increased late >45 mmHg. Calculate $AaDO_2$.	• Most closely reflect effectiveness of gas exchange. • Extensive right-to-left shunting causes the hypoxaemia to be refractory to oxygen therapy. • Tachypnoea and dyspnoea cause carbon dioxide to be eliminated, predisposing to hypocapnia. • Alveolar-arterial gradient <250-300 mmHg with an FIO_2 of 100 per cent; a classic hallmark of ARDS.
			• Haematology: Haematocrit, haemoglobin.	• Maintenance of normal physiologic levels of haemoglobin ensures maximal oxygen transport and release of oxygen to the tissues. Increased haemoglobin levels increase blood viscosity.
			• Administer prescribed humidified oxygen therapy.	• Oxygenation is the mainstay of treatment of ARDS; a large right-to-left shunt predisposes to a hypoxaemia refractory to administration of even high concentrations ($FIO_2 > 50\%$) of oxygen. • Oxygen is administered in conjunction with mechanical ventilation and PEEP therapy • Precautions associated with oxygen therapy: – Oxygen is a potent drug necessitating cautious use.

Contd...

Contd...

Problem	*R*	*Objective*	*Nursing interventions*	*Rationales*
				– Oxygen concentration should be kept to a minimum to maintain PaO_2 > 60 mmHg. – Duration of oxygen therapy should be kept to a minimum ◆ Prolonged administration of high oxygen concentrations predisposes to oxygen toxicity. ◆ Use of an FIO_2 > 50% over a period of 6-30 hr has been associated with oxygen toxicity. ◆ Maintenance of a PaO_2 > 60 mmHg can produce a haemoglobin saturation of ~90%.
			◆ Monitor for signs/symptoms of oxygen toxicity: Retrosternal chest pain; paresthesias in extremities; fatigue, lethargy, malaise, restlessness; anorexia, nausea, vomiting; dyspnoea, coughing.	◆ Signs and symptoms of oxygen toxicity are often subtle and may be easily overlooked: meticulous and thorough ongoing assessment and evaluation of patient's responses to therapy assist in determining effectiveness of therapy and prevention of complications.
			◆ Late symptomatology: Progressive respiratory distress; dyspnoea, cyanosis; asphyxia; increasing $AaDO_2$; decreased compliance and lung volumes.	
			◆ Monitor serial arterial blood gas measurements.	◆ Frequent monitoring of arterial blood gases is a mandatory safety measure when an FIO_2 > 40% is used.
			• Implement positive end-expiratory pressure (PEEP) therapy in conjunction with mechanical ventilatory support. ◆ Dosage: Early non-cardiogenic pulmonary oedema; 5-15 cm H_2O pressure; severe ARDS 15-30 cm H_2O pressure.	• PEEP therapy maintains airway opening pressure at end expiration above atmospheric pressure. This distending airway pressure increases lung volumes including FRC, it prevents airway collapse; it enhances gas exchange and oxygen transport; and it functions to reduce right-to-left shunting.
			◆ Criteria used to determine effective PEEP level: Arterial blood gas analysis; mixed venous oxygen tension; lung compliance; haemodynamic parameters: pulmonary artery pressure; PCWP; cardiac output.	◆ Use of PEEP therapy increases PaO_2 without requiring an increase in FIO_2. ◆ Lung compliance is determined by dividing the peak inspiratory pressure (PIP) into the tidal volume (V_T).
			◆ PEEP is usually increased in increments 3-5 cm H_2O pressure until "best PEEP" is achieved.	◆ "Best PEEP" is achieved when the inherent "stiffness" of the lungs prevents further distention of air spaces; it is

Contd...

Contd...

Problem	*R*	*Objective*	*Nursing interventions*	*Rationales*
				the level at which maximal benefit of PEEP is realised (i.e., PaO_2 > 60 mmHg on FIO_2 50%).
			◆ Monitor for complications of PEEP therapy: Reduction in venous return to the heart and cardiac output; reduction in cerebral perfusion—Assess mental status.	◆ Positive intrathoracic pressure generated by PEEP is applied to the great veins within the chest, reducing venous return to the right heart.
			◆ Barotrauma.	◆ Overdistention and rupture of alveoli are major complications of PEEP therapy.
			◆ Monitor fluid status.	◆ Overly vigorous administration of fluids may aggravate the pulmonary oedema; the increased capillary hydrostate pressure favours movement of fluid into lung interstitium. ◆ Excessive fluid accumulation increases total lung water, causing an increase in ventilation/perfusion mismatching
Nursing Diagnosis #2 Breathing pattern, ineffective: Tachypnoea, hyperventilation.		Patient will: 1. Achieve effective minute ventilation. • Tidal volume (V_T) > 5-7 ml/kg. • Respiratory rate < 30/min 2. Achieve a vital capacity (V_C) > 12-15 ml/kg. 3. Verbalise ease of breathing. • Breath sounds audible throughout anterior/posterior chest. • Reduced to absent adventitious sounds.	• Assess respiratory function: ◆ Rate, rhythm, depth, and pattern of breathing.	◆ Tachypnoea is the compensatory mechanism for hypoxaemia. ◆ Hyperventilatory effort is responsible for the hypocapnia observed during the edge course of the illness.
			◆ Symmetry of chest wall and diaphragmatic excursion: Use of accessory muscles; flaring of nares. – Monitor for fatigue, exhaustion.	
			◆ Lung compliance.	◆ Accumulation of fluid, oedema, and secretions within the lungs, with lung consolidation, reduces lung compliance.
			◆ Pulmonary lung volumes: – Total minute ventilation (V_E). – Tidal volume (V_T). – Respiratory rate (f). – Vital capacity (V_C).	◆ Maximal respiratory effort is made to facilitate optimum ventilation. ◆ A minimal volume of ventilation is necessary to ensure adequate alveolar ventilation; this minimal volume of gas enlarge gas exchange to occur during the phase of the respiratory cycle when no new gas inspired (expiratory and end-expiration phases).
			• Assist patient into position of comfort to allow for best lung expansion. • Implement mechanical ventilation.	• Expansion of lungs facilitates more even distribution of ventilation; increases ventilation/perfusion matching.

Contd...

Contd...

Problem	*Objective*	*Nursing interventions*	*Rationales*
Nursing Diagnosis #3 Airway clearance, ineffective, related to increased tracheobronchial secretions.	Patient will: 1. Be alert and oriented to person, place, time. 2. Maintain effective alveolar ventilation: • Breath sounds audible throughout anterior/posterior chest. • Reduced to absent adventitious sounds. • Arterial blood gas values stabilized as follows: pH 7.35-7.45. $PaO_2 > 60$ mmHg. $PaCO_2$ 35-45 mmHg.	• Assess respiratory function with emphasis on status of pulmonary secretions and the patient's ability to handle secretions. ◆ Presence of adventitious sounds. – Rales (crackles) wheezes. • Assess fluid status. ◆ Intake and output; daily weight. • Implement chest physiotherapy and bronchial hygiene measures.	• Patients with ARDS often have increased secretions, which impair adequate ventilation further compromising the hypoxaemia. • Excessive intrapulmonary accumulation fluid reduces compliance and further vates underlying right-to-left shunting ventilation/perfusion mismatching. • Pooling of secretions within the trancho-bronchial tree compromises ventilation predisposes to infection. • In patients receiving PEEP therapy adapter should be used to maintain the reative and end-expiratory pressure. • Even the slightest interruption of therapy can significantly increase the poxemia.
Nursing Diagnosis #4 Cardiac output, alteration in: Decreased (diminished) venous return. *Nursing Diagnosis #5* Tissue perfusion, alteration in: Cardiopulmonary. *Nursing Diagnosis #6* Tissue perfusion, alteration in: Cerebral.	For specific patient outcomes related to these nursing diagnoses, see Table 33-2, Nursing Diagnosis #4, #5, and #6.	For specific nursing interventions and their rationales, See Table 33-2, Nursing Diagnoses #5 and #6.	
Nursing Diagnosis #7 Fluid and electrolytes, alteration in.	For specific patient outcomes related to this nursing diagnosis, see Table 33.2, Nursing Diagnosis #7.	• Administer prescribed intravenous therapy.	• Because of the alveolar-capillary ability defect in ARDS, the fluid of .... intravenous administration is cry rather than colloid. Colloids would be of intravascular space to equilibrate interstitial fluid.
Nursing Diagnosis #8 Acid-base balance, alteration in: Respiratory alkalosis (tachypnoea, hyperventilation).	The patient's arterial blood gas values will stabilize as follows: pH 7.35-7.45. $PaO_2 > 60$ mmHg. $PaCO_2$ 35-45 mmHg.	• Assess for signs and symptoms of respiratory alkalaemia: ◆ Neurologic function: Light headedness, weakness, muscle cramps, twitching; paraesthesias; hyperactive deep tendon reflexes, seizure activity; tetany. ◆ Cardiovascular function: Cardiac dysrhythmias. ◆ Serum calcium levels. ◆ Serial arterial blood gases. • Implement supportive therapy to maintain adequate ventilation and optimal gas exchange.	• Respiratory failure in the patient is associated with tachypnoea and hypolation as the body tries to compensation severe hypoxemia. ◆ Hyperventilation reduces $PaCO_2$ consequent rise in pH. ◆ A rise in pH reduces the serum conection of freely ionized calcium by can increase in the calcium that is bound. The consequent hypocal sufficiently severe, may predispose romuscular alterations.

Contd...

Contd...

Problem	R	Objective	Nursing interventions	Rationales
			♦ Increase tidal volume. ♦ Decrease respiratory rate. ♦ If mechanically ventilated, increase dead-space ventilation; decrease minute ventilation.	♦ Increasing tidal volume and decreased respiratory rate decreases total minute ventilation; reduced ventilation enables the alveolar PCO_2 and, thus, the $PaCO_2$ return to an acceptable physiologic rate (35-45 mmHg).
Nursing Diagnosis #9 Nutrition, alteration in: Less than body requirements (see Chap. 53).		For specific patient outcomes related to this nursing diagnosis, see Table 33-2, Nursing Diagnosis #9.	For specific nursing interventions and their rationales, see chapter having NCP with similar nursing diagnosis.	
Nursing Diagnosis#10 Infection, potential for.		For specific patient outcomes related to this nursing diagnosis, see Table 33-2, Nursing Diagnosis #10.	For specific nursing interventions and their rationales, see chapter having NCP with similar nursing diagnosis.	
Nursing Diagnosis#11 Pulmonary mechanics, alterations in, related to respiratory muscle weakness and atrophy (immobility, mechanical ventilation).		Patient will: 1. Perform deep breathing exercises hourly. 2. Achieve maximum pulmonary function: • Tidal volume >7-10 ml/kg. • Vital capacity >15 ml/kg. • Respiratory rate <30/min. • Maximal expiratory flow.	• Teach deep-breathing exercises: ♦ Assess emotional and physiologic readiness for such teaching. ♦ Allow patient to demonstrate deep breathing exercises. ♦ Combine deep-breathing therapy with other chest physiotherapy manoeuvres. • Assess pulmonary volumes to determine effectiveness of therapy.	• Use of positive-pressure ventilation for a prolonged period predisposes to atrophy of the respiratory musculature. ♦ Breathing exercises mobilise secretion improve ventilation, stimulate circulation and increase muscle tone.
Nursing Diagnosis#12 Skin integrity, impairment of related to immobility.		For specific patient outcomes related to this nursing diagnosis, see Table 33-2, Nursing Diagnosis #12.	For specific nursing interventions and their rationales, see chapter having NCP with similar nursing diagnosis.	
Nursing Diagnosis#13 Coping, ineffective individual/family.		Patient/family will: 1. Verbalize knowledge and understanding of the illness. 2. Verbalize feelings as to what this potentially life-threatening illness means to each family member, individually and collectively. 3. Verbalize strengths and coping capabilities. 4. Identify family resources. 5. Make decisions regarding matters of importance to patient and family.	• Assess patient/family perceptions regarding a potentially life-threatening illness. ♦ Develop a trusting relationship with patient and family. ♦ Establish a caring rapport: Patient advocacy; accessible to patient/family. ♦ Encourage verbalization of perceptions, concerns, and feelings. • Assist patient/family to identify past coping capabilities: ♦ Emphasize strengths. ♦ Assist patient/family in defining areas requiring problem-solving and decision-making.	• Knowledge of patient and family perception of the illness assists in identifying coping pabilities and potential coping problem. ♦ A trusting, caring, supportive relation facilitates verbalization of concerns fears. ♦ A definitive, dependable support system insists patient/family to assume responsibility for decision-making. ♦ Unexpressed and unresolved fears and concerns may compromise ability to do effectively.

Contd...

Contd...

Problem	*R*	*Objective*	*Nursing interventions*	*Rationales*
			– Support patient/family in this regard. ◆ Involve in decision-making regarding care. – Offer praise for accomplishments. – Encourage development of new coping mechanisms. – Assist patient/family to explore and identify options and the consequences of the options. Assist patient/family to implement chosen options.	◆ Active participation in self-care assistant individual/family to gain a new sense of dignity, self-worth, and self-esteem.
			• Initiate referrals to intrahospital and community resources for special needs: Psychiatric social worker, family pastor, home care.	Additional resources may assist patient potentially to gain increased awareness of self interactions among patient, family, he care providers, and environment.

Table 6.3: Nursing care plan for the patient with pulmonary embolism

Problem	*R*	*Objective*	*Nursing interventions*	*Rationales*
Nursing Diagnosis #1 Anxiety, related to: 1. Sudden, acute respiratory insufficiency with disruption of lifestyle. 2. Pain; haemoptysis. 3. Knowledge deficit regarding illness and its prognosis. 4. Intensive care setting.		Patient will: 1. Verbalise feeling less anxious. 2. Demonstrate a relaxed demeanor. 3. Perform relaxation techniques with assistance. 4. Verbalise familiarity with ICU routines and protocols.	• Assess for signs/symptoms of anxiety: Restlessness, agitation, diaphoresis; tachypnoea, sighing; tachycardia, palpitations; anorexia, nausea, diarrhea; presence of anxiety-related behaviours: nailbiting, insomnia, finger tapping; uncooperative or noncompliant behaviours; verbalisation of fears and concerns.	• Thorough assessment assists in discerning underlying cause of anxiety and provides a basis for intervention. *Examples:* (1) Relief of pain with medication often alleviates its anxiety-related symptomatology, (2) coping with the fear of dying with a listening ear and caring attitude may assist in reducing the patient's anxiety.
			• Examine the circumstances underlying the anxiety. ◆ Manipulate ICU environment to provide calm, restful periods.	• Removal of precipitating factors may reduce anxiety. ◆ Reduction in stimuli is essential to assist patient/family to relax and avoid useless dissipation of compromised energy stores.
			• Assess patient/family coping behaviours and their effectiveness in dealing with current stressors.	
			◆ Provide positive reinforcement when desired response is achieved.	◆ Positive feedback nurtures self-confidence.
			• Initiate interventions to reduce anxiety: ◆ Relieve pain or other discomfort. – Medication for pain. – Comfort measures: Turning, positioning, mouth care, skin care, and so forth.	◆ Pain precipitates and/or aggravates anxiety.
			◆ Monitor effectiveness of ventilatory support and oxygen therapy if these therapies are indicated. – Serial arterial blood gas values.	◆ Inadequate gas exchange, hypoxaemia and/or hypercapnia precipitate symptomatology that contributes to the patient "sense of doom."
			◆ Listen attentively, encourage verbalisation, provide a caring touch.	◆ These nursing activities reassure the patient that he/she is not alone.

Contd...

Contd...

Problem	*R*	*Objective*	*Nursing interventions*	*Rationales*
			◆ Let patient know it's okay to feel anxious or to experience fear of dying. ◆ Remain with patient during periods of acute stress.	◆ Reassurance helps patient focus on his/her feelings, work them through, and, eventually, accept them.
			◆ Assess readiness to learn and implement the following when appropriate:	◆ Readiness to learn facilitates meaningful learning and a sense of accomplishment.
			– Orient to environment, ICU equipment, routines, and staff. – Explain all procedures and activities involving the patient.	◆ Knowing what to expect helps to reduce anxiety.
			◆ Involve in decision-making regarding care when possible and appropriate.	◆ Helps patient maintain some degree of control over his/her body and health care.
			◆ Help in establishing short-term goals that can be attained.	◆ Builds and reinforces self-confidence.
			◆ Instruct in relaxation techniques.	◆ Energy-release techniques allow an out for pent-up feelings; enable the patient have some control over anxiety.
Nursing Diagnosis #2 Gas exchange, impaired, related to: 1. Right-to-left shunting. 2. Ventilation/perfusion mismatch. *Nursing Diagnosis #3* Breathing pattern, ineffective, related to tachypnoea, dyspnoea.		For specific patient outcomes and related to these Nursing Diagnoses.	For specific nursing interventions and their rationales pl. see chapters having NCP with similar nursing diagnosis.	
Nursing Diagnosis #4 Cardiac output, alteration in: decreased, related to: 1. Pulmonary arterial hypertension. 2. Right-sided congestive heart failure (cor pulmonale). 3. Decrease in left ventricular end-diastolic pressure (LVEDP). 4. Systemic arterial hypotension/hypovolemic shock.		Patient will: 1. Maintain stable haemodynamics: • Heart rate < 100 beats/min. • CVP 0-8 mmHg. • Pulmonary artery pressure <25 mmHg. • PCWP 8-12 mmHg. • Cardiac output ~5 liters/min. • Systemic arterial blood pressure within 10 mmHg of baseline.	• Assess for signs/symptoms of right-sided congestive heart failure: ◆ Weight gain; fluid intake/output. ◆ Haemodynamic changes: – Tachycardia (> 100 beats/min). – Jugular neck vein distention. – Peripheral (dependent) oedema. – CVP > 8-12 mmHg. – Extra heart sounds; S_3, S_4; systolic murmur. – Fatigue; mottled appearance of skin, cool to touch; cyanosis of nailbeds.	• The major haemodynamic disturbance associated with pulmonary embolism is pulmonary arterial hypertension (>25-30 mm) which may predispose to right ventrical failure. ◆ Hypoxaemia, acidaemia, and a reduced cross-sectional area of the pulmonary cular bed all contribute to the development of pulmonary hypertension. ◆ Right ventricular failure causes alteration in systemic haemodynamics; left ventricular failure alters pulmonary hemody namics. Commonly, failure in one ventricle causes failure of the other.
			◆ Breath sounds may be clear and without adventitious sounds; or breath sounds may be diminished with localized rales (crackles) or wheezing. A pleural friction rub may be detected. Breathing pattern may reflect tachypnoea, dyspnoea.	◆ A massive pulmonary embolism with ac........... cor pulmonale may be characterized by dyspnea, cyanosis, and hypovolemic shock.

Contd...

Contd...

Problem	*R*	*Objective*	*Nursing interventions*	*Rationales*
			◆ Hepatic involvement: – Hepatomegaly, positive hepatojugular reflex; abdominal distention; ascites. ◆ Gastrointestinal: Anoraexia, nausea/vomiting; abdominal distention. ◆ Oliguria. ◆ Mental status changes.	
			• Monitor diagnostic tests/studies: ◆ Laboratory studies: BUN, creatinine, hematocrit, serum albumin; electrolytes; arterial blood gases. ◆ ECG may reflect signs of ischaemia; dysrhythmias (atrial). ◆ Chest X-rays frequently reflect cardiomegaly, pleural effusion, and possibly, pulmonaryoedema (left-sided heart failure).	• Serum sodium values reflect hydration status. ◆ Serum potassium needs to be carefully monitored especially during diuretic therapy.
			• Administer prescribed medication regimen to treat cor pulmonale, a consequence of pulmonary hypertension.	• Therapies are directed toward decreasing myocardial oxygen consumption and demand.
			◆ Vasopressor therapy (e.g., dopamine in the presence of heart failure and hypovolemic shock).	◆ A pulmonary embolic episode may reflexly trigger systemic peripheral arteriolar vasodilation with a consequent "relative" volume depletion, which, if severe, can cause hypotension or hypovolemic shock.
			◆ Cardiac glycosides (digoxin). – Positive inotropic agent - improved contractility. – Negative chronotropic agent - reduced heart rate. – End result-improved cardiac output.	
			◆ Morphine. – Induces systemic venous vasodilation. – Reduces chest pain frequently associated with pulmonary embolism. Decreases anxiety and helps to reduce the work of breathing. Exerts a sedative effect, which assists in relaxing the patient.	◆ Increased pooling of blood in the periphery reduces venous return to the right heart, which helps to decrease the work of the right ventricle.
			◆ Diuretics (e.g., furosemide).	◆ A reduction in total blood volume reduces venous return (preload) while also reducing systemic arterial blood pressure (after load). The end result is a decrease in myocardial work. ◆ Use of diuretics requires the maintenance of fluid volume.
			◆ Vasodilator therapy may be initiated especially in the setting of left ventricular compromise.	◆ Vasodilators function to decrease preload and after-load and thus, decrease the work of the heart.
			◆ Anticoagulant therapy. Heparin, coumadin derivatives. Aspirin (antiplatelet agent).	◆ Major focus of therapy in the patient experiencing a pulmonary embolic episode is to *prevent* recurrent embolisation; anticoagulants function effectively in this capacity.

Contd...

Contd...

Problem	*Objective*	*Nursing interventions*	*Rationales*
Nursing Diagnosis #5 Fluid volume, alteration	Patient will: 1. Maintain body weight within 5% of baseline. 2. Balance fluid intake with output. 3. Have: • Good skin turgor. • Absence of peripheral oedema. • Absence of jugular vein distention. • Absence of rales (crackles) on auscultation. Serum electrolytes, BUN, creatinine, total, protein, will stabilize within acceptable physiologic range.	• Maintain fluid and electrolyte balance. ◆ Administer prescribed fluid volume. ◆ Document intake and output, urine specific gravity. ◆ Record daily weight. ◆ Monitor electrolytes. • Monitor haemodynamic parameters. ◆ Systemic arterial blood pressure, CVP, pulmonary artery pressure, PCWP, cardiac output. • Administer oxygen therapy as prescribed and monitor arterial blood gases to evaluate patient's response to therapy. • Implement nursing measures to improve and/or maintain cardiac output. ◆ Manipulate environment to reduce stressors and promote rest and relaxation. ◆ Plan frequent rest periods. ◆ Maximize patient activities in accordance with the acuity of the illness. ◆ Place in high fowler's position. ◆ Assist with frequent position changes. ◆ Provide special care to back and to skin over joints and pressure points. ◆ Assist with passive range-of-motion exercises.	• Fluid therapy is directed towards reducing the work of the heart while still maintaining adequate tissue perfusion. ◆ Close monitoring of urine output helps to evaluate renal perfusion/function; a reduction in cardiac output may reduce renal perfusion, which is manifested clinically by a decrease in hourly urine output. • These measures best reflect the patient's response to therapy, and insertion of a pulmonary artery flotation catheter is commonly indicated in the setting of massive pulmonary embolism. • Hypoxaemia in pulmonary embolism is a consequence of ventilation/perfusion mismatching and right-to-left shunting. • A quiet, calm environment decreases anxiety, and reduces sympathetic nervous system stimulation. The overall net effect is to reduce the work of the heart. ◆ A reduction in cardiac workload reduces myocardial oxygen consumption and demand. ◆ Nursing interventions are implemented to maximize circulation, prevent pooling or stasis of blood, maintain venous return, and promote comfort. ◆ Facilitates breathing pressure on the diaphragm is reduced; less effort exerted - decrease in oxygen demand. ◆ Compromised circulation predisposes to tissue ischemia; statsis or pooling of blood predisposes to venous thrombosis; reduce venous return, which decreases cardiac output.
Nursing Diagnosis #6 Tissue perfusion, alteration in, related to: 1. Thromboembolic disorder. 2. Deep venous thrombosis. 3. Pulmonary embolism.	Patient will: 1. Remain without recurrent pulmonary embolism as reflected by: • Absence of pain. • Stable vital signs (see Nursing Diagnosis #4 above).	• Assess for signs/symptoms of venous thrombosis: ◆ Tenderness, warmth, pain, and peripheral (pitting) oedema of lower extremities. – Evidence of oedema is best assessed and monitored by determining the circumference of the limb at a designated point using a tape measure.	• Ninty-five per cent of all pulmonary emboli arise in the deep veins of the lower extremities. ◆ Oedema is a characteristic manifestation when alteration in tissue perfusion is due to venous interference.

Contd...

Contd...

Problem	*R*	*Objective*	*Nursing interventions*	*Rationales*
		• Stable arterial blood gases (within acceptable physiologic range) pH 7.35-7.45. $PaCO_2$ 35-45 mmHg. PaO_2 > 60 mmHg.	◆ Skin colour and temperature. – Observe extremities in both dependent and elevated positions.	◆ In the presence of altered tissue perfusion or venous obstruction a bluish-red colour of the skin may be observed. ◆ Temperature of skin is assessed by use of touch; usually warm temperatures in the lower extremities are commonly associated with venous thrombosis.
			◆ Bleeding/bruising tendency, petechiae, ecchymosis, haematuria, occult blood in stool.	◆ Hypercoagulable state is often reflected by bleeding tendency.
			◆ Complaints of pain: – Pain associated with deep venous thrombosis may be described as heavy, aching, or cramping. – Pain associated with arterial insufficiency is characteristically sudden and sharp; the presence of cool skin temperatures suggests decreased arterial blood flow.	◆ Pain occurs when there is an alteration in tissue perfusion.
			• Monitor for signs/symptoms indicative of extended or recurrent pulmonary embolism. ◆ Sudden occurrence of persistent or exacerbated chest and/or shoulder pain. ◆ Onset of respiratory difficulties: Tachypnoea, dyspnoea, cough with haemoptysis. ◆ Alterations in cardiopulmonary function: Tachycardia, hypotension, cyanosis. ◆ Neurologic findings: Restlessness, lethargy, confusion.	• The presence of deep venous thrombosis places the patient at increased risk of pulmonary embolism.
			• Monitor laboratory data: ◆ Arterial blood gas values. ◆ Haematologic studies: Complete blood count, hematocrit, haemoglobin. ◆ Coagulation studies: aPTT; prothrombin time; clotting time. ◆ Platelet count. Implement prescribed anticoagulant therapy.	
			• Implement prescribed anticoagulant therapy.	
			• Implement measures to reduce the risk of recurrent pulmonary embolism. ◆ Maintain hydrated state as prescribed.	◆ Dehydration increases blood viscosity. The consequent disturbed blood flow may predispose to endothelial injury within blood vessels, and/or a hypercoagulable state.
			◆ Apply antiembolic hose to both lower extremities; remove hose once per shift. ◆ Assist patient to perform active range-of-motion exercises; active/passive foot and leg exercises should be performed hourly unless otherwise contraindicated.	◆ Exercise enhances "skeletal-muscular pump," which functions to prevent pooling of blood in the lower extremities (venous stasis) and maintains venous return to the heart.

Contd...

Contd...

Problem	*R*	*Objective*	*Nursing interventions*	*Rationales*
				◆ If a thrombosis is suspected, the involved extremity should not be massaged or exercised to prevent possible dislodgement of thrombi with consequent pulmonary embolism.
			◆ Instruct patient to avoid positions that compromise blood flow in the extremities (e.g., gatch knees, pillow under knees, crossing of legs, prolonged sitting in one position).	◆ Positions that compromise blood flow can cause circulatory stasis.
			◆ Encourage deep breathing hourly.	◆ Expands lungs and minimizes areas of atelectasis.
			◆ Caution patient to avoid activities that involve a Valsalva's manoeuvre (e.g., straining to defecate, breath holding).	◆ Such activities increase risk of dislodging thrombi.
Nursing Diagnosis #7 Comfort, alteration in: Pain associated with compromised pulmonary perfusion.		Patient will: 1. Verbalize pain relief. 2. Exhibit relaxed demeanor: • Relaxed facial expression and body posturing. • Ease of breathing.	• Determine how patient usually copes with pain. ◆ Pain tolerance. ◆ Willingness to discuss pain; or stoically "keeping it within" himself or herself. ◆ Willingness to use medication for pain.	
			• Assess for nonverbal clues as to the presence of pain (e.g., restlessness, or reluctance to move; tense facial features; clenched fists; diaphoresis; rapid, shallow breathing).	
			• Assess complaints of pain including severity, location/radiation; influencing factors (e.g., what precipitates, aggravates, or ameliorates the pain; and associated signs and symptoms such as diaphoresis), pain duration and the quality of pain (e.g., sharp, dull, "knifelike).	• To assist in comprehensive assessment.
			• Implement measures to alleviate pain: ◆ Assist patient into comfortable position (e.g., high Fowler's).	◆ Upright position favours better lung expansion; improves alveolar ventilation.
			◆ Enclurage deep breathing hourly.	◆ Minimizes atelectasis and improves distribution of ventilation.
			◆ Teach/assist patient to splint chest with hands or pillow when coughing, deep breathing, or repositioning.	◆ Splinting may help to reduce discomfort.
			◆ Stay with patient until pain is relieved.	◆ Providing support can reduce anxiety and help the patient relax.
			• Provide a listening ear and caring touch; encourage verbalization; explain procedures, routines, tests, and so forth.	◆ Keeping the patient informed may help to alleviate anxieties, which may potentiate pain.
			◆ Refrain from non-essential activities.	◆ Reducing patient's activities decreases oxygen consumption and demand.
			◆ Provide comfort measures (e.g., position change, back care, reducing environmental stimuli).	◆ Comfort measures and touch therapy are often sufficient to alleviate pain.
			• Administer analgesic medication therapy as prescribed.	

Contd...

Contd...

Problem	*R*	*Objective*	*Nursing interventions*	*Rationales*
			◆ Encourage to request medication when pain is first realized rather than waiting until it gets unbearable. ◆ Evaluate effectiveness of pain medication in relieving the patient's pain.	◆ Pain medication administered early on may be more effective.
Nursing Diagnosis #8 Knowledge deficit, related to: 1. Thromboembolic disease 2. Follow-up care 3. Prevention		Patient/family will: 1. Identify risk factors of significance in thromboembolic disease. 2. Identify activities that promote venous blood flow and reduce risks of venous thrombosis. • Importance of individualized exercise programme. 3. Explain the prescribed treatment regimen and the importance of complying with it: • Rationale for anticoagulant therapy. • Medicatioan routine, dosage, and side effects. • Signs/symptoms to report to health-care provider. • Measures to minimize risks of bleeding during anticoagulant therapy. • Importance of follow-up care.	Patient/family educatioan, for information essential to the patient/family's understanding of and compliance with, the prescribed therapeutic regimen.	

PROCEDURE 6.1: **ASSISTING WITH ARTERIAL PUNCTURE FOR BLOOD GAS ANALYSIS.*

Equipment Commercially available blood.
gas kit
or
2-or 3 ml syringe
23-9r 25-gauge needle
0.5 ml sodium heparin (1:1,000)
Stopper or cap
Lidocaine
Sterile germicide
Cup or plastic bag with crushed ice
Gloves.

STEPS OF PROCEDURE

Nursing action	*Rationale*
Preparatory Phase	
1. Record patient's inspired oxygen concentration	1. Changes in inspired oxygen concentration alter the change in PaO_2. Degree of hypoxaemia cannot be assessed without knowing the inspired oxygen concentration.

Contd...

Nursing action	*Rationale*
2. Take patient's temperature	2. May be taken into consideration when results are evaluated. Hyperthermia and hypothermia influence oxygen release from haemoglobin.
If not using a commercially available blood gas kit. 3. Heparinize the 2 ml syringe.	3.
a. Withdraw heparin into the syringe to wet the plunger and fill dead space in the needle.	a. This action coats the interior of the syringe with heparin to prevent blood from clotting.
	b. Air in the syringe may affect measurement of PaO_2. Heparin in the syringe may affect measurement of the pH

PERFORMANCE PHASE (BY PHYSICIAN, NURSE, OR RESPIRATORY THERAPIST WITH SPECIAL INSTRUCTION)

1. Wash hands
2. Don gloves

Contd...

Nursing action	Rationale
3. Palpate the radial, brachial or femoral artery.	The radial artery is the preferred site of puncture. Arterial puncture is performed on areas where a good pulse is palpable.
4. If puncturing the radial artery, perform the Allen test.	4. The Allen test is a simple method for assessing collateral circulation in the hand. Ensures circulation if radial artery thrombosis occurs.
In the conscious patient:	
a. Obliterate the radial and ulnar pulses simultaneously by pressing on both blood vessels at the wrist.	a. Impedes arterial blood flow into the hand.
b. Ask patient to clench and unclench fist until blanching of skin occurs	b. Forces blood from the hand.
c. Release pressure on ulnar artery (while still compressing radial artery). Watch for return of skin colour within 15 seconds.	c. Documents that ulnar artery alone is capable of supplying blood to the hand, because radial artery is still occluded.

Note: If the ulnar does not have sufficient blood flow to supply the entire hand, another artery should be used.

Nursing action	Rationale
In the unconscious patient:	
a. Obliterate the radial and ulnar pulses simultaneously at the wrist.	
b. Elevate patient's hand above heart and squeeze or compress hand until blanching occurs.	
c. Lower patient's hand while still compressing the radial artery (release pressure on ulnar artery) and watch for return of skin colour.	
5. For the radial side, place a small towel roll under the patient's wrist.	5. To make the artery more accessible.
6. Feel along the course of the radial artery the palpate for maximum pulsation with the middle and index fingers. Prepare the skin with germicide. The skin and subcutaneous tissues may be infiltrated with a local anaesthetic agent (lidocaine).	6. The wrist should be stabilized to allow for better control of the needle.
7. The needle is at a 45-60 degree angle to the skin surface and is advanced into the artery. Once the artery is punctured, arterial pressure will push up the hub of the syringe and a pulsating flow of blood will fill the syringe.	7. The arterial pressure will cause the syringe to be filled within a few seconds.
8. After blood is obtained, withdraw needle and apply firm pressure over the puncture with a dry sponge.	8. Significant bleeding can occur because of pressure in the artery.

Contd...

Nursing action	Rationale
9. Remove air bubbles from syringe and needle. Insert needle into rubber stopper.	9. Immediate capping of the needle prevents room air from mixing with the blood specimen.
10. Place the capped syringe in the container of ice.	10. Icing the syringe will prevent a clinically significant loss of O_2.
11. Maintain firm pressure on the puncture site for 5 minutes. If the patient is on anticoagulant medication, apply direct pressure dressing.	11. Firm pressure on the puncture site prevents further bleeding and haematoma formation.
12. For patients requiring serial monitoring of arterial blood, an arterial catheter (connected to a flush solution of heparinised saline) is inserted into the radial or femoral artery.	12. All connections must be tight to avoid disconnection and rapid blood loss. The arterial line also allows for direct blood pressure monitoring in the critically-ill patient.
Follow-up phase	
1. Send labelled, iced specimen to the laboratory immediately.	1. Blood gas analysis should be done as soon as possible, because PaO_2 and pH can change rapidly.
2. Palpate the pulse (distal to the puncture site, and assess for cold hand, numbness, tingling or discolouration.	2. Haematoma and arterial thrombosis are complications following this procedure.
3. Change ventilator settings, inspired oxygen concentration or type and setting of respiratory therapy equipment if indicated by the results.	3. The PaO_2 results will deter mine whether to maintain, increase or decrease the F_IO_2. The PaO_2 and pH results will detect if any changes are needed in tidal volume of rate of patient's ventilator.

PROCEDURE 6.2: ****ASSISTING WITH TRANSTRACHEAL ASPIRATION***

Equipment Sterile Transtracheal Set:

- No 14, No 16 and No 18 gauge needles
- Polyethylene catheter
- Syringe
- Skin preparation solutions
- Local anaesthetic
- Sterile gloves, masks
- Specimen containers
- Atropine
- ECG monitoring equipment
- Endotracheal tube
- Suction apparatus with catheters
- Cardiac resuscitation equipment

SETPS OF PROCEDURE

Nursing action	Rationale
Preparatory Phase	
1. Explain the procedure and give reassurance by skilled and empathetic attention to the patient's needs. Instruct the patient to breathe quietly and to remain still.	1. Inform the patient that the procedure will cause coughing and that there will be an unpleasant sensation of breathe a foreign body in the lower airway.

Contd...

Nursing action	*Rationale*
2. Administer supplemental oxygen, as directed during the procedure if the patient's arterial oxygen tension is below normal while the patient is breathing room air.	2. This prevents worsening of hypoxaemia.
3. Extend the patient's neck and place a pillow under shoulders.	3. This is the optimum position for cricothyroid puncture.
Performance phase	
The cricothyroid membranc is identified by palpation.	
1. The skin over the cricothyroid area is cleansed and the area is infiltrated with local anaesthetic.	1. The cricothyroid membrane is less vascular and offers more safety in preventing posterior wall puncture than other areas.
2. A no 14, 16, or 04 18 gauge needle is inserted through the cricothyroid membrane into the trachea, and a polyethylene catheter is threaded through the needle into the lower trachea. Caution the patient against swallowing or talking while the needle is introduced through the cricothyroid membrane.	
3. The needle is withdrawn, leaving the catheter in place.	3. The catheter's passage usually stimulates vigorous coughing.
4. A syringe is attached to the catheter and secretions may be aspirated back into the syringe as the patient coughs. Request the patient to turn head while coughing.	4. Sterile saline (2 to 5 ml) may be injected into catheter to reduce coughing if necessary.
5. Air is removed from the syringe, and the syringe is capped or the sample is injected into an anaerobic transfer vial. The specimen is sent to the laboratory for immediate processing.	5. This ensures anarobic conditions cytologic, mycobacterial and other studies are carried out.
6. The catheter is withdrawn and pressure is applied over the puncture site.	6. Gentle firm pressure over the site for about 5 minutes helps prevent bleeding and reduces subcutaneous emphysema.
Follow-up phase	
1. Instruct the patient to rest quietly for about an hour.	
2. Observe for the following complications: local bleeding, puncture of posterior tracheal wall, subcutaneous emphysema, vasovagal reactions, cardiac dysrhythmias.	2. Assess for hoarseness after the procedure: this may be from a submucosal tracheal haematoma, which can cause suffocation, inform the patient that minor blood streaking of sputum almost always occurs after this procedure.

PROCEDURE 6.3: **ASSISTING THE PATIENT UNDERGOING THORACENTESIS*

Equipment Thoracentesis tray (if available)
or
Syringes, 5-, 20-, 50-mL
Needles No 22, No 26, No 16 (7.5 cm long)
Three-way stopcock and tubing
Haemostat
Biopsy needle
Germicide solution
Local anaesthetic (e.g. lidocaine 1%)
Sterile gauze sponges (4 × 4 and 2 × 2)
Sterile towels and drape
Sterile specimen containers
Sterile gloves

STEPS OF PROCEDURE

Nursing action	*Rationale*
Preparatory Phase	
1. Ascertain in advance if chest X-ray and/or other tests have been prescribed and completed. These should be available at the bedside.	1. Localisation of pleural fluid is accomplished by physical examination, chest roentgenogram, ultrasound localisation, or fluoroscopic localization.

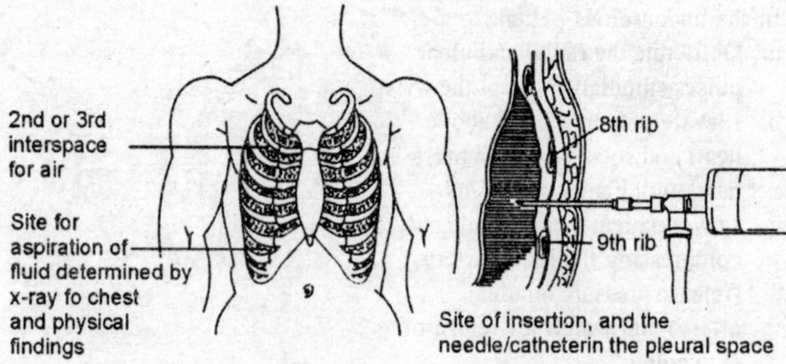

Fig. 6.3: Technique of Thoracentesis

Nursing action	*Rationale*
Technique of thoracentesis.	
2. See if consent form has been explained and signed.	
3. Determine if the patient is allergic to local anaesthetic agent to be used. Give sedation if prescribed.	
4. Inform the patient about the procedure and indicate how he or she can be helpful. Explain.	4. An explanation helps orient the patient to the procedure, assists with coping and provides an opportunity to ask questions and verbalise anxiety.
a. The nature of the procedure.	
b. The importance of remaining immobile.	
c. Pressure sensations to be experienced.	
d. That no discomfort is anticipated after the procedure.	

Contd...

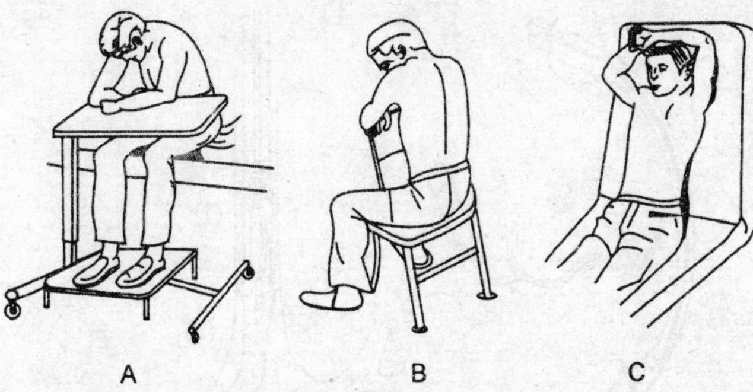

Fig. 6.4: Positioning the patient for a thoracentesis. The nurse assists the patient to one of three positions, and offers comfort and support throughout the procedure. (A) Sitting on the edge of the bed with head and arms on and over the bed table. (B) Straddling a chair with arms and head resting on the back of the chair. (C) Lying on unaffected side with the bed elevated 30 to 45 degrees.

Nursing action	*Rationale*
5. Make the patient comfortable with adequate supports. If possible, place upright (see accompanying figure and help patient maintain position during procedure.	5. The upright position ensures that the diaphragm is most dependent and facilitates the removal of fluid that usually localises at the base of the chest. A comfortable position helped reduce.
6. Support and reassure the patient during the procedure. a. Prepare the patient for sensations of cold from skin germicide and for pressure and sting from infiltration of local anaesthetic agent. b. Encourage the patient to refrain from coughing. c. Be prepared to monitor patient's condition throughout the procedure.	6. Discomfort by the patient can cause trauma to the visceral pleura with resultant trauma to the lung. A local anaesthetic inhibits nerve conduction and is used to prevent pain during the procedure.
Performance Phase	
1. The site for aspiration is determined from chest X-rays, by percussion, or by fluoroscopic of ultrasound localisation. If fluid is in the pleural cavity the thoracentesis site is determined by study of the chest X-ray and physical findings, with attention to the site of maximal dullness on percussion.	1. If air is in the pleural cavity, the thoracentesis site is usually in the 2nd or 3rd intercostal space in the midclavicular line. Air rises in the thorax because the density of air is much less than the density of liquid.
2. The procedure is done under aseptic conditions. After the skin is cleansed, the healthcare provider slowly injects a local anaesthetic with a small-caliber needle into the intercostal space.	2. An intradermal wheal is raised slowly, rapid intradermal injection causes pain. The parietal pleura is very sensitive and should be well infiltrated with anaesthetic before the thoracentesis needle is passed through it.

Contd...

Nursing action	*Rationale*
3. The thoracentesis needle is advanced with the syringe attached. When the pleural space is reached, suction may be applied with the syringe.	
a. A 20 ml or 50 ml syringe with a three way adapter (stop-cock) is attached to the needle. (one end of the adapter is attached to the needle and the other end to the tubing leading to a receptacle that receives the fluid being aspirated.)	a. When a larger quantity of fluid is withdrawn, a three-way adapter serves to keep air from entering the pleural cavity. The amount of fluid removed depends on clinical status of the patient and absence of complications during the procedure.
b. If a considerable quantity of fluid is to be removed, the needle is held in place on the chest wall with a small hemostat.	b. The haemostat steadies the needle on the chest wall and prevents too deep a penetration of pleural space. Sudden pleuritic pain or shoulder pain may indicate that the visceral or diaphragmatic pleura are being irritated by the needle point.
c. A pleural biopsy may be performed	
4. After the needle is withdrawn, pressure is applied over the puncture site and a small sterile dressing is fixed in place.	4. This is done to prevent air entry into pleural space.
Follow-up Phase	
1. Place the patient on bedrest A chest X-ray is usually obtained after thoracentesis.	1. Chest X-ray varifies that there is no pneumothorax.
2. Record vital signs every 15 minutes for one hour.	
3. Administer oxygen, as directed, if patient is suffering from cardiorespiratory disease.	3. Pulmonary gas exchange may worsen after thoracentesis in patients with cardiorespiratory disease.
4. Record the total amount of fluid withdrawn and the nature of the fluid, its colour and viscosity. If prescribed, prepare samples of fluid for laboratory evaluation (usually bacteriology, cell count and differential determinations of protein, glucose, LDH specific gravity). A small amount of heparin may be needed for several of the specimen containers to prevent coagulation. A specimen container with preservative may be needed if a pleural biopsy is to be obtained.	4. The fluid may be clear, serous bloody, or purulent.
5. Evaluate the patient at intervals for increasing respiration's faintness, vertigo, tightness in the chest, uncontrollable cough blood-tinged mucus, and rapid pulse and signs of hypoxaemia.	5. Pneumothorax, tension pneumothorax, haemothorax, subcutaneous emphysema, or pyogenic infection may result from a thoracentesis.

PROCEDURE 6.4: **ENDOTRACHEAL INTUBATION*

Equipment Laryngoscope with curved or straight blade and working light source (check batteries and bulb periodically).

Endotracheal tube with low-pressure cuff and adapter to connect tube to ventilator or resuscitation bag.

.... to guide the endotracheal tube.

Oral airway (assorted sizes) or bite block to keep patient from being into and occluding the endotracheal tube. Adhesive tape or tube fixation system.

Sterile anaesthetic lubricant jelly (water-soluble)

10 ml syringe

Suction source

Suction catheter and tonsil suction

Resuscitation bag and mask connected to oxygen source

Sterile towel

Gloves

Goggles or other eye protection.

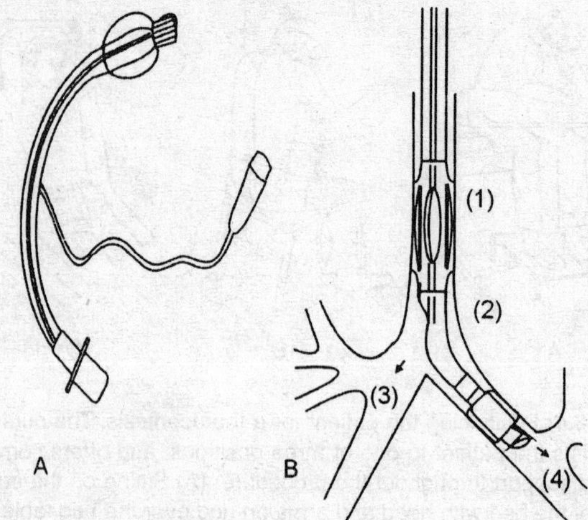

Fig. 6.5: (A) Single lumen endotracheal tube, (B) Double lumen endotracheal tube. When the double lumen tube is used, two cuffs are inflated. One cuff (1) is positioned in the tracks and the second cuff (2) in the left mainstem bronchus. After inflation, air flows through an opening below the tracheal cuff (3) to the right lung and through an opening below the bronchial cuff (4) to the left lung. This permits differential ventilation of both lungs, lavage of one lung, or selective inflation of either lung during thoracic surgery

STEPS OF PROCEDURE

Nursing action	*Rationale*
Preparatory Phase	
1. Assess the patient's heart rate, level of consciousness, and respiratory status.	1. Provide a baseline to estimate patient's tolerance of procedure.
Performance Phase	
1. Remove the patient's dental bridgework and plates.	1. May interfere with insertion. Will not be able to remove easily from patient once intubated.
2. Remove headboard of bed (optional).	
3. Prepare equipment	3.
a. Ensure function of resuscitation bag with mask and suction.	a. Patient may require ventilatory assistance during procedure. Suction should be functional, because gagging and emesis may occur during procedure.
b. Assemble the laryngoscope. Make sure the light bulb is tightly attached and functional.	
c. Select an endotracheal tube of the appropriate size (6.0 to 9.0 mm for average adult).	
d. Place the endotracheal tube on a sterile towel.	d. Although the tube will pass through the contaminated mouth or nose, the airway below the vocal cords is sterile, and efforts must be made to prevent iatrogenic contamination of the distal end of the tube and cuff. The proximal end of the tube may be handled, because it will reside in the upper airway

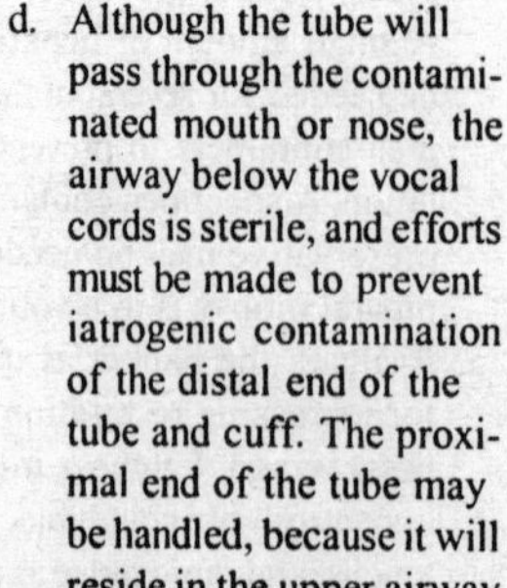

Contd...

Nursing action	*Rationale*
e. Inflate the cuff to make sure it assumes a symmetric shape and holds volume without leakage. Then deflate maximally.	e. Malfunction of the cuff must be ascertained before tube placement occurs.
f. Lubricate the distal end of the tube liberally with the sterile anaesthetic water-soluble jelly.	f. Aids in insertion.
g. Insert the stylet into the tube (if oral intubation is planned). Nasal intubation does not employ use of the stylet.	g. Stiffens the soft tube, allowing it to be more easily directed into the trachea.
4. Aspirate stomach contents if nasogastric tube is in place.	
5. If time allows, inform the patient of impending inability to talk and discuss alternate means of communication.	5. Discuss alternate means of communication.
6. If the patient is confused, it may be necessary to apply soft, wrist restraints.	6. Restraint of the confused patient may be necessary to promote patient's safety and maintain sterile technique.
7. Put-on goggles and gloves or other eye protection system.	7. Prevent contact with patient's oral secretions.
8. During oral intubation cervical is not injured, place patient's head in a position (i.e. extended at the junction of the neck and flexed at the junction of the spine and skull.	8. Upper airway is open maximally in this position.

Contd...

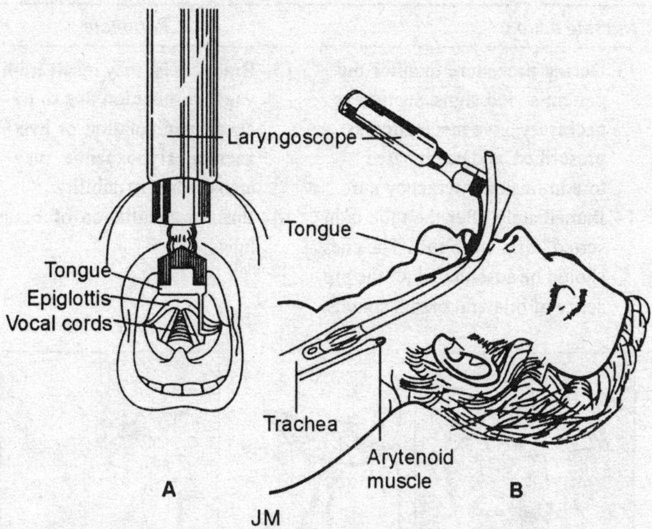

Fig. 6.6: Endotracheal intubation: (A) The primary glottic landmarks for tracheal intubation as visualized with proper placement of the laryngoscope, (B) Positioning the endotube

Nursing action	*Rationale*
9. Spray the back of the patient's with anaesthetic spray if time is available.	9. Will decrease gagging.
10. Ventilate and oxygenate the patient with the resuscitation bag and mask before.	10. Preoxygenation decreases the likelihood of cardiac dysrhythmia or respiratory distress secondary to hypoxemia.
11. Hold the handle of the laryngoscope in the left hand and hold the patient's mouth with the right hand by placing crossed fingers on the thumb	11. Leverage is improved by crossing the thumb and index fingers when opening of the patient's mouth (scissor-twist technique).
12. Insert the curved blade of the laryngoscope along the right side of the tongue to the left and use right thumb and index finger to pull patient's lower lip away from lower.	12. Rolling the lip away from teeth prevents injury by being caught between teeth and blade.
13. Lift laryngoscope forward to expose the epiglottis.	13. Do not use teeth as a fulcrum, this could lead to dental damage.
14. Lift laryngoscope upwards 45-degree angle to expose glottis.	14. This stretches the hypoepiglottis ligament, folding the epiglottis upwards and exposing the glottis.
15. As the epiglottis is lifted towards ceiling, the vertical opening of the vocal cords will come into view.	15. Do not use wrist. Use shoulder and arm to lift the epiglottis.

Contd...

16. Once vocal cords are visualised into the right corner of the mouth and keeping vocal cords in constant view.	16. Make sure you do not insert tube into esophagus; the esophageal mucosa is pink and the opening is horizontal rather than vertical.
17. Gently push the tube through triangular space formed by the vocal cords and back wall of trachea.	17. If the vocal cords are in spasm (closed), wait a few seconds before passing the tube.
18. Stop insertion just after the tube cuff has disappeared from view beyond the cords.	18. Advancing tube further may lead to its entry into a mainstem bronchuse causing collapse of the unventilated lung.
19. Withdraw laryngoscope while holding endotracheal tube in place. Disassemble mask from resuscitation bag, attach bag to ET tube, and ventilate the patient.	
20 Inflate cuff with the minimal amount of air required to occlude the trachea.	20. Listen over the cuff area with a stethoscope. Occulusion occurs when no air leak is heard during ventilator inspiration or compression of the resuscitation bag.
21. Insert bite block if necessary.	21. This keeps patient from biting down on the tube and obstructing the airway.
22. Ascertain expansion of both sides of the chest by observation and auscultation of breath sounds.	22. Observation and auscultation help in determining that tube remains in position and has not slipped into the right mainstem bronchus.
23. Record distance from proximal end of tube to the point where the tube reaches the teeth.	23. This will allow for detection of any later change in tube position.
24. Secure tube to the patient's face with adhesive tape or apply a commercially available endotracheal tube stabilization device.	24. The tube must be fixed securely to ensure that it will not be dislodged. Dislodgement of a tube with an inflated cuff may result in damage to the vocal cords.
25. Obtain chest X-ray to verify tube position.	
Follow-up Phase	
1. Record tube type and size, cuff pressure, and patient tolerance of the procedure. Auscultate breath sounds every 2 hours or if signs and symptoms of respiratory distress occur. Assess ABGs after intubation if requested by the physician.	1. ABGs may be prescribed to ensure adequacy of ventilation and oxygenation. Tube displacement may result in extubation (cuff above vocal cords), tube touching carina (causing paroxysmal coughing) or intubation of a mainstem bronchus (resulting in collapse of the unventilated lung).
2. Measure cuff pressure with manometer, adjust pressure. Make adjustment in tube placement on the basis of the chest X-ray results.	2. The tube may be advanced or removed several centimeters for proper placement on the basis of the chest X-ray results.

PROCEDURE 6.5: ****ASSISTING WITH TRACHEOSTOMY INSERTION*

Equipment Tracheostomy tube (Sizes 6.0 to 9.00 mm form most adults).
Sterile instruments, haemostat, scalpel and blade, for suture material, scissors.
Sterile gown and drapes, gloves
Cap and mask
Antiseptic prepared solution
Gauze sponges
Shave prepared kit.
Sedation
Local anaesthetic and syringe
Resuscitation bag and mask with oxygen source
Suction source and catheters
Syringe for cuff inflation
Respiratory support available for post-tracheostomy (mechanial ventilation, tracheal oxygen mask, CPAP, T-piece)
Goggles or other eye protection device.

STEPS OF PROCEDURE

Nursing action	*Rationale*
Preparatory Phase	
1. Monitor vital signs (heart rate, respiration, blood pressure, temperature) before insertion.	1. Provide baseline for assessment of progress or complications.
Tracheostomy Tube Placement *Performance Phase*	
1. Explain the procedure to the patient. Discuss a communication system with the patient.	1. Apprehension about inability to talk is usually a major concern of the tracheostomised patient.
2. Obtain consent for operative procedure.	
3. Shave neck region.	3. Hair and beard may harbour micro-organisms. If beard is to be removed, inform the patient or family.
4. Assemble equipment. Using aseptic technique, inflate tracheostomy cuff and evaluate for symmetry and volume leakage. Deflate maximally.	4. Ensures that the cuff is functional before the insertion.
5. Position the patient (supine with head extended, with a support under shoulders).	5. This position brings the trachea forward.
6. Apply soft wrist restraints if patient is confused.	6. Restraint of the confused patient may be necessary to ensure patient safety and preservation of aseptic technique.
7. Give medication if ordered.	7.
8. Position light source.	8.
9. Assist with antiseptic preparation.	9.
10. Assist with gowning and gloving.	10. To prevent infection and maintain aspectic technique.
11. Assist with sterile draping.	
12. Put on goggles.	12. Spraying of blood or airway secretions may occur during this procedure.

Contd...

Nursing action	*Rationale*
13. During procedure monitor the patient's vital signs, suction as necessary, give medication as prescribed, and be prepared to administer emergency care.	13. Bradycardia may result from vagal stimulation due to tracheal manipulation or hypoxaemia. Hypoxaemia may also cardiac irritability.
14. Immediately after the tube is inserted, inflate the cuff. The chest should be auscultated for the presence of bilateral breath sounds.	14. Ensures ventilation of both lungs.

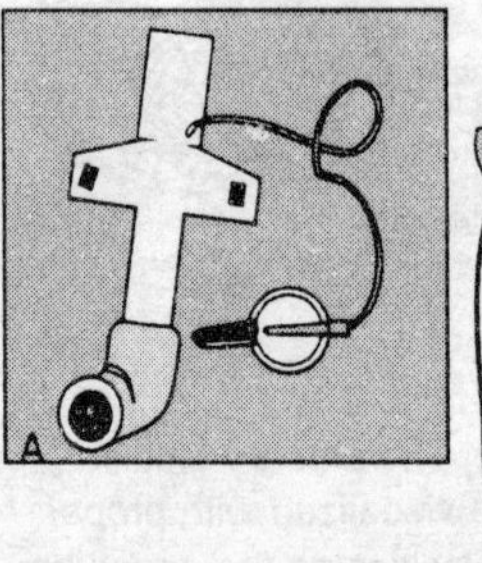

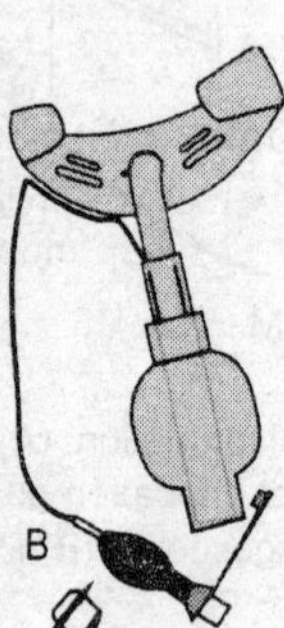

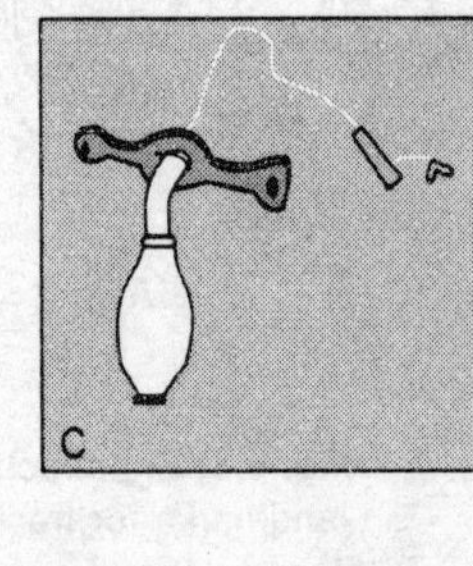

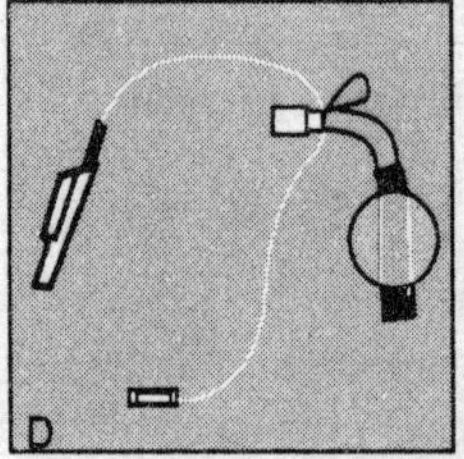

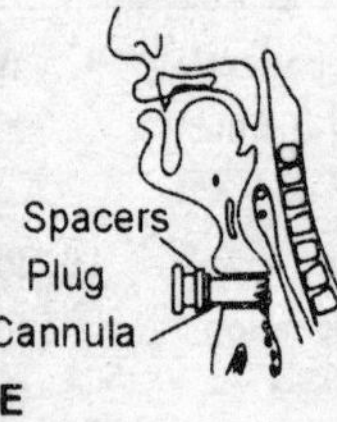

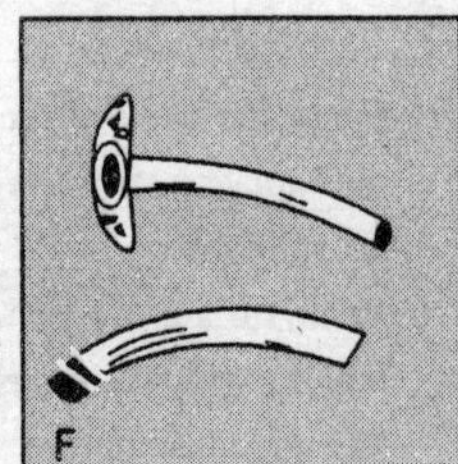

Fig. 6.7: Types of tracheostomy tubes. (A) Low pressure cuff (Shiley), (B) Fenestrated tube (Portex), (C) Polyurethane foam-filled cuff (FOME-Cuff), (D) Pitt speaking tube (National Catheter Corporation), (E) Tracheal button, (F) Silver tube

Nursing action	*Rationale*
15. Secure the tracheostomy tube which will tapes or other securing device and apply dressing.	
16. Apply appropriate respiratory assistive device (mechanical ventilation, tracheostomy, oxygen mask (Pap, T-piece adapter).	
17. Check the tracheostomy tube cuff pressure.	17. Excessive cuff pressure may cause tracheal damage.
18. "Tie sutures" or "stay sutures" of 00 silk may have been placed through either side of the tracheal cartilage at the incision and brought out through the wound. Each is to be taped to the skin at a 45-degree angle laterally to the sternum.	18. Should the tracheostomy tube become dislodged, the stay sutures may be grasped and used to spread the tracheal cartilage apart, facilitating placement of the new tube.

Contd...

Nursing action	Rationale
Follow-up Phase	
1. Assess vital signs and ventilatory status, note tube size used, physician performing procedure, type, dose, and route of medications given.	1. Provides baseline.
2. Obtain chest X-ray.	2. Documents proper tube placement.
3. Assess and chart condition of stoma.	3.
a. Bleeding	a. Some bleeding around the stoma site is not uncommon for the first few hours. Monitor and inform the physician of any increase in bleeding. Clean site aseptically when necessary. Do not change tracheostomy ties for first 24 hours, because accidental dislodgement of the tube could result when the ties are loose, and tube reinsertion through the as yet unformed stoma may be difficult or impossible to accomplish.
b. Swelling	
c. Subcutaneous air.	c. When positive pressure respiratory assistive devices are used (mechanical ventilation, (CPAP) before the wound is healed, air may be forced into the subcutaneous fat layer. This can be seen as enlargement of the neck and facial tissues and felt as crepitus of "cracking" when the skin is depressed. Report immediately.
4. An extra tube, obturator, and haemostat should be kept at the bedside. In the event of tube dislodgement, reinsertion of a new tube may be necessary. For emergency tube insertion.	4. The haemostat will open the airway and allow ventilation in the spontaneously-breathing patient. Avoid inserting the tube horizontally, because the tube may be forced against the back wall of the trachea.
a. Spread the wound with a haemostat or stay sutures.	
b. Insert replacement tube (containing the obturator) at an angle.	
c. Point cannula downward and insert the tube maximally.	
d. Remove the obturator.	

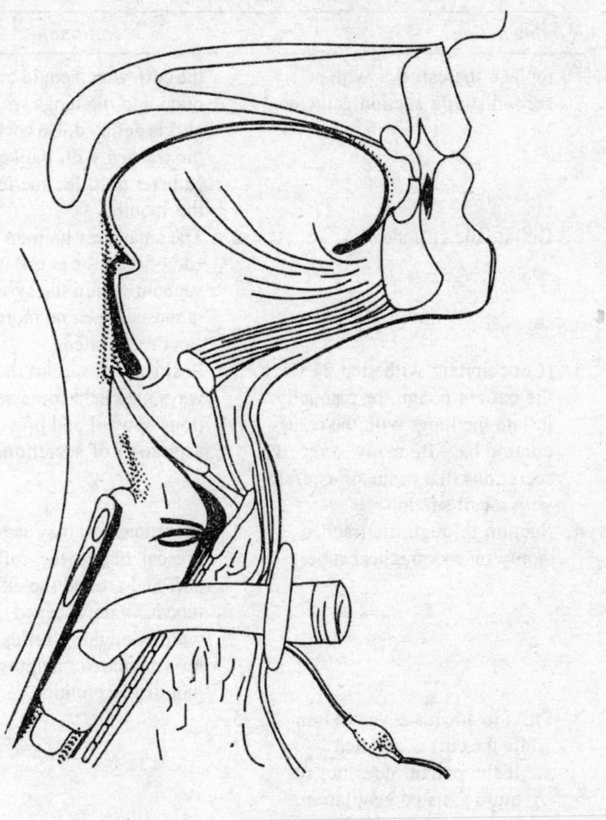

Fig.6.8: Tracheostomy tube placement

PROCEDURE 6.6: ****ARTIFICIAL AIRWAY CUFF MAINTENANCE*

Equipment Suction catheter
Tonsil suction
Suction source
10 ml syringe
Pressure manometer (mercury or aneroid)
Manual resuscitation bag with reservoir, connected to 100 per cent O_2 at 10 to 15 l/min
Goggles or other eye protection device

STEPS OF PROCEDURE

Nursing action	Rationale
Preparatory Phase	
1. Note degree of air leakage around cuff by listening over the cuff area with a stethoscope.	1. Provides a baseline. Air leakage is heard as a crowing sound at peak, airway pressure.
2. Auscultate breath sounds.	2. Provides data baseline.
Performance Phase	
1. Explain procedure to the patient.	1. Decrease the patient's anxiety and promotes cooperation.
2. Put on goggles.	2. Spraying of secretions may occur.
Deflating the Cuff	
1. Suction the trachea, then the oral and nasal pharynx. Then	1. Remove secretions collected above the cuff, which could

Contd...

Nursing action	*Rationale*
replace the catheter with a second sterile suction catheter.	the cuff, which could be aspirated into the lungs when the cuff is deflated. Do not reenter the trachea with the same catheter used for suctioning the mouth.
2. Deflate the cuff slowly.	2. The small test balloon at the end of the tube is inflated. A vacuum within the syringe is sensed when no more air can be aspirated.
3. (Concomitant with step 2) Have the patient cough, or manually inflate the lungs with the resuscitation bag. Be ready to receive secretions in a tissue or aspirate with tonsil suction.	3. Positive pressure in the airways may help force secretions upward and prevent aspiration of secretions.
4. Suction through the tracheostomy or endotracheal tube.	4. Secretions that may have been present above the inflated cuff and around the exterior tube have now seeped downward. Coughing reflex may be stimulated, helping to mobilize secretions.
5. Provide adequate ventilation while the cuff is deflated	5.
a. If the patient does not require assisted ventilation, maintain humidified oxygen as directed.	
b. If the patient requires assisted ventilation, provide manual ventilation via a resuscitation bag. Leave cuff deflated for as long as the tube repositioning requires, then reinflate.	b. Monitor patient closely for tolerance. Loss of tidal volume or PEEP may promote hypoxaemia and hypocarbia. Cuff should not be deflated for more than 30 to 45 seconds.
Inflating a Cuff	
1. No leak technique	1. Air leakage will be heard when the intra-airway pressure is most positive (maximum peak airway pressure). For the spontaneously patient, air leakage will be heard on exhalation. For the patient on positive pressure ventilation, air leakage will be heard at maximum ventilator inspiration.
a. Attach air-filled syringe to cuff injection port	
b. Slowly inject air until no air escapes from the patient's lungs around the cuff.	
c. Note the amount of air injected to provide a seal.	
2. Minimal leak technique (for mechanical ventilation).	2. Inflates cuff at lowest possible pressure while still maintaining an adequate seal. Prevents tracheal necrosis from excessive or prolonged cuff pressure.
a. Attach air-filled syringe to cut off injection port.	
b. Slowly inject air until no leak is heard at maximum peak airway pressure.	

Contd...

Nursing action	*Rationale*
c. Slowly remove air from cuff until a small air leak is heard at maximum peak airway pressure.	c. Adjustment in tidal volume setting may be necessary to compensate for the leak.
d. Note amount of air injected.	
3. Measurement of minimal occluding volume.	
Determination of minimal occluding volume and cuff inflation pressure. A stopcock is inserted into the cuff injection port. When the stopcock is opened to the manometer, cuff pressure is registered on the manometer. An aneroid manometer can also be used.	
a. Inject sufficient air into the manometer tubing to raise the dial reading 1 cm H_2O above the zero reading.	a. This "pressurizes" the tubing and prevents loss of air from the cuff to the tubing when the reading is taken.
b. Insert male part of three way stopcock into cuff injection port. One female port of stopcock holds the air filled syringe, and one port holds the pressure manometer.	b.
c. Inject air into cuff until desired intracuff pressure is reached at maximum peak airway pressure.	c. Aneroid manometer measures cuff pressure in cm H_2P. A pressure of 20 to 25 cm H_2O is desired. Mercury manometer pressure should be 15 to 20 mm Hg pressure greater than upper limit may cause compression of tracheal vessels, resulting in decreased blood flow to tissue. Pressure less than lower limit may allow aspiration of gastric or oral secretions.
d. Note amount of air needed to achieve the desired intracuff pressure.	d.
e. Remove the stopcock from the injection port.	e. Most injection ports have self-sealing valves. If not, a cap or closed stopcock may be left in the injection port (clamping of the inflation tubing is discouraged, because it may result in cracking or kinking of the line permanently.
Monitoring Cuff Pressure	
1. While the cuff is inflated, monitor cuff pressure every 4 hours. Maintain cuff pressure between 15 and 20 mm Hg or 20 and 25 cm H_2O.	1. Excessive pressure will decrease blood flow to the tissue, resulting in tracheal necrosis, insufficient cuff pressure predisposes to aspiration.

Contd...

Nursing action	*Rationale*
2. Document the amount of air required to maintain cuff pressure at this level.	2. Establishes a baseline for evaluation of change in pressure.
Inability to Maintain a Seal	
1. Assess the degree of leakage and length of time elapsed since cuff volume was replenished.	1. If an inflated cuff leaks air within 10 minutes, assessment is necessary. Possibilities may be: a. Cuff positioned above the vocal cords (direct visualization necessary for repositioning). b. Incompetence of self-sealing valve on injection port. c. Tracheal dilatation (requiring larger size tube). d. Cuff may be ruptured, requiring a new tube.
2. Inflate the cuff to desired level.	
3. Disconnect syringe (and manometer if used).	
4. Assess for leakage.	
5. If leakage..........place three way stopcock between syringe and close stopcock. Remove syringe and manometer if used) leaving closed stopcock on port.	5. Closed stopcock left in injection port acts as "plug" if selfsealing valve is incompetent.
6. If air..........tube or replacement may be consult with appropriate personnel.	
Follow-up Phase	
1. Note and...........amount of air used for adequate seal, intercut and inability to achieve seal. Document intervention necessary to.......or change tracheostomy tube to obtain a desired seal.	
2. While the cuff is inflated, assess cuff-pressure every 4 hours. The cuff pressure manometer is useful for this.	2. Leakage of air from the cuff or cuff injection port may occur. Assess the inflation status and adjust as needed.

PROCEDURE 6.7: *TRACHEOSTOMY (ROUTINE)

Equipment Assemble the equipment or obtain a prepackaged tracheostomy care kit.

- Sterile towel
- Sterile gauze
- Sterile cotton
- Sterile gloves
- Hydrogen peroxide
- Sterile water
- Antiseptic solution and ointment (optional)
- Tracheostomy tie tapes or commercially available tracheostomy securing device.
- Goggles or other eye protection devices.

STEPS OF PROCEDURE

Nursing action	*Rationale*
Preparatory Phase	
1. Assess area of stome before tracheostomy care (redness, swelling, character of secretions, presence of pure.	1. The presence of skin breakdown or infection must be monitored. Culture of the site may be warranted by appearance of these signs.
Performance Phase	
1. Suction the trachea and pharynx thoroughly before tracheostomy care.	1. Removal of secretions before tracheostomy care keeps the area clean longer.
2. Explain procedure to the patient.	2. For co-operation of client
3. Wash hands neately.	3. Prevent infection
4. Assemble equipment.	4.
a. Place sterile towel on patient's chest under tracheostomy site.	a. Provides sterile field.
b. Open four sterile sponges and pour hydrogen peroxide on them.	b. For removal of mucus and crust, which promotes bacterial growth.
c. Open 2 gauze sponges and pour antiseptic.	c. May be applied to fresh stoma. Not necessary for clean, healed stoma.
d. Open 2 gauze sponges. Keep dry.	d.
e. Open 2 gauze sponges and pour sterile water on them.	e.
f. Place tracheostomy tube tapes on field.	f.
g. Put on goggles and sterile gloves.	g. Goggles prevent spraying of secretions into the nurse's eyes. Sterile gloves prevent contamination of the wound by nurse's hands and also protect the nurse's hands from infection.

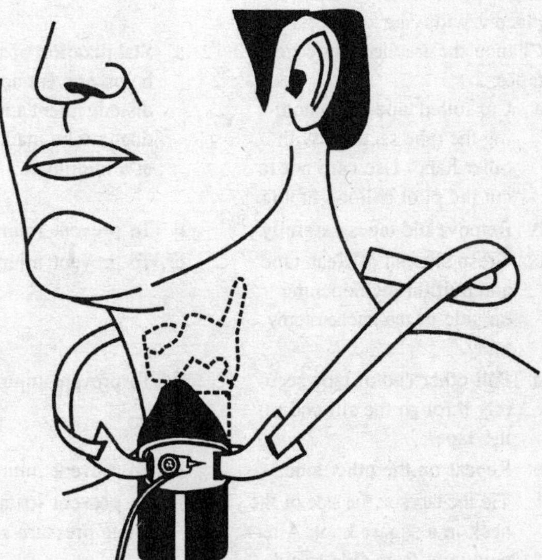

Fig. 6.9: Placement of tracheostomy tube tapes and elective gauze pad

Nursing action	*Rationale*
5. Clean the external end of the tracheostomy tube with 2 gauze sponges with hydrogen peroxide; discard sponges.	5. Designate the hand you clean with as contaminated and reserve the other hand as sterile for handling sterile equipment.
6. Clean the stoma area with 2 peroxide soaked gauze sponges. Make only a single sweep with each gauze sponge before discarding.	6. Hydrogen peroxide may help loosen dry-crusted secretions.
7. Loosen and remove crust with sterile cotton swabs.	
8. Repeat step 6 using the sterile water-soaked gauze sponges.	8. Ensures that all hydrogen peroxide is removed.
9. Repeat step 6 using dry sponges.	9. Ensures dryness of the area. Wetness promotes infection and irritation.
10. (Optional). An infected wound may be cleansed with gauze saturated with an antiseptic solution, then dried. A thin layer of antibiotic ointment may be applied to the stoma with a cotton swab.	10. May help clear wound infection.
11. Change a disposable inner cannula, touching only the external portion, and lock it securely into place. If inner cannula is reusable remove it with your contaminated hand and clean it in hydrogen peroxide solution, using brush or pipe cleaners with your sterile hand. When clean, drop it into sterile saline solution and agitate to rinse thoroughly with your sterile hand. Tap it gently to dry it and replace it with your sterile hand.	11. Because cannula is dirty when you remove it, use your contaminated hand. It is considered sterile once you clean it, so handle it with your sterile hand.
12. Change the tracheostomy tie tapes:	
a. Cut soiled tape while holding the tube securely with other hand. Use care not to cut the pilot balloon tubing.	12. a. Stabilization of the tube helps prevent accidental dislodgement and keeps due to tube manipulation at a minimum.
b. Remove old tapes carefully.	b. To prevent injury.
c. Grasp slit end of clean tape and pull through opening on side of the tracheostomy tube.	c. To prevent injury.
d. Pull other end of tape securely through the slit end of the tape.	d. To prevent injury.
e. Repeat on the other side.	e. To prevent injury.
f. Tie the tapes at the side of the neck in a square knot. Alternate knot from side to side each time tapes are changed.	f. To prevent irritation and rotate pressure site.

Contd...

Nursing action	*Rationale*
g. Tape should be tight enough to keep tube securely in the stoma, but loose enough to permit two fingers to fit between the tapes and the neck.	g. Excessive tightness of tapes will compress jugular veins, decrease blood circulation to the skin under the tape and result in discomfort for the patient.

Note: If only one clinician is available, the stoma is new (less than 2 weeks), or the patient's condition is unstable, follow steps c through f before removing old tape. Two set(s) of ties will be in place at the same time. After completing step f, cut and remove the old tapes. Also a tracheostomy-securing device can be used instead of the tracheostomy ties

13. Place a gauze pad between the stoma site and the tracheostomy tube to absorb secretions and prevent irritation of the stoma according to institution policy (see accompanying figure). Many clinicians feel that gauze should not be used around the stoma. In their opinion, the dressing keeps the area most and dark, promoting stomal infection. They believe the stoma should be left open to the air and the surrounding area kept dry. A dressing is used only if secretions are draining on to subclavian or neck IV sites or chest incisions	
Follow-up Phase	
1. Document procedure performance observations of stoma (irritation redness, oedema, subcutaneous air) and character of secretions (colour, purulence). Report changes in stoma appearance or secretions	1. Provides a baseline.
2. Cleaning of the fresh stoma should be performed every 8 hours, or more frequently if indicated by accumulation of secretions. Ties should be changed every 24 hours or more frequently if soiled or wet.	2. The area must be kept clean and dry to prevent infection or irritation of tissues.

PROCEDURE 6.8: ****INSERTION OF A TRACHEOSTOMY BUTTON*

Equipment: Tracheostomy button kit (includes cannula, solid closure plug, spacers, universal adapter)
Water-soluble lubricant
Syringe for deflation of tracheostomy cuff
Replacement tracheostomy tube.

STEPS OF PROCEDURE

Nursing action	*Rationale*
Preparatory Phase	
1. Assess whether patient meets teria for use of tracheostomy button. (Criteria include: able to be adequately oxygenated with nasal	1. If patient does not meet these criteria, use of tracheostostomy tube as airway must be continued.

Contd...

Nursing action	Rationale
cannula or face mask; able to swallow and protect the airway; able to cough up secretions; and a non-infected, nonirritated tracheal stoma.	
2. Determine vital signs, level of consciousness, SaO_2 of ABG.	2. Provides baseline for future assessment.
Performance Phase	
1. Elevate the head of the bed 45 degrees, suction the airway, deflate the tracheostomy tube cuff and remove the tube.	1. Protects against aspiration.
2. Determine the distance from anterior tracheal wall to the outer edge of the stoma (skin surface) using a probe with a right angle bend (contained in the kit).	2. Insert the angled end of the probe into the stoma, pull gently until the probe touches the anterior wall, then mark the probe at the outer edge of the stoma (skin) surface.
3. Compare the length of the tracheostomy button cannula with this measurement. If the cannula is too long, it can be sized to fit by adding spacers included into the kit.	3. Spacer rings can be slipped over cannula to size it for individualised patient requirements.
4. Coat the cannula with water-soluble lubricant. Ask the patient to relax and take several deep breaths. Insert the cannula into the stoma.	4. The cannula should pass easily into the stoma. If insertion is difficult, recheck cannula size. Several sizes are available.
5. Insert the closure plug into the cannula. Ties may be used to hold the button in place until the stoma closes round the button.	5. A slight snap will be heard as the plug enters the cannula. The plug causes the proximal end of the cannula to flare, holding in place.
6. Remove button two times a week, clean with antibacterial soap, and replace it.	6. Periodic removal helps to keep tissue from granulating into distal portion of the cannula.
Follow-up Phase	
1. Observe immediate patient response and obtain SaO_2 or ABG after insertion. Report changes.	1. Use of the button increases dead space, which may increase work of breathing or cause a decrease in SaO_2.
2. Determine ability of patient to cough out secretions and swallow with button in place.	2. Confirms patient will not retain secretions or be at risk for aspiration with use of this device.

PROCEDURE 6.9: *NASOTRACHEAL (NT) SUCTIONING

Equipment: Assemble the following equipment or obtain a prepackaged kit

- Disposable curved-tipped suction catheter
- Sterile towel
- Sterile disposable gloves
- Sterile water
- Anaesthetic water-soluble lubricant jelly
- Suction source at 80 to 120 mm Hg
- Resuscitation bag with face mask. Connect 100 per cent O_2 source with flow of 10 L/min.

STEPS OF PROCEDURE

Nursing action	Rationale
Preparatory Phase	
1. Monitor heart rate, respiratory rate, colour, ease of respirations. If the patient is on monitor, continue monitoring heart rate or arterial blood pressure. Discontinue the suctioning and apply oxygen if heart rate decreases by 20 beats per minute or increases by 40 beats per minute. If blood pressure increases, or if cardiac dysrhythmia is noted.	1. Suctioning may cause the occurrence of: a. Hypoxaemia—initially resulting in tachycardia and increased blood pressure, and later causing cardiac ectopy, bradycardia, hypotension, and cyanosis. b. Vagal stimulation resulting in bradycardia.
Performance Phase	
1. Ascertain that the suction apparatus is functional. Pace suction tubing within easy reach.	1. The procedure must be done aseptically, because the catheter will be entering the trachea below the level of the vocal cords and introduction of bacteria is contraindicated.
2. Inform and instruct the patient regarding procedure. a. At a certain interval, the patient will be requested to cough to open the lung passage, so the catheter will go into the lungs and not into the stomach. The patient will also be encouraged not to try to swallow, because this will also cause the catheter to enter the stomach. b. The postoperative patient can splint the wound to make the coughing produced by NT suctioning less painful.	2. A thorough explanation will decrease patient's anxiety and promote patient's co-operation.
3. Place the patient in a semi-Fowler's or sitting position if possible.	3. NT suctioning should follow chest physical therapy, postural drainage and/or ultrasonic nebulization therapy. The patient should not be suctioned after eating or after a tube feeding is given (unless absolutely necessary) to decrease the possibility of emesis and aspiration.
4. Place sterile towel across the patient's chest. Squeeze small amount of sterile anaesthetic water-soluble lubricant jelly on to the towel	
5. Open sterile pack containing curved tipped suction catheter	
6. Aseptically glove both hands. Designate one hand (usually the dominant one) as "sterile" and	6. The contaminated hand must also be gloved to ensure that organisms in the sputum do

Contd...

Nursing action	*Rationale*
the other hand as "contaminated.	not come in contact with the nurse's hand, possibly resulting in infection of the nurse.
7. Grasp sterile catheter with sterile hand.	
8. Lubricate catheter with the anaesthetic jelly and pass the catheter into the nostril and back into the pharynx.	8. If obstruction is met, do not for the catheter. Remove it and try the other nostril.
9. Pass the catheter into the trachea. To do this, ask the patient to cough or say "ahh" If the patient is incapable of either, try to advance the catheter on inspiration. Asking the patient to stick out tongue or hold tongue extended with a gauze sponge, may also help to open the airway. If a protected amount of time is needed to position, the catheter in the trachea, stop and oxygenate the patient with face mask or the resuscitation bag-mask unit at intervals, if three < attempts to place the catheter are unsuccessful, request assistance.	9. These manoeuvres may add in opening the glottis and allowing passage of the catheter into the trachea. To evaluate proper placement, listen at the catheter end for air, or feel, for air movement against the cheek. An increase in intensity of breath sounds or more air movement against cheek indicates nearness to the larynx. Gagging or sudden lessening of sound means the catheter is in the hypopharynx, Drawback and advance again. The presence of the catheter in the trachea is indicated by: a. Sudden paroxysms of coughing b. Movement of air through the catheter c. Vigorous bubbling of air, when the distal end of the suction catheter is placed in a cup of sterile water d. Inability of the patient to speak.
10. Specific positioning of catheter for deep bronchial suctioning: a. For left bronchial suctioning, turn the patient's head to the extreme right, chin up. b. For right bronchial suctioning, turn the patient's head to the extreme left, chin up.	10. Turning the patient's head to one side elevates the bronchial, passage on the opposite side, making catheter insertion easier. Suctioning of a particular lung segment may be of value in patients with unilateral pneumonia, atelectasis or collapse.

Note: The value of turning the head as an aid to entering the right or left mainstem bronchi is not accepted by all clinicians.

Nursing action	*Rationale*
11. Never apply suction until catheter is in the trachea. a. Once correct position is ascertained, apply suction and gently rotate catheter while pulling it slightly upward. Do not remove catheter from the trachea.	11. a. Because entry into the trachea is often difficult, less change in arterial oxygen may be leaving the catheter in the trachea than by repeated insertion attempts.

Contd...

Nursing action	*Rationale*
12. Disconnect the catheter from the suctioning source after 5 to 10 seconds. Apply oxygen by placing a face-mask over the patient's nose, mouth and catheter and instruct the patient to breathe deeply.	12. Ensure that adequate time is allowed to reoxygenate the patient as oxygen is removed, as well as secretions, during suctioning.
13. Reconnect suction source. Repeat as necessary.	13. Not more than three to four suction passes should be made per suction episode.
14. During the last suction pass, remove the catheter completely while applying suction and rotating the catheter gently. Apply oxygen when catheter is removed.	14. Never leave the catheter in the trachea after the suction procedure is concluded, because the epiglottis is splinted open and aspiration may occur.

Placement of nasotracheal tube for suctioning the tracheobronchial tree.

Follow-up Phase

1. Dispose of disposable equipment.	
2. Measure heart rate and blood pressure. Record the patient's tolerance of procedure, type and amount of secretions removed, and complications.	2. Record any patient intolerance of procedure (changes in vital signs, bleeding, laryngospasm, upper airway noise).

PROCEDURE 6.10: **STERILE TRACHEOBRONCHIAL SUCTION BY WAY OF TRACHEOSTOMY OR ENDOTRACHEAL TUBE (SPONTANEOUS OR MECHANICAL VENTILATION)*

Equipment: Assemble the following equipment or obtain a prepackaged suctioning kit.

Sterile suction catheters—No 14 or 16 (adult) No 8 or (child). The outer diameter of the suction catheter should be no greater than one half of the inner diameter of the artificial airway.
Two sterile gloves
Sterile towel
Suction source at 80 to 120 mm Hg
Sterile water
Resuscitator bag with a reservoir connected to 100 per cent oxygen source (if patient is on PEEP or CPAP, add positive end expiratory pressure (PEEP) valve to valve on resuscitation bag in an amount equal to that on the ventilator or CPAP device).
Normal saire solution (in syringe or single-dose packet)
Sterile cup for water
Alcohol swabs
Sterile water soluble lubricant jelly
Goggles or other eye protection device

STEPS OF PROCEDURE

Nursing action	*Rationale*
Preparatory Phase	
1. Monitor the heart rate and auscultate breath sounds. If the patient is monitored, continuously monitor heart rate and arterial blood pressure, progressing to blood pressure. If arterial blood	1. Suctioning may cause a. Hypoxaemia, initially resulting in tachycardia and increased blood pressure, progressing to cardiac ectopy, bradycardia,

Contd...

Nursing action	*Rationale*
gases are done routinely, know baseline values (it is important to establish a baseline because suctioning should be discontinued and oxygen applied or manual ventilation reinstituted if, during the suction procedure, the heart rate decreases by 20 beats per minute or increases by 40 beats per minute, blood pressure drops, or cardiac dysrhythmia is noted).	hypotension and cyanosis. b. Vagal stimulation which may result in bradycardia.
Performance Phase	
1. Instruct the patient how to "spling" surgical incision, because coughing will be induced during the procedure. Explain the importance of performing the suction procedure in an aseptic manner.	
2. Assemble equipment. Check function of suction and manual resuscitation bag connected to 100% O_2 source. Put on goggles.	2. Make sure that all equipment is functional before sterile technique is instituted to prevent interruption once the procedure is begun. Use of 100% O_2 will help to prevent hypoxaemia.
3. Wash hands properly.	
4. Open sterile towel. Place in a biblike fashion on patient's chest. Open alcohol wipes and place on corner of towel. Place small amount of sterile water-soluble jelly on towel.	
5. Open sterile gloves. Place on towel.	
6. Open suction catheter package.	
7. If the patient is on mechanical ventilation, test to make sure disconnection of ventilator attachment may be made with one hand.	
8. Don sterile gloves. Designate one hand as contaminated for disconnecting, bagging, and working the suction control. Usually the dominant hand is kept sterile and will be used to thread the suction catheter.	8. The hand designated as sterile must remain uncontaminated to organisms are not introduced into the lungs. The contaminated hand must also be gloved to prevent sputum from contacting the nurse's hand, possibly resulting in an infection of the nurse.
9. Use the sterile hand to remove carefully the suction catheter from the package, curling the catheter around the gloved fingers.	
10. Connect suction source to the suction fitting of the catheter with the contaminated hand.	

Contd...

Nursing action	*Rationale*
11. Using the contaminated hand, disconnect the patient from the ventilator, CPAP device, or other oxygen source (Place the ventilator connector on the sterile towel and flip a corner of the towel over the connection to prevent fluid from spraying into the area).	11. Prevents contamination of the connection.
12. Ventilate and oxygenate the patient with the resuscitator bag compressing firmly and as completely as possible approximately four to five times (try to approximate the patient's tidal volume). The procedure is called "bagging" the patient, in the spontaneously breathing patient, coordinate manual ventilations with the patient's own inspiratory effort.	12. Ventilation before suctioning helps prevent hypoxaemia. When possible two nurses work as a team to suction. Attempting to ventilate against the patient's own respiratory efforts may result in high airway pressures predisposing the patient to barotrauma (lung injury due to pressure).
13. Lubricate the tip of the suction catheter. Gently insert suction catheter as far as possible into the artificial airway without applying suction. Most patients will cough when the catheter touches the carina.	13. Suctioning on insertion would unnecessarily decrease oxygen in the airway.
14. Withdraw catheter 2 to 3 cm and apply suction. Quickly rotate the catheter while it is being withdrawn.	14. Failure to withdraw and rotate catheter may result in damage to tracheal mucosa. Release suction if a pulling sensation is felt.
15. Limit suction time to not more than 10 seconds. Discontinue if heart rate decreases by 20 beats per minute or increases by 40 beats per minute, or if cardiac ectopy is observed.	15. Suctioning removes oxygen as well as secretions and may also cause vagal stimulation.
16. Bag patient between suction passes with approximately four to five manual ventilations.	16. The oxygen removed by suctioning must be replenished before suctioning is attempted again.
17. At this point, sterile normal saline may be instilled into the trachea by way of the artificial airway if secretions are tenacious.	17. Some clinicians believe secretion removal may be facilitated with saline instillation. Others believe saline does not mix with mucus and that suctioning of the saline just instilled is the only effect produced by performing this step. It is now thought that the greatest benefit of instilling sterile normal saline is to initiate a cough.
a. Open prepackaged container and instill 3 to 5 ml normal saline into the artificial airway during spontaneous inspiration.	a. Instillation of the saline during inspiration will prevent the saline from being blown back out of the tube.
b. Bag vigorously and then suction.	b. Bagging stimulates cough and distributes saline to loosen secretions.

Contd...

Nursing action	*Rationale*
18. Rinse catheter between suction passes by inserting tip in cup of sterile water and applying suction	
19. Continue making suction passes bagging the patient between passes, until the airways are clear of accumulated secretions. Not more than four suction passes should be made per suctioning episode.	19. Repeated suctioning of a patient in a short time interval predisposes to hypoxaemia, as well as being tiring and traumatic to the patient.
20. Give the patient four to five "sigh" breaths with the bag.	20. Sighing is accomplished by dropping the bag slowly and completely with two hands to deliver approximately 1½ times the normal total volume to the patient, allowing for maximal lung expansion and prevention of atelectasis.
21. Return the patient to the ventilator or apply CPAP or other oxygen-delivery device	
22. Suction oral secretions from the oropharynx above the artificial airway cuff	
23. Clean elbow fitting of resuscitation bag with alcohol; cover with a sterile glove or 4 × 4	
Follow-up Phase	
1. Note any change in vital signs patient's intolerance to the procedure. Record amount and consistency of secretions.	1. Evaluate the effectiveness of procedure and patient response.
2. Assess need for further suctioning at least every 2 hours, or more frequently if secretions are copious.	

Note: A closed system for suctioning may be in place in the ventilator circuit that allows suctioning without removal from the ventilator.

Teach caregivers to suction in the home situation using clean technique, rather than sterile. Wash hands well before suctioning and reuse catheter after rinsing it in warm water.

PROCEDURE 6.11: **TEACHING THE PATIENT BREATHING EXERCISES*

STEPS OF PROCEDURE

Nursing action	*Rationale*
Preparatory Phase	
Instruct the patient as follows.	
Diaphragmatic Breathing	
1. Place one hand on stomach just below the ribs and the other hand on the middle of the chest.	1. This helps the patient become aware of the diaphragm and its function in breathing.
2. Breathe in slowly and deeply through the nose, letting the abdomen protrude as far as it will. The abdomen enlarges during inspiration and decreases in size during expiration.	2. Slow inhalation provides ventilation and hyperinflation of the lungs.
3. Breathe out through pursed lips while contracting (tightening) the abdominal muscles. Press firmly inward and upward on the abdomen while breathing out.	3. Contracting the abdominal muscles assists the diaphragm in rising to empty the lungs. The hand generates pressure, on the abdomen to facilitate more complete expiration.
4. The chest should not move, attention is directed at the abdomen, not the chest.	4. Contraction of the abdominal muscles should take place during expiration.
5. Repeat for 1 minute (followed by a rest period of 2 minutes). Work upto 10 minutes, four times daily	
6. Learn to do diaphragmatic breathing while lying, then sitting, and ultimately standing and walking.	6. Diaphragmatic breathing helps the patient breathe in a controlled manner during activities that produce dyspnoea. If shortness of breach occurs, advise stopping the exercises until breathing pattern comes under control.
Pursed Lip Breathing	
1. Inhale through the nose.	1.
2. Exhale slowly and evenly against pursed lips while contracting (tightening) the abdominal muscles. (Avoid exhaling forcefully)	2. Pursing the lips increases intrabronchial pressure (helps maintain the branch in an open position) as well as intra-alveolar pressure. The pursed lips manoeuvre also prolongs the expiratory phase of breathing, makes it easier to empty the air in the lungs, and promotes carbon dioxide elimination.
3. Sit in a chair. Fold arms across the abdomen	3. a.
a. Inhale through the nose	
b. Bend over and exhale slowly through pursed lips while counting up to 7.	b. Leaning forward pushes the abdominal organs upward.
4. While walking	4. Try any similar combinations according to breathing tolerance of patient.
a. Inhale while walking two steps.	
b. Exhale through pursed lips while walking four steps.	

Contd...

Lower Side Rib Breathing

1. Place hands on sides of lower ribs.
2. Inhale deeply and slowly while sides expand moving hands outward.
3. Exhale slowly through pursed lips and feel the hands and the ribs move inward.
4. Rest.

Lower back and ribs breathing

1. Sit in a chair. Place hands behind back; hold flat against lower ribs.
2. Inhale deeply and slowly while rib cage expands backward; the hands will move outward.
3. Keep hands in place. Blow out slowly; hands will move in.

SEGMENTAL BREATHING

1. Place hands on sides of lower ribs.
2. Inhale deeply and slowly while concentrating on moving the right hand outward by expanding the right rib cage.
3. Ensure that the right hand moves outward more than the left hand.
4. Keeping hands in place, exhale slowly, and feel the right hand and ribs moving in.
5. Repeat concentrating on expanding left side more than the right side.
6. Rest.

Patient Education

Instruct patient to:

1. Always inhale through the nose. This permits filtration, humidification and warming of air.
2. Breathe slowly in a rhythmic and relaxed manner. This permits more complete exhalation and emptying of lungs; helps overcome anxiety associated with dyspnoea and decreases oxygen requirement.
3. Avoid sudden exertion.
4. Practice in several positions; air distribution and pulmonary circulation vary according to position of the chest.

PROCEDURE 6.12:**PERCUSSION (CLAPPING) AND VIBRATION*

Equipment Pillows
Tilt table
Emesis basin
Sputum cup
Paper tissues

STEPS OF PROCEDURE

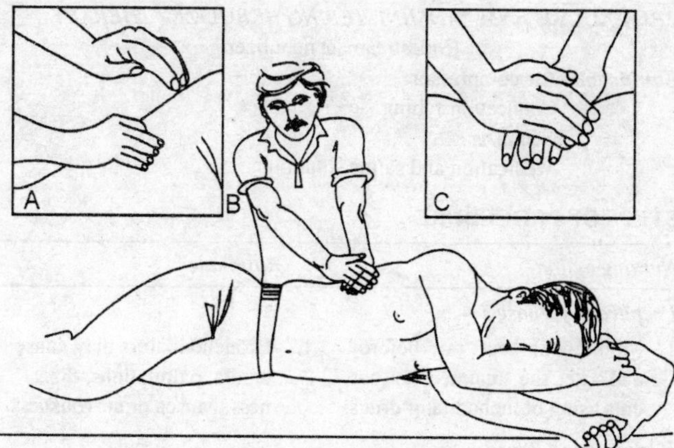

Fig. 6.10: Percussion and vibration: (A) Proper hand positioning for percussion, (B) Proper technique for vibration. Note that the wrists and elbows are kept stiff and the vibrating motion is produced by the shoulder muscles, (C) Proper hand position for vibration.

Nursing action	*Rationale*
Performance Phase	
1. Instruct the patient to use diaphragmatic breathing.	1. Diaphragmatic breathing helps the patient relax and helps widen airways.
2. Position the patient in prescribed postural drainage position/s. The spine should be straight to promote rib cage expansion.	2. The patient is positioned according to the area of lung that is to be drained.
3. Percuss (or clap) with cupped hands over the chest wall for 1 or 2 minutes from: a. The lower ribs to shoulders in the back. b. The lower ribs to top of chest in the front.	3. This action helps dislodge mucous plugs and mobilize secretions towards the main branch and trachea. The air trapped between the operator's hand and chest wall will produce a characteristic hollow sound.
4. Avoid clapping over the spine, liver, kidneys, spleen, breast, scapula, clavicle, or sternum.	4. Percussion over these areas may cause injuries to the spine or internal organs.
5. Instruct the patient to inhale slowly and deeply. Vibrate the chest wall as the patient exhales slowly through pursed lips.	5. This sets up a vibration that carries through the chest wall and helps free the mucous.
a. Place one hand on top of the other over-affected area or place one hand on each side of the rib cage.	a.
b. Tense the muscles of the hands and arms while applying moderate pressure downward and vibrate hands and arms.	b. This manoeuvre is performed in the direction in which the ribs move on expiration.
c. Relieve pressure on the thorax as the patient inhales	c.
d. Encourage the patient to cough and using abdominal muscles, after three or four vibrations.	d. Contracting the abdominal muscles while coughing increases cough effectiveness coughing aids in the movement and expulsion of secretions.
6. Allow the patient to rest for several minutes	6.
7. Listen with a stethoscope for changes in breath sounds.	7. The appearance of crackles and rhonchi indicate movement of air around mucous in the bronchi.
8. Repeat the percussion and vibration cycle according to the patient's tolerance and clinical response, usually 15 to 30 minutes.	8.

Contd...

PROCEDURE 6.13: ******ADMINISTERING NEBULIZER THERAPY*

(Sidestream jet nebulizer)

Equipment Air compressor
Connection tubing
Nebulizer
Medication and saline solution.

STEPS OF PROCEDURE

Nursing action	*Rationale*
Preparatory Phase	
1. Monitor the heart rate before and after the treatment for patients using bronchodilator drugs.	1. Bronchodilators may cause cardia, palpitations, dizziness, nausea or nervousness.
Performance Phase	
1. Explain the procedure to the patient. This therapy depends on patient effort.	1. Proper explanation of the procedure helps to ensure the patient's co-operation and effectiveness of the treatment.
2. Place the patient in a comfortable sitting of semi Flowler's position.	2. Diaphragmatic excursion and lung compliance are greater in this position. This ensures maximal distribution and deposition of aerosalized particles to basilar area of the lungs.
3. Add the prescribed amount of medication and saline to the nebulizer. Connect the tubing to the compressor and set the flow at 6 to 18 L/min.	3. A fine mist from the device should be visible.
4. Instruct the patient to exhale.	
5. Tell the patient to take in a deep breath from the mouthpiece hold breath briefly, then exhale.	5. This encourages optimal dispersion of the medication.
6. Nose clips are sometimes used if the patient has difficulty breathing only through the mouth.	6.
7. Observe expansion of chest to ascertain that patient is taking deep breaths.	7. This will ensure medication is deposited below the level of the oropharynx.
8. Instruct the patient to breathe slowly and deeply until all the medications is nebulized.	8. Medication will usually be nebulized within 15 minutes at a flow of 6 to 8 L/mn.
9. On completion of the treatment encourage the patient to cough after several deep breaths.	9. The medication may dilate airways, facilitating expectoration of secretions.
Follow-up Phase	
1. Record medication used and description of secretions.	1.
2. Disassemble and clean nebulizer after each use. Keep this equipment in the patient's room. The equipment is changed every 24 hours.	2. Each patient has own breathing circuit (nebulizer, tubing, and mouthpiece). Through proper cleaning, ing, sterilization and storage of equipment, organisms can be prevented from entering the lungs.

Nebulizer tubing and mouthpiece can be reused at home repeatedly. Recommend thorough rinsing with hot water after each use and periodic washing with liquid soap and hot water.

PROCEDURE 6.14: ******ADMINISTERING OXYGEN BY NASAL CANNULA*

Equipment Oxygen source
Plastic nasal cannula with connecting tubing (disposable)
Humidifier filled with distilled water
Flowmeter
No smoking signs

STEPS OF PROCEDURE

Nursing action	*Rationale*
Preparatory Phase	
1. Determine current vital signs level of consciousness, and most recent ABG.	1. Provides a baseline for future assessment. Nasal cannula oxygen administration is often used for patients prone to CO_2 retention. Oxygen may depress the hypoxic drive of these patients (evidenced by a decreased respiratory rate, altered mental status, and further $PaCO_2$ elevation).
2. Assess rise of CO_2 retention with oxygen administration.	2. If $PaCO_2$ is decreased or normal, the patient is not experiencing CO_2 retention and can use oxygen without fear of the above consequences.
Performance Phase	
1. Paste no smoking signs on the patient's door and in view of patients and visitors	
2. Show the nasal cannula to the patient and explain the procedure	
3. Make sure the humidifier is filled to the appropriate mark.	3. Humidification may not be ordered if the flow rate is ≤ 4 L/min.
4. Attach the connecting tube from the nasal cannula to the humidifier outlet	
5. Set flow rate at prescribed liters/minute. Feel to determine if oxygen is flowing through the tips of the cannula.	5. Because a nasal cannula is a low-flow system (patient tidal volume supplies part of the inspired gas), oxygen concentration will vary, depending on the patient's respiratory rate and tidal volume. Approximate oxygen concentrations delivered are: 1 L = 24 to 25% 2 L = 27 to 29% 3 L = 30 to 33%

Contd...

Nursing action	*Rationale*
	4 L = 33 to 37% 5 L = 36 to 41% 6 L = 39 to 45% Patient's who require low constant concentrations of oxygen and whose breathing pattern varies greatly may need to use a venturi mask, particularly if they are carbon dioxide retainers.
6. Place the tips of the cannula in the patient's nose and adjust straps around ears for snug comfortable fit.	6. Inspect skin behind ears periodically for irritation or breakdown.
	Administering oxygen by nasal cannula. Patient's inspiration consists of a mixture of supplemental oxygen supplied via the nasal cannula and room air. Oxygen concentration is variable and depends on patient's tidal volume and ventilatory pattern.
Follow-up Phase	
1. Record flow rate used and immediate patient response.	1. Note the patient's tolerance of treatment. Report any intolerance noted.
2. Assess patient's condition ABG or SaO_2 and the functioning of equipment at regular intervals.	2. Depression of hypoxic drive is most likely to occur within the first hours of oxygen use. Monitoring of SaO_2 with oximetry can be substituted for ABG if the patient is not retaining CaO_2.
3. Determine patient comfort with oxygen use.	3. Flow rates in excess of 4 L/min may cause irritation to the nasal and pharyngeal mucosa.

Nursing Focus: Avoid use of petroleum jelly to lubricate nares, because it may clog openings of cannula.

PROCEDURE 6.15: *ADMINISTERING OXYGEN BY SIMPLE FACE MASK WITH/WITHOUT AEROSOL

Equipment Oxygen source
Humidifier bottle with distilled water, if high humidity is desired
Plastic aerosol mask
Large-bore tubing (high humidity) or small-bore tubing
Flowmeter
No smoking signs
For heated aerosol therapy humidifier heating element.

STEPS OF PROCEDURE

Nursing action	*Rationale*
Preparatory Phase	
1. Determine current vital signs, level of consciousness, and SaO_2 or ABG, if patient is at risk for CO_2 retention.	1. Because the aerosol face mask is a low-flow system (patient's tidal volume may supply part of inspired gas). Oxygen Oxygen concentration will vary depending on the patient's respiratory rate and rhythm. Oxygen delivery may be inadequate for tachypnoeic patients (flow does not meet peak inspiratory demand) or excessive for patients with slow respirations.
2. Assess viscosity and volume of sputum produced.	2. Aerosol is given to assist in mobilizing retained secretions.
Performance Phase	
1. Paste no smoking signs on patient's door and in view of the patient and visitors	1.
2. Show the aerosol mask to the patient and explain the procedure	2.
3. Make sure that the humidifier is filled to the appropriate mark.	3. If the humidifier bottle is not sufficiently full, less moisture will be delivered.
4. Attach the large-bore tubing from the mask to the humidifier in the heating element, if used	4.
5. Set desired oxygen concentration of humidifier bottle and plug in the heating element, if used.	5. The inspired oxygen concentration is determined by the humidifier setting. Usual concentrations are 35 to 50 per cent.
6. If the patient is tachypnoeic and concentration of 50% oxygen or greater is desired, two humidifiers and flow meters should be yoked together.	6. The aerosol mask is a low-flow system. Yoking two humidifiers together doubles humidifier flow but does not change the inspired oxygen concentration.
7. Adjust the flow rate until the desired mist is produced (usually 10 to 12 L/min).	7. This ensures that the patient is receiving flow sufficient to meet inspiratory demand and maintains a constant accurate concentration of oxygen.
8. Apply the mask to the patient's face and adjust the straps so the mask fits securely.	8.
9. Drain the tubing frequently by emptying condensate into a separate receptacle, not into the humidifier. If a heating element is used, the tubing will have to be drained more often.	9. The tubing must be kept free of condensate allowed to accumulate in the delivery tube will block flow and alter oxygen concentration. If condensate is emptied into the humidifier, bacteria may be aerosolized into the lungs.
10. If a heating element is used, check the temperature. The humidifier bottle should be warm, not hot to touch.	10. Excessive temperatures can cause airway burns; patients with elevated temperature should be humidified with an unheated device.

Contd...

Simple face mask. Oxygen concentration varies with patient's tidal volume and respiratory rate.

Nursing action	*Rationale*
Follow-up Phase	
1. Record FiO_2 and immediate patient response. Note the patient's tolerance of treatment. Notify the physician if intolerance occurs.	
2. Assess the patient's condition and the functioning of equipment at regular intervals.	2. Assess the patient for change in mental status, diaphoresis, changes in blood pressure, and increasing heart and respiratory rates.
3. If the patient's condition changes, assess SaO_2 or ABG.	3. If the patient has a high air flow from the mask, may not be sufficient to meet inspiratory needs without pulling in room air. Room air will dilute the oxygen provided and lower the inspired oxygen concentration, resulting in hypoxaemia. A change in mask or delivery system may be indicated.
4. Record changes in volume and tenacity of sputum produced.	4. Indicates effectiveness of humidification.

PROCEDURE 6.16: ***ADMINISTERING OXYGEN BY VENTURI MASK*** (High air flow oxygen entrainment (HAFOE))

Equipment Oxygen source
Flowmeter
Venturi mask for correct concentration (24%, 28%, 31%, 35%, 40%, 50%) or correct concentration adapter if interchangeable colour-coded adapters are used.
If high humidity desired: Compressed air source and flowmeter humidifier with distilled water. Large bore tubing.
No smoking signs.

STEPS OF PROCEDURE

Nursing action	*Rationale*
Preparatory Phase	
1. Determine current vital signs, level of consciousness, and most recent ABG.	1. Provides a baseline for future assessment. Venturi masks are used for patients prone to CO_2 retention. Oxygen may depress the hypoxic drive of these patients (evidenced by a decreased respiratory rate, altered mental status and further $PaCO_2$ elevation).
2. Assess risk of CO_2 retention with oxygen administration.	2. Risk is greater if the patient is experiencing an exacerbation of illness.
Performance Phase	
1. Paste no smoking signs on the door of the patient's room and in view of the patient and visitors.	1.

Contd...

Nursing action	*Rationale*
2. Show the venturi mask to the patient and explain the procedure.	2.
3. Connect the mask diaphragm tubing to the oxygen source.	3.
4. Turn on the oxygen flowmeter and adjust to the prescribed usually inscribed on the mask. Check to see that oxygen is flowing out the vent holes in the mask.	4. To ensure the correct air/oxygen mix, oxygen must be set at the prescribed flow rate. Prescribed flow rates differ for different oxygen concentrations. Usually this information is printed on the mask or interchangeable colour-coded source.
5. Place venturi mask over the patient's nose and mouth and Adjust flow.	5.
6. Check entries are not obstructed by the patient's bearings.	6. Proper mask function depends on mixing of sufficient amount of air and oxygen.
7. If high air flow is used: a. Connect the humidifier to a compressed air source. b. Attach the mask and connect the tubing to the at the base of the venturi mask.	7. When a venturi mask is used with high humidity, both an oxygen source and compressed air source are required. The compressed air source provides air for the air/oxygen mix. Excessive oxygen would be inspired if both tubings were connected to an oxygen sources.
Ventury mask constant concentrations of oxygen can be delivered.	
Follow-up Phase	
1. Record flow rate used and immediate patient response. Note the patient's tolerance of treatment. Report if intolerance occurs.	1. Depression of hypoxic drive is most likely to occur within the first hours of oxygen use.
2. If Co_2 retention is present, assess ABG every 30 minutes for 1 to 2 hours or until PaO_2 is > 50 mm Hg and the $PaCO_2$ is no longer increasing. Monitor pH. Report if the pH decreases below normal assessment value.	2. A modest (5 to 10 mm Hg) increase in $PaCO_2$ may occur after initiation therapy. A decreasing pH indicates failure of compensatory mechanisms. Mechanical ventilation may be required.
3. Determine patient comfort and oxygen use.	Venturi masks are best tolerated for relatively short periods because of their size and appearance. They also must be removed for eating and drinking. With improvement in patient condition, a nasal cannula may often be substituted.

PROCEDURE 6.17: ***ADMINISTERING OXYGEN BY PARTIAL REBREATHING OR NONREBREATHING MASK***

Equipment: Oxygen source
Plastic face mask with reservoir bag and tubing
Humidifier with distilled water
Flowmeter
No smoking signs.

STEPS OF PROCEDURE

Nursing action	Rationale
Preparatory Phase	
1. Determine current vital signs, level of consciousness.	1. Provide a baseline for evaluating patient response. Typically used for short-term support of patients who require a high-inspired oxygen concentration.
2. Determine most recent SaO_2 or ABG.	
Performance Phase	
1. Paste no smoking signs on the patients door and in view of the patient and visitors.	1.
2. Fill humidifier with distilled water.	2. If the humidifier is not sufficiently full, less moisture will be delivered.
3. Attach tubing to outlet on humi difier.	3.
4. Attach flowmeter.	4.
5. Show the mask to the patient and explain the procedure.	5.
6. Flush the reservoir bag with oxygen to inflate the bag and adjust flowmeter to 6 to 10 L/min.	6. Bag serves as reservoir, holding oxygen for patient inspiration.
7. Place the mask on the patient's face.	7. Be sure the mask fits snugly, because there must be an airtight seal between the mask and the patient's face.
8. Adjust liter flow so the rebreathing bag will not collapse during the inspiratory cycle, even during the deep inspiration.	8. With a well-fitting rebreathing bag adjusted so that the patient's inhalation does not deflate the bag, inspired oxygen concentration of 60 per cent to 90 per cent can be achieved. Some patients may require flow rates higher than 10 L/min to ensure that the bag does not collapse on inspiration.

Nursing Focus

1. Adjust the flow to prevent collapse of the bag, even during deep inspiration.
2. A partial rebreathing mask does not have a one-way valve between the mask and reservoir bag, if the bag is allowed to collapse on inspiration, more exhaled air can enter the reservoir and the patient can inhale high concentrations of CO_2.
3. A non-breathing mask will deliver a lower concentration of O_2 if the bag is allowed to collapse on inspiration. O_2 from the bag will be diluted by room air drawn in through the side holes of the mask.

Nursing action	Rationale
9. Stay with the patient for a time to make the patient comfortable and observe reactions.	9.
10. Remove mask periodically if the patient's condition permits) to dry the face around the mask. Powder skin and massage face around the mask.	10. These actions reduce moisture accumulation under the mask. Massage of the face stimulates circulation and reduces pressure over the area.

Contd...

Nursing action	Rationale
Follow-up Phase	
1. Record the flow of air and immediate patient response. Note the patient's tolerance of treatment. Report if tolerance occurs	
2. Observe the patient for change of condition. Assess equipmentary malfunctioning and low water level in humidifier.	2. Assess the patient for change in mental status diaphoresis, change in blood pressure, and increasing heart and respiratory rates.

PROCEDURE 6.18: *ADMINISTERING OXYGEN BY TRANSTRACHEAL CATHETER

Equipment Oxygen source
Transtracheal catheter with connecting tubing
Flow-meter
No smoking signs

STEPS OF PROCEDURE

Nursing action	Rationale
Preparatory Phase	
1. Determine current vital signs level of consciousness and .... if patient is at risk for CO_2 retention.	1. Provides a baseline for future assessment.
2. .... evidence of infection warmth, redness, swelling at infection site or temperature elevation.	2. The transtracheal catheter provides a direct communication between the skin and trachea, if the insertion site is not kept clean and dry, infection can develop.
3. Assess catheter patency, construction is indicated by a decreased SaO_2, whistling of the humidifier, high pressure of the delivery tubing, or stimulation of a cough.	3. Mucus can form on the end of the catheter and restrict oxygen delivery. This increases pressure in the delivery tubing and humidifier. The mucus may touch the back of the trachea, stimulating a cough.
Performance Phase	
Stent Phase	
1. Paste no smoking signs on the patient's door and in view of the patient and visitors.	1.
2. Instruct the patient in purpose of stent.	2. The stent is used to maintain a patent tract during the first week after catheter insertion. It facilitates breathing and allows gradual adjustment to use of the catheter. It is not used for oxygen delivery.
3. Teach that care of stent involve daily cleaning of the site with cotton-tipped applicators and observation for signs of infection. A 4×4 may be placed over the stent.	3. Until the tract heals, the patient is at increased risk of infection. Because the stent is open to the trachea, muscus, may be coughed from the stent.

Contd...

Nursing action	*Rationale*
• Immature Tract (Stent is removed and transtracheal catheter inserted)	
1. Instruct patient in cleaning and irrigation procedure. The patient should inject one half (1.5 mL) ampule of the sterile normal saline into the catheter, insert and remove the cleaning rod three times, and inject the remaining sterile normal saline two to three times a day (morning, noon and evening).	1. The catheter cannot be removed from the tract for cleaning until the tract completely heals (about 2 months). Cleaning in place helps to prevent mucus from forming on the end of the catheter and obstructing oxygen delivery.
2. Teach the patient use of the staged cough technique (i.e., sit with feet on floor, pillow over abdomen, inhale three to four times in through the nose and out through the mouth, on the last exhalation cough while bending forward with pillow against abdomen).	2. Use of this cough technique helps to increase airflow during coughing. Higher airflows help to dislodge any mucus that has formed on the outside of the catheter and cannot be removed by the cleaning technique).
3. Instruct the patient to clean the insertion site daily with cotton-tipped applicators and report signs of infection.	3. Mucus may form at the insertion site. Keeping the tract clean and dry decreases infection risk. Do not use hydrogen peroxide because it can dry mucous membrane.
4. Teach the patient to place two small strips of transparent tape over the chain on either side of the catheter for the first 2 weeks of catheter use.	4. This helps to keep the catheter in place during the night when the patient is sleeping. Serves as a second security system to keep the catheter from being inadvertently pulled from the tract during the initial adjustment phase.
5. Instruct the patient to replace the nasal cannula and call for instruction if the catheter is displaced from the tract or if symptoms of subcutaneous emphysema develop (swelling insertion site, tight chain, change in voice).	5. If the catheter comes out of the tract before it is mature, reinsertion may be difficult. If the tract is not completely healed, O_2 may enter the tissues around the insertion site. The patient may need to return to the clinic for assistance in replacing the or catheter or delay in using it until the tract is fully healed.
• Mature Tract (catheter is removed for cleaning)	
1. Instruct the patient in steps involved, in removing the tract for cleaning. Two catheters are used. The catheter in the tract is removed and replaced with a second catheter. The catheter removed from the tract is cleaned with antibacterial soap under warm running water, it then is air-dried and stored for reuse.	1. The catheter should easily enter the tract. Practicing while looking in a mirror helps to develop skill in removing and reinserting the catheter. This step should be performed twice daily if a catheter with multiple side holes (SCOOP 2) is used. Removal daily, or less often, is necessary with a single end hole catheter (SCOOP 1).
2. Instruct the patient to report immediately signs of infection and difficulty replacing the catheter.	2. These problems are less common with a mature tract, but can still occur.
Follow-up Phase	
1. Record flow rate of oxygen and patient response.	1. Transtracheal oxygen delivery is more efficient. The same SaO_2 is typically maintained at one half of the former flow rate.
2. Determine patient's ability to perform care independently.	2. Repeat demonstration of care may be required before the patient masters selfcare skills.
3. Ensure patient is able to demonstrate appropriate use of oxygen and attachment of oxygen to transtracheal catheter	3.
4. Discuss with patient signs and symptoms of oxygen toxicity and carbon dioxide retention. carbon dioxide retention	4. Too much carbon dioxide retention could lead to confusion, decreased level of consciousness or somnolence.

PROCEDURE 6.19: **ADMINISTERING OXYGEN BY CONTINUOUS POSITIVE AIRWAY PRESSURE* **(CPAP) MASK**

Equipment: Oxygen blender
Flowmeter
CPAP mask
Valve for prescribed PEEP (2, 5, 5, 57, 3, 10 cm H_2O)
Large bore tubing
Nasogastric tube
Sealing pad to accommodate nasogastric tube and
No smoking signs.

STEPS OF PROCEDURE

Nursing action	*Rationale*
Preparatory Phase	
1. Assess the patient's level of consciousness and gag reflex.	1. CPAP mask may lead to aspiration unless the patient is breathing spontaneously and is able to protect the airway.
2. Determine current ABG.	2. Document that patient meets criteria for use of this mask (normal or decreased $PaCO_2$) and provides baseline to evaluate whether therapy results in CO_2 retention.

Nursing Focus:
1. CPAP is used when patients have not responded to attempts to increase PaO_2 with other types of masks.
2. The patient will require frequent assessment to detect changes in respiratory status, cardiovascular status and level of consciousness.
3. If the patient's level of consciousness decreases or ABGs deteriorate, intubation may be necessary.

Contd...

Nursing action	*Rationale*
Performance Phase	
1. Paste no smoking signs on the patient's door and in view of the patient and visitors.	
2. Show the mask to the patient and explain the procedure.	
3. Make sure humidifier is filled to the appropriate mark.	
4. Insert nasogastric tube.	With CPAP, the patient may swallow air, causing gastric distensions or emesis. Prophylactic nasogastric suction diminishes this risk.

Note: Some clinicians do not believe a nasogastric tube is needed if the PEEP level is less than 10 cm H_2O.

Nursing action	*Rationale*
5. Attach nasogastric tube adapter.	5. Use of adapter may increase air leak around the mask.
6. Set desired concentration of oxygen blender and adjust flow rate so it is sufficient to meet the patient's inspiratory demand.	6. O_2 blenders are devices that mix air and O_2 using a proportioning valve. Concentrations of 21 per cent to 100 per cent may be delivered depending on the model. Because the patient will be receiving all minute ventilation from this "closed system", it is essential that the flow rate be adequate to meet changes in the patient's breathing pattern.
7. Place the mask on the patient's face, adjust the head strap, and inflate the mask cushion to ensure a tight seal.	7. To maintain CPAP, an airtight seal is required. Head straps and the inflatable cushion help to ensure that difficult areas, such as the nose and chin, are sealed with greater comfort to the patient.
8. Organize care to remove the mas as infrequently as possible.	8. If mask is removed (for coughing, suctioning) CPAP is not maintained and inspired oxygen concentration drop.

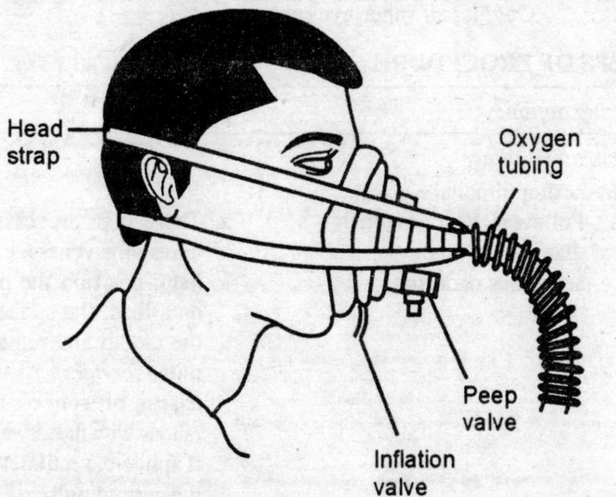

Fig. 6.11: Administering oxygen by face mask with continuous positive airway pressure (CPAP)

Nursing action	*Rationale*
Follow-up Phase	
1. Assess ABGs, haemodynamic status, and level of consciousness frequently.	1. Provides objective documentation of patient response, CPAP may increase work of breathing, resulting in patient's tiring and inability to to maintain ventilation without intubation CPAP may also decrease venous return (PEEP effect), resulting in decreased cardiac output.
2. Immediately report any increase in $PaCO_2$.	2. An increase in $PaCO_2$ suggests hypoventilation, resulting from tiring of the patient or inadequate alveolar ventilation. Need for intubation and mechanical ventilation should be evaluated.
3. Assess patency of nasogastric tube at frequent intervals.	3. May become obstructed, causing gastric distention.
4. Assess patient comfort and functioning of the equipment frequently.	4. Tight fit of the mask may predispose to skin breakdown. System may develop leaks, resulting in air escaping between the patient's face and mask.
5. Record patient's response. With improvement, oxygen therapy without positive airway pressure can be substituted. With deterioration intubation and mechanical ventilation may be required. Note the patient's tolerance of treatment. Report if intolerance occurs.	5. Face mask CPAP is usually continued only for short periods (72 hours) because of patient tiring and the necessity to remove mask for suctioning and coughing.

PROCEDURE 6.20: **ADMINISTERING OXYGEN VIA ENDOTRACHEAL AND TRACHEOSTOMY TUBES WITH A T-PIECE (BRIGGS) ADAPTER*

Equipment: Oxygen
Oxygen blender
Flowmeter
Humidifier with distilled water (heating element may be used as described in aerosol masks)
Large-bore tubing
T-piece and reservoir tubing
No smoking signs.

STEPS OF PROCEDURE

Nursing action	*Rationale*
Preparatory Phase	
1. Assess patient's SaO_2, haemodynamic status, and level of consciousness frequently. If patient's condition changes, assess ABGs.	1. Provide baseline to assess response.

Contd...

Nursing action	*Rationale*
2. Assess viscosity and volume of sputum produced.	2. Aerosol is given to assist in mobilizing retained secretions.
Performance Phase	
1. Paste no smoking signs on the patient's door and in view of the patient and visitors.	1. Provides baseline to assess response.

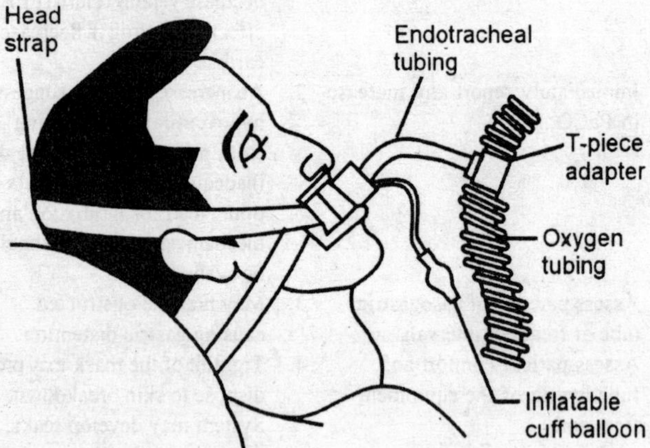

Fig. 6.12: Administering oxygen via endotracheal tube with a T-piece adapter. A T-piece adapter is attached to the endotracheal tube and large-bore tubing, which serves as a source of oxygen and humidity.

Nursing action	*Rationale*
2. Show the T-tube to the patient and explain the procedure.	2.
3. Make sure that the humidifier is filled to the appropriate mark led to the appropriate mark.	3. If humidifier is not sufficiently fulless aerosol will be delivered.
4. Attach the large-bore tubing from the T-tube to the humidifier outlet.	4.
5. Set desired oxygen concentration of O_2 blender or humidifier bottle and plug in heating element if used.	5. O_2 blenders are devices that mix air and O_2 using a proportioning valve. Concentrations of 21 to 100% may be delivered at flows of 2 to 100 L/min, depending on the model. Used in situation when precise control is required.
6. Adjust the flow rate until the desired mist is produced and meets the patient's inspiratory demand.	6. The aerosol mist in the reservoir, tubing attached to the T-tube should not be completely withdrawn on patient inspiration. If mist is withdrawn (does not extend from reservoir tubing), on inspiration, room air may be inspired and O_2 concentration decreased.
7. Drain the tubing frequently by emptying condensate into a separate receptacle, none into the humidifier, if a heating element is used the tubing will have to be drained more often.	7. The tubing must be kept free of condensate allowed to accumulate in the delivery tube will block flow and alter oxygen concentration. If condensate is emptied into the himidifier, bacteria may be aerosolized into the lungs.
8. If a heating element is used, check the temperature. The humidifier bottle should be warm, not hot, to touch.	8. Excessive temperatures can cause airway burns, patients with elevated temperatures will be better humidified with an unheated device.
Follow-up Phase	
1. Record FiO_2 and immediate patient response. Note the patient's tolerance of treatment. Report if intolerance occurs.	1.
2. Assess the patient's condition and the functioning of equipment at regular intervals.	2. Assess the patient for change in mental status, diaphoresis, perspiration, changes in blood pressure, and increasing heart and respiratory rates.
3. If the patient's condition changes, assess SaO_2 or ABGs and vital signs. Note changes suggesting increased work of breathing (diaphoresis, intercostal muscle retraction).	3. If the patient is being weaned, return to the ventilator if changes suggesting inability to tolerate spontaneous ventilation occur.
4. Record changes in volume and city of sputum produced.	4. Indicates effectiveness of humidification therapy.

PROCEDURE 6.21: **ADMINISTERING OXYGEN BY MANUAL RESUSCITATION BAG*

Equipment: Oxygen source
Resuscitation bag and mask
Reservoir tubing or reservoir bag
O_2 connecting tubing
Nipple adapter to attach flowmeter to connecting tubing
Flowmeter
Glovee and
Goggles or other eye protection

STEPS OF PROCEDURE

Nursing action	*Rationale*
Preparatory Phase	
1. In cardiopulmonary arrest.	1.
a. Follow steps to establish that a cardiopulmonary arrest has occurred.	a. These steps are: establish unresponsiveness, call for help, position the patient on a firm, flat surface, open the mouth and remove vomitus for debris. If visible; assess presence of respirations with the airway open; if apnoeic, ventilate; palpate the cartoid pulse; if absent, deliver chest compressions.

Contd...

Contd...

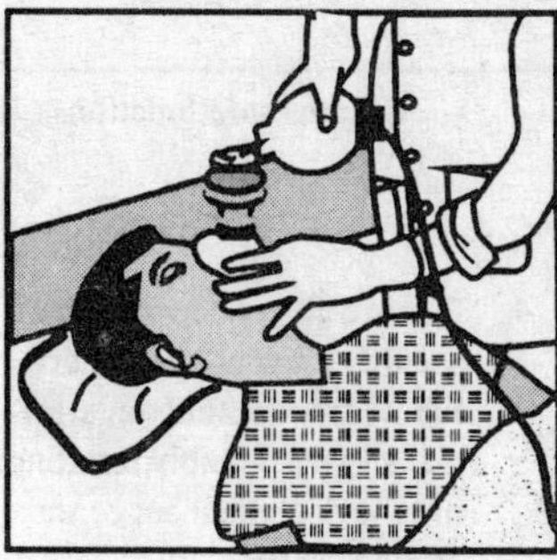

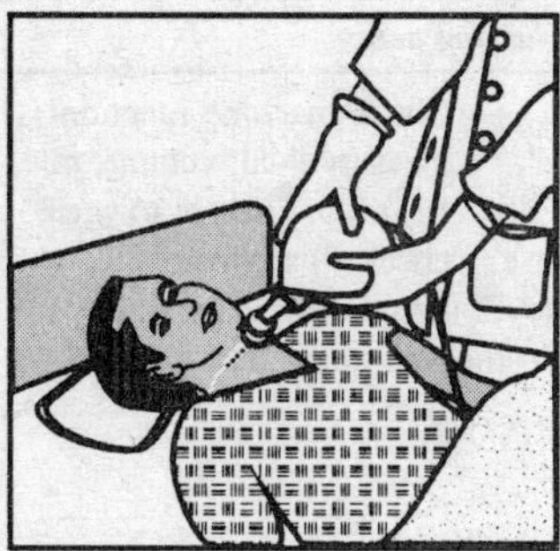

Fig. 6.13: Using a manual resuscitation bag, with mask (left), or connected to an artificial airway (right)

b. Use caution not to injure or increase injury to the cervical spine when opening the airway.	b. If cervical spine injury is a potential, the modified jaw thrust should be used. In other situations, the headtilt/chin-lift method can be used. These manoeuvres lift the tongue off the back of the throat and, in some situations, may be all that is needed to restore breathing.
2. In suctioning or transport situation. Assess patient's heart rate level of consciousness and respiratory status.	2. Provides a baseline to stimulate patient's tolerance of procedure.
Performance Phase	
1. Attach connecting tubing from flowmeter and nipple adapter to resuscitation bag.	1. A humidifier bottle is not used, because the high flow rates of oxygen required would force water into the cubing and clog it.
2. Turn flowmeter to "flush" position.	2. A high flow rate or "flush" position is necessary to meet the minute ventilation of the patient.
3. Attach reservoir tubing or reservoir bag to resuscitation bag.	3. A high inspired O_2 concentration is required. Without a reservoir inspired O_2 concentration wi'l be low (28 to 56%) because inspired gas will be air/O_2 mix. With a reservoir, manual resuscitation bags can achieve a FiO_2 of > 96 at a flow rate of 15/L/min.
4. Put-on goggles and gloves.	

Ensure that good seal is maintained between the face and mask. So volume delivered through compression of bag is noticed cardiopulmonary arrest. Follow steps given below:

Contd...

1. If respirations are absent after the airway is open, insert an oropharyngeal airway and ventilate twice with slow, full breaths of 1 to 1.5 seconds each. Allow 2 seconds between breaths.	1. The airway helps prevent obstruction from the tongue in an unconscious patient. If ventilation is difficult, confirm that airway is unobstructed. Airways are not appropriate in a conscious patient or patients with a gag reflex because stimulation of the propharynx could cause vomiting and aspiration.
2. Breaths will have to be quickly interposed between cardiac compressions if the patient needs only respiratory assistance, watch for chest expansion and listen with the stethoscope to ensure adequate ventilation.	2. Squeeze resuscitation bag with sufficient force and at the rate necessary to maintain adequate minute ventilation.
3. A rate of approximately 12 to 15 breaths per minute is used unless the patient is being given external cardiac compressions.	3. Continue squeezing bag at appropriate interval until CPR is no longer required.
Preoxygenation and Suctioning	
1. If hyperinflation is being used with suctioning ventilate the patient before and after each before and after each suctioning pass including after the last suction pass.	1. Hyperinflation before suctioning helps prevent hypoxaemia. Hyperinflation after suctioning replaces O_2 removed during the procedure and helps to prevent atelectasis. The larger tidal volumes may also assist in mobilizing secretions and promote surfactant secretion.
Transport	
1. If hyperinflation is used in transport, suction patient before disconnection for transport, monitor heart and respiratory rates and level of consciousness during procedure.	1. Establishes a patient airway before patient is moved. Provides information for assessing tolerance of transport.
2. Ventilate at rate of 12 to 15 breaths per minute.	2.
Follow-up Phase	
1. In cardiopulmonary arrest, verify return of spontaneous pulse and respirations initiate further support as needed.	1. Establishes patient's need for definitive therapy (drugs, defibrillation, intensive care).
2. In suctioning or transport, return to previous support. Note patient tolerance of procedure.	2. Note SaO_2, heart rate, rate and ease of respirations, arterial blood pressure (if monitored), level of consciousness. Report if tolerance occurs.

PROCEDURE 6.22: **MANAGING THE PATIENT REQUIRING MECHANICAL VENTILATION*

Equipment: Artificial airway
Mechanical ventilator
Ventilation circuitry
Humidifier
See manufacturer's directions for specific machine

STEPS OF PROCEDURE

Nursing action	*Rationale*
Preparatory Phase	
1. Obtain baseline samples for gas determinations (pH, PaO_2, $PaCO_2$, HCO_3) and chest X-ray.	1. Baseline measurements blood serve as a guide in determining progress of therapy.
Performance Phase	
1. Give a brief explanation to the patient.	1. Emphasize that mechanical ventilation is a temporary measure. The patient should be prepared psychologically for weaning at the time if the ventilator is first used.
2. Establish the airway by means of a cuffed endotracheal or tracheostomy tube.	2. A closed system between the ventilator and patient's lower airway is necessary for positive pressure ventilation.
3. Prepare the ventilator (respiratory therapist does this in many institutions)	
a. Set up desired circuitry	
b. Connect oxygen and compressed air source.	
c. Turn on power	
d. Set tidal volume (usually 10 to 15 ml/kg body weight).	d. Adjusted according to pH and $PaCO_2$.
e. Set oxygen concentration.	e. Adjusted recording to PaO_2.
f. Set ventilator sensitivity.	
g. Set rate at 12 to 14 breaths per minute (variable).	g. This setting approximates normal ventilation. These machines settings are subject to change according to the patient's condition and response, and the ventilator type being used.
h. Adjust flow rate (velocity of gas flow during inspiration). Usually set at 40 to 60 L/min. Is dependent on rate and tidal volume set to avoid inverse inspiratory expiratory (IE) ratio usual IE ratio is 1:2.	h. The slower the flow, the lower will be the peak air way pressure resulting from set volume delivery. This results in lower intrathoracic pressure and less impedance of venous return. However, a flow that is too low for the rate selected may result in inverse inspiratory or expiratory ratios.
i. Select mode of ventilation.	

Contd...

Nursing action	*Rationale*
j. Check machine function- measure tidal, volume, rate, IE, ratio, analyze oxygen, check all alarms.	j. Ensures safe function.
4. Couple the patient's airway to the ventilator.	4. Be sure all connections are secure. Prevent ventilator tubing from pulling on artificial airway, possibly resulting in tube dislodgement or tracheal damage.
5. Assess patient for adequate chest movement and fate. Do not depend on digital rate readout of ventilator. Note peak airway pressure and PEEP. Adjust gas flow of necessary to provide safe IE ratio.	5. Ensures proper function of equipment.
6. Set airway pressure alarms according to patient's baseline	6.
a. High pressure alarm.	a. High airway pressure or 'Pop off' pressure is set at about 20 cm H_2O above peak airway pressure. An alarm sounds if airway pressure selected is exceeded. Alarm activation indicates decreased lung compliance (Worsening pulmonary disease), decreased lung volume (such as pneumothorax, tension pneumothorax, haemothorax, pleural effusion). Increased airway resistance (secretions, coughing, breathing out of phase with the ventilator), loss of patency of airway (mucous plug, airway spasm, biting or kinking of tube)
b. Low pressure alarm.	b. Low airway pressure alarm set at 5 to 10 cm H_2O below peak airway pressure. Alarm activation indicates inability to build up airway pressure because of disconnection or leak, or inability to build up airway pressure because of insufficient gas flow to meet patient's inspiratory needs.
7. Assess frequently for change in respiratory status via ABGs, pulse oximetry, spontaneous rate, use of accessory muscles, breath sounds, and vital signs. (Other means of assessing are through the use of exhaled carbon dioxide. If change is noted, notify appropriate personnel.	7.

Contd...

Nursing action	Rationale
8. Monitor and troubleshoot alarm conditions. Ensure appropriate ventilation at all times.	8. Priority is ventilation and oxygenation of the patient. In alarm conditions that cannot be immediately corrected, disconnect the patient from mechanical ventilation and manually ventilate with resuscitation bag.
9. Positioning	9. Positioning.
a. Turn patient from side to side every 2 hours or more frequently if possible.	a. For patients on long-term ventilation, this may result in sleep deprivation. Evolve a turning schedule best suited to a particular patient's condition.
b. Lateral turns are desirable from right semiprone to left semizone	
c. Sit the patient upright at regular interval if possible.	c. Upright posture increases lung compliance.

Nursing focus

For patients in severe compromised respiratory state or who are unstable haemodynamically, consider use of specialty bed with rotational therapy. New versions may also have built in vibration and percussion as adjunct therapy options

Nursing action	Rationale
10. Carry out passive range–motion exercises of all extremities for patients.	10.
11. Assess for need of suctioning least every 2 hours.	11. Patients with artificial airways on mechanical ventilation are unable to clear secretions on their own. Suctioning may help to clear secretions and stimulate the cough reflex.
12. Assess breath sounds every 2 hours.	12.
a. Listen with stethoscope to the chest from bottom to top on both sides.	a. Auscultation of the chest is a means of assessing airway patency and ventilatory distribution, it also confirms the proper placement of the endotracheal or tracheostomy tube.
b. Determine whether breath sounds are present on absent, normal or abnormal and whether a change has occurred.	b.
c. Observe the patient's tachragmatic excursions and use of accessory muscles of respiration.	c.
13. Humidification.	13.
a. Check the water level in the humidification reservoir to ensure that the patient is never ventilated with dry gas. Empty the water the ordences in the delivery and exhaliation tubing into a scarate receptacle not into the humidifier. Airways were hands after emptying fluid from ventilator circuit humidifier must be changed every 24 hours.	a. Water condensing in the inspiratory tubing may cause increased resistance to gas flow. This may result in increased peak airway pressures. Warm, moist tubing is a perfect breeding area for bacteria. If this water is allowed to enter the humidifier, bacteria may be aerosolized into the lungs. Emptying the tubing also prevents introduction of water into the patient's airways.
14. Assess airway pressure adequate intervals.	14. Monitor for changes in compliance or onset of conditions that may cause airway pressure to increase or decrease.
15. Measure delivered tidal volume and analyze oxygen concentration every 4 hours to more frequently if indicated	
16. Monitor cardiovascular function. Assess for depression.	16.
a. Monitor pulse rate and arterial blood pressure, intra-arterial pressure monitoring may be carried out.	a. Arterial catheterization for intra-arterial pressure monitoring also provides access for ABG samples.
b. Use Swan-Ganz catheter to monitor pulmonary capillary wedge pressure mixed venous oxygen, and cardiac output.	b. Intermittent and continuous positive pressure ventilation may increase the pulmonary artery pressures and decrease cardiac output.
17. Monitor for pulmonary injection	17.
a. Aspirate tracheal secretions into a sterile container and send to laboration for culture and sensitivity testing. This is done immediately after endotracheal intubation and in some distances on an every other day basis.	a. This technique allows for the earliest detection of infection or change in infecting organisms in the tracheobronchial tree.
b. Daily Gram's staining of secretions may also be done in some institutions.	b.
c. Monitor for systemic signs and symptoms of pulmonary infection (pulmonary physical examination findings, increased heart rate, increased temperature, increased WBC count).	c.
18. Evaluate need for sedation or muscle relaxants.	18. Sedatives may be prescribed to decrease anxiety, or to relax the patient to prevent "competing" with the ventilator. At times, pharmacologically-induced paralysis may be necessary to permit mechanical ventilation.

Contd...

Nursing action	*Rationale*

Nursing Focus

Never administer paralyzing agents until the patient is intubated and mechanical ventilation sedatives should be prescribed in conjunction with paralyzing agents.

Nursing action	*Rationale*
19. Report intake and output precisely and obtain and accurate daily weight to monitor fluid balance.	19. Positive fluid balance resulting in increase in body weight and interstitial pulmonary oedema is a frequent problem in patient's requiring mechanical ventilation, prevention requires early recognition of fluid accumulation. An average adult who is dependent on parenteral nutrition can be expected to lose 0.25 kg (½ lb)/ day; therefore, constant body weight indicates positive fluid balance.
20. Monitor nutritional status.	20. Patients on mechanical ventilation require inflation of artificial airway cuffs at all times. Patients with tracheostomy tubes may eat, if capable, or may require enteral feeding tubes or parenteral nourishment. Patients with endotracheal tubes are to be NPO (the tube splints the epiglottis open) and must be entirely tube fed or parenterally nourished.
21. Monitor GI function.	21. Mechanically ventilated patients are at risk for development of stress ulcers.
a. Test all stools and gastric drainage for occult blood.	a. Stress may cause some patient's requiring mechanical ventilation to develop GI bleeding.
b. Measure abdominal girth daily.	b. Abdominal distention occurs frequently with respiratory failure and further hinders respiration by elevation of the diaphragm. Measurement of abdominal girth provides objective assessment of the degree of distention.
22. Provide for care and communication needs of patient with an artificial airway.	
23. Provide psychological support a. Assist with communication b. Orient to environment and function of mechanical ventilator. c. Ensure that the patient has adequate rest and sleep.	23. Mechanical ventilation may result in sleep deprivation and loss of touch with surroundings and reality.

Contd...

Nursing action	*Rationale*
Follow-up Phase	
1. Maintain a flowsheet to record ventilation patterns, ABGs, venous chemical determinations, haemoglobin and haematocrit, status of fluid balance, weight, and assessment of the patient's condition. Notify appropriate personnel of changes in the patient's condition.	1. Establishes means of assessing effectiveness and progress of treatment.
2. Change ventilator circuitry 24 hours, assess ventilator's function every 4 hours or more frequently if problem occurs.	2. Prevents contamination of lower airways.

PROCEDURE 6.23: ****WEANING THE PATIENT FROM MECHANICAL VENTILATION*

Equipment: Varies according to technique used
Briggs T-piece
IMV or SIMV (set up in addition to ventilator or incorporated in ventilator and circuitry)
Pressure support

STEPS OF PROCEDURE

Nursing action	*Rationale*
Preparatory Phase	
1. For weaning to be successful, the patient must be physiologically capable of maintaining spontaneous respirations. Assessments must ensure that a. The underlying disease process is significantly reversed, as evidenced by pulmonary examination, ABGs, chest X-ray b. The patient can mechanically perform ventilation, should be able to generate a negative inspiratory force (NIF) – 20 cm H_2O1 have a vital capacity (VC) 10 to 15 ml/kg, have a resting minute ventilation (Ve) 10 l/min, and be able to double this, have a spontaneous respiratory fate of 25 breaths per minute, without significant tachycardia, not be hypotensive, have optimal haemoglobin for condition which have adequate nutritional status.	1. Provides baseline, ensure that patient is capable of having adequate neuromuscular control to provide adequate ventilation.
2. Assess for other factors, that cause respiratory insufficiency. a. Acid-base abnormality b. Nutritional depletion	2. Weaning is difficult when these conditions are present.

Contd...

Nursing action	*Rationale*
c. Electrolyte abnormality d. Fever e. Abnormal fluid balance f. Hyperglycaemia g. Infection h. Pain i. Sleep deprivation j. Decreased level of consciousness.	
3. Assess psychological readness weaning.	3. Patient must be physically and psychologically ready for weaning.

Performance Phase

Nursing action	*Rationale*
1. Ensure psychological preparation. Explain procedure and that weaning is not always successful on the initial attempt.	1. Explaining procedure to patient will decrease patient anxiety and promote cooperation. The patient should not be discouraged if weaning is unsuccessful on the first attempt.
2. Prepare appropriate equipment.	
3. Position the patient in sitting or semi-Fowler's position.	3. Increase lung compliance, decreases work of breathing.
4. Pick optimal time of day, preferably early morning.	4. The patient should be rested
5. Perform bronchial hygiene necessary to ensure that the patient is in best condition (postural drainage, suctioning) before weaning attempt.	5. The patient should be in best pulmonary condition for weaning to be successful.

T-piece Weaning

This system provides oxygen enrichment and humidity to a patient with an endotracheal or tracheostomy tube while allowing completely spontaneous respirations.

Nursing action	*Rationale*
1. Discontinue mechanical ventilation and apply T-piece adapter.	1. Stay with the patient during weaning time to decrease patient anxiety and monitor for tolerance of procedure.
2. Monitor the patient for factors indicating need for reinstitution of mechanical ventilation. a. Blood pressure increase of decrease greater than 20 mm Hg systolic or 10 mm Hg diastolic. b. Heart rate increase of 20 beats/min or greater than 110. c. Respiratory rate increase greater than 10 breaths/mine of rate greater than 30. d. Tidal volume less than 250 to 300 ml (in adults). e. Appearance of new cardiac ectopy or increase in base-line ectopy.	2. Indicates intolerance of weaning procedure

Contd...

Nursing action	*Rationale*
f. PaO_2 less than 60, $PaCO_2$ greater than 55, or pH less than 7.35 (may accept lower PaO_2 and pH 1 and higher $PaCO_2$ in patients with (OPD).	
3. Increase time of ventilator with each weaning attempt as the patient's condition indicates. Evaluate for toleration before moving to the next increment.	3. The patient will progress as he or she becomes mentally and physically, able to perform adequate spontaneous ventilation.
4. Institute other techniques, helpful in encouraging weaning. a. Mental stimulation b. Biofeedback c. Participation in care d. Provision of rewards e. Contact with successfully weaned patients	4. Provides motivation and positive feedback.
5. When patient tolerates 40 to 60 minutes of continuous weaning, weaning increments can increase rapidly	
6. When the patient can maintain spontaneous ventilation throughout day, begin night weaning.	

CPAP Weaning

Nursing action	*Rationale*
1. The principles and techniques CPAP weaning are the same as for T-piece weaning.	1. This weaning technique preferred for patient prone to atelectasis, when placed on a T-piece.
2. The patient breathes with CPAP at low level (2.5 to 5 cm H_2O_2) rather than with the T-piece for periods that increase in length.	

IMV or SIMV Weaning (Synchronised Intermittent Mandatory Ventilation)

Nursing action	*Rationale*
1. Set ventilator to IMV or SIMV mode.	
2. Set rate interval	2. This determines the time interval between machine-delivered breaths during which the patient will breathe on own.
3. If the patient is on continuous, flow IMV circuitry, observe reservoir bag to be sure that it remains mostly inflated during all phases of ventilation.	3. The gas flows rate into the the bag must be adequate to prevent the bag from collapsing during inspiration. Flow rates of 6 to 10 L/min are usually adequate.
4. If gas for the patient's spontaneous breath is delivered via a demand valve regulator, ensure that machine sensitivity is at maximum setting.	4. Aids in decreasing work of breathing necessary to open demand valve.

Contd...

Nursing action	*Rationale*
5. Evaluate for tolerance of procedure. Monitor for factors indicating need for increase or decrease of mandatory respiratory rate (See step 3 of T-piece adaptor section above). In rapid weaning, changes may be made approximately every 20 to 30 minutes.	5. If the patient does not tolerate the procedure, the $PaCO_2$ will rise and pH will fall.
6. If $PaCO_2$ and pH levels remain stable, then continue to decrease mandatory rate as patient tolerates.	6. May be done as frequently as every 20 to 30 minutes with ABG monitoring, pulse oximetry documentation of successful weaning.

Pressure Support

1. May be beneficial adjunct to IMV or SIMV weaning
2. The amount of pressure support (cm H_2O) provided to the airway is progressively decreased overtime, allowing the patient to increase role in supporting own spontaneous ventilation.

Follow-up Phase

Nursing action	*Rationale*
1. Record at each weaning interval heart rate, blood pressure, respiratory rate, FiO_2, ABG, pulse oximetry value, respiratory and ventilator rate (if IMV or SIMV), or length of time off ventilator if T-piece weaning.	1. Provides record of procedure and assessment of progress.

Note: It is not within the scope of this manual to establish criteria for the use of one weaning modality as opposed to another

PROCEDURE 6.24: *EXTUBATION

Equipment: Tonsil suction (surgical suction, instrument)
10 ml syringe
Resuscitation bag and mask with oxygen flow
Face mask connected to large bore tubing, humidifier, and oxygen source.
Suction catheter.
Suction source
Gloves, goggles, or other eye protection devices.

STEPS OF PROCEDURE

Nursing action	*Rationale*
Preparatory Phase	
1. Monitor heart rate, lung expansion, and breath sounds before extubation, Record VI, VC, NIF.	1. VI, VC and NIF are measured to assess respiratory muscle functions and adequacy of ventilation.
2. Assess the patient for other signs of adequate muscle power.	2. Adequate muscle strength is necessary to ensure maintenance of a patient airway.
a. Instruct the patient to tightly squeeze the index and middle fingers of your hand. Resistance to removel of your fingers from the patient's grasp must be demonstrated.	
b. Ask the patient to lift head from the pillow and hold for 2 to 3 seconds.	

> *Nursing Focus*
>
> Keep in mind that patient's underlying problems must be improved or resolved before extubation is considered. Patient should also be free from infection and malnutrition.

Nursing action	*Rationale*
Performance Phase	
1. Obtain orders for extubation and postextubation oxygen therapy.	1. Do not attempt extubation until postextubation oxygen therapy is available and functioning at the bedsides.
2. Explain the procedure to the patient. a. Artificial airway will be removed. b. Suctioning will occur before extubation. c. Deep breath should be taken on command. d. Instruction will be given to cough after extubation.	2. Increases patient cooperation.
3. Prepare necessary equipment. Have ready for use tonsil suction, suction catheter, 10 ml syringe, bag mask unit and oxygen via face mask.	
4. Place patient in sitting or semi-Flowler's position (unless contraindicated).	4. Increased lung compliance and decreased work of breathing facilitates coughing.
5. Put on goggles.	5. Spraying of airway secretions may occur.
6. Suction endotracheal tube.	
7. Suction oropharyngeal airway above the endotracheal cuff as thoroughly as possible.	7. Secretions not cleared from above the cuff will be aspirated when the cuff is deflated.
8. Put on gloves, loosen type or endotracheal tube-securing device.	
9. Extubate the patient	9.
a. Ask the patient to take as deep a breath as possible (if the patient is not following commands, give a deep breath with the resuscitation bag).	a. At peak inspiration, the traches and vocal cords will dilate, allowing a less traumatic tube removal.
b. At peak inspiration, deflate the cuff completely and pull the tube out in the direction of the curve (out and downward).	
10. Once the tube is fully removed ask the patient to cough or exhale forcefully to remove secretions. Then suction the back of	10. Frequently, old blood is seen in the secretions of newly extubated patients. Monitor for the appearance of bright

Contd...

Nursing action	Rationale
the patient's airway with the tonsil suction.	red blood due to trauma occurring during extubation.
11. Evaluate immediately for any signs of airway obstruction, stridor, or difficult breathing. If the patient develops any of the above problems, attempt to ventilate the patient with the resuscitation bag and mask and prepare for reintubation. (Nebulized treatments may be ordered to avoid having to reintubate patient).	11. Immediate complication: a. Laryngospasm may develop, causing obstruction of the airway. b. Oedema may develop at the cuff site. Signs of narrowing airway lumen are high-pitched crowing sounds, decreased air movement and respiratory distress.
Follow-up Phase	
1. Note patient tolerance of procedure, upper and lower airway sounds postextubation, description of secretions.	1. Establishes a baseline to a assess improvement/development of complications.
2. Observe patient closely postextubation for any signs and symptoms of airway obstruction or respiratory insufficiency.	2. Tracheal or laryngeal oedema develop postextubation (a possibility for up to 24 hours). Signs and symptoms include high pitched, crowing upper airway sounds and respiratory distress.
3. Observe character of voice.	3. Hoarseness is a common postextubation complaint. Observe for worsening hoarseness or vocal cord paralysis.

Evaluation

A. Respirations 24 shallow, lungs clear. ABGs within normal limits.
B. Blood pressure, CVP, and pulse stable.
C. Coughing and turning independently; reports reliefs of pain.
D. Performing active range of motion of affected arm and shoulder.

PROCEDURE 6.25: **ASSISTING THE PATIENT USING AN INCENTIVE SPIROMETER*

Equipment: According to the type of device used

STEPS OF PROCEDURE

Nursing action	Rationale
Preparatory Phase	
1. Measure the patient's normal VI and auscultate the chest.	1. The patient's baseline is established.
Performance Phase	
1. Explain the procedure and its purpose to the patient.	1. Optimal results are achieved when the patient is given pretreatment instruction, preoperative instruction is also beneficial for the surgical patient.
2. Place the patient in a comfortable sitting or semi-Fower's position.	2. Diaphragmatic excursion is greater in this position; however, if the patient is medically unable to be in this position, the exercise may be done in any position.
3. For the postoperative patient, try as much as possible to avoid discomfort with the treatment administration. Try to Co-ordinate treatment with administration of pain relief medications. Instruct and assist the patient with splinting of incision.	3. More likely to have best results is in using incentive spirometry when patient suffers from as little pain as possible.
4. Set the incentive spirometer VI indicator at the desired goal the patient is to reach or exceed (500 ml, is often used to start). The V1 is set according to the manufacturer's instructions.	4. The initial V1 may be prescribed, but the purpose of the device is to establish a baseline, V1 and provide insentive to achieve greater volumes progressively.

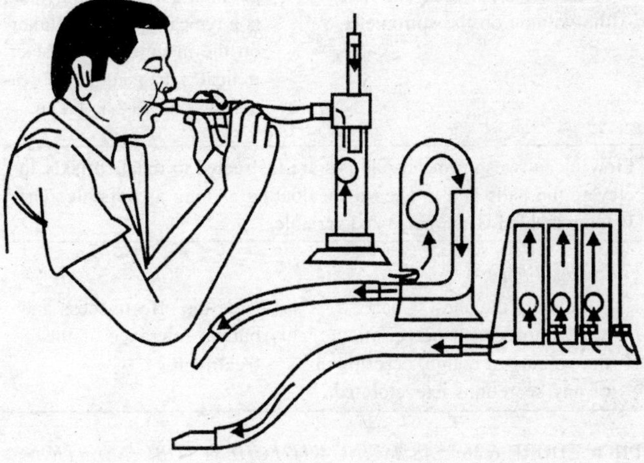

Fig. 6.14: Flow incentive spirometer. Patients are instructed toinhale briskly to elevate the balls and to keep them floating as long as possible. The volume inhaled is estimated and variable

Nursing action	Rationale
5. Demonstrate the technique to the patient.	
6. Instruct the patient to exhale fully.	

Contd...

Nursing action	*Rationale*
7. Tell the patient to take in a slow, easy deep breath from the mouthpiece.	7. Nose clips are sometimes used if the patient has difficulty in breathing only through mouth. This will ensure full credit for each breath measured.
8. When the desired goal is reached (lungs fully inflated), ask the patient to continue the inspiratory effort for 3 seconds, even though the patient may not actually be drawing in more air.	8. Sustaining the inspiratory effort helps to open closed alveol.
9. Instruct the patient to remove the mouthpiece, relax and passively exhale, patient should take several normal breaths before attempting another one with the incentive spirometer.	9. Usually one incentive breath per minute minimizes patient fatigue. No more that four to five manoeuvres should be performed per minute to minimize hypocarbia.
10. Continue to monitor the patient's spirometer breaths, periodically increasing the tidal volume as the patient tolerates.	10.
11. At the conclusion of the treatment, encourage the patient to cough after a deep breath.	11. The deep lung inflation may loosen secretions and enable the patient to expectorate them.
12. Instruct the patient to take 10 sustained maximal inspiratory manoeuvres per hour and note the volume on the spirometer.	12. A total of 10 sustained maximal inspiratory manoeuvres per hour during waking hours is a typical order. A counter on the incentive spirometer indicates the number of breaths the patient has taken.

Flow incentive spirometer patients are instructed to inhale briskly to elevate the balls and to keep them floating as long as possible. The volume inhaled is estimated and variable.

Follow-up Phase

1. Auscultate the chest. Chart any improvement or variation, the volume of cough, description of any secretions expectorated.	1. Note the effectiveness and patient tolerance of the treatment.

PROCEDURE 6.26: **ASSISTING WITH CHEST TUBE INSERTION*

Equipment:

The thoracostomy tray	Suture material
Syringes	Local anaesthetic
Needles/trocar	Chest tube (appropriate size), connector
Basins skin germicide	Chest drainage system-connecting tubes and tubing.
Sponges	Collection bottles or commercial system, vacuum pump (if required)
Scalps/sterile drape/ gloves.	
Two large clamps.	

Contd...

STEPS OF PROCEDURE

Nursing action	*Rationale*
Preparatory Phase	
1. Assess patient for pneumothorax, haemothorax, presence of a respiratory distress.	1.
2. Obtain a chest X-ray. Other means of localization of pleural fluid include ultrasound and/or fluoroscope localization.	2. To evaluate extent of lung collapse or amount of bleeding in pleural space.
3. Assemble drainage system.	3.
4. Reassure the patient and explain the steps of the procedure. Tell the patient to expect a needle prick and a sensation of slight pressure during infiltration anaesthesia.	4. The patient can cope by remaining immobile and doing relaxed breathing during tube insertion.
5. Position the patient as for an intercostal nerve block, or according to physician preference.	5. The tube insertion site depends on the substance to be drained, the patient's mobility, and the presence/absence of coexisting conditions.
Performance Phase	
Needle or Intracath Technique.	
1. The skin is prepared and anaesthetized using local anaesthetic with a short 25 gauge needle. A larger needle is used to infiltrate the subcutaneous tissue, intercostal muscles, and parietal pleura.	1. The area is anaesthetized to make tube insertion and manipulation relatively painless.
2. An exploratory needle is inserted.	2. To puncture the pleura and determine the presence of air/blood in the pleural cavity.
3. The intracath catheter is inserted through the needle into the pleural space. The needle is removed, and the catheter is pushed several centimeters into the pleural space.	3.
4. The catheter is taped to the skin.	4. To prevent it from being pushed out of the chest during patient movement or lung expansion.
5. The catheter is attached to a connector/tubing and attached to a drainage system (under water-seal or commercial system).	5.

TROCAR TECHNIQUE FOR CHEST TUBE INSERTION

A trocar catheter is used for the insertion of a large-bore tube for removal of a modest to large amount of air leak or for the evacuation of serious effusion.

1. A small incision is made over the prepared, anaesthetized site. Blunt dissection (with a	1. To admit the diameter of the chest tube.

Contd...

Nursing action	Rationale
haemostat) through the muscle planes in the interspace to the parietal pleura is performed.	
2. The trocar is directed into the pleural space, the cannula is removed, and a chest tube is inserted into the pleural space and connected to a drainage system.	2. There is a trocar catheter available equipped with an indwelling pointed rod for ease of insertion.

HAEMOSTAT TECHNIQUE USING A LARGE BORE CHEST TUBE

A large bore chest tube is used to drain blood or thick effusions from the pleural space

Nursing action	Rationale
1. After skin preparation and anaesthetic infiltration, an incision is made through the skin and subcutaneous tissue.	1. The skin incision is usually made one interspace below proposed site of penetration of the intercostal muscles and pleura.
2. A curved haemostat is inserted into the pleural cavity and the tissue is spread with the clamp.	2. To make a tissue tract for the chest tube.
3. The tract is explored with an examining finger.	3. Digital examination helps confirm the presence of the track and penetration of the pleural cavity.
4. The tube is held by the haemostat and directed through the opening up over the ribs and into the pleural cavity.	4.
5. The clamp is withdrawn and the chest tube is connected to a chest drainage system.	5. The chest tube has multiple openings at the proximal and for drainage of air/blood.
6. The tube is sutured in place and covered with a sterile dressing.	6.

Chest tube (tube thoracostomy) inserted via haemostat technique.

Follow-up Phase

Nursing action	Rationale
1. Observe the drainage system for blood/air. Observe for fluctuation in the tube on respiration.	1. If a haemothorax is draining through a thoracostomy tube into a bottle containing sterile normal saline, the blood is available for autotransfusion.
2. Secure a follow-up chest X-ray.	2. To confirm correct chest tube placement and re-expansion, of the lung.
3. Assess for bleeding, infection, leakage of air and fluid around the tube.	3.

PROCEDURE 6.27: **MANAGING THE PATIENT WITH WATER-SEAL CHEST DRAINAGE*

Equipment: Closed chest drainage system
Holder for drainage system (if needed)
Vacuum motor
Sterile connector for emergency use

STEPS OF PROCEDURE

Nursing action	Rationale
Performance Phase	
1. Attach the drainage tube from the pleural space (the patient) to the tubing that leads to a long tube with end submerged in sterile normal saline.	1. Water-seal drainage provides for the escape of air and fluid into a drainage bottle. The water acts as a seal and keeps the air from being drawn back into the pleural space.
2. Check the tube connections periodically. Tape if necessary.	2. Tube connections are checked to ensure tight fit and patency of the tubes.
a. The tube should be approximately 2.5 cm (1 inch) below the water level.	a. If the tube is submerged too deep below the water level, a higher intrapleural pressure is required to expel air.
b. The short tube is left open to the atmosphere.	b. Venting the short glass tube lets air escape from the bottle.
3. Mark the original, fluid level with tape on the outside of the drainage bottle. Mark hourly/daily increments (date and time) at the drainage level.	3. The marking will show the amount of fluid loss and how fast fluid is collecting in the drainage bottle. It serves as a basis for blood replacement, if the fluid is blood. Grossly bloody drainage will appear in the bottle in the immediate postoperative period and, if excessive, may necessitate reoperation. Drainage usually declines progressively after the first 24 hours.
4. Make sure that the tubing does not loop or interfere with the movements of the patient.	4. Fluid collecting in the dependent segment of the tubing will decrease the negative pressure applied to the catheter, kinking looping or pressure on the drainage tubing can produce back pressure, thus, possibly forcing drainage back into the pleural space or impeding drainage from the pleural space.
5. Encourage the patient to assume a position of comfort. Encourage good body alignment. When the patient is in a lateral position, place a rolled towel under the tubing to protect it from the weight of the patient's body. Encourage the patient to change position frequently.	5. The patient's position should be changed frequently to promote drainage and body kept in good alignment to prevent postural deformity and contractures. Proper positioning helps, breathing and promotes better air exchange. Pain medication may be indicated to enhance comfort and deep breathing.
6. Put the arm and shoulder of the affected side through range of	6. Exercise helps to avoid ankylosis of the shoulder

Contd...

Nursing action	*Rationale*
motion exercises several times daily. Some pain medication may be necessary.	and assist in lessening post-operative pain and discomfort.
7. "Milk" the tubing in the direction tion of the drainage bottle as often as ordered (Many institutions do not advocate milking because of the increased intrapleural pressure it causes.	7. "Milking" the tubing prevents it from becoming plugged with clots of fibrin. Constant attention to maintaining the patency of the tube will facilitate prompt expansion of the lung and minimize complications.
8. Make sure there is fluctuation ("tidaling") of the fluid level in the long glass tube.	8. Fluctuation of the water level in the tube shows that there is effective communication between the pleural space and the drainage bottle, provides a valuable indication of the patency of the drainage system, and is a gauze of intrapleural pressure.
9. Fluctuation of fluid in the tubing will stop when: a. The lung has re-expanded b. The tubing is obstructed by blood clots or fibrin c. A dependent loop develops (see step 4) d. Suction motor or wall suction is not operating properly.	9.
10. Watch for leaks of air in the drainage system as indicated by constant bubbling in the water seal bottle.	10. Leaking and trapping of air in the pleural space can result in tension pneumothorax.
a. Report excessive bubbling in the water-seal change immediately.	a.
b. "Milking" of chest tubes in patients with air leaks should be done only if requested by surgeon.	b.
11. Observe and report immediately signs of rapid, shallow breathing, cyanosis, pressure in the chest, subcutaneous emphysema, or symptoms of haemorrhage.	11. Many clinical conditions may cause these signs and symptoms, including tension pneumothorax, mediastinal shift, haemorrhage, severe incisional pain, pulmonary embolus, and cardiac tamponade. Surgical intervention may be necessary.
12. Encourage the patient to breathe deeply and cough at frequent intervals. If there are signs of incisional pain, adequate pain medication is indicated.	12. Deep breathing and coughing help to raise the intrapleural pressure, which allows emptying of any accumulation in the pleural space and removes secretions from the tracheobronchial tree so that the lung expands.
13. If the patient had to be transported to another area, place the drainage bottle below the chest (as close to the floor as possible).	13. The drainage apparatus, must be kept at a level lower than the patient's chest to prevent backflow of fluid into the pleural space.

Contd...

Nursing action	*Rationale*
14. If the tube becomes disconnected, cut off the contaminated tips of the chest tube and tubing. Insert a sterile connector in the chest tube and tubing, and reattach to the drainage system. Otherwise, do not clamp the chest tube during transport.	14.
15. When assisting with removal of the tube. a. Administer pain medication 30 minutes before removal of chest tube. b. Instruct the patient to perform a gently Valsalva manoeuvre or to breathe quietly. c. The chest tube is clamped and removed. d. Simultaneously, a small bandage is applied and made airtight with petroleum gauze covered by a 4 × 4. Inch gauze and throughly covered and sealed with tape.	15. The chest tube is removed as directed when the lung is re-expanded (usually 24 hours to several days). During the tube removal, avoid a large sudden inspiratory effort, which may produce a pneumothorax.
Follow-up Phase	
1. Monitor patient's pulmonary status for signs and symptoms of decompensation.	1. Patient could have reformation of pneumothorax upon removal.

PROCEDURE 6.28: *TUBERCULIN SKIN TEST

Equipment: Purified protein derivative (PPD) tuberculin antigen, intermediate strength
Tuberculin syringe
Short 1.25 cm (½ inch) 26-94 27-gauze steal needle
Alcohol sponge.

STEPS OF PROCEDURE

Nursing action	*Rationale*
Preparatory Phase	
1. Determine if the patient has ever BCG vaccine, recent viral disease, immunosuppression by disease, drugs, or steroids.	1. Any of these may cause had false readings.
Performance Phase	
1. Draw up PPD-tuberculin into tuberculin syringe.	1. Follow the manufacturer's directions each 0.1-ml oz should contain 5 tuberculin units (TU of PD-tuberculin). Use the antigen immediately to avoid absorption on to the plastic/glass syringe.
2. Cleanse the skin of the inner aspect of forearm with alcohol. Allow to dry.	2.
3. Stretch the skin taut.	3.
4. Hold the tuberculin syringe close to the skin so the hub of	4. This reduces the needle angle at the skin suites and

Contd...

Nursing action	*Rationale*
the needle touches it as the needle is introduced, bevel up.	facilitates the injection of tuberculin just between the surface of the skin.
5. Inject the tuberculin into the superficial layer of the skin to form a wheal 6 to 10 mm in diameter.	5. If no wheal appears (because the injection was made too deep) inject again at another site. East 5 cm (2 inches) away.
Follow-up Phase	
To read the test	
1. Read the test within 48 to 72 hours when the induration in most evident.	1. Tuberculin skin tests are tests of delayed hypersensitivity.
2. Have a good light available. Flex the forearm slightly at the elbow.	2.
3. Inspect for the presence of induration inspect from a side view against the light inspect by direct light.	3. Induration refers to hardening or thickening of tissues.
4. Palpate lightly rub the fingure across the injection site from the area of normal skin to the area of induration outline the diameter of induration.	4. Erythema (redness) without induration is generally considered to be of no significance.
5. Measure the maximum transverse diameter of induration (not erythema) in millimeters with a flexible ruler.	5. The extent of induration is measured in two diameters and recorded.
Interpretation	
1. Induration of 5 mm or more in diameter.	1. Considered positive in a. Persons with known HIV or unknown HIV but with risk factors for HIV. b. Persons who have had recent contact with active tuberculosis. c. Persons who have fibrotic changes or chest X-ray, consistent with healed TB.
2. Induration of 10 mm or more in diameter.	2. Considered positive in all persons who do not meet above criteria but who have other risk factors in tuberculosis, such as homelessness, alcoholism malnutrition, and health-care work.
3. Induration of 15 mm or more in diameter.	3. Considered positive in persons who do not meet the above criteria.

PROCEDURE 6.29: *ASSISTING WITH AN INTERCOSTAL NERVE BLOCK.

Equipment: Syringes, 10-ml Luer-Lok
Needles No. 22 to 30 gauge
Anaesthetic solution (lidocaine, bupivacaine, procaine)
Skin germicide, sterile gloves.

STEPS OF PROCEDURE

Nursing Action	*Rationale*
Preparatory Phase	
1. Inform the patient that he or she will experience the prick of the needle and a slight sensation of pressure.	1.
2. Position the patient as directed. a. Have the patient sit up, bend forward and hug a pillow. or b. Place the patient prone with pillow under chest. or c. Have the patient on unaffected side with upper arm hanging over the side of the table.	2. a. This posture moves the scapulae forward and out of the way. b. The prone position helps immobilize the patient. c. This pulls the scapula out of the way.
3. Ask the patient to identify the site of pain.	3. To determine which intercostal nerves are to be injected.
Performance Phase (by the physician)	
1. After the skin is prepared, the lower margin of the rib is palpated and a small skin wheal is raised, using a 25 to 30 gauge needle.	1. This is infiltration anaesthesia.
2. Usually nerve blocks are done at the posterior angle of the ribs between the posterior axillary line and the spine.	2. The posterior angle is the most prominent and accessible, and an injection at this area produces a block of the entire distal nerve.
3. A fine needle is advanced through the wheal and directed downward so it slips under the edge of the rib into the upper portion of the interspace.	3.
4. The syringe (needle in place) is aspirated.	4. To ensure that the needle has not punctured the lung or that an intercostal vessel has been entered.
5. The local anaesthetic (usually 3-5 ml) is injected into the area.	5. Usually the local anaesthetic is injected above and below the painful rib to obtain complete relief of pain, as the sensory fields or intercostal nerves overlap.
Follow-up Phase	
1. Assess for relief of pain and less painful coughing.	1. This is the expected outcome.
2. Obtain a chest X-ray.	2. To ensure that a pneumothorax has not occurred.
3. Complications: a. Intravascular injection. b. Puncture of the lung with pneumothorax. c. Hypotension.	

Alimentary Nursing or Gastrointestinal Nursing

GASTROINTESTINAL NURSING

The gastrointestinal (GI) system, also termed as the digestive system and alimentary canal, consists of the GI tract and its accessory organs. The GI tract or alimentary canal is a hollow muscular tube that extends from mouth to the anus. Its principal function is to provide the body with fluid, nutrients, and electrolyte. This is accomplished through the processes of ingestion (taking food), digestion (breakdown of food) and absorption (transfer of food products into circulation). Another main function of the GI system is the storage and final excretion of the solid waste products of digestion, i.e. elimination.

The GI system consists of the GI tract, and its associated organs and glands, which includes mouth, oesophagus, stomach, small intestine, large intestine, rectum, and anus. The associated organs are the liver, pancreas, and gallbladder. Proper functioning of the GI system is essential to the maintenance of proper nutrition and health. Psychological or emotional factors such as stress and anxiety influence GI functioning in many persons. Stress may be manifested as anorexia, epigastric and abdominal pain or diarrhoea. However, GI problems should never be solely attributed to psychological factors. Organic and psychologically-based problem can exist independently or concurrently. Physical factors such as dietary intake, ingestion of alcohol, and cafeine–containing products, cigarette smoking, and fatigue may affect GI function. Some organic diseases of the GI system such as peptic ulcer, ulcerative colitis may be aggravated by stress. These both physical and emotional factors affect the GI functions. So it is very essential for the nurses to understand the disorders of GI system, because they will come across such clients, and to provide proper nursing services.

Assessment of GI System

Assessment of GI system involves a detailed health history as well as a comprehensive physical examination of the oral cavity, abdomen, rectum and anus. And a review of the client's demographic data.

Demographic Data

A review of the patient's demographic data such as age, sex, culture, religion and occupation is helpful when assessing GI system, because many GI disorders are associated with it. For example, many GI cancers occur more frequently in the elderly and in males, whereas others are more common in females. Sexual abuse may play role in GI problems in some women. Reproductive cycling in females contribute to other GI manifestations. Duodenal ulcers develop in younger adults, whereas gastric ulcers are more common in middle-aged and older adults.

Past Health History

The nurse collects data about previous hospitalizations, major illness, surgery, use of medications and allergies as a part of past health history.

- Informations should be gathered from the patients about the history or existence of the following diseases or problems related to GI functioning: abdominal pain, gastritis, nausea, and vomiting, diarrhoea, and constipation, hepatitis, colitis, peptic ulcer, abdominal distension, jaundice, anaemia, haital hernia, gallbladder disease, dysphagia, heartburn, dyspepsia, changes in appetite, haematemesis, food intolerance, indigestion, excessive gas, bloating, melena, haemorrhoids, hernia, or rectal bleeding. In addition, nurse should ask whether the client currently has or previously had a change in bowel habits, GI bleeding, jaundice, ulcers, colitis, or unexplained weight loss or gain.
- The health history should include an assessment of the patient's past and current use of medications, particularly in relation to liver problems. Because many chemicals and drugs are potentially haepatotoxic (E.g. alcohol, arsenic, carbon tetrachloride, gold compounds, mercury, phosphorous, anabolic steroids, halothane, isoniazed, propylthiouracil, sulfonamides, thiazide diurectics, metho-trextate, acetominephen). The nurse should ask the patient if laxatives or antacids are taken, including the kind and frequency. The use of prescription or over the counter appetite suppressant drug should be noted including name, duration, frequency and also any allergies to medication should be noted.
- Information should be obtained about the hospitalization for any problems related to the GI system, including abdominal surgery, rectal surgery, reasons for surgery, postoperative course and possible blood transfusion, etc.
- The nurse should also have the knowledge about the patient's health practices relted to GI system, such as

maintenance of normal body weight, attention to proper dental care, maintenance of adequate nutrition and effective elimination habits and patient should be asked about exposure to hepatotoxic chemicals and exposure to hepatitis or parasitic infection. And also patient should be assessed in relation to certain habits like consumption of alcohol and cigarette smoking, which may delay healing of ulcers and lead to liver problems.

- Thorough *nutritional* assessment is essential. The nurse should ask open-ended questions that will allow the patients to express beliefs and feelings about the diet. The nurse may need to ask the patient to do a 24-hours dietary recall to analyse the adequacy of diet and *find out whether patient is taking adequate* diet or not.

The patient should be questioned about any changes in appetite food tolerance and weight. Anorexia and weight loss may indicate carcinoma. The nurse should ask the patient about allergies to any food and determine what GI symptoms show allergic response cause.

- A detailed account of the patient's bowel *elimination* pattern should be elicited. The frequency, time of the day, and usual consistency of stool should be noted. The use of laxatives and enema, including type, frequency, and results should be documented. Any recent changes in bowel pattern should be investigated.
- *Activity and Exercise* may affect GI motility. Immobility is risk for constipation. So the patient's ambulatory status may be assessed to determine if the patient is capable of securing and preparing food. any limitation in it should be noted.
- The patient should be asked if GI symptoms affect *sleep or rest*. For example, a patient with a hiatal hernia may be awakened because of burning pain, sleep may be improved by elevating the head of the bed for such patients. Hunger can prevent sleep and should be relieved by a light, easily digested snack unless contraindicated. A patient often has bed time ritual that involves the use of a particular food or beverages, e.g. warm milk, herbal tea, etc. should be noted.
- *Cognitive-perceptual pattern*. i.e. decrease in sensory adequacy can result in problems related to the acquisition, preparation and ingestion of food. For example changes in taste or smell can affect appetite and eating pleasure. The nurse should assess the patient in this pattern to judge the effect of deficiencies on adequate nutritional intake and pain in another area that requires careful assessment related to its effect on GI system and nutrition. The possible effects of pain medication related to constitution, sedation and appetite suppressive should be assessed.
- Self-perception-Self-concept pattern should be assessed because many GI and nutritional problems can have a serious effect on the patient's self-perception, for example: (1) Overweight and underweight persons often have problems related to self-esteem and body image. (2) The altered physical changes often associated with liver disease can be problematic for the patient, e.g., jaundice, ascitis.
- It is important that the nurse should be aware of the role-relationship pattern of patient. For example, problem related to the GI system such as: cirrhosis, alcoholism, hepatitis, ostomies, obesity, and carcinoma can have a major impact on the patient's ability to maintain usual roles and relationships.
- It is also important that nurse should ask sensitive questions to determine sexuality-reproductive pattern of the patient, changes related to sexuality and reproductive status on result from problems of the GI system. For example, obesity, jaundice, anorexia, could decrease the acceptance of a potential sexual partner. Chronic alcoholism decreases meaningful sexual relationship. The presence of an ostomy could affect the patient's confidence related to sexual activity. Anorexia can affect the reproductive status of a female patient. Alcoholism can affect the reproductive status of both men and women.
- The nurse should try to determine the coping stress tolerance pattern of the patient, because GI symptoms such as epigastric pain, nausea, and diarrhoea develop in many individuals in response to stressful or emotional situations. Some organic GI problems such as peptic ulcers are aggravated by stress. The nurse should also assess the value-belief pattern of the patients, i.e. the patient's spiritual and cultural belief regarding food and food preparations which helps for prescribing food and medication accordingly.

Physical Examination of GI System

The physical examination of the GI system include examination of the oral cavity, abdomen, anus and rectum.

Oral cavity Assessment of oral cavity involves inspection and palpation. The nurse puts on gloves, faces the client and begins by inspecting the lips. For observation of abnormalities of colour, lesions, nodules and symmetry. The abnormalities of lips include pallor, or cyanosis, cracking ulcer, or fissure using a tonge blade. The nurse should inspect the buccal mucosa and not the colour, any areas of pigmentation or any lesion. In assessing teeth and gums, nurse should look for caries, look teeth, abnormal shape and position of teeth, and swelling, bleeding, discoloration or inflammation of gingivae. Any distinctive breath odour should be noted. The pharynx should be inspected for any abnormalities. Abnormalities of mouth include thrush, leukoplakia, white plaques with red patches, cancer sore, etc.

The nurse should palpate any suspicious area in the mouth such as ulcer, nodules, indurations and areas of tenderness should be palpated. It should be noted that if patient having any dentures or partial appliances should be removed when examining the oral cavity.

Abdomen

To assess the patient's abdomen, have the client lie in a supine position with the arms at the sides. Bending the knees slightly helps to relax the abdomen muscles. Begin in the patient's right lower quadrants and proceed in clockwise manner. When assessing the abdomen, the nurse proceeds the following sequence: inspection, auscultation, percussion and palpation. The sequence may vary according to situations.

- *Inspection*. The nurse should inspect the abdomen for skin changes (colour, texture, scars, striae, dilated veins, rashes and lesions), umbilicus (location and contour) symmetry, contour (flat, rounded, carved, concave, protuberant, distention), observable mass (hernias or other masses) and movement (pulsations and peristalsis).
- *Auscultation* of the abdomen begins by listening with the diaphragm of the stethoscope, which provides information on bowel and vascular sounds. The stethoscope is lightly pressed on the abdominal wall in all four quadrants. Begin in the right lower quadrant at the ilecaecal valve area because bowel sounds are normally present there. Normal bowel sounds occur 5 to 35 times per minute and sound like high-pitched clicks or gurgles. The nurse should listen for bowel sounds for 2 to 5 minutes. Bowel sounds cannot be described as absent until no sound is heard for 5 minutes in each quadrant. The frequency and intensity of the bowel sounds vary depending on the phase of digestion. Loud gurgles indicate hyperperistalsis termed as 'borborygoni (stomach growling). Terms used to describe bowel sounds include, present, absent, increased, decreased, high pitched, tinkling, gurgling, and rushing.
- The nurse uses the bell of the stethoscope to ausculcate vascular sounds. Three abnormal sounds should be listened for: a bruit, a venous hum, or a friction rub. The nurse listens over the aorta, renal arteries, and iliac arteries. A bruit is heard over the aorta which indicates presence of aortic aneurysm. A continuous venous hum heard in preumbilical area indicates engorged liver circulation. Friction rub indicates hepatic tumour or splenic infarction.
- *Percussion* of the abdomen is to determine the size and location of the abdominal organs and to detect fluid, air and masses. The nurse uses percussion in all four quadrants and compare sounds. Normally, percussion sounds over the abdomen are tympanic (high-pitched loud or musical over gas) or dull (thud-like sounds over fluid or solid organs).

To percuss the liver the nurse should start below the umbilicus in the right midclavicular line and percuss lightly upward until dullness is heard, thus determining the lower border of liver dullness. After the lower border of the liver has been determined, the nurse should start the nipple line in the midclavicular line and percuss downward between ribs to the area of dullness indicating the upper border of the liver. The height or vertical space between two areas should be measured to determine the size of the liver. Dull sounds normally occur over the liver and spleen or a bladder filled with urine. Abnormal findings occur because of the presence of ascitis or abnormal masses.

Table 7.1: Location of organs in each abdominal quadrant

• RIGHT UPPER QUADRANT (RUQ). – Liver – Gallbladder – Duodenum – Right kidney – Hepatic flexure of colon	• RIGHT LOWER QUADRANT (RLQ). – Cecuem – Appendix – Right ovary and tube
• LEFT UPPER QUADRANT (LUQ) – Stomach, spleen – Left kidney, pancreas, – Splenic flexure of colon	• LEFT LOWER QUADRANT (LLQ) – Signoid colon – Left ovary and tube

Interpretation of Common Finding of Inspection

- *Scars on strials* may be result of pregnancy, obesity, ascitis, tumours oedema, surgical procedure, or healed burned areas.
- *Engorged veins* may be caused by obstruction of vena cava or portal vein and circulation from abdomen.
- *Skin colour* observe for evidence of jaundice, or inflammation (Redness).
- *Visible peristalsis* may be caused by pyrolic or intestinal obstruction; normally peristalsis not visible except the slow waves in thin persons.
- *Visible Pulsation* normally slight pulsation of aorta is visible to epigastric region.
- *Visible masses and altered contour* observe for hernia, distension of ascitis, and obesity; instructing patient to cough may bring hernia 'bulge or elicit pain or discomfort in the abdomen, marked concavity may be caused by malnutrition.
- *Spider angioma* appear on the upper portion of the body and blanch with pressure: commonly result from liver disease.

Interpretation of Common Findings from Auscultation

- *Absence from Sounds in 5 minutes* may be due to peritonitis, paralytic ileus, pneumonia, and hypokalaemia.
- *Repeated, high-pitched sounds occurring at frequent intervals.* Increased peristalsis heard in gastroenteritis, early pyloric obstruction, early intestinal obstruction, and diarrhoea.
- *Bruit* presence of abnormal sounds (turbulence of blood flow through partially occluded or diseased aorta or renal artery).
- *Hum and friction rub* heard over liver and splenic areas, indicating an increased venous blood flow, possibly related to peritoneal inflammation.

- *Palpation* is of value in determining the outlines of the abdominal organs, determining the presence and characteristics of any abdominal masses, and identifying the presence of direct tenderness, guarding, rebound tenderness and muscular rigidity.

Light palpation is used to detect tenderness or cutaneous hypersensitivity, muscular resistance, masses, and swelling. The nurse uses the pads of the fingertips with the finger together, and press gently, depressing the abdominal wall about 1 cm. All quadrants are palpated using smooth movement.

Deep palpation is used to delineate abdominal organs and masses. The palmar surface of the fingers should be used to press more deeply. Again all quadrants should be palpated. When palpating masses, the nurse should note the location, size, shape and presence of tenderness. The patient's facial expression should be observed during these manoeuvre, because it will give non-verbal cues of discomfort or pain.

An alternate method for deep abdominal palpation is the two-hand method. One hand is placed on the top of the other. The fingers of the top hand apply pressure to the bottom hand. The fingers of the bottom hand feel for organs and masses.

To palpate nurse's left hand is placed behind the patient to support the right eleventh and twelth rib. The patient may relax on nurse's hand. The nurse should press the left hand forward and place the right hand on the patient's right abdomen lateral to the rectus muscle. The finger tips should be below the lower border of liver, dullness and pointed towards the right costal margin. The nurse should gently press in and up. The patient should take deep breath with the abdomen so that liver drops and is in a better position to be palpated. The nurse should try to feel the lower edge as it comes down to the fingertips. The liver edge should be firm, sharp and smooth. Any abnormality should be noted.

To palpate spleen, the nurse moves to the left side of the patient. The nurse places the left hand under the patient and supports and presses the patient's left lower rib cage forward. The right hand is placed below the left costal margin and pressed it in towards the spleen. The nurse should ask the patient to breathe deeply. The tip or edge of an enlarged spleen will be felt by the fingertips. The spleen is normally not palpable.

RECTUM AND ANUS

Examination of the anus and rectum is potentially embarrassing and uncomfortable for the patient. The nurse uses a gentle approach and a matter-of-fact manner. The client's position depends on the circumstances of the examination. A female client may be examined while in the lithotomy position immediately following assessment of the genitalia, in the Sim's position or in a dorsal recumbent position. A male client may be examined in the Sim's position or while standing and leaning across the examination table, a position which facilitates palpation of the prostate gland.

Clients are draped accordingly. For the digital examination of the rectum the gloved lubricated index finger is placed against the anus while the patient strains (Valsalva manoeuvre). Then as the sphincter relaxes, the finger is inserted. The finger is pointed towards the umbilicus. The nurse should try to get the patient to relax. The finger inserted into the rectum as far as possible, and all surfaces are palpated. Nodules, tenderness or any irregularities should be assessed. A sample of stool can be removed with the gloved finger and should be checked for occult blood. Abnormal findings may include pruritus ani, coccygeal or pilonidal sinus, tract openings, fistulas, fissures, external haemorrhoids, rectal prolapse, and internal haemorrhoids, etc.

DIAGNOSTIC STUDIES IN GI SYSTEM

Number of examinations and tests performed for diagnosis of problems of the GI system are both consuming and unpleasant. Several tests are intrusive procedures that are uncomfortable and embarassing for the patient which results in added stress for the patient. It remains the nurse's responsibility to meet the educational and psychological needs of the patient by answering questions concerning the test procedure, rationale for its use and specific test preparation in a caring manner.

Laboratary Tests

Numerous tests may be used as a part of the evaluation of the GI biliary, and exocrine pancreas function. The main blood and urine tests are as follows.

A. Blood tests

- *Stomach gastrin test*: Gastrin is a gastric hormone that is a powerful stimulus for gastric acid secretion. Elevated levels are found in those with pernicious anaemia and Zollinger-Ellison syndrome. The normal gastrin value is less than 200 dg/ml (200 mg/L)
- *Helicobacter pylori* detected in serum is a highly sensitive but less-specific indicator of an active infection. H. pylori infection predisposes to peptic ulcer disease.
- *Total bilirubin test.* Bilirubin is exerted in the obstruction in the biliary tract contribute primarily to a rise in conjugated (direct) values. The normal value 0.1 to 1.0 mg/dl, conjugaged 0.1-0.3 mg/dl, unconjugated 0.1-0.8 mg/dl.
- *Alkaline phosphate.* It is found in many tissues with high concentration in bone, liver and biliary tract epithelium. Obstructive biliary tract disease and carcinoma may cause significant elevations. The normal value is 30-85 1nu/ml.
- *Amylase.* It is secreted normally by the acinar cells of the pancreas. Damage to these cells or obstruction of

the pancreatic duct causes the enzyme to be absorbed into the blood is significant quantities. It is a sensitive yet non-specific test for pancreatic disease. The normal value is 80-150 Somogyl units.

- *Lipase*. It is a pancreatic enzyem normally secreted into the duodenum. It appears in the blood when damage occurs to the acinor cells. It is a specific test for pancreatic disease. The normal value 0-110 units/L.
- *Calcium* levels may be low in cases of severe pancreaticis or steatorrhoea because calcium soaps are formed from the sequestration of calcium by fat necrosis. The normal value is 9.0-11.5 mg/dl.
- *Total protein* of blood includes albumen and globulin. Although primarily a reflection of liver function, serum protein level is also a meausre of nutrition. Malnourished patients have greatly decreased levels of blood protein. The normal protein is 6.8 g/dl (Albumin 3.2-4.5 g/dl, Globulin 2.3-3.4 g/dl).
- *D-xylose absorption test*. D-xylose is a monosaccharide that is easily absorbed by the normal intestine but not metabolized by the body. D-xylose is administered orally and assists in the diagnosis of malabsorption. Normally blood levels of 25-40 mg/dl 2 hr after ingestion.
- *Lactose tolerance test*. An oral dose of lactose is administered. In the absence of intestinal lactase, the lactose is neither broken down nor absorbed and plasma glucose levels do not rise. The test assists in the diagnosis of lactose intolerance. Normally rise in blood glucose level is more than 20 mg/dl.
- *CEA test*. Carcinoembryonic antigen is a protein normally present in fetal gut tissue. It is typically elevated in persons with colorectal tumours. It is useful in determining prognosis and response to therapy. The normal value is less than 5 mg/ml.

B. Urine tests

- *5-Hydroxindoleacetic Acid (5-HIAA)*. Carcinoid tumours are serotin in secreting and are derived from neuroectoderm tissue, e.g. the appendix and intestine. These neurohormones are metabolised to 5-HIAA by the liver and excreted in urine. The normal value is 2-5 mg/2 hr.
- *Urine Bilirubin*. Bilirubin is not normally excreted in the urine. Biliary structure, inflammation, or stones may cause its presence.
- *Urobilinogen*. A sensitive test for hepatic or biliary diseases. Decreased levels are seen in those with biliary obstruction and pancreatic cancer. In 24-hour collection, urobilinogen is 0.2-1.2 units and 0.05-2.5 mg.
- *Urine Amylase*. Normally 10-80 amylase units/hour. A rise in levels usually minimises the rise in serum amylase. The level remains elevated for 7-10 days; however, which allows for retrospective diagnosis.

C. Stool examination

Stool specimens are collected primarily for culture, determination of fat content, and examination for the presence of ova, parasites, and fresh or occult blood. Stools to be analyzed for the presence of bacteria, i.e. Salmonella, Shigella, Staphyloccus ureas. Detection of occult blood in the stool is useful in identifying bleeding in the GI Tractoccult blood may be identified by one of the three tests-guiac test (hemoccult), benzidine, or orthotobrdine (occultest).

The colour of the stool also indicates few cues for the following:

- Brown - Presence of fecal urobilinogen.
- White - Barium.
- Gray, tan (clay) - Lack of bile, biliary obstruction.
- Black - Tarry-Upper GI bleeding.
  - Dry-Rapid peristalsis with bile presence.
- Green - Rapid peristalsis with bile presence.

RADIOLOGICAL STUDIES

i. Upper GI or barium swallow

It is a X-Ray study with fluoroscopy with contrast medium. This is used to diagnose structural abnormalities of the oesophagus, stomach and duodenal bulb. The nurse's responsibility in this procedure includes.

- Explain procedure to patient and that patient will need to drink contrast medium and assume various positions on X-ray table.
- Keep patient NPO (nil per oral) for 8-12 hours before procedure.
- Tell the patient to avoid smoking after midnight, the night before the study.
- After X-ray test, take measures to prevent contrast medium impaction (fluids, laxatives).
- Tell patient that stool may be white upto 72 hours after test.

ii. Small bowel series

In this contrast medium is ingested and flat film taken q 20 min until medium reaches terminal ileum. Here the nurse's responsibilities are as stated in barium swallow.

These procedures are used to identify oesophageal and stomach disorder such as strid varices, polyps, tumours, hiatal hernia and peptic ulcers.

iii. Lower GI or barium enema

It is fluoroscopic X-ray examination of colon, used contrast medium, which is administered rectally (enema). Double contrast or air contrast barium enema is test of choice. Air is infused after barium is evacuated. The nurse's responsibility in barium enema includes:

- Before the procedure, administer laxatives and enema until colon is clear of stool evening before procedure.
- Administer clear liquid diet evening before procedure.
- Keep patient NPO for 8 hours before test.
- Instruct patient about being given barium by enema.
- Explain that cramping and urge to defecate may occur during procedure and that patient may be placed in various positions on tilt table.
- After the procedure give fluids, laxatives or suppositories to assist in expelling barium.
- And observe stool for passage of contrast medium.

This procedure identifies polyps, tumours and other lesion in colon.

iv. Oral cholecytogram (Gallbladder series)

It is X-ray examination visualizes gallbladder (GB) after radio-opaque dye such as iopanoic acid (Telepaque) has been ingested orally. It is used to determine the GB ability to concentrate and store dye and to observe the patency of the biliary duct system. It also may be used to detect gallstones, obstructions of the biliary tract, and other GB disorders. In this procedure, the nurse's responsibilities will include:

- Assess patient for sensitivity to iodine, (telepaque contains iodine).
- Administer radiopaque dye evening before test.
- Give 6 tablets (3q) 1q 5 minutes.
- Explain that patient may need 2 consecutive days of dye ingestion.
- Keep patient NPO after ingestion of dye.
- Observe for side effects of dye, such as nausea, vomitting, diarrhoea.
- May give fatty test meal after X-ray test to check for GB emptying.
- Assess patient's medication for possible contraindications, precautions or complications with the use of dye.

v. Cholangiography

Cholangiogram: In the X-rays are used to visualize biliary duct system after IV injection of radiopaque dye, the nurse's responsibilities in the procedure will include:

- Keep patient NPO for 8 hours prior to procedure.
- Assess sensitivity to iodine dye.
- During injection of dye, assess for urticaria, extreme flushing and respiratory distress.
- Assess patient's medications for possibly contraindication, complications, with the use of dye.

Percutaneous transhepatic cholangiogram. This is performed after local anaesthesia. Liver is entered with long needles (under fluoroscopy) bile duct is entered, bile withdrawn and radiopaque dye injected. Fluoroscopy is used to determine filling of hepatic and biliary ducts. The nurse's responsibilities are:

- Observe patient for signs of haemorrhage or bile leakage.
- Assess patient's medications for possible contraindications precautions or complications with the use of dye.

Surgical cholangiogram is performed during surgery on biliary structure such as gallbladder, contrast medium is injected into common bile duct. The nursing responsibilities are:

- Explain the patient that anaesthetic will be used.
- Assess patient's medications for possible contraindications, precautions, or complications with the use of dye.

vi. Ultrasound

This non-invasive procedure uses high frequency sound waves (ultrasound waves), which are passed into body structures and recorded as they are reflected (bounded). A conductive gel (lubricant jelly) is applied to the skin and a transducer is placed on the area. In these procedures nurses should be aware that patient's bowel must be cleaned, because of the presence of solid material in GI tract causes change in reflected sounds and that ultrasound is not transmitted well through gas or air. Schedule test before upper GI or barium enema.

a. Abdominal ultrasound study detects abdominal masses (tumours and cysts) and is also used to assess ascitis.
b. Hepatobiliary ultrasound study detects subphrenic abscesses, cysts, tumours, cirrhosis and is used to visualize biliary ducts.
c. GB ultrasound study detects gallstones (high degree of accuracy) and can be used for a patient with jaundice, or allergic reaction to GB contrast media. The nurse's responsibilities include:
    - Administer clear liquids for 24 hours before examination.
    - Give laxatives evening before and cleansing enema morning of examination.
    - Keep patient NPO 8 hours prior to procedure.

vii. Nuclear imaging scans

The purpose of nuclear imaging scans is to show size, shape, and position of organ. Functional disorders and structural defects may be identified. Radionuclide (radioactive isotope) is injected IV and a counter (scanning) device picks up radioactive emission, which is recorded on paper. Only tracer doses of radioactive isotopes are used. In these procedures, nurses use to:

- Tell patients that substances contain only traces of radioactivity and pose little to no danger.
- Schedule no more than one radionuclide test on the same day.

- Explain to patient need to lie flat during the scanning.
  a. *Gastric emptying studies*: A Radionuclide study is used to assess ability of stomach to empty solids or liquids. In solid emptying study, egg white containing Tc 99m is eaten. In liquid emptying study, orange juice with Tc 99 m is drunk. Sequential images from gamma camera are recorded q2 minutes for upto 60 minutes. Study is used in patients with emptying disorders from peptic ulcer, ulcer surgery, diabetes and gastric malignancy.
  b. *Liver and spleen scan*: Here patient is given LV injection of Tc 99m and positioned under camera to record distribution of radioactivity in liver and spleen. In normal person, intensity of liver and spleen images is equal. Test is useful in detecting hepatomegaly hepatocellular diseases, hepatic malignancy and splenomegaly.

viii. Computed tomography (CT)

Computed tomography (CT) is a non-invasive radiological examination combines special X-ray machine used for CT (exposures at different depth) with computer. This study detects mainly biliary tract, liver and pancreatic disorders. Use of contrast medium accentuates density differences and helps detect biliary problems. In this procedure, nurses are used to explain procedures to patient and determine sensitivity to iodine if contrast material is used.

ix. Magnetic resonance imaging (MRI)

MRI is a non-invasive procedure using radiofrequency waves and a magnetic field. This procedure is used to detect hepatic metastasis, sources of GI bleeding, and to stage colorectal cancer. The nurse's responsibilities in MRI includes

- Keep patient NPO for six hours prior to procedure.
- Explain procedure to patient.
- This procedure contraindicated in patient with metal implants (e.g. pacemaker), or who is pregnant.

ENDOSCOPIC EXAMINATION

Endoscopy refers to the direct visualization of a body structure through a lighted instrument (scope). Most of the GI tract can be visualised by endoscopy, especially with the flexible fibroptic scopes. The fiberscope is an instrument channel through which biopsy forceps and cytology brushes may be passed. Cameras may be attached and pictures taken. Endoscopy is frequently done in combination with the biopsy and cytologic studies. The major complication of GI endoscopy is perforations through the structure being scooped. All endoscopic procedures required informed, written consent.

i. Esophago-gastro-duodenoscopy

Esophago-gastro-duodenoscopy is a technique directly visualizes mucosal lining of esophagus, stomach and duodenum with flexible, fibroptic endoscope. Tests may use video imaging to visualize stomach motility, inflammations, ulcerations, tumours, varices, or Mallory-weiss tear may be detected. The nursing responsibility in this procedure includes:

- Keep patient NPO for 8 hours prior to the procedure.
- Make sure signed consent is on chart.
- Give pre-operative medication if ordered (diazepam, midazolam, or meperidine).
- Explain to patient that local anesthetic may be sprayed on throat before insection of scope and that patient will be sedated during procedure.
- After procedure, keep patient NPO until gag reflex returns.
- Gently tickle back of throat to determine reflex.
- Use warm saline gargles for relief of sore throat.
- Check temperature q 15-30 minutes for 1-2-hours (sudden temperature spike is sign of perforation).

ii. Colonoscopy

Study directly visualizes entire colon upto iliocecal valve with flexible fiberoptic scope. Patient's position is changed frequently during procedure to assist with advancement of scope to cecum. Test is used to diagnose inflammatory bowel disease, detect tumours, and dilate strictures. Procedure allows for removal of colonic polyps without laparotomy. The nursing responsibilities in this procedure will include:

- Before the procedure, keep patient on clear liquids 1-3 days.
- Keep patient NPO for 8 hours prior to procedure.
- Make sure signed consent is on chart.
- Administer laxatives 1-3-days before and enema night before.
- Explain to patient some information regarding insertion of scope as for sigmoidoscopy.
- Explain to patient that sedation will be given.
- Administer alternate preparation of 1 glass of golytely or colyte evening before (8 oz glass q 10 min).
- On morning of procedure, allow clear liquids.
- After the procedure, be aware that patient may experience abdominal cramps caused by stimulation of peristalsis because the patient's bowel is constantly inflated with air during procedure.
- Observe for rectal bleeding and signs of perforation (e.g. malaise, abdominal distentions.

iii. Endoscopic retrograde cholangiopancreatography (ERCP)

In ERCP fiberoptic endoscope is inserted through the oral cavity into descending duodenum, then common bile and pancreatic ducts are cannulated. Contrast medium is injected into ducts and allows for direct visualisation of structures. Technique can also be used to retrieve a gallstone from distal GBD, dilate structures, biopsy tumours diagnose pseudocysts. In this procedure, the nursing responsibilities will include the following:

- Before the procedure, explain procedure to patient including patient's role.
- Keep patient NPO 8 hours prior to procedure.
- Ensure consent form is signed.
- Administer sedation immediately before and during procedure.
- Administer antibiotics if ordered.
- After the procuedure, check vital signs.
- Check for signs of perforation or infection.
- Be aware that pancreatitis is most common complication.
- Check for return of gag reflex.

iv. Peritoneoscopy (Laparoscopy)

Peritoneal cavity and contents are visualized with laparoscope. Biospy specimen may also be taken. Double puncture peritoneoscope permits better visualization of abdominal cavity, especially liver. This technique can eliminate need for exploratory laparotomy in many patients. In this, following are the nursing responsibilities".

- Make sure signed permit is on chart.
- Keep patient NPO 8 hr before study.
- Administer preoperative sedative medication.
- Ensure that bladder and bowel are emptied.
- Instruct patient that local anaesthesia is used before scope insertion.
- Observe for possible complications of bleeding and bowel perforation after the procedure.

LIVER BIOPSY

It is an invasive procedure; uses needle inserted between sixth and seventh or eighth and ninth intercostal spaces on the right side to obtain specimens of hepatic tissue. The nurse's responsibilities include:

- Check patient's coagulation status (PT, CT, BT) prior to procedure.
- Ensure patient's blood is typed and cross matched.
- Take vital signs as baseline data.
- Explain holding breath after expiration when needle is inserted.
- Ensure that informed consent has been signed.
- After the procedure, check vital signs to detect internal bleeding, q 15 min × 2, q 30 min × 4, q 1 hr × 4.
- Keep patient lying on right side for minimum 2 hours to splint puncture site.
- Keep patient on bed in flat position for 12-14 hours.
- Assess patient for complications such as bile peritonitis, shock pneumothorax.

PROBLEMS OF MOUTH

Ingestion is the process of taking food and fluids into the body via the GI tract. It begins in the mouth with mastication of food by teeth. Food then passes down the oesophagus and into the stomach. It is important that sufficient nutrient is ingested to meet bodily requirements. Oral problems, such as poor dental health, infections and inflammation and cancer interfere with ingestion.

Dental Problems/Tooth and Gum Disorder

Tooth decay is by far the most common problem affecting the teeth termed as "dental caries". It is the result of a pathological process that causes the gradual destructions of the enamel and dentin of the teeth. Caries development starts when 'plaque' builds up and adheres to the teeth. Plaque is a gelationous substance consisting of bacteria, saliva and epithelial cells.

Pathophysiology of Dental Decay

Dental plaque is a soft mass composed of proliferation bacteria in a matrix of polysaccharides and salivery glycoproteins. It adheres to the teeth and its both transparent and colourless. Acids produced by the bacteria slowly decalcify the inorganic tooth enamel. Food, particularly carbohydrates, stimulates bacterial acid production. Simple sugars have the greatest effect. The plaque begins to collect on the teeth within 2 hours of eating and the longer or more frequently carbohydrates are ingested, the longer it takes for the pH of the mouth returns to normal cavity formation is the visible clinical evidence of the progression of the decay process.

Pathophysiology of Periodontal Disease

The periodontium is the tissue surrounding and supporting the teeth. It is composed fo the gingive (gums), cementum, alveolar bone and the periodontal ligament, which helps to fix the tooth firmly in its bony socket. Periodontal disease is the major loss of tooth in adults. Gingevitis is the earliest form of periodontal disease, it is characterised by colour alterations in the gums, swelling, and easy bleeding. Inflammation causes gingivae to separate from the tooth surface. Pockets form in the gingivae that can collect bacteria, food particles and pus. As the process is gradually worsens over a period of time, the gum recedes, the alveolor bone is resorbed, and the teeth loosen. Bleeding of the gums with normal tooth brushing is a common early sign. There is usually no pain.

Aetiology of Periodontal Disease

- Dental Plaque, when dental plaque calcifies, it forms calculus, which is hard, tenacious mass on the crowns of teeth.
- Malocclusion—faulty relationship between the teeth when the jaws are closed, margins of over-extended fillings, impacted food.
- Systemic conditions such as:
  - Poorly, controlled diabetes mellitus,
  - Thyroid diseases, pregnancy, HIV infections,
  - Vitamins and nutritional deficiencies, and
  - Certain drugs, smoking also.

Management of Dental Problem

- Prevention is the most appropriate management of dental problem, which includes:
  - Widespread fluoridation of water supplies reduces dental decay. Fluoride makes tooth enamel more resistant to acids and is commonly added to drinking water in many localities. It is widely available in toothpastes, dental rinses and mouthwashes.
  - Early treatment of periodontal disease consists of scaling and root planning.
  - Scaling is the removal of calculus and root planning is the smoothening of root surfaces. Gingivectomy and gingivoplasty may be necessary.

Nursing Assessments

- The patient's mouth should be assessed for tooth caries, missing teeth displaced teeth and dental appliances.
- The face should be assessed for symmetry and the jaw should be palpated for lumps.
- The gingivae should be assessed for redness, pallor, bleeding, recession and ulcers.

Nursing Diagnosis

- Altered oral mucous membrane related to
  - caries, ineffective and hygienic, periodontal disease or ill-fitting dentine.
- Altered nutrition less than body requirement related to inability to ingest adequate nutrients (ill-fitting dentures, displaced teeth, gingival discs, dental caries).
- Body image disturbance related to change in appearance of or unattractive teeth, difficulty with eating or *Halitosis*.
- Non-compliance related to altered perception, lack of motivation, inadequate finance or lack of knowledge of consequence of non-compliance.

Planning

The objectives of the nursing management is

- To decrease dental caries through improved oral hygiene.
- Able to identify and reduce risk factors (Caries and periodontium).
- To have a balanced diet intake.

Implementation

- Advise or assist in maintaining proper oral hygiene.
- Advise and assist for regular periodic dental examination.
- Reduce sugar intake and brush teeth after 30 minutes of eating sugar to reduce plaque formation.
- Increase intake of vitamin C.
- Advise use of fluoride content toothpaste.
- Advise for fluoridation of drinking water in the community.
- Referrals made for acute dental problem cases, such as:
  i. Local manifestation of pain that is caused by sensitivity to heat cold stimulation, dull and continuous pain, facial swelling, halitosis and bleeding or drainage of pus from the mouth.
  ii. Systematic manifestation of fever, nausea, vomiting and malaise.

Evaluation: Check the objective of care will be met or not.

ORAL INFECTIONS AND INFLAMMATION

Any of the structures of the mouth may develop infections when oral infections and inflammations are present, they can severely or seriously affect the ability of the patient to adequately and comfortably ingest food and fluids by mouth. These infections are inflammations; may be specific mouth disease or they may occur in the presence are inflammation may be specific mouth disease or they may occur in the presence of some systemic disease such as leukaemia or vitamin deficiency.

Pathophysiology

The structure of the mouth causes many ulcerative diseases to have similar signs and symptoms. The mucus throughout the mouth is thin, and evolving vesicles and bullae break open rapidly into ulcers. The ulcers are typically further traumatized by the teeth and can become readily infected by the abundant oral flora. Many of the causative organisms are the same on those that cause common skin infections. The common inflammation and infections of the oral cavity are as follows. With this aetiology, there comes clinical manifestation and treatment.

1. *Gingivitis*: Inflammation of the gingivae in the early form of periodontal disease. It may occur due to neglected oral hygiene, malocclusion, missing or irregular teeth, faulty dentistry, eating of soft rather than fibrous foods.

The clinical manifestation include inflammed gingivae and interdental papillae, bleeding during toothbrushing, development of pus, formation of abscess with loosening teeth (Periodontitis).

Treatment include prevention through health teaching, dental care, gingival massage, professional cleaning of teeth, nonfibrous foods, conscientious brushing habits with flossing.

2. *Vincent's angina* (Necrotizing ulcerative gingivitis, Trench mouth).

It is an acute bacterial infection of the gingivae, caused by a tremendous proliferation of normal mouth flora, such as spirochetes and fusiform bacilli. It is commonly triggered by poor oral hygiene, nutritional deficiencies (B and C vitamins), alcoholism, infections, or immunocompromise.

The clinical manifestations are, painful bleeding gingivae, eroding necrotic lesions of interdental papillae, ulceration than bleed, increased saliva with metallic taste, fetid mouth odour, anorexia, fever and general malaise.

The nursing measure will include- advising the patient to take rest (physical & mental), avoidance of smoking and alcoholic beverages, advice soft nutritious diet, correct oral hygiene habits, topical application of antibiotics, mouth irrigations with H_2O_2 and saline solutions.

3. *Oral candidiasis (monilasis or thrush)* is caused by an increase in the level of *Candida albicans*, a yeast-like fungus is normally found in the skin, GI tract, vagina and oral cavity. Overgrowth of the organism may result from antibiotic depletion of normal flora (prolonged high dose of antibiotics) or immunosuppress from steroid therapy, chemotherapy or HIV infections.

The clinical manifestations are pearly, bluish white (creamy white) "milk-curd" membranous lesions on mucosa of mouth and larynx, sore mouth, yeasty halitosis. The conditions is painful and if widespread, can interfere with oral nutrition. When mucosa bleeds, and ulcerates when patches are scraped off.

Treatments include nystatin, or amphotericin B as oral suspension or buccal tablets, good oral hygiene. Oral nystatin, ketoconazole, clotrimazole; amphotericin for the immunocompromized person.

4. *Herpes simplex stomatitis.* (cold sore, fever-blister): It is an externally common viral infection that produces characteristic blisters commonly called 'cold sore' or fever blister. It is caused by herpes simplex virus, type I or II, predisposing factors of upper respiratory infections, excessive exposure to sunlight, food allergies, emotional tensions, onset of menstruation.

The virus is harboured in a dormant state by cells in the sensory nerve ganglia. Reactivation of the virus can occur with emotional stress, fever, exposure to cold or ultraviolet rays. The lesion appears most commonly on the mucus membranous border junction of the lips in the form of small vesicles, which then erupt and form painful, shallow ulcers. Vesicle formation may be single or clustered. Painful vesicles and ulceration of mouth, lips or edge of nose; may have prodromal itching or burning, fever, malaise, lymphadenopathy may occur.

Treatment is palliative, which include mild antiseptic mouthwash. Application of spirits of camphor, corticosteroid cream, viscous lidocaine, removal or control of predisposing factors, topical or systemic antiviral agents, e.g. acyclovir (zovirax) in severe cases.

5. *Aphthous stomatitis (Cancer sore):* It is a recurrent and chronic form of infection secondary to systemic disease, trauma, stress or unknown causes. It produces well-circumscribed ulcers on the soft tissues of the mouth, including lips, tougue, insides of the cheeks, pharynx and soft palate. Ulcers of the mouth and lips causing extreme pain, ulcers surrounded by erythematous base. Painful small ulceration on oral mucosa heals in 1 to 3 weeks.

Treatment is palliative; includes mouthwashes, hydrocortisone, antibiotic ointment, fluocinonide (Lidex ointment in orabase. Corticosterdoid (topical or systemic) tetracycline oral suspension for children.

6. *Parotitis* is an inflammation of the salivary or parotid glands. The viral inflammation known as "mumps" in children.

Parotitis usually caused by staphylococcus species, streptococcus species, occasionally. Acute bacterial parotitis typically occurs in debilitated or elderly patients in whom dehydration, minimal oral intake, or medication have resulted in chronic dry mouth. Poor oral hygiene also causes parotitis. Acute parotitis occurs in postoperation patient called "surgical mumps".

The clinical manifestations are: Pain in the glands with an abrupt onset, i.e., pain in area of gland and ear, absence of salivation, purulent exudate from duct of gland, fever and swelling.

Treatment includes application of heat and cold, frequent oral hygiene, adequate hydration, broad spectrum antibiotics, occasionally needed. Nursing measures are mouthwashes, warm compresses, preventive measures such as chewing gum, sucking on hard candy (Lemon drops) adequate fluid intake.

7. *Stomatitis* is the inflammation of the mouth caused by trauma, pathogens, irritants (tobacco, alcohol) renal, liver and nematologic disorders, side effects of many cancer chemotherapentic drugs.

The clinical manifestation is excessive salivation, halitosis, sore mouth.

Treatment includes, removal or treatment of cause, oral hygiene with soothing solutions, topical medication, soft, bland diet.

ORAL CANCER

Carcinoma of the oral cavity may occur on the lips or anywehre within the mouth which includes tongue, floor of the mouth, buccal mucosa, hard palate, soft palate, pharyngeal walls and tonsils.

Aetiology

The development of oral cancer is clearly linked to a history of smoking and alcohol consumption and the risk increases strongly with heavy use. The exact cause of oral cancer is not clear, but there are number of predisposing factors which includes:

- Constant over-exposure to ultraviolet radiation from the sun, for cancer lips.
- Tobacco usage (smoking and chewing) i.e, pipe and cigar smoking, snuff, chewing tobacco.
- Chronic alcohol intake (excessive use of alcohol).
- Chronic irritation (jagged tooth, ill-fitting prosthesis, chemical or mechanical irritants).

- Ruddy fair complexion leads to lip cancer.
- Syphilis, immunosuppresion leads to lip cancer.
- Recurrent herpetic lesions.
- Poor oral hygiene.
- Hot and spicy foods or drinks.
- Malnutrition.
- Cirrhosis of the liver.
- Age over 45 years.
- Family history of oral cancer.

Pathophysiology

The vast majority of oral cancer arise from the squamous cells, which line the surface, oral epithelium, epidermoid, basal cell and other carcinoma may arise. The majority of tumours arise on the lateral or ventral surfaces of the tongue, although rarely on the dorsal surface, and commony go unnoticed by the patients. A single ulcer is the typical pattern. The tongue has an abundant vascular supply and lymphatic drainage channels, and spread of the cancer to adjacent structures may be rapid. Metastasis to the neck has already occurred in 60% of patients at the time of the diagnosis is made. The mortality rate is high, early metastasis is rare, although rapid extension to the mandible or floor of the mouth is possible. Tumours that involve the parotid gland are usually benign, although those arising submaxillary glands have a high rate of malignancy and tend to grow rapidly.

Clinical Manifestations

Many oral cancers are asymptomatic in the early stages. The premalignant lesions of the oral cavity are:

- *Leukoplakia*—is a potentially precancerous, yellow-white or grey white lesions may occur in any region of mouth also called "white patch" or "smoker's patch". Leukoplakia is the result of chronic irritation usually from the smoking and Candida infection.
- The patch becomes keratonical (hard and leathery) is sometimes described as hyperkaratosis.
- *Erythroplasia*—is a red, velvety-appearing patch that is often indicative of early squamous cell carcinoma occur on the mouth or tongue. These may turn to malignant.

Cancer of the lip usually appears as an indurated, painless ulcer on the lip. The first sign of carcinoma of tongue is ulcer or area of thickening. Soreness or pain of the tongue may occur, especially on eating hot or highly-seasoned foods. Cancer lesions are most likely to develop in the proximal half of the tongue. Later symptoms of cancer of the tongue include increased salivation, slurred speech, dysphagia, toothache, and earache.

Approximately 30% of oral cancer present with an asymptomatic neck mass. Anyhow, the common clinical manifestation of oral cancer are as follows:

- Masses in the mouth or neck.
- Chronic ear pain.
- Enlarged lymp nodes (cervical nodes are commonly affected).
- Discomfort or burning.
- Ulcer on lateral or ventral surface of the tongue or elsewhere.
- Dysphagia.
- Visible lesions on lips or elsewhere.
- Presence of erythroplasia (bright red, velvety leisions).

Diagnostic Study

- Biopsy of the suspected lesion with cytologic examination. It may be used to evaluate lymph nodes, leukoplakia or erythroplasia.
- Ultrasonography is an excellent adjust to evaluate masses that are closed to the surface.
- Computed tomography (CT) scans may be used to evaluate deeper, less definite masses.
- Magnetic resonance imaging (MRI) is most useful in the effort to evaluate deep masses of the inconclusive structure.

Treatment

Treatment of oral cancer depends on the location and staging of the tumour. Early-stage cancer is usually treated by either radiation or surgery, depend upon the size and accessibility of the tumour. More invasive cancers may require both modalities and advanced cancers are treated palliatively.

Radiation Therapy for Oral Cancer

Early lesions are highly curable with radiation, if they are confined to the mucosa, and the use of radiation prevents widespread tissue destruction. Radiation may be delivered by external beam or through the insertion of needle. If both radiation and surgery are planned, the radiation therapy is usually administered after the surgery because irradiated tissue is more susceptible to infection and breakdown. Care of the patient with implanted radioactive needles in oral tissue includes the following:

- *Implant care*
  - Do not pull on the strings. Any movement could alter the placement or direction of the radiation or cause the needles to loosen.
  - Check needles-patency several times each day.
  - Monitor linens, bed areas, and emesis basin, for needles that may dislodge.
  - Ensure that a protective container is present in the room to contain any needles that might dislodge.
- *Patient care*
  - Be familiar with gentle oral hygiene q 2h while awake.
  - Encourage the patient to avoid hot and cold foods and beverages as well as smoking.

- If the patient has dentures, encourage their removal at night, for comfort. Assess gums for irritations and bleeding whenever dentures are removed.
- Provide viscous Lidocaine (Xylocaine) solution or lozenges as needed, when oral discomfort interferes with nutrition.
- Provide the patient with an alternate means of communication, talking around implanted needles is usually difficult or impossible.
- Assist the patient to implement the mouth care regimen prescribed by the physician.
- The side effects of radiation therapy to the mouth and neck include mucositis, xerostomia, and dental decay should be reported and managed accordingly.

Surgical Management

Surgical management of oral cancers range from local excision of small tumours to expensive surgery for invasive tumours. Some examples are partial mandibulectomy, hemiglossectomy, resection of the buccal mucosa and floor of the mouth and radical neck dissection, etc. Chemotherapy and radiation therapy also may be used along with surgical measures wherever indicated in palliative purposes. Because of depression, alcohol or presurgery radiation treatment patient may be malnourished even before surgery and after the surgery also there may be chance to become malnourished. For which nurse must observe for tolerance of the feedings and adjust the amount, time and formula if nausea, vomiting, diarrhoea or distension occurs. The patient usually instructed about the tube feedings. When the patient can swallow, small amount of water is given. Close observation for choking is essential. Suction may be necessary to prevent aspiration. While managing the patient undergoing for *surgery* for oral cancer, the nurse can follow the undermentioned guidelines for care.

- *Preoperative*
  - Clarify the patient's knowledge of changes expected after surgery.
  - Explain expected postoperative measures including suctioning, nasogastric tube, etc.
  - Provide opportunities for the patient to begin to express feelings about changes in body image.
- *Postoperative*

1. *Monitoring*
   - Assess facial movement for facial nerve damage (if parotid gland excised); ask the patient to raise the eyebrows, frown, smile, show the teeth, pucker the lips.
   - Assess the degree and character of drainage.
     - Amount of drainage and presence of blood should be mentioned.
     - Haemorrhage may occur with wide resection of tongue.
2. *Maintaining an adequate airway*
   - Place the patient in sidelying position initially.
   - Place the patient in Fowler's position when fully alert.
   - Suction the mouth (except for lop surgery).
   - Gauze wick may be used to direct salive into an emesis basin.
   - Maintain patency of drainage tubes if used.
3. *Promoting oral hygiene and comfort*
   - Clean involved areas of the mouth with a cotton applicator moistened with H_2O_2 and saline.
   - Mouth irrigations.
     - Use sterile equipment.
     - Use a solution of sterile water, diluted H_2O_2, normal saline, or sodium bicarbonate.
     - Avoid commercial mouthwashes.
     - Protect any dressings from getting wet.
     - A catheter may be inserted along the side of the cheek and the solution injected with gentle pressure; a spray may also be used.
     - Give analgesics as indicated (pain is not usually severe).
4. *Promoting nutrition*
   - Tube feedings will be used initially with hemiglossectomy.
   - Oral fluids: place in back of throat with asepto syringe or feeding up with attached tubing.
   - Eating soft foods.
     - Encourage the patient to feed self when possible.
     - Teach the patient to drink clear water after all meals to cleanse the mouth.
     - Avoid using a fork, which may traumatize new tissue.
     - Avoid very hot or cold foods (hot foods may irritate new tissue cold foods may cause facial pain or paralyze oral function.
5. *Promoting speech*
   - Limit patient's response intitially to yes or no, which can be answered by gestures.
   - When ability speech returns, encourage patient to speak slowly.
   - Listen carefully and validate communication before acting on requests.
   - Speak in a soft, clear voice.
   - Refer the patient to a speech therapist if needed.
6. *Promoting body image*
   - Prepare all visitors for visible outcomes of surgery.
   - Include the family in all teaching.
   - Encourage the patient to ventilate feelings about changes.
   - Encourage socialization with others.

Nursing Management of Oral Cancer

Nursing assessment

Subjective and objective data should be collected as follows: The subjective data include:

- Important health information. i.e.,
  - Past health history: Recurrent herpetic lesions, syphilis, exposure to sunlight.
  - Medications: Use of immunosuppressants.
  - Surgical or other treatment—Removal of prior tumours.
- Functional health patterns:
  - Health perception—health management: Use of alcohol and tobacco, pipe smoking; Poor oral hygiene.
- Nutritional metabolic: Reduction in oral intake, weight loss, difficulty in chewing, increased salivation, intolerance to certain foods and temperatures of foods.
- Cognitive-perceptual: Mouth or tongue soreness or pain, toothache earache, neck stiffness, dysphagia, difficulty in speaking.

The objective data includes:

- Integumentary: indurated, painless ulcer on lips painless neckmasses
- Gastrointestinal: Areas of thickening or roughness, ulcers, leukoplakia, or erythroplasia on the tongue, increased salivation, drooling, slurred speech, foul breath odour.

Nursing Diagnosis

Nursing diagnosis for the patients with oral cancer may include the following:

Altered nutrition: less than body requirement related to oral pain, difficulty in chewing, and swallowing, surgical resection, and radiation therapy.

- Pain related to tumour and surgical radiation.
- Anxiety related to diagnosis of cancer, uncertain future, potential for disfiguring surgery, recurrence bronchoscopy.
- Ineffective individual coping related to body image change, smoking and alcohol cessation.
- Altered health maintenance related to lack of knowledge of disease process and therapeutic regimen, and unavailability of support systems.

Planning

The objective of oral cancer patient will include that the patient will:

- Have a patent airway.
- Be able to communicate.
- Have adequate nutritional intake to promote healing.
- Have relief of pain and discomfort.

Implementation

The nurse should take preventive measures such as:

- Teach clients to avoid excessive use of tobacco, alcohol, hot and spicy foods and drinks.
- Encourage use of sunscreen during exposure to sunlight.
- Screen smokers and drinkers of alcohol and teach them to stop smoking and to limit alcohol intake.
- Ensure that client fix broken teeth and improperly-fitting dentures.
- Teach persons at risk to observe for manifestation of cancer.
- Ensure that client's tumour is excised and followed with chemotherapy and radiation as indicated.
- Provide nutritional support with tube feedings or feedings through precaution endoscopic gastrostomy and gastrostomy tube.

Evaluation

The expected outcomes (objectives) that the patient with oral cancer will:

- Maintain airway.
- Be able to communciate.
- Have adequate nutritional intake.
- Have relief of pain and discomfort.

NAUSEA AND VOMITING

Nausea and vomiting are the most common symptoms of GI diseases, which most often occur together but may occur independently. They are part of the body's protective mechanisms and are usually a response to chemical, bacterial, or viral insults to the body's integrity. They are present in a wide array of disorders and if persistent can lead to serious consequences.

Nausea is a feeling of discomfort in the epigastrium with a conscious desire to vomit. Anorexia usually accompanies nausea and is brought on by unpleasant stimulation involving any of the five senses. Generally, nausea occurs before vomiting and is characterized by contraction of the duodenum and by slowing of gastric motility and emptying.

Vomiting is the forceful ejection of partially digested food and secretions from the upper GI tract. It occurs when the gut becomes overly irritated, excited, or distended. It can be a protective mechanism to rid the body of spoiled or irritating foods and liquids. Immediately before the act of vomiting, the person becomes aware of the need to vomit. The autonomic nervous system is activated resulting in both parasympathetic and sympathetic nervous systems, stimulation sympathetic activation produces tachycardia, tachypnoea and diaphoresis. Parasympathetic stimulation causes relaxation of lower oesophageal sphincter, an increase in gastric motility and a pronounced increase in gastric motility and a pronounced increase in salivation.

Vomiting is a complex act that requires coordinated activities of several structures, closure of the glottis, deep inspiration with contraction of the diaphragm in the inspiratory position, closure of the glottis relaxation of the stomach and lower oesophageal spincter, and contraction of the abdominal muscles with increasing abdominal pressure. These stimulation activities force the stomach contents up through the oesophagus into the pharynx and out of the mouth.

Aetiology

Nausea and vomiting are the most common manifestations of the *Gastrointestinal* disorders. They are also found in a wide variety of conditions that are unrelated in GI disease. These include:

- Pregnancy.
- Infectious diseases.
- CNS disorders (e.g. meningitis, CNS lesion).
- Cardiovascular problem (e.g. digitalis, antibiotics).
- Metabolic disorders (e.g. uraemia, diabetic acidosis, etc.
- Psychological factors (d.g. stress, fear, unpleasant nights and odours).

Pathophysiology

Nausea may be accompanied by weakness, hypersalivation, and diaphoresis. Gastric tone and peristalsis are typically slowed or absent. The neural pathways that control nausea are not well identified but probably are the same general pathways that control vomiting. The vomiting center is located in the medulla (brain stem) adjacent to the respiratory and salivary control centers and can be stimulated by the vagus nerve and sympathetic nervous system. Receptors can be found throughout the GI tract and internal organs that, when triggered by spasm or inflammation, can directly produce vomiting. Indirect stimulation can come from the chemoreceptor trigger zone (CTZ) which is located on the floor of the fourth ventricle and appears to act as an emetic chemoreceptor responding to chemical stimuli in the blood. A wide variety of medication and other substances can act on the CTZ in this manner. The CTZ also mediate the response to nonchemical stimuli such as radiation and motion sickness. There is a strong evidence that dopamine receptors in the CTZ play a role in mediating vomiting.

When nausea and vomiting are prolonged, dehydration can rapidly occur. In addition to water, essential electrolytes, (e.g. potassium) are also lost. As vomiting persists, there may be severe electrolyte imbalances, loss of extra cellular fluids (ECF) volume, decreased plasma volume and eventually circulatory failure. Metabolic alkosis can result from loss of gastric HCL. When contents from the small intestine are vomited. Weight loss is evident in a short time when vomiting is severe. The threat of aspiration is constant concern when vomiting is severe.

Nursing Management

Nursing assessment

The nurse has to obtain the important health information which include:

- *Past health history*: GI disorders, chronic indigestion, food allergies, pregnancy, infection, CNS disorders, recent travel, bulimia, metabolic disorders, cancer, cardiovascular disease, renal disease.
- *Medications*: Use of antiemetics, digitalis, opiates, ferrous sulphate aspirin, aminophylline, alcohol, antibiotics, general anaesthesia, chemotherapy.
- *Surgery of other treatment*: Recent surgery.

And also functional health pattern like amount, frequency, character and colour of vomitus, dry heaves, anorexia, weight loss, abdominal tenderness, weakness, fatigue, stress, fear, etc.

And also objective data include observing for lethargy, sunken eyeballs, pallor, dry mucus membrane, poor skin turgor, GI symptoms like amount frequency, character (e.g. projectile, or regurgitation) content (undigested food, bloody bile, feces) and colour of vomitus (red, coffee ground, green-yellow) and decreased output of urine, concentrated urine to locate causes.

Nursing Diagnosis

- Selfcare deficiency related to fatigue and discomfort and prolonged nausea and vomitus.
- Altered oral mucus membrane related to persistent vomiting and inadequate oral hygiene.
- Vomiting related to multiple aetiologies.
- Fluid volume deficient R/T prolonging.
- Anxiety R/T lack of knowledge of cause.
- Altered nutrition less than body requirements.

Planning

The overall goals of the patient with nausea/vomiting will

- Experience minimal or no nausea and vomiting.
- Have normal electrolyte levels and hydration status.
- Return to normal pattern of fluid balance and nutrition intake.

Nursing Implementation

The patient with nausea and vomiting should be managed with following guidelines for:

1. *Safety and comfort*
   - Keep head of the bed elevated and emesis basin handy.
   - Protect airway with suction and positioning if patient is not alert.
   - Provide frequent mouth care.
   - Control sights and odours in room.

- Reduce anxiety if possible.
- Provide quiet or distraction on the basis of patient response.
- Modify environmental stimuli (cool cloth, dim light) and evaluate response.
- Provide ongoing patient support. Exploreany strategies.

2. *Diet modification*
   - Maintain NPO if vomiting is severe.
   - Explore use of clear liquids:
     - Serve liquid cool or room temperature.
     - Try effervescent drinks and evaluate effect.
     - Avoid fatty foods.
     - Avoid highly sweetened foods and milk products.
     - Encourage adequate, fluids to prevent dehydration.
     - Keep meals small, avoid overdistention.
3. *Drugs/medications*
   - Administer medication before vomiting occurs, if possible.
   - Evaluate the patient response to medication.
   - Maintain patient safety and assess for sedation or confusion.

Generally the drugs used for nausea and vomiting and their nursing intervention are as follows:

i. *Antihistamines* are believed to act on neurons in the vomiting center and in the vescibular pathways. They are effective in motion sickness and morning sickness management, but have little known effect in GI disorders. These drugs cause drowsiness and sedation. The nurse has to monitor drowsiness and sedation and instruct patient to use caution with all activities that require alertness. Driving may be hazardous, so should be avoided. The example of antihistaminer are bucilizine hydrochloride, cyclizine hydrochloride, meclizind, promemethazine (all genric names).

ii. *Antidopamineroics* are believed to act by antagonizing dopamine receptors in the CTZ. They also have antihistamine and anticholenergic effects. They are effective in managing mild symptoms and often first lane therepies. The examples of antidopamergics are prochlorperazine, ethylperazine, fluphenazine droperidol. The nursing measures in this therapy include:

Monitor severity of drowsiness and sedation.

Teach patient to avoid all hazardous activities and driving during use.

Avoid alcohol and sun exposure.

iii. *Anticholenergics* reduce neuron transmission and are useful in the management of motion sickness and postoperative nausea. But the common side effects of dry mouth, urinary retention and drowsiness limit their use. During use, nurse should instruct patient to apply dry surfaces behind the ear. Use in advance anticipated need, e.g. scopalamine (Transderm-Scop).

iv. *Benzyamides* have complex action in both CNS and GI tract and useful in preventing vomiting associated with anaesthetics and chemotherapeutic agents.

Metadopramide stimulates gastric emptying.

Domoperidone does not cross blood-brain barrier. Here nurse has to monitor side effects. Diarrohea and mild sedation.

v. *Serotonin antagonists* like ondanserton (Zofran) and Granisertron bind serotonin receptor sites along GI tract and afferent nerves. They are useful in controlling severe chemotherapy induced and postoperative vomiting.

vi. *Cannabis derivatives*. The antiemetic site of action is uncertain but the active ingredient in marijuana is often useful in controlling chemotherapy related nausea and vomiting. In such cases, the nurse has to instract patient to alert on mood and behavioural changes. Drowsiness is common, so driving should be avoided. Avoid concurrent alcohol use while using this drug.

GASTRO-OESOPHAGEAL REFLUX DISEASE (GERD)

Gastro-oesophageal reflux diseases (GERD) is not a disease but a heterogenous syndrome resulting from oesophageal reflux. Most cases are attributed to the inappropriate relaxation of lower oesophageal spincter (LES) in response to unknown stimulus.

Aetiology

The common cause of GERD is Haital Hernia, the presence of which displaces the LES into the thorax and number of environmental and physical factors have been identified that appear to influence the tone and contractility of the LES and these may play an aetiological role in some cases of GERD. The pressure of the LES is lowered by fatty acids. chocolate, peppermint, cola, coffee and tea; nicotine, alcohol, drugs such as calcium channel blockers, the theophylline, and possible non-steroidal anti-inflammatory drugs (NSAID), elevated levels of oestrogen and progestrone; and that conditions that elevate intrabdominal pressure such as obesity, pregnancy or heavy lifting.

Pathophysiology

There are two zones of high pressure, one at each end of the oesophagus, normally prevent the reflux of gastric contents. The zones maintain a constant pressure and relax only during swallowing. Although they are termed as LES, they are not really distinct anatomical structures. Esophageal reflux occurs when either gastric volume or intra-abdominal pressure is elevated or when LES tone is decreased. Periodic reflux occurs normally in most persons and is usually asymptomatic. The normal physiologic response to occasional reflux is immediate swallowing one or more rapid swallows induce peristatic

Table 7.2: Nursing care plan of patient with nausea and vomiting

Problem	*Reason*	*Objective*	*Nursing intervention*	*Evaluation*
Vomiting R/T multiple aetiologies.	As manifested by episodes of nausea & vomiting.	• Minimal or No nausea and vomiting. • Verbalization of satisfaction with care.	• Assess duration, frequency and nature of vomitus and aggravating and alleviating factors to plan appropriate action. • Offer reassurance and explanations to increase patient cooperation. • Remove visual stimuli and source of odours to avoid precipitating factors of nausea and vomiting. • Provide mouth care; change soiled gown and linen to ensure patient comfort. • Use diversional activities (if appropriate) to decrease awareness of nausea. • Maintain quiet environment, restrict visitors and avoid unnecessary procedures to minimize triggering of vomiting. • Administer antiemetics as ordered. • Instruct patient to take several deep breaths, prevent sudden changes in position. • Keep head of bed elevated to decrease stimulation of the vomiting center. • Instruct patient to avoid foods and beverages that stimulate nausea and vomiting.	
Fluid volume deficit R/T – prolonged vomiting. – inability to ingest, digest or absorb food and fluids.	As manifested by decreased urine output and increased urine concentration, increased pulse rate, postural hypotension, decreased intake, decreased skin turgor, dry skin and mucous.	No signs of dehydration.	• Assess for signs of dehydration to plan appropriate care. • Administer and monitor amount and type of IV fluids to maintain fluid and electrolyte balance. • Administer antiemetic as prescribed. • Provide small amounts of clear liquids when vomiting stops for maintaining hydration. • Record amount and frequency of vomitus. • Maintain accurate intake and output records. • Weight daily in acute phase to accurately monitor fluid balance. • Monitor lab results of serum sodium, potassium and chloride as indicators of electrolyte balance.	
Anxiety R/T – Lack of knowledge of the cause of it – Treatment plan and follow-up care.	As manifested by verbalization of lack of knowledge apprehension.	• Decrease in anxiety. • Verbalization of understanding of causation factors and the repeutic interventions.	• Explain rationale for plan of care and diagnosis tests to increase patient understanding to reduce anxiety. • Justruct about relationships between nausea and vomiting and foods, medications, treatment regimens and psychosomal factors to elicit patient cooperation and avoiding potential causative factors.	
Altered nutrition body requirement R/T nausea and vomiting.	As manifested by lack of interest in or aversion to food perceived or actual inability to ingest food weight loss.	Gradual return to usual eating habits and weight.	• Assess the patients interest in food, ability to ingest food, and weight to determine if a problem is present. • Assure patient that appetite will return when nausea and vomiting are controlled. • Maintain IV fluids or TPN until oral intake is possible, provide fluids, electrolytes, calories, and protein intake. • Instruct patient to resume eating cautiously with bland, non-irritating foods.	

contractions to clear the reflux and neutralize the acid with bicarbonate-rich saliva. However, the oesophagus has only a limited ability to withstand the damaging effects of acid reflux and GERD will develop when frequent episodes of reflux break-down the mucosal barrier and initiate an inflammatory response.

The degree of oesophageal inflammation related to the number, duration and acidity or alkalinity of the reflux episodes. The effectiveness and efficiency of oesophageal clearance also are important. Oesophageal clearance is particularly important at night when the swallowing rate and salivation decrease by two thirds and recumbent position interferes with clearance. An inflammed oesophageal gradually loses its ability to clear reflexed material quickly and efficiently, and the duration of each episode gradually lengthens. Hyperemia and erosion occur in the face of chronic inflammation. Minor capillary bleeding is common, although frank bleeding is rare. Repeated episodes of inflammation and healing can gradually produce a change in the epithelial tissue, which makes it more resistant to acid. Over-time, fibrotic tissue changes can also result in oesophageal stricture, which can progressively impair normal swallowing.

Clinical Manifestation

- *Heartburn* is caused by irritation of the oesophagus by the gastric secretion. It is a burning, tight sensation that appears intermittently beneath the lower sternum and spreads upward to the throat or jaw. It occurs following ingestion of substances that decrease LES pressure. It is relieved with milk, alkaline substance or water.
- *Pulmonary symptoms* including wheezing, hoarseness, coughing, (nocturnal cough), dyspnoea are secondary to microaspiration of gastric contents into the pulmonary system.
- *Gastric symptoms* including early satiety, prostating bloating, nausea, and vomiting, are related to gastric stasis.
- *Regurgitation* is effortless return of material from stomach into oesophagus or mouth, oftenly described as hot, bitter or sour liquid coming into the throat or mouth. This taste is perceived in the Pharynx.
- *Water brash* a reflex, hypersecretion that does not have a bitter taste.
- *Frequent belching* and *flatulence* and feeling of lump in the throat or food stopping.
- *Dysphagia* difficulty in swallowing.
- *Odynophagia* painfull swallowing.
- *Bleeching.*

In addition GERD patients may experience complication of respiratory system - bronchospasm, laryngospasm, circopharyngal system and other complications include:

- Esophageal stricture (due to repeated episodes),
- Esophageal metaplasia (Barretts esophages),
- Pneumonia (due to aspiration of gastric contents to pulmonary system).

Management of GERD

Patients with GERD are rarely admitted to the acute care setting unless they require surgery or experience serious complications. The problem is self-managed in the out-patient setting. The goal of treatment is to decrease the incidence of reflux and eliminate the symptoms.

The *diagnostic studies* are performed to determine the causes are:

- Barium swallow for determining the protrusion of upper part of the stomach (gastric cardia).
- Radio-nuclide tests - to detect reflux of gastric contents and the rate of oesophageal clearance.
- Oesophagioscopy - to detect the incompetence of LES and the extent of inflammation, potential scarring and strictures.
- Biopsy and cytologic tests to differentiate heital hernia, carcinoma and Barret's oesophagus.
- Oesophageal motility (manometry) studies to measure pressure in the oesophagus and GES.
- pH monitoring for presence of acid or alkaline.

Pharmocologic management is focussed on improving LES function, increasing oesophageal clearance, decreasing volume or acidity reflux, and protecting oesophageal mucosa.

- Antacids are used to relieve heartburn by their neutralizing effect on hydrochloric acid. (For example, Gelucil, Maalox, Mylanta).
- Antacids plus alginic acid (Gaviscon) are used to neutralize gastric acid and reacts with sodium bicarbonate and forms a viscous solution that floats to the surface of the gastric contents and coats the esophagus acting on mechanical barrier to reflux.

When clientis an antacid and alginic acid the nurse should evaluate the effectiveness of the drug, monitor frequency of use and monitor for constipation ro diarrhoea and assist patient to adjust product use as needed.

Anti-secretory drugs: i.e. histamine (H_2) receptors are used to reduce the gastric acid secretion and supports tissue healing which include ranitidine, cimetidine, famotidine, nizaoidine. During use of these, the nurse should instruct patient to take drugs with meals if ordered at intervals, and monitor for common side effects, fatigue, headache, diarrhoea.

- Prokinetic drugs are used to increase LES pressure and enhance gastrointestinal motility, which includes cisapride (Propulsid). Here the nurse has to instruct patient to take drug no more than 15 minutes before eating and monitor levels of drugs that require useful titration.
- Proton pump inhabitors are used to inhabit enzyme system of gastric parietal cells and suppress gastric acid secretions by more than 90 per cent. Here the nurse has to instruct patient to take the drug before meals and monitor for side

effects, abdominal cramping, headache, diarrhoea. For example, omeprazole, lansoprazole are PP inhibitors.

Surgical management. Antireflux surgery is usually performed in patient with severe GERD who do not respond to aggressive medical management which includes:

- Nissen fundoplication
- Hill gastropexy
- Belseys fundoplication
- Antireflux prosthesis.

Nursing Management

The nurse by using nursing process, assesses the client on the basis of clinical manifestation stated above and take body weight, ascultate for signs for reflux aspirates and observe for hoarseness or wheezing-day or night.

The nursing diagnosis are made from analysis of patient's data. The diagnoses are not limited to pain and knowledge deficit. The objectives of nursing care will include reports, minimal or no episodes of heart burn and list diet and life style changes. GERD is typically managed by using a combination of drug therapy, diet, and life style modification and assisting surgical therapies if needed.

The nurse discusses the medication regimen with the patient and ensures that written information about the safe use and expected side effects of all meciations is provided, and administer the ordered medication and observe for response and side effects; Antacids that contain aluminium tend to cause constipation, where as those contain magnesium tend to cause diarrhoea. Several of the antacids are combination of aluminium and magnesium designed to minimize these effects. If the patient is taking bethenechol (cholenergic) side effects to observe for urinary urgency, increased salivation, abdominal cramping with darrhoea, nausea, vomiting, and hypotension. Side effects of metadopramide (dopamine antogonist) a prokinetic drug includes restlessness, anxiety and insomnia. Side effects of sucralfate (acid-protective) include drowsiness, dizziness, nausea, vomiting, constipation, urticaria and rash.

When nursing the patient with GERD the nurse has to use the following Diet and life style modifications to manage the same:

- In relation to diet patient are encouraged to
  - Eat 4-6 small meals daily.
  - Follow a low-fat, adequate protein diet.
  - Reduce intake of chocolate, tea and all foods and beverages that contain caffeine.
  - Limit or eliminate alcohol intake.
  - Eat slowly and chew food thoroughly.
  - Avoid evening snacking and do not eat for 2-3 hours before bed time.
  - Remain upright for 1-2 hours after meals when possible and never eat in bed.
  - Avoid any food that directly produces heart burn.
  - Reduce over all body weight if indicated.
- The nurse has to promote lifestyle of the patient by encouraging to:
  - Eliminate or drastically reduce smoking.
  - Avoid evening smoking, and never smoke in bed.
  - Avoid constrictive clothing over the abdomen.
  - Avoid activities that involve straining, heavy lifting or working in a bent-over position.
  - Elevate the head of the bed at least 6-8 inches for sleep using wooden blocks or a thick foam wedge.
  - Never sleep flat in bed.
- For prevention of GERD, the nurse should use the following teaching guidelines for patient and family.
  - Explain the rationale for a high-protein, low-fat diet.
  - Encourage the patient to eat small, frequent meals to prevent gastric distention.
  - Explain the rationale for avoiding alcohol, smoking (causes an almost immediate, marked decrease in LES pressure) and beverage that contains caffeine.
  - Instruct the patient not to lie down for 2 to 3 hours after eating, wear tight clothing around the waist, or bend over (especially after eating).
  - Encourage the patient to sleep with head of bed elevated on 4-6 inch blocks (gravity fosters oesophageal emptying).
  - Teach regarding medication including rationale for their use and common side effects.
  - Discuss strategies for weight reduction if appropriate.
  - Encourage patient and family to share concerns about lifestyle changes and living with a chronic problem.

HIATAL HERNIA

Hiatal hernia is herniation of a portion of the stomach into the esophagus through an opening, or hiatus, in the diaphragm. It is also referred to as 'diaphragmatic hernia and oesophagial hernia.'

Hiatal hernias are common in older adults and occur more frequently in women than in men. They are classified into two types (1) Sliding hiatal hernia (2) Paraoesophagical h.h.

- *In sliding*. The junction of the stomach and oesaphagus is above the hiatus of the diaphragm and a part of the stomach slides through the hiatal opening in the diaphragm. It "slides" into the thoracic cavity when the patient is supine and usually goes back into the abdominal cavity when the patient is standing upright.
- In paraoesophageal or rolling, the oesophagogastric junction remains in the normal position, but the fundus and the greater curvature of the stomach roll up through the diaphragm forming a pocket alongside the oesophagus.

Aetiology

The actual cause of hiatal hernia is unknown. Many factors contribute to the development of hiatal hernia. Structural changes, such as weakening of the musceles in the diaphragm around the oesophagogastric opening are usually contributing factors. Factors that increase intra-abdominal pressure, including obesity, pregnancy, ascitis, tumours, tight corsets, intense physical exertions, and heavy lifting on a continued basis, may also predispose to development of a hiatal hernia. Other predisposing factors are increased age, trauma, poor nutrition, and forced recumbent position, as when a prolonged illness confines the person to bed. In some cases, congenital weakness is a contributing factor.

Pathophysiology

A hiatal hernia involves herniation of part of the stomach through weakness in the diaphragm. The resulting regurgitations and motor dysfunction cause the major manifestation of the hiatal hernia. With *sliding* hernias the problems are rarely anatomical. The problems relate directly to the functional consequences of chronic reflux. Reflux occurs from the ongoing exposure of the LES to the low pressure environment of the thorax where spincter function is significantly impaired. Reflux is rarely a concern with *rolling* hernias, because the LES remains anchord below the diaphragm. However, the anatomical risks of volvulus, strangulation and obstructions are high. In addition, venous obstruction in the herniated portion of the stomach causes the mucosa to become engorged and to ooze. Slow bleeding leads to the development of iron deficiency anaemia, but significant bleeding is rare.

Clinical Manifestation

Manifestation of hiatal hernia varies in kind and severity. In sliding hiatal hernia, clients may have heartburn 30 to 60 minutes after meals. In addition, reflux may result in substernal pain. The clients with a rolling hernia does not have manifestation of reflux but client may complain of a feeling of fullness after eating or have difficulty in breathing. some clients experience chest pain similar to that of anginal pain. Pain is usually worse when the client assumes a recumbent position. Bending over may cause a severe burning pain which is usually relieved by sitting or standing. The other common factors of pain includes large meals, alcohol, and smoking. Nocturnal attacks are common especially if the person has eaten before going to sleep.

The complication that may occur with hiatal hernia includes problems such as haemorrhage from erosion, stenosis, ulceration of the herniated portion of the stomach, strangulation of the hernia, and regurgitation with tracheal aspiration. Severe chronic oesophagitis may follow reflux problem.

Diagnostic Studies

A barium swallow is an important diagnostic measure that may show the protrusion of gastric mucosa through the oesophageal hiatus in the patient with hiatal hernia. The other tests are similar that are performed in the GERD.

Management of Hiatal Hernia

Conservation therapy of hiatal hernia includes administration of antacids, and antisecretory agents, elimination of constricting garments, avoidance of lifting and straining, elimination of alcohol and smoking, and elevation of the head of the bed. Elevation of the bed on 4 to 6 inch blocks assists gravity in maintaining the stomach in the abdominal cavity and also helps prevent reflux and trachial aspiration. If obese, the client is encouraged to lose weight.

Surgical corrections of rolling hernias is mandatory because the risk of serous complications is significant. The objective of surgical interventions for hiatal hernia is to reduce reflux by enhancing the integrity of the LES. Surgical procedures are termed "Vulvoloplastics or antireflux" procedures. There are three slightly varied procedures namely:

i. The Hill gastropexy
ii. The Nissen fundoplications and
iii. The Belseys fundoplication.

The diet and activities of hiatal hernia are as discussed in GERD.

Surgical Nursing Management of Hiatal Hernia

Preoperative teaching focus on instructing the patient in deep breathing, the correct use of an incentive spirometer and splinting the incision effectively, for coughing. The surgical approaches all involve the diaphragm, and pulmonary hygiene is essential in preventing respiratory complications. Individuals who are overweight are encouraged to lose weight if possible before surgery and smokers are encouraged to significantly reduce or eliminate their use of tobacco. The nurse also teaches the patient about nasogastric tube that will be inserted during surgery with open procedures and planned time frame for restarting oral feedings.

Postoperative care focuses on concern related to prevention of respiratory complications, maintenance of fluid and electrolytic balance, and prevention of infection. If thoracic approach is used, a chest tube is inserted. Assessment and management related to closed chest drainage are important. After surgical intervention, there should be no symptoms of gastric reflux. The patient should be instructed to report symptoms such as heartburn and regurgitation. A normal diet can be resumed within 6 weeks. The patient should avoid foods that are causing gas problems and should try to prevent gastric distension. Food should be thoroughly chewed.

Table 7.3: Nursing care plan for client undergoing hiatal hernia repair

Problem	*Reason*	*Objective*	*Nursing Intervention*	*Evaluation*
Ineffective airway clearance R/T • Incisional pain, and • Limited mobility	Due to surgery	Maintains clear breath sounds effectively coughs up secretion	• Maintain head of bed in semi-Fowler's position. (at least 30 degrees). (drugs diaphragm and lungs to facilitate ventilation). • Perform pulmonary assessment Q2-4hr. (assess for atelectasis and retained secretions). • Monitor PCA pump or provide adequate narcotic analgesia (adequate pain control facilitates pulmohygiene and motility). • Supervise pulmonary hygiene q4 Hr. – Incentives spir metry. – Chest percussion and vibration. – Deep breathing q1-2 hours. (Prevents atelectasis and facilitates expulsion of secretions). • Assist with position changes and ambulation. (It facilitates expulsion of secretion and prevent atelectasis) • Splint incisions for movement and position changes (facilitate ability to deeply breathe and cough).	
Impaired swallowing R/T functional changes.	Due to fundoplication surgery.	Successfully progress from clear liquids to a normal diet without aspiration and discomfort.	• Maintain initial NPO status and monitor patency of NG tube. • Do not irrigate or reposition the NG Tube (stomach must remain decompressed to prevent vomiting). • Report the incidence of any fresh blood in the drainage after 8 hours of postoperatively (fresh blood indicates incisional complication). • Offer frequent oral and nasal hygiene. • Initiate feedings with 30 ml of clear liquids once peristalisis is reoestablished. • Evaluate presence and severity of desophagia. • Advance to multiple small feedings. • Progress from liguids to solid as patient tolerates. • Encourage thorough chewing of small food boluses. • Teach patient to avoid air swallowing and gas bloat. • Avoid carbonated beverages, using straws, and gas-producing foods. • Eat slowly and chew thoroughly. • Always eat in sitting up position. • Avoid over talking while eating. • Ambulate after meals.	

Contd...

Contd...

Problem	*Reason*	*Objective*	*Nursing Intervention*	*Evaluation*
Altered health maintenance R/T lack of knowledge.	Lack of knowledge concerning measures to prevent reflux.	Correctly identifies dietary and lifestyle changes to reduce the incidence of reflux.	• Provide patient with instructions about diet modifications: – Follow a low fat diet and avoid excessive tea, coffee, chocolate, and other such foods. – Strictly eliminate or limit alcohol intake. – Eat 4-6 small meals daily. – Eat slowly and chew food thoroughly. – Remain upright 1-2 hours after meals. – Never eat on bed. – Avoid evening snacking. – Reduce over 11 body weight. – Avoid any food that induce heartburn. – Discuss lifestyle modifications that can reduce incidence of reflux. – Enroll in smoking cessation program. – Avoid activities such as straining, lifting and stopping. – Avoid constrictive clothing. – Never sleep flat in bed. – Elevate the head on a 6-inch foam wedge for sleep. – Use antacids for occasional heartburn- Report frequent or severe episodes.	

ACHALASIA

Achalasia is a primary motility disorders of the oesophagus are conditions in which the normal function of the oesophagus is disturbed which problem may be primary in the oesophagus or secondary to another systemic disease (neuromuscular disorders, i.e. cerebrovascular accident, multiple sclerosis, myasthenia grans, amyotrophic lateral sclerosis, myopathiccranial nerve disease or traum 5th, 9th, 10th). The classic motility disorder is a failure of the oesophageal muscle to relax in sychrony, which can result in mechanical or functional obstruction of good passage. Failure to close adequately after swallowing can also occur, resulting in chronic reflux or regurgitation. Oesophageal spasm is common component of motility disorder and the spasm is usually intense enough to mimic angina.

As stated above *Achalasia* is the predominant primary disorder in which the lower oesophageal muscles and spincter fail to relax appropriately in response to swallowing.

Aetiology

The cause of the achalasia is unknown, although a familial link is possible. It usually develops in early or middle adulthood and one-third of cases develop after age of 60 years and both sexes are affected equally.

Pathophysiology

Achalasia (cardiospasm) results from a neuromuscular defect that is localized in the inner circular muscle layer of the oesophagus. Degeneration of ganglion cells causes both a failure of peristalsis and severe muscle spasm. Here the peristalsis of the lower third (smooth muscle) of the oesophagus is absent. Pressure in the LES is increased, along with incomplete relaxation of the LES. As the disease progresses, the portion of the oesophagus around the constriction becomes dilated and the muscle walls hypertrophy. Obstruction of oesophagus at or near the diaphragm occurs. Food and fluid accumulate in the lower oesophagus. Although the severity of achalasia varies widely, the spasms may be so severe that little or no food can enter the stomach. In extreme cases, the oesophagus may hold a liter or more food and fluid above the constricted area. The altered peristalsis is a result of impairment of the autonomic nervous system innervating the oesophagus.

Chronic and progressively worsening dysphagia is the classic symptom and occurs more frequently with liquids. Spasm may be provoked by cold or hot liquids or foods and worsened by stress or overeating. Substernal chest pain (similar to pain of angina) occurs during or imemdiately after a meal. Halitosis and the inability to erucate are other symptoms. Another common symptom is regurgitation of sour tasting food and liquids especially when the patient is in horizontal position weight loss is typical. A foul mouth odour from retension of food and the oesophagus may be a chronic problem.

Diagnostic Studies

The classic 'bird's beak narrowing plus dilation are readily observed with barium studies. Oesophageal manometry reveals an elevated resting LES pressure, combined with diminished or absent peristaltic waves.

Management of Achalasia

Treatment of achalasia consists of dilation, surgery and use of drugs.

All these therapies are directed at relieving the stasis caused by the increased LES pressure, non-relaxing LES, and aperistaltic oesophagus. The aim of management is to relieve symptoms. Symptomatic treatment consists of semi-soft bland diet, eating slowly and drinking fluid with meals and sleeping with the head elevated.

Oesophageal dilation (bougienage) is an effective treatment measure for many patients. Pneumatic dilation of LES with a balloon-tipped dilator passed orally is usually used. The commonly used dilators for pneumatic dilation are the Mosherbag, the Tucker mercury dilator, and Browne-McHardy dilator. They all depend on forcible expansion of a balloon in the LES. The forceful dilation does not restore normal oesophageal motility, but it does provide for emptying of the oesophagus into the stomach.

Surgical measures that may be necessary in the "Oesophago myotomy". In this procedure, the muscle fibers that enclose the narrowed area of the oesophagus are divided. This allows the mucosa to pouch out through the division in the muscle layer to allow food to be swallowed without obstruction. Measure similar to this procedure is Heller's Myotomy (cardiomyotomy) which disrupts the LES in a similar manner and reduces LES Pressure. An antiregina procedure is frequently done with myotomy. This procedure can be performed laparoscopically, reducing the potential for postoperative complications.

Various classes of medications are used in the treatment of achalasia include anticholenergics and calcium channel blockers (e.g. nifedipine Procardia), but none of them proved to be effective. Analgesics may be needed when pain is severe. Recent studies indicated that "botulinum toxin injection which relaxes oesophageal muscle delivered endoscopically in the management of achalasia.

Health Education

The nurse works with the patient and family to explore diet and lifestyle modifications that will best control dysphagia, which is prominent in achalasia. Education begins with careful assessment of the scope and severity of dysphagia, which includes.

- Swallowing ability with liquids v/s solids.
- Response to foods of differing textures and temperature.
- Variability of the dysphagia (intermittant or constant).
- Response to stress, fatigue and other activities.

- Approaches used by the patient to manage the dysphagia and the degree of success.

The nurse encourages the person to experiment with various types and consistency of foods and meal sizes to evaluate their influence on swallowing. Small, frequent semi-soft meals, are usually best tolerated. Warm liquids are recommended, and extremes of temperature should be avoided because they usually worsen the spasm. The nurse also advises the patient to experiment with changing positions during eating. Some individuals can swallow more effectively if they arch their back. Use of the valsalva, a manoeuvre (bearing down with a closed glottis) while swallowing may help proper food beyond the LES. Nocturnal reflux of retained food and fluid presents a significant risk for aspiration. The nurse should instruct the patients to sleep on a foam wedge or with the head of the bed elevated. And suitable advices also should be given to the patient who has undergone surgical procedures.

OESOPHAGEAL CARCINOMA

Carcinoma of the oesophagus is unique in its geographic distribution. Both benign and malignant tumours occur in the oesophagus. Benign tumours are usually leiomyomas, and extremely rare and usually asymptomatic. They require no intervention unless symptoms necessitate local excision. Malignant tumours of the oesophagus are not common, but they assume increased importance because of their virulence.

Aetiology

The cause of cancer of the oesophagus is unknown. Possible predisposing factors are cigarette smoking, excessive alcohol intake chronic trauma, poor oral hygiene, and spicy foods. The most important risk factors include exposure to asbestos and metal and low intake of fresh fruits and vegetables.

Pathophysiology

Tumours may develop any point along the length of the oesophagus, but the majority occur in the middle and lower two-thirds of the oesophagus. *Squamous cell* tumours have typically predominated. They tend to develop in the middle third and clearly related to the risk factors of smoking and alcohol use. *Adenocarcinomas* represent the remaining minoitry of tumours. These tend to develop in the lower third of the oesophagus and may evolve from the Barret's epithelium. It is an acquired condition in which changes occur in response to acid irritation over a period of 1 to 2 years and its presence increases the risk of cancer.

Oesophageal tumours of all types appear to emerge as a part of an initially slow process that begins with benign tissue changes. Local growth of the tumour is rapid, however, the early spread is common because of the rich lymphatic supply found in the oesophagus. Tumours are characteristically intraluminal and ulcerating. With a tendency to encircle the oesophageal wall, as well as extend upon down the length. The spread of cancer is by local invasion or through the blood stream or lymphatics. Neoplasm of the upper and middle oesophagus may extend into the pulmonary system and those of the lower oesophagus into the diaphragm, vertebral or heart.

The common clinical manifestation of oesophageal cancer are as follows:

- Early disease is largely asymptomatic.
- Gradually progressive dysphagia.
- Odynophagia-typically steady, dull, substernal pain.
- Regurgitation- foul breath, from retained food in oesophagus.
- Heartburn, anorexia, weight loss.

The on set of symptoms is usually late in relation to the extent of the tumour. Progressive *dysphagia* is the most common symptom and may be expressed as a substernal feeling as if food is not passing. Initially the dysphagia occurs only with meat, then soft foods and eventually with liquids. *Pain* develops late and it is described as occurring in the substernal, epigastric, or back areas and usually increases with swallowing. The pain may radiate to the neck, jaw, ears, and shoulders. If the tumour is in upper third of oesophagus symptoms such as sore throat, choking, and hoarseness may occur. Weight loss is fairly common. When oesophageal stenosis is severe, regurgitation of blood-flecked oesophageal contents is common.

The complication of the oesophageal cancer will include the following.

- Haemorrhage may occur if the cancer erodes through the oesophagus and into the aorta.
- Oesophageal perforation with fistual formation into the lung or trachea may develop.
- Oesophageal obstruction due to enlargement of the tumour.

Diagnostic Studies

- Barium swallow with fluoroscopy may demonstrate a narrowing of the oesophagus at the site of tumour. Creater may be visible.
- Oesophagoscopy with biopsy is necessary to make a definitive diagnosis of carcinoma by identification of malignant cells.
- Endoscopy-ultrasonography is also used to detect tumour invasion to muscle layer.
- Bronchoscopic examination may be performed to detect malignant involvements of the trachea.
- Computerized tomography scanning and magnetic resonance imaging are also used to assess the extent of disease.

Management

Treatment of oesophageal cancer are based on the location and size of the tumour, degree of metastasis and the individual health status.

Non-surgical options are usually selected where the individual is unable or unwilling to undergo radical surgery. Surgery may not be performed if the patient is an older adult or in poor physical health. Palliative therapy consists of restoratioan of the swallowing function and maintenance of nutrition and hydration. Dilation, stent replacement or both can relieve obstruction. Laser therapy or vaporization with *neodymium, yttrium aluminium-garnet* (-Nd:YAG) by means of endoscopy may be used in combination with dilation. Dilation is done with various types of dilators (celestin tube) to relieve dysphagia and allows for improved nutrition. Placement of a stent or prosthesis may help when dilation is no longer effective. The prosthesis are composed of silicone rubber or nylon-reinforced latex tubes with distal and proximal cellars.

Radiation therapy is the treatment of choice for palliation. It reduces tumour size and gives consistent long-term symptom relief. But it may lead to debilitating stricture or stenosis because oesophageal tissue is extremely sensitive to radiation. The best results of oesophageal cancer treatment have been obtained by the surgery and radiation.

Radical surgery is the only definitive treatment of oesophageal cancer. The types of surgical procedures that can be performed are:

- *Oesophagectomy*: Removal of part or all of the oesophagues with the use of a dacrongraft to replace the resected pain.
- *Oesophagogastrostomy*: Resection of a portion of the oesophagus and anastomosis of the remaining portion of the oesophagus.
- *Oesophagoenterostomy*: Resection of a portion of the oesophagus and anastomosis of a segment of colon to the remaining portion.

After surgery parenteral fluids are given. When fluids are allowed after bowel sounds have returned 30 to 60 ml water are given hourly with gradual progression to small, frequent, bland meals. The patient should be in an upright position to prevent regurgitation of the fluid. The patient is observed for signs of intolerance to the feeding or leakage of the feeding into the mediastinum. Symptom of leakage (pain, temperature, dyspnoea) and food intolerance (vomiting and abdominal distension) should be monitored and suitable measures to be taken accordingly.

GASTRITIS AND DYSPEPSIA

Gastritis, an inflammation of the gastric mucosa, is one of the most problems affecting the stomach. The terms gastritis and dyspepsia are used in a highly non-specific manner by both lay persons and health care professionals. *Gastritis* refers to a diffuse of localized response of the gastric mucosa to injury or infection. The *dyspepsia* refers to a symptom complex of fullness, heartburn, bloating and possibly nausea that is typically experienced after eating and may not be accompanied to any histological changes in the stomach or duodenum.

Dyspepsia Syndrome

Dyspepsia syndrome: is a syndrome of chronic dyspepsia, one of the most common GI complaints encountered in primary practice. The person experiences persistent or recurrent discomfort centered in the upper abdomen. There is no evidence of structural or biochemical abnormality and the cause is unknown. Study findings to date indicate that individual with dyspepsia syndrome have:

- Normal rates of acid secretion.
- Post-prondial hypomotility and delayed gastric emptying, and 25 to 50 per cent cases. Cause is unknown.
- Increased sensitivity of gastric distention, cause is unknown.
- No identified link with life stress or personality profiles.

Symptoms

- Epigastric discomfort or pain.
- Feeling of fullness or flatulence.
- Early satiety.
- Bloating or nausea.

Treatment of Dyspepsia Syndrome

There is no approved drug treatment, but

- Histamine receptor antagonists may be used for ulcer-like pain.
- Antacids may be used for occasional heartburn or bloating syndrome.
- Prokinetic agents (Cispride) are helpful in many cases.
- Diet and lifestyle changes are suggested will include:
  - Reducing dietary fat (it prolongs digestion, worsen bloating).
  - Avoiding foods that precipitate symptoms.

Gastritis may be acute or chronic and may be diffused or localized.

ACUTE GASTRITIS

Aetiology of Acute Gastritis

Acute gastritis is short-term inflammatory process that can be initiated by numerous factors such as excess alcohol ingestion, drug effects. aspirin, NSAID, corticosteroids, etc.) severe physical stress or trauma, ingestion of caustic noxious substances, and bacterial contaminated water or food (staphylococcus, salmonella or staphylococci).

Pathophysiology

Acute gastritis develops when the protective mechanism of the mucosa are overwhelmed by the presence of bacteria or irritating substances. In other words, gastritis occurs as the result of

Table 7.4: Nursing care plan for the patient with cancer of the esophagus treated by surgery

Problem	*R*	*Objective*	*Nursing interventions*	*Rationales*
Nursing Diagnosis #1 Alteration in cardiac output: decreased, related to: 1. Altered hemodynamics associated with thoracic/abdominal surgery. *Nursing Diagnosis#2* Alteration in tissue perfusion: cardiopulmonary.		Patient will: 1. Maintain presurgical cardiovascular function as manifested by: A. Stable haemodynamics. • Blood pressure within 10 mmHg of baseline. • Heart rate < 100 beats/minute. • Cardiac output ~5 liters/minute. • CVP: 0-8 mmHg. • CWP: 8-12 mmHg. B. Absence of: Extreme weakness or fatigue, peripheral oedema, neck vein distention or chest pain. C. Absence of cardiac dysrhythmias.	• Perform ongoing cardiovascular assessment: ◆ Continuous cardiac monitoring, Establish baseline rate, rhythm and ectopy. ◆ Continuous haemodynamic monitoring when indicated. Establish baseline CVP and PCWP measurements. ◆ Auscultate lungs q 4 hr. ◆ Auscultate heart sounds•-presence of S3. ◆ Assess for fatigue, neck vein distention? sacral oedema? ◆ Monitor arterial blood gases.	• Chest surgery may cause cardiac irritability. Many patients develop atrial fibrillation. This dysrhythmia may decrease cardiac output by 20-30 per cent. ◆ Rales (crackles) are an indication of fluid overload. ◆ Diagnostic sign for congestive heart failure.
		2. Maintain intact neurological status: • Mental status: Alert and oriented.	• Perform neurological assessment. ◆ Level of consciousness. ◆ Behaviour.	• Compromised haemodynamics and hypoxemia predispose to cerebral hypoxia with altered cerebral function.
		3. Maintain fluid and electrolyte balance. • Stable body weight. • Balanced intake and output. • Hourly urine output >30 cc/hr.	• Assess fluid and electrolyte status. ◆ Daily weight. ◆ Intake and output with hourly urine outputs. ◆ Serum electrolytes, BUN, creatinine.	• Reduced blood volume will further compromise venous return and cardiac output; blood volume may need to be expanded with use of colloids or fluids. ◆ Reduced cardiac output may diminish renal perfusion, placing patient at risk of developing acute renal failure.
Nursing Diagnosis #3 Impaired gas exchange, related to: 1. Pulmonary congestion associated with surgical manipulation of intrathoracic structures and altered by lymphatic drainage. 2. Atelectasis.		Patient will: 1. Maintain effective respiratory function: • Rate <25/minute • Rhythm eupneie. • Breath sounds clear on auscultation. • Mental status: Alert and oriented. • Usual skin colour. • Arterial blood gases at baseline.	• Monitor and report signs and symptoms of altered respiratory function: ◆ Presence of rapid, shallow, or irregular respirations; dyspnoea, orthopnea; use of accessory muscles. ◆ Presence of adventitious breath sounds on auscultation. ◆ Presence of restlessness, irritability, confusion, or somnolence. ◆ Presence of dusky red, mottled, or cyanotic skin colour. • Monitor arterial blood gas values and report abnormal results. • Monitor pulse oximetry. Obtain ABGs for saturation of haemoglobin. • Monitor haemoglobin/haematocrit.	• Monitors the oxygen saturation of available haemoglobin. • Anaemia provokes tissue hypoxia.

Contd...

Contd...

Problem	*R*	*Objective*	*Nursing interventions*	*Rationales*
			• Implement measures to maintain adequate respiratory function: ◆ Maintain semi-Fowler's position. ◆ Maintain prescribed O_2 therapy and monitor resposne. ◆ Encourage coughing and deep breathing q 1-2 hr. ◆ Assist in turning q 2 hr. ◆ Instruct to splint incision when coughing. ◆ Encourage use of pain medication as prescribed and monitor response.	◆ Due to extent of surgery, patient will "guard" incision, which leads to decreased lung expansion, atelectasis and poor gas exchange.
Nursing Diagnosis #4 Alteration in bowel elimination, related to: 1. Surgical trauma, stress, and enteral tube feedings.		Patient will: 1. Regain peristaltie activity and presurgical bowel function.	• Maintain nasogastric tube to low suction. Irrigate with 30 cc normal saline solution q 4 hr or as prescribed.	• Maintains patency and prevents gastric distention which may cause stress to suture line and lead to an anastomotic leak.
			◆ Do not reposition or reinsert	◆ The tube is placed during surgery. Care must be taken to avoid harm to the anastomosis. Physician will determine benefit risk, and method of replacement.
			• Assess for presence of abdominal distention and auscultale for bowel sounds every shift.	• Distention may indicate malfunctioning NG and stress to the anastomosis. • Bowel sounds indicate that the intestines have regained peristaltic activity.
			• Inquire as to the presence or absence of flatulence. ◆ Encourage ambulation when indicated.	
			• Monitor daily intake and output, weight, and electrolyte balance.	• Fluid loss after gastrointestinal surgery may approach 2 liters or more. Fluid and electrolyte replacement may be required with the loss of large amounts of fluids.
			• Assess character and frequency of stool.	• Diarrhoea may result in wasting of Mg^{++} and Ca^{++}. Observe for muscle weakness or tetany.
Nursing Diagnosis #5 Impairment of skin integrity, related to: 1. Surgical incision with potential for impaired wound healing due to: A. Preoperative radiation therapy. B. Poor nutrition. C. Infection. 2. Irritation or breakdown related to: A. Contact of skin with wound drainage. B. Stress from drainage tubes. C. Use of tape.		Patient will: 1. Experience normal healing of surgical wounds.	• Position patient to reduce stress on suture lines.	
			• Maintain NG tube patency.	• Prevents gastric distention.
			• Splint wounds while coughing.	• Equalizes pressure to the wounds. Reduces the possibility of dehiscence.
			• Change dressings frequently and perform aseptic wound care. • Note type and amount of drainage. Obtain culture if indicated and monitor results.	• Minimizes skin irritation from drainage and prevents nosocomial infections.
			• Note drainage tube sites. Provide anchoring tape to prevent tensions or "pulling" at insertion sites. ◆ Consider use of Montgomery straps.	◆ Prevents skin abrasions due to frequent tape changes.
			• Monitor laboratory values for signs of anaemia, decreased albumin levels, or an increased leukocyte count.	• Anaemia will results in decreased oxygenation. Low albumin level: Indicates a decrease in the colloidal osmotic pressure, which will lead to oedema and interference with healing. A leukocytosis may indicate an infectious process.

Contd...

Contd...

Problem	*R*	*Objective*	*Nursing interventions*	*Rationales*
Nursing Diagnosis #6 Alteration in comfort level: pain, related to: 1. Surgical procedure.		Patient will: 1. Utilize measures effective in managing pain. 2. Verbalize pain relief. 3. Exhibit relaxed demeanor: • Relaxed facial expression and body posturing. • Ease of breathing.	• Determine pain "tolerance." Assess patient's willingness to use pain medication vs. stoic behaviour. • Assess for physical manifestations of pain. ◆ Restlessness, reluctance to move, guarding incision, clenched fist. ◆ Diaphoresis, rapid shallow breathing, tachycardia, hypertension. • Assess complaints of pain including severity, location/radiation, duration, and quality (i.e. sharp, dull, knifelike). • Collaborate with physician and patient in titrating pain medication as needed. • Suggest alternate position changes.	• Many people fear they will become addicted to narcotics.

a breakdown in the normal gastric mucosal barrier. This mucosal barrier normally potects the stomach tissue from autodigestion by acid and the enzyme pepsia. When the barrier is broken, acid can diffuse back into the mucosa. This allows hydrochloric acid (HCl) to enter. The HCL acid stimulates the conversion of pepsinogen to pepsin and stimulates the release of histamine from mast cells. The combined results of these occurrences is tissue oedema, disruption of capillary walls with loss of plasma into the gastric lumen and possible haermorrhage.

Regeneration of the gastric mucosa after injury is both prompt and efficient, however, and the disorder usually is self-limiting once the irritating agent is removed. The common symptoms of acute gastritis include anorexia, nausea, and vomiting, abdominal cramping or diarrhoea, epigastric pain and fever. Painless GI bleeding, may occur and in persons using aspirin and NSAIDs.

Management

Acute gastritis cases are managed by removing the causative agent and supporting the patient while the mucosa heals itself. The person is usually put on nothing by mouth (NPO) status to support healing of the mucosa and then slowly advanced to liquids and a return to a normal diet. antacids and histamine 2 (H_2) receptor antagonists may be administered to reduce acid secretion and increase comfort. Temporary IV fluid and electrolyte replacement may be indicated in severe cases and the patient is monitored carefully for signs of bleeding.

The nurse also should give health instruction to prevent bacterial food-borne illness and concerning safe good handling and preparation. The nurse will educate the individual and family to take general measures to prevent food-related illness as follows:

- Wash hands before handling food.
- Do not thaw foods in the kitchen counter.
- Keep meats, fish, poultry, mayonnaise and cream-filled food, refrigerated.
- Wash hands and utensils after contact with raw meat or poultry.
- Never leave perishable foods unrefrigerated for more than 2 hours- less in hot weather.
- Use a meat thermometer when cooking large pieces of meat especially pork.
- Stuff poultry immediately before roasting (warm stuffing is a good medium for bacterial growth.
- Avoid slow cooling of meat and poultry.
- Freeze or refrigerate leftovers promptly.
- Can low-acid food (foods other than tomatoes or fruits) under pressure to prevent botulism.
- Discard any can that bulges.

CHRONIC GASTRITIS

Gastritis can occur from reflux of bile salts from the duodenum into the stomach as a result of anatomical changes following surgical procedures such as gastroduodenostomy and gastrojejunostomy. Prolonged vomiting may also cause reflux of bile salts, inflammation of the mucosal lining as a result of hypersecretion of HCL acid. The chronic gastritis can result from repeated episodes of acute gastritis.

Pathophysiology

Chronic gastritis is a separate clinical entity that can be further subdivided into Type A and Type B. Its presence is usually a sign of some underlying disease process.

- Type A is believed to be autocimmune in nature and involves all of the acid-secreting gastric tissue, particularly the tissue in the fundus. Circular antibodies are produced that attack the gastric parietal cells and eventually may cause pernicious anaemia from loss of the intrinsic factor.
- Type B is related to the presence of helicobacter pylori (H-pylori). It primarily involves the antrum of the stomach. There is less reduction in the acid secretions, gastrin levels remain normal, and vitamin B_{12} absorption is rarely impaired. As the condition progresses, the mucosa increasingly atrophies, and acid secretion is reduced. The presence of

H. pylori has been correlated with the presence of other gastric disorders including gastric and duodenal ulcer and gastric cancer.

The clinical manifestation of chronic gastitis are similar to those described for acute gastritis. In addition eventually the body's storage of cobalmin (B_{12}) in the liver is depleted and a deficiency state exists. Lack of this leads to important vitamins which is essential for the growth and development of RBC result in development of anaemia, i.e., cobalmin deficiency anaemia.

Diagnostic studies include endoscopic examination with biopsy. Breath, urine, serum or gastric tissue biopsy tests are available for the determination of H. pylori. CBC for presence of anaemia, gastric analysis for presence of HCl acid and stool test for occult blood. Cytologic examination of carcinoma.

Management

The treatment of chronic gastritis focuses on evaluating and eliminating the specific cause (e.g. cessaction of alcoholic intake abstinence from drugs), currently double and triple antibiotic combinations are used to eradicate infection with H.pylori. Original triple therapy consists of tetracycline + metronidaole + bismuth sub-salicylate × 14 days. New triple therapy includes amoxcilin + clarithromycin + omeprozole × 7 days.

For the patient with pernicious anaemia, regular injection of cobalmin (vit. B_{12}) are needed. An individualized bland diet and use of antacids are recommended.

UPPER GASTROINTESTINAL BLEEDING

Upper gastrointestinal bleeding is serious problem. The severity of bleeding depends on whether the origin is venous, capillary or arterial. The bleeding may be obvious or occult.

An *obvious bleeding* are:

- *Haematemesis* refers to bloody vomitus appearing as fresh, bright red blood or 'coffee ground' appearance (dark, grain-digested blood).
- *Melena* refers to a black, tarry stools (often foul smelling) caused by digestion of blood in the GI tract. The black appearance is from the presence of iron.
- *Occult bleeding* refers to small amount of blood in gastric secretions. Vomitus or stools not apparent by appearance detectable by guaiac test.

Bleeding from arterial source is profuse and the blood is bright red. It indicates that blood has not been contacted with gastric secretions. In contrast 'coffee ground' vomitus reveals that the blood and other contents have been in the stomach and have been changed by contact with gastric secretions. A massive upper GI bleeding is generally defiend as a loss of more than 1500 ml of blood of 25 per cent of intravascular blood volume.

Aetiology

The common causes of upper gastrointestinal bleeding includes:

- Drug induced: Some medications prescribed are self-administered and prolonged use causes bleeding which includes salicylates, corticosteroids, NSAIDS.
- Chronic oesophagitis, Mallory-Weiss tear or syndrome, or oesophageal varices, leads to upper GI bleeding.
- Peptic ulcer disease, stress ulcer, haemorrhagic gastritis, Ca. Polyps.
- Systemic diseases such as blood dyscrasiasis, leukaemea and uramea.

Management

As the nurse begins care of the patient admitted with upper GI bleeding, a thorough and accurate assessment is made by taking important health informatioan including past health history. Use of medication as mentioned in the aetiology and observe for signs of fever, shock, etc. Sometimes, patient experiencing upper GI bleeding may not be able to provide specific information about the cause of bleeding until the immediate physical needs are met.

An immediate nursing assessment should be performed while getting the patient ready for initial treatment. The assessment should include the patient's level of consciousness, vital signs, appearance of neck veins, skin colour, and capillary refill. The abdomen should be checked for distension, guarding and peristalsis. Immediate determination of vital signs indicate whether the patient is in shock from blood loss and also provides a baseline blood pressure and pulse by which to monitor the progress of treatment. Signs and symptoms of shock include, low blood pressure, rapid, weak pulse increased thirst, cold, clammy skin, and restlessness. Vital signs should be monitored every 15 to 30 minutes and concerned doctor should be informed of any significant changes. treatment of shock should be initiated promptly.

The patient should be approached in a calm and assured manner to help decrease the level of anxiety. Once an infusion has been started, the IV Line must be maintained for fluid or blood replacement. An accurate intake and output record is essential so that the patient's hydration status can be assessed. When the NG tube is inserted, the nurse pays her attention to keep it in proper position and observing the aspirate for blood. Care of nasogastric tube to be taken promptly.

Antacids are sometiems used after upper GI bleeding to reduce the acidity of gastric content. Anticipating the effect of prescribed preparations can be helped in providing better care. The expected outcomes of such bleeding cases will

- Have no further GI bleeding.
- Have the cause of the bleeding identified and treated.
- Experience a return to a normal haemodynamic stage.
- Experience minimal or no symptom of pain or anxiety.

Table 7.5: Nursing care plan for the patient with acute upper gastrointestinal haemorrhage and hypovolemic, haemorrhagic shock

Problem	*R*	*Objective*	*Nursing interventions*	*Rationales*
Nursing Diagnosis#1 Fluid volume deficit, actual, related to: 1. Acute blood loss•- haematemesis, haematochezia. 2. Gastric drainage (continuous).		Patient will: 1. Maintain an effective circulating blood volume and stable haemodynamic functions: • Heart rate (resting) <100 beats/min. • Central venous pressure 0-8 mmHg. • Pulmonary artery pressure <25 mmHg. • Pulmonary capillary wedge pressure 8-12 mmHg. • Cardiac output ~5 liters/min. • Systemic arterial blood pressure within 10 mmHg of baseline, without orthostatic hypotension. 2. Remain alert, and oriented to person, place and time, without weakness and dizziness. 3. Maintain urine output >30 ml/hour. 4. Remain without signs of rebleeding: • No haematemesis; haematochezia. • Gastric aspirate blood-free. 5. Maintain body weight within 5 per cent of baseline. 6. Balance intake with output. 7. Exhibit good skin turgon moist mucous membranes; minimal thrist. 8. Maintain laboratory parameters within acceptable physiological range: • Haematocrit 37-52 per cent. • Haemoglobin 12-18 g/100 ml. • RBC and WBC counts. • BUN, electrolytes, calcium.	• Assess for signs and symptoms of hypovolemic, haemorrhagic shock: ♦ Observe for signs of acute or subacute haemorrhage; haematemesis, haematochezia; melena; abdominal distention, epigastric pain.	• A baseline assessment is necessary to establish the stage of shock-initial compensatory, progressive or final, and emergent measures indicated; it serves as a measure of the patient's response to therapy. (See Chapter 46 for a discussion of hypovolemic haemorrhagic shock, including the stages of shock.)
			♦ Assess cardiovascular function: – Hypotension (orthostatic).	♦ A drop in blood pressure of 10-15 mmHg from supine to sitting position suggests blood loss of ~1 liter.
			– Resting pulse >100 beats/min. Characteristics-faint, rapid, thready.	♦ Blood loss and enhanced peripheral vaso-constriction underlie diminished to absent pulses, coolness of the extremities, and pallor of conjunctiva, mucous membranes and nailbeds.
			– Skin colour-pallor, cyanosis; skin temperature; delayed capillary refill time (>3 sec.)	
			– Signs of dehydration–poor skin turgor; weakness, fatigue.	♦ Skin turgor is best assessed over forehead or sternum.
			– Cardiac monitoring: rate and rhythm.	♦ Reflect effect of blood loss on cardiac function.
			• Assess renal function: ♦ Urine output > 30 ml/hour.	• Reduced circulating blood volume and hypotensive state compromises renal perfusion. The consequent reduction in glomerular filtration underlies the reduced urine1 output associated with hypovolemic shock.
			• Establish baseline abdominal assessment data: ♦ Presence or absence of bowel sounds (timing and characteristics).	
			♦ Pain and tenderness (location, radiation, quality, severity, duration).	♦ Abdominal pain with muscle guarding and rebound tenderness is highly suggestive of peptic ulcer perforation, especially if preceded by an episode of severe abdominal pain, followed by sudden, but temporary relief, in patients at risk.
			♦ Hepatomegaly, ...	♦ Suggestive of elrrhosis with portal hypertension.
			♦ Abdominal mass or bruit.	♦ Questionable abdominal aneurysm.
			• Insert at least one, or more (if bleeding is massive) large gauge angiocatheters for rapid administration of blood and blood products, volume expanders, and fluids (Ringer's lactate, and normal saline).	• A single peripheral intravenous catheter may not be sufficient to provide adequate blood replacement in a profusely bleeding patient.
			♦ Obtain blood samples for baseline laboratory data.	

Contd...

Contd...

Problem	R	Objective	Nursing interventions	Rationales
				◆ A central venous line or pulmonary artery catheter is indicated to closely monitor the patient's response to volume replacement:
			• Monitor Hct, Hgb; RBC, WBC counts; electrolytes, serum calcium; blood glucose levels.	• In patients bleeding profusely, there may be insufficient time for the blood volume to equilibrate. Thus, Hct and Hgb may not be reliable indicators of the patient's status. In such patients, changes in blood pressure and pulse are better indicators for replacement of blood and blood products.
				◆ Rapid fluid shifts during GI bleeding, and subsequent infusion of blood, blood products and other fluids, require frequent assessment of serum electrolytes-sodium, potassium, chloride, bicarbonate, and serum calcium. The serum calcium level may become depressed after several units of anticoagulate (cltrate)-containing blood have been administered.
			◆ Monitor BUN and creatinine levels.	◆ Metabolism of blood by intestinal bacteria, coupled with compromised liver perfusion, causes the BUN level to rise. – A rising BUN in the presence of a normal creatinine is highly indicative of a massive upper GI bleed.
			◆ Obtain blood samples for type and cross-match.	◆ Even in acute emergencies, there is usually sufficient time to type and cross-match blood for infusion properly. This reduces the incidence of blood incompatibility and transfusion reactions.
			◆ Monitor prothrombin time, clotting factors, fibrin degradation products.	◆ Patients receiving massive fluid and blood replacement therapy are at risk of developing a dilutional coagulopathy; patients with profuse haemorrhaging are at high risk of developing consumptive congulopathles (e.g., disseminated intravascular coagulation, DIC).
			• Initiate aggressive infusion of electrolytes, and volume expanders until blood is ready for administration.	
			• Insert nasogastric tube:	• To decompress the stomach and assist (in conjunction with endoscopy) in determining site, amount, and rate of bleeding); to test gastric aspirate for blood, and pH; and to administer antacids, iced saline lavage (as prescribed).

Contd...

Contd...

Problem	*R*	*Objective*	*Nursing interventions*	*Rationales*
			• Check for tube placement:	• Inadvertent placement of the nasogastric tube into the respiratory passage is always a potential complication of this procedure.
			◆ Auscultate over the gastric area while injecting 50 ml air into the nasogastric tube.	◆ A rush of air should be heard if the tube is properly placed.
			• Assess gastric aspirate: ◆ Presence of fresh blood, or a large amou-nt of old blood (coffee-ground material) are indications for gastric lavage.	• Removal of as much clot and intragastric material as possible is important; it assists in evaluating continuous bleeding; an empty stomach will allow the walls to collapse and may contribute to haemostasis.
			• Implement gastric lavage as prescribed.	• Irrigation with iced saline causes vasoconstriction of bleeding vessels; the efficacy of this treatment has yet to be substantiated.
			◆ Maintain patency of tube by irrigation and repositioning if necessary.	◆ Use saline rather than water for lavage to minimize saline depletion via gastric mucosa.
			• Maintain the patient NPO, and implement continuous gastric suction, as prescribed. ◆ Monitor amount and characteristics of gastric drainage. • Maintain a strict intake and output. ◆ Include amount of fluid lavaged, and that removed via gastric suction. ◆ Document amount and characteristics of any emesis.	• Continuous gastric suctioning enables close monitoring of bleeding; it minimizes the amount of blood passing into the intestine; where the action of the intestinal bacteria metabolizes blood to ammonia.
			• Provide comfort measures:	
			◆ Provide quiet, calm environment with frequent rest periods; minimize stimull.	◆ To promote physical and mental rest; stimulation may provoke vomiting, bleeding.
			◆ Provide mouth care with oral suctioning as necessary.	◆ Aspiration is a potential complication.
			◆ Secure tube to patient's gown with adeauate sluck.	◆ This prevents tugging on tube when patient moves, which can injured nose.
			◆ Lubricate nares; assess nares for pressure areas caused by nasogastric tube.	
			◆ Monitor body temperature. – Provide extra blankets if appropriate.	◆ Continuous Iced saline lavage can lower body temperature.
			• Transfuse blood and blood products as prescribed. ◆ Consider unit procedure and protocols for: – Administering blood therapy. – Monitoring patient's response to blood therapy. – Recognizing early signs of adverse effects and transfusion reactions. – Procedure to follow in the event of transfusion reaction.	• See Tables 49-2, 49-3, and 49-4 for nursing care considerations, precautions, and summary of adverse reactions (respectively) in the administration of blood and blood products.
			• Insert Foley catheter to measure hourly urine output.	• Hourly urine outputs assist in monitoring renal perfusion and function.
			• Assist with insertion of haemodynamic pressure monitoring lines.	• Insertion of systemic arterial and pulmonary artery flotation (Swan-Ganz) catheters are indicated in the setting of massive upper GI haemorrhage, and massive blood and fluid replacement therapy.

Contd...

Contd...

Problem	*R*	*Objective*	*Nursing interventions*	*Rationales*
			◆ Monitor haemodynamics: arterial, and pulmonary artery pressures-CVP, pulmonary artery and pulmonary capillary wedge pressures (PCWP); and cardiac output. • Monitor hydration status during fluid replacement therapy.	◆ PCWP i a useful parameter for monitoring for fluid overload, a potential complication of massive, aggressive fluid replacement therapy.
			◆ Assess respiratory function: respiratory rate and rhythm; presence of adventitious sounds.	◆ The detection of rales in previously clear lungs suggest possible overhydration.
			◆ Assess signs/symptoms of fluid overload. ◆ Monitor daily weight.	◆ Should be maintained within 5 per cent of baseline.
			• Assist with insertion of Sengstaken-Blake-more tube in setting of persistent varical bleeding.	
Nursing Diagnosis #2 Gas exchange impaired: Ventilation/perfusion imbalance, related to: 1. Reduced circulating volume and compromised haemodynamics.		Patient will: 1. Be alert and oriented to person, place, time. 2. Exhibit appropriate behaviour. 3. Maintain effective cardiovascular function: • Blood pressure within 10 mmHg of baseline. • Cardiac output:~5 liters/min. 4. Maintain arterial blood gas parameters within acceptable physiological range: • pH 7.35-7.45 • PaO_2 > 60 mmHg • $PaCO_2$ 35-45 mm Hg 5. Maintain hematologic values within acceptable range. • Hematocrit 37-52 per cent. • Haemoglobin 12-18 g/100 ml. • Red blood cell count.	• Perform neurological assessment. ◆ Mental status; orientation to person, place, time; level of consciousness; appropriateness of responses/behaviour.	• Hypoxaemia coupled with hypovolemic shock can predispose to cerebral tissue hypoxia.
			• Monitor cardiovascular function: ◆ Cardiac dysrhythmias.	◆ Hypoxaemia is commonly associated with myocardial irritability.
			◆ Tachycardia; rapid, thready peripheral pulses.	◆ Commonly associated with blood loss, and consequent reduced circulating blood volume and peripheral vasoconstriction.
			◆ Cyanosis.	◆ Late sign reflecting desaturation of at least 5 gm/100 ml of haemoglobin; commonly associated with ventilation/perfusion mismatch, and right to left shunting.
			• Monitor respiratory function: ◆ Respiratory rate and pattern, breath sounds: normal and adventitious breath sounds.	◆ Presence of rales (crackles) may be indicative of fluid overload.
			◆ Arterial blood gases: pH, PaO_2, $PaCO_2$; alveolar-arterial gradient ($AaDO_2$).	◆ Most closely reflect effectiveness of gas exchange.
			◆ Monitor haematologic profile: haematocrit, haemoglobin, red blood cell count.	◆ Reflects haemoglobin oxygen-carrying capacity within blood; reduced haemoglobin levels can compromise oxygen delivery to tissues.
			• Administer prescribed humidified oxygen therapy. ◆ Monitor arterial blood gas and haematologic parameter as indicated.	• Tissue hypoxia is a common consequence of hypovolemic, haemorrhagic shock due to depleted blood volume, and reduced number of RBCs.
			◆ Provide frequent rest periods. ◆ Evaluate effectiveness of oxygen therapy: assess neurological function and vital signs.	◆ To reduce oxygen demand by tissues.
Nursing Diagnosis #3 Anxiety, related to: 1. Acute upper gastrointestinal haemorrhage (haematemesis). 2. Abdominal pain. 3. Transfusion therapy.		Patient will: 1. Verbalize feeling less anxious. 2. Demonstrate relaxed demeanor. 3. Perform relaxation techniques with assistance.	For specific nursing interventions and their rationales, please see related nursing diagnosis appeared in earlier or carring chapters.	

Contd...

Contd...

Problem	*R*	*Objective*	*Nursing interventions*	*Rationales*
4. Intensive care setting.		4. Verbalize familiarity with ICU routines and protocols.		
Nursing Diagnosis #4				
Comfort, alteration in epigastric pain, related to: 1. Enhanced gastric acidity. 2. Reflex muscle spasm.		Patient will: 1. Verbalize pain relief. 2. Exhibit relaxed demeanor: • Relaxed facial expression and body posturing. Gastric aspirate: pH > 4.5	• Assess complaints of pain including: severity: location/radiation; influencing factors (e.g., what precipitates, aggravates or ameliorates the pain?; what signs and symptoms are associated with the pain?). • Assess for nonverbal clues as to the presence of pain (e.g., restlessness, irritability, agitation, diaphoresis, tense facial features; rapid, shallow breathing). • Implement measures to reduce pain: ◆ Administer the following medications as prescribed:	• Use of the "SLIDT" tool assists in elicifing specific informatioan about the nature of the complaints.
			◆ Antacids.	◆ Antacids neutralize gastric acidity.
			◆ Histamine, antagonist—cimetidine (Tagamet) or ranitidine (Zanatac).	◆ Inhibit gastric acid secretion. The combination of antacids/histamine antagonist therapy is more efficacious than either therapy alone in reducing the harmful effects of acid and pepsin on the bleeding lesion.
			◆ Analgesics. – Encourage patient to request medication when pain is first perceived, rather than waiting until it becomes severe. – Evaluate the effectiveness of medication in relieving patient's pain.	
			◆ Mild sedation.	◆ It is absolutely essential to assist the patient to rest and relax, mentally and physically, to reduce danger of continued bleeding, or rebleeding.
			• Determine how patient usually copes with pain or stress: ◆ Pain tolerance. ◆ Willingness to discuss pain; or stoically "keeping it within." ◆ Willingness to use medication for pain. ◆ Behaviour used to reduce level of stress.	• Details elicited at this time regarding patient/family attitudes about pain and stress may help lay the foundation for patient/family educatiaon in this regard.
Nursing Diagnosis #5				
Nutritin, alteration in: less than body requirements, related to: 1. Maintenance on NPO with continuous gastric suctioning		Patient will maintain: 1. Body weigth within 5 per cent of baseline. 2. Total serum proteins 6.0-8.4 g/100 ml. 3. Laboratory data within acceptable physiological range: • BUN, serum creatinine. • Electrolytes, serum calcium.	• Consult with nutritionist in assessing overall nutritional status; and signs and symptoms of malnutrition. ◆ Major considerations: General state of health—weakness; body weight; physiological factors—age, height, triceps skin fold; mid-upper arm circumference; food intolerance; allergies. ◆ Laboratory data: BUN, serum creatinine; fasting blood glucose; serum electrolytes, total protein (serum albumin); cholesterol; transfusion levels, haematology profile.	• Catabolic state associated with critical illness rapidly depletes body stores of nutrients.

Contd...

Contd...

Problem	*R*	*Objective*	*Nursing interventions*	*Rationales*
		• Blood glucose levels. • Serum albumin 3.5-5.5 g/100 ml. • Haematology profile. 4. Triceps skinfold measurements within normal range.	• Maintain adequate nutrition with prescribed enteral and/or parenteral nutrition.	• The purpose of total parenteral nutrition (TPN) is to provide sufficient nutrients intravenously, to achieve anabolism, and to promote weight gain.
			◆ Order prescribed feeding from pharmacy.	◆ Solution should be prepared in pharmacy under a laminar airflow unit to minimize danger of contamination.
			◆ Assist with placement of TPN central intravenous catheter. – Explain purpose of parenteral therapy. – Explain procedure for insertion: ❑ Use of Trendelenburg position and valsalva maneouvre.	◆ Helps to avoid air embolism upon insertion.
			– Apply dressing. – Prepare patient for chest x-ray.	◆ To confirm correct placement of catheter and rule out potential pneumothorax.
			– Assess patient for signs and symptoms of respiratory distress: Dyspnoea, decreased breath sounds; chest pain; haematoma formation.	◆ Pneumothorax, haemothorax, air embolism, and sepsis are major complications.
			– Initiate prescribed parenteral feedings. ❑ Begin infusion at slow rate (60-80 ml/hour); increase infusion by 25 ml/day.	◆ Allows for physiological adjustments in pancreatic insulin secretion; helps to avoid glucose intolerance.
			❑ Use flow control device or pump to administer feeding. ❑ Weight patient daily; record intake and output. ❑ Monitor serum glucose; monitor for signs of hyperglycaemia (polyuria, glycosuria, elevated serum glucose).	◆ This helps to prevent fluid or glucose overload.
			❑ Wean from TPN therapy slowly.	◆ This avoids danger of hypoglycaemic reaction as pancreatic secretion of insulin is allowed to decline accordingly.
			• Ongoing monitoring/maintenance: ◆ Maintain catheter asepsis. Monitor body temperature at regular intervals and report any temperature elevation to physician, Follow unit protocol in obtaining specimens for culture and sensitivity.	◆ Consistent monitoring is necessary because there is no single febrile pattern associated with TPN sepsis. Temperature elevation may be low-grade, constant, or intermittent, or characterized by daily spiking.
			◆ Never use TPN catheter for anything other than parenteral feedings.	◆ If catheter is used as a central access line in an emergency, it should not be resued for TPN.
			◆ Provide catheter site care as per unit protocol.	◆ Cleansing of catheter site minimizes potential complications of sepsis, or mechanical disruption of catheter placement; it helps to preserve skin integrity at insertion site.
Nursing Diagnosis #6 Infection, potential for, related to:		Patient will: 1. Maintain body temperature within acceptable physiological range.	For specific nursing interventions and their rationales, see other chapters included similar nursing diagnosis in nursing care plan.	

Contd...

Contd...

Problem	*R*	*Objective*	*Nursing interventions*	*Rationales*
1. Invasive procedures. 2. Malnutrition.		• ~98.6°F (37°C). 2. Maintain white blood count: • 5000-10,000/mm³. 3. Remain without signs and symptoms of infection; urine free of infection.		
Nursing Diagnosis# 7				
Sleep pattern disturbance, related to: 1. Frequent interruption for assessment and treatments. 2. Intensive care environment and protocols. 3. Psychologic stress.		Patient will: 1. Verbalize underlying concerns regarding inability to sleep. 2. Verbalize familiarity with ICU protocols and environmental stimuli. 3. Assist in planning for undisturbed rest periods within the constraints of ongoing monitoring and essential patient care. 4. Report a sense of well-being and restfulness.	• Assess sleep pattern and difficulty sleeping: ◆ Encourage patient to verbalize concerns regarding sleeplessness. ◆ Monitor the amount of time the patient is sleeping or napping. – Identify times and circumstances during which sleep seems most restful. – Identify factors particularly disturbing to the patient. – Observe for signs and symptoms of fatigue, restlessness, apprehension.	• To minimize bleeding and prevent rebleeding, it is essential to provide a clinical milieu that is as calm and quiet as possible, and conductive to patient rest and relaxation.
			• Administer prescribed medications for pain and sedation. ◆ Monitor effectiveness of medications in relieving pain, and relaxing the patient.	• Pain and anxiety undermine efforts to rest and relax.
			• Provide comfort measures: ◆ Include personal hygiene; back massage, position changes. ◆ Minimize room noise; dim lighting during rest periods (if possible); maintain comfortable room temperature.	• Comfort measures aid muscle relaxation.
			• Assist patient to establish a pattern conducive to sleep. ◆ Explain ICU protocols and procedures. ◆ Encourage patient to verbalize feelings; provide an attentive, listening ear.	◆ Understanding what to expect, and what is expected of the patient, may help to relieve concerns and apprehension.
			◆ Stay with patient at times that are especially stressful. ◆ Provide reassurance.	◆ Demonstration of caring, concern, and acceptance may be reassuring to patient.
			◆ Allow patient to make some decisions regarding his/her care (e.g., when to rest; or when to have visitors).	◆ Enables patient to assume responsibility for some aspects of overall care.
Nursing Diagnosis #8				
Fear, related to: 1. Possibility of bleeding to death.		Patient will: 1. Verbalize fear of dying. 2. Verbalize knowledge of clinical status and proposed course of therapy. 3. Demonstrate behaviours indicative of lessened fear (e.g., relaxed facies and posture).	• Assess degree of fear and patient's perceptions as to the reality of the possibility of dying. ◆ Encourage patient/family to discuss their perceptions and feelings regarding the patient's health status; to share subjective experiences. ◆ Observe nonverbal and verbal responses.	• An episode of massive upper GI haemorrhage can be perceived by patient/family as an imminent threat that the patient is going to bleed to death.
			◆ Assess for accompanying changes in patient's physiological status. – Vital signs	◆ Recognize that sympathetic response to fear may actually aggravate bleeding, and needs to be minimized.
			◆ Assess for accompanying changes in patient's psychological status. – Evidence of denial, anger, depression.	◆ These responses may assist patient/family to cope at least temporarily until patient/family have learned ways to reduce the threat.

Contd...

Contd...

Problem	*R*	*Objective*	*Nursing interventions*	*Rationales*
			• Assist patient/family to deal with fear: ◆ Stay with patient/family. ◆ Allow time for, and encourage expression of feelings and concerns. ◆ Assist patient/family to identify feelings. ◆ Clarify questions or misconceptions regarding illness or treatment.	
			• Assist patient/family to learn from this experience and to problem solve: ◆ Identify strength of family members, individually and collectively. ◆ Acknowledge usefulness of fear, denial, anger, in coping. ◆ Promote honest and open communication between family members. ◆ Involve patient/family in problem-solving and decision-making.	• Recognize that fear can be a motivating factor for learning only if the arousal of fear is accompanied by steps/actions to reduce the threat. ◆ Assists patient/family in coping; this may help to increase self-confidence in their own capabilities.
			• Referral to psychiatric liaison nurse and/or social worker as indicated, and/or requested by patient and/or family.	• Patient/family may feel reassured that other resources are available to lend assistance and support.

PEPTIC ULCER DISEASE (PUD)

Peptic ulcer is an erosion of the gastrointestinal (GI) mucosa resulting from the digestive action of hydrochloric acid (HCl) and pepsin. Any portion of the GI tract that comes into contact with gastric secretions is susceptible to ulcer development, including the lower oesophagus, stomach, duodenum and margin of gastrojejunal anastomasis after surgical procedure.

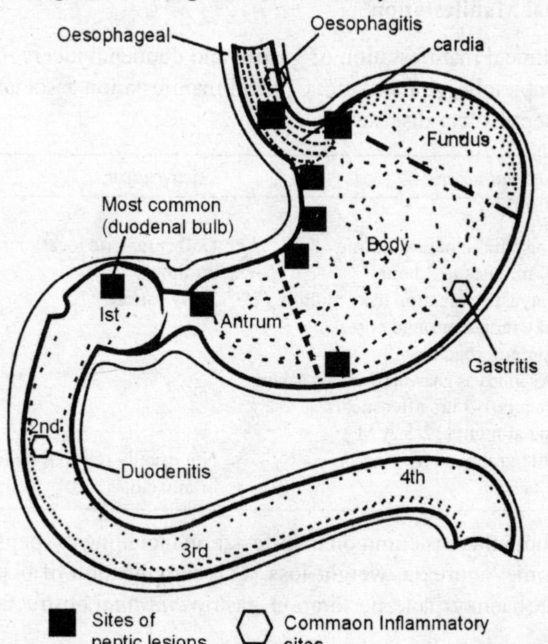

Fig. 7.1: The stomach is divided on the basis of its physiologic functions into two main portions. The proximal two thrids, the fundic gland area, acts as a receptacle for ingested food and secretes acid and pepsin. The distal third, the pyloric gland area, mixes and propels food into the duodenum and produces the hormone gastrin. "Peptic" lesions may occur in the esophagus (esophagitis), stomach (gastritis), or duodenum (duodenitis). Note peptic ulcer sites and common inflammatory sites.

Classification of PUD

Peptic ulcers can be classified as acute or chronic depending on the degree of mucosal involvement and gastric or duodenal according to the location.

i. The *acute ulcer* is associated with superficial erosion and minimal inflammation. It is of short duration and resolves quickly when the cause is identified and removed.
ii. A chronic ulcer is one of long duration, eroding through the muscular wall with the formatioan of fibrous tissue. It is present continuously for many months or intermittently throughout the person's life time. A chronic ulcer is at least four times as common as acute erosion.

Gastric and duodenal ulcer although defined as peptic ulcer are distinctly different in their aetiology and incidence, but generally treatment of all types of ulcer, is almost quite similar.

The differences between *Gastric* and *Duodenal ulcers* as given below.

Gastric ulcer	*Duodenal ulcer*
1. *Lesion*	
• Superficial; smooth margins round, oval, or cone shaped	• Penetrating (associated with deformity of duodenal bulb from healing of recurrent ulcers.
• Predominantly antrum, also in body and fundus of stomach.	• First 1-2 cm of duodenum.

Contd...

Gastric ulcer	*Duodenal ulcer*
2. *Gastric Secretion incidence*	
• Normal to decreased	• Increased.
– Greater in women	– Greater in men, but increasing in women in post-menopausal.
– Peak age fifth to sixth decade.	– Peak age 35-45 years.
– More common in persons of lower socio-economic status and in unskilled labourers.	– Associated with psychologic stress.
– Increased with smoking, drug and alcohol use.	– Increased with smoking, alcohol and drug use.
– Increased with incompetent pyloric spincter.	– Associated with other disease, e.g. COPD pancreatic disease hyperparathyroidism zollinger ellison syndrome, chronic renal failure.
– Increased with stress ulcers after severe burns, head trauma and major surgery.	
3. *Clinical manifestations*	
• Burning or gaseous pressure in high left epigastrium and back and upper abdomen.	• Burning, cramping, pressure like pain across midepigastrium and upper abdomen; backpain with posterior ulcers.
• Pain 1-2 hour after meals; if penetrating ulcer, aggravation of discomfort with food.	• Pain 2-4 hours after meals and midmorning, midafternoon, middle of night, periodic and episodic.
• Occasional nausea and vomiting, weight loss.	• Pain relief with antacids and food; occasional nausea and vomiting.
4. *Recurrence Rate complications*	
• High	• High
• Haemorrhage, perforation outlet obstruction, intractability.	• Haemorrhage, perforation obstruction.

Aetiology

Peptic ulcers were once believed to be the direct result of acid over secretion in response to stressful events. This assumption is reflected in the traditional treatment, approaches, which emphasized acid neutralization and acid reduction. Although it is true that ulcers will not develop in the absence of acid, it is increasingly apparent that the primary aetiological factors relate to:

- Infection by the organism Helicobacter Pylori (H.pylori) which produces a chronic gastritis:
- The *side effects* of NSAIDs administration.

These factors target the mucosal defenses of the stomach and duodenum and can eventually lead to ulceration. The other factors which are related: decreasing or increasing of gastrical secretions lead to peptic ulcer included in the page no 264, i.e. difference between gastric and duodenal ulcer.

Pathophysiology

The integrity of the gastric mucosa is maintained when a balance exists between the acid-secreting functions and mucosal protective functions of the stomach and duodenum. Peptic ulcers develop only in the presence of an acid environment. It has been well established that the patient with pernicious anaemia and achlorhydria rarely has gastric ulcers. An excess of gastric acid may not be necessary for ulcer development. The typical person with gastric ulcer has normal to less than normal gastric acidity compared with person with a duodenal ulcer. However, some intraluminal acid does seen to be essential for gastric ulcer to occur.

The stomach is normally protected from autodigestion by gastric mucosal barrier. Under specific circumstances, the mucosal barrier can be impaired and back-diffusion of acid can occur. When the barrier is broken, HCl acid freely enters the mucosa and causes injury to the tissue, this results in cellular destruction and inflammation. Histamine is released from the damaged mucosa, resulting in vasodilation and increased capillary permeability. The release of histamine is then capable of stimulating further secretion of acid and pepsin. Variety of agents are known to destroy the mucosal barrier, by generating ammonia in the mucus layer *H.pylori* may create a chromic inflammation. Ulcerogenic drugs inhibit synthesis of mucus, e.g. aspirin cause abnormal permeability, e.g. prostaglandin, decrease the rate of mucous renewal (Corticosteroids), and destroy the broncosal barrier (Cytotoxic drugs). When the mucosal barrier is disrupted, there is compensatory increase in blood flow. This phenomenon can occur in several ways.

Clinical Manifestation

The clinical manifestation of gastric and duodenal ulcers may be completely symptomatic. Clinical manifestation associated with peptic ulcer disease are:

Duodenal ulcer	*Gastric ulcer*
1. *Pain*	
• Episodic in nature lasting 30 minutes to 2 hours.	• Dull epigastric location near midline.
• Epigastric location near midline, may radiate around costal border to back.	• Early satiety.
• Described as gnawing, burning aching.	
• Occurs 1-3 hrs after meals and at night (12-3 A.M.)	
• Often relieved by food or antacid.	• Not usually relieved by food or antacid.

In both there is common manifestation including dyspepsia, syndrome, anorexia, weight loss. The complication of peptic ulcer are haemorrhage, perforation, gastrio *intestinal* obstruction.

Diagnostic Studies

The diagnostic measures used to determine the presence and location of peptic ulcers are:

- Complete blood count.
- Urinalysis
- Fibroptic endoscopy with biopsy.
- Upper GI barium-contrast study.

- Liver enzymes
- Gastric cytology.
- H-pylori testing of breath, urine, blood, stool.

Management

When the patient's clinical manifestations and health history suggest the diagnosis of a peptic ulcer and diagnostic studies confirm its presence, a medical regimen is instituted. The regimen consists of adequate rest, dietary modifications, medications, elimination of smoking and long-term follow-up-care.

- Adequate rest benefits the patient to elimination of stressors, help decrease the stimulus for overproduction of HCl acid.
- Dietary modification may be necessary so that foods and beverages irritating to the patient can be avoided or eliminated (alcohol & caffeine contents). A bland diet consisting of six small meals may be suggested.
- Smoking has an irritating effect on the mucosa, increases gastric motility, and delays mucosal healing. So it should be eliminated.
- Medications have major role in the treatment of peptic ulcers.
  - Antacids are weak bases that neutralize free hydrochloric acid to prevent irritation and permit mucosal healing.
  - Histamine receptor antagonists inhibit HCl secretion by binding to the H_2 receptor on stomach cells and blocking, the release of histamine which is a secretagogue for HCl. Gastrict emptying is unaffected by their use. Eg cimetedine, ranitidine, famotidine, nizatidine.
  - Bosom pump inhibitors more effective than H_2 receptor antagonists, e.g. omeprazole, lansoprasole, pantaprazole.
  - Mucosol protective agents, sucralfate, misoprostol.
  - Antibiotic therapy is instituted for patients verified with H. pylori.

The nurse has to teach the following points for the patient and family members for self-care management to the patients with peptic ulcer disease.

1. *Medication*
   - Know the dosage, administration, action and side effects of all drugs in use.
   - Take all the prescribed drugs, even when pain is relieved. It is essential to complete the full treatment.
   - Keep antacids available for use as needed, but do not take them at the same time as H_2 receptor antagonists. Antacids should be taken 1 to 3 hours after meals, at bed time and as needed for pain.
   - Avoid the use of over-the-counter H_2 receptor antagonists.
   - Use acetaminophen for routine pain relief during treatment if needed. Avoid the use of all NSAIDs including aspirin, ibuprofen.
   - If the treatment of arthritis or other chronic illness require the ongoing use of NSAIDS, explore the use of misoprostol with health care provider.
   - Know the symptoms of ulcer recurrence and report them promptly to the health care provider.
2. *Diet*
   - Eat three balanced meals a day.
   - Eat between meal snacks if this helps control pain.
   - Avoid bed time snacking because it increases night time acid secretion.
   - Eat slowly and chew food thoroughly. Do not overeat.
   - Avoid any foods that increase discomfort.
   - Avoid the use of alcohol during treatment if possible. Never drink alcohol on an empty stomach.
3. *Smoking*
   - Stop smoking if possible.
   - Explore community support for smoking cessation or use of nicotine withdrawal patches.
4. *Stress Reduction*
   - Participate in recreation and hobbies that promote relaxation.
   - Participate in a moderate aerobic exercise program for promotion of well-being.
   - Provide for increased rest during healing.

   And explain the importance of reporting of any of the following:
     - Increased nausea and/or vomiting.
     - Increase in epigastric pain
     - Bloody emesis or tarry stools.

The nursing care plan of patient with peptic ulcer disease is as follows (Table 7.5).

Surgical Management of Peptic Ulcer

When the medical therapy has been tried and proved unsuccessful the surgery is indicated. The following criteria are used as general indication for surgical intervention.

- Intractibility: failure of the ulcer to heal or recurrence of the ulcer after therapy.
- History of haemorrhage or increased risk of bleeding during treatment.
- Prepyloric or pyloric ulcers, both have high recurrence rates.
- Concurrent conditions, such as severe burns, trauma, or sepsis.
- Multiple ulcer sites.
- Drug-induced ulcers, especially when withdrawal from the drug may put the person at risk.
- Possible existence of a malignant ulcer.
- Obstruction.

Usually the surgical procedure performed to treat ulcer disease are partial gastrectomy, vagotomy or pyloroplasty.

i. *Partial gastrectomy* with removal of the distal two thirds of the stomach and anastomosis of the gastric stump to the duodenum is called "gastroduodenostomy" or Billroth's operation. Partial gastrectomy with removal of the distal two-thirds of the stomach and anastomosis of the gastric stump to the jejunum is called as "gastrojejunostomy" or Billroth's II operation. In both procedures the antrum and pylorus are removed, because the duodenum is bypassed. The Billroth's II operation is preferred to prevent recurrence of duodenal ulcers.

Table 7.5: Nursing care plan for patient with peptic ulcer

Problem	*Reason*	*Objective*	*Nursing intervention*	*Evaluation*
Pain R/T – Increased gastric secretion – Decreased mucosal protection – Ingestion of gastric irritants.	As manifested by burning cramp-like pain in epigastrium and abdomen. – Pain onset 1-2 hours after meals with gastric ulcer. – Pain onset 2-4 hours after meals.	Verbalization of satisfaction with pain control.	• Determine pain characteristics from verbal description and physical assessment data. • Administer antacids, H_2 antagonists, PP inhibition, anticholenergic, protective agents on prescribed to reduce pain. • Teach the patient to avoid smoking and ingesting spicy, hot or cold foods, coffee, tea, and cold drinks and alcoholic beverages to prevent increasing acid production. • Teach patients stress reduction as relaxation results in decrease acid products and reduction in pain.	(Write the responses and progress of ulcers)
Ineffective management of therapeutic regimen R/T – Lack of knowledge of management of peptic ulcer. – Not following treatment plan – Unwillingness to modify lifestyles.	As manifested by request question about home care, incorrect responses to questions about disease. Noncompliance with medical regimen.	Verbalization of plan to modify lifestyle and incorporate the rapeutic regimen into lifestyle.	• Explain ulcer disease process at patient level to faster understanding. • Help patient to identify stressors and initiate modification in daily routine as stress causes hypersecretion of HCl and pepsin which can alter mucosal barrier. • Discuss diet plan and assist with implementation at home and in work setting. • Explain rationale for the elimination of alcohol, spicy foods, coffee, tea and cola from diets. • Explain harmful effects of smoking which directly irritates gastric mucosa. • Inform patient what to do if symptoms related to ulcer recur to ensure early initiation of treatment.	
Pain related to acute exacerbation of disease process and inadequate comfort measures.	As manifested by verbalization of increase in pain, nonverbal indication of pain, e.g. moaning, crying, doubling up.	Expression of satisfaction with pain management.	• Encourage bed rest or light activity to conserve energy and promote comfort. • Provide quiet, relaxed environment and limit visitors to decrease stress and other factors that increase secretion. • Administer medication as ordered to relieve pain.	
Vomiting R/T acute exacerbation of disease process.	As manifested by increase in nausea and vomiting.	Decrease in or absence of nausea and vomiting.	• Maintain NPO status to prevent irritation of GI mucosa. • Maintain NG tube to suction to keep stomach empty and remove any stimulus for HCl acid and pepsin secretion. • Check vomitus or aspirate for occult blood to assess haemorrhage.	
Potential for haemorrhage R/T R/T eroded mucus tissue.		• Monitor for signs of haemorrhage. • Carry out medical and nursing interventions if haemorrhage occurs.	• Assess for evidence of haematemesis, bright red melena stool, abdominal pain or discomfort. Symptoms of shock to pain appropriate action. • If ulcer is actively bleeding, observe NG tube aspirate or emesis for amount and colour to assess degree of bleeding. • Take vital signs every 15 to 30 minutes to determine haemodynamic status and an indication of shock. • Maintain IV infusion line to provide ready access for blood and fluid replacement. • If RBC infusion given, observe for transfusion reaction for appropriate action.	

Contd...

Contd...

Problem	*Reason*	*Objective*	*Nursing intervention*	*Evaluation*
			• Monitor haematocrit and haemoglobin as indicators for severity, fluid and blood replacement. • Record intake and output to monitor fluid balance. • Reassure patient and family to decrease anxiety. • Remain calm and confident in plan of care to faster confidence in patient and family.	
Potential for perforation of GI mucosa R/T impaired mucosal tissue integrity.	–	• Monitor signs of perforation. • Report deviations from expected parameters. • Carry out appropriate medical and nursing intervention.	• Observe the manifestatiaon of perforation to ensure early recognition and treatment ie., – Sudden severe abdominal pain – Rigid board-like abdomen – Pain to shoulder – Increasing distension – Decreasing bowel sounds. • Monitor vital signs every 15 to 30 minutes as indicator of shock. • Maintain NG tube to suction to provide continuous aspiration and gastric decompression to prevent further leakage of gastric fluid through perforation. • Administer pain medication to promote comfort and reduce anxiety. • Prepare patient for emergency diagnostic tests and possible surgical interventions to foster timely intorvention.	

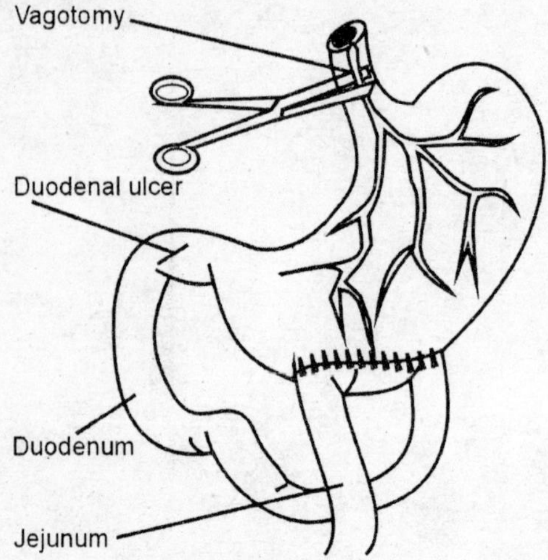

Fig. 7.2: A. Gastrojejunostomy and vagotomy. The jejunum is anastomosed to the stomach to provide a second outlet of gastric contents. The severed vagus nerve reduces secretions and movements of the stomach (90% good results).

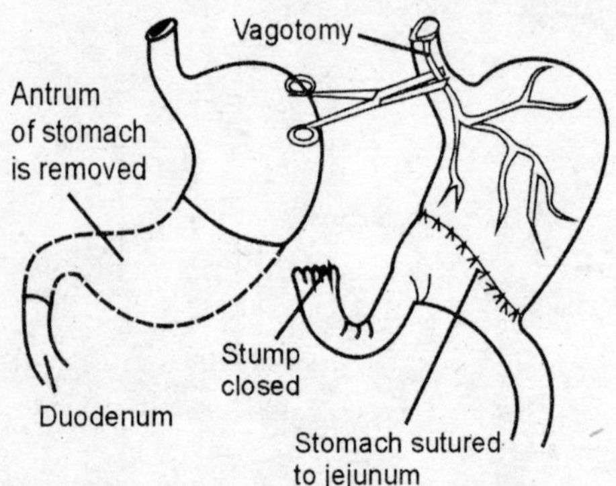

Fig.: B. Antrectomy and vagotomy. The resected portion includes a small cuff of duodenum, the pylorus, and the antrum (about one half of the stomach). The stump of the duodenum is closed by suture, and the side of the jejunum is anastomosed to the cut end of the stomach.

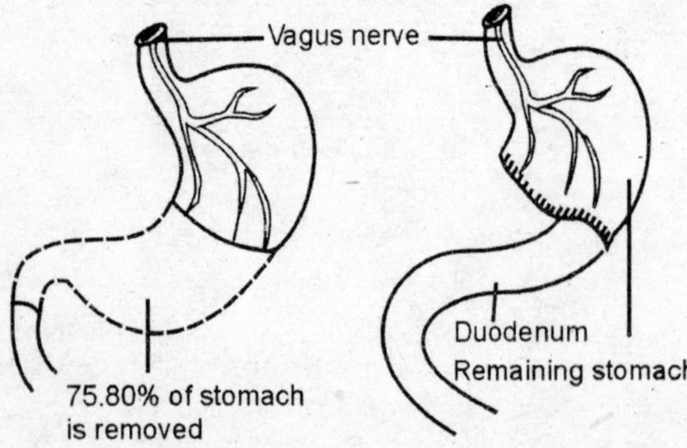

Fig.: C. Subtotal gastrectomy. The resected portion includes a small cuff of the duodenum, the pylorus, and from two thirds to three quarters of the stomach. The duodenum or side of the jujunum is anastomosed to the remaining portion of the stomach.

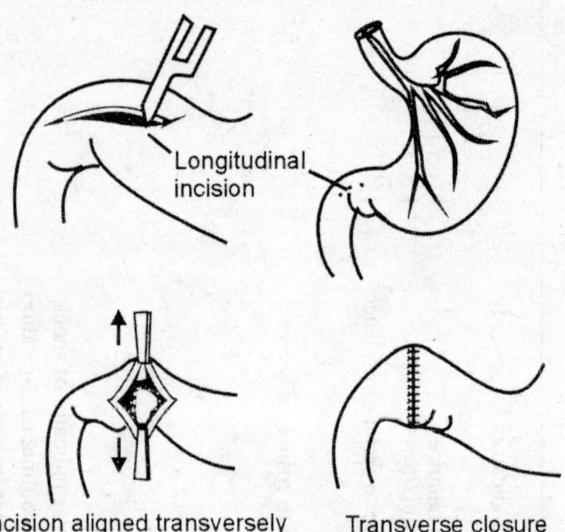

Fig.: D. Vagotomy and pyloroplasty. A longitudinal incision is made in the pylorus, and it is closed transversely to permit the muscle to relax and to establish an enlarged outlet. This compensates for the impaired gastric emptying produced by vagotomy.

ii. *Vagotomy* is the severing of the vagus nerve, either totally (truncal) or selectively at some point in its innervation to the stomach. In a *truncal* vagotomy the nerve is severed bilaterally in both the anterior and the posterior trunk. *Selective* vagotomy consists of cutting the nerve at a particular branch of the vagus nerve, resulting in denervation of only a portion of the stomach, such as the antrum or the parietal cell mass.
iii. *Pyloroplasty* consists of surgical enlargement of the spincter to facilitate the easy passage of contents from the stomach. It is most commonly done after vagotomy or to enlarge an opening that has been constricted from scar tissue. A vagotomy causes decreased gastric motility. A pyloroplasty accompanying vagotomy increases gastric emptying.

The combination of a Billroth I or II operation with vagotomy has the advantage of eliminating the ulcer and the stimulus for acid secretion. Surgical removal of the antrum results in removal of the source of gastrin secretion. Vagotomy eliminates the stimul of HCl acid and gastrin hormone secretion caused by vagal stimulation.

The postoperative complication of peptic ulcer surgery.

Dumping Syndrome

Dumping Syndrome is the term used for a group of unpleasant vasomotor and gastrointestinal system that occurs after surgery. It is associated with meals having a hyperosmalar composition. The onset of symptoms occurs at the end of a meal or within 15 to 30 minutes after eating. The patient usually describes feeling of generalized weakness, sweating, palpitations and dizziness. These symptoms are attributed to the sudden decrease in plasma volume. The patients complain of abdominal cramps, borborygmi and the urge to defecate. In addition, diaphoresis, tachycardia, feeling of fullness or discomfort, nausea, diarrhoea, may be present. These manifesttions usually last for longer than an hour after meal.

For which, prevention is the key and its management which includes small frequent meals, moderate fat, high-protein diet, limited carbohydrates, no simple sugars, minimal liquids with meals, avoiding very hot or very cold foods and beverages, and rest on left side for 20-30 minutes after eating. Anticholinergic or antispasmodic medication are useful.

Postprandial Hypoglycaemia

Postprandial hypoglycaemia is considered a variant of the dumping syndrome, since it is the result of uncontrolled gastric emptying of a bolus of fluid high in carbohydrate into the small intestine. The bolus of fluid concentrated carbohydrate results in hypoglycaemia and the release of excessive amounts of insulin into the circulation. The symptoms experienced are sweating, weakness, mental confusion, palpitations, tachycardia, and anxiety.

The immediate ingestion of sugared fluids or candy relieves the hypoglycaemic symptoms.

Bile Reflux Gastritis

Bile reflux gastritis occurs when surgery that involves the pylorus. Prolonged contact with bile damage, the gastric mucosa may cause bile reflux gastritis. The symptoms associated with epigastric distress that increases after meals. Vomiting relieved the distress but only temporarily. The administration of cholestyramine (Questran) either before or with meals are helpful to relieve bile reflux gastritis.

CANCER OF THE STOMACH

Cancer of the stomach is the most common malignant disease more prevalent among the lower economic class primarily living in urban areas. The male: female ratio is about 2:1. Gastric Cancer is rare before the age of 40, and the incidence increases sharply with age.

Aetiology

The cause of cancer of the stomach remains unknown yet it is highly erratic. Worldwide incidence pattern suggests the involvement of multiple environmental, genetic and possibly cultural factors. Diet and living conditions appear to be the most significant aspects in aetiology and early life exposure is critical. The risk factors of gastric cancer will include the following.

- Diet high in smoked preserved foods which contain nitrites and nitrates.
- Diet low in fresh fruits and vegetables.
- High nitrate content in the soil and water.
- Presence of chronic gastritis and achlorhydria.

Pathophysiology

Gastric cancers are virtually all primary adenocarcinoma that are derived from the epithelium. They have been found traditionally in the pyloric and antral regions, particularly along the lesser curvature. There are numerous ways to classify gastric cancers, which manifest in a variety of forms. Histologically, the cancer is classified as diffused or intestinal. The intestinal form is associated with the presence of intestinal metaplasia in the stomach. The diffuse forms have believed to begin locally in the mucosa and exhibit a long latency.

Gastric cancers may spread directly through the stomach wall into adjacent tissues; to the lymphates, to the regional lymph nodes of the stomach; to the oesophagus, spleen, pancreas and liver or through the blood stream to the lungs or bones. Involvement of regional lymph nodes occur early. Prognosis depends on the depth of invasion and extent of metastasis.

Gastric cancer has an insidious onset. It is accompanied by vague non-descript dyspeptic symptoms that overlap with multiple benign disorders, including non-ulcer dyspepsia and peptic ulcer.

The possible clinical manifestations of gastric cancer are:

- Dyspepsia: early satiety, bloating, anorexia.
- Epigostric pain or burning (usually mild and relieved by antacids).
- Mild nausea.
- Weight loss (may be rapid and severe).
- Fatigue and weakness.
- Change in the bowel habits; constipation or diarrhoea.
- Marked cachexia and a palpable mass in the abdomen.

Diagnostic Studies

- Biopsy
- Endoscopy
- Barium meal
- CT Scanning.
- Lab analysis of blood, stool, gastric secretion.
- Blood Chemistry studies.
- Carcinoembryonic antigen (CEA) test.

Management

When the diagnosis of gastric malignancy has been confirmed, the treatment of choice is surgical removal of the tumour. The preoperative management of the patient with gastric cancer focuses on the correction of nutritional deficits, treatment of anaemia, and replacement of blood volume.

The nursing care of the patient undergoing gastric surgery (a total gastrectomy for gastric cancer–total gastrectomy with oesophagojejunostomy) are as follows:

Preoperative

- Teach deep breathing exercises.
- Explain special postoperative measures; Nasogastric tube and parenteral flids until peristalsis returns.

Postoperative Care

i. *Promote pulmonary ventilation*
- Position patient in mid or high Fowler's position.
- Encourage patient to turn and breathe deep at least q2h (or more frequently until ambulating well); Splint or support incision with hands or folded towel during coughing if needed to clear secretions.
- Provide adequate analgesics during first few days. Patient-controlled analgesia (PCA) is effective.
- Encourage ambulation.
- Provide good mouth care until oral fluids can be resumed.

ii. *Promote Nutrition*
- Measure NG drainage accurately, monitor for blood in drainage. Do not irrigate or reposition tube unless ordered.
- Monitor for signs of leakage of anastomosis (dyspnoea, pain, fever) when oral fluids are resumed.
- Add food in small amounts at frequent intervals until well tolerated.
- Monitor for early satiety and regurgitation.
- If regurgitation occurs, tell patients to eat less food at a slower pace.
- Report signs of dumping syndrome to doctor (weakness, faintness, palpitations, diaphoresis, nausea and darrhoea.
- Monitor weight.

iii. *Provide patient/family education*
- Gradually increase amount of food each meal until able to eat 3 to 6 meals per day if possible.
- If discomfort occurs after eating, decrease size of meals and amount of fluids with meals; eat more slowly.
- Avoid eating simple carbohydrates and concentrated sweets.
- Avoid stress during and immediately after meals; plan a rest period after eating. Lie on left side.
- Elevate the head when lying down (if cardia of stomach removed).
- Monitor weight regularly.
- Report signs of complications: vomiting after meals, increasing feeling of abdominal fullness or weakness, haematemesis, tarry stools and persistent diarrhoea.

IRRITABLE BOWEL SYNDROME (IBS)

Irritable bowel syndrome (IBS) is a symptom of complex characterized by intermittent and recurrent abdominal pain associated with an alteration in bowel function (diarrhoea and constitpation). Other symptoms commonly found include abdominal distention, excessive flatulence, urge to defecate, and sensation of incomplete evacuation.

Aetiology

The cause is unknown. Much more common in women. Related to stress and excessive intake of food. Often linked to a history of physical or sexual abuse. Onset typically during late adolescence to mid-thirties. Most frequently encountered GI condition in Medical practice.

Pathophysiology

Major findings are rarely present. Lab tests are typically normal but colon spasticity can be visualized by X-Ray and endoscopy. Increased small bowel motility plus increased frequency and amplitude of large bowel contraction occurs. Symptom patterns include:

- Spastic Colon: Colicky abdominal pain, periodic constipation and diarrhoea.
- Painless urgent diarrhoea after meals.

Management

Treatment involves lifestyle modification and supportive care i.e. Diet modification includes avoiding rich fatty foods, gas producing foods, gastric stimulants (alcohol & smoking) using medication such as bulk forming, antispasmodic, antidiarrhoeal and motility agents. In addition, adequate rest, stress management and regular aerobic exercises are advised.

DIARRHOEA

Diarrhoea is not a disease but a symptom. It is commonly used to denote an increase in stool frequency or volume and an increase in the looseness of stool. Diarrhoea may be acute or chronic. Acute diarrhoea, most commonly results from infection diarrhoea is considered chronic when it persists for atleast 2 weeks or when it subsides and returns more than 2 to 4 weeks after the initial episode. Chronic diarrhoea is usually related to changes in the GI tract, that alter the fluid and electrolyte balance.

Aetiology

Causes of diarrhoea can be divided into the general classification of decreased fluid absorption, increased fluid secretion, motility disturbances or a combination of them. The causes of diarrhoea are:

i. *Decreased fluid absorption.*
- Oral intake of poorly absorbable solutes (eg. Laxatives)
- Maldigestion and malabsorption
  - Mucosal damage: tropical sprue, Crohn's disease, radiation injury, ulcerative colitid, ischemic bowel disease.
  - Pancreatic insufficiency.
  - Intestinal enzyme deficiency (eg. Lactase)
  - Bile Salt deficiency.
  - Decreased surface area. eg. intestinal resection).

ii. *Increased fluid secretion.*

- Infections: Bacterial endotoxin (e.g. cholera, E.Coli, Shigella Salmonella, staphylococcus, Clostridium, Campylobacter jejuni).
  - Viral agents (Rotavirus, HIV).
  - Parasitic agents, giardia lambia, cryptosoridium, trichinella, hookworm).
  - Drugs: Laxatives, antibiotics, suspension or elixirs containing sorbitol (eg. acetaminophen).
  - Hormonal : Vasocative intestinal polypeptide (VIP) secretion from adenoma of the pancreas, gastrin secretion caused by Zollinger-Ellison syndrome, calcitonin secretion from carcinoma of thyroid.
- Tumour: Villus adenoma.

iii. *Motility disorders*

- Irritable bowel syndrome
- Diabetic enteropathy
- Visceral scleroderma
- Carcinoid syndrome
- Vagotomy.

The risk factors of acute diarrhoea are:

- Recent travel to developing nations.
- Outdoor camping.
- Ingestion of raw meat, seafood, or shellfish.
- Eating at banquets, restaurants, picnics, or fast food centres.
- Day care placement of employment.
- Residence in institutions, nursing homes, prisons or mental institutions.
- Prostitution.
- Intravenous drug abuse.

Pathophysiology

Large-volume diarrhoea is caused by hypersecretion of water and electrolytes by the intestinal mucosa. This secretion occurs in response to the osmotic pressure exerted by non-absorbed food partices in the chyme or from direct irritation of the mucosa. Peristalsis increased, and the transit time through the intestine is significantly decreased. Increased peristalsis may result from inflammation as mucosal cells hypersecrete water in the presence of infectious organisms. Diarrhoea may be accompanied by severe abdominal cramping, tenesmus (persistent spasm) of the anal area, abdominal distension and borborygmns (loud bowel sounds).

Fluid and electrolyte imbalances can quickly result from diarrhoea, depending on its severity. Mild diarrhoea in adults can lead to losses of sodium and potassium (causing metabolic alkalosis). Severe diarrhoea causes dehydration, hyponatraemia, hypokalaemia, and metabolic acidosis (from the loss of large amounts of bicarbonate). Malnourished or elderly persons tolerate severe diarrhoea less well than do younger or well-nourished persons. Persistent diarrhoea also readily leads to skin breakdown in the perianal region.

Clinical Manifestations

Bacterial or viral infection of the intenstine may result in explosive water diarrhoea, tenesmus (spasmotic contraction of anal spincter with pain and persistent desire to defecate) and abdominal cramping pain, perianal skin irritation may also develop. Systemic manifestations include fever, nausea, vomiting and malaise, leukocytes blood and mucus may be present in the stool depending on the causative agent as given below:

i. *Viral (Rotavirus Norwalk)*

Onset is 18-24 hours and duration 24-48 hours shows signs and symptoms include explosive, water diarrhoea, nausea, vomiting and abdominal cramps.

ii. *Bacterial*

- Escherichia coli-onset 4 to 24 hours duration 3-4 days, signs and symptoms are four or five loose stools per day, nausea, malaise, low-grade fever.
- Enterohaemorrhagic E.Coli: Onset 4-24 hours, duration 4-9 days signs and symptoms are bloody diarrhoea, severe cramping, fever.
- Shigella-' Onset 24 hours duration 7 days, signs and symptoms are watery stool containing blood and mucus, tenesmus, urgency severe cramping and fever.
- Salmonella-onset 6-48 hours duration 2-5-days. Signs and symptoms are watery diarrhoea, nausea, vomiting, abdomenal cramps and fver.
- Compylobacter species - Onset 24 hours duratiaon less than 7 days. Signs and symptoms are profuse watery diarrhoea, malaise, nausea abdominal cramps, low-grade fever.
- Clostridium perfringens - Onset 8-12 hours duration 24 hours. Signs and symptoms are watery diarrhoea, abdominal cramps, vomiting.
- Clostridum defficila - Onset 4 days after start of antibiotics, duration 24 hours. It is associated with antibiotic treatment, symptoms range from mild, watery diarrhoea to severe abdominal pain, fever, leucocytosis and leucocytes in stool.

All these are treated with proper antibiotics and antidiarrheal drugs.

iii. *Parasitic*

- Entamoeba histolytica leads to amebiasis - Onset 4-day duration weeks to months. Here ingested cyst releases active trophozite that invades and ulcerates intestinal mucosa. It can migrate to liver and cause abscesses.

Clinical manifestations are: abdominal cramping, frequent soft stools with blood and mucus (in severe cases watery stools), flatulence, distention fever, leucocytes in stool and reappearance of symptoms. It is treated by metronidazole for 5-10 days often in combination with other amebicides.

- Giardia Lamblia leads to Giardiasis- Here infested cyst releases active trophozoite that infects the small intestine and onset is 1-3 weeks and duration is a few days to 3 months shows sudden onset, malodorous, explosive, watery diarrhoea, abdominal cramping and bloating, malabsorption in severe cases. Treatment self limiting in 2-6 weeks but may recur. Quinacrine (Atabrin or flage for at least 2-10 cases).
- Cryptosporidium leads to cryptosporidiosis. The parasite is present in birds, fish, cattle, sheet and spread by persons to person contact and contaminated water. In which organism is ingested and primarily affects the small intestine. It can affect the entire GI tract in immunocompromised persons. It causes massive watery diarrhoea, which exceeds 4L/day, if persistent malabsorption may develop-nausea and fatigue. Abdominal cramps, weight loss in AIDS for which no effective therapy is available. Supportive treatment, replacement of fluid and electrolyte.
- Trichinella spiralis causes trichinosis. It is due to ingestion of undercooked pork and pork products. In which larvae of round worms infect the meat and mature in the intestine. Larvae are then released into blood and lymphatics and pass into striated muscle of the host where they encyst. Early state symptoms include nausea, anorexia, cramping and diarrhoea, muscle pain and fever develop in 2-8 weeks can involve jaw, eyes diaphragm and heart, for which only symptomatic treatment can be available. Use of mebondazole or thiabendazole is helpful.

Diagnostic Studies

Accurate diagnosis and management require a thorough history, physical examination and when indicated Lab tests.

Management

The management of diarrhoea involves the prevention of fluid and electrolyte imbalance, controlling the symptoms and treating the underlying cause if possible. Aggressive rehydration with oral replacement solutions is used if the person is alert and able to take oral fluids. Solutions such as the WHO solution, pedialyte, resol, and rehydralate are preferred to fruit juices, soda or even gatorade because they have balanced electrolyte composition plus glucose. Clear liquids are provided along with diets low in fibre but rich in sodium and glucose. Oral rehydration therapy with available standard ORS can be instituted.

The use of antidiarrheal agents are variable. Common medication for treatment of acute diarrhoea are:

i. *Local acting*

- Bismuth sub salicylate (Pepto Bismol) mechanism not known may bind bacterial *toxin*.
- Kaolin and pectin (Kao pectate) which soothes the intestinal mucosa and increases absorption of water, nutrients and electrolytes.

These are in liquid form. So shake well before using. Bismuth product may turn the stool black. No significant side effects with Kaolin and pectin.

ii. *Systemic acting drugs*

Include loperamide (imodium, tincture of opium (Paregoric), Diphenoxylate hydrochloride with atrophine (Lomotil). These drugs act systematically to reduce peristalsis and GI motility. Be aware that these drugs are part of the narcotic family; potential for addiction exists with paregoric. Loperamide has few side effects and no associated physical dependence. Lomotil has a low potential for dependency. So, monitor patient response, can enhance bacterial invasion and prolong excreation of the pathogen. Monitor for narcotic side effects-CNS depression or respiratory depression.

FECAL INCONTINENCE

Fecal incontinence or the involuntary passage of stool may be due to multiple causes.

Aetiology

The causes for the fecal incontinence are:

i. Traumatic
- Obstetric
- Post-surgical
- Haemorrhoidectomy
- Anterior resection
- Fistulectomy
- Anorectal surgery
- Spinal cord injury.

ii. Neurologic
- Stroke
- Tumour
- Degenerative diseases
- Iatrogenic drug intoxication
- Multiple sclerosis
- Diabetes mellitus
- Dementia

iii. Inflammatory
- Infections
- Trauma
- Radiation

iv. Other
- Pelvic floor relaxation
- Perineal descent
- Loss of elasticity of rectum
- Decreased spincter tone (age relaxation)
- Rectal prolapse
- Focal impaction
- Diarrhoea
- Medications.

Table 7.6: Nursing care plan of patient with acute infectious diarrhoea

Problem	*Reason*	*Objective*	*Nursing intervention*	*Evaluation*
1. Diarrhoea R/T acute infectious process.	As manifested by frequent loose, watery stools.	• Normal bowel elimination	• Monitor frequency, amounts, colour, consistency of stools to determine severity and need for intervention. • Record intake and output to monitor fluid balance. • Follow hospital procedure for infection control precautions, use strict aseptic technique, while handling bedpan, linens or patient to prevent the spread of infection. • Monitor vital signs 4th hourly as changes can indicate hypovolaemia. • Administer anti-infective and anti diarrheal medication as ordered.	
2. Fluid volume deficit R/T excessive fluid loss and decreased fluid intake secondary to diarrhoea.	As manifested by dry skin and mucus membrane, poor skin turgor, hypotension, tachy cardia, urine output, electrolye imbalance.	• Normal vital signs and • Skin turgor • Moist mucus membrane. • Urine output >0.5 ml/kg/hr • Normal serum electrolytes.	• Assess skin turgor changes, sunken eyes, rapid pulse and anorexia, as indicator of fluid volume deficit. • Monitor intake and output. • Monitor serum Na. K. level. • Monitor vital signs 4th hourly. • Weight patient daily to monitor fluid loss. • Administer IV fluid as ordered. • Assess dehydration, administer ORS. Medicate with antidiarrheal drugs as ordered.	
3. Impaired skin integrity R/T perianal contact with diarrheal stools and inadequate perianal hygiene.	As manifested by redness, irritation swelling, possible ulceration of skin pain during elimination.	• No evidence of skin breakdown in perianal area.	• Assess skin perianal area to plan appropriate interventions. • Cleanse area with warm water each bowel movement rinse well and dry with a soft towel to prevent skin excoriation. • Apply ointment (e.g. Alo, Zinc Oxide) to protect skin and promote healing. • Use an anoesthetic ointment or spray foam to decrease local discomfort.	
4. Risk for infection transmission R/T lack of knowledge about prevention of reinfection or transmission of infectious disase.	–	• No recurrence of symptoms • Knowledgeable about disease process and preventive measures.	• Teach the patient to be alert for recurrence of diarrhoea, fever, and other presenting symptoms in family members. • Assist patient in identifying factors that precipitated diarrhoea to avoid cause of reinfection of self. • Stress importance of seeking medical care where diarrhoea and other symptoms present for early treatment.	

Pathophysiology

Normally fecal contents pass from the signoid colon into the rectum, causing rectal distention. Sensory (stretch) receptors in the muscles surrounding the rectum provide the sensation of rectal filling. This causes a reflex relaxation of the internal anal spincter and contraction of the external anal spincter. Sensory receptors in the epithelium of the anal canal can usually distinguish among solid, liquid, and gas. The combination of contraction of the abdominal muscles, relaxation of the pelvic muscles, squatting (which straightens the anorectal angle) and voluntary relaxation of the external anal spincter allows for elimination of feces.

Management

The diagnosis and effective management of fecal incontinence require a thorough health history and physical examinations with appropriate diagnostic studies (as per causes stated above.) The nurse should identify normal bowel habits and current symptoms, including frequency and nature of the stools. The nursing diagnosis of the patient with fecal incontinence are:

- Impaired skin integrity R/T incontinence of stool and irritation in perianal area.
- Social isolation R/T embarrassment and odour.
- Self-esteem disturbance R/T inability to manage bowel evacuation independently.

The overall goal is that patient with fecal incontinence will have normal bowel control.

- Maintain perianal skin integrity and
- Not suffer any selfesteem problem.

Preventions and treatment of fecal incontinence may be managed by implementing a bowel-training program. The patient should be put on a bedpan, assisted to a bedside commode, or walked to the bathroom at a regular time daily to assist with re-establishment of bowel regularity. Bowel training is the major approach used with patients who have cognitive and neurological problems resulting from stroke or other chronic diseases. If a person can sit on a toilet, it may be possible to achieve automatic defecation when a pattern of consistent timing, familar surroundings, and controlled diet and fluid intake can be achieved. This approach allows many patients to defecate predictable and remain continent throughout the day. Surgical correction is possible for small groups of patients whose incontinence is related to structural problems of the rectum and anua. Perianal pouching is an alternative in the management of fecal incontinence. Pouching provides skin protection and fecal containment as well as comfort and dignity. Since odour is a problem deodarant spray and room deodars can be used.

CONSTIPATION

The term 'Constipation' refers to an abnormal infrequency of defecation or the passage of abnormally hard stools or both. It may be defined as a decrease of frequency of bowel movement from what is "normal" for the individual, hard, difficult-to-pass stools, a decrease in stool volume, and retention of feces in the rectum.

Aetiology

Frequently constipation may be due to insufficient dietary fibres, inadequate fluid intake, medication use, and lack of exercise. It may be due to socio-cultural beliefs. chronic laxative abuse, and multiple organic causes as given below.

i. *Colonic disorders*
   - Luminal or extra-luminal obstructing lesions.
   - Inflammatory strictures
   - Volvolus
   - Intussusception
   - Irritable bowel syndrome
   - Diverticular disease
   - Rectocele.

ii. *Drug induced*
   - Antacids (calcium and alluminiuum)
   - Antidepressants
   - Anticholenergics
   - Anticonvulsives
   - Antipsychotics
   - Antihypertensives
   - Barium sulfate
   - Iron supplements
   - Bismuth
   - Calcium supplements
   - Laxative abuse.

iii. *Systemic disorders*
   - Metabolic disorders: Diabetes mellitus, hypothyroidism, pregnancy, hypercalcaemia, hyperparathyroidism.
   - Collagen vascular disease: Scleroderma, amyloidosis.
   - Neurogenic disorders:
     - Hirshsprungs megacolon
     - Neurofibromatosis
     - Autonovic neuropathy (psudoobstruction)
     - Multiple sclerosis
     - Parkinson's disease
     - Spinal cord lesion or injury
     - Cerebrovascular accident.

Pathophysiology

Constipation may result from decreased motility of the colon or from retention of feces in the laser portion of the colon or rectum. Dietary fiber increases the water content of the stool, and colonic motility is enhanced through the bacterial degradation of the fiber.

The longer the feces remain in the colon, the greater the amount of water reabsorbed and the drier the stool becomes. The stool is then more difficult to expel. Occassionally constipation is not detrimental to health, but habitual constipation leads to decreased intestinal muscle tone, increased use of valsalvas manoeuvre as the person bears down in the attempt to pass the hardened stool, and an increased incidence of haemorrhoids, id mass complication of chronic constipation. Diverticulosis is other complication.

The clinical manifestation of constipation are

- Hard, dry stool
- Abdominal distention
- Decreased frequency of bowel movement
- Abdominal pain
- Straining
- Rectal pressure
- Tenesmus
- Increased flatulence
- Nausea
- Anorexia
- Headache
- Palpable mass
- Stool with blood
- Urinary retention
- Dizziness.

Management of Constipation

A thorough history and physical examination should be performed so that the underlying causes of constipation can be identified and treatment started. Usual diagnostic studies can be followed accordingly.

Most causes of constipation can be managed by/with the diet therapy including dietary fiber and fluid and an exercise program. Laxatives should always be used cautiously because with chronic overuse, they may become a cause of constipation. The common cathartic agents used in constipation are:

i. *Bulk forming* agents absorb water, increase bulk, thereby stimulating peristalsis in which polysaccharides and cellulose derivatives mix with intestinal fluids, swell and stimulate peristalsis. Eg psyllium, methyl cellulose. During its use, ensure adequate fluid intake to prevent impaction or obstruction. Take separately from presribed drugs to avoid problems with absorption.

ii. *Emollients* are stool softeners and lubricants, which lubricate intestinal tract and soften feces, making hard stools easier to pass, do not affect peristalsis. Eg. Docusate sodium, Docusate calcium. These docusate salts act as a detergent in the intestine, reducing surface tension, which facilitates the incorporation of liquid and fat, softening the stool. The preparations lose effectiveness with long-term use. Discontinue if abdominal cramping occurs.

iii. *Lubricants* i.e. mineral oils, soften fecal matter by lubricating the intestinal mucosa, facilitating easy stool passage. Excessive use interfere with absorption of fat soluble Vitamin ADE and K. leading to deficiency. These mineral oils should not take with meals or drugs, because oils can impair absorption, swallow carefully to prevent lipid aspiration.

iv. *Hyperosmalar laxatives* like lactulose, polyethyline glysol, sorbitol, which nonabsorbable sugars are degraded by colonic bacteria and increase stool osmolarity. Fluid is drawn into the intestine, stimulating peristalsis. When these are used, adjust the dose and frequency of administration to control side effects and regulate defection. Monitor for fluid and electrolyte imbalance if response is severe.

v. *Saline laxatives* cause osmotic retention of fluid which distends the colon and increases peristalsis. eg. magnesium citrate, Mg. sulfate, Mg. hydroxide. The liquids preparations are more effective than tablets. Take with full glass of water. Monitor for fluid and electrolyte imbalance if response is severe.

vi. *Stimulants* increase peristalsis by irritating colon wall and stimulating enteric nerves eg. cascara sagroda, senna, Bisacodyl (Bulcolax), castor oil. Cramps and diarrhoea can occur. Monitor for fluid and electrolyte imbalance if reaction is severe.

Nursing management should be based on the patient symptoms and the assessment of the patient. An important role of the nurse is teaching the patient the importance of dietary measures to prevent constipation. The following are teaching guidelines for the patient with constipation:

i. Eat dietary fiber.
   - Eat 20 to 30 grams of fiber per day. Gradually increase amount of fiber eaten over 1 to 2 weeks. Fiber softens hard stools and add bulk to stool, promoting, evacuation - Food high in fiber: Raw vegetable and fruits, beans.

ii. Drink fluids
   - Drink 3 quarts per day. Drink water or fruit juice, avoid coffee, tea and cola.

iii. Exercise regularly
   - Walk, swim, or bike at least three times per week.
   - Contract and relax abdominal muscles when standing or by doing sit-ups to strengthen muscles and prevent straining.
   - Exercises stimulates bowel motility and moves stools through the intestine.

iv. Set a regular time to defecate.

v. Do not delay defecations.
   - Respons to the urge to have bowel movement as soon as possible.
   - Delaying defecation results in hard stools and decreased 'urge' to defecate.
   - Water is absorbed from stool by the intestine over time.
   - The intestine becomes less sensitive to the presence of stool in the rectum.

vi. Record your bowel eliminating time.

Develop a habit of recording when you have a bowel movement on your calender. Regular monitoring of bowel movement will assist in early problem identification.

vii. Avoid laxatives and enemas.
Do not overuse laxatives and enemas as they can actually cause constipation. The normal motility of the bowel is interrupted and bowel movements slow or stop.

ACUTE ABDOMEN

The patient with an acute abdomen has an acute onset of abdominal pain requiring prompt decision making. Many disorders must be ruled out before a diagnosis is confirmed.

Aetiology

Causes of an acute abdomen are varied as follows:

- Abdominal penetrating trauma
- Acute ischemic bowel
- Appendicitis
- Bowel obstruction with perforation or necrosis
- Cholecystitis
- Crohn's disease
- Diverticulosis with peritonitis
- Foreign body perforation
- Gastritis
- Gastroenteritis
- Mesentric adenitis
- Pancreatitis
- Pelvic inflammatory disease
- Perforated gastrointestinal malignancy
- Peritonitis
- Ruptured abdominal aneurysm
- Ruptured ecopic pregnancy
- Ruptured ovarian cyst
- Ulcerative colitis
- Uterine rupture
- Volvulus.

Clinical Manifestation

- Pain is the most common presenting symptom. The patient also complains abdominal tenderness, vomiting, diarrhoea, constipation, flatulence, fatigue, fever, and increase in abdominal girth.

Management

Assessment begins with a complete history and physical examination including rectal and pelvic examination. CBC, urinalysis abd. X-ray, ECG, pregnancy test (for ladies) are also performed to get some clue for causes of acute abdomen. An assessment finding will include:

- Diffuse, localized, dull, burning or sharp, abdominal pain and tenderness.
- Rebound tenderness
- Abdominal distention
- Abdominal rigidity
- Nausea, vomiting
- Diarrhoea
- Haematemesis
- Melena

In addition, signs and symptoms of hypovolumic shock

- Decreased blood pressure
- Decreased pulse pressure
- Tachycardia
- Cool, clammy skin
- Decreased level of consciousness.

Acute abdomen requires an emergency management. The goal of which is to identify and treat the cause. Because many causes of which do not require surgery. An initial intervention will include:

- Ensure patent airway
- Administer oxygen via nasal cannula or nonbreather mask.
- Establish IV access with large bore catheter and infuse warm normal saline or lactated Ringer's solution.

Insert additional large bore catheter if shock is present.

- Obtain blood for CBC; electrolytes.
- Anticipate order for amylase, pregnancy test, clotting studies and type and crossmatch as appropriate.
- Obtain urinalysis.
- Insert nasogastric (NG) tube as needed.
- Monitor vital signs, level of consciousness, O_2 saturation, intake and output.
- Assess quality and amount of pain.
- Anticipate surgical intervention.
- Keep NPO.

ABDOMINAL TRAUMA

Injuries to the abdominal area most often occur as a result of blunt trauma or penetration injuries. (i) *Blunt trauma* usually occurs due to falls, motor vehicle collisions, pedestrian event, assault with blunt object, crash injuries and explosions. (ii) *Penetrating* injuries are due to stab, knife, gunshot wounds and other reasons. Regardless of whether it is blunt or penetration injury, the result is often the same damage to/or alteration of the internal organs.

Common injuries of the abdomin includes lacerated liver, ruptured spleen, pancreatic trauma, mesentric artery tears, diaphragmatic rupture, urinary bladder rupture. These injuries may result in massive blood loss and hypovolemic shock. Surgery (laparotomy) is performed as early as possible to repair the damaged organs and to stop bleeding. Common sequale of intrabdominal trauma are peritonitis and massive infection, particularly when the bowel is perforated.

Table 7.7: Nursing care plan for patient following laparotomy

Problem	*Reason*	*Objective*	*Nursing intervention*	*Evaluation*
1. Pain R/T surgical incision and inadequate pain control measures	As manifested by complaints of pain, body post-uring, unwillingness to move in bed or ambulate	Satisfactory level of pain control.	• Assess for pain and give pain medications every 3 to 4 hours, as ordered for first 72 hours. • Splint incision with pillow during coughing, deep breathing and moving to relieve pain while performing these activities. • Position patient comfortable to relieve pain.	
2. Nausea and vomiting R/T decreased GI motility, GI distention and narcotics.	As manifested by nausea, vomiting, lack of diminished bowel sounds. Abdominal distentions.	• Relief of nausea, vomiting.	• Administer antiemetic as ordered. • Assess response to pain medication. • Maintain patency of NG tube. • Assess for bowel sounds and abdominal distention. • Keep patient on NPO status until bowel sound returns. • Limit unpleasant sights smells and stimuli to prevent initiate episodes of nausea and vomiting.	
3. Constipation R/T immobility, pain medication and GI motility.	As manifested by decreased or absent bowel sounds, abdo pain abd. distention inability to pass flatus or stool.	• Normal bowel sounds within 72 hours • Soft-formed bowel movement within 4 days.	• Assess abdomen for bowel sounds every shift to determine need for intervention. • Administer cathartic as ordered if patient has not had bowel movement in 4 days. • Encourage frequent position changes and ambulation as tolerated to increase peristalsis. • Encourage increased fluid intake as tolerated to soften fecal material.	

Clinical Manifestation

The clinical manifestations of abdominal trauma are:

- Guarding and splinting of the abdominal wall
- A hard, distended abdomen (indicating intra-abdominal bleeding).
- Decreased or absent bowel sounds.
- Contusions, abrasions or bruising over abdomen.
- Abdominal pain.
- Pain over the scapula caused by irritation of the phrenic nerve by free blood in the abdomen.
- Haematemesis of haematuria and so.
- Signs of hypovolemic shock.
- An ecchymotic discoloration around the umbilicus (collens sign) can indicate intra-abdominal or retroperitoneal haemorrhage.

Intra-abdominal injuries are often associated with rib fractures, feactured femur, fractured pelvis, and thoracic injury. If any of these injuries are present, the patient should be observed for abdominal trauma.

Management

Routine diagnostic procedures include CBC, urinalysis, X-ray of abdomen, CT Scan and peritoneal lavage. For emergency management of the abdomenal trauma focuses on establishing a patent airway, and adequate breathing fluid replacement and prevention of hypovolemic shock. The nursing intervention will include:

- Ensure patent airway.
- Administer oxygen via non-breather mask.
- Control external bleeding with direct pressure or sterile pressure dressing.
- Establish IV access with large bore catheters and infuse warm normal saline or lactated Ringers solutions.
- Obtain blood for type and crossmatch and CBC.
- Remove clothing.
- Stabilize impaled objects with bulky dressing do not remove.
- Cover-protruding organs or tissue with sterile, saline dressing.
- Insert indwelling urinary catherter if there is no blood at the meatus, pelvic fracture, or boggy prostate.
- Obtain urine for urinalysis.
- Insert NG tube if no evidence of facial trauma.
- Anticipate diagnostic peritonical lavage.
- Monitor vital signs, level of consciousness, O_2 saturations and urine output.
- Maintain patient's warmth using blankets, Warm IV fluids or Warm humidified oxygen.

Regardless of the mechanism of injury, physical evidence of abdominal trauma in a patient who is haemodynamically unstable mandates immediate laparotomy, for which routine preoperative procedure and postoperative intervention will be followed in addition to specific intervention.

APPENDICITIS

Appendicitis is an inflammation of the vermiform appendix, a narrow blind tube that extends from the inferior part of the ceacum usually just below the ileocecal valve.

Aetiology

The most common causes of appendicities are obstructions of the lumen by a fecalith (accumulated feces), foreign bodies, tumour of the cecum or appendix, or intramural thickening caused by lymphoid hyperplasia.

Pathophysiology

The inflammatory process of the appendicitis can involve all or part of the appendix. Intraluminal pressure increases, leading to occlusion of the capillaries and venules and vascular endorgement. Bacterial invasion follows and microabscesses may develop in the appendiceal wall or surrounding tissue, which, unless treated, can progress to gangrene and perforation within 24 to 36 hours. If the inflammatory process develops fairly, slowly the infection may be successfully be walled off in a local abscess. In more rapidly developing cases, the risk of rupture and acute peritonitis is quite high.

Clinical Manifestations

The clinical manifestations of appendicits is abdominal pain that comes in waves. The pain is persistent and continuous, eventually shifting to the right lower quadrant and localizing at McBurney's point (located half way between the umbilicus and the right iliac crest). It typically begins with periumbilical pain, followed by anorexia, nausea, and vomiting. Further assessment of the patient reverals localized tenderness, rebound tenderness and muscle guarding. The patient usually prefers to lie still, often with right leg flexed. Low-grade fever may or may not be present, and coughing aggravates pain. Rovsing's sign may be elicited by palpation of the left lower quadrants, cauing pain to be felt in the right lower quadrant, complications of acute appendicities are performation, peritonitis and abscesses.

Management

The diagnosis of appendicits is made from the classic physical and laboratory indicators when they are present. The patient with abdominal pain is advised to see physician and to avoid self treatment. Until then the patient is advised to take anything by mouth. (NPO) to ensure that stomach is empty in the event of surgery is needed. An icebag may be applied to the right lower quadrant to decrease the flow of blood to the area and impede the inflammatory process. Heat is never used because it may cause appendix to rupture.

Surgery is usually performed as soon as a diagnosis is made. Pre and postoperative nursing management is similar to that of patients after laparotomy or any surgical treatment. In addition, patient should be observed for evidence of peritonitis.

PERITONITIS

Peritonitis involves either a local or generalized inflammation of the peritoneum, the membranous lining of the abdomen, that covers the viscera. Peritonitis may be primary or secondary, aseptic or septic and acute or chronic.

Aetiology

Primary peritonitis usually caused by bacterial infection, bloodborne organism, genital tract organism and cirrhosis with ascitis. Where as secondary peritonitis often results from trauma, surgical injury or chemical irritations, which includes ruptured appendix, perforated peptic ulcer, diverticulitis, pelvic inflammatory disease, urinary tract infections, or trauma, bowel obstructions and surgical complications.

Peritonitis may appear in acute or chronic forms, and trauma or rupture of an organ containing chemical irritants or bacteria, which are released into peritonial cavity eg. gastric ulcer perforations and ruptured ectopic pregnancy. Bacterial peritonitis can be caused by a traumatic injury (eg. gunshot wound ruptured appendix) or it can be secondary to other diseases or conditions (eg. pancreatitis, peritoneal dialysis).

Pathophysiology

The peritoneal lining serves as a semipermeable membrane lining that allows the flow of water and electrolytes between the blood stream and peritoneal cavity. When peritonitis occurs, fluid can shift into the abdominal cavity at a rate of 300 to 500 ml/hr in response to acute inflammation. The inflammatory process also shunts extra blood to the inflammed areas of the bowel to contract the secondary bacterial infection and peristalsis typically ceases. The bowel increasingly becomes distended with gas and fluid. The circulatory fluid and electrolyte changes can rapidly become critical. Local reaction of the peritoneum include redness and inflammation and the production of large amounts of fluid that contains electrolytes and proteins. Hypovolaemei, electrolyte imbalance, dehydration, and finally shock can develop. This loss of circulatory volume is proportional to the severity of peritoneal involvement. The fluid usually becomes purulent as the condition progresses and as the bacteria becomes more numerous. The bacteria also may enter the blood and cause septicaemia.

Clinical Manifestation

Abdominal pain is the most common symptom of peritonitis. A universal sign of peritonitis is tenderness over the involved area. Rebound tenderness, muscular rigidity, and spasm are other major signs of irritation of the peritoneum. Abdominal distentions, or ascitis, fever, tachycardia, tachypnoea, nausea, vomiting, altered bowel habits may also be present. These manifestations vary depending on severity and acuteness of the underlying cause. Complications of peritnonitis include hypovlaemic shock, septicaemia, intra-abdominal abscess, formation, paralytic ileus, and organ failure.

Diagnostic Studies

- CBC
- Serum electrolytes
  Abdominal X-Ray
- Abdominal paracentesis and culture of fluid
- CT Scan or ultrasound and
- Peritonoscopy.

Management

The goal of management of peritonitis are to identify and eliminate the cause, combat infection, and prevent complications. Patients with milder cases of peritonitis or those who are poor surgical risks may be managed non-surgically. Treatment consists of antibiotics, NG suction, analgesics, and IV fluid administration.

Patient who requires surgery need preoperative preparation as described earlier. Those patiens may need total parenteral nutrition (TPN) because of increased nutrition requirement. Post-operative nursing management is similar to that provided for any surgical patient who has undergone abdominal surgery.

DIVERTICULITIS

Diverticula are small outpouchings or herniation of the mucosal lining of the gastrointestinal track. Diverticulosis has been described as a disease of west because its higher incidence in developed countries. The incidence of the disease should wide geographic variatioan that are at least partly attributable to the quantity of non-absorbable dietary fiber. Low-fiber diets have been shown to increase intraluninal pressure in the bowel but aging also appears to change the composition of the bowel which decreases its tensile strength.

Pathophysiology

Diverticula tend to form at point in the colon wall where blood vessels penetrate the mucosal and muscular layers, creating points of relative weakness. The increased muscular contractions in the signoid colon that are generated to push stool in the rectum increase both the thickness of the muscle and the intraluminal pressure. The weaker connective tissue then herniates between the circular muscle and the intraluminal pressure, the weaker connective tissue then herniates between the circular muscle band and forms the diverticula.

Diverculitis frequently develops in a single diverticulum in response to irritation initiated by trapped foecal material. Blood supply to the area decreases, and bacteria proliferates in the obstructed diverticulum. Perforation of the dome may occur, which, if small is usually quickly and effectively walled off. Large perforation may progress to abscess formatioan orgeneral peritonitis. Generalaized inflammation can result in thickening and scarring of the bowel wall.

Clinical Manifestations

Usually diverticular disease is asymptomatic, but mild inflammation can trigger a nonspecific bowel dysfunction that resolves in a matter of hours or days. The clinical manifestations of diverculitis reflect the inflammation of the diverticula or the developments of complication. Cramps lower left quadrant abdominal pain accompanied by low grade fever in classic sign.

The pain is triggered by muscle spasms of the sigmoid colon and is acute and persistent in nature. Nausea, vomiting, and a feeling of bloating are also common. The inflammatory process also frequently involves the bladder and cause urinary symptoms. The development of abscess initiates the symptoms of localised peritonitis. Diverticular disease is one of the most common cause's of GI bleeding. Meckel's diverticulum is a congenital abnormality in which a blind tube, similar in structure to the appendix is present, which is usually open into the distal ileum near the ileocaecal valve. The tube may be attached to the umbilicus by a fibrous band.

Management

The preliminary diagnosis of divertuclitis may be made from the history and presenting symptoms. CT scan, barium enema reveals presence of abscess and diverticular pouches respectively.

An episode of diverticulitis is managed by resting the bowel. Hospitalization may be required in acute episodes. The patient is given nothing by mouth and regimen of IV fluids, antibiotics, anticholinergic (Probanthine) is started to reduce bowel spasm. Mild cases managed at home environment. Acute diverticulitis usually subsides with conservative medical management. However, surgical intervention may be needed to deal with complications.

Nursing care during an acute episode is largely supportive and focussed on patient comfort. The nurse teaches rationale for bed rest and bowel rest and the role of there interventions play in bowel healing. The nurse monitors fluid and electrolytes balance and status of the pain. The patient is regularly assessed for complications. Asymptomatic divericulosis is managed by prevention of constipation through the use of a high-fiber diet. Encourage mere fluid intake (2500 ml to 3000 ml/day). Diet modification may be made by allowing foods high in fiber with emphasis on cellulose and haemocellulose type (wheat, whole grain breads and cereals, peas, carrots, seedless grapes, lettuce, peaches, prunes) and avoiding foods containing nuts and seeds, or indigestible strings or threads (cucumbers, celery, tomatoes, cornpop, strawberries, rasoberries, peanuts and seeds). The patient is also encouraged to avoid activities that increase intra-abdominal pressure. Weight loss may be recommended in the attempt to lower the baseline levels of intra-abdominal pressure.

INFLAMMATORY BOWEL DISEASE (IBD)

Inflammatory is an umbrella term used to describe conditions that are characterised by bowel inflammation Crohn's disease and ulcerative colitis are the two major forms of IBD. They have distinctly different pathological characteristics but share among overlapping features.

Aetiology

Exact cause is unknown. The passive causes include

- An infectious agent (bacteria, virus)
- An autoimmune reaction from the presence of immune-related disorder
- Food allergies and
- Heredity.

ULCERATIVE COLITIS

Ulcerative colitis characterized by inflammation and ulceration of the colon and rectum. It may occur at any age but peaks between the ages of 15 and 25 years. There is a second, smaller peak onset between 50-80 years. It affects both sexes but has higher incidence in women.

Pathophysiology and Clinical Manifestation

The inflammation of ulcerative colitis is diffuse and involves the mucosa and submucosa. With alternate periods of exacerbations and remissions the disease is usually begun in the rectum and signoid colon and spreads up the colon in a continuous pattern. The mucosa of the colon is hyperemic and endematous in the affected area. Multiple abscesses develop in the crypts of the Lieberkuhn (intestinal gland). As the disease advances the abscesses break through the crypts into the submucosa, leaving ulceration. These ulcerations also destroy the mucosal epithelium, causing bleeding and diarrhoea. Losses of fluid and electrolytic occur because of the diseased mucosal surface area of absorption. Breakdown of cells results in protein loss through the stools. Areas of inflammed mucosa form pseudopolyps, tongue-like projection and the bowel lumen. Grannulation tissue develops and the mucosa musculature becomes thickened, shortening in colon.

Clinical Manifestations

- Anorexia, nausea, and weight loss.
- Weakness and malaise
- Fever and leucocytosis (High fever and WBC more than 15000/mw suggest abscess).

- Iron deficiency anaemia.
- Profuse diarrhoea (15-20 stool/day).
- Stools containing blood, mucus and possibly pus.
- Abdominal cramping can be present before the bowel movements.
- Loss of fluid, sodium, calcium, potassium and bicarbonate.

The complications of ulcerative colitis be classified into those that are intestinal and those that are extraintestinal. Intestinal include haemorrage, strictures perforation, toxic mega colon and colonic dilation. An extra-intestinal complication of ulcerative colitis are:

- Joints involvement large joints, hips, ankles, wrists, elbows, periperal arthritis, ankylosing, spondylitis, sacroilitis and finger clubbing.
- Skin Erythema nodosum, Pyoderma gangrenosum.
- Mouth Apthous ulcers.
- Eye-conjunctivitis, uvetis, episcleritis.
- Hepato—Cholethiasis, fatty liver, cirrhosis, cholengitis
- Renal kidney stones, ureteral obstruction.

Diagnostic Studies

- Fiberoptic colonoscopy
- Sigmoidoscopy
- Barium enema
- CBC and
- Stool for blood, culture and sensitivity.

Management of Ulcerative Colitis

The goals of treatment are to rest the bowel, control the inflammatioan, combat infection, correct malnutrition, alleviate stress and symptomatic relief using drug therapy. The common drugs used for IBD are:

i. *Aminosalicylates* (oral) are converted in colon to sulfapyridine and 5-amino salicylic acid, which may exert an anti-inflammatory effect, possibly through prostaglandine inhibition (eg. azulfidine, oslazine, mesalamine). During this medications, nurse has to assess for allergy to sulfanamides or aspirins. Monitor for common side effects, anorexia, nausea, vomiting and headache and teach patients to take the drug in divided doses with full glass of fluid or with food. Maintain a liberal intake and report incidence of sit in rash or other adverse effects.
ii. *Aminosalicylates* (Rectal) has same actions as stated in oral. Drugs used are mesalamine in suspension for retention enema and mesalamine suppository. Administer enema while patient is positioned on left side and teach patient to retain as long as possible.
iii. *Corticosteroids* (oral/IV) has potent systemic anti-inflammatory action eg prenisolone/prednisone. During medication, teach patient to; take with food or fluid, monitor weight gain; assess for oedima; Be alert to signs of infection and report promptly, discontinue drug. Maintain good personal hygiene and keep perianal area clean and dry.
iv. *Corticosteroid* (Rectal) has same effect in oral or IV eg hydrocortisone intrarectal foam (Cort-foam), retentive enema (cortenema). Budesonide enema has rapid presystemic metabolism minimises absorption in addition to above actions. Hence, administer enema while patient is positioned on left side and teach patient to retain as long as possible. Other interventions as stated above, side effects should be less.
v. *Immunosuppressive agents* have potent systemic suppressors of immune response; may take 4-6 months for full effect. eg. mercaptopurine (parinethol), azathioprine (imuran). During these medications, teach patient to report any signs of infection; be alert to easy bruising. Return for lab work as scheduled. Maintain liberal daily fluid intake with food or after meals. Another drug cyclosperine (Sandimmun) is oral solution. It may be mixed in glass and given with milk or orange juice at room temperature. Avoid refrigeration. Teach patient to monitor blood pressure; report haematuria or any change in urinary infection.

Surgical intervention may be selected for patients with incurable colitis whose disease cannot be satisfactorily controlled with standard medical management. This procedure is curative in nature and involves removal of the entire colon. i.e., Brook ileostomy, Dr. Nils Kocks, continent ileostomy, Sleoanal anastomasis, or ileorectostomy, ileoanal resurr.

The drugs used are:

- Sulfasalazine
- Corticosteroids and
- Immunosuppressive agents (6-MP, azathioprine)

The dosage and the routes of administeration depend on the severity of the illness and the area involved.

The elemental diet and parenteral nutrition may be used. Parentaral nutrition for severe cases, small bowel fistulas, small bowel syndrome. It is given to promote healing and reduce complications. The elemental diet provides a high caloric, high nitrogen, fat free, no residue sustrate that is absorbed in the proximal small bowel. Vitamin deficiency may develop. Vitamin B_{12} injection may be used.

Surgical intervention is avoided in Crohn's disease as much as possible because of recurrence of the disease process in same region is virtually inevitable.

The nurse should educate the patient and family to take care of the person with inflammatory bowel disease as given below.

i. *Diet and Fluids.*
    - Eat a high caloric and well-balanced diet.
    - Avoid any food that increases symptoms (eg. fresh fruits, and vegetables, fatty foods, spicy foods and alcohol).

Table 7.8: Nursing care plan of patient with ulcerative colitis

Problem	*Reason*	*Objective*	*Nursing intervention*	*Evaluation*
1. Diarrhoea R/T irritated bowel; intestinal hyper-activity.	As manifested by frequent diarrhoeal stools more than 10 per day.	• Fewer firmer stool.	• Monitor frequency and character of stools. • Maintain food and fluid restrictions to rest bowel. • Teach patient to avoid caffeine and food or fluids that are irritating to bowel. • Rarely administer antidiarrhoeal medications, as they may precipitate colonic dilation.	
2. Anxiety R/T Possible social embarassment. Unfamiliar environment, diagnostic test and treatment.	As manifested by expression of concern about effect of disease on social relationships, questions about disease and treatment.	• Less anxious feelings.	• Monitor signs of anxiety. • Encourage open discussions of feelings about diagnosis. • Explain disease, treatments, diagnostic tests and medication. • Provide privacy to reduce embarrassment.	

In addition, NCP also incldue *problem* of altered nutritions; less than body requirements, impaired skin integrity, ineffective individual coping, ineffective management of the rapeutic regimen and hypovolaemia and electrolyte imbalance can be looked for and proper nursing intervention be taken as stated earlier.

- Assess the effect of dairy products on disease symptoms and limit use if appropriate.
- Take multivitamins/mineral supplements daily.
- Ensure a lieberal fluid intake - 2500-3000 ml. per day. Drink electrol or other commercial products if tolerated during flare-ups, to replace lost electrolytes.
- Use salt liberally during disease flare-ups.

ii. *Elimination*
- Take medication as prescribed.
- Keep rectal area clean and dry; use analgesic rectal ointment or sitz baths for rectal discomfort.
- Consult with physician about the appropriateness of antidiarrhoeal agents or bulk laxatives when diarrhoea is present.
- Monitor weight daily disease flare-ups.

iii. *Rest and coping*
- Maintain a regular sleep schedule.
- Schedule daily activities to avoid fatigue, take rest periods as needed.
- Use relaxation strategies when stress levels rise.
- Discuss concern with family or support person.
- Attend local IBD support group if available.

CROHN'S DISEASE

Crohn's disease is a chronic, nonspecific inflammatory bowel disorder of unknown origin that can affect any part of the GI tract. It may occur at any age. But occurs most often between the age of 25 and 30 years. Both sexes are affected with slighly high incidence in women.

Pathophysiology

Crohn's disease can affect any part of the GI tract, but is most often seen in the terminal ileum, jejunum and colon. The inflammation involves all layers of the bowel wall (ie. transmural). Area of involvements are usually discontinuous with segments of normal bowel occurring between diseased portions. Typically ulcerations are deep and longitudinal and penetrate between islands of inflammed oedematous mucosa causing the classic cobblestone appearance. Thickening of bowel wall occurs as well as narrowing of the lumen with stricture development. Abscesses or fistuala tract, that communicates with other loops of bowel, skin, bladder, rectum or vagina may develop.

Clinical Manifestation

The manifestations depend largely on the anatomical site of involvement, extent of the disease process and presence or absence of complications. The onset of Crohn's disease is usually insidious. With non-specific complaints such as diarrhoea, fatigue, abdominal pain, weight loss, and fever. Fever diagnosis is difficult than ulcerative colitis. The principal symptoms are diarrhoea and abdominal pain. Other manifestations include abdominal cramping, anal tenderness, abdominal distention, fever and fatigue. Extraintestinal manifestation such as arthritis, finger clubbing, may precede the onset of disease. As the disease progresses, there is weight loss, malnutrition, dehydration, electrolyte imbalances, anaemia, increased peristalsis and pain around the umbilicus and right lower quadrant. The complitations are fistulas, strictures, anal abscesses, perforation, toxic megacolon.

Diagnostic Studies

- Complete blood cell count
- Serum chemistries
- Stool for occult blood
- Barium enema of small and large intestine
- Procosigmoidoscope examination and
- Sigmoidoscopy and colonoscopy with biopsy.

Management

The goal of management is to control the inflammationary process, relieve symptoms, correct metabolic and nutritional problems and promote healing. Drug therapy and nutritional support are the main-stays of treatment.

iv. Health maintainance
- Report signs requiring medical attention:
  - Change in pattern or severity of abdominal pain or diarrhoea
  - Development of constipation
  - Change in stool character
  - Unusual discharge from rectum and
  - Fever
- Plan for regular follow-up care.

INTESTINAL OBSTRUCTION

Normal functioning of the small and large intestine depends on an open lumen for the movement of intestinal content, as well as adequate circulation and nervous innervation to sustain rhythmic peristalsis. Any factor or condition that either narrows the intestinal passage way or interfere with peristalsis can result in bowel obstruction.

Intestinal obstruction occurs when intestinal contents cannot pass through the GI tract, and it requires prompt treatment. The obstruction may either be partial or complete.

Aetiology

The intestinal obstruction can be classified as mechanical and non-mechanical.

The causes of mechanical obstruction are:

i. *Adhesions* may form after abdominal surgery for unknown reasons; perhaps related to inflammatory responses in the healing bowel. In some cases, the adhesion may become massive. The fibrous bands of scar tissue can loop over bowel segments, either causing the bowel to kink or compress the loop.

ii. *Hernias*. A hernia is a protrusion of an organ or structure from its normal cavity through a congenital or acquired defect usually in the muscle of the abdominal wall. Depending on its location, hernia may contain peritone uro-omentum, a loop of bowel or a section of bladder. Inguinal and umbilical hernias usually result from congenital weakness of the muscle, whereas incisional hernias for usually complications of surgery. Hernia can result in bowel obstruction if the abdominal wall defect through which the hernia protrudes becomes so tight that the bowel segments become strangulated. The lumps or swellings may always be present or may have appeared suddenly after coughing, straining, lifting and other vigorous exertion.
iii. *Tumour*. Tumour mass will gradually restrict the internal tumours of the bowel as it enlarges. Eventually a fecal mass may be unable to pass through the constriction, leading to partial or complete obstruction.
iv. *Volvulus*. A twisting of the bowel upon itself, usually at least a full 180°, obstructing the intestinal lumen both proximally or distally, is called 'Volvulus'. The acute obstruction can quickly result in bowel infarction and can be life-threatening as a result of necrosis, perforation and peritonitis.
v. *Intussusception*. Intussusception involves a telescoping of the bowel in itself. In invagination occurs with peristalsis and in the adult often is triggered by the presence of tumour mass. The bowel segment containing the mass is propelled by peristalsis and adjacene bowel segment. Constriction is immediate and strangulation of the trapped segment can develop.

The other possible causes of mechanical obstruction will include foecal impaction, gallstones and stricture resulting from the diverticulitis and IBD.

The causes of nonmechanical obstruction may result from a neuromuscular or vascular disorder.

i. *Paralytic ileus* (or Adynamic ileus) results from a lack of peristaltic activity, usually as a result of neurogenic impairment. Ileus is a common temporary problem after abdominal surgery particularly if the bowel has been extensively handled. Other causes of paralytic ileus include inflammatory responses (Eg. appendicitis, pancreatitis), electrolyte abnormalities, and thoracic and lumbar spinal fractures.
ii. *Vascular distinctions* are rare and are due to an interference with the blood supply to a position of the intestines. The common causes are emboli; and ather osclerosis of mesentric arteries, thrombosis of the mesentric arteries.

Pathophysiology

Intestinal obstruction triggers a series of GI tract events whose clinical manifestation depends largely on the location of the obstruction and the degree of circulatory compromise. Normally 6 to 8 litres of fluid enters the small bowel daily. Most of the fluid is absorbed before it reaches the colon. Approximately 75 per cent of the intestinal gas is swallowed air. Bacterial metabolism produce methane and hydrogen gases fluid and intestinal content accumulates proximal to the intestinal obstruction. This causes distention and the distal bowel may collapse. The distention reduces the absorption of the fluids and stimulates intetinal secretion. As the fluid increases. So does the pressure in the lumen of the bowel. The incresaed pressure leads to an increase in capillary permeability and extravasation of fluids and electrolytes into the peritoneal cavity. Oedema, congestion and necrosis from imparied blood supply and possible rupture of the bowel may occur. The retention of fluid in the intestine and peritoneal cavity can lead to a severe reduciton in circulating blood volume and result in hypotension and hypovolaemic shock.

Vascular compromise is the most serious aspect of obstruction. Bowel ischemia breaks down the normal barrier to bacteria and the stagnant and distended bowel becomes increasingly permeable to bacteria. Organism can enter the peritoneal cavity and lead to peritonitis. Bacteria are normally sparse in the small bowel but accumulated rapidly during obstruction. E. Coli, klebsiella prevalent and the release of toxins can result in septic shock. The ischaemic process can progress to gangrene and perforation. Submucosal haemorrhage and sloughing can also be a source of substantial blood loss.

Clinical Manifestation

The clinical manifestations of intestinal obstructions very based on the exact site of obstruction and include nausea, vomiting, abdominal pain, distensiton, inability to pass flatulence and constipation (fecal impaction secondary to constipation, colonar perforation).

Obstruction located high in the small intestine produces rapid onset, sometimes projective vomiting with bile containing vomitus. Vomiting from more distal obstruction of the small intestine is more gradual in onset. The vomitus may be orange-brown and foul-smelling because of bacterial growth. Vomiting may be entirely absent in large bowel obstruction if the iliocecal valve is competent. Otherwise, the patient may eventually vomit facalent material.

Abdominal pain is fairly universal symptom. Simple obstruction produce cramy and poorly localized pain. Its onset parallels the initial increase in peristalsis that raises intraluminal pressure in an attempt to clear the obstruction. Frequent loud, high pitched bowel sounds are often heard on ausculation. The pain typically lessens as the obstructions worsen. Smooth muscle atony decreases peristalsis and bowel sounds are diminshed. The pain associated with bowel strangulation is constant and severe vomitings usually relieve abdominal pain in high intestinal obstruction. persistent, colicky abdominal pain is seen with lower intestinal obstruction.

Abdominal distention usualy develops slowly although obstipation is common. Rising fever usually indicates the presence of dying bowel. Laboratory values typically reflect the progressive nature of the dehydration. There is decreased urine output, haemoconcentration, hypokalaemia and hyponatraemia.

Management

Intestinal obstruction is a potentially life-threatening condition. Assessment must begin with a detailed patient's history and physical examination. The type of location of obstruction usually causes characteristic symptoms. The nurse should determine the location, duration, intensity and frequency of abdominal pain and whether abdominal tenderness or rigidity is present. Onset, frequency, colour; odour and amount of vomitus should be recroded. Bowel funciton, including passage of flatus should be determined. this should ausculatate for bowel sounds and document character and location, irrespective the abdomen for scars, palpable mass, and distention, and observe for muscle guarding and tenderness. The usual diagnosis measures taken are abdominal X rays, barium enema, as these given, e.g. clues for locating obstruciton. Lab tests are also helpful, CBC, serum-electrolyte, amylase, BUN. The nurse should prepare the patient for such measures.

Treatment is directed towards decompression of the intestine by removal of gas and fluid, correciton and maintenance of fluid and electrolyte balance, and relief or removal of the obstruction. NG or intestinal tube may be used to decompress the bowel. NG tubes should be inserted before surgery to empty the stomach and relieve distention. They are also used instead of nasointestinal tubes to treat partial or complete small-bowel obstrucitons. Intestinal tubes such as the Center or Miller-Abbot or Dennis tubes are passed into the small intestine. They are 10 fect (9300 cm) long and mercury-weighed.

The patient should be monitored closely for signs of dehydrations and electrolyte imbalance. A strict intake and output record should be maintained. All vomitus and tube drainage should be included. IV fluids should be administered. Serum electrolyte levels should be monitored. A patient with high obstruction is more likely to have metabolic alkalosis. A patient with low obstruction is at greater risk of metabolic acidosis. The patient is often restless and cosntantly changes position to releive the pain. Analgesics may be with held until the obstruction is diagnosed because they may mask other signs and symptoms and decrease intestinal motility. The nurse should provide comfort measures to promote a restful environment, and keep distraction and visitors to a minimum. Nursing care of the patient after surgery for an intestinal obstruciton is similar to the care of the patient after laparotomy.

COLORECTAL CANCER

Colorectal cancer has been widely spread by the turn of the last millenmium. The causes of colorectal cancer remain unclear. Groups at high risk of colorectal cancer have been identified are:

- Age (after 40 years) is a risk time for both men and women.
- Colorectal polyps.
- Chronic inflammatory bowel disease (H/o ulcerative colitis).
- Family history of colerectal cancer or adenomas.
- Previous history of colorectal cancer.
- History of genital or breast cancer (woman).
- High caloric, high fat/or low-fiber diet.
- Cigarette smoking.
- Obseity (Nature of the risk currenlty unknow).

Pathophysiology

Adenocarcinoma is the most common type of colon cancer. Most colorectal cancers appear to arise from adenomatous polyps. All tumours tend to spread through the walls of the Intestine and into the lymphatic system. Tumours commonly spread to the liver because the venous blood flow from the colorectal tumour is through the portal vein. Since the cancer of the colon may spread by direct extension or through the lymphatic or circulatory systems it may seed at distant point in the peritonium or at distant points in the colon. The liver and lungs are the major organs of metastasis.

Clinical Manifestation

The clinical manifestation of the colon cancer varies with the location of the tumour. There are usually no early symptoms and the disease is often diagnosed incidentally. Cancer in distal colon and rectum typically produces symphony related to partial obstruciton. The lesiosn are more likely to be annular, and they grow circumferentially, encircling the colon wall. The lumen becomes narrow and constricted. Obstruction occurs when formed stool is unable to pass through the narrowed lumen.

- The patient may experience a change in bowel habits, a feeling of incomplete bowel emptying, or rectal bleeding. The clinical manifestation of bowel cancer are as followed:
- Frequently a symptomatic and diagnosed incidentaly,
- Symptoms of partial bowel obstruction.
  - Change in bowel habits, e.g. constipation or diarrhoea and
  - Pencil or ribbon-shaped stool.
  - Sensation of incomplete bowel emptying.
- Gas or bloating
- Occurs blood in the stool or rectal bleeding
- Weakness, fatigue, malaise, anorexia and anaemia.
- Weight loss usually accompany with metastasis.
- Abdominal pain (usually accompanies in larger lesions).

Diagnostic test: Rectal examination. sigmoidoscopy, colonoscopy, Barium enema, CBC, LFT, Ocult blood test, CEA test, CT scan and ultrasound.

Management

Prognosis and treatment correlates with pathological staging of the disease. Several methods of staging currently being used are:

1. Duke's classification 2. TNM classification.

1. *Duke Staging* system for colorectal cancer.
   - A Negative nodes, limitations of lesion to mucosa.
   - B_1 Negative nodes, extension of lesion through mucosa but still within the bowel wall.
   - B_2 Negative nodes extention through entire bowel wall.
   - C_1 Positive nodes, limitation of lesion to bowel well.
   - C_2 Positive nodes, extension of lesion through entire bowel wall.
   - D Presence of distant unresectable metastasis.

This staging is used to establish the appropriates level of intervention and treatment.

The most recent classifications of colorectal cancer is the tumour, node, metasis, (TNM) system which is based on pathologic assessment and includes data from the history and physical examination and presurgical and Lab evaluation.

- T – *Primary Tumours*
- T_x – Primary tumour can not be assessed.
- T_0 – No evidence of primary tumour.
- Tis – Carcinoma in situ
- T_1 – Tumour invades submucosa.
- T_2 – Tumours invades muscularis propria.
- T_3 – Tumour invades through the msculari propriat into the subserosa or into the non-peritonealized pericalic or perirectal tissue.
- T_4 – Tumour perforates the visceral peritoneum or directly invades other organs or structures.

N-REGIONAL LYMPH NODE INVOLVEMENT

N_x – Regional lymph node cannot be assessed.
N_o – No regional lymph node metastasis.
M_I – Disticnt metastasis.

After diagnosis has been confirmed, treatment may initiated by radiation and chemotherapy.

Radiation may be used preoperatively or as a palliative measure for patients with advanced lesions. It is primary objective is to reduce tumour size and provide symptomatic relief.

Chemotherpay is recommended when a patient has a positive lymph node at the time of surgery or has metastatic disease. No drug is available that can cure malignant colon or rectal tumours.

Surgery is the only curative treatment of colorectal cancer. Success of surgery depends on resection of the tumour with an adequate margin of healthy bowel and resection of the reginoal lymph nodes. the usual surgical procedure includes.

i. Right hemicolectomy is performed when the cancer is located in the cecum, ascending colon, hepatic flexure, or transverse colon to the right of the middle artery. A portion of the terminal ileum, the appendix are removed, and an ileotransverse anastomosis is performed.
ii. A left hemicolectomy involves resection of the left transferes colon, the splenic flexure, the descending colon, the sigmoid colon and the upper portion of the rectum and abdominal-perinal resection, laparascopy colectomy is also performed.

Pre and postoperative care are similar to that of any laparatomy within specific activities is initiated accordingly (See Ostomy Surgery).

OSTOMY SURGERY

An ostomy is a surgical procedure in which an opening is made to allow the passage of intestinal contents from the bowel to an incision trauma. The stoma which is the opening on the surface of the abdomen is created when the intestine is brough through the abdominal wall and sutured to the skin. It may be permanent or temporary. Fecal matter is diverted through the stoma to the outside of the abdominal wall.

- An *ileostomy* is opening from the ileum through the abdominal wall and is also referred to as a covnentional or Brooke's ileostomy. It is most commonly used in surgical treatment of ulcertative colitis crohn's disease and familial polyp.
- A *Cecostomy* is an opening between the cecum and the abdominal wall. They are usually temporary most often used for fecal diversion before surgery or for palliation.
- A *colostomy* is an opening between the colon and abdominal wall. The proximal end of the colon is sutured to the skin. Temporary colostomy is usually performed to protect an end-to-end anastomosis after a bowel resection or in an emergency measure following bowel obstruction. (Eg. malignant tumour), abdominal trauma (Gunshot wound) or a perforated diverticulum. Loop colostomy and double barrel colostomy are more commonly performed as temporary colostomy, but they may be permanent.

Preoperative Care

Preoperative care focuses on patient teaching.

The nurse assesses the patient's knowledge and understanding of the proposed surgery and its outcomes. This inlcudes brief overview of GI tract structure and functioning and the nature of functioning of the ostomy. Emotional preparation for ostomy surgery is extremely important. The nurse encourages the pateint to verbalize feelings related to the radical change to body image and function. Validating the appropriateness of these concerns lays in the family for an effective working relationship with patient.

The patient may need to progress through the grieving process, and if the person is in the shock state, specific factual teaching may be ineffective. The nurse offers acceptance of all feelings and reinforces the importance of open communication.

The preparation phase may include nutritional support and possibly total parental nutrition (TPN), if the patient's nutitional state is inadequate for surgery. The patient should know what to except in the postoperative period. The nurse discusses the management of postoperative pain. The nature and apperance of all incisions and drains.and the purpose of the NG tube and IV lines. Bowel cleansing is also performed and may include the use of enemas, laxatives, and antibiotics to reduce intestinal bacterial flora.

Postoperative Care

Postoperative nursing care should focus on assessing the stoma protecting the skin, selecting the pouch, and assisting the patient to adapt psychologically to a changed body. In addition, maintenance of fluid and electrolyte balance, stoma monitoring and managing the wound are important.

(Further please see Ng Careplan of patient with colostomy (ileostomy Table 7.9).

The following guidelines should be kept in mind while changing the ostomy pouch.

i. *Stoma measurement*

- Use the measuring guide and sample diameters and cut the ostomy appliances to fit pattern should be 1/8 to 1/4 inch larger than stoma.
- Use the same procedure to prepare the skin barrier.
  Note: The pouch opening is cut slightly larger than that of the skin barrier to prevent paper from cutting the stoma.

ii. *Removing Pouch*

- Empty drainable pouch to prevent spills.
- Disconnect pouch from skin wafer if two-piece system is used.
- Gently peel the wafer away from the skin beginning at the top.

iii. *Skin Care*

- Cleanse the skin with warm water and dry thoroughly. Use soap only stool adheres to skin. Rinse thoroughly with water.
- Assess peristomal skin and stoma carefully for signs of irritation or infection.
- Pat peristoma skin dry thoroughly.

iv. *Applying New Pouch*

- Center the pouch opening over the stoma. Ask patient to abdominal muscle to make application easier.
- Gently press into place and hold for at least 30 seconds to seal special emphasis will be on ostomy skin care as follows:
- When a pouch seal leaks, the pouch should be immediately changed, not taped. Stool held against the skin quickly results in severe irritation.
- Pouches are removed gently, with one hand holding the skin in place to decrease pulling.
- The skin should be gently but thoroughly cleansed, rinsed and patted dry.
- A skin should be gently but thoroughly cleansed, rinsed and patted dry.
- Peristomal hair should be trimmed but not shaved to prevent folliculitis.
- A skin barrier should be used to protect the peristomal skin from liquid stools.
- A skin sealant should be used under all types.
- The patient should consult special nurse for specific care if available.

An ostomy irrigation is an enema given through the stoma to stimulate bowel emptying at a regular and convenient time for which the following guidelines are helpful.

- Assemble all euqipment: Water container, irrigating sleeve and belt, skin care, items, new pouch system, ready for use.
- Remove old pouch and dispose.
- Clean the stoma and peristomal skin with water and assess.
- Apply the irrigating sleeve and belt. Place open end of sleeve in toilet.
- Fill irrigating container with 500 ml to 1000 ml of lukewarm tap water, and suspend container at shoulder height.
- Run water through the tubing to remove air.
- Gently insert the irrigating cone into stoma, and slowly start the flow of water. Cathetors are inserted no more than 2 to 4 inches. Do not fork. If cramping occurs, stop the irrigation and wait.
- Allow approximately 15 to 20 minutes for stool to empty.
- Rinse sleeves, dry the bottom, roll it up and close off the end. Patient should go about regular activities for 30 to 45 minutes.
- Remove sleeve, clean stoma, and apply new pouch.
- Clean and store the irrigating equipment.

ANORECTAL DISORDERS

A variety of common disorders can affect the perianal area. Persons who experience anorectal disorders typically seek medical care for symptoms such as pain, tenderness, itching or the development of rectal bleeding. Many of them will be treated on outpatient basis. They include haemorrhoid, fissure, abscesses, fistula, pilonideal sinus.

Haemorrhoids are masses of dilated blood vessels that lie beneath the lining of the skin in the anal canal. They are dilated haemorrhoidal veins. They may be internal or external. Internal occurring about the internal spincter, external occurring

Table 7.9: Nursing care plan of patient with a colostomy/ileostomy

Problem	*Reason*	*Objective*	*Nursing intervention*	*Evaluation*
1. Risk for impaired skin integriety R/T irritation and lack of knowledge of skin.	• Irritations from fecal drainage. • Irritation of pouch.	• Normal skin *integrity* • Intact pouch seal	1• Have special nurse (ET Nurse) see before surgery to mark stoma site if possible. • After surgery, assess peristoma skin for erythema with burning, itching, poorly fitting appliances with leakage, lack of adequate skin care and failure to use skin barrier. • During pouch change, assess skin for signs of breakdown. • Clean area with milk soap and water and dry thoroughly. • Apply skin barrier to protect skin and to prevent direct contact to intestinal contents. • Teach patient proper skin and pouch care. • Plan home visit for outpatient for continued teaching. • Empty pouch when it is one-third full prevent seal from leaking.	
2. Body image disturbance R/T presence of stoma, and malador.	As manifested by verbalization of embarrassessment of shame due to stoma and odour.	• Adjustment to altered body image. • Satisfactory plan for control odour.	• Assessment the patient atitude towards stoma. • Instruct patient to measure for odour control, use of odour of pouch, pouch deodarant, and use of room deodarant when, pouch is opened/ emptied. • Teach patient to use loose clothing to conceal pouch. • Discuss normal emotional response to stoma and encourage patient to excpress feeling. • Encourage family members to be active in care. • Provide patient with information on resoruces supporint ostomy patients. • Prepare patient to do own stoma and pouch care.	
3. Altered nutrition more than body requirement R/T lack of knowledge of appropriate foods and decreased appetite.	• As manifested by weight loss. Vitamin and mineral deficiency, inability to tolerate certain foods.	• During intake to maintain weight at approved level.	• Assess nutritional intake. • Gradually introduce foods one at a time and begin with low-residue diet. • Teach patient to chew food slowly and properly and make digestion and earlier and prevent gas. • Give list of foods to be avoided.	
4. Altered sexuality pattern R/T Perceived loss of sexual appeal and possibilit of accidental seepage of fecal materal during sexual activity.	• As manifested by verbalization of concern about intimate relation with spous or significant others.	• Confidence in ability to resume avoid sexual activity.	• Assess patient's attitude about impact of astomy on sexual functioning. • Encourage discussion on meaning of sexuality to patient and his nears and dear in a non-threatening manner • Discuss way to avoid seepage and conceal stoma and/or pouch during intimate relation to avoid embarrassments.	
5. Risk for fluid volume deficit R/T excessive fluid loss.	• Fluid loss from ileostomy or diarrhoea with colostomy and inadequate oral intake	• Normal serum electrolytes • Normal vital signs • Good skin turger • Urine output more then 0.5 ml/kg/hr	• Assess for signs of weakness, poor skin turgor sunken eyes, hypotension, tachycardia, hypokalaemia, hyponatnaemia, oliguria. • Record intaken and output and include ileostomy drainage to have an accurate record for replacement. • Ensure fluid intake of at least 3000 ml/day in the initial postoperative period. • Instruct patient to maintain high fluid intake and increase it during hot weather, patient is perspiring excessively and during diarrhoeal episode. • Monitor serum electrolyte • Instruct the patients on signs and symptoms of sodium, potassium and fluid deficit.	

outside the external spincter. Symptoms of haemorrhoids include bleeding, pruritis, prolapse and pain are common in all age groups.

Haemorrhoids affect the person of all ages, but they typically cause more problems with increasing age. Pregnancy is common condition for initiating or aggravating haemorrhoids. Other conditions associated with the development of haemorrhoids include obesity, congestive herat failure, and chronic liver disease which result in portal hypertension. These conditions are associated with persistent elevation in intra-abdominal pressure. Sedentary occupations that involve long period of sitting or standing also implicated though exact mechanism is unknown.

The diagnosis of haemorrhoids is done by inspection, digital examination, proctoscopy or examination with the flexible sigmoidoscopy.

Conservative management of haemorrhoids includes a high-fiber diet, bulk laxatives warm sitz baths, and gentle cleansing. A high fever diet and increased fluid intake prevent constipation and reduce straining, which allows engorgement of the veins to subside. Ointments such as Nupercaine, creams, suppositories and impregnated pads that contain anti-inflammatory agents, (hydrocortisone) or astrigent and anaesthesia may be used to shrink the mucus membrane and relive discomfort. Stool softeners may be ordered to keep the stool soft and sitz bath may be ordered to relieve pain.

Application of ice packs for few hours followed by warm packs may be used for thrombosed haemorrhoids. If severe pain, bleeding or thrombosis are present, more definitive treatment may be indicated. A variety of options have been used over time including sclerotherapy, cryotherapy, binolar diathermy, rubber band ligation and surgical haemorrhoidectomy.

The following guidelines are helpful for persons undergonig anal/rectal surgery.

i. *Preoperative care*
   - Bowel preparation is standard, but an enema may not be prescribed if rectal pain is actue.
   - Stool softeners may given to promote a soft stool before surgery.

ii. *Postoperative care*
   - Administer analgesics as prescribed, especially before initial defeclation (considerable rectal discomfort may be present).
   - Provide emotional sport before and after first defecation.
   - Suggest side-lying position.
   - Provide sitz baths as ordered (monitor for hypotension secondary to dilation of pelvic blood vessels in early postoperative period).

iii. *Promotion of Elimination*
   - Administer prescribed stool softeners.
   - Encourage patient to defectate as soon as the inclination occurs (prevents strictures and preserves normal anal lumen considerable anxiety is usually personal.)
   - Monitor for hypotension, dizziness, and faintness during first defecation.
   - If an enema must be given, use small bore rectal tube.

iv. *Patient Teaching*
   - Clean rectal area after each defecation until healing is complete. (sitz bath is recommended).
   - Avoid constipation with a high-fiber diet, high-fluid in-take, regular exercise, and regular time for defecation.
   - Use stool softeners until healing is complete.
   - Seek medical consultation for rectal bleeding, suppurative drainage, continued pain on defecation, or continued constipation despite preventive measures.

Anal Fissure

An anal fissure or fissure in and around the anus is a skin ulcer or a crack in the lining of the anal walt that is caused by trauma or local infection. It is frequently associated with constipation and subsequent stretching of the anus from hard feces. The most common clinical manifestations are painful spasm of the anal spincter and severe, burning pain during defecation. Some bleeding may occur and constipation resutls becasue of pain assocaited with bowel movements.

Conservative treatment consists of bowel regulations with mineral oil and stool softeners. Sitz bath and anal anaesthetics suppositories (Anusol) are also ordered. Surgical treatment usually consists of excision of fissure. Postoperative care is similar to that of haemorroidectomy.

Anorectal Abscess

Anorectal abscesses are defined as undrained collections of perianal pus. They are due to perirectal infections in patient who have compromised local circulation or active inflammatory disease. The most common causative organism are E. coli, Staphylococci and Streptococci. Clinical manifestation includes local pain, swelling, foul-smelling, drainage, tenderness and elevated temperature and sepsis can occur.

Surgical therapy consists of drainage of abscess of packing is used. It should be allowed to heal by granulation. The packing is changed every day and moist and hot compresses are applied to the area. Care must be taken to avoid soiling the dressing during urination and defecation. A low-residue diet is given. The patient may leave the hospital with area open. Teaching, should include wound care, the importance of sitz-bath, thorough cleaning after bowel movement and periodic check-up.

Anorectal Fistula

An anorectal fistula is an abnormal tunnel leading out from the anus or rectum. It is a hollow tract leading through anal tissue from anorectal canal through skin near anus. It may extend to the outside the skin, vagina or buttocks. Anorectal fissures are complications of Crohn's disease. This condition often precedes an anorectal abscess.

Feces may enter the fistula and cause an infection. There may be persistent, blood stained, purulent discharge, or stool leakage from the fistula. The patient may have to wear a pad to prevent staining of clothes.

Surgical therapy involves a fistulotomy or a fistulectomy, Gauze packing is inserted and the wound is left to heal by granulation. Care is the same after haemorrhoidectomy.

Pilonidal Sinus

A pilonidal sinus is a small tract under the skin between the buttocks in the sacrococcygeal area. It is thought to be congenital origin. It may have several openings and is lined with epithelium and hair, thus the name pilonidal (a nest of hair).

The skin is moist and movement of the buttocks causes the short wiry hair to penetrate the skin. The irritated skin becomes infected and forms a pilonidal cyst or abscess. There are no symptoms unless there is an infection. If it becomes infested, the patient complains of pain and selling at the base of the spine.

The formed abscess requires incision and drainage. The wound may be closed or left open to heal by secondary intention. This wound is packed and sitz bath are ordered. Nursing care includes hot moist, heat application when an abscess is present. The patient is usualy more comfortable lying on the abdomen or side. The patient should be instructed to avoid contamination of dressing during urination or defecation and to avoid straining whenever possible.

PROCEDURE 7.1: **ASSISTING WITH AN A PROTOSIGMOIDOSCOPY.*

Equipment

Fleet type enema used at least 1 hour before before the sigmoidoscopy	Specimen bottles containing 10 per cent. Formmalin culture tubes.
Oral laxative	4 × 4 gauze sponges.
Water soluble lubricant.	Cytology brush.
Sigmoidoscopy	Glass eyepiece to fit on scope during insufflation of air.
Biposy forceps.	Disposable gloves for preliminary examination.
Culture swap.	Suction machine.
Long applicator sticks (cotton).	Microscopic slides with fixative or 95 per cent ethyl alcohol.
Drapes or sheets.	Specimen labels.

Nursing Focus

1. Emergency resuscitation equipment needs to be available, because the vagus nerve is often stimulated and can tentiate a vagal reaction (pallor, diaphoresis, dizziness, weakness, unconsciousness, decrease in blood pressure, pulse rate, sometimes causing these vital signs to be unobtainable).
2. If giving enemas before the procedure, do not advance the the tube too high into the colon, and administer the some slowly. If rectal bleeding or abdominal pain occur, stop at once and call the physician.

Inform the health care provider of any known allergies and current medications certain medications, such as anticoagulants, may be held before the test.

Obtain prior X-rays and studies and send with the patient.

STEPS OF PROCEDURE

Nursing action	*Rationale*
Preparatory Phase	
1. Record baseline vital signs. Leave the blood pressure cuff in place. An Automatic blood pressure machine may be used, however, a manual cuff is preferred in the event the patient has a vagal reaction (See nursing alert above).	1. Monitoring of the blood pressure and pulse throughout the procedure will be necessary.
2. Have the patient assume the knee-chest or sims lateral position.	2. The position used depends on physician preference, patient condition, and nature of examining table (or bed).
a. Knee-Chest position. 1. Knees are spread comfortable apart. 2. Thighs are perpendicular to table. 3. Feet are extended over the edge. 4. Head is turned sideways to right (head shares pillow with chest). 5. Left arm is flexed to side of chest. 6. Right arm may rest above head.	a. This position permits the sigmoid to hang forward, diminishing the angle at the rectosigmoid junction.
b. Sims lateral position. 1. Place, patient on left side with left leg partially flexed at hip and knee, right leg should be fully flexed. 2. Pelvis to be perpendicular to table.	b. Used for elderly, ill, or arthritic patients or those who are reluctant to assume the knee-chest position.
3. Drape the patient so that only perineum is visible.	3. A disposable large sheet with a circular opening is practical. This will minimize embarrassment.
4. Explain to the patient to take slow deep breaths as the physician examines the rectum by digital examination.	4. The physician is examining for tenderness, mucus, blood fistula, inflammation, ulceration and fexes. The digital examination also indicates the direction

Contd...

Nursing action	Rationale
	of the anal-canal, its patency, and the presence of any abnormality, if promotes anal relaxation and helps to lubricate the orifice.
5. Warm sigmoidoscope in tap water or sterilizer to slightly above body temperature, lubricate tip of scope.	5. A Cold scope would cause discomfort and promote contraction rather than relaxation of perianal muscles. Water soluble lubricant permits easier passage of scope. It also minimizes the urge to defecate at tube insertion.
6. Physician spreads buttocks and anal margins with left hand and inserts instrument with right hand (or vice versa). Have the patient breathe deeply.	6. Keep instrument out of view of patient. Breathing slowly and deeply will help relax abdominal muscles and minimize cramping.
7. Nurse encourages relaxation and explain each step in advance.	7. Reassuring the patient promote relaxation.
8. Physician may use a glass eye piece over viewing end of scope, an insufflation bulb and tubing are attached. A small quantity of air may be pumped into the bowel. Tell patient as the air moves down the bowel he may experience flatulence. This is normal.	8. The purpose of inflating lower bowel with air is to expand the area viewed so that vision is not obstructed by mucosal folds and to facilitate passage into the sigmoid colon.
9. Examination of the sigmoid, rectum, and mucosa are done while the scope is being removed. If a rigid scope is used, passage of a large cotton swab through the scope may be done to remove blood, mucus, and feces. If a flexible scope is used, only suction is necessary to clear the field. Turn suction to lowest setting initially.	9. This clears the field of vision.
10. Passage of biopsy forceps, cytology brush, or culture swab through the scope is done to collect specimens.	10. Specimens will be placed in 10 per cent formalin and labelled. A specimen for cytology is placed in a container of 95 per cent ethyl alcohol or affixed to a microscopic slide with slide fixative. Specimens for cultures will be sent in specimen tubes.
11. Relay to the physician any expressions or complaints of pain by the patient.	11. Tenderness and pain may be experienced by the patient with a history of abdominal surgery procedure may have to be terminated in order to risk perforation.
Follow-up Phase	
1. On withdrawl of scope, assist patient into gradually assuming a relaxed position.	1. To promotes comfort.
2. Wipe perianal area.	2. Prevent soilage of garments.

Contd...

Nursing action	Rationale
3. If disposable scope is used, rise and discard in proper receptacle. Reusable scopes are properly cleaned with solution and water, per protocol. Sterilizable parts are sterilized before scope is stored.	3. Prevents contamination and infection.
4. Record the procedure, preparation of the patient, reaction of the patient, and patient's vital signs.	
5. Label all specimens immediately and send to the laboratory.	5. Minimize error, allow fresh samples for evaluation.
6. Observe the patient for complications haemorrhage (increased pulse, decreased blood pressure, weakness, pallor, rectal bleeding and possible abdominal pain), perforation (sudden, severe abdominal pain), fever, malaise, changes in vital signs, bloody or mucoid rectal drainage, and possible abdominal distention.	
7. Instruct the patient on these signs and symptoms and advise to notify health care provider immediately should they occur, ever after discharge.	7. Prevent risk of complications.

PROCEDURE 7.2: ***ADMINISTERING AN ENEMA.**

Equipment

Prepackaged enema or enema container.
Disposable gloves.
Water-soluble jelly.
Water-proof pad.
Bath blanket.
Bedpan or commode.
Washcloth and towel.
Basin.
Toilet tissue.

STEPS OF PROCEDURE

Nursing Action	Rationale
Preparatory Phase	
1. Asses the patient's bowel habits (last, BM, laxative usage, bowel patterns) and physical condition (haemorrhoids, mobility, external sphincter control).	1. Enema should not be given if there is a suspicion of appendicitis or bowel obstruction.
2. Provide for privacy and explain procedure to patient.	2. Provide comfort.
Performance Phase	
1. Wash hands.	1. Promote hygiene.
2. Place patient on left side with rigth knee fixed (Sims' position), place waterproof pad underneath patient and cover with bath blanket.	2. Allow for enema solution to flow by gravity along the natural curve of the sigmoid colon and rectum.
3. Place bedpan or bedside commode in position for patients who	3. Allow for easy accessibility.

Contd...

cannot ambulate to the toilet or who may have difficulty with sphincter control.	
4. Remove plastic cover over tubing and lubricate tip of enema tubing 3-4 in. (7.5-10 cm) unless prepackaged (tip is already lubricated). Even prepackaged enema may need more lubricant.	4. Prevent trauma and eases application.
5. Apply disposable gloves.	
6. Separate buttocks and locate rectum.	
7. Instruct patient that you will be inserting tubing and to take slow, deep breaths.	7. Allows for patient relaxation and readiness.
8. Insert tubing 3-4 in for adult patients.	8. Prevents tissue trauma of rectum.
9. Slowly instill the solution using a clamp and the height of the container to adjust flow rate if using an enema bag and tubing for high enemas, raise enema container 12-18 in, above anus; for low enemas, 12 in. If using a prepackaged enema, slowly squeeze the container until all solution is instilled.	9. Rapid infusion can cause colon distention and cramping container elevated past 12-18 in., and controller on tubing not regulated contribute to rapid infusion.
10. Lower container or clamp tubing if patient complains of cramping.	
11. Withdraw rectal tubing after all enemas solution has been instilled or until clear (usually not more than three enemas).	11. "Until Clear" means until results do not contain fecal matter and are clear.
12. Instruct patient to hold solution as long as possible and that a feeling of distention may be felt.	12. Promotes better results.
13. Discard supplies in the appropriate trash receptacle.	13. Maintains hygiene, minimizes patient embarrassment.
14. Assist patient on the bedpan or to the beside commode or toilet when urge to defecate occurs.	
15. Observe enema return for amount, fecal content. Instruct patient not to flush toilet until the nurse has seen the results.	

Nursing Focus

> Enemas should not be given routinely to treat constipation because they disrupt normal defecation reflexes and the patient becomes dependent.

Follow-up Phase

1. Document the type of enema given volume and results on the appropriate chart forms.
2. Assess and document presence or absence of abdominal distention after enema was given.
3. Assist the patient with washing perineum and rectal area, if indicated, may also need a clean gown or linen change.

NASOGASTRIC/NASOINTESTINAL INTUBATION

Nasogastric intubation refers to the insertion of a tube through the nasopharyns into the stomach. See procedure 7.3.

Nasointestinal intubation is performed by inserting a small bore-weighted tube that is carried via peristalsis into the duodenum or jejunum. It is primarily used for administering feedings and maintaining nutritional intake. See procedure 7.4; nasointestinal intubation.

Purposes of Nasogastric Intubation

1. Remove fluids and gas from stomach (decompression).
2. Prevent or relieve nausea and vomiting after surgery or traumatic events by decompressing the stomach.
3. Determine the amount of pressure and motor activity in the GI tract (diagnostic studies).
4. Irrigate the stomach for active bleeding or poisoning.
5. Treat mechanical obstruction.
6. Administer medications and leeding (gavage) directly into the GI tract.
7. Obtain a specimen of gastric contents for laboratory studies when pyloric or intestinal obstruction is suspected.

PROCEDURE 7.3: **NASOGASTRIC INTUBATION AND REMOVAL.*

Equipment

Nasogastric tube is usually levin or double lumen Salem, sump tube.	Hypoallergenic tape "1/2 and 1" Bio-occlusive transparent dressing irrigating set with 20-ml syringe of a 50-ml catheter-tip syringe.
Water soluble lubricant.	
Suction equipment.	
clamp for tubing.	Stethoscope.
towel, tissues, and emesis basin	Tongue blade.
Glass of water and straw.	Penlight.
Tincture of benzoin.	Disposable gloves.
	Normal saline.

Follow-up Equipment

Insertion Procedure

Lip pomade

Mouth hygiene materials.

Intubation Procedure

Preparatory Phase

1. Ask the patient if he or she has ever had nasal surgery, trauma, or a deviated septum.
2. Explain procedure to the patient and tell how mouth breathing, panting, and swallowing will help in passing the tube.
3. Place the patient in a sitting or high. Fowler's position, place a towel accross chest.
4. Determine with the patient what sign he or she might use, such as raising the index finger, to indicate "Wait a few moments" because of gagging or discomfort.
5. Remove dentures, place emesis basin and tissues within the patient's reach.
6. Inspect the tube for defects, look for partially closed holes or rough edges.

7. Place rubber tubing in ice-chilled water for a few minutes to make the tube firmer. Plastic tubing may already be firm enough, if too stiff, dip in warm water.
8. Determine the length of the tube needed to reach the stomach by placing the end of the tube at the tip of the patient's nose. Then extend it to the earlobe and down to the xiphoid process (see figure). Mark this distance with hypoallergenic tape. (Measurement range for the average-size adult is 55-66 cm (22-26 in).
9. Have the patient blow nose to clear nostrils.
10. Inspect the nostrils with a penlight, observing for any obstruction, occlude each nostril and have the patient breathe. This will help determine which nostril is more patient.
11. Wash your hands. Put on disposable gloves.

General Procedures/Treatment Modalities

1. Mark the nasoglastric tube at a point 50 cm from the distal tip; call this point 'A'.
2. Have the patient sit in a neutral position with head facing forward place the distal tip of the tubing at the tip of the patient's nose (N), extend tube to the tragus (tip) of his ear (E), and then extend the tube straight down to the tip of his xiphoid (X). Mark this point 'B' on the tubing.
3. To locate point C on the tube, find the midpoint between points A and B. The nasogastric tube is passed to point C to the ensure obtimum placement in the stomach.

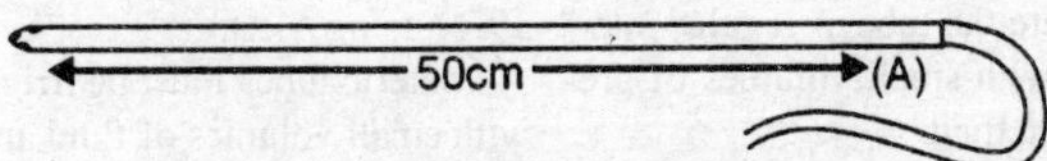

Fig. 7.3: Mark the nasogastric tube at a point 50 cm. from the distal tip; call this point 'A'.

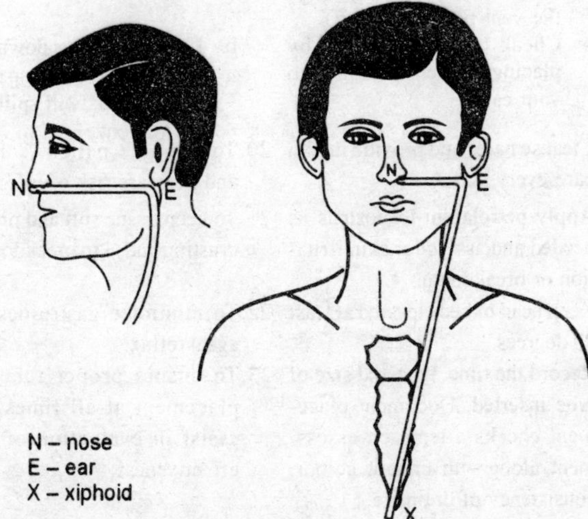

Fig. 7.4: Have the patient sit in a neutral position with head facing forward. Place the distal tip of the tubing at the tip of the patient's nose (N); extend tube to the tragus tip) of his ear (E), and then extend the tube straight down to the tip of his xiphoid (X). Mark this point 'B' on the tubing.

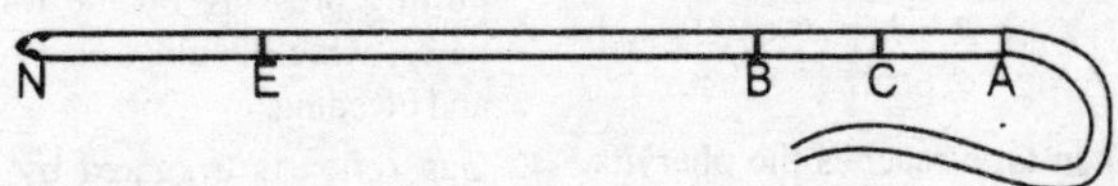

Fig. 7.5: To locate point C on the tube, find the midpoint between points A and B. The nasogastric tube is passed to point C to ensure optimum placement in the stomach.

The above diagram and steps (1, 2, 3) indicate how far a nasogastric tube is passed for optimal placement in the stomach.

STEPS OF PROCEDURE

Nursing action	*Rationale*
1. Coil the first 7-10 cm (3-4 in) of the tube around your fingers.	1. This curves tubing and facilitates tube passage.
2. Lubricate the coiled portion of the tube with water soluble lubricant. Avoid occluding the tube's holes with lubricant.	2. Lubrication reduces friction between the mucous membranes and tube and prevents injury to the nasal passages. Using a water soluble lubricant prevents oil aspiration pneumonia if the tube accidently slips into trachea.

Anatomical sites

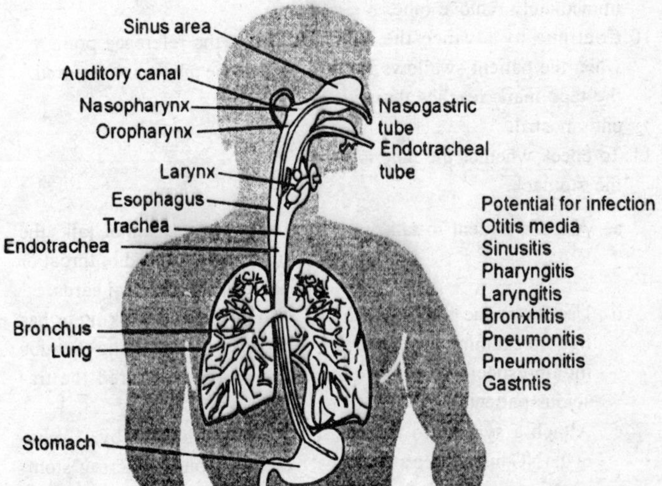

Fig. 7.6: All along the upper respiratory tract and upper digestive system, there is the potential for abnormal areas of colonization (infection) when various tubes are in place (i.e., tracheostomy, nasogastric or endotracheal tube). In addition, there is the potential for aspiration of secretions that may cause bronchitis and/or pneumonitis.

3. Tilt back the patients head before inserting tube into nostril and gently pass tube into the posterior nasopharynx, directing downward and backward the ear.	3. Passage of the tube is facilitated by following the natural contours of the body. The slower the advancement of the tube at this point, the lesser likelihood of

	putting pressure on the torbinates, which could cause pain and bleeding.
4. When tube reaches the pharynx, the patient may gag; allow patient to rest for a few moments.	4. Gag reflex is triggered by the presence of the tube.
5. Have the patient tilt head slightly forward offer several sips of water sipped through a straw or permit patient to suck on ice chips, unless contraindicated. Advance tube as patient swallows.	5. Flexed head position partially occludes the airway and the tube is less likely to enter frachea, Swallowing closes the epiglotus over the trachea and facilitates passage of tube into the esophagus. Actually, once the tube passes the cricopharyngeal sphincter into the oesophagus, it can be slowly and steadily advanced even if the patient does not swallow.
6. Gently rotate the tube 180 degrees to redirect the curve.	6. This prevents the tube from entering the patient's mouth.
7. Continue to advance tube gently each time the patient swallows.	7.
8. If obstruction appears to prevent tube from passing, do not use force. Rotating tube gently may help, if unsuccessful, remove tube and try other nostril.	8. Avoid discomfort and trauma to patient.
9. If there are signs of distress such as gasping, coughing or cyanosis, immediately remove tube.	9. May have entered the trachea.
10. Continue to advance the tube when the patient swallows until the tape mark reaches the patient's nostril.	10. This is the reference point where the tube was measured.
11. To check whether the tube is in the stomach.	11.
a. Ask the patient to talk.	a. If the patient cannot talk, the tube may be coiled in throat or passed through vocal cards.
b. Use the tongue blade and penlight to examine the patient's mouth-especially an unconscious patient.	b. If the patient is choking or has difficulty in breathing the tube has probably entered the trachea.
c. Attach a syringe to the end of the NG tube. Place a stethoscope over the left upper quadrant of the abdomen and inject 10-20 cc of air while auscultating the abdomen.	c. Air can be detected by a "Whooshing" sound entering stomach rather than the bronchus. If bel-ching occurs, the tube is probably in the oesophagus.
d. Aspirate contents of stomach with a 50-ml catheter tip Syringe. If stomach contents cannot be aspirated, place the patient on left side and advance the tube 2.5-5cm (1-2in) and try again.	d. Aspirated stomach contents indicate that the tube is in the stomach.
	e. X-rays may be done to confirm tube placement.
12. After tube is passed and the correct placement is confirmed, attach the tube to suction or clamp the tube.	12. Clamping can be done using a clamp, plastic plug, of folding the tube over and slipping the bend into the tube end.
13. Apply tincture of benzoin to the area where the tape is placed.	13. This helps make the tube adhere, especially with diaphoretic patients.
14. Anchor tube with: a. Hypoallergenic tape; split lengthwise and only half way attach unsplitend of tape to nose and cross split ends around tubing. Apply another piece of tape to bridge of nose. b. Bio-occlusive transparent dressing where it exits the nose.	14. Prevents the patient's vision from being distrubed; prevents tubing from rubbing against nasal mucosa. This will ensure tape being secure.
15. Anchor the tubing to the patient's gown. Use a rubber band to make a slip-knot to anchor the tubing to the patient's gown. Secure the rubber band to the patient's gown using a safety pin.	15. To permit mobility of patient. This prevents tugging of the tube when the patient moves.
16. Clamp the tube until the purpose for inserting the tube takes place.	16. See = 12.
17. Attach the tube to suction equipment of prescribed.	
18. Assure the patient that most discomfort he or she feels will lessen as he or she gets used to the tube.	
19. Irrigate the tube at regular intervals with small volumes of prescribed fluid.	19. Nursing Alert: All enteric tubes must be irrigated with small volumes of fluid and at regular intervals to ensure patency.
a. If the tube is a Salem sump, it will require periodic placing of 10-20 ml of air through the vent port (blue port).	a. A soft hissing sound is heard if the tube is patient.
b. Check the tube patency by placing the vent port next to your ear.	b. If the port hangs downward and the tube backs up stomach contents will spill over the patient.
20. Cleanse nares and provide mouth care every shift.	20. To promote patient comfort and decrease risk of infection.
21. Apply petrolatum to nostrils as needed and assess for skin irritation or breakdown.	21. To keep tissue soft and prevent crusting and skin breakdown.
22. Keep head of bed elevated at least 30 degrees.	22. To minimize gastro-oesophageal reflux.
23. Record the time, type and size of tube inserted. Document placement checks after each assessment, along with amount, colour, consistency of drainage.	23. To ensure proper tube and placement at all times, and assist in evaluation of tube effectiveness.

Contd...

Nursing Focus

If the patient has a nasal condition that prevents insertion through the nose, the tube is passed through the mouth. Remove denture, slide the tube over the tongue, and proceed the same way as a nasal intubation. Make sure to coil the end of the tube and direct it downward at the pharynx.

Other Nursing Patient Care Considerations

1. If the patient is unconscious, advance the tube between respirations to make sure it does not enter the traches. You will need to stroke the unconscious patient's neck to facilitate passage of the tube down the oesophagus.
2. Watch for cyanosis while passing the tube in an unconscious patient, cyanosis indicates the tube has entered the trachea.
3. Never place the end of the tube in a container of fluid while checking for placement. If the tube is in the trachea the patient could inhale the water.
4. Do not tape the tube to the forehead; it can cause necrosis of the nostril.
5. a. Sucralfate (Carafate) may be ordered after NG tube insertion to provide a protective barrier against gastric acid, pepsin and bile. After administering carafate, clamp tube for half on hour, then unclamp and reconnect to suction (if ordered).
   b. Clotrimazole (Mycelex) may be ordered as prophylactic treatment for candida albicans.
6. Pain or vomiting after the tube is inserted indicates tube obstruction or incorrect placement.
7. The air vent on the Salem sump tube should not be used for irrigation.
8. If the air vent (Salem sump tube) is draining fluid or is not drawing air, instill 20cc of air through the vent.
9. Irrigate the NG tube every 2 hours unless otherwise ordered.
10. If the NG tube is not draining, the nurse should reposition tube by advancing or withdrawing it slightly (with a physician order). After repositioning, always check for placement.
11. Recognize the complications when the tube is inside for prolonged periods; nasal erosion, sinusitis, oesophagitis, oesophagus, tracheal fistula, gastric ulceration, and pulmonary and oral infections (see figure).

All along the upper respiratory tract and upper digestive system, there is the potential for abnormal areas of colonization (infection) when various tubes are in place. (i.e., tracheostomy, nasogastric or endotracheal tube). In addition, there is the potential for aspiration of secretions that may cause bronchitis and/or pneumonitis.

12. Notify the health care provider of any continuous problems.

REMOVAL PROCEDURE

Preparatory Phase

1. Be certain that gastric or small bowel drainage is not excessive in volume.
2. Ensure by ausculation that audible peristalsis is present.
3. Determine whether the patient is passing flatus, this indicates peristalsis.
4. There is a physician's order for removal.

Removing Nasogastric Tubing

Steps of Procedure

Nursing action	*Rationale*
1. Place a towel across the patient's chest and inform him of her that the tube is to be withdrawn.	1. No doubt, the patient will be happy to have progressed to this stage.
2. Apply disposable gloves.	2. Provides protection from contaminated body fluids.
3. Turn off suction, disconnect and clamp tube.	3. Prevents fluids from leaking from tube.
4. Remove the tape from the patient's nose.	
5. Instruct the patient to take a deep breath and hold it.	5. This manoeuvre closes the epiglottis.
6. Slowly but evenly withdraw tubing and cover it with a towel as it emerges. (As the tube reaches the nasopharynx, you can pull quickly).	6. Covering the tubing helps dispel patient's nausea.
7. Provide the patient with materials for oral care and lubricant for nasal dryness.	7. Mouthwash and a nasal lubricant will be appreciated for the patient.
8. Dispose of equipment in appropriate receptacle.	
9. Document time of tube removal and the patient's reaction.	
10. Document tube removal and colour, consistency, and amount of drainage in suction canister.	
11. Continue to monitor the patient for signs of GI difficulties.	11. Recurrence of nausea or vomiting may require reinsertion of nasogastric tubing, changes in vital signs may suggest infection.

PROCEDURE 7.4: ***NASOINTESTINAL INTUBATION***

Small Bore-Feeding Tubes)

Equipment

1. Type of tube ordered by health care provider.
2. 30cc or 60cc Luer-Lok or tip Syringe.
3. Water soluble lubricant.
4. Tape, rubber band, clamp and safety pin.
5. Glass of water.
6. Stethoscope.

Nursing Focus

All tubes and endoscopes should be routinely pre-tested for patency and function before passage.

STEPS OF PROCEDURE

Nursing action	*Rationale*
1. Tube preparation.	
a. Do not ice plastic tubes.	a. Become too stiff to work with.
b. Inject 10cc of water into the tube.	b. Aidee in insertion.
c. Insert guidewire or stylet into tube, making sure it is positioned snugly against tube.	c. Prevent trauma.
d. Dip weighted tip into glass of water.	d. Activate lubricant.
2. Similar to passing a short nasogastric tube and taping to patient (See procedure guidelines, 16-3).	
3. After the tube enters the stomach, it passes by peristalsis and gravity into the small intestine.	3. This will assist in advancing the tubing to and through the pylorus; tilting to the right is helpful.
a. Change patient's position from Fowler's to a position in which the patient is leaning forward.	
4. Obtain an x-ray of the abdomen after tube insertion.	4. Confirm placement.
5. Stylet should remain in place until position is confirmed.	

Nursing/Patient Care Considerations

1. Beware of risk of aspiration in an unconscious patient.
2. Instruct patient on complications associated with tube feedings, such as nausea, vomiting and diarrhoea.

PROCEDURE 7.4: ***CHANGING A TWO-PIECE DRAINABLE FECAL POUCHING SYSTEM.***

Equipment: Duplicate wafer and pouch
Tail closure
Washcloth and towel
Mid non-oily soap (optional)
Accessory products prescribed for patient.

STEPS OF PROCEDURE

Nursing action	*Rationale*
Preparatory Phase	
1. Explain the details of this activity.	1. Encourages patient understanding and participation to learn self-care.
2. Gather equipment and place within easy reach.	2. Minimizes distractions and fasters organization.
3. Have the patient assume a relaxed position and provide privacy. The best position may be sitting, reclining, or standing.	3. Patient must see stoma site to learn care.
Performance Phase	
1. To remove pouching system.	
a. Wear nonsterile gloves.	a. Maintain universal precautions.
b. Push down gently on skin while lifting up on the wafer (ostomy adhesive remover may be used).	b. Minimize skin trauma.
c. Discard soiled pouch and wafer in odorproof plastic bag. Save tail closure for reuse.	c. Removes room odor and maintains universal precautions.
2. To Cleanse skin;	
a. Use toilet tissue to remove feces from stoma and skin if needed.	a. Stoma may function during the change.
b. Cleanse stoma and peristomal skin with soft cloth and water, soap optional. The patient may shower with or without pouching system in place. Clip or shave peristomal hair if appropriate.	b. Minimizes skin breakdown and promotes hygiene.
c. Raines and dry skin throughly after cleansing. It is normal for the stoma to bleed slightly during cleansing and drying.	c. Removes residue, which may interfere with adhesion of wafer.
3. To apply wafer.	
a. Use measuring guide or stomal pattern to determine stoma size.	a. This step is omitted when stomal shrinkage is complete about 2 months postop.
b. Trace correct size pattern onto back of wafer and cut to nearly stoma size. It is acceptable to cut 1/16-1/8 in larger than stoma.	b. Avoids wafer rubbing stoma, omit this step if the wafer is precut.
c. Apply a line of skin barrier paste around stoma or on lip of wafer opening. Allow to set according to manufacturers instructions (other barrier may be used in place of paste, such as strips or washer, because some patients are allergie to the alcohol in paste).	c. Extra skin protection is imperative for ileostomy and right sided colostomy. A left sided colostomy may not need secondary barrier because formed stool is less harmful to skin, paste acts as "Caul King" to prevent undermining of feces.
d. Remover paper backing(s) from the wafer, center opening over stoma, and press wafer down onto peristomal skin.	d. Ensures adherence.
4. Snap pouch onto the flange of the wafer according to manufacturer's directions (See accompanying figure).	4. If attached properly, there will be no leakage or odor.
5. Apply till closure to pouch tail.	5. Proper closure controls odor.

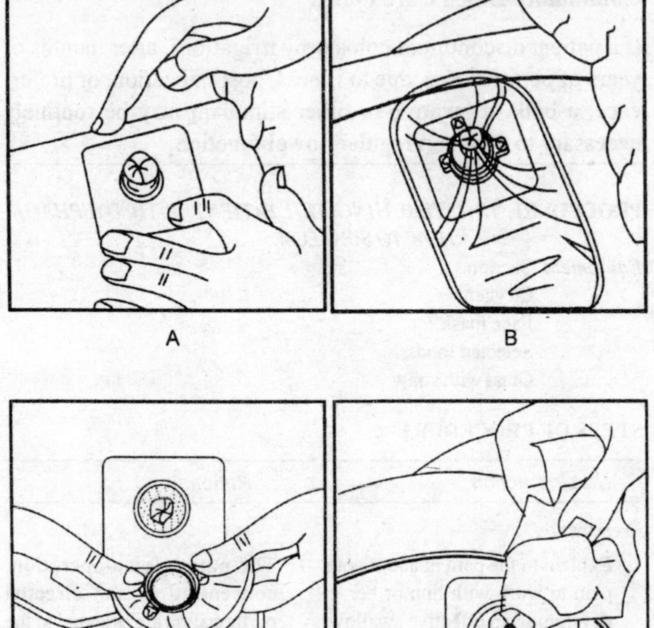

Fig.7.7: (A) A wafer with flange (1 1/2", 1 3/4", 2 1/4", 2 3/4", 4") is applied after cleaning and drying of peristomal skin. (B) A transparent or opaque drainable pouch is positioned over stoma at desired angle. (C) Pouch may be removed without removal of wafer. (D) Stoma may be assessed without removing wafer. (Adapted by permission from Convatec, A Bristol-Myers, Squibb Company).

PROCEDURE 7.5: ***CHANGING A TWO-PIECE DRAINABLE FECAL POUCHING SYSTEM (CONTINUED).***

STEPS OF PROCEDURE

Nursing action	*Rationale*
Follow-up Phase	
1. Dispose of plastic bag with waste materials.	
2. Clean drainable pouch with soap and water, if appropriate Drainable pouches may be reused several times.	2. Controls odor, reduces cost.
3. A commercial deodorant can` be placed in the pouch to reduce odor.	
4. Gas can be released from the pouch by releasing the tail closure or by snapping off an area on the pouch flange. Never make a pinhole in the pouch to release gas.	4. Destroys the odorproof seal.

PROCEDURE 7.6: ***IRRIGATING A COLOSTOMY***

Equipment

1. Reservoir for irrigating fluids, irrigator bag or enema bag if irrigator bag not available.
2. Irrigating fluid 500-1,500 ml lukewarm water or other solution prescribed by health care provider. (Volume is titrated based on patient tolerance and results, average amount is 1,000 ml).
3. Irrigating tip cone tip or soft rubber catheter 22 or 24 with shield to prevent backflow of irigating solution. (Use only if cone not available. The cone is the preferred method to avoid possibility of bowel perforation).
4. Irrigation sleeve (long large capacity bag with opening at top to insert cone or catneter into stoma) Available in different styles snap-on, self-adhering to skin, orheld in place by belt.
5. Large tail closure.
6. Water-soluble lubricant.

Preparatory Phase

1. Explain the details of the procedure to the patient and answer any questions.
2. Select a consistent time, free from distractions. If the patient is learning to irrigate for bowel control, choose the time of day that will best fit into the patient's lifestyle.
3. Have the patient sit in front of the commode on chair or on the commode itself providing privacy and comfort.
4. Hang irrigating reservoir with prescribed solution so that the bottom of the reservoir is approximately at the level of the patient's shoulder and above the stoma.

STEPS OF PROCEDURE

Nursing action	*Rationale*
Performance Phase	
1. Remove pouch or covering from stoma and apply irrigation sleeve, directing the open tail into the commode.	1. Allows wafer and feces to flow directly into commode.
2. Open tubing clamp on the irrigating reservoir to release a small amount of solution into the commode.	2. Removes air from the setup: avoids air from being introduced into the colan, which can cause crampy pain.
3. Lubricate the tip of the cone/catheter and gently insert into the stoma. Insert carneter no more than 3 in. Hold cone/shield gently, but firmly against stoma to prevent backflow of water.	3. Prevents intestinal perforation and irritation of mucous membranes.
4. If catheter does not advance easily, allow water to flow slowly while advancing catheter. Never Force Catheter.	4. Slow rate relaxes bowel to facilitate passage of catheter.

Contd...

Contd...

Nursing action	Rationale
Dilating the stoma with lubricated gloved pinky finger may be necessary to direct cone/catheter properly.	
5. Allow water to enter colon slowly over a 5-10 minute period. If cramping occurs, slow flow rate or clamp tubing to allow cramping to subside, removed cone/catheter to release contents.	5. Cramping may occur from too rapid flow, cold water excess solution, or colon ready to function.
6. Hold cone/shield in place 10 seconds after water is instilled, then gently remove cone/catheter from stoma.	6. Discourages premature evacuation of fluid.
7. As feces and water flows down sleeve, periodically rinse sleeve with water. Allow 10-15 minutes for most of the returns, then dry sleeve tail and apply tail closure.	7. Ecophageal disorders.
8. Leave sleeve in place for approximately 20 more minutes while patient gets up and moves around.	8. Ambulation stimulates peristalsis and completion of irrigation return.
9. When returns are complete, clean stomal area with mild soap and water pat dry; reapply pouch or covering over stoma.	9. Cleanliness and dryness promote comfort.
Follow-up Phase	
1. Clean equipment with soap and water, dry and store in wellventilated area.	1. This will control odour and mildew prolonging the life of equipment.
2. If applicable, the patient should use a pouch until the colostomy is sufficiently controlled.	2. It may take several months to establish control. The patient can then use minipouch stoma cap, or gauze covering as desired.

Other Nursing/Patient Care Considerations

1. It is a patient preference whether colostomy irrigations are attempted for control irrigation may occur every day or every other day depending on bowel pattern. It usually takes 1-2 months to establish control, patients with a preoperative history of regular, formed bowel movements are more likely to realize success.
2. Disadvantages to the colastomy irrigation approach for control include (a) It is a time-consuming procedure requiring consistency which may not fit into a patient's lifestyle. (b) Bowel dependency can occur with the irrigation as the stimulus for evacuation of bowel movements.
3. Only a patient with a descending or sigmoid colostomy is an irrigation candiadate for foecal control. A colostomy more proximal than descending has too liquid and higher volume of foecal output to be managed through irrigation.

Community-Based Care Points

If a patient discontinues colostomy irrigations, after months or years of performance, due to illness, hospitalization, or preference, a bulk of laxative or other stimulant may be routinely necessary to maintain regular bowel function.

PROCEDURE 7.7: ****TEACHING TEH PATIENT WITH DYSPHAGIA HOW TO SWALLOW.***

Equipment Suction
Oxygen
Face mask
Selected foods
Glass with straw.

STEPS OF PROCEDURE

Nursing action	Rationale
Preparation	
1. Explain to the patient about your plan to work with him or her in developing an effective swallow.	1. The patient's co-operation, concentration, and directed participation are essential to the success of the learning experience.
2. Ensure that emergency equipment is available at the bedside-suction, oxygen and face mask.	2. For use in the event that the patient chokes, vomits, or aspirates.
3. Place the patient in an upright sitting position in a chair or support with pillows in high-Fowler's position if unable to get out of bed for about 200 minutes before and 45-60 minutes after meals.	3. This will allow time to adjust and relax in this position before meals; allows gravity to assist the swallowing procedure during meals, helps prevent reflux or regurgitation after meals.
4. Provide mouth care before meals. Suction the patient of secretions are present. If the patient's mouth is dry, provide a lemon wedge or pickle to suck on.	4. This will increase patient's ability to taste and enjoy the sensation of eating.
5. Prepare an environment that is pleasant, peaceful, and without interruptions. Remove distracters, such as TV and radio.	5. Patient must be able to concentrate on the process of swallowing in a relaxed manner.
Food and Fluid Selection	
6. Food should be chosen that hold some shape, most enough to prevent crumbling but dry enough to hold a bolus shapecasseroles, custards, scrambled eggs.	6. Foods that crumble may be aspirated when they false apart foods that are too moist may be drooled through the lids.
7. Mugs and glasses with spouts or a straw should be used for liquids.	7. These utensils help prevent liquids from leaking out of corners of patient's mouth.
8. Avoid sticky foods, peanut butter, chocolate, milk and ice cream.	8. These foods stimulate thick mucos and will make swallowing more difficult.
9. Dry foods can be moistened with margarine, gravy, or broths, If liquids are a problem, juices can be thickened with sherbets.	9. Foods need to be of a consistency that will hold a bolus form until swallowed.

Contd...

Contd...

Nursing action	Rationale
10. Avoid tepid or room temperature foods.	10. Hot and cold foods are thought to be maximally stimulate receptors that activate swallowing mechanism.
Instructions During Meals	
11. Have patient position head in the midline and forward, chin pointed toward chest.	11. Improve ability to consciously swallow without food falling down the posterior pharynx. Support patient's forehead with a hand if the patient lacks neck control.
12. Instruct the patient to smell the food before each bite, hold each bite for a few seconds; hold lips together firmly; concentrate on swallowing; then swallow.	12. Concentrating on each step before swallowing will increase the effectiveness of the swallow.
13. If the patient has an increase in saliva during the meal, instruct the patient to collect the saliva with the tongue and consciously swallow it between bites throughout the meal.	13. This will help prevent aspiration of saliva between mouthfuls.
14. If the patient complains of a dry mouth during meals, instruct the patient to move the tongue in a circular form against the insides of the cheeks.	14. This will help stimulate salivation.
15. Caution the patient against talking during the meal or with the mouth full of food.	15. Talking or laughing during eating is a common cause of airway obstruction.
Follow-up Care	
16. Provide mouth care after meals.	16. Food particles may collect in the mouth or cheeks.
17. Record the amount of intake, the patient's taste and food preferences, progress, and any special tactics that were effective in helping the swallowing process.	17. Progress notes will assist in moving toward self care.
18. Encourage family members to participate in the patient's feeding program.	18. This will help provide continuity on discharge.

Feeding the Patient with an Affected Side of the Mouth (Facial Paralysis, Hemiplegia).

Nursing action	Rationale
1. Turn the patient to the unaffected side.	1. This helps prevent food from falling down the weaker/paralyzed part of the oral cavity, a possible cause of aspiration.
2. Place food on the unaffected side of mouth rather than in the middle of the mouth.	2. Permits food to be managed more effectively.
3. Encourage the patient to form a bolus by moving the food around the mouth with the tongue.	3. This assists in placing food in a proper position for swallowing rather than permitting food to collect near the cheek.

Hepatobiliary Pancreatic Nursing

Hepatobiliary pancreatic nursing refers to the nursing care of the disorders of liver and pancreas. In this chapter difference disorder related to liver and pancreas and them nuring management discussed.

JAUNDICE

Jaundice, a yellowish discoloration of body tissues, resulting from an alteration in normal bilirubin metabolism or flow of bile into the hepatic or biliary duct systems. It is a symptom which results when the concentration of bilirubin level has to be approximately three times normal level (2 to 3 mg) for jaundice to occur. The three types of jaundice are classified in haemolytic, hepatocellular and obstructive.

i. Haemolytic jaundice (prehepatic) is due to an increased breakdown of red blood cells which produces an increased amount of unconjugated bilirubin in the blood. The liver is unable to handle this increased load. Causes of this type include blood transfusion reaction, sickle cells crisis, and haemolytic anaemia.
ii. *Haepatocellular jaundice* (hepatic) results from the liver's altered ability to take up bilirubin from the blood or to conjugate or excrete it. Both unconjugated and conjugated bilirubin serum levels increase. Because conjugated bilirubin is water soluble; it is excreted in the urine. The most common cause of this type are hepatitis, cirrhosis, and hepatocarcinoma.
iii. *Obstructive jaundice* (Posthepatic) is due to impeded or obstructed flow of bile through the liver or biliary duct system. The obstruction may be intrahepatic or extrahepatic. Intrahepatic obstructions are due to swelling or fibrosis of the liver's caliculi and bile ducts. This can be caused by damage from liver tumors, hepatitis, or cirrhosis. Causes of extrahepatic obstructions include common bile duct obstruction from a stone, sclerosing cholangitis and carcinoma of the head of the pancreas. Here moderate elevation is both conjugated and unconjugated bilirubin and urine bilirubin.

Jaundice is a major problem in patients with diffuse hepatocellular disorder, which includes hepatitis, cirrhosis and hepatic carcinoma.

HEPATITIS

Hepatitis is an inflammation of the liver. Although the term hepatitis is most often used in conjunction with viral hepatitis, the disease can also be caused by the bacteria or toxic injury to the liver. Although some differences exist in the pathological and clinical phenomena of viral, bacterial, and toxic hepatitis, the clinical management of the person with any of these types of hepatitis is quite similar.

Toxic Hepatitis

Since liver has a primary role in the metabolism of foreign substances, many agents including drugs, alcohol, industrial toxins and persons can cause toxic hepatism. Many health care workers are concerned about hepatic injury caused by adverse drug reactions from the drugs they handle.

Aetiology

The agents that produce hepatic injury are categorized into two major groups. Predictable (intrinsic) hepatotoxins and non-predictable (idiosyncratic) hepatotoxins.

i. Predictable hepatotoxic agents cause toxic hepatitis with predictable regularity and produce injury in a high percentage of persons exposed to them. Occurrence of toxic hepatitis is dose dependent. The predictable hepatotoxins are further divided into two subgroups—direct or indirect.
   - The direct predictable hepatotoxin agents have direct effect on hepatic cells and organelles, producing structural changes that lead to metabolic defects. For example
     - Carbon tetrachloride and other chlorinated hydrocarbon (Ind-toxin).
     - Yellow phosphorous (Industrial toxin).
     - Mushroom poisoning (Plant toxin).
   - The indirect predictable hepatotoxins are mostly; Drugs such as ethanol, tetracycline, methotrexate, L-asparaginase, puromycin, 6-merca topurine, acetaminophine, mictramycin, urethane, halothane, cholecystographic dyes, rifamycin B. These are agents which first interfere with normal metabolic function and this alteration in metabolic function produces structural change.

ii. Non-predictable hepatoxic agents produce hepatic injury only in unusually susceptible persons and in only a small percentage of persons exposed to them. Occurrence is not dose-dependent. These drugs such as phenytoin, PAS, INH, chloropromazin and androgens and anabolic steroids, chloropropmide, imipramine, methyldopa, monoamino oxidase (MAO) inhibitors, oral contraceptives, sulfanamides, allupurionl, cindamycin, erythromycin, esters, nitrofurantoin, oxacillin and oestrogen steroid.

Pathophysiology

The morphological changes produced in the liver by the toxin vary, depending on the specific hepatotoxin. For example, carbon tetrachloride, tetracycline, and ethanol cause fatty infiltration and/or necrosis, oral contraceptives, cholecystographic dyes and chloropromazine produces cholestasis and portal inflammation. The alterations may result in only minimal manifestations of altered liver function such as slightly-elevated serum enzymes or major manifestation associated with terminal liver failure.

Clinical Manifestation

Early manifestation includes anorexia, nausea, vomiting, lethargy, elevated ALT and AST levels. Later manifestations are icterus, hepatomegaly, hepatic tenderness, dark urine, elevated serum bilirubin level and urine bilirubin level.

Management

Proper attention is focussed on identifying the toxic agents and removing or eliminating it. Gastric lavage, and cleansing of the bowel may be indicated to remove the hepatotoxins from the intestinal tract. There are specific treatments for particular hepatotoxins. (Follow as prescribed). In most instances of toxic hepatitis, medical treatment is supportive and focussed on particular manifestation such as treatment of cirrhosis, portal-systemic encephalophathy or accompanying renal failure. Nursing care includes maintaining fluid and electrolyte balance, promoting a well-balanced diet, when food and fluids are allowed, and promoting rest and treating complications.

Nurses also should teach patient's family to use only prescribed medication with precaution to the liver injury.

Viral Hepatitis

Viral hepatitis is by far the most important liver infections. The term viral hepatitis is used to refer to several clinically similar but aetiologically and epidemiologically distinct infections.

Aetiology

Viral hepatitis can be caused by one of the five major viruses A,B,C,D and E, ie., HAV, HBV, HCV, HDV, HEV. Two other forms of hepatitis—hepatitis F and hepatitis G have been identified but occur rarely.

- HAV is a RNA virus transmitted through feco-oral route. Incubation period is 15-50 days (average 28 days). Crowded condition, poor personal hygiene, poor sanitation, contaminated food, milk water and shell-fish, persons with subclinical infections, infected food handlers, and sexual contacts are the sources of infection and spread of disease. Most infections during 2 weeks before onset of symptoms; infectious until 1-2 weeks after symptoms start.
- HBV is a DNA virus that is transmitted by percutaneous (IV drug use, accidental needle-strick punctures or permucosal exposure to infective blood, blood products, or per mucosal exposure to infectious blood, blood products or other body fluids (semen, vaginal secretions, saliva) Perinatal transmission is also possible. The source and spread of disease are caused by contaminated needle, syringes and blood products, sexual activities with infected partners and asymptomatic carriers eg. Tattoo/body piercing bite, most infections before and after symptoms appear for 4-6-months in carriers it continues through patients' lifetime, incubation period is 45-18 days.
- HCV is RNA virus that is primarily transmitted percutaneously. Thus, the major risk factor for infection is direct percutaneous exposure such as injecting drugs, transfusion of blood products, haemodialysis, tattooing, high-risk sexual behaviour, organ transplantation and exposure to blood and blood products by health workers. Less frequent routes are sexual and perinatal.

  HDV also called delta virus, is defective RNA virus that cannot survive on its own. So it can cause infections only together with HBV; routes of transmission same as for HBV. Blood is infectious at all stages of HDV infections. Incubation period is 2-26 weeks. Chronic carriers of HBV are always at risk.
- HEV is an RNA virus, that is transmitted by the fecal-oral route. The most common mode of transmission is drinking contaminated water.
- HGV is an RNA virus which is found in some blood donors and can be transmitted by transfusion. It frequently coexists with other hepatitis virus, e.g. HCV.

Pathophysiology

Viral hepatitis causes diffuse inflammatory infiltrations of hepatic tissue with mononuclear cells and local spotty or single cell necrosis. The liver cells may be very swollen. With typical viral hepatitis, there is no collapse of lobules, no loss of lobular architecture, and minimal or no fibrosis. Inflammation degeneration and regeneration occur simultaneously, distorting the normal lobular pattern and creating pressure within and around the portal vein areas and obstructing the bile channels. These changes are associated with elevated serum transminase levels, prolonged prothrombin time and slightly elevated bilirubin level. The outcome of viral hepatitis is affected by such factors as the following:

- Virulence of the virus.
- Amount of hepatic damage sustained.

- Natural individual barriers to damage and disease of the liver such as immune status, nutritional status, and overall health of the individual.

Most patients recover normal level functions but the disease can progress to atypical life-threatening variants.

- Fulminant viral hepatitis—sudden, severe, degenerated and atrophy of liver, resulting in hepatic failure.
- Subacute viral hepatitis—severe, but slower degeneration of livers.
- Confluent hepatic necrosis—submassive or massive destruction of substantial groups of adjacent cell with necrosis of portions of a lobule (submassive) or entire lobule (massive), can result in chronic active disease or cirrhosis but most patients will recover.

Clinical Manifestations

The clinical manifestation of viral hepatitis may be classified into three phases (1) Preicteric or prodramal phase. (2) Icteric phase (3) Posticteric phase or convalescent phase.

Preicteric	*Icteric*	*Posticteric*
• Anorexia	• Jaundice	• Malaise
• Nausea, vomiting	• Pruritis	• Easy fatigability
• Right upper quadrant discomfort	• Dark urine	• Hepatomegally
• Constipation or diarrhoea	• Bilirubinuria	
• Decreased sense of taste and smell	• White stool	
Malaise	Fatigue	
• Headache	Continual hepatomegaly with tenderness	
• Fever	• Weight loss	
• Arthralgia		
• Urticaria		
Hepaticmegaly		
• Splenomegaly		
• Weight loss.		

Complications that can occur include chronic persistent hepatitis, chronic active hepatitis, fulminant viral hepatitis and cirrhosis of the liver.

Diagnostic Studies

- Liver function studies.
- Hepatitis serology.
  HGs Ag
  Anti-HBs
  Anti-HBs-IgH and IgG
  Anti-HAV Igh and IgG
  Anti-HCV.

Management

There is no specific treatment or therapy for viral hepatitis. Most patients can be managed at home. Emphasis on measures to rest the body and assist the liver in regenerating needs to be stressed. Adequate nutrients and rest seem to be more beneficial for healing and liver cell (hepatocyte) regeneration. Rest reduced the metabolic demands on the liver and promotes cell generation. The degree of rest depends on the severity of symptoms. Dietary emphasis is on a well-balanced diet that the patient can tolerate. A low fat, high carbohydrate diet may be better tolerated. Protein and sodium are restricted. Alcohol should be avoided.

Vitamin K is given if the prothromb in time is prolonged. Antihistamines are given for pruritis associated with jaundice, and antiemetics are given for nausea. Most patients of hepatitis are not hospitalized. Those requiring hospitalization include persons with serum bilirubin concentration 10 mg or greater than 10 times normal. In persons with fulminating hepatitis, hospitalization and bedrest are indicated. Unnecessary medication including sedatives are discontinued. Coagulation defects may be treated with administration of fresh frozen plasma. The patient's intake and output is carefully monitored, and intravenous fluid continuously. Electrolytes administered in vomiting and diarrhoea may cause electrolyte imbalance, particularly hypokalaemia.

Hepatitis A vaccine and immonologlobulins are used in the prevention of viral hepatitis. Hepatitis B vaccine and immunoglobulin is the first line of defence against hepatitis B.

The possible nursing diagnosis of viral hepatitis are:

- Fatigue R/T imbalance between energy level and demand, decreased rest, feeling of malaise.
- Activity intolerance R/T fatigue, weakness.
- Fluid volume deficit R/T vomiting, sweating, decreased intake, increased temperature.
- Infection (Risk for) R/T length of infectivity through blood and body fluids.
- Nutrition, altered R/T anorexia, inadequate intake, increased metabolic needs.
- Pain R/T arthralgia, pruritis, headache, abdominal tenderness.
- Health maintenance, altered. R/T lack of knowledge, indifference to "safe sex" practice and needle.
- Skin integrity (F/F) R/T jaundice, pruritis, scratching.
- Injury R/T altered clothing or prothrombic time.

Preventive Measures for Viral Hepatitis

All patients with hepatitis require precautions to prevent spread of virus. For patients with hepatitis A virus (HAV), the following transmission-based precautions are necessary.

- Proper handwashing by patient and staff.
- Wearing gloves when handling feces and urine.
- Wearing a glove when soiling of uniform is likely.
- Cleansing the toilet daily and use private toilet.
- Having a private room (only if patient cannot take care of selfregarding proper disposal of urine and feces).

- Proper cleansing, bagging, and labelling of contaminated items such as bed linens and bedpan.
- Discarding contaminated items such as rectal thermometer.

For the patients with HBV, transmission-based precautions are used and include the following.

- Good handwashing by patient and staff.
- Wearing gloves when handling blood and body fluids.
- Wearing gown, goggles and/or mask when splattering of blood and body fluid is likely.
- Proper cleansing, bagging and labelling of contaminated equipments and linens.
- Proper disposing of needles or any items exposed to the patient's blood or body fluids.
- Careful labelling of blood specimen and protect personnel working with them.
- Avoiding contamination of open cuts and mucus membranes with patient's blood and body fluids.
- Teaching patients to avoid sexual contact until results of liver function tests have returned to normal.

Similar precaution is to be followed in other hepatitis. At times, the nurse in the hospital and particularly nurse in the community are also involved in identifying patient's contacts who will require prophylactic therapy.

CIRRHOSIS OF LIVER

Cirrhosis of the liver is the term applied to chronic disease of the liver characterised by diffuse inflammation and fibrosis resulting in drastic structural changes and significant loss of liver function in which extensive degeneration and destruction of the liver parenchymal cells. The liver cells attempt to regenerate but the regenerative process is disorganized, resulting in abnormal blood vessels and bile duct relationships from the fibrosis. The overgrowth of new and fibrous connective tissue distorts lever's normal lobular structure resulting in lobules of irregular size and shape with impeded vascular flow. Cirrhosis may be insidious and prolonged course.

Aetiology and Pathophysiology

Cirrhosis of the liver can be classified in various ways. The major types of cirrhosis based on pathological classification are:

i. *Alcoholic* Previously called "Laennecs Cirrhosis" also called portal or nutritional cirrhosis is usually associated with alcohol abuse or malnutrition. The first change in the liver from excessive alcohol intake is an accumulation of fat in the liver cells. Uncomplicated fatty changes in the liver are potentially reversible if the person stops drinking alcohol. If the alcohol abuse continues, widespread scar formation occurs in the liver.
ii. *Postnecrotic cirrhosis* is a complication of viral toxic or idiopathic (autoimmune) hepatitis due to massive necrosis from hepatotoxins. Broad bands of scar tissue from within liver.
iii. *Biliary cirrhosis* is associated with inflammation of intra-hepatic bile-ductules resulting in biliary obstruction in liver and common bile duct. Cholangitis (destruction of the ntrahepatic bile ducts) of unknown aetiology may occur. There is chronic impairment of bile drainage occurs. Liver is first large, then becomes firm and nodular, Jaundice is a major symptom. Pruritis, hypercholestraemia, cholestrasis (blockage of bile flow) and malabsorption are common manifestation due to diffuse fibrosis of liver.
iv. *Cardiac cirrhosis* results from long-standing, severe, right-sided heart failure in patient with corpulmonale, constrictive pericarditis and tricuspid insufficiency.
v. *Nonspecific metabolic* cirrhosis are due to metabolic problems, infectious diseases, infiltrative diseases and GI diseases in which portal and liver fibrosis may develop, liver is enlarged and firm.

Clinical Manifestation

The onset of cirrhosis is usually insidious. GI disturbances are common, early symptoms include anorexia, dyspepsia, flatulence, nausea and vomiting and change in bowel habits (constipation or diarrhoea)-due to altered metabolism of carbohydrate, fats and proteins. Pain may be due to swelling and stretching of the capsule and spasm of biliary ducts, other symptoms include, fever, lassitude, slight weighlessness and enlargement of liver and spleen. Liver may be palpable. Later symptoms may be severe and result from liver failure and portal hypertension, jaundice, peripheral, oedema, and ascites develop gradually. Other late symptoms are as follows:

Gastrointestinal

- Anorexia
- Dyspepsia
- Nausea
- Vomiting
- Change in bowel habits
- Dull abdominal pain
- Factor hepatitis
- Oesophageal and gastric varices
- Haematemesis
- Haemorrhoidal varices
- Congestive gastritis

Haematologic

- Anaemia
- Thrombocytopnoea
- Leukopnoea
- Coagulation disorder
- Splenomegally.

Endocrine disturbance/metabolic

- Potassium deficiency
- Hyponatraemia
- Hypoalbuminaemia.

Cardiovascular

- Fluid retention
- Peripheral oedema
- Ascitis.

Integumentary/skin lesions

- Jaundice

Neurologic

- Hepatic encephalopathy

- Spider angioma
- Palmar erythema
- Purpura
- Petechea
- Caput medusae
- Peripheral neuropathy
- Asterixis
- Rynoductre
- Amenorrhoea
- Testicular atrophy
- Gynecomastia
- Impotence.

The major complications of cirrhosis of liver are portal hypertension with resultant oesophageal varices, peripheral oedema and ascitis, hepatic encephalopathy (coma) and hepatorenal syndrome.

Diagnostic Studies

- Liver function studies.
  - Alkaline phosphatase
  - Asparate amino transferase (AST)
  - Alumine amino transferase (ALT)
  - Serum glutamic pyruvic transaminase (SGPT)
  - Y-glutamyl transferase
- Liver biopsy (Percutaneous needle)
- Esophago gastroduodeneoscopy
- Angiography
- Liver scan
- Serum electrolyte
- Prothrombin time
- Serum albumin
- CBC
- Stool for ocult blood
- Upper GI barium swallow.

Management

Although there is no specific therapy for cirrhosis, certain measures can be taken to promote liver cell regeneration and prevent or treat complications.

Rest is significant in reducing metabolic demands of the liver and allowing for recovery of liver cells. At various times, during the progress of cirrhosis the rest may have to take the form of complete bedrest. Avoidance of alcohol and aspirin and administration of B-complex vitamin are helpful.

For *ascitics*, sodium restriction, diuretics and fluid removal are indicated. Administration of 3000-calories high carbohydrate, protein (depends on stage), low-fat diet, low sodium diet are advised. The diuretics used for ascitics are spirono-factone (Aid-actine), amiloride (Midamor) triamferene (Dyrenium), Furosemide (Lasix). In some cases, paracentesis, or peritoneo-venous shunts are indicated.

For *Oesophageal varices* β-adrenorgic blockers, vasopnersion are used. And endoscopic sclerotherapy or ligation, balloon tampanode, somatostatin, surgical shunting procedures, transjugular intrahepatic portosystematin shunt may be indicated accordingly.

For *hepatic encephalopathy*, sterilization of GI tract with antibiotics, and levodopa are used.

Nursing assessment will include eliciting complete history focussing on recent history of fever, infected weakness, fatigue, changes in the sclera, edema, itching, muscle wasting, use of alcohol, change in appetite, weight loss, anorexia, nausea, vomiting, indigestion, flatulence, abdominal tenderness, change in the movement of bowel and bladder, sexuality (erectile dysfunction decreased libido or changes in menstrual pattern assessing vital signs, other manifestation and the need for nursing management see NCP of patient with cirrhosis of liver.

The usual nursing intervention of cirrhosis is supporting respiration (by using Fowler's position), controlling fatigue (with bedrest), maintaining fluid and electrolyte balance (IV or oral fluid if no restriction) helping the patient to avoid alcohol, preventing infection, preventing bleeding and falls, promoting nutrition, controlling pruritis, promoting positive self-esteem. The factors which are supposed to monitor in the person with cirrhosis are:

- Monitor urine and stool for blood.
- Check up patient's body daily for purpura, haematoma and petechea.
- Check mouth especially gums, carefully for signs of bleeding.
- Check vital signs at least every 4 hours.
- Monitor prothrombintime, portal thromboplastin, and thrombocyte count frequently.

Following are the guidelines for decreasing the risk of bleeding.

- Avoid all intramuscular and subcutaneous injections if possible.
- Use the smaller-gauge needle possible while giving an injection.
- Apply pressure to injection site and venous puncture sites for at least 5 minutes and arterial punctures for 10 minutes.
- Give Vitamin K as ordered.
- Use or instruct patient to use a soft bristle tooth brush or cotton swabs for oral hygiene.
- Instruct patient to avoid foods (Eg. spicy, hot or raw) that can traumatize oesophageal varices.
- Provide assistance to avoid falling.
- Make sure that room is free of clutters, that floors are dry, and shoes or slippers are worn to avoid injuries.

PROBLEMS OF GALLBLADDER

The biliary system is affected by stones and obstructions, inflammation and infection. The most common disorders of the biliary system is cholelithiasis (Stone in the gallbladder).

Cholelithiasis

Gallstones can occur at anywhere in the biliary tree. The *cholelithasis* refer to stone formation in the gallbladder. Either acute or chronic inflammation termed as "*Cholecytitis*" can result precipitated by the presence of stones. When stones form in or migrate to the common bile duct the condition is termed as *Choledochole lithasis*.

Table 8.1: Nursing care plan for patient with cirrhosis of liver

Problem	*Reason*	*Objective*	*Nursing intervention*	*Evaluation*
Fatigue R/T muscle wasting blood loss.	Featuring potential anaemia.	No, fatigue or reduced fatigue.	• Ensure or maintain bedrest in acute phase. • Encourage increased activity gradually after acute phase. • Restrict visitors. • Make sure that patient is getting balanced prescribed diet.	
Altered nutrition more than body requirement R/T anorexia, impaired utilization and storage of nutrients, nausea vomiting	As manifest by lack of interest in food, aversion to eating, inadequate food intake.	• Adequate intake of food. • Maintenance of normal body weight.	• Monitor weight to evaluate nitrogen balance. • Provide oral care before meals to remove foul taste and improve taste. • Administer antiemetics as ordered. • Provide small, frequent meals with nourishment. • Determine food preferences and allow these whenever possible.	
Impaired skin integrity R/T oedema, ascitis Pruritis	As manifested by complaints of itching, areas of excoriation from scratching, taut, shining skin over edematus areas of skin breakdown.	• Maintain skin integrity. • No pruritus.	• Restrict sodium intake and fluids to reduce oedema. • Administer prescribed diuretics. • Monitor intake and output. • Assess location and extent of oedema by weighing, taking daily measurement of exteremities and abdominal girth. • Provide meticulous skin care. • Reposition patient at least with the intervels of two hours. • Elevate edematous area to promote venous drainage. • Have patient use special mattresses to reduce skin breakdown. • Clip patient's nails short and keep clean. • Administer antipruritic medication as ordered. • Provide diversions and distractions.	
Ineffective breathing pattern R/T pressure on diaphragm and reduced-lung volume. Secondary to ascitis.	As manifested by dyspnoea, cyanosis, changes in pulse, respn. depth or pattern.	• Able to breathe with minimised difficulty.	• Place the patient in semi-Fowler's or Fowler's position. Support the arms and chest with pillows. • Auscultale chest for crakes to identifying fluid in lungs. • Assess respiratory rate and rythm to know dyspnoea.	
Risk injury R/T diminished perception secondary to peripheral neuropathy.	Peripheral neuropathy.	No injury due to decreased perception.	• Assess numbness and tingling of lower extremities, decrease sensation in lower extremities. • Prevent excess stimulation or trauma to extremities. • Do not use restrictive bedlining. • Instruct patient to avoid tight clothing. • Use care with heat and cold application. • Assist with ambulation.	

Note: There may be problems of liver activity intolerance, risk for infection, ineffective airway clearance, potential for hepatoencephality and take nursing measures accordingly.

Aetiology

Cholecystitis is most commonly associated with stones. When it occurs in the absence of stones it is thought to be caused by bacteria reaching gall bladder via the vascular or lymphatic route or chemical irritant in the bile. E.coli, streptococci, and salmonellae are common bacteria. Other causative factors include adhesions, neoplasms, extensive fasting, frequent weight fluctuations, anaesthesia and narcotics.

The actual cause of cholelithiasis is unknown. It develops when the *valarice* that keeps cholestrol, bile salts and calcium in solutions is altered so that precipitation of these substances occurs. Conditions that upset this balance include infection and disturbance in the metabolism of cholestrol. A high percentage of gallstones are precipitated of cholestrol. Other components of bile that precipitates into stone are bile salts, bilirubin, calcium and proteins. Stones sometimes are mixed. The risk factors for cholestrol gallstones are obesity, middle age, pregnancy, multiparity, use of oral contraceptives, rapid weight loss, diseases of the ileum and hypercholestrolaemia.

Pathophysiology

Bile is primarily composed of water plus conjugated bilirubin, organic and inorganic ions, small amounts of proteins and three lipids bile salts, lecithin, and cholestrol. When the balance of these three lipids remain intact, cholestrol is held in solution. If the balance is upset cholestrol can be precipitated. Cholestrol gall stone formation is enhanced by the production of a mucin glycoprotein, which traps cholestrol particles. Supersaturation of the bile with cholestrol also impairs gallbladder mobility and contributes to statis.

Cholestrol stones are hard, white or yellow-brown in colour, radiolucent and can be quite large upto 4 cm. Black-pigmented stones form as the result of an increase of unconjugated bilirubin and calcium with a corresponding decrease in bile salts. Gall bladder motility may also be impaired. Brown stones develop in the intra and extrahepatic ducts and are usually preceded by bacterial invasion.

Clinical Manifestations

Manifestation of cholecystitis varies from indigestion and moderate to severe pain, fever and jaundice. Initial symptoms of acute cholecystitis include indigestion and pain and tenderness in the right upper quadrant (RUQ), which may be referred to the right shoulder and scapula. The pain may be accompanied by anorexia, nausea and possibly vomiting, restlessness and diaphoresis. Manifestation of inflammation are such as leukocytosis and fever.

Physical findings include RUQ tenderness and abdominal rigidity. Symptoms of chronic cholecystitis include history of fat intolerance, dyspepsia, heart burn and flatulence.

Cholelithiasis may produce severe symptom or none at all. The severity of symptoms depends on whether the stones are stationary or mobile and whether obstruction is present. The clinical manifestations caused by obstructed blood flow are:

- Obstructive jaundice due to no bile flow into diodenum.
- Dark amber urine which forms when shaken are due to soluble bilirubin in urine.
- No urobilirubin in urine due to no bilirubin reaching small intestine to be converted to urobilirubin.
- Clay-coloured stools urobilirubin.
- Pruritis due to deposition of bile salts in skin tissues.
- Intolerance for fatty foods- No bile in small intestine for fat digestion.
- Bleeding tendencies—Lack or decreased absorption of Vitamin K resulting in decreased production of prothrombins.
- Steatorrhoea—No bile salts in duodenum, preventing fat emulsion and digestion.
- Billary colic—Murphy sign—i.e. Pain colicy and more flow steady. Complications of cholecystitis include subphrenic absess, pancreatitis, cholangitis (inflammation of bile ducts), biliary cirrhosis, fistulas, and rupture of gallbladder which can produce bile peritonitis.

Diagnostic Study

- Ultrasound
- Cholecystogram or IV cholengiogram
- Liver function studies
- WBC counts and
- Serum bilirubin.

Management

During an acute episode of cholecystitis the focus of treatment is on control of pain, control of possible infection with antibiotics and maintenance of fluid and electrolyte balance. Treatment is mainly supportive and symptomatic. conservative therapy includes:

- IV fluids.
- NPO with NG tube later progressing to low fat diets.
- Antiemetic to prevent nausea and vomiting.
- Analgesics to relieve pain (i.e. meperidine) as prescribed.
- Administration of Fat - soluble vitamins (A B E/C).
- Anticholenergic to decrease secretions which prevents biliary contraction.
- Antispasmodic counteracts smooth muscle spasm.
- Hydrocholetic drugs - Dehydrocholic acid, Florantyrone (Zanchal).
- Antibiotics.
- ETCEP with spincterotomy (Pillotomy).
- Cholestrol solvents.
- Extracorporeal shock-wave lithotripsy (ESWL).
  The dissolution therapy incldues-
- Ursodeoxycholic acid (UDCA).
- Ursodial.
- Chenodeoxycholic acid (CDCA).
- Any medication prescribed by the physician.

Surgical intervention for cholelithiasis is frequently indicated and may consider any one of the several procedures as follows:

- Cholecystectomy – Removal of gallbladder.
- Cholecystostomy – Incision of gallbladder for removal of stones.
- Choledocholithotomy – Incision to common bile duct for removal of stones.
- Cholicystogastrotomy – Anastomosis between stomach and gallbladder.
- Choledecysoduodenostomy – Anastomosis between gall bladder and duodenum to relieve obstruction to distal end of common bile duct.
- Laparoscopic cholecystectomy – Removal of gallbladder via Laproscopy using a dissecting laser.

The nurse has to follow the undermentioned guidelines for the patient undergoing open cholecysteatomy in addition to general guidelines.

Preoperative

- Patient with complete preoperative preparations at home before their arrival on the day of surgery. The nurse will verify that the patient has had NPO and completed any required bowel preparation. Preoperative teaching includes.
- Teach patient the importance of frequent breathing and use of incentive spirometer because the high incision and RUQ pain predispose the patient to atelectasis and right lower lobe pneumonia.
- Explain the types of biliary drainage tubes which are anticipated if any.
- Teach the patient about the pain control plan to be used in the postoperative period.

Postoperative

- Place the patient in low-Fowler's position, assist to change position frequently.
- Urge patient to deep by breathe at regular intervals (every 1 to 2 hrs) and to cough if secretions are present until ambulating well. Assist patient to effectively splint the incision. Encourage use of incentive spirometer.
- Give analgesics fairly liberally for the first 2 to 3 days.
- Use patient-controlled analgesia if possible. Meperidine has been the drug of choice because it is believed to minimize spasms in the bile ducts, but morphine is being used with increasing frequency.
- Maintain a dry, intact dressing, usually a drain is inserted near the stump of the cyst duct; Some serous fluid drainage is normal initially.
- Encourage progressive ambulation when permitted.
- Increase diet gradually to be regular with fat content as tolerated (appetite and fat tolerance may be diminished if there is external biliary drainage).

Biliary drainage

- Connect any biliary drainage tubes to be closed gravity drainage.
- Attach sufficient tubing so the patient can move without restriction.
- Explain to patient the importance of avoiding kinks, clamping or pulling of the tube.
- Monitor the amount and colour of drainage frequently, measure and record drainage at least every shift.
- Report any signs of peritonitis (abdominal pain, rigidity or fever) to the concerned doctor.
- Monitor colour of urine and stools; stools will be grayish-white if the bile is flowing out a drainage tube, but the normal colour should gradually reappear as external drainage diminishes and disappears.

PRIMARY SCLEROSING CHOLANGITIS (PSC)

Inflammation and scarring of the biliary tree occur more commonly as a result of gallstones and bile duct infection. Parasites are most common source of infections. When no cause for the bile duct injury can be found, the process is called ideopathic or primary sclerosing cholangitis. It has closest link with inflammatory bowel disease.

Pathophysiology

PSC causes changes in and around the large bile ducts from inflammation obstruction and intra and extrahepatic fibrosis. Strictures can usually be found in multiple locations. These strictures are short and diffusely distributed and alternate with normal or dilated segments of the ducts to create a bead-like appearance in X-ray. It is unusual for the gallbladder or cystic ducts to be involved.

Clinical Manifestation

Many patients are symptomatic in early stages. Others are seen with combination of fatigue, fever, jaundice, abdominal pain and weight loss. Persistent severe pruritis can be a particularly difficult aspect of the disease. Patient may experience recurrent attacks of cholangitis.

Diagnostic studies of other liver and biliary disorders.

Management

Drug therapy aimed at reducing biliary tree inflammation and preventing the scarring that leads to obstruction. The drug ursodeoxycholic acid has shown promise. surgical procedures other than transplant have been effective for diffuse disease. Endoscopic treatment to remove stones, relieve obstruction, dilate ducts, and place stout tubes in ongoing but primarily in the form of clinical trials.

The uncertain nature of PSC is one of its most difficult characteristics. Patients are instructed about the disease and its possible outcome and are prepared for the possibility of the eventual need for liver transplant. Persistent jaundice may negatively affect body image, and chronic severe pruritis may be a daily nightmare. Some patients are responding to cholestyramine resin (Drug), which theoretically binds the itching triggering elements in the bile. The nurse also suggests that patient experiments with common intervention that may lessen his/her itching. A low fat diet is recommended to patient who develops problems with diarrhoea or steatorrhoea and the fat restriction usually promptly corrects the problems. Fat-soluble vitamin replacement is often needed.

The following strategies to control pruritis are helpful.

- Avoid irritating clothing (Wool or restrictive clothing).
- Use tepid water for bathing rather than hot.
  - Experiment with nonirritating soaps and detergents
  - Pat skin dry after bathing or showering; do not rub.
- Apply emollient creams and lotions to dry skin regularly.
- Avoid activities that increase body temperature or cause sweating.
- Experiment with treatments such as oatameal baths.
- Keep the fingernails short and consider use of cotton gloves at night to minimize skin damage from scratching.
- Use antipruritic medications as ordered.

ACUTE PANCREATITIS

Acute pancreatitis is an acute inflammatory process of the pancreas. The degree of inflammation varies from mild oedema to severe haemorrhage necrosis.

Aetiology

Acute pancreatitis is most common in middle-aged men and women, but affects more men than women. Many factors can cause injury to the pancreas. The primary aetiological factors are *biliary tract disease* and *alcoholism*. The other less common causes are:

- Acute pancreatitis include trauma (postsurgical, abnormal).
- Viral infections (mumps, coxsakie virus B).
- Pancreating duodenum ulcer.
- Abscesses.
- Cystic fibrosis.
- Kaposis sarcoma.
- Certain drugs (corticosteroids, thiazetic diurectics, oral contraceptives sulfanamide and NSAIDS).
- Metabolic disorders: (hyperlipidaemia, renal failure).
- After surgical procedure (of pancreas, stomach, duodenum and biliary tract).
- After ERCP.
- Ideopathic.

Pathophysiology

The most common pathogenic mechanism is believed to be autodigestion of the pancreas. the two major pathological varieties of acute pancreatitis are (1) acute intestinal form and (2) acute haemorrhagic form. Although either can be fatal, intestinal form is often a milder form. The defining characteristics of *acute intestinal pancreatitis* is a diffusely swollen and inflammed pancreas, which retains its anatomical features. There are minimal or no area of haemorrhage or necrosis in gland. The intestitial spaces becomes grossly swollen by extracellular oedema and the ducts may contain purulent material. The acute haemorrhage disease presents with a different picture. The gland readily shows acute inflammation, haemorrhage, and marked tissue necrosis. Extensive fat necrosis is present in patients with fulminant disease not just in the pancreas but throughout the abdominal and thoracic cavities and subcutaneous tissues. Necrosis of vessel can cause significant loss of blood and abscesses and infections form in areas of walled-off necrotic tissue. Systemic complications such as fat emboli, hypotension, shock and fluid overload are common.

The aetiologic factors cause injury to pancreatic cells or activation of the pancreatic enzymes in the pancreas. Trypsionogen is an inactive proteolytic enzyme produced by pancreas. Activation fo pancreatic enzymes before they reach the duodenum has long been recognized as a major component of the disease process. Enzyme activation overwhelms all of the normal protective mechanisms of the pancreas and initiates a massive attack on the pancreatic tissues. Pancreatic autodigestion is initiated. Other systemic effects of the activated enzymes include:

- Activation of complement and kinin-producing increased vascular permeability and vasodilation.
- Increased stickness of the inflammatory leucocytes with formation of emboli, which plug the microvasculature.
- Initiation of consumptive coagulopathy, leading to disseminated intravascular coagulation.
- Increased permeability causing massive movement of fluids which leads to circulatory insufficiency.
- Release of myocardial-depressant factor, which further compromises cardiac function.
- Activation of the renin-angiotensin network, which impairs renal function in conjunction with circulatory insufficiency.

Clinical Manifestations

Pain

- Steady and severe in nature, excruciating in fulminant cases.
- Located in the epigastric or umbilical region, may radiate to the back.
- Worsened by lying supine; may be lessened by flexed knee, curved back positioning.

Vomiting

- Varies in severity but is usually protracted.
- Worsened by ingestion of food or fluid.

- Does not relive the pain.
- Usually accompanied by nausea.

Fever

- Rarely exceeds 39°C.

Abdominal Findings

- Rigidity, tenderness, guarding.
- Distension.
- Decreased or absent peristalsis.

Additional Features of Fulminanal Disease

- Symptoms of hypovolumic shock.
- Oliguria; acute tubular necrosis.
- Ascites.
- Jaundice.
- Respiratory failure.
- Grey Turner's sign (bluish discoloration along the flanks).
- Cullen's sign (bluish discoloration around the umbilicus).

(These signs indicate the accumulation of blood in these areas and represent the presence of haemorrhagic pancreatitis).

The significant local complications of acute pancreatitis are pseudocyst and absess. The main systemic complication as pulmonary (plueral effusion, atelectasis and pneumonia) and tetany and hypotension hypovolumea, hypoalbuminea, leukocytosis, ARDS, GI bleeding, pseudocyst, hyperglycemea, hypocalcemia, and hyperlipidemea.

Diagnostic Studies

The primary diagnostic tests are serum amylase, lipase and urinary amylase level. usually there is elevation. The secondary tests are blood glucose, (hyperglycemic due to impaired carbohydrate metabolism due to E.-Cell damage and release of glucagon). Serum calcium (hypocalcemea) and serum triglycerides (Hyperlipidemia) and also CTS, ERCEP.

Management

The main objective of the management of acute pancreatitis are: relief of pain; prevention and alleviation of shock; reduction of pancreatic secretions, control of fluid and electrolyte imbalance, prevention and treatment of infections and removal of precipitatory cause for which the measures to be taken according to the following.

- Administer meparidin (analgesics) to relieve pain.
- NPO with NG tube to suction and reduce secretions.
- Cimetidine or rantidine IV.
- Administer antibiotics as prescribed.
- Lactated Ringer's solution for fluid and electrolyte valancy and bedrest and proper diet, good oral hygiene should be maintained and take measures to treat complications accordingly.

And teach patients to avoid alcohol.

CHRONIC PANCREATITIS

Chronic pancreatitis is progressive destruction of the pancreas with fibrotitic replacement of pancreatic tissue structure and calcification may also occur in the pancreas.

Aetiology

Chrome pancreatic may follow acute pancreatitis. The two major types are chronic-obstructive pancreatitis and chronic-calcifying pancreatitis. Chronic obstructive pancreatis is associated with biliary disease. The most common cause is inflammation of the spincter associated with cholelithiasis. Cancer of the ampules of valex duodenum, or pancreas also can cause this type. The chronic calcifying pancreatitis there are inflammation and sclerosis mainly in the head of the pancreas and around the pancreatic duct. It is associated with alcohol. These are also called "alcohol-induced pancreatitis.

Pathophysiology

The basic pathological change of chronic pancreatitis is destruction of the exocrine parenchymas and replacements with fibrous tissue. This process is associated with varying degrees of duct dilation. Scarring and fibritic changes may occur throughout the pancreas or be limited to the selected areas. Calcium salts may be deposited in both the ducts and the parenchyma, usually in areas of fat necrosis. Ductal obstructions occur secondarily. The factors which influence the solubility on the calcium-rich pancreatic secretions are not well-identified. As the process becomes increasingly severe the islets of langerhans are also involved and destroyed.

Clinical Manifestation

As with acute pancreatitis, a major manifestation of the chronic pancreatic is abdominal pain. The patient may have episodes of acute pain, but it is usually chronic (recurrent attack at intervals of months or years). The attacks may become more and more frequent until they are almost constant, or they may diminish as the pancreatic fibrosis develops. The pain is located in the same area as in the acute pancreatitis, but it is usually described as heavy, gnawing feeling and sometimes a burning and cramp like. The pain is not relieved by food or antacids. The other manifestations are pancreatic insufficiency including malabsorption with weight loss, constipation, mild jaundice with dark urine, steatorrhoea and diabetes mellitus. The steatorrhoea may become severe with voluminous, foul, fatty stools. Urine and stools may be frothy. Some abdominal tenderness may be present.

Diagnosis: (Diagnostic studies as in acute pancreatitis).

Management

When the patient with chronic pancreatitis is experiencing an acute attack, the therapy is identical as that for acute pancreatitis. At other times, the focus is on prevention of further attacks, relief of pain, and control of pancreatic exocrine and endocrine insufficiency. It sometimes takes large, frequent doses of analgesics to relieve pain. And diet, pancreatic enzyme replacement, and control of diabetes are measures used to control pancreatic insufficiency. The diet is a bland, low-fat, high-carbohydrate and high protein diet. The patient does not tolerate fatty, rich and stimulating foods and these should be avoided to decrease pancreatic secretions and demands on the pancreas. Alcohol must be totally eliminated. Antacids and anticholenising drugs may be given to decrease HCl acid. Where stimul .... Pancreatic is active, i.e. cemetidine and rantidine pancreatic enzymes such as pancreatin, pancrealipase are used to replace enzymes. For diabetes insulin is giving as per instruction of the medical doctors. When pseudocysts or obstruction develops, surgery may be indicated and treated accordingly.

Table 8.2: Nursing care plan for the patient with severe acute pancreatitis

Problem	*R**	*Objective*	*Nursing interventions*	*Rationales*
Nursing Diagnosis#1 Tissue perfusion, alteration in related to hypovolemic shock.		Patient will: 1. Maintain stable haemodynamics: • Blood pressure within 10 mmHg of baseline. • Heart rate < 100 beats/min. • Central venous pressure 0-8 mmHg. • Pulmonary capillary wedge pressure 8-12 mmHg. • Cardiac output ~5 liters/min. • Skin warm with usual colour.	• Perform ongoing cardiovascular assessment: ◆ Continuous cardiac monitoring. – Establish baseline rate, rhythm, ectopy. ◆ Continuous haemodynamic pressure monitoring: – Establish baseline values: Central venous pressure, pulmonary capillary wedge pressure. ◆ Assess peripheral pulses: Rate, rhythm, quality. ◆ Assess skin temperature, moisture, colour, turgor.	• Establishing baseline data assists in evaluating subsequent responses to therapy. ◆ Cardiac tissue hypoxia may predispose to dysrhythmias. ◆ Offers significant data regarding cardiopulmonary status; affords *trending*, i.e., frequent serial measurements; trending more accurately reflects changes occurring in patient's condition and the patient's response to therapeutic measures. ◆ Presence of cool, moist skin with pallor or cyanosis reflects compensatory peripheral vasoconstriction response to permit blood to be shunted to vital organs.
		2. Demonstrate alert mental status, appropriate behaviour and neurological function: • Oriented to person, place, time. • Cranial nerves intact. • Deep tendon reflexes brisk.	• Assess ongoing neurological function: Mental status; level of consciousness; behaviour—appropriate?; cranial nerves; deep tendon reflexes.	• Compromised haemodynamics (hypotension) and hypoxemia predispose to cerebral hypoxia, reflected by alterations in cerebral function, level of consciousness, responsiveness of cranial nerves, and deep tendon reflexes.
		3. Maintain renal function: • Urine output >30 ml/hr. • Balanced intake and output. • BUN, serum creatinine within acceptable physiological range.	• Monitor renal function: Hourly urine output; intake and output. ◆ Daily weight.	• Reduction in urine output suggests decreased renal perfusion commonly associated with hypovolemic shock. Acute renal failure is a major complication of acute pancreatitis. ◆ Most closely reflects hydration status.
Nursing Diagnosis #2 Fluid volume deficit (intravascular), actual, related to: 1. Haemorrhage. 2. Third-spacing (pancreatic ascites). A. Hypoalbuminaemia. 3. Dehydration. A. NPO.		Patient will: 1. Achieve resolution of oedema/ascites: • Body weight within 5% of baseline. • Abdominal girth at baseline measurement.	• Assess gastrointestinal function: ◆ Abdominal assessment: Abdomen—soft, rigid; rebound tenderness; presence of Cullen or Grey-Turner signs; abdominal girth. ◆ Nausea/vomiting/constipation, haematemesis, melena.	• Compensatory vasoconstriction of splanchnic circulation (sympathetic response), may result in decreased peristalsis, and ischemia of the gastric and intestinal mucosa, – Cullen sign; Bluish umbillcus or family blue discoloration of skin associated with haemoperitoneum from any cause.

*'R' refers to "Reason" ie. key points obtained in subjective and objective data to support the problem "identified".

Contd...

Contd...

Problem	*R**	*Objective*	*Nursing interventions*	*Rationales*
B. Nasogastric suctioning. C. Vomiting.				– Grey-Turner sign: Ecchymoses on abdomen and flanks possibly associated with infiltration of extraperitoneal tissues with blood.
Nursing Diagnosis #3 Electrolyte balance, alteration in related to: 1. Diuretic therapy. 2. Acid-base imbalance.		Patient will: 1. Restore/maintain laboratory parameters within acceptable physiological range: • Serum osmolality 285-295 mOsm/Kg. • Serum sodium>135 <148 mEq/liter. • Serum potassium 3.5-5.5 mEq/liter. • Serum albumin 3.5-5.5 g/100 ml. • Haematocrit 37-52 per cent. • Haemoglobin 12-18 g/100 ml. • CBC. • Urine electrolytes and specific gravity.	• Assess for signs and symptoms of electrolyte imbalance: ◆ Hypokalaemia—cardiac dysrhythmias; hypotension; weakness; fatigue; nausea, vomiting; lethargy, muscle weakness; paresthe-sias, hyporeflexia. ◆ Hyponatraemia—nausea, vomiting, headache, lethargy, confusion, seizures, coma. ◆ Hypocalcaemia—tremors, paresthesias, tetany laryngospasm, convulsions, positive Chvostek's and Trousseau's signs. ◆ Hypochloraemia: Alkalaemia.	• Acute pancreatitis usually predisposes to electrolyte imbalance. Nasogastric suctioning, vomiting, diarrhoea, and extravasation of fluid account for much of the loss of sodium, potassium, and chloride. – It is important to establish baseline blood chemistry values so that replacement therapy may be guided by serial studies, which should include total protein and serum osmolality in addition to electrolytes.
			• Implement prescribed measures to re-establish and maintain normovolaemia and electrolyte balance.	
			◆ Administer blood products and intravenous fluids.	◆ To reverse hypovolaemia/hypotension. Re-establishing intravascular volume improves circulation, tissue perfusion and oxygenation. Replace fluid losses associated with NPO, vomiting, and nasogastric suctioning. – Irrigating and inflammatory effects of acute pancreatitis on the pancreatic parenchyma and surrounding tissues cause extravasation of fluids, electrolytes, and protein into the interstitium and peritoneal cavity (third-spacing).
			◆ Replace serum albumin.	◆ Loss of plasma proteins from the intravascular space disrupts colloidal osmotic pressure, predisposing to even greater fluid loss with interstitial oedema and ascites.
			◆ Monitor for signs of circulatory overload: Generalized (dependent) oedema, weight gain, increased blood pressure, bounding pulses; signs of pulmonary congestion—dyspnoea, rales (crackles), elevation of central venous and pulmonary artery pressures; neck vein distention.	◆ Fluid overload is a complication of aggressive fluid volume replacement.
			◆ Monitor for signs of hypovolaemia: Hypotension, tachycardia, decreased central venous and pulmonary artery pressures; decreased urine output, increase in urine-specific gravity; signs of dehydration—elevated body temperature, poor skin turgor, sunken eyeballs, and dryness of mucous membranes.	
			◆ Administer prescribed inotropic and vasopressor therapy. – Dopamine hydrochloride.	◆ Increases cardiac output by increasing preload (venous return) and cardiac contractility; enhances tissue perfusion.
			◆ Replace serum electrolytes:	

Contd...

Problem	*R**	*Objective*	*Nursing interventions*	*Rationales*
			• Sodium. – Hyponatraemia/hypernatraemia: monitor hydration status, monitor serum/urine sodium levels.	• Hyponatraemia is a frequent occurrence in acute pancreatitis. – A decrease in total body sodium predisposes to hypovolaemia. – Intravenous replacement of sodium needs to be carefully monitored to prevent sodium excess (hypernatraemia) with consequent fluid overload.
			• Potassium. – Hypokalaemia/hyperkalaemia: Monitor ECG for dysrhythmias, monitor arterial blood gases (acid-base status), monitor serum potassium levels.	• Potassium, an intracellular ion, is closely associated with acid-base balance: – Acidemia—hydrogen ions are driven into cells in exchange for potassium; this increases serum potassium levels. – Alkalaemia—hydrogen ions move out of cells in exchange for potassium; this decreases serum potassium levels. – This reciprocal relationship between potassium and hydrogen ions also occurs in the distal tubules, necessitating that kidney function be closely monitored.
			• Calcium. – Hypocalcaemia.	• Deposition of calcium into areas of fatty necrosis occurs frequently in acute pancreatitis and requires close monitoring of serum calcium levels. Calcium replacement therapy requires careful administration to prevent complications: – Patent intravenous line needs to be maintained because tissue sloughing and necrosis can occur with extravasation of calcium preparations.
			• Monitor ECG for dysrhythmias.	• Potentiation of digitalis effect by calcium can occur in patients receiving digitalis; this can predispose to digitalis toxicity. Continuous ECG monitoring is essential.
			• Monitor total serum protein and serum albumin levels.	• Calcium is highly bound to serum proteins; alkalaemia increases percent calcium bound to protein, thus reducing fraction of ionized calcium.
			• Chloride.	• Chloride is necessary for gastric production of HCl; it plays a major role in acid-base balance.
			– Hypochloraemia: monitor acid-base status, monitor serum chloride.	• Hypochloremia is associated with vomiting, and nasogastric suctioning; it predisposes to metabolic alkalosis.
Nursing Diagnosis#4 **Breathing pattern, Ineffective, related to:** 1. Hypoventilation associated with severe abdominal pain.		Patient will: 1. Demonstrate effective minute ventilation: • Tidal volume (Vr) > 5-7 ml/Kg.	• Assess respiratory function: • Rate, rhythm, depth and pattern of breathing. • Symmetry of chest wall and diaphragmatic excursion.	• Abdominal pain causes splinting and hypoventilation; hypoventilation predisposes to hypercapnia and atelectasis; atelectasis predisposes to ventilation/perfusion inequality.

Contd...

Contd...

Problem	*R**	*Objective*	*Nursing interventions*	*Rationales*
2. Atelectasis. 3. Pleural effusion. *Nursing Diagnosis #5* Airway clearance, ineffective, related to: 1. Cough suppression and failure to deep breathe because of severe abdominal pain. 2. Immobility.		• Respiratory rate < 25-30 per min. 2. Achieve vital capacity (Vc) > 12-15 ml/Kg. 3. Verbalize ease of breathing. 4. Demonstrate deep-breathing techniques and effective secretion-clearing cough. 5. Maintain arterial blood gases within acceptable physiological range: • $PaO_2 > 60$ mmHg. • $PaCO_2$ 35-45 mmHg. • pH > 7.35 < 7.45. • Base excess +2/-2. 6. Maintain appropriate responses on respiratory examination: • Tactile fremitus present on palpation. • Resonance throughout lung fields on percussion. • Vesicular breath sounds throughout peripheral lung fields on auscultation. 7. Demonstrate an absence of atelectasis and pleural effusion.	◆ Use of accessory muscles. ◆ Auscultation of breath sounds. ◆ Pulmonary lung volumes: Total minute ventilation; tidal volume, respiratory rate; vital capacity. ◆ Assess quantity, quality, colour, odour and consistency of sputum. ◆ Assess arterial blood gases.	– Abdominal pain predisposes to cough suppression and immobility; pooling of secretions predisposes to pneumonia.
			• Implement measures to improve respiratory function: ◆ Administer prescribed medication for abdominal pain and monitor response.	◆ Relief of pain encourages patient to breathe more deeply and to cough more vigorously.
			◆ Meperidine is drug of choice.	◆ Meperidine causes less spasm of Oddi's sphincter than does morphine.
			◆ Perform measures to reduce anxiety: – Encourage verbalization of fears and concerns. – Provide a caring touch and listening ear. – Provide explanations and feedback regarding care and health status. – Identify patient/family coping strengths and resources.	◆ A reduction in the level of anxiety or stress may help to reduce the level of pain, and facilitate breathing.
			◆ Perform measures to facilitate chest wall expansion and diaphragmatic excursion: – Minimize abdominal distention associated with gastrointestinal gas and fluid accumulation.	◆ Help to improve ventilation and oxygenation, and prevent atelectasis and pooling of secretions.
			◆ Maintain proper placement and patency of nasogastric tube.	◆ Nasogastric suction helps to reduce gastric distention.
			◆ Encourage frequent position changes. – Maintain patient in semi to high-Fowler's position unless contraindicated.	◆ Patient is inclined to assume a position of greatest pain relief and to remain in that position. Coughing, deep breathing, and position changes may best be performed following administration of analgesics.
			◆ Encourage patient to expel flatus whenever the urge arises.	◆ Deep breathing and position changes may stimulate peristalsis and flatulence.
			◆ Monitor for signs and symptoms of pleural effusion: Shortness of breath; pleuritic pain; splinting to reduce chest excursion; dullness on percussion; and diminished to absent breath sounds over the affected area on auscultation.	

Contd...

Problem	R*	Objective	Nursing interventions	Rationales
			◆ Perform measures to minimize pancreatic secretory activity.	◆ The pancreas is stimulated by gastric juice in the duodenum; a patent nasogastric tube with suction reduces delivery of HCl to duodenum.
			◆ Administer anticholinergic drugs cautiously, if prescribed.	◆ Blocking parasympathetic stimulation (via vagus) decreases amount of gastric HCl secretion; use of anticholinergics in a patient with paralytic ileus may actually worsen the patient's condition by suppressing pancreatic secretion and allowing enzymes to accumulate within the pancreas.
			◆ Prepare patient and assist with thoracentesis (see Table 36-2).	◆ Decompression of pleural effusion facilitates greater lung expansion.
			◆ Prepare patient and assist with paracentesis (see Table 50-4, Nursing Diagnosis#1).	◆ Decompression of peritoneal fluid increases diaphragmatic excursion.
			◆ Implement prescribed respiratory support therapy: ◆ Oxygen therapy. ◆ Intermittent positive pressure breathing (IPPB).	
Nursing Diagnosis #6 Comfort, alteration in: Acute pain.		Patient will: 1. Verbalize relief of pain. 2. Exhibit relaxed demeanor: • Relaxed facial expression and body posturing. • Ease of breathing. 3. Identify effective pain relief and coping mechanisms.	• Implement measures to reduce pancreatic stimulation.	• Stimulation of inflamed pancreatic acinar cells aggravate pain. ◆ Pain and anxiety increase pancreatic secretory activity via enhanced parasympathetic stimulation.
			◆ Maintain the patient NPO.	◆ It is necessary to minimize gastric secretions as they stimulate secretion of the hormones secretin and cholecystokinin, both of which stimulate pancreatic secretion.
			◆ Maintain patency of nasogastric tube with continuous nasogastric suction. – Confirm tube placement every two hours.	◆ Nasogastric suction also relieves nausea, vomiting, and intestinal distention.
			◆ Administer prescribed medications: – Meperidine is usual analgesic of choice. Evaluate the effectiveness of the prescribed analgesic.	◆ Morphine is avoided because it causes a greater degree of spasm of the sphincter of Oddi than does meperidine.
			– Anticholinergics, papaverine:	◆ These drugs function to relax smooth muscle which may help to reduce pain.
			Provide frequent oral care.	◆ Anticholinergic drugs suppress salivary secretion; oral mucous membranes become dry.
			– Monitor urine output.	◆ Urinary retention and paralytic ileus are also associated with anticholinergic therapy.
			◆ Provide frequent comfort measures: – Mouth care; position changes; time periods of quiet and sleep; spending more time with patient: – Provide a listening ear.	
			◆ Involve patient/family in quiet recreational activities.	◆ This may help to distract the patient from thoughts of food and to avoid parasympathetic

Contd...

Contd...

Problem	*R**	*Objective*	*Nursing interventions*	*Rationales*
				stimulation associated with the cephalic phase of digestive activity.
			♦ Minimize visitors.	♦ Increased activity may aggravate pain.
			♦ Instruct family members friends not to take food into the patient's room.	♦ Sight of food can stimulate pancreatic secretory activity (cephalic phase of digestion)
Nursing Diagnosis #7 Nutrition, alteration in, less than body requirements (inalnutri-tion), related to: 1. Nausea and vomiting. 2. NPO status. 3. Malabsorption (altered fat metabolism). 4. Altered carbohydrate and protein metabolism. A. Hypoglycaemia. B. Hypoalbumi-naemia.		Patient will: 1. Maintain body weight within 5% of baseline. 2. Maintain serum albumin within physiological range: • 3.5-5.0 g/100 ml. 3. Demonstrate unimpaired integrity of skin and mucous membranes. 4. Verbalize feeling of increased strength. 5. Triceps skinfold within acceptable range. 6. Laboratory parameters within acceptable range: • Haematology profile. • Cholesterol. • BUN, creatinine.	Refer to Table nutritional support of the critically III patient, for details related to treatment and prevention of malnutrition.	
Nursing Diagnosis #8 Oral mucous membranes, alteration in, related to: 1. Altered fluid and electrolyte imbalance (dehydration). 2. Mouth breathing with nasogastric tube. 3. Reduced salivation associated with dehydration and medication regimen (e.g., narcotics, anticholinergics).		Patient will: 1. Maintain integrity of mucous membranes: • Mucous membranes moist. • Lips without cracking or fissures.	• Assess and monitor status of mucous membranes: Monitor daily weight, intake and output; monitor dietary intake. • Implement measures to prevent drying and cracking of mucous membranes: ♦ Maintain hydration. ♦ Provide frequent oral hygiene, rinsing mouth frequently. ♦ Keep lips well lubricated. ♦ Assess lips, mouth and pharynx for lesions, fissures, or bleeding. • Implement measures to treat dryign and cracking or oral membranes: Apply topical ointment to keep mucous membranes moist.	• When nutritional intake is less than body requirements, the patient becomes at risk of infections, and healing capabilities become compromised. ♦ Adequate hydration is necessary to keep mucous membranes moist. ♦ Prevent cracking and fissure formation. ♦ Ongoing assessment assists in determining changes in the mucosa, and the effectiveness of therapy.
Nursing Diagnosis #9 Infection, potential for, related to: 1. Malnutrition. 2. Invasive procedures. 3. Peritonitis associated with autodigestion of adjacent tissues by pancreatic juices.		Patient will: 1. Maintain body temperature within acceptable physiological range ~98.6°F. 2. Maintain white blood count: ~5000-10,000/mm^3. 3. Remain without signs and symptoms of infection: Pain, erythema, oedema, increased temperature (peripheral sites).	Monitor • Check for WBC visul signs • Administry antibiotics as orderd. • Provide nourishments as prescribed • Observe for complications	

Contd...

Problem	*R**	*Objective*	*Nursing Interventions*	*Rationales*
Nursing Diagnosis#10 Knowledge deficit regarding: 1. Convalescence and follow-up care. 2. Impact on lifestyle. • Alcoholism • Stress		Patient will: 1. Verbalize importance of strict adherence to prescribed dietary regimen: • Total abstinence from alcohol. • High carbohydrate and protein diet; low-fat intake. 2. Verbalize alternatives in pain relief: • Medication therapy. • Relaxation exercises. 3. Identify effective coping mechanisms in stress management.	• Establish a trusting rapport with patient and family members. ◆ Verbalize fears and concerns for patient and family.	• An environment of mutual respect and trust can enhance the learning process. Often a long convalescence follows recovery from acute pancreatitis. Discharge planning should begin as early as possible. ◆ While the patient may be too ill initially to participate in learning, involvement of family members in the patient's overall care may impact on the progress made by patient and family members alike towards level of health and well-being desired.
			• Assess patient/family baseline knowledge and readiness to learn. ◆ Encourage patient/family to assist in identifying needs and learning objectives.	• An informed patient/family can participate in care and make necessary adjustments in lifestyle.
			• Assist patient/family in problem-solving techniques. ◆ Help to identify family strengths and weaknesses.	◆ Assisting patient/family to cope increases self-confidence in their own capabilities.
			• Determine appropriate teaching strategies to facilitate learning: ◆ Encourage open discussions regarding illness and impact on family lifestyle. – Consider role of alcohol in lifestyle if appropriate.	• Learning should occur at a rate that is meaningful to participants.
			• Initiate health teaching concerned with the following: "Diet management: Emphasis importance of strict adherence to prescribed diet; abstinence from alcohol and high-fat intake. ◆ Consider who in the family is responsible for meal preparation.	◆ It is essential for the family member who cooks to appreciate the patient's diet and its preparation.
			◆ Pain management: Advise patient as to alternatives in pain relief: Medication therapy; surgery; relaxation exercises, recreational therapy. – Support patient/family in their decision. – Include the following in teaching: purpose, action(s), dosage, frequency and route of administration and drug interactions for prescribed medications.	
			◆ Management of stress: Assist patient/family to: Identify sources of stress; identify effective and ineffective coping mechanisms and their usefulness; assist patient/family to become in touch with their feelings, and to communicate these feelings to each other.	◆ Effective stress management may be helpful in reducing pain.
			• Initiate referrals to appropriate resources: ◆ Nutritionist. ◆ Social worker. ◆ Psychiatric liaison nurse. ◆ Other.	• Successful recovery of all members of the family from the stress of acute illness, and continued health maintenance requires timely and ongoing support. No one lives in a vacuum.

Table 8.3: Care plan for the patient with hepatic failure and hepatic encephalopathy

Problem	*R*	*Objective*	*Nursing interventions*	*Rationales*
Nursing Diagnosis #1 Fluid volume deficit (intravascular, actual), related to: 1. Ascites and anasarca ("third spacing"). A. Hypoalbuminaemia. B. Portal hypertension. C. Hyperaldosteronism (secondary). D. Capillary fragility/increased permeability. 2. Bleeding. A. Bleeding varices (haematemesis). B. Erosive gastritis. C. Coagulopathy. *Nursing Diagnosis #2* Electrolyte balance, alteration in: hypokalaemia, related to: 1. Diuretic therapy. 2. Hyperaldosteronism (sodium retention).		Patient will: 1. Maintain stable haemodynamics: • Heart rate (resting) <100 beats /min. • Central venous pressure 0-8 mmHg. • Pulmonary artery pressure<25 mmHg. • Pulmonary capillary wedge pressure 8-12 mmHg. • Cardiac output ~5 liters/min. • Systemic arterial blood pressure within 10 mmHg of baseline. 2. Maintain baseline mental and neurological status; deep tendon reflexes brisk. 3. Achieve resolution of ascites and anasarca. • Body weight within 5% of baseline. • Abdominal girth at baseline measurement. • Functioning peritoneovenous shunt (if inserted). 4. Balance intake and output. 5. Maintain urine output >30 ml/hour. 6. Maintain laboratory parameter as follows: • Serum osmolality 285-295 mOsm/Kg. • Serum sodium > 135 and < 148 mEq/liter. • Serum potassium 3.5-5.5 mEq/liter. • Serum albumin 3.5-5.5 g/100 ml. • Haematocrit 37-52 per cent. • Haemoglobin 12-18 g/100 ml. • RBC count > 4.7-5.9 million/mm3. • Platelet count > 150,000 mm^3.	• Assess for signs and symptoms of hypovolaemia: ◆ Assess cardiovascular function:	• Establish baseline assessment data with which to evaluate the patient's response to therapy.
			– Heart rate (resting).	◆ An increase in heart rate reflects a compensatory response to maintain cardiac output.
			– Hypotension (orthostatic).	◆ A decrease in blood pressure of more than 10-15 mmHg from a supine to sitting position reflects a reduced circulatory (intravascular) volume.
			– Skin colour—pallor, mottled appearance; cyanosis; cool to touch; peripheral oedema (anasarca).	◆ Compensatory peripheral vasoconstriction shunts blood from skin and nonvital organs to the heart and brain.
			– Assess for ascites—abdominal assessment: – Inspect for bulging of flanks or a protruding, misplaced umbilicus; skin tautness; new striae. – Percuss for shifting dullness. – Palpate for fluid wave.	◆ Ascites results from a combination of low intravascular colloidal osmotic pressure (hypoalbuminaemia), portal hypertension, overproduction of hepatic lymph, and secondary retention of sodium and water. – When forces favouring movement of fluid from the intravascular space into the interstitium (portal hypertension) exceed forces favouring movement of fluid in the opposite direction (e.g., decreased intravascular colloidal osmotic pressure), fluid accumulates. When the capacity of the lymphatic system to return fluid to the circulating blood is exceeded, ascites results. Of central importance to the formation of ascites is renal sodium and water retention.
			– Measure abdominal girth daily using markings indicated on abdomen.	◆ Measurement of abdominal girth assists in evaluating the status of the ascites. Markings made on the abdomen help to assure that repeated measurements are made at the same circumference; measure with patient in same position. Clinical findings of ascites are usually demonstrable after more than 1500 ml of ascites fluid has accumulated.
			– Determine body weight.	◆ Daily measurement of body weight most closely reflects total body fluid volume.
			– Assess serum albumin levels.	◆ Serum albumin is largely responsible for maintaining serum colloidal osmotic pressure.

Contd...

Problem	*R**	*Objective*	*Nursing interventions*	*Rationales*
			◆ Cardiac monitoring.	◆ Cardiac dysrhythmias may occur in response to ischaemia or electrolyte imbalance.
			◆ Haemodynamic pressure monitoring parameters: Central venous pressure; pulmonary artery pressure; pulmonary capillary wedge pressure: cardiac output; arterial pressure monitoring.	◆ Monitoring of these parameters is indicated in the setting of hypovolaemic shock, haemodynamic instability, and during massive fluid, albumin, and blood replacement, to monitor patient's response to therapy and prevent fluid overload.
			◆ Assess neurological function: Mental status, orientation; thought processes; motor responses; deep tendon reflexes.	◆ See Nursing Diagnosis #7, Thought processes, alteration in (below).
			◆ Assess renal function: Intake and output; hourly urine output; monitor creatinine and BUN.	◆ Hypovolaemia can cause a decrease in renal perfusion; patients with hepatic failure are at risk of developing hepatorenal failure. Renal function is best monitored by serum creatinine; BUN may be altered by GI bleeding and impaired liver function.
			◆ Assess for signs and symptoms of electrolyte imbalance: Hypokalaemia—general malaise, fatigue, anorexia, nausea, vomiting, diarrhoea; abdominal cramps; muscle weakness hyporeflexia; cardiac dysrhythmias. ◆ Monitor serum electrolytes.	◆ Excessive sodium reabsorption and retention associated with increased aldosterone secretion, and diuretic therapy can predispose to hypokalemia and metabolic alkalaemia.
			• Implement prescribed measures to re-establish normovolaemia:	• Therapeutic goal is to gradually mobilize fluid back into the intravascular compartment and prevent further third-spacing.
			◆ Maintain fluid restriction (~1000-1500 ml/day).	◆ To decrease ascites and generalized oedema.
			◆ Maintain sodium restriction (200-500 mg/day). – Avoid use of saline for intravenous therapy gastric lavage or other irrigation.	◆ To reduce fluid retention as ascites and anasarca, and enhance mobilization of excessive fluids from the tissues.
			◆ Administer diuretic therapy with necessary potassium replacement therapy.	◆ Controlled diuresis decreases water load with consequent reduction in ascites and oedema: it minimizes the risk of renal failure.
			◆ Furosemide, thiazide diuretics.	◆ Require monitoring of serum potassium with concomitant potassium replacement therapy.
			◆ Spironolactone therapy.	◆ A potassium-sparing diuretic, it inhibits the action of aldosterone on the distal tubular cells, thereby increasing excretion of sodium chloride and water, while retaining potassium.
			◆ Administer inotropic agents and vasopressors (e.g., low-dose dopamine).	◆ To increase cardiac output and maintain effective renal perfusion.
			◆ Administer protein supplementation.	◆ To restore intravascular colloidal osmotic pressure to within acceptable physiological range;

Contd...

Contd...

Problem	*R**	*Objective*	*Nursing interventions*	*Rationales*
				and enhance movement of ascitic and oedema fluid into the intravascular space, promoting diuresis.
			◆ Administer salt-poor albumin intravenously.	◆ Replaces albumin levels, restores intravascular volume and maintains renal perfusion. Monitor for fluid overload.
			• Assist with abdominal paracentesis: ◆ Key nursing considerations:	• In patients with severe ascites, paracentesis may be necessary to relieve dyspnoea and compromised respiratory excursion, and/or urinary frequency.
			– Have patient urinate prior to procedure.	◆ Reduces risk of nicking bladder with needle.
			– Provide necessary explanations. – Position appropriately and as comfortably as possible.	◆ May help patient to relax.
			– Note that fluid removal should not exceed 1-1.5 liters. – Removal of fluid should be done slowly.	◆ Sufficient quantity of fluid is removed to decrease intra-abdominal pressure; altered haemodynamics including phypotension and shock can be precipitated by the removal of too large a volume of fluid.
			– Monitor vital signs pre-, peri- and post-paracentesis.	◆ Assists in assessing possible intra-abdominal bleeding.
			– Measure abdominal girth pre- and post-paracentesis, and daily thereafter.	◆ Assists in assessing for further fluid accumulation.
			– Assess insertion site; monitor for complications of hypotension, bleeding, protein depletion, and infection.	
			• Implement ongoing monitoring:	• Assists in evaluating the patient's response to therapy; reduces risk of complications.
			◆ Cardiovascular status: – Monitor heart rate, pulses, blood pressure, haemodynamic parameters.	◆ Patients with cirrhosis, ascites and bleeding potential are at high risk of complications.
			◆ Respiratory status. ◆ Monitor respiratory rate and pattern; respiratory excursion, breath sounds (normal and adventitious).	◆ Respiratory embarrassment caused by ascites can lead to pulmonary complications; e.g., compromised alveolar ventilation with CO_2 retention (CO_2 narcosis may causes hepatic encepha-lopathis the patic encephalopathy); and pneumonia.
			– Monitor arterial blood gases.	◆ Assists in evaluating effectiveness of ventilation; and acid-base balance.
			◆ Renal status: Assess urine output (hourly); BUN, creatinine. ◆ Assess fluid and electrolyte status: Assurate intake and output; daily weight; daily measurement of abdominal girth. ◆ Serum studies: Electrolytes; protein (albumin/globulin ratio); osmolality, glucose. ◆ Urine studies: Electrolytes, specific gravity.	◆ Assists in evaluating the patient's response to therapy.
			• Assist in preparation of patient for peritoneovenous shunt (e.g., LeVeen and Denver shunts): ◆ Monitor for effectiveness of shunt post-surgery. ◆ Maintain bedrest as indicated.	• This procedure may be indicated for the treatment of intractable ascites. It allows ascitic fluid to flow from the peritoneal cavity through

Contd...

Problem	*R**	*Objective*	*Nursing interventions*	*Rationales*
			◆ Enhance flow through shunt using abdominal binder and teaching patient to perform breathing exercises. ◆ Monitor for complications: haemodilution; congestive heart failure; gastrointestinal bleeding: leakage of ascitic fluid from incision site; infection, sepsis, coagulopathy (DIC); shunt occlusion/malfunction.	a catheter tunneled under subcutaneous tissues, into the jugular vein or superior vena cava. The patient's own breathing triggers the shunt: On inspiration, the diaphragm descends, increasing intra-abdominal pressure while reducing intrathoracic pressures. This differecne in pressure allows the fluid to flow from the peritoneal cavity into the thoracic veins.
Nursing Diagnosis #3 Breathing pattern, Ineffective, related to: 1. Ascites (abdominal distention). 2. Weakened, debilitated state.		Patient will: 1. Maintain baseline mental status. 2. Maintain effective respiratory function: • Respiratory rate <25-30/min. • Tidal volume (Vr) >5-7 ml/Kg. • Vital capacity (Vc) > 12-15 ml/Kg.	• Assess respiratory function: Assess specific parameters—rate, pattern, depth of breathing; symmetry of chest wall and diaphragmatic excursion.	• Ascites causes pressure on diaphragm, limiting respiratory excursion and contributing to decreased alveolar ventilation, and atelectasis. The end result is hypoxaemia.
			◆ Assess use of accessory muscles; breath sounds, evidence of adventitious sounds (rales, wheezes); dyspnoea, tachypnoea, orthopnoea.	◆ Weakened, debilitated status may compromise patient's respiratory effort, reducing alveolar ventilation and predisposing to hypoxaemia.
			◆ Assess effectiveness of cough; sputum production. ◆ Assess pulmonary volume/capacity; tidal volume (Vr); vital capacity (Vc).	◆ Accumulation of fluids and secretions reduces ventilation and predisposes to infection.
			◆ Monitor arterial blood gases: PaO_2, $PaCO_2$ pH.	◆ Reflect effectiveness of ventilation and gas exchange.
			• Assess tissue perfusion and oxygenation. ◆ Assess cerebral function: mental status—restlessness, apprehension, confusion; drowsiness. ◆ Assess cardiovascular function: evidence of cyanosis—lips, mucous membranes, nailbeds; vital signs: heart rate, blood pressure, peripheral pulses, cardiac dysrhythmias. ◆ Assess fluid status: intake and output; body weight. ◆ Laboratory data: haematocrit, haemoglobin, serum electrolytes; BUN; serum osmolality.	• These signs and symptoms may be reflective of hypoxaemia and tissue hypoxia.
			• Assist patient to semi-Fowler's position.	• This position allows for maximal respiratory excursion and lung expansion. Adequate lung expansion facilitates more even distribution of ventilation; it enhances ventilation/perfusion matching.
Nursing Diagnosis #4 Airway clearance, ineffective, related to: 1. Compromised cough reflex. 2. Immobility, with decreased mobilization of secretions.		Patient will: 1. Verbalize ease of breathing. • Breath sounds audible throughout anterior and posterior chest. • Reduced to absent adventitious sounds. 2. Maintain arterial gases: • pH 7.35-7.45. • PaO_2 > 60 mmHg. • $PaCO_2$ 35-45 mmHg.	• Monitor quality, quantity colour, odour consistency of sputum. ◆ Obtain sputum for culture as indicated.	
			◆ Assess secretions for state of hydration.	◆ Maintaining hydration keeps secretions thin and easily mobilized.
			◆ Monitor body temperature, sputum production, and white blood count profile. ◆ Obtain baseline cultures: sputum, urine, blood, wounds, IV sites when changed.	◆ Early detection of an infectious or inflammatory process affords prompt intervention to minimize the effect of the insult on pulmonary and other organ functions.

Contd...

Contd...

Problem	*R**	*Objective*	*Nursing interventions*	*Rationales*
			• Initiate chest physiotherapy—bronchial hygiene (as appropriate). ◆ Encourage coughing and deep breathing: use incentive spirometry if appropriate.	• These activities help to loosen and dislodge secretions and facilitate movement towards trachea from where they are accessible to removal via cough and/or suctioning.
			◆ Turn and position every 2 hours. – Position so as to minimize risk of aspiration, especially in lethargic or semicomatose patient.	◆ Turning and deep breathing assist to mobilize secretions, enhance ventilation and prevent areas of atelectasis.
			◆ Provide necessary pharyngeal and tracheal suctioning if patient is unable to handle pulmonary secretions.	
			• Consider endotracheal intubation and mechanical ventilation in the following settings: ◆ Hypoxaemia: $PaO_2 < 60$ mmHg on $FIO_2 >$ 40 per cent. ◆ Cerebral oedema, as a complication of fulminant hepatic failure. ◆ High risk of aspiration (e.g., patient unable to handle secretions; absent or compromised gag reflex).	◆ Tissue hypoxia predisposes to lactic acldosis. ◆ Carbon dioxide retention ($PaCO_2$ > 45 mmHg) may precipitate cerebral vasodilation and aggravate existing cerebral oedema.
			• Administer prescribed oxygen therapy. ◆ Humidify inspired oxygen.	• Assists in relieving hypoxaemia. ◆ Humidification liquefies secretions.
			• Maintain hydrated state. ◆ Monitor intake and output; weigh daily.	• Adequate hydration moistens, loosens, and liquefies sectretions.
Nursing Diagnosis #5 Potential for infection: pneumonia, related to: 1. Prolonged immobility. 2. Compromised cough reflex. 3. Compromised immune response.		Patient will: 1. Remain without signs/ symptoms of pulmonary infection: • Body temperature 98.6°F. • WBC at baseline. • Lungs resonant to percussion. • Vesicular breath sounds over peripheral lung fields. 2. Demonstrate effective cough	• Monitor patient's environment for potential sources of infection ◆ Visitors, staff, other patients. • Administer prescribed antibiotic therapy: ◆ Obtain necessary cultures prior to initiation of antibiotic therapy.	• Depression of immune response associated with liver disease places patient at increased risk of infection.
Nursing Diagnosis #6 Acid-base balance, alteration in: metabolic alkalemia, related to: 1. Hypokalaemia 2. Diuretic therapy. 3. Nausea/vomiting or continuous nasogastric decompression (suctioning). 4. Secondary hyperaldosteronism. 5. Poor nutrition.		Patient will: 1. Maintain serum electrolyte levels: • Sodium > 135<148 mEq/liter. • Potassium 3.5-5.5 mEq/liter. • Chloride 100-106 mEq/liter. 2. Maintain serum pH 7.35-7.45 (arterial blood gas). 3. Maintain serum ammonia within acceptable physiological range: 80-110 μg/100 ml.	• Monitor laboratory data: ◆ Serum electrolytes. – Sodium, potassium, chloride. ◆ Arterial blood gas—pH. ◆ Serum ammonia levels. ◆ Blood urea nitrogen.	• Patients with cirrhosis have depleted stores of potassium related to nausea, vomiting, poor nutrition, diuretic usage, and secondary hyperaldosteronism. Hypokalaemia contributes to metabolic alkalaemia. ◆ Alkalaemia shifts the ammonia-ammonium ion dissociation equilibrium in favour of ammonia: $NH_3 + H^+ - NH_4^+$ ↑ pH ◆ Ammonia easily crosses blood-brain barrier; high ammonia levels in the setting of liver disease are associated with hepatic encephalopathy. ◆ It is necessary to titrate patient's

Contd...

Problem	*R**	*Objective*	*Nursing interventions*	*Rationales*
				protein intake so as to keep serum ammonia and BUN at acceptable levels. ◆ In hepatic failure the liver is unable to convert ammonia, a by-product of protein metabolism, to urea for elimination.
			• Administer prescribed potassium replacement therapy.	• Use of furosemide and thiazide diuretics should be accompanied by potassium therapy.
			• Administer spironolactone therapy.	• This drug is a potassium-sparing diuretic.
			• Titrate dietary protein intake.	• Excess dietary protein is an excellent substrate for the generation of NH_3.
Nursing Diagnosis #7 Thought process, alteration in, related to: 1. Hepatic encephalopathy associated with high serum ammonia levels caused by the inability of the liver to convert ammonia to urea.		Patient will: 1. Maintain baseline mental status: • Level of consciousness: arousable; oriented to person, place and time. • Mentation: memory intact; able to concentrate; performs simple calculations; demonstrates abstract reasoning. • Usual personality. • Appropriate behaviour.	• Assess for signs and symptoms of hepatic encephalopathy ◆ Mental status: level of consciousness; arousable; comatose. ◆ Mentation: Memory lapses, shortened attention span; confusion; ability to perform simple calculations; abstract reasoning. ◆ Behaviour: Appropriate or inappropriate. – Agitatuion, combativeness; incoherent; drowslness, lethargy.	• Signs and symptoms of hepatic encephalopathy are categorized into stages; familiarity with the stages of hepatic coma assists in bedside assessment, and in evaluation of response to therapy. • Establishing a baseline and ongoing monitoring is essential to determine the clinical course and the patient's response to therapy.
		2. Maintain baseline neurological function: • Able to write name and draw simple figures/numbers. • Speech intact, without slurring. • Absence of asterixis; deep tendon reflexes brisk. • Without seizure activity.	◆ Personality changes. ◆ Neurological status: Status of speech—evidence of slurring; asterixis; tremors; deep coma—unarousable, unresponsive to painful stimuli; pupillary responses, oculocephalic reflexes, decorticate/decerebrate posturing: hyperactive deep tendon reflexes, bilateral Babinski sign. ◆ Electroencephalogram (EEG).	◆ Family and friends may assist in establishing baseline data, ◆ There is a characteristic but not pathogenic slowing of EEG. These changes may precede clinical deterioration, but are not usually present early in the course.
		3. Maintain serum ammonia levels within acceptable range.	• Monitor serum ammonia levels.	• Increase in circulating serum ammonia levels predisposes to hepatic encephalopathy as ammonia is toxic to cerebral tissues. However, hepatic encephalopathy can occur in the absence of elevated ammonia levels, and mechanisms of toxicity remain undefined. ◆ Possible toxic effects of ammonia on cerebral tissues include: Alteration in cerebral energy metabolism; disruption of resting membrane potentials; and altered neurotransmission.

Contd...

Contd...

Problem	*R**	*Objective*	*Nursing interventions*	*Rationales*
			• Implement anti-ammonia regimen:	
			◆ Initiate and/or assist with measures to prevent or control bleeding.	◆ Blood in the gastrointestinal tract is metabolized by intestinal bacteria with the production of ammonia. In liver disease, with intrahepatic and portal hypertension, ammonia absorbed from gut bypasses liver and enters the systemic circulation. Ammonia easily traverses the blood-brain barrier.
			◆ Initiate gastric decompression with iced gastric lavage (as prescribed).	◆ Evacuates blood and allows assessment of the extent of bleeding.
			◆ Assist with insertion of Sengstaken-Blakemore tube.	◆ Inserted to control oesophageal and variceal bleeding.
			◆ Assist with selective angiography with continuous vasopressin (pitressin) influsion (as prescribed).	
			◆ Assist with selerotherapy.	◆ This therapy may be prescribed for patients with uncontrollable bleeding who are poor surgical risks.
			◆ Initiate prescribed therapy to reduce gastric acidity: – Combination of parenteral ranitidine or cimetidine (histamine, antagonists) and antacid therapy via nasogastric tube.	◆ Gastric acidity plays a key role in the pathogenesis of upper gastrointestinal bleeding.
			◆ Serial monitoring of gastric pH.	◆ Ideally gastric pH should be maintained at > 4.5.
			◆ Cautiously administer blood replacement therapy: Packed RBCs should be administered in conjunction with massive blood replacement with stored whole blood. – Monitor haematology profile, prothrombin time, clotting factors.	◆ Stored whole blood is deficient in some clotting factors and can predispose to dilutional coagulopathy.
			◆ Implement nursing measures to prevent/control bleeding.	◆ See Nursing Diagnosis #10, Injury, potential for: bleeding diathesis (below).
			• Initiate lactulose (cephulic) therapy. ◆ Initial dosage: 30-45 ml/hourly (orally or via nasogastric tube) until first bowel movement. ◆ Maintenance dose: 30-45 ml 3-4 times daily. Overdose can cause diarrhoea.	• Lactulose, in conjunction with the action of intestinal bacteria, creates an acidic milieu within the colon that favours conversion of ammonia to ammonium, which is speedily evacuated by the cathartic action of lactulose. $\downarrow$ pH $NH_3 + H^+ - NH_4^+$
			◆ Monitor serial serum glucose.	◆ Lactulose contains galactose and glucose; it may elevate glucose levels; use with caution with diabetes; contraindicated in patients requiring a low-galactose diet.
			• Initiate antibiotic therapy: ◆ Aminoglycosides used: Neomycin (most commonly) and Kanamycin.	• Antibiotics reduce intestinal bacterial flora, thereby reducing bacterial ammonia production. Note: Lactulose and neomycin should not be administered concurrently. Lactulose requires bacteria for its action;

Contd...

Problem	*R**	*Objective*	*Nursing interventions*	*Rationales*
				neomycin destroys intestinal bacteria flora.
			◆ Avoid use with other aminoglycosides, or other nephrotoxic or ototoxic drugs.	◆ The nephrotoxic and ototoxic effects may be potentiated.
			◆ Contraindicated in the setting or renal insufficiency and hepatorenal failure.	◆ Approximately 1 3 per cent of drug is absorbed; in the presence of renal failure, the drug can accumulate, predisposing to nephrotoxicity and ototoxicity.
			◆ Monitor renal function: BUN, creatinine, urine output (hourly); intake and output.	
			• Avoid constipation. ◆ Lactulose is a good cathartic. ◆ Administer stool softeners as prescribed.	• Intestinal bacteria have a longer exposure and greater bulk to convert to ammonia.
			• Restrict or eliminate protein dietary intake.	• To reduce ammonia production and consequent increase in serum ammonia levels.
			◆ Administer high carbohydrate diet (~1400 calories); or intravenous infusion of 10% glucose.	◆ Glucose provides the primary source of energy for cerebral tissues; prevents gluconeogenesis (protein catabolism).
			◆ Provide potassium supplements. – Cautious use of diuretic therapy.	◆ Hypokalaemia predisposes to metabolic alkalaemia which favours the conversion of ammonium to ammonia. $NH_3 + H^+ - NH_4^+$ $\downarrow K^+$
			◆ Maintain fluid and electrolyte balance.	◆ Refer to Nursing Diagnosis #1 above.
			• Prevent hepatotoxicity: ◆ Avoid use of sedatives, hypnotics and other drugs normally metabolized by the liver, or containing ammonia.	• Compromsied hepatocellular function may cause accumulation of drug; some drugs may be toxic to the liver. Such drugs, or combination of drugs, may precipitate or aggravate encephalopathy or mask signs of developing coma.
			◆ Review patient's entire drug regimen: – Dosage may need to be revised in presence of hepatocellular failure. – Potential for adverse drug reactions and toxicity should be monitored. – Assess effect of newly prescribed drugs on neurological function.	
			• Implement nursing interventions in caring for the patient with hepatic encephalopathy: ◆ Monitor neurologic function hourly (if in coma). ◆ Monitor serial laboratory studies: Serum ammonia; BUN, creatinine, electrolytes. • Implement specific measures:	◆ Specific parameters are listed under nursing interventions at the beginning of Nursing Diagnosis #7, in the section on assessing for signs and symptoms of hepatic encephalopathy, neurological status.
			◆ Maintain safe environment: Remove hazardous objects from bedside; use padded rails; keep rails in up position; provide close supervision; initiate seizure precautions. ◆ Reorient patient to person, place, time. ◆ Explain procedures clearly.	◆ A confused, agitated, or unrellable patient is at greater risk of injury (e.g., falling out of bed).

Contd...

Contd...

Problem	*R**	*Objective*	*Nursing interventions*	*Rationales*
			◆ Obtain feedback from family and friends regarding mental status, personality and behaviour.	
			◆ Plan for same staff members to care for the patient (if possible).	◆ This affords continuity of care, and facilitates very close monitoring of the patient's response to therapy.
			◆ Provide comfort measures: Oral hygiene, back care, gentle passive range of motion exercises.	◆ Relaxes tired muscles; a caring touch may help to relieve anxiety and apprehension.
			◆ Plan for undisturbed rest periods. ◆ Use calm, reassuring approach: Anticipate patient/family needs for support; be accessible; offer directions and explanations; allow patient/family to verbalize fears and concerns.	◆ All efforts should be directed towards keeping the patient relaxed and quiet to prevent bleeding or rebleeding.
			◆ Involve patient/family in decision-making process regarding care when possible.	◆ Enables patient/family to assume some control and responsibility for their well-being.
Nursing Diagnosis #8 Nutrition, alteration in, less than body requirements, related to: 1. Malnutrition associated with insufficient dietary protein intake. 2. Avitaminosis associated with impaired absorption of fat-soluble vitamins. 3. Vitamin B_{12} deficiency associated with liver disease. 4. Anorexia, nausea/vomiting, weakness and fatigue associated with elevated serum ammonia levels.	•	Patient will: 1. Maintain stable body weight within 5 per cent of baseline. 2. Maintain the following laboratory parameters within acceptable physiologic range: • Total serum protein; serum albumin. • Serum ammonia levels. • Serum cholesterol; fasting serum glucose. • Haematology profile. • Vitamin B_{12}, folate. • Transferrin levels. 3. Verbalize an increase in strength and improved appetite.	• Collaborate with nutritionist to perform comprehensive nutritional assessment. ◆ Assess the following parameters: Total serum protein; serum albumin; fasting serum glucose; serum cholesterol; haematology profile, vitamin B_{12}, folate; transferin levels; body weight (dry), height; skin-fold measurements. ◆ Assess for anorexia, nausea, vomiting, diarrhoea, dyspepsia.	• Assists in determining basic caloric requirements sufficient to meet the energy needs of the body, while limiting protein to that amount which the liver can effectively metabolize.
			• Implement nutritional plan: ◆ Acute phase (hepatic encephalopathy) dietary requirements include: – Restriction of protein, sodium and fluid.	• Goal of diet therapy is to reduce dietary protein so that a minimum of protein will remain in the gastrointestinal tract for conversion to ammonia.
			– Protein 20 to 60 gm/day.	◆ The degree of protein restriction will depend upon patient's level of consciousness and clinical status. – Except in advanced coma, it is seldom necessary to reduce daily protein intake to less than 20 gm. Further reduction of protein offers little benefit because of consequent catabolism of endogenous proteins.
			– Sodium 250 to 500 gm/day.	◆ Sodium restriction is necessary because of sodium and water retention associated with secondary hyperaldosteronism.
			– Fluids ~ 1000 ml/day.	◆ Degree of fluid restriction depends on degree of third-spacing (ascites and anasarca).
			◆ High carbohydrate intake.	◆ Glucose prevents hypoglycaemia and breakdown of energy reserves.
			◆ Vitamin supplementation: – Fat-soluble vitamins: A, D, E, and K.	◆ Hepatocellular dysfunction alters bilirubin metabolism and bile synthesis; inadequate bile secretion impairs absorption of fat, and fat-soluble vitamins.

Contd...

Problem	*R**	*Objective*	*Nursing interventions*	*Rationales*
			– Folate B_9 (parenterally).	♦ Hepatic stores depleted in liver disease.
			– Vitamin B_{12} (parenterally). – Thiamine (vitamin B_1) (parenterally). ♦ Minerals and trace elements supplementation (refer to Table 53-13). ♦ Methods of dietary intake: ♦ Oral: Provide mouth care; pleasant environment; assist to comfortable position. – Minimize nausea/vomiting; eliminate noxious stimuli.	♦ Used to correct anorexia, and neuritis associated with alcoholism (Wernicke-Korsakoff's syndrome).
			– Offer frequent smaller meals; avoid fatigue; plan rest period prior to meal-time. – Consider patient's preference for food choices. – Encourage visit by family at meal times if patient desires so.	♦ Large meals may precipitate nausea.
			♦ Enteral feedings.	♦ Enteral approach to feeding may be necessary for patients unable to ingest food normally; bleeding varices necessitate enteral feedings.
			– Assess gag reflex prior to feeding. – Confirm tube placement in stomach prior to feeding. – Assess for signs of gastrointestinal intolerance of feeding (e.g., nausea, vomiting, abdominal distention, hyperactive bowel sounds).	♦ To avoid pulmonary aspiration.
			♦ Total parenteral nutrition. – Provides for nutritional needs including: Hypertonic glucose.	♦ If adequate intake of nutrients is impossible via oral or enteral feedings, total parenteral nutrition may be indicated.
			– Amino acids; high concentration branched chain amino acids; low concentration aromatic amino acids. – Electrolytes; minerals, vitamins, trace elements; lipid therapy (when indicated).	♦ Amino acid imbalance may predispose to synthesis of false neurotransmitters that may be responsible for neurologic changes seen in hepatic encephalopathy. Aromatic amino acids are precursors to false neurotransmitters (e.g., octopamine).
			♦ Document: Type of feeding, amount; how tolerated by patient; adverse effects, if any. ♦ Monitor: Weight, intake and output; laboratory data (see "Assess the following paramters" under nursing interventions at the beginning of Nursing Diagnosis #8).	
Nursing Diagnosis #9 Tissue perfusion, alteration in, hepatorenal syndrome, related to: 1. Hypovolaemia associated with ascites (third-spacing).		Patient will: 1. Maintain adequate haemodynamics: • Systemic arterial blood pressure within 10 mmHg of baseline. 2. Maintain adequate renal function:	• Assess for signs and symptoms of hepa-torenal syndrome: ♦ Specific features: Oliguria (urine output < 30 ml/hr); azotemia; specific gravity > 1.015; low urinary sodium; increasing ascites; peripheral oedema; weight gain; rising BUN, serum creatinine; hyperphosphatemia; hyperkalemia.	• Hepatorenal syndrome describes development of progressive functional renal failure in the setting of advanced liver disease.

Contd...

Contd...

Problem	*R**	*Objective*	*Nursing interventions*	*Rationales*
2. Renal arteriolar vasoconstriction.		• Urine output > 30 ml/hour. • Urine specific gravity: 1.010-1.025. • BUN, serum creatinine, urinary sodium within acceptable range. 3. Maintain body weight within 5 per cent of baseline.	• Implement prescribed measures to re-establish normovolaemia: ◆ Specific measures: Restrict fluids and sodium; administer prescribed diuretic therapy and potassium replacement therapy; administer inotropic agent/vasopressor (e.g., low-dose dopamine); administer protein supplementation. ◆ Assist with abdominal paracentesis (if indicated). • Monitor patient's response to therapy. • Prepare for dialysis if indicated.	
Nursing Diagnosis#10 Injury, potential for, bleeding diathesis, related to: 1. Massive blood transfusion for treatment of bleeding varices (dilutional coagulopathy). 2. Decreased synthesis of clotting factors related to impaired hepatocellular function, and impaired vitamin K absorption. 3. Thrombocytopeina associated with splenomegaly (portal hypertension).		Patient will: 1. Maintain stable vital signs: • Systemic arterial pressure within 10 mmHg of baseline. • Heart rate (resting) < 100 beats/min. • Respiratory < 25-30/min. 2. Maintain baseline mental status: • Level of consciousness; mentation intact. 3. Maintain stable haematologic profile: • Haematocrit; haemoglobin, platelets. 4. Maintain stable coagulation profile.	• Assess for signs/symptoms of bleeding: ◆ Vital signs: Blood pressure (orthostatic), heart rate, peripheral pulses; respiratory rate. ◆ Physical signs: petechiac, ecchymosis; gingival bleeding; epistaxis; haematemesis, melena, hematochezia expanding aboaominal girth; unusual joint swelling; haematuria; oozing from wounds, venipuncture and invasive sites. ◆ Neurological signs: Headache, dizziness, confusion, lethargy; deep tendon reflexes. ◆ Haematologic profile: Haematocrit, haemoglobin, platelet count. ◆ Coagulation profile: Prothrombin time; activated partial thromboplastin time; platelet count; bleeding time. • Implement measures to prevent or minimize bleeding:	• Increased risk of bleeding in hepatic failure is associated with reduced hepatocellular synthesis of clotting factors (including vitamin K dependent factors II, VII, IX, X) and reduced inactivation of activated clotting factors. ◆ In the setting of profuse bleeding with massive blood transfusions, bleeding may be associated with dilutional coagulation.
		5. Remain without signs of bleeding: • No petechiae, ecchymosis. • No haematuria; no occult blood in stool, vomitus, gastric drainage. • No unusual joint pain/swelling. 6. Maintain stable abdominal girth.	◆ Specific measures: Use smallest gauge needle possible for venipuncture and subcutaneous injection. ◆ Avoid intramuscular injections; apply firm, prolonged pressure to venipuncture and injection sites. ◆ Avoid activities with the potential to cause bleeding: Avoid use of straight razor, use electric razor; avoid gingival bleeding associated with vigorous tooth brushing; pad bedrails for confused, restless or agitated patients; provide close supervision.	◆ Minimizes tissue trauma. ◆ There is a greater tendency to bleed with intramuscular injections.
			• Administer prescribed therapy to improve haemostasis. ◆ Vitamin K (parenterally).	◆ Necessary for synthesis of clotting factors A, D, E, K.
			◆ Bile salts.	◆ Necessary for absorption of vitamin K.
			◆ Administration of fresh, frozen plasma or packed red blood cells.	◆ Stored whole blood lacks some of the clotting factors; citrate, used as a blood preservative (anticoagulant) may not be metabolized by hepatocytes.

Contd...

Problem	*R**	*Objective*	*Nursing interventions*	*Rationales*
			• Consider the following if bleeding occurs: ◆ Apply firm, prolonged pressure to bleeding site if possible.	
			◆ Administer fluids and blood products as prescribed.	◆ To maintain haemodynamic parameters and haematologic profile within acceptable limits.
			◆ Administer prescribed oxygen therapy.	◆ Maximizes arterial blood oxygenation.
			◆ Maintain gastric decompression. ◆ Initiate iced gastric lavage (as prescribed).	◆ To determine presence of upper gastrointestinal bleeding, and the extent of bleeding.
			◆ Prepare to assist with insertion of Sengstaken-Blakemore tube; if tube is in place, assess its position, balloon inflation, and catheter patency.	◆ For specific nursing care considerations of patients with a Sengstaken-Blakemore tube.
			◆ Provide reassurance and support to patient and family.	◆ Profuse haemorrhage can be a frightening experience for patient and family.
			◆ Monitor vital signs, neurological status, hourly urine output.	
Nursing Diagnosis#11				
Skin integrity, impairment of, potential, related to: 1. Increased skin fragility associated with generalized oedema (anasarca and ascites). 2. Malnutrition. 3. Immobility associated with stupor and oedema. 4. Pruritus associated with hyperbilirubinaemia.		Patient will: 1. Maintain skin intact, no breaks, lesions, irritation or infection; good skin turgor.	• Assess skin, especially reddened areas over bony prominences where skin is thin. ◆ Assess generalized oedema, especially dependent areas (e.g., sacrum, extremities). • Initiate measures to prevent skin breakdown. ◆ Mobilize extracellular fluid accumulation, especially in dependent areas. – Turn patient at least every 2 hours; administer backrubs.	◆ Promotes circulation and relieves muscle tension; helps to prevent decubiti.
			◆ Provide supportive measures and pressure-relief device: – Utilize alternating pressure or egg carton mattress; provide sheepskin; change linen frequently.	– If reddened areas at pressure points do not blanch within less than 30 minutes, avoid using the position except for shorter periods at less frequent intervals.
			◆ Keep skin well lubricated. If pruritus is present, apply calamine lotion with 1% phenol, or use cholestyramine or cool baking soda bath (as prescribed).	
			◆ Assist with range of motion exercises. Handle limbs gently. Apply support stockings.	◆ Exercise promotes circulation and prevents venostasis, a contributing factor to the development of a coagulopathy (e.g., disseminated intravascular coagulation, DIC).
			◆ Assist with personal hygiene. – Provide oral hygiene frequently, especially when a nasogastric tube or Sengsaken. Blakemore tube is in place. – Provide perineal care, keeping buttacks clean and dry restrich use of soap. Keep nails trimmed and clean. – Instruct patient to apply firm pressure over pruritic areas rather than scratching.	◆ To minimize trauma from scratching. Patient may need gloves or mittens at night while asleep.

Contd...

Contd...

Problem	*R**	*Objective*	*Nursing interventions*	*Rationales*
Nursing Disgnosis#12 Self concept, disturbance in, related to: 1. Altered physical appearance associated with jaundice, ascites, alopecia, gynecomastia, and other changes associated with chronic liver disease.		Patient will: 1. Express feelings about self. 2. Participate in decision-making process regarding care. 3. Initiate self-care activities.	• Establish a trusting rapport and working relationship: ◆ Spend time to get to know patient. ◆ Explain all procedures simply and clearly. ◆ Allow patient participation in procedures whenever possible. ◆ Encourage patient to participate in decision-making process whenever appropriate. – Assess readiness for decision-making. ◆ Encoruage patient to talk about the illness and how it impacts on self, family and others. – Explain that jaundice, oedema, and ascites are usually temporary. ◆ Help patient to identify strengths, weaknesses, and coping capabilities. – Utilize time during direct patient care to involve patient in discussion of needs, priorities, and how to cope. Encourage patient to ventilate feelings; provide listening car and "sounding board." ◆ Call attention to areas of improvement in the patient's condition. ◆ Offer immediate praise and feedback for patient's accomplishments no matter how small.	• It is important to encourage/assist the patient to verbalize concerns, to acknowledge and cope with the illness, and to achieve independence in self-care. ◆ Emphasis is focused on assisting the patient/family to get in touch with their feelings, to identify them, and to begin to deal with them. ◆ It is important to assist the patient to acknowledge his/her perceptions, and how they differ from those of others, or from the actual situation. ◆ Praise helps to build self-confidence.
Nursing Diagnosis#13 Grieving, dysfunctional, related to: 1. End-stage liver disease. 2. Altered appearance and lifestyle associated with chronic liver disease.		Patient will: 1. Verbalize feelings about liver disease and how it impacts on patient/family. 2. Demonstrate progress in dealing with stages of grieving at own pace. 3. Participate in self-care activities and in decision-making process regarding care.	• Assess patient's perception of liver disease and how it impacts on patient/family lifestyle. • Identify the stage of grief being experienced by patient/family. ◆ Assist patient/family to acknowledge that grieving is a process and experiencing the stages of grief is most appropriate and necessary. – Assist patient to acknowledge bodily changes and consequent changes in lifestyle so that the process of grieving can begin. • Assist patient/family to develop a plan for discharge and follow-up care. ◆ Be honest and forthright in discussing disease and its ramifications both with patient and family. ◆ Help patient and family to identify resources. – Assist with referrals to counseling services and support groups.	• Stages of grief include denial, anger, bargaining, depression, and acceptance. ◆ The nurse must be aware that not every stage is experienced or expressed by each individual; and some individuals will remain in one stage longer than others. In chronic disease, the grief may recur.

PROCEDURE 8.1: **ASSISTING WITH ABDOMINAL PARACENTESIS*

Equipment:

Sterile paracentesis tray and gloves.	Collection bottle (vaccum bottle)
Local anaesthetic	Skin preparation tray with antiseptic.
Drape or cotton blankets	Specimen bottles and laboratory forms.

STEPS OF PROCEDURE

Nursing action	*Rationale*
Preparatory Phase	
1. Explain procedure to the patient.	1. This may reduce the patient's fear and anxiety.
2. Record the patient's vital signs.	2. Provides baseline values for later comparison.
3. Have the patient void before treatment is begun. See that consent form has been signed.	3. This will lessen the danger of accidentally piercing the bladder with the needle or trocar.
4. Keep the patient in Fowler's position with back, arms, and feet supported (sitting on the side of the bed is a frequently used position).	4. The patient is more comfortable and a steady position can be maintained.
5. Drape the patient with sheet exposing abdomen.	5. Minimizes exposure of patient and keeps patient warm.
Performance Phase	
1. Assist in preparing skin with antiseptic solution.	1. This is considered a minor surgical procedure, requiring aseptic precautions.
2. Open sterile tray and package of sterile gloves; provide anaesthetic solution.	
3. Have collection bottle and tubing available.	
4. Assess pulse and respiratory status frequently during procedure; watch for pallor, cyanosis, or syncope (faintness).	4. Preliminary indications of shock must be watched for keeping emergency drugs available.
5. Physician administers local anaesthesia and introduces needle or trocar.	
6. Needle or trocar is connected to tubing and vaccum bottle or syringe, fluid is slowly drained from peritoneal cavity.	6. Drainage is usually limited to 1-2L to relieve acute symptoms and minimize risk of hypovo-laemia and shock.
7. Apply dressing when needle is withdrawn.	7. Elasticized adhesive patch is effective, serving as waterproof adhering dressing.
Follow-up Phase	
1. Assist the patient to a comfortable position after treatment.	
2. Record amount and characteristics of fluid removed, number of specimens sent to laboratory, the patient's condition during treatment.	
3. Check blood pressure and vital signs every half an hour for 2 hours, every hour for 4 hours, and every 4 hours for 24 hours.	3. Close observation will detect poor circulatory adjustment and possible development of shock.

Contd...

Nursing action	*Rationale*
4. Usually, a dressing is sufficient, however, if the trocar wound appears large, the physician may close the incision with sutures.	
5. Watch for leakage or scrotal oedema after paracentesis.	5. If seen, report at once.

PROCEDURE 8.2: **USING BALLOON TEMPONADE TO CONTROL OESOPHAGEAL BLEEDING (Sengstaken-Blakemore tube method, Minnesota tube method).*

Oesophageal balloon (Sengstaken-Blackmore or Minnesota).	Glass of water and straw.
Basin with cracked ice.	Adhesive tape.
Clamps for tubing.	device to apply traction (eg. foot-ball helmet).
Water soluble lubricant.	Large scissors (for emergency deflation).
Syringe (50 ml with catheter tip).	Manometer (to measure balloon pressure).
Towel and emesis basin.	

STEPS OF PROCEDURE

Preparatory Phase

1. Provide support and reassure the patient that this procedure will help to control bleeding.
2. Explain procedure to the patient and explain how breathing through the mouth and swallowing can help in passing the tube (See accompanying figure).
3. Elevate head of bed slightly unless the patient is in shock.

Oesophageal varices and their treatment by a compressing balloon tube (Sengstaken-Blakemore). (A) Dilated veins of the lower oesophagus. (B) The tube is in place in the stomach and the lower oesophagus but is not inflated. (C) Inflation of the tube causing compression of the veins. It may be necessary to pass an additional tube through the other nostril to aspirate.

Note: The Minnesota fourlumen oesophagogastric tamponade tube has an additional outlet for aspiration of the oesophagus.

Nursing action	*Rationale*
Preparatory Phase	
1. Check balloons by trial inflation to detect leaks.	1. This is best done under water because it is easier to see escaping air bubbles.
2. Chill the tube, then lubricate it before the physician passes it via mouth or nose (preferable).	2. Chilling makes the tube more firm and lubrication lessens friction.
3. Provide the patient with a few sips of water.	3. This will help pass the tube more easily.
4. After the tube has entered the stomach, verify its placement by irrigating the gastric tube with air while auscultating over the stomach.	4. It is imperative to be certain that the tube is in the stomach so that the gastric tube is not treated in the oesophagus.

Contd...

Contd...

Nursing action	Rationale
5. After obtaining an X-ray film of the lower chest and upper abdomen to verify placement in the stomach, inflate gastric balloon (200-250 ml) with air and gently pull tube back to seat balloon against gastro-oesophageal junction.	5. This is to exert force against the cardia.

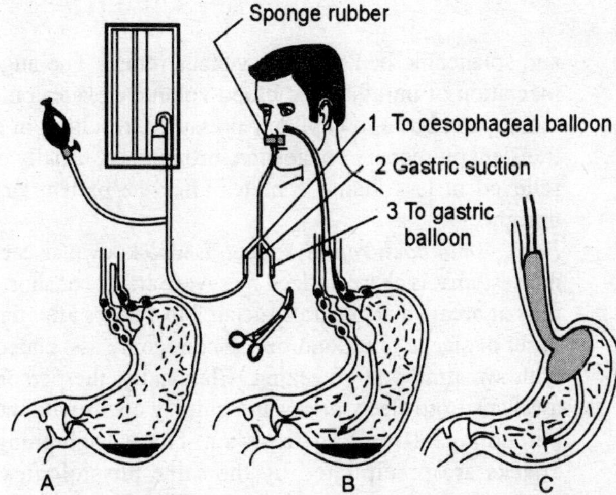

Fig.8.1: Oesophageal varices and their treatment by a compressing balloon tube (Sengstaken-Blakemore). (A) Dilated veins of the lower oesophagus. (B) The tube is in place in the stomach and the lower oesophagus but is not inflated. (C) Inflation of the tube causing compression of the veins. It may be necessary to pass an additional tube through the other nostril to aspirate. Note: The Minnesota four-lumen oesophagogastric tamponade tube has an additional outlet for aspiration of the oesophagus.

Nursing action	Rationale
6. Clamp gastric balloon, mark tube locatioan at nares.	6. This prevents air leakage and tube migration. The mark on the tube allows for easy visualization of movement of the tube.
7. Apply gentle traction to the balloon tube and secure it with a foam rubber cube at the nares or tape it to the faceguard of a football helmet.	7. This prevents the tube from migrating with peristalsis and assists in exerting proper pressure.
8. Attach Y connector to oesophageal balloon opening attach syringe to one arm of the Y connector and manometer to the other. Inflatc oesophageal balloon to 25-35 mm Hg. Clamp oesophageal balloon.	8. Maintains enough pressure to temponade bleeding while preventing oesophageal necrosis.

Contd...

Contd...

Nursing action	Rationale
9. Apply suction to gastric aspiration opening irrigate at least hourly.	9. Suctioning and irrigating the tube can remove old blood from the stomach and prevent hepatic encephalopathy allows, monitoring of bleeding status.
10. (If using Sengstaken-Blakemore tube). Insert a nasogastric tube, positioning it above the oesophageal balloon and attach to suction. (If using a Minnesota tube) Attach fourth port, oesophageal suction port, to suction.	10. To Suction saliva accumulated above the oesophageal balloon, which may be aspirated, and to check for bleeding above the oesophageal balloon.
11. Label each port.	11. To prevent accidental deflation or irrigation.
12. Tape scissors to hcad of bed.	12. Airway occlusion may occur if the oesophageal balloon is pulled into the hypopharynx. If this occurs, the oesophageal balloon tube must be cut and removed immediately.

Nursing Responsibilities

1. Maintain constant vigilance while balloons are inflated in the patient.
2. Keep balloon pressures at required level to control bleeding. (Clamp help to maintain pressure).
3. Observe and record vital signs, monitor colour and amount of nasogastric lavage fluid (Subtracting lavage input) for evidence of bleeding.
4. Be alert for chest pain—may indicate injury or rupture of oesophagus.
5. Irrigate suction tube as prescribed, observe and record nature and colour of aspirated material.
6. Keep head of bed elevated to avoid gastric regurgitation and to diminish nausea and a sensation of gagging.
7. Maintain nutritional and electrolyte levels parenterally.
8. Maintain nasogastric suction or suction to oesophageal suction port to aspirate any collected saliva.
9. Note nature of breathing; if counterweight pulls the tube into oropharynx, the patient may be asphyxiated.

Nursing Focus

Keep a pair of scissors laped to the head of the bed in the event of acute respiratory distress, use the scissors to cut across tubing (to deflate both balloons) and remove tubing.

Note: This procedure should be reserved for patients who are known, without a doubt, to be bleeding from oesophageal varices and in whom all forms of concervative therapy have failed.

Cardiovascular Nursing

CARDIOVASCULAR ASSESSMENT

Systematic cardiovascular assessment provides the nurse with baseline data useful in identifying the physiological and psychosocial needs of the patient and for planning appropriate nursing interventions to meet these needs.

A careful history and physical examination should help the nurse in differentiating symptoms that reflect a cardiovascular problem from problems of other body systems. Many illnesses affect the cardiovascular system directly or indirectly. The patient should be questioned about a history of chest pain, shortness of breath, alcoholism, or excessive drinking, anaemia, rheumatic fever, streptococcal sore throat, congenital heart disease, stroke, syncope, hypertension, thrombophlebitis, intermittent claudications, varicositis and oedema.

The classic symptoms of heart disease include dyspnoea, chest pain, or discomfort, oedema, syncope, palpitations and excessive fatigue. Cardiovascular function, which may be adequate at rest may be insufficient during exercise or exertion. Therefore, careful attention is directed to the effect of activity on the patient's symptoms.

i. Dyspnoea

Dyspnoea is an abnormally uncomfortable awareness of breathing, in which patient complains of shortness of breath. It is a subjective experience associated with anxiety and variety of disease processes.

- Exertional Dyspnoea: Dyspnoea on exertion is a common symptom of cardiac dysfunctions. In the early stages of heart failure, dyspnoea usually is provoked only by effort and is relieved promptly by rest. It is important to identify the amount of exertion necessary to produce dyspnoea, because the lower the cardiac reserve (heart's ability to adjust and adapt to increased demands), lesser the effort is required to precipitate dyspnoea.
- Orthopnoea refers to dyspnoea in the recumbent position. It is usually a symptom of more advanced heart failure that is exertional dyspnoea. Patients insist that they require two or more pillows to sleep restfully. When the person assumes the recumbent position, gravitational forces redistribute blood from the lowest extremities and splanchnic bed increase venous return. The augmentation of intrathoracic blood volume elevates pulmonary venous and capillary pressures, resulting in a transient pulmonary congestion, orthopnoea, usually is relieved in less than 5 minutes after the patient sits upright.
- *Paraxysmal nocturnal dyspnoea* is also known as cardiac asthma, is characterized by severe attacks of shortness of breath that generally occur 2 to 5 hours after the onset of sleep. This condition is commonly associated with sweating and wheezing. Classically, the person awakens from sleep, arises and quickly opens with the perception of needing fresh air. These frightening attacks are precipitated by the same physiological mechanism that causes orthopnoea. The diseased heart is unable to compensate for this increase in blood volume by pumping extra fluid into the circulatory system and pulmonary congestion results. Paraxysmal nocturnal dyspnoea is relieved by sitting on the side of the bed or getting out of the bed. For relief of dyspnoea, 20 minutes or more is needed. The cues to dyspnoea are air hunger, especially after exertion, pillows or upright chair necessary for sleep.

ii. Chest Pain

Although pain or discomfort in the chest is one of the cardinal symptoms of cardiac disorder, chest pain can be precipitated by various conditions. For example, chest pain may be caused by anxiety, ischemia, heart disease, acute dissection of the aorta, acute pericardia, pulmonary disorders, (pleurisy and pul-embolism) oesophageal spasm, or reflux, and peptic ulcer disease. The cues for chest pain-related heart disorders are indigestion, burning, numbness, tightness or pressure in midchest, epigastric or substernal pain, radiating to shoulder, neck, and arms.

iii. Syncope

Syncope is dyspnoea as a generalized muscle weakness with an inability to stand upright, accompanied by loss of consciousness. The most common cause of syncope is decreased perfusion to the brain. Any condition that results in a sudden reduction of Cardiac output (CO) and therefore reduced cerebral blood flow could potentially cause a syncopal episode. In patients with cardiovascular disorders, conditions such as orthostatic hypotension, hypovolaemia, or variety of dysrhythmias may precipitate syncope.

iv. Palpitation

Palpitation is a common subjective phenomenon defined as an unpleasant awareness of the irregular heart beat. It may be precipitated by a change in cardiac rate or rhythm i.e., by an increase in myocardial contractivity. Patient may experience sensation of heart in throat or skipped beat, racing heart, and dizziness. Patients may describe that heart beat as "pounding", "racing" or skipping. Palpitation that occurs either during or after strenuous activity are considered physiological. Palpitations that occur during mild exertion may suggest the presence of heart failure, anaemia or thyrotoxicosis. Other non-cardiac factors may precipitate palpitation include, nervousness, heavy meals, lack of sleep and a large intake of Caffene-containing beverage, alcohol or tobacco.

v. Fatigue

Fatigue refers to no energy, needs more rest than usual, normal activities result in tiring. Fatigue and lassitude have many causes, but it has direct consequence of heart failure. The exact physiological mechanism is not known. But probably, it is a consequence of an inadequate cardiac output. Such fatigue can occur during effort or at rest and generally worsens as the day progresses. Fatigue that occurs after mild exertion may indicate a low cardiac reserve if the heart is unable to meet even small increase in metabolic demand.

vi. Dizzy

Dizzy, light headedness: Dizzy with change of position; woozy, unstable and week.

vii. Oedema (fluid retention)

The cues for oedema are: Weight gain, bloated feeling, swelling, tightening of clothing, shoes no longer fitting comfortably, marks or identification left from constricting garments.

viii. Tenderness in Calf of Legs

The cues for tenderness of calf of legs are–inability to bear weight, swelling of the involved extremity; inflamed warm skin over vein; distended, discoloured, tortuous veins in calves of legs, ache in lower extremities after standing for short periods.

PHYSICAL EXAMINATION

Physical examination of the CVS includes the standard assessment techniques of inspection, palpation, percussion and auscultations.

1. Inspection

Inspection of the patient includes skin colour, neck vein distension, respiration, pulsations and clubbing and capillary refill.

The inspection of the *skin colour*, hair distribution and venous blood flow provide information about arterial blood flow. A person's normal colour depends on race, ethnic background and lifestyle and is an indication of adequate cardiac output (CO) and circulation. Pallor may indicate anaemia, hypoxia, or peripheral vasoconstriction. Cyanosis (cerebral), a bluish discoloration of the skin is most easily observed by examining the earlobes, the oral mucosa at the base of the tongue, legs and the nailbeds. Peripheral cyanosis results from low CO and generally is accompanied by decreased skin temperature and mottling. In contrast to central cyanosis, no cyanosis of the tongue is present. Central cyanosis is caused by low arsenal oxygen saturation, (ex. congenital heart defects). Skin colour and the extremities also be assessed for noting any erythema or pigmentation changes as well as the shiny, or dry, scaly skin, which may indicate vascular disorders.

A general estimate of *venous pressure* can be obtained by observation of the neck veins. Normally, when a person is supine, the neck veins are distended. However, when the head of the bed is elevated to a 45 degree angle, the neck veins are collapsed. If jugular distention is present, assess the jugular venous pressure by measuring from the highest point of visible distention to the sternal angle. Measurements above 3 cms area considered elevated. The Jugular veins reflect venous tone, blood volume and right atrial pressure. Therefore, distended neck veins suggest increased venous pressure, which may be caused by right-sided heart failure, circulatory volume load, superior venacaval obstructions or tricuspid valve regurgitation.

The rate and character of the patients' respirations are important to assess. Normally an adult breathes comfortably at a rate of 12 to 20 times per minute. Particular attention is paid to the case of difficulty in breathing and patient's general demeanour.

Inspection of the anterior chest is best accomplished with the patient lying supins, either flat or with the head slightly elevated. Observe the pericardium for the apical inpulse, which is a *pulsation* of the chest wall caused by the forward thrustings of the left ventricle during systole. When visible, the apical impulse occupies the fourth or fifth intercostal space at or inside midclavicular line. The apical impulse was formerly known as the point of maximal impulse. The apical inpulse is not always visible, but it is palpable in about half of adults.

The nails are assessed for clubbing and capillary refill. The exact cause is unknown. However, clubbing of the finger in the fistulas with right to left shunting. Capillary filling or blanching (whitening) is an indicator of peripheral circulation to the fingers and toes and can be tested in all nailbeds. The examiner presses a thumbnail against the edge of a patient's finger nails or toe nail and quickly releases it and notes the blanching resposne and observes for the returning colour within three seconds.

2. Palpations

Palpations of the pulses in the neck and extremities also provides information on arterial blood flow. One method of evaluating arterial flow of the vascular system is to palpate the extremities simultaneously to determine skin temperature. A second method is to palpate the peripheral pulses, which are evaluated bilaterally on the basis of their absence or presence, rate, rhythm, amplitude, quality and equality. Each pulse, except the carotids should be palpated on the left and right sides simultaneously to evaluate the contralateral symmetry.

A scale may be used to document pulse volume or amplitude by rating on a scale of 0 to +4 as follows:

0 = Absent
+ = Palpable, but diminished
++ = Normal or average
+++ = Full and risk
++++ = Full and bounding, often visible.

Several abnormalities may be detected during palpation of pulses.

- A *hypokinetic* (weak) pulse signifies a narrowed pulse pressure, that is decreased differences between systolic and diastolic pressure. It is usually produced by a low CO and is associated with often detected in such conditions as severe LVF, hypovolaemia, or mitral and aortic valve stenosis.
- A *hyperkinetic* (Bounding) pulse represents a widened pulse pressure. It is usually associated with increased left ventricular stroke volume and a decreased peripheral vascular resistance. This is found in hyperkinetic circulatory state caused by exercise, fever, anaemia or hyperthyroidism.
- *Pulsus alternans* is a condition in which the heart beats regularly, but the pulses vary in amplitude. It is caused by an alternating left ventricular contractile force and usually indicates severe depression of myocardial infarction, pulsus alternans can be detected by palpation and accurately by auscultation.
- *Pulsus paradoxus* signifies a reduction in the amplitude of the arterial pulse during inspiration. Variation in pulse strength can be palpated and also readily detected by sphygmomanometry. Pulsus paradoxus is a result of decreased left ventricular stroke volume and the transmission of negative intrathoracic pressure to the aorta. It may occur in conditions such as cardiac temponade and constrictive pericarditis and also COPD.

Oedema is defined as an accumulation of fluid in the interstitial spaces. It may be localized to one particular body part, organ or tissue or that may be generalized distribution. An important indicator for card ovascular function in the presence of absence of peripheral oedema, especially in the feet, ankles, legs and the sacrum. This is caused by gravity flow or by interruption of the venous return to the heart as a result of constricting clothing or pressure on the veins of the lower extremities. Oedema often disappear on elevation of the body part. In contrast, pitting oedema does not disappeear with elevation of the extremity of body part, and it may indicate fluid overload or pathological condition (Eg. congestive heart failure). Pitting oedema is present if an indication is left in the skin after a thumb or finger has been used to apply gentle pressure.

3. Percussion

The borders of the right and left sides of the heart can be estimated by percussion. The use of percussion for detecting cardiac enlargement generally has been replaced by chest X-Ray which is much more accurate. The nurse stands to the right of the recumbent patient and percusses along the curve of the rib in the fourth and the fifth intercostal spaces (ICS), starting at the midaxillary line. The percussion note over the heart is dull in comparison with the resonance over the lung and is recorded in relation to midclavicular line. Cardiac dullness is the characteristics of cardiac hypertrophy.

4. Auscultation

The movement of the cardiac valves creates some turbulence in the blood flow. The vibration of the blood causes normal heart sounds. These sounds can be heard through a stethoscope placed on the chest wall. The first heart sound (S_1) which is associated with the closure of the tricuspid and mitral valve (AV) has a soft "lubb" sound. S_1 is longer and lower pitched than the second heart sound (S_2). The second heart sound (S_2) which is associated with the closure of the aortic and pulmonic (semilunar) valve, has a sharp "dubb" sound. The first and second heart sounds together are referred to as "lub-dub". S_1 corresponds to the beat of the carotid pulse. As stated earlier S_2 is caused mainly by the closure of the semilunar valves. S_2 is usually loudest at the base of the heart and is described as shorter, higher pitched and "snappier" than S_1. S_1 signals the beginning of systole, S_2 signals the beginning of diastole. The nurse should listen to the auscultatory areas in sequence with both the diaphragm and bell of the stethoscope.

The first and second heart sounds are heard best with diaphragm of the stethoscope because they are high-pitched. Extra heart sounds (S_3 or S_4) if present, are heard best with the bell of the stethoscope because they are low-pitched. The nurse listens at the apical area with diaphragm of the stethoscope while simultaneously palpating the radial pulse. If fewer radial than apical pulse are counted, a pulse deficit is present. A patient with a pulse deficit should have the apical and radial pulse taken often to monitor this abnormality. A judgement about the rhythm (regular or irregular) is also made when listening at the apex.

Normally no sounds are heard between S_1 and S_2 during the periods of systole and diastole. Sounds that are heard during these periods probably represent abnormalities and should be described. An exception to this is normal splitting of S_2, which is best heard at the pulmonic area during inspiration. Splitting of this heart sound can be abnormal if S_1 is heard during expiration or if it is constant (fixed) during the respiratory cycle.

If an abnormal sound is heard, it should be documented. This description should include the timing (during systole or diastole), location (the site on the chest where it is heard the loudest), pitch (heard best with the diaphragm or bell of the stethoscope), position (heard best when the patient is recumbent, sitting, leaning forward, or in the left lateral cubitus position). Characteristic (harsh, musical, soft, short, long) and any abnormal findings (irregular cardiac rhythms or palpable chest wall heaves) associated with sound.

The abnormal sound, occurring during diastole and systole are classified as either murmurs or extra sound (S_3 and S_4). Murmurs are sounds produced by turbulent blood flow through the heart or the walls of large arteries. Most murmurs are the result of cardiac abnormalities, but some occur in normal cardiac structures. Murmurs are graded on six point scale of loudness and recorded as Roman numeral ratio, the numerator is intensity of the murmur and denominator is always VI which indicates the six point scale sued.

DIAGNOSTIC STUDIES OF CVS

A number of diagnostic procedures add to the information obtained from the history and physical examination of the cardiovascular system. These procedures are usually classified as noninvasive or invasive. If only needle insertion for withdrawal of blood or injection of dye is used these studies are usually considered noninvasive. Catheter insertion for angiography is considered as invasive procedure. Certain responsibilities of the nurse remains the same regardless of whether patient is to undergo invasive or noninvasive procedure. First, the nurse must see that the procedure is scheduled and that any necessary preliminaries (e.g. special diets or changes in medication) are completed. Appropriate safety measures, such as the use of bedside rails after administration of preprocedure medicatioan or identification of patient allergies should be instituted. Comfort measures such as oral care before procedure are important. The nurse must also check to see to it that in obtaining consent the procedure should be explained skillfully, relieving the anxiety of patrents and significant ones of the patient. These are the most common diagnostic measures to be carried out by nurses to assess the cardiovascular system and main nursing responsibility required for the same is presented as follows:

1. Chest X-ray

A radiograph of the chest may be taken to determine overall size and configuration of the heart in which patient is placed in two upright positions to examine the lung fields and size of the heart. The two common positions are anterior/posterior (AP) and left lateral. Normal heart size and contour for the individual age, sex and size are noted. Most abnormalities of heart size and calcification of the heart muscle, valves and great vessels can be detected with a standard posterior anterior and lateral view of the chest.

The nursing responsibilities incldue inquiring about the frequency of recent X-Rays and possibility of pregnancy (of female). Provide lead shielding to the areas not being viewed, remove any jewellery or metal objects that may obstruct the view of the heart and lungs.

2. Cardiac Fluoroscopy

It facilitates the observation of the heart from varying view while the heart is in motion. Fluoroscopy can be used to detect ventricular aneurysms, monitor prosthetic valve movement, or assess the position of cardiac calcification during the cardiac cycle. Because of the radiational risk associated with fluoroscopy, most of them are not used in this procedure. Nursing responsibility is the same as for Chest-X-Rays.

3. Electrocardiogram (ECG)

The ECG is a graphic representation of the electrical forces produced within the heart. The ECG is an essential tool for cardiac evaluation, but it must be combined with other data sources for an accurate diagnosis. An ECG may be normal even in the presence of heart disease. Conversely, abnormal variance may be seen in the ECG of a normal heart. The ECG may be used for a variety of diagnostic purposes as given below.

- Tachycardia, bradycadia, dysrhythmia.
- Sudden onset of dyspnoea.
- Pain occurring in the upper portion of the trunk and in the extremities.
- Syncopical episodes.
- Shock state or coma.
- Preoperative status.
- Postoperative hypertention.
- Hypertension, murmurs, or cardiomegaly.
- Artificial pacemaker function.

In taking ECG, electrodes are placed on the chest and extremities, allowing the ECG machine to record cardiac electrical activity from differcnt views by using standard 12-lead ECG machine. ECG can detect rhythm of heart, site of pace maker, conduction abnormalities, position of the heart, size of atria and ventricles and presence of injury.

The nurse has to inform the patient step-by-step procedure and assures of its safe, painless nature and comfortability. Instruct the patient to avoid moving to decrease muscle motion artifact.

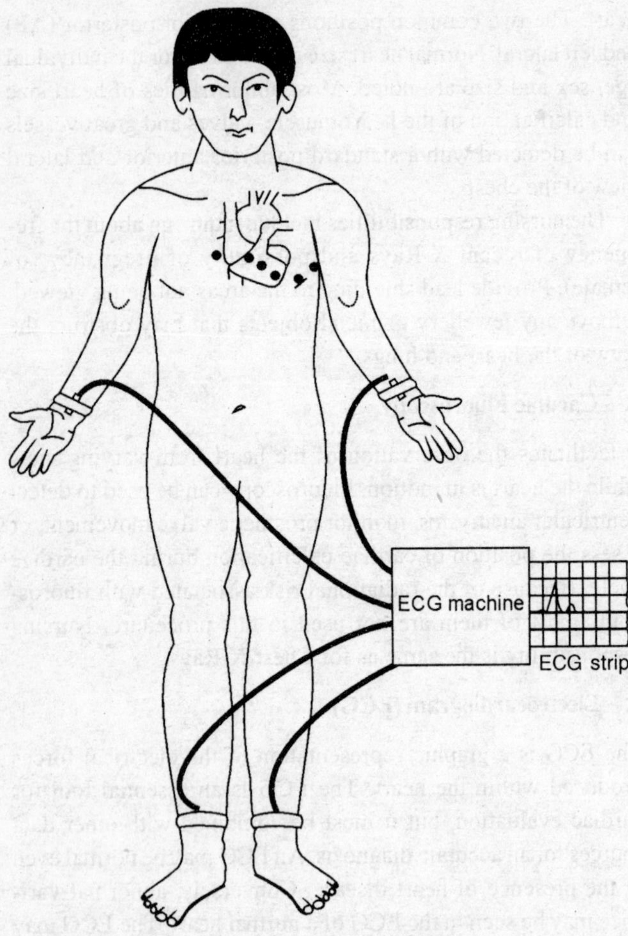

Fig.9.1: Transmission of heart's impulse to a graphic display by ECG machine. The electrodes that are capable of conducting electrical activity from the heart to the ECG machine are placed at strategic positions on the extremities and chest precordium.

4. Ambulatory ECG Monitoring

i. *Holter monitoring*

It is used to obtain a continuous graphic tracing of patient's ECG during daily activities, in which recording of ECG rhythm for 24-48 hours and then correlating rhythm changes with symptoms recorded in diary. Normal patient activity is encouraged to stimulate conditions that produce symptoms. Electrodes are placed on chest and a recorder is used to store information until it is recalled, printed, and analysed for any rhythm disturbance. It can be performed on an inpatient or outpatient basis.

In this procedure, nurse has to prepare skin and apply electrodes as leads. Explain importance of keeping an accurate diary of activities and symptoms. Tell the patient that no bath or shower can be taken during monitoring. Skin irritations may develop from electrodes. Take care of it.

ii. *Stress testing (ECG during exercise)*

It may be performed for a variety of reasons and often combined with ECG to obtain additional information about heart functions. Indications for performing a stress test are:

- Evaluation of the patient with symptoms suggestive of coronary artery disease.
- Determination of the patient's physical work capacity and aerobic capacity.
- Determination of the patient's functional capacity after a myocardial infarction and as an aid in planning and exercise rehabilitation program.
- Evaluation of the exercise-induced dysrhythmias.
- Evaluation of the symtom-free person older than 40 years of age who is at risk for coronary artery disease.
- Evaluation of pharmacological intervention for dysrhythmias, angina or ischemia.

Various protocols are used to evaluate the effect of exercise tolerance on myocardial function. A common protocol uses 3 minutes, stages at speeds and elevation of the treatmill belt. Continued monitoring of vital signs and ECG rhythms or ischemic changes are important in the diagnosis of left ventricular function and coronary artery disease. An exercise bike may be used if the patient is unable to walk on the tread mill. Stress test is designed to progressively increasing myocardial oxygen demand. Some patient may experience untoward effects (ventricular tachycardia, change in systolic BP, chest pain, etc. So test may be terminated at any point of test.

Adequate preparation for stress testing is important. Although procedure is not painful. It can be fatiguing. Patient may become anxious because they will be exercising at a level that may produce symptoms such as dyspnoea, palpitations and chest pain. The nurse may review the purposes and method of stress testing and encourage the patient to do the following.

- Avoid coffee, tea and alcohol on the day of test.
- Avoid smoking and taking nitroglycerine during the 2 hours immediately before the test.
- Wear comfortable, loose-fitting clothes (women should be advised to wear a brassiere for support).
- Wear sturdy, comfortable walking shoes.
- Consult the physician about taking any medication before the test.

And the nurse should:

- Instruct the patient about procedure and application of lead placements.
- Monitor vital signs and obtain 12-lead ECG before exercise, during each stage of exercise, and after exercise until all vital signs and ECG changes have returned to normal.
- Monitor patient's symptoms throughout procedure.

iii. *Trans-telephonic event recorders*

Allow more freedom than regular Holter Monitor. It records rhythm disturbances that are not frequent enough to be recorded in a 24-hours period. Some units have electrodes that are attached to the chest and have a loop of memory that captures the onset and end of an event. Other types are placed directly on patient's wrist, chest, or fingers have no loop memory, but records the patient's ECG in real time. Recordings are transmitted over the phone to a receiving unit, and the recordings are printed out for review. Tracings can then be erased and the unit can be reused.

The nurse has to instruct the patient in the use of equipment for recording and transmitting transient events. Teach the patient about skin preparation for lead placement or steddy skin contact for units not requiring electrodes. This will ensure the reception of optimal ECG tracings for analysis.

5. Sonic Studies

i. *Echocardiogram (M-mode-two-dimensional)*
Echocardiography uses ultrasound to assess cardiac structure and mobility noninvasively. It is useful in the diagnosis of a variety of cardiac conditions as follows:

- Abnormal pericardial fluid.
- Vulvular disorders including prosthetic valves.
- Ventricular aneurysms.
- Cardiac chamber size.
- Stroke volume and cardiac outputs.
- Some myocardial abnormalities, such as idiopathic hypertrophic subaortic stensosis (IHSS).
- Wall motion abnormalities.

In this, a small transducer is placed on the chest of the patient at the level of third or fourth intercostal space near the left lower sternal border. The transducer transmits high frequency sound waves then receives these waves back from the patient as they are reflected from different structures. The ultrasonic beam that is reflected back from the patient's heart produces "echoes" that are viewed as lines and spaces on an oscilloscope. These lines and spaces represent bone, cardiac chambers and valves, the septum and the muscle. A copy of echocardiogram is recorded on paper.

Here, the nursing responsibility is to place the patient in supine position on left side facing equipment. Instruct patient and family about procedure and sensations (pressure and mechanical movement from head of transducer). No contraindication to procedure exists.

ii. *Stress echocardiogram*
It is the combination of exercise, treadmill test and echocardiogram. Resting images of the heart are taken with ultrasound and then the patient exercises. Postexercise images are taken immediately after exercise (which 1 minute of stopping exercises). Differences in left ventricular wall motion and thickening before and after exercise is evaluated. Here the nurse has to instruct and prepare patient for exercise tread mill. Make the patient aware that ultrasound is not harmful and the importance of speed in returning to examination table for imaging after exercise. Contraindication includes any patient unable to reach peak exercise. Take precautions.

iii. *Dobutamine echocardiogram*
It is used as a substitute for the exercise stress test in individual unable to walk on a treadmill. Dobutamine (a positive in-strophic agent) is infused IV and dosage is increased in 5 minutes intervals while echocardiogram is performed to detect wall motion abnormalities in each stage. In this, nursing responsibilities include—starting IV infusion, administering debutamine, monitoring vital signs before, during and after test until baseline is achieved. Monitor patient for signs and symptoms of distress during procedure.

iv. *Transesophageal echocardiogram (TEE)*
Cardiac doppler, colour-flow imaging.
TEE allows high resolution ultrasonic imaging of the cardiac structure and great vessels via the oesophagus. The clinical indications for TEE are:

- Mitral valve prosthetic dysfunction.
- Mitral valve regurgitation.
- Infective endocarditis.
- Congenital heart disease.
- Intracardial thrombi. (especially left atrium and left atrial appendage).
- Cardiac tumour.
- Intraoperative assessment: left ventricle functions, adequacy of valve repair and replacement.

This technique uses a probe with an ultrasound transducer at the tip is swallowed. This procedure can be performed at the bedside without contrast dye. It is performed under local anaesthetic and sedation. Usually the physician controls the angle of and depth of oesophagus with transducer. As it passes down the oesophagus, it sends back clear images of heart size, wall motion, valvular abnormalities, and possible source of thrombi without interference from lungs or chest ribs. A contrast medium may be injected IV for evaluating direction of blood flow if an atrial or ventricular septal defect is suspected. Doppler ultrasound and colour flow imaging can also be used concurrently.

In this procedure, nursing responsibility will include the following:

- Instruct patient to be NPO for at least 6 hours before test.
- A tranquilizer will be given and throat locally anaesthetized. So, if done as an outpatient, a designated driver is needed.
- Monitor vital signs and oxygen saturation levels and perform suctioning continually during procedure.
- Explain to patient the proper procedure for easy passage of transducer.

- Assist patient to relax.
- Patient may not eat or drink until gag reflex returns.

6. Scintigraphic Studies

Nuclear cardiological study involves IV injection of radioactive isotopes. Radioactive uptake is counted over the heart by scintillation camera. It supplies information about myocardial contractility, myocardial perfusion and acute cell injury. The common nuclear cardiological at:

i. *Thallium 201 scan*
Thallium 201 is injected IV and used to evaluate blood flow in different parts of heart. Cold spots correlate with area of infarction. For stress testing, IV thallium is given 1 minute before the patient reaches maximum heart rate on bicycle or treadmill. Patient is then required to continue exercise for 1 minute to circulate the radioactive isotopes. Actual scanning is done within 5-10 minutes after exercise. A second testing scan performed 2-4 hours later and compared to postexercise scan. Instruct patient to eat only a light meal between scans.

ii. *Dypyridomole thallium scan*
As with thallium exercise test, depyridamole (Persantine) is also injected. This drug acts as a powerful vasodilator and will increase blood flow to well-perfused coronary arteries. Scanning procedure is same as with thallium scan. In this, instruct the patient to hold all caffeine products for 12 hours before procedure.

iii. *Teahnetium 99 m sestamibi scan*
In this technetium 99 m sestamibi is injected IV and taken up area of MI, producing hot spots. Maximum results are produced when performed 1-6 days after suspected MI waiting period after injection is 1-1/2-2 hours.

iv. *Blood pool imaging*
In this technetium 99 m per technetate injected intravenously. Single injection allows sequential evaluation of heart for several hours. Study is indicated for patient with recent MI or congestive heart failure, especially if not recovering well. It can be used to measure effectiveness of various cardiac medications and can be done at the patient's bedside.

v. *Posterior emissiontomography (PET)*
PET is a radionuclide-based imaging technique that uses short-lived radio nuclides as tracers to report both perfusion and metabolic events. Here uses two radionuclides. Nitrogen-13-ammonia is injected intravenously and scanned to evaluate myocardial perfusion. A second radioactive isotope. Fluoro-18-1deoxyglucose is then injected and scanned to show myocardial metabolic function. In the normal heart, both scans will match, but in an ischaemic or damaged heart, they will differ. The patient may or may not be stressed. A baseline resting scan is usually obtained for comparison. Here the nurse has to

- Instruct the procedure.
- Explain that patient will be scanned by a machine and will need to stay still for a period of time.
- Patient's glucose level must be between 6 and 140 mg/dl. for accurate metabolic activity.
- If exercise included as part of testing, patient will need to be NPO and refrain from tobacco and caffeine for 24 hours prior to test.

In general, in all studies related to IV injection of isotopes, nurse has the responsibility to:

- Explain procedure to patient.
- Establish IV line for injection of isotopes.
- Explain that isotopes used in small diagnostic and will loss most of its radioactivity in a few hours.
- Patient's glucose level must be between 60 and 140 mg/dl, for accurate metabolic activity.
- If exercise is included as a part of testing, patient will need to be NPO and refrain, from tobacco and caffeine for 24 hours prior to test.

In general in all studies related to IV injection of isotopes nurse has the responsibility to:

- Explain procedure to patient.
- Establish IV line for injection fo isotopes.
- Explain that isotopes are used in small diagnostic quantities and will lose most of their radioactivity in a few hours.
- Inform the patient that he or she will be lying down on back with arm extended overhead for period of time.
- Repeated scans are performed within a few minutes to hours after the injection.

7. Magnetic Resonance Imaging (MRI)

It is a noninvasive imaging technique which obtains information about cardiac tissue integrity, aneurysms, ejection factions, cardiac output, and patency of proximal coronary arteries. It does not involve ionizing radiations and is an extremely safe procedure. It provides images in multiple planes with uniformly good resolution. It has limited use in critical care patients, because of access and equipment problem. It cannot be used in persons with any implanted metallic devices. In this procedure, the nurses will explain the procedure to patient, inform the patient that the small diameter of the cylinder along with loud nose of the procedure may cease panic or anxiety. Antianxiety medications and music may be recommended.

8. Blood Studies

The important blood studies are followed in diagnosis are:

- Creatinine kinase (CK)
- CK-MB fraction
- AST (SGOT)

- (Myoglobin)
- Troponin
- Lactic dehydrogenase (LOH)
- Serum lipids- Cholestrol, Tryglycerides, Lipoproteins.
- Drug levels- Digoxin, Quinidine, Inderol (propronolol).

9. Cardiac Catheterization

It is an extremely valuable diagnosis tool used for obtaining detailed information about the structures and functions of the cardiac chambers, valves and coronary arteries. This diagnostic study involves insertion of catheter in the heart. Information can be obtained about O_2 saturation and pressure readings within chambers. Dye can be injected to assist in examining structure and motion of heart. Procedure is done by insertion of catheter into a vein for right-sided heart or an artery for left-sided heart.

The nursing responsibilities before procedure are:

- Obtain written permission.
- Withhold food and fluids for 6-18 hours before procedure.
- Give sedation if ordered.
- Inform patient about use of local anaesthesia, insertion of catheter and feeling of warmth and fluttering sensation of heart as catheter is passed.
- Note that patient may be instructed to cough or take a deep breathing when catheter is inserted.
- See that the patient is monitored by ECG throughout procedure.

After the procedure, nurse has the responsibility to:

- Assess circulation to extremity used for catheter insertion.
- Check peripheral pulses, colour and sensation of extremity, every 15 minutes for 1 hour and then with decreasing frequency.
- Observe injection site for swelling and bleeding.
- Place sand bag over arterial site if indicated.
- Monitor vital signs.
- Assess for abnormal heart rate, arrythmias and signs of pulmonary emboli (resporatory difficulty).

In addition to above diagnostic tests, the following should also be performed.

- Coronary angiography.
- Intracoronary ultrasound.
- Haemodynamic monitoring.
- Electrophysiology study.
- Peripheral arteriography and venography.
- Digital subtraction angiography and
  General routine blood tests, urinalysis, etc.

HYPERTENSION

Hypertension is defined as a consistent constant elevation of the systolic or diastolic pressure above 140/90 mm Hg. It is sustained deviation of blood pressure (BP). In adults, hypertension exists when systolic blood pressure (SBP) is equal to or greater than 140 mm Hg or distolic blood pressure (DBP) is equal to or greater than 90 mm Hg for extended periods of time. The diagnosis of hypertension requires that elevated readings be present on at least three occasions during several weeks.

High blood pressure (HBP) means that the heart is working harder than normal, putting both the heart and the blood vessels under strain. HBP may contribute to myocardial infarctions, cerebrovascular accidents, (CVA), renal failure and atherosclerosis. Hypertension causes no symptoms to motivate a person to seek treatment. When symptoms do occur, they signify either secondary causes of hypertension or effects of sustained elevation of BP on target organs (coronary artery disease, left ventricular hypertrophy, cerebrovascular disease, peripheral vascular disease, or renal insufficiency).

Aetiology

The aetiology of hypertension can be classified as either primary (essential) or secondary.

Primary (Essential) hypertension accounts for more than 90 per cent of all cases and has no known cause, although it is theorized that genetic factor, hormonal changes, and alterations in sympathetic tone all may play a role in its development. Although the exact cause is unknown, several contributing factors including increased SNS activity, overproduction of sodium retaining hormones and vasoconstrictors, increased sodium intake, more than ideal body weight, diabetes mellitus and excessive alcohol intake. The identified risk factors in primary hypertension are as follows:

- Age: Blood pressure rises progressively with advancing or increasing age—Elevated BP is present in approximately 50 per cent of people over 65 years of age, and with onset usually between the ages of 30 and 50 years.
- Sex: Hypertension is more prevalent in men and young adulthood and early middle age. After the age of 55, hypertension is more prevalent in women.
- Race: Incidence of HBP is twice as great in African-Americans as in Caucasians.
- Family History: Level of BP is strongly familial. Risk of hypertension increases for those with a close relatives having hypertension.
- Obesity: Weight gain is associated with increased frequency of hypertension. The risk is greater with central abdominal obesity.
- Smoking: Smoking greatly increases the risk of cardiovascular disease. Nicotine constricts blood vessels. Hypertensives who smoke are at even greater risk.
- High salt diet: Sodium causes water retention, increasing blood volume. Excessive dietary sodium

intake can contribute to hypertension in some patients, and decreases the efficacy of certain anti-hypertensive medication.

- Elevated serum lipids: Elevated levels of cholesterol and triglycerides are primary risk factors in atherosclerosis. Narrowing of arteries increases blood pressure. Hyperlipidemia is more common in hypertensives.
- Alcohol: Alcohol increases plasma catecholamines. Excessive alcohol intake is strongly associated with hypertension. Hypertensives should limit their daily intake of ethanol to 1 Oz.
- Sedantary life styles: Regular physical activity can help control weight and reduce cardiovascular risk. Physical activity may decrease.
- Diabetes mellitus: Hypertension is more common in diabetics. Where hypertension and diabetes coexist, complications are more severe.
- Socioeconomic status: Hypertension is more prevalent in low socioeconomic groups and among the less educated.
- Emotional stress: Stress stimulates sympathetic nerve systems. People exposed to repeated stress may develop hypertension more frequently than others. People who become hypertensive may respond differently to stress from those who do not become hypertensive.

Secondary Hypertension

It develops as a consequence of a particular underlying disease or condition. It is elevated BP with a specific cause that often can be identified and corrected. This type of hypertension accounts for less than 5 per cent of hypertension in adults but more than 80 per cent of hypertension in children. If a person below the age of 20 or over the age of 50 suddenly develops hypertension, if it is severe, a secondary cause should be suspected. Clinical findings suggest that secondary hypertension include unprovoked hypokalaemia, abdominal bruit, variable pressure with tachycardia, sweating and tremor, or family history of renal diseases. Causes of secondary hypertension include the following:

- Coarctation or congenital narrowing of the aorta.
- Renal disease such as renal artery stenosis parenchymal disease (Glomerulonephritis, renal failure) and renovascular disease.
- Endocrine disorders such as pheochromocytoma (Excessive secretion of catecholamines). Cushing syndrome (Blood volume), hyperaldosteronism, primary aldosteronisms (increase in aldosterone causing sodium and water retention and increase blood volume).
- Neurologic disorders such as brain tumour, quadriplegia and head injury.
- Sleep apnoea.
- Medications such as sympathetic stimulants (including cocaine) monamino oxidase inhibitors taken with tyramine containing foods, oestrogen replacement therapy, oral contraceptive pills, and nonsteroidal anti-inflammatory drugs (NSAIDS).
- Pregnancy-induced hypertension: cause is unknown, generalized vasospasm may be a contributing factor.

Pathophysiology

Blood pressure is the force exerted by the blood against the walls of the blood vessels and must be adequate to maintain tissue perfusion during activity and rest. The maintenance of normal BP and tissue perfusion requires the integration of both systemic factors and local peripheral vascular effects. Arterial BP (ABP) is primarily a function of cardiac output (CO) and systemic vascular resistance (SVR). The relationship is summarized by following equation

$$ABP = CO \times SVR$$

Cardiac output (CO) is the total blood flow through the systemic or pulmonary circulation per minute. CO can be described as the stroke volume amount of blood pumped out of the left ventricle per beat (approximately 70 ml) multiplied by the heart rate (HR) for one minute. Systemic vascular resistance (SVR) is the force opposing the movement of blood within the blood vessels. Radius of the small arteries and arterioles is the principal factor determining vascular resistance. A small change in the radius of the arterioles create a major change in the SVR. If SVR is increased and CO remains constant or increases ABP will increase.

The mechanism that regulate BP can affect either CO or SVR or both. Regulation of BP is a complex process involving nervous, cardiovascular, renal and endocrine functions. BP is regulated by both short-term (seconds to hours) and long-term (days to weeks mechanisms). Short-term mechanisms including autonomic nervous system and vascular endothelium, one active within a few seconds. Long-term mechanisms include renal and hormonal process that regulates arteriolar resistance and blood volume.

The regulation of blood pressure is a complex process involving renal control of sodium and water retention and nervous system control of vascular tone. The two primary regulatory factors are blood flow and peripheral vascular resistance refers to size of the peripheral blood vessels. The more constricted the vessel, the greater the resistance to flow and the more dilated the vessel, the lesser is resistence. As peripheral vessels become more constricted, the blood pressure becomes more elevated. Dilation and constriction of the peripheral blood vessels are controlled by primarily by the SNS in stimulated, catecholamines such as epinephrine and nonepinephrine are released. These chemical causes increased vasoconstriction, increased cardiac output, and increased strength of ventricular contraction. Likewise, when the renin-angiotension system is activated, angiotension causes vasoconstriction of the blood vessels. Long-term vasoconstriction of renal vessels causes permanent renal damage and may lead to kidney failure. Other important organs such as the brain and heart also suffer long-term damage from untreated hypertension.

Clinical Manifestation

Hypertension is called the "SILENT KILLER", because it is a disease that usually occurs without any symptoms. It is frequently asymptomatic until it becomes severe and target organ disease has occurred. A patient with severe hypertension may experience a variety of symptoms secondary to effects on blood vessels in the various organs and tissues or to the increased work load of the heart. These secondary symptoms include fatigue, reduced activity tolerance, dizziness, palpitations, angina, and dyspnoea. The most advanced disease may produce symptoms such as early morning headache, blurred vision, and spontaneous nose-bleed, and depression. However, these symptoms are not more frequent in people with hypertension than in the general population.

The most common complications of hypertension are target organ disease occurring in the heart (hypertensive heart disease), brain (cerebrovascular disease), peripheral vasculature (Peripheral vascular disease), kidney (nephrosclerosis) and eyes (retinal damages).

Diagnostic Studies

The initial diagnosis of hypertension is made on the basis of two or more elevated blood pressure readings, supine and sitting, obtained on at least two separate occasions. If the first two readings differ more than 5 mm Hg additional readings should be obtained. Postural changes in BP and pulse should be measured in older adults, people taking antihypertensive drugs and when orthostatic hypertension is suspected.

Specific diagnostic test will be ordered to rule out an underlying cause or evaluate the extent of organ damage. A comprehensive physical examination is performed, including careful evaluation of blood vessels of the retina and as typically supplemented with laboratory tests, that will evaluate the neurological, cardiovascular and renal system for evidence of target organ damage. The laboratory studies that are performed in a person with sustained hypertension, routine urinalysis, BUN and serum creatinine levels are used to screen for renal involvement. Measurement of serum electrolytes, especially potassium levels is important to detect hyperaldesteronim. Fasting blood glucose level (diabetes) serum cholesterol and triglyceride level provide information about additional risk factors that predispose to atherosclerosis. Complete blood count, ... serum chemistry, ECG to know cardiac status.

Management

The management of hypertension does not involve any specific treatment but management is usually improved when the patient is able to make targeted lifestyle adjustment that support the drug therapy. Two important measures are abstaining from smoking and stress reduction management. Smoking has a direct vasoconstrictive effect on the blood vessels and should be given up it at all possible costs. The role of stress is less clear but the use of relaxation and stress management strategies are often helpful in blood pressure control.

Lifestyle modifications should be used in all hypertensive patients either as definitive or adjunctive therapy. These modifications directed toward reducing BP and overall cardiovascular risk. Modifications include:

1. Dietary changes.
2. Limitation of alcohol intake.
3. Regular physical activity.
4. Avoidance of tobacco use (smoking and chewing).

Based on assigned risk group, lifestyle modifications are usually continued upto one year before drug therapy is used. Patients with hypertension are encouraged to develop a pattern of regular aerobic exercise, which may help control their hypertension and also contributes to weight loss and reduces cardiac risk factors. Patients are cautioned to avoid strenuous exercises, particularly activities involve heavylifting or the Valsalva's maneuver. Weightlifting should be avoided and sustained moderate exertion is preferable to bursts of efforts.

Drug Therapy

This is the primary treatment of essential hypertension. The drug currently available for treating hypertension have two main actions reduction of ever and volume of circulating blood. The drugs used in the treatment of hypertension include diuretics, adrenergic (sympathetic) inhibitors, vasodilators, angiotension inhibitors and calcium channel blockers. The details of medications used for hypertension are as follows:

A. *Diuretics*

1. *Thiazide/thiazide-like diuretics*

Thiazide/Thiazide-like diuretics blocks or inhibits sodium reabsorbtion in the distal convulted tubule, in the portion of ascending tubule; Water exerted with sodium, producing decreased volume. They will be increased in Na+ and Cl. Initial decrease in ECF and sustained decrease in SVR lowers BP moderately in 2 to 4 weeks. The technical terms used for these drugs are bendroflumethiazide, bebzythiazide, chlorothiazide, chlorothiazide, cyclothiazide, hydrochlorothiazide, (Esidrex), hydroflumethazide indapamide, methyl chlorothiazide, metalazine, polythiazyde, quinethiazone and trichlomethiazide, Thiazides are ineffective in Renal failure.

The side effects of thiazides are:

- Fluid and electrolyte imbalances:
  Volume depletion, hypocalaemia, hyponatraemia, hypercalcaemia, hyperuricaemia, metabolic alkalosis.

- CNS effects: Vertigo, headache, weakness.
- GI effects, anorexia, nausea, vomiting, diarrhoea, constipation and pancreatitis.
- Sexual problems: importence and decreased libido.
- Blood dyscreas and dermatologic effects; photosensitivity and skin rash.
- Decreased gluco tolerance.

During this treatment nurses have to monitor the following:

1. Check vital signs before administering in early days of treatment.
2. Monitor lab value of electrolytes, particularly potassium.
3. Monitor patient weight.
4. Teach patients to:
   - Take drug early in the day.
   - Maintain liberal fluid intake.
   - Take drug with food if GI upsets occur.
   - Eat potassium-rich diet (eg. fruits, legumes, whole grains, cereals and potato).
   - Expect an increased frequency and volume of urination.
   - Report the incidence of muscle weakness. Cramping, fatigue and nausea.
   - Change positions slowly.

2. *Loop diuretics*

It blocks sodium and water reabsorption in medullary portion of ascending tubule, cause rapid volume depletion. The drugs used are bumetanide, ethacrynic acid, furosemide (Lasix). The side effects are fluid and electrolyte imbalance as with thiazides except hypercalcaemia, ototoxicity (hearing impairment, deafness, vertigo) that is usually reversible. Metabolic effects including hypeuricaemia, hyperglycaemia, increased LDL cholesterol and triglycerides with decreased HDL cholesterol. Nursing intervention are as same as with thiazides, but potassium loss can be severe. So, nurse has to monitor

- Daily weight to assess response to treatment.
- Lab values for increase in uric acid and glucose BUN.

3. *Potassium sparing diuretics:*

It inhibits aldosterone; sodium excreted in exchange of potassium. The drugs are amiloride, spironolactone, and triamaterine. The side effects are hyperkalaemia, nausea, vomiting, diarrhoea, headache, leg cramps and dizziness. Nursing intervention includes:

- Monitor lab value for potassium excess.
- Weigh patient daily.
- Teach patient to:
  - Expect an increased volume of urine.
  - Avoid potassium-rich foods.
  - Report any incidence of drowsiness or GI side effects.

B. *Adrenergic inhibitors*

1. *Centrally acting alpha blockers:*

These activate central receptors that suppress vasomotor and cardiac centers causing decrease in peripheral resistance. They reduce sympathetic outflow from CNS and peripheral sympathetic tone produces vasodilation and decreases SVR and BP. Commonly used are cloridine, gunabenz, guantacine, methyldopa (Aldomat) ... The side effects of these drugs are, dry mouth, sedation, impotence, nausea, dizziness, sleep disturbance, nightmares, restlessness, and depression. There is symptomatic bradycardia in patient wth conduction disorder. In this, nursing intervention includes.

- Change position slowly.
- Teach patient to:
  - Change position slowly.
  - Avoid hot baths, steam rooms, saunas.
  - Use gum or hard candies to counteract dry mouth.
  - Be cautious in driving or operating machinery if drowsiness or sedation occurs.
  - Report any decline in sexual responsiveness.

2. *Peripheral acting adrenergic antagonists:*

It depletes catecholamine, in peripheral sympathetic post-ganglionic fibers and blocks norepinephrine release from adrenergic nerve endings. Usually used are guanadrel, guanethedine (ismelin) rauwolfin, serpentina, reserpine (texpasil).. The side effects include marked orthostatic hypertension, diarrhoea, cramps bradycardia, retrograde or delayed ejaculation, sodium and water retention sedation and inability to concentrate, depression, nasal stuffiness with reserpine. The nursing intervention is as with the above (1) drug and report incidence of oedema in hands and feet.

3. *Beta-adrenergic blockers:*

Beta-adrenergic blockers block beta-adrenergic receptors of sympathetic nervous system, decreasing heart rate and blood pressure. Please note that beta blockers should not be used in patients with asthma. COPD, CHF and heart block. Use with caution in diabetes and peripheral vascular disease. Commonly used betablockers are acebutolol, atenolol, betaxolol, carteolol, metaprolol, nadolol, petbutolol, pindolol, propranolol, timolol and essmolol (IV). The side effects of these drugs are bronchospasm, atrioventricular conduction block, impaired peripheral circulation, nightmares, depression, weakness, reduced exercise capability. It can be included in exacerbate symptom of ischaemic heart disease. The nursing intervention include:

- Establish baseline vital signs and lab values before treatment.
- Check blood pressure and pulse before administration.
- Teach patients to:
  - Change position slowly.

- Take drug as prescribed.
- Avoid abruptly discontinuing the use.
- Report any decline in sexual responsiveness.
- Report incidence of fatigue, drowsiness, difficulty in breathing.
- Be alert to the signs of hypoglycaemia if diabetic drug masks the symptoms.

4. *Combined alpha and beta-adrenertic blockers:* Labetalol is a common drug used as combined one. Action and nursing actions are as same as beta blockers.

C. *Vasodilators*

Vasodilators such as diazoxide, hydralazine, minoxidil, nitroglycerine (tridil) dilate peripheral blood vessels by directly relaxing vascular smooth muscle. These are usually used in combination with other antihypertensives as they increase sodium and fluid retention and cause reflex cardiac stimulation.

Diazoxide direct arterial vasodilation reduces SVR and BP. It is used intravenously for hypertensive crisis in hospitalized patients. It should be administered only into peripheral veins. The side effects include reflex sympathetic activation producing increased HR, CO and salt and water retention. Hyperglycaemia is especially in type 2 diabetes.

Hydralazine has same effect as diazoxide; it should be given IV in hypertensive crisis in hospitalized patients. Also use 2 oral doses per day. The side effects are headache, nausea, flushing, palpitation bradycardia, angina, haemolytic anaemia, vasculitis and rapidly progressive glomerulonephritis.

Minoxidil (Leniten) used in severe hypertension associated with renal failure. It may cause reflex tachycardia, fluid retention and ECG changes and tridol administered intravenously in case of hypertensive crisis with myocardial ischaemea.

The nursing intervention during the use of vasodilator in hypertension clients are as follows:

- Check BP and pulse before each dose. Palpitation and tachycardia are common during first week of therapy.
- Teach patients to:
  - Change in position slowly because dizziness is common.
  - Avoid hot baths, steam rooms, saunas.
  - Take drug with meals.
  - Be prepared for nasal congestion and excess lacrimation.
  - Report incidence of constipation or peripheral oedema.

D. *Angiotens in inhibitors*

1. *ACE (Angiotensin converting enzyme) Inhibitors*

These inhibit conversion of angiotensin to angiotensin II, thus blocking the release of aldosterone, thereby reducing sodium and water retention commonly used are Benazepril, Captopril, Clazapril, Enlapril, Fosionopril, Lisionopril, Moexpril, Perindopril, Ramipril, Ouinapril, Trandolapril, Enalaprila (injectable). The side effects are hypotension, loss of taste, cough, hyperkalaemia, acute renal failure, skin rash angionuerotico-edema. The nursing interventions are:

- Monitor for first-dose syncope in patients with CHF.
- Monitor renal function through lab work and potassium levels.
- Check BP before administering.
- Teach patient to change position slowly, report any incidence of fatigue, skin rash, impaired taste and chronic cough.

2. *Angiotensin II receptor antagonist*

It selectively blocks the binding angiotensin I to the angiotensin II receptors found in many tissues and vascular smooth muscle, which blocks its vasoconstrictive and aldosterone-secreting effects. The commonly used are Candisartan, Irbesartan, Losartan, Tasosartan, Valsartan. The side effects are hyperkalaemia and decreased renal function. These drugs prevent action of angiotensin II and produce vasodilative and increasing salt and water excretion. The nursing intervention are as in (1 ACE inhibitors).

E. *Calcium channel blockers*

Calcium channel blockers inhibit influx of calcium into muscle cells; act on vascular smooth muscles (Primary arteries) to reduce spasms and promote vasodilation. Here it blocks movement of extracellular calcium into cells causing peripheral vasodilation and decreased SVR. The commonly used calcium channel blockers are Amlodipine, Diltiazem, Felodipine, Istadipine, Mibefradil, Nicrandipine. Nifedipine, Nisoldipine, Verapamol (Isoptin) and Verapanil SR. The side effects are nausea, headache, dizziness, peripheraloedema, reflex tachycardia. Reflex disease in HR (with ditiacem), constipation (with verapamil). The nursing interventions include:

- Check vital signs before administering (Bradycardia is common)
- Monitor renal and liver function tests.
- Teach patient to take drugs before meals, change positions slowly, report any incidence of peripheraloedema, fatigue and headache.

In addition to the above, the patient and family especially the members who prepare the meals should be educated about sodium-restricted diet.

The primary nursing responsibilities for long-term management of hypertension are to assist the patient in reducing BP and complying with the treatment plan. Nursing actions include patient and family education, detection and reporting of adverse treatment effects, compliance assessments, enhancement and evaluatioan of therapeutic effectiveness. Patient education includes diet therapy, drug therapy, physical activity, home monitoring of BP (if appropriate) and avoidance of tobacco (if applicable). When presenting information to the patient or family, the nurse should do the following.

- Provide the numerical value of the patient's BP and explain that it exceeds normal limits.
- Inform the patient that hypertension usually asymptomatic and symptoms do not reliably indicate BP levels.
- Explain that long-term follow-up and therapy are necessary.
- Explain that therapy will not cure but should control hypertension.
- Tell the patient that controlled hypertension is usually compatible with an excellent prognosis and a normal lifestyle.
- Explain to the patient about dangers of uncontrolled hypertension.
- Be specific about the names, actions, dosages and side effects of prescribed medication.
- Tell the patient to plan regular and convenient times for taking medications.
- Tell the patient not to discontinue drugs abruptly because withdrawal may cause a severe hypertensive reaction.
- Tell the patient not to double upon doses when a dose is missed.
- Instruct the patient that if BP increases, not to take an increased medication dosage before consulting a health care provider.
- Tell the patient not to take a medication belonging to someone else.
- Make aware the patient that side effects of medication often diminish with the passage of time.
- Tell the patient to consult the health care provider about changing drugs or dosage if impotence or other sexual problems develop.
- Tell the patient to supplement diet with foods high in potassium (eg citrus fruits, and green leafy vegetables) if he/she is taking potassium-losing diuretics.
- Tell the patient to avoid hot baths, excessive amounts of alcohol, and strenuous exercises within 3 hours of taking medication that promote vasodilation.
- Explain to decrease orthostatic hypotension, the patient should arise slowly from bed, sit on side of bed for a few minutes, stand slowly, not stand still for a long time, do leg exercises to increase venous return, sleep with head of bed raised or on pillows, and lie or sit down when dizziness occurs.

CORONARY ARTERY DISEASE (CAD)

Coronary artery disease is a type of blood vessel disorder that is included in the general category of atherosclerosis. The term *Atherosclerosis* is derived from two Greek Words. '*Athero*' meaning '*Fatty Mish*' and '*Skleros*' meaning "*Hard*". This word-combination indicates that atherosclerosis begins as soft deposits of fat, that hardens with age. Atherosclerosis is often referred to as 'hardening of the arteries'. Although this condition can occur in any artery in the body, the atheromas (fatty deposits) have a preference for the coronary arteries. Patients with CAD often seek health care after experiencing angina or myocardial infarction (M.I.). Vascular diseases such as dysrhythmia, heart failure, and cardiomyopathy. All nurses need to be familiar with the management of coronary artery diseases.

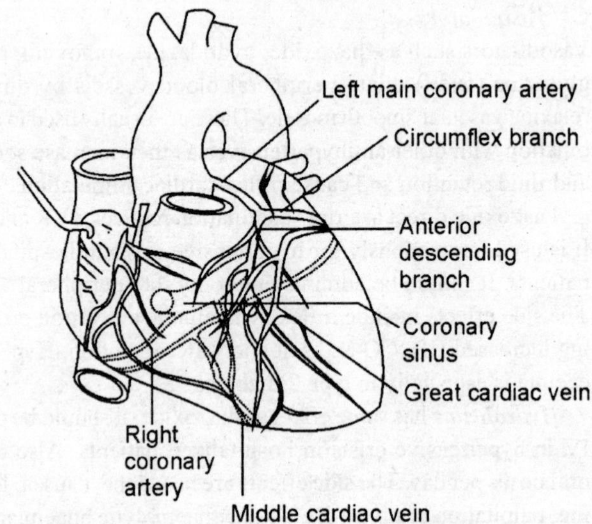

Fig.9.2: Diagram of the coronary arteries arising from the aorta and encircling the heart. Some of the coronary veins also are shown.

Aetiology

Atheroclerosis is the major cause of coronary artery diseases. It is characterised by a focal deposit of cholesterol and lipids, primarily within the wall of the artery. Many risk factors have been associated with CAD are:

- *Age and gender*

Incidence of CAD occurs in men between 35 to 45 years age. After the age of 65 incidence of men and women equalizes; although there is evidence suggesting that more women are being seen with CAD earlier because of increased stress, increased smoking, presence of hypertension and use of birth control pills. For both decrease in elasticity of arteries with age. Oestrogen in females lowers serum cholesterol.

- *Heredity*

Genetic predisposition is an important factor in the occurrence of CAD, but exact mechanism is not yet known.

- *Diabetes*

Incidence of CAD is two-three times more in diabetes. This may be due to elevated levels of circulating insulin helps to form atheroma and damaged arterial intima and insulin also modifies lipid metabolisms.

• *Hypertension*

Hypertension affects the ability of blood vessels to constrict or dilate. Decreased elasticity of blood vessels, tearing affect on arteries, and increased resistance of ejection of ventricular volume may lead to CAD.

• *Smoking and tobacco use*

The unifying factor promoting CAD is nicotine. Nicotine has the following physiological effects and may cause CAD.

- Decreased high-density lipoproteins (HDL).
- Displacement of oxygen from haemoglobin.
- Increased catecholamine in response to nicotine, increasing heart rate and blood pressure.
- Increased platelet adhesiveness.
- Accelerates atheroma formation.
- Accelerates atheroma formation.
- Coronary spasm.

• *Sedentary lifestyle*

This alters lipid metabolism and decrease in HDLS. Physical inactivity may lead to CAD.

• *Diet*

Dietary intake of more cholesterol and fat, provides more substance for lesion formation. Hypercholesterdaemia, familial hyperlipidaemia, increased levels of low density lipoproteins, and increasing atherogenesis.

• *Obesity*

Obese persons are more prone to diabetes, hypertension, and hyperlipidemias. In addition, they often demonstrate other behaviours such as sendentary lifestyles, that are known as risk factors for CAD.

• *Stress and behaviour pattern*

Catecholamine, released during stress response, increases platelet aggregation and may also precipitate vasospasm. It was generally agreed that individuals with type 'A' behaviour had a higher incidence of CAD than individuals who were more relaxed. The type 'A' personality characters include the following (Freidman & Rosanna 1960).

- Perfectionistic
- Competitive
- Aggressive
- Constantly time-oriented
- Has hurry sickness
- Never says 'no'
- Compulsive
- Impatient
- Always tense
- Unduly irritable
- Obsessed with number of sale made, articles written Patients seen, forms completed.
- Holds in feelings
- Never has leisure time
- Never takes a relaxing vacation or day offs.

There are three major clinical manifestations in coronary artery disease, which include anginapectoris, acute myocardial infarction and hidden cardiac death. They are stages of the continum and CAD. The detailed description of these three are as follows:

ANGINA PECTORIS

Angina Pectoris is literally translated as pain (angina) in the chest (pectoris). Myocardial ischaemia is expressed symptomatically as angina. More specifically, angina pectoris is transient chest pain caused by myocardial ischaemia. It usually lasts for only few minutes (3 to 5 min), and commonly subsides when the precipitating factor (usual exertion) is relieved. Typical exertional angina should not persist longer than 20 minutes after rest and administration of nitroglycerine.

Aetiology

Myocardial ischaemia develops when the demand for myocardial oxygen exceeds the ability of the coronary arteries to supply it. The below given are the primary reasons for insufficient blood flow in narrowing of coronary arteries by atherosclerosis. Extracardiac factors may precipitate myocardial ischaemia and anginal pain. They include:

- *Physical exertion*: increases the heart rate (HR) Increasing heart rate decreases the time the heart spends in diastole, which is the time of greatest coronary blood flow. Walking outdoors is the most common form of the exertions that produce an attack. Isometric exertions of the arms as on raking leaves, painting or lifting heavy objects also causes exertional angina.
- *Strong emotions* stimulate the sympathetic nervous system and increase the work of the heart. This results in an increase in HR, BP and myocardial contractility.
- *Consumption of heavy meal* (especially if the person exerts afterwards) can increase the work of the heart. During the digestive process, blood is diverted to the GI system, causing a low flow rate in the coronary arteries.
- *Temperature extremes* it may be either hot or cold. Increases the work load of the heart (blood vessels contstrict in response to the cold climate; blood vessels dilate and blood pools in the skin in response to a hot stimulus). Cold weather also causes increased metabolism to maintain internal temperature regulation.
- *Cigarette smoking* causes vasoconstriction and an increased HR because of nicotine stimulation of the catecholamine release. It also diminishes available oxygen by increasing level of carbon monoxide.
- *Sexual activity* increases the workload and sympathetic stimulation. In a person with severe CAD, the resulting extra workload of the heart may precipitate angina.

- *Stimulants*, such as cocaine, cause increased HR and subsequent myocardial demand. Stimulation of catecholamine release is the precipitating factor.
- *Circadian rhythm* have been related to the occurrence of the stable angina, unstable angina, MI and cardiac death. These manifestations of CAD tend to occur in the early morning after awakening.

Pathophysiology

Coronary artery disease refers to the development and progression of plaque accumulation in the coronary arteries. This process has three stages along the continum viz., stable angina, unstable angina and myocardial infarction.

Normally the endothelium of the coronary artery allows for unrestricted blood flow to the myocardium. Any kind of trauma or irritant can disrupt this protective endothelium. The body's response to injury is a complex interplay of chemical mediators designed to protect the area. Endothelial injury causes the release of thromboxane, which minimizes the extent of injury through local vasoconstriction and by stimulating platelet aggregation. The intima releases prostacyclin in response to the effects of thromboxane. Prostacycline works to restore equilibrium through local vasodilation and by opposing platelet aggregation. With repeated injury, the deteriorated intima cannot produce enough prostacycline and platelet aggregation forces predominate.

Platelets and accumulating monocytes release powerful growth factors into the arterial wall. These factors stimulate the proliferation and migration of medial smooth muscle cells into the intima. This structural changes cause an increased permeability of the vessel wall to the cholesterol. The accumulation of cholesterol produces a fatty streak that protrudes into the lumen of the artery. Smooth muscle cells and fibrous tissue form a fibrous cap over the fatty streak. The fatty streak continues to grow, invading both the intima and media. Involvement of the media affects the ability of the vessel wall to vasodilate and vasoconstrict. The artery may continue to maintain the supply of oxygen and nutrients to the myocardium as long as the blockage is less than 70 per cent of the arterial lumen. Concomitant conditions such as anaemia, smoking and hypovolaemia further compromise the delivery of oxygen to the myocardium.

The presence of risk factors accelerate atherogenesis, thereby decreasing oxygen supply. Risk factors can also increase the myocardium's demands for oxygen. The demand of the myocardium for oxygen can be met only by an adequate blood supply. As long as supply is greater than or equal to demand, aerobic metabolism occurs. When demand is greater than that of supply, the myocardium must switch to anaerobic metabolism for nourishments. Anaerobic metabolism produces lactic acid which is believed to be responsible for ischaemic anginal pain. The pain is the most common initial symptom of CAD. With *stable angina* the patient is usually experiencing a known threshold beyond which myocardial oxygen demand exceeds supply. Myocardial oxygen demand increases with any condition causing an increase in heart rate, an increase in resistance to ejecting blood volume, and an increase in myocardial size.

When atherosclerosis progresses beyond 70 per cent, pressure within the lesion (plaque) can increase to the point of plaque rupture. Rupture of the fibrous cap exposes the inner plaque to the circulating blood. In an effort to heal, collagen accumulates, smooth muscle cells proliferate and clotting factors are activated. Aggregating platelets activate the coagulation system immediately to seal the rupture. With plaque disruptions stable angina becomes *unstable angina*. Risk factors like nicotine from tobacco use increases platelet adhesion and increases the potential for clotting at the site of disruption. Catecholamines released during the stress response also increase platelet aggregation. The third stage that occurs is complete obstruction of the coronary artery with a fibrous cloth called coronary thrombosis or acute MI.

Clinical Manifestation

The following may occur with stable angina, unstable angina or acute MI.

- Chest pain or anginal equivalent (Jaw pain, left arm pain).
- Non-verbal indicators of pain: clutch, rub, stroke and the chest.
- Increase or decrease in heart rate.
- Dysrhythmias.
- Increase or decrease in blood pressure.
- Angina that occurs with predictable level of exertion (in stable angina).
- Angina not necessarily associated with activity and ST depression. (or unstable angina).

In addition to the unique feature of myocardial infarction which includes:

- Angina not relieved by rest or nitroglycerin therapy.
- Associated with symptoms: dizziness, dyspnoea, nausea, vomiting feeling of impending doom.
- Altered neurological status, if decreased output.
- Rales, if decreased contractility creates left ventricular function.
- Presence of S3 or S4 gallop.
- Diminished pulses.
- Pallor.
- ECG ST elevation, Q-waves, J-wave abnormalities.
- Elevated ESR.

Management

When a patient has a history indicating coronary artery disease, thorough physical examination should be carried out and physician may order several diagnostic studies, which the nurse has to promptly attend and assist. Those studies include Chest-X-Ray, ECG, serum enzyme level (CK-LDH) cardiac troponin, serum lipid level. Exercise stress test. Nuclear imaging studies, Position emission tomography (PET), coronary angiographic studies and echocardiography.

(CK = Creatinine kinase.

LDH = Lactic dehydrogenase.)

Nursing assessment made on the basis of present subjective and objective data. Nursing diagnosis for the patient with angina may include chest pain, anxiety, decreased cardiac output, activity intolerances related to myocardial ischaemia. The main nursing objectives for the patient with angina are pain assessment, evaluation of treatment and reinforcement of appropriate therapy. Because chest pain may be caused by many factors other than ischaemia (eg. Pericarditis, valvular disease, pulmonary artery stenosis, MI Congestive cardiomyopathy). It is important to have a clear understanding of the patient's chest pain.

The nurse should determine whether breathing in or out of changing positions makes the patients chest pain better or worse. Anginal pain does not vary with body positions or respiration. In contrast, the pain is deep or superficial, mild or intense, diffuse or localized. Cardiac pain usually is deep or intense and diffuse. The patient may rub the entire chest to explain as to where the pain is occurring. If the nurse is present during anginal attack, the following measures should be taken.

- Administration of oxygen.
- Determination of vital signs.
- 12-Lead ECG.
- Prompt pain relief Ist with a nitrate followed by narcotic analgesic if needed.
- Physical assessment fo the chest.
- Comfortable positioning of the patient.

The patient will more likely appear distressed and have pale, cool, clammy skin. The blood pressure and heart rate will probably be elevated and an atrial gallop (S_4) sound may be heard. If a ventricular gallop (S_3) is heard, it may indicate LV decompensation. A murmur may be heard during an anginal attack secondary to ischaemia of a papillary muscle. The murmur is likely to be transient and abates with the cessation of symptoms. Supportive and realistic assurance and a calm, soothing manner help reduce the patient's anxiety.

The patient should be instructed in the proper use of nitroglycerine tablets. Nitrates decrease myocardial oxygen demand by venodilate (decrease preload), peripherally vasodilated (decrease after load), increase myocardial oxygen supply and coronary vasodilate. Nitroglycerine should be easily accessible to the patient at all times. However, patients should be taught not to carry nitroglycerine in their pockets because heat from the body can cause loss of potency of the tablet. For protection from degradation. It should be kept in a tightly closed dark glass bottle. The patient should be instructed to place a nitroglycerine tablet beneath the tongue and allow it to dissolve. This should cause a fizzing or slightly warm feeling locally. The patient should be warned that heart rate may increase and pounding headache, dizziness, or flush may occur. The patient should be cautioned against quickly rising to standing position, because postural hypertension may occur after nitroglycerine ingestion. If pain has not been relieved after 5 minutes ask him/her to repeat the dose, but not to exceeded three tablets. If pain persists after three doses, the patient should be referred to seek immediate proper medical attention.

The patient should be reassured that a long, productive life is possible even with angina. The patient should be educated regarding coronary artery disease and angina, precipitating factors, risk factors and medication. Educating the patient and family about diet that are low in sodium and reduced in saturated fat may be appropriate. Maintaining ideal body weight is important in controlling angina because weight above the level increase myocardial workload, and may cause pain. Several small meals in place of three meals per day may be suggested. Application of topical nitrates over the chest may be taught to patient.

NURSING MANAGEMENT

Nursing diagnosis will be made thorough nursing assessment by asking the patient to describe the anginal attack (when, where, how often, how long, and other associative symptoms and signs), family history, previous history and their habits, etc. The main nursing diagnosis which needs nursing interventions are:

- Pain related to an imbalance in O_2 supply and demand.
- Decreased cardiac output related to reduced preload, overload, contractility and HR secondary to the haemodynamic effects of drugs.
- Anxiety related to chest pain, uncertain prognosis and threatening environment.

In addition, control of angina pectoris is achieved through the:

- Review information on low-fat/low cholesterol diet with patient.
- Inform patient of available cardiac rehabilitation programs, that offer structured classes on exercise, smoking cessation and weight control.
- Avoid excessive caffeine intake (coffee, cola drinks) that can increase the heart rate and produce angina.
- Avoid the use of alcohol or drink only in moderation.
- Avoid use of 'diet pills', nasal decongestants or any over the counter medication that can increase the HR or stimulate HBP.

Table 9.1: Nursing care-plan of (CAD) corunary artery disease

Problem	*Reason*	*Objectives*	*Nursing intervention*	*Evaluation*
1. Pain R/T imbalance of O_2 supply	(Write Subjective and objective data highlighting related key points)	Pain will be reduced.	• Determine the intensity of the patient's angina. • Observe the other signs and symptoms. – Diaphoresis – Shortness of breath. – Protective body posture. – Dusky facial colour. – Changes in level of consciousness. – Place the patient in comfortable position. • Administer oxygen if prescribed. • Obtain blood pressure, AHR respiration. • Obtain a 12-lead ECG as directed. • Administer anti-anginal medication as prescribed. • Report findings to physician. • Note duration of anginal pain episode. • Take vital signs until pain relief. • Monitor progression of stable angina to unstable angina. • Determine the level of activity that precipitated anginal episode. • Identify specific activities patient may engage in, that are below the level at which pain occurs. • Reinforce the importance of notifying nursing staff whenever angina pain is experienced.	Patient verbalizes relief of pain.
2. Decreased cardiac output R/T reduced preload after load in	"	Improving cardiac output.	• Monitor patient response to drug therapy. – Take BP and HR in sitting and lying positions. – Recheck vital signs as indicated. – Note patient's complaints for headache and dizziness. – Administer analgesics as prescribed. – Encoruage supine position for dizziness. • Institute continuous ECG monitoring as directed. • Evaluate the development of heart failure. (When beta-blockers-calcium channel blocker advised). – Obtain serial weights. – Auscultate lung fields for crakles. – Monitor the presence of oedema. • Be sure to remove previous nitrate patch or paste before applying new paste or pad (prevents hypotension). • Be alert to adverse reaction related to abrupt discontinuation of beta-blockers and others. • Report all untoward drug effects to physician.	Blood pressure and heart status are stable.
3. Anxiety R/T chest pain and others	"	Alleviation of anxiety.	• Explain to the patient and family, reasons for hospitalization, diagnostic tests and therapies. • Encourage the patient to verbalize fears and concerns regarding illness, by good listening. • Answer the patient's questions with concise explanations.	Patient verbalizes lessening anxiety ability to cope.

Contd...

Contd...

Problem	*Reason*	*Objectives*	*Nursing intervention*	*Evaluation*
			• Explain to the patient the importance of anxiety reduction to assist in angina. • Teach relaxation techniques. • Discuss measure to be taken when angina episode occurs.	
4. Knowledge deficit R/T coronary artery disease.	Patient and family do not have proper knowledge of CAD	Educate the patient and family regarding CAD.	• Instruct the patient and family about CAD (anatomy and physiology and heart warning signals of angina). • Identify suitable activity level to prevent angina: – normal activities do not produce discomfort to chest. – Avoid activities known to cause angina. – Rest after meals. – Try to avoid cold weather. – Reduce weight if necessary. • Instruct about appropriate use of medications and side effects. – Carry nitroglycerine at all times. – Demonstrate how to administer nitroglycerin – Place nitroglycerin under the tongue. – Teach side effects of other medications Constipation – Verapanel Ankle oedema – Nifedipine Heart failure – Beta or calcium blockers. dizziness – Vasodilators.	

MYOCARDIAL INFARCTION

Myocardial infarction occurs when ischaemic intracellular changes become irreversible and necrosis results. Angina as a result of ischaemia causes reversible cellular injury, and infarction in the result of sustained ischaemia causing irreversible cellular death.

Pathophysiology

Cardiac cells can withstand ischaemia condition for approximately 20 minutes before cellular death (necrosis) begins. Contractile function of the heart stops in the area of myocardial necrosis. The degree of altered function depends on the area of the heart involved the LV. A transmural MI occurs when the entire thickness of the myocardium in a region involved. A subendocardial MI (non-transmural) exists when the damage has not penetrated through the entire thickness of the myocardial wall. Infarction is described as the area of occurrence, as anterior, inferior, lateral, or posterior wall infarctions, common combination and anteriolateral or anterioseptal MI. An inferior MI also called diaphragmatic MI. The location and area of the infarct correlates with the part of the coronary circulation involved. The degree of pre-established collateral circulation also determines the severity of infarction. The clot extends into lumens, completely obstructs lumen. Complete obstruction of the coronary artery with the fibrous clot is termed as coronary thrombosis or coronary occlusion. Coronary occlusion creates a rapid series of physiological events. The first of these events is immediate myocardial ischaemia distal to the occlusion. Ischaemia alters the integrity and permeability of the myocardial cell membranes to vital electrolytes. This instability depresses myocardial contractility and predisposes the patients to sudden death from dysrhythmias.

The body responses to cell death is inflammatory process within 24 hours, leukocytes infiltrate the area. Enzymes are released from the dead cardiac cells and important diagnostic indicators of MI.

Clinical Manifestation

- *Chest pain* very severe immobilizing chest pain not relieved by rest or nitrate administration is the hall mark of MI. This pain is usually described as a heaviness, tightness, or constrictions. Common locations are substernal or retrosternal, radiating to the neck, jaw and arms or to the back. It may occur when patient is active, or at rest, awake or during sleep and it commonly occurs at early morning hours. It lasts for 20 minutes or more.
- *Nausea and vomiting* as a result of vasovagal reflexes initiated from the area of the infarcted myocardium.
- *Sympathetic nervous system* stimulation is increased due to release of increased catecholemine (norephinephrine) and epinephrine leads to ashen cool and clammy skin (cold sweats).

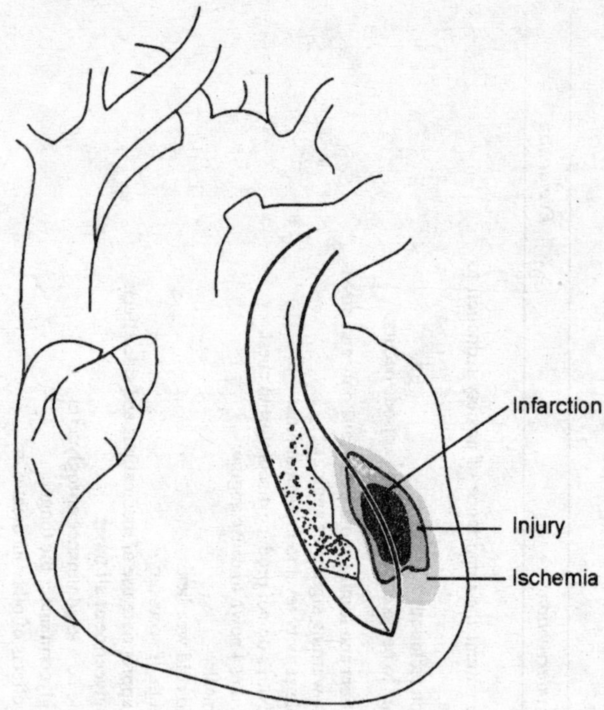

Fig.9.3: Different degrees of damage occur to the heart muscle after a myocardial infarction. The diagram shows the zones of necrosis, injury, and ischemia.

- *Fever*: The temperature may increase upto 38°C.
- Cardiac vascular manifestation includes elevated BP and HR. Later, BP may drop as decreased cardiac output, urinary output may be decreased. Crackles may be noted in the lungs. Later hepatic engorgement and peripheral oedema occurs which indicates cardiac failure.

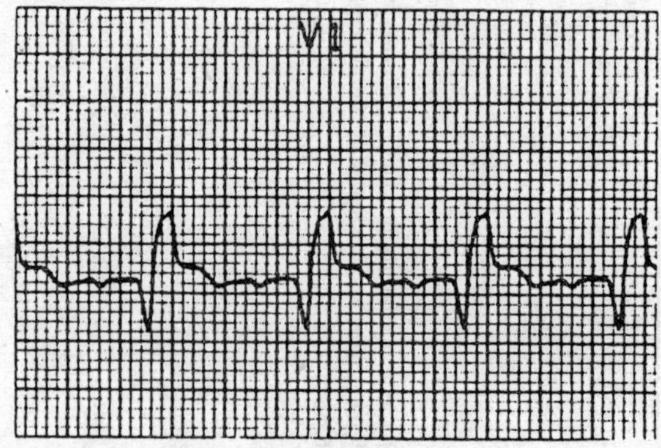

Fig. 9.4: Abnormal Q wave.

In addition, following complications may develop.

- Arrythmias (Abnormal wave)
- Congestive heart failure.
- Cardiogenic shock.
- Papillary muscle dysfunction.
- Ventricular aneurysm.

- Pericarditis.
- Dressler's syndrome.
- Right ventricular infarction.
- Pulmonary embolism.

Management

Common diagnostic parameters used to determine whether a person has sustained an acute MI include (1) The patient's history of pain. Risk factors and health history (2) 12-lead ECG. Consistent with acute MI. (ST-T wave elevated by greater than 1 mm or more in two continuous leads and (3) Serious measurement of myocardial serum enzyme and comparison of the pain with angina as given below:

Angina	*Myocardial infarction*
1. *Precipitating factors*	*Precipitating factors*
• Stress, either physiologic (Exertion or psychology.	• Exertion or rest.
• Digestion of heavy meal	• Physical or emotional stress.
• Valsalva's maneuver during micturation or defecation	• Often no precipitation factors are associated with angina.
• Extremity of weather.	
• Hot baths or showers.	
• Sexual excitation.	
2. *Location*	
• Midanterior chest	• Midanterior chest.
• Substernal	• Substernal.
• Abdominal with radiation to neck, back arms, fingers.	• Diffuse.
• Diffuse, nor easily located.	• Radiation to neck and jaw or down left arm or both arms to fingers.
3. *Description*	
• Deep sensation of tightness or squeezing feeling.	• Severe pressure, squeezing or heaviness with a crushing oppressive quality.
• Mild to moderate in severity or pressure.	• Report of such severe pain that the patient would rather than experience pain again.
• Similar attack each time.	
• Twinges or dullness in thoracic arc.	• Residual 'soreness' of several days following MI.
4. *Onset and duration*	
• Gradual or sudden onset.	• Sudden onset.
• Usual duration of 15 minutes or less (usually less than 30 minutes).	• Duration of 30 min to 2 hours.
• Relief by nitroglycerine	• No relief from rest or nitroglycerine.
5. *Associated clinical manifestations:*	
• Apprehension.	• Apprehension.
• Dyspnoea.	• Nausea and vomiting.
• Diaphoresis.	• Dyspnoea.
• Nausea.	• Diaphoresis.
• Desire to void.	• Extreme fatigue.
• Belching.	• Dizziness or faintness (after abatement of pain).

Acute nursing interventions for patient with MI are best done in a specialized unit (ICCU). Such nursing includes the initial ICCU stay for 1 to 2 days and the rest of hospitalization for 4 to 6 days. Priorities for nursing intervention in the initial stage of recovery after MI includes pain assessment and relief, physiologic monitoring, promotion of rest and comfort, alleviation of stress and anxiety and understanding of the patient's emotional and behavioural reactions. In initial stages, of emergency management, the nursing responsibility includes:

- Ensure patent airway.
- Administer oxygen by nasal cannula or non-rebreather mask.
- Insert two IV catheters.
- Obtain 12-lead ECG.
- Determine location of pain-Assess severity using pain scale (0-10).
- Medicate for pain as ordered (eg. Morphine, nitroglycerin).
- Identify underlying rhythm.
- Obtain cardiac enzyme levels.
- Assess need for thrombolytic therapy as appropriate.
- Administer asprin and beta-adrenergic blockers for cardiac-related chest pain unless contraindicated.

Ongoing monitoring by nurses include the followıng.

- Monitor vital signs, level of consciousness, cardiac rhythm, and O_2 saturation.
- Monitor pain and remedicate as needed.
- Reassure patient.
- Anticipate need for intubation if respiratory distress is evident.
- Prepare for CPR, defibrillation, transcutaneous pacing, or cardioversion.

And nurses should keep in mind that common medication used for coronary artery disease and nursing intervension during their administration as follows:

1. *Antiplatelet agents* (asprin, ticlopidine) inhibits platelet aggregation. Aspirn should be prescribed unless a true hypersensitivity reaction is present or the patient has a severe risk of bleeding.
2. *Nitrates* (Isosorbide denitrate, Isosorbide mononitrate, nitroglycer) Nitrate decreases myocardial oxygen by venodilate, peripherally vasodilate, increase myocardial oxygen supply and coronary vasodilate. Patient should be lying or sitting with administration of sublingual nitrates. Intravenous nitroglycerin is titrated to relief of symptoms or limiting side effects such as headache or systolic BP less than 90 mm Hg. IV preparations are usually replaced with oral or topical preparation when the patient has been symptom-free for 24 hours. Cautiously use with known aortic stenosis. Anticipate headache develop within 24 hours. A nitrate-free interval of 6 to 8 hours may improve responsiveness to therapy.

Topical nitrates must be cleaned from the skin surface before applying new dose. Appropriate areas of application include any hair-free area, preferably in noticeable areas when the initial dose is being determined. Application areas should be rotated. Gloves should be worn when applying topical preparation.

3. *Beta blockers*. (Atenolol, metoprolol, timlol, esmolol, propranolal) Betablocker decreases myocardial oxygen demand by decreasing contractility, slow heart rate, slow impulse conduction, decreased BP. They also increase myocardial O_2 supply, slow heart rate, thereby increasing diastolic filling time and coronary perfusion and decreases incidence of morbidity and mortality after MI. IV Metoprolol is given in 5 mg increments over 1 to 2 minutes. Other beta blockers may be prescribed IV instead metoprolol. All IV preparations are followed by oral preparations after patient is stabilized. Monitor for atrioventricular block including PR interval, symptomatic bradycardia hypotension, left ventricular failure (rales, decerease CO) and brock spasm. Beta 1 Cardio selective agents are the profound drugs. Beta 2 agents should be avoided in patients with respiratory or peripheral vascular disease. Target heart rate for betablockade is 50 to 60 beats per minute.
4. *Calcium channel blockers* (Amidolpin, dilitiagen, verapanil, nifedepin) which decrease myocardial oxygen demand and increase in myocardial oxygen supply by inhibiting the influx of calcium through the slow calcium channels. Heart rate decreases and conduction through the AV node slows (decreases demand indirectly increases supply). Inhibition of calcium influx into the arterial cell also promotes vasodilation of peripheral arteries (decreased demand) and coronary arteries (increased supply).

They often prescribed when vasospasm is considered as the part of the pathology or if significant hypertension exists. Monitor for symptomatic bradycardia, prolonger PR intervals, advanced heart blocks, hypotension, congestive heart failure and peripheraloedema.

5. *Heparin* (intravenous) prevents propogation of established thrombus by rapidly inhibiting thrombin. Nursing intervention here includes that heparin PTTs should be measured 6 hours after any change in dose. Dose is weight based. Therapeutic levels should be maintained between 1.5 and 2.5 times patient's control. Haemoglobin, haematocrit, and platelets should be followed for heparin-induced thrombocyteopnoea. Recurrent ischaemia, active bleeding and hypotension may signify sub-therapeutic or supratherapeutic dosages should be evaluated immediately.
6. *Thrombolytics* (Streptokinase, tissue plasminogen activator). They are given in acute myocardial infarction to activate plasmin for lysis of obstructive clots specific, therefore, systemic lysis may occur. Patients must be carefully screened before administration of thrombolytic agents. The nurse monitors for reperfusion, reocclusion and bleeding complications with thrombolysis administration. Interventions are directed towards preventing bleeding complications.
7. *Morphine sulphate* blunts the deleterious consequences of sympathetic stimulation with pain, and vasodilates creating decreased preload. Here, nurse should establish base-line vital signs, level of consciousness and orientation. Monitor for hypotension, respiratory depression changes in level of consciousness. Doses are usually given in increments of 2 to 5 mg.
8. *Oxygen* increases arterial O_2 saturation. Monitor for adequate arterial oxygenation with finger pulse oximetry. Maintain saturation level by about 90%.
9. *Cholesterol lowering agent* (Atorvastatin, Lovastatin, Pravastatin Simvastatin, Cremfibrozil, Nicotinic acid) they reduce the substance for lipid deposition in the coronary artery. Side effects vary with drug class. Insolence of side may limit the usefulness of certain medications. Lipid levels should be obtained at regular intervals to monitor for success in effecting charges. Patients must be educated that cholesterol-lowering agents do not substitue for dietary modification.
10. Angiotensin-converting enzyme inhibitor (Captabril, Enalapril, Beneapril, Lisinopril, Posinopril). They decrease after load and preload, thereby decreasing the workload of the heart. This prevents remodelling of the left ventricle (Remodelling refers to hypertrophy of the unaffected left ventricle to compensate for the infarcted area). Long-term consequences of remodelling are increased oxygen demand and heart failure. During their administration, nurse monitors for adverse affects: angioneurotic oedema, cough, hypotension, hyperkalaemia, pruritic rash, renal failure. First dose requires taking BP before and 30 minutes after administration. NPO (-Nil per Os-nil orally) in coronary artery diseases may be treated with following procedures.

- Intra-aortic balloon (IABP).
- Percutaneous transluminal coronary angioplasty (PTCA).
- Intracoronary stunting.
- Coronary artery bypass graft (CABP).

Health teaching for patients with coronary artery disease include use and storage of nitroglycerin in case of angina and guidelines for sexual activity after MI, risk factors, modification and resumption of activities.

1. *Use and storage of nitroglycerin.*
   - Sit or lie down at onset of angina/chest pain.
   - Place tablet under the tongue and allow tablet to dissolve, don't chew.
   - If pain not relieved within 5 minutes, take a second tablet. A third tablet can be used after an additional 5 minutes if pain persists. Continuing pain after 3 tablets and 15 minutes indicate need to receive immediate medical attention.
   - Tablet will cause tingling sensation under the tongue.

- Rest for 15 to 20 minutes after taking nitroglycerin to avoid faintness.
- A tablet with the physician's permission may be taken 10 minutes before an activity known to trigger an anginal attack.
- Anticipate the occurrence of hypotension, tachycardia, and headache in response to the medication. Headache may persist for 15 to 20 minutes after administration.
- Keep a record of number of anginal attacks experienced, the number of tablets needed to obtain pain relief and precipitating factors if known.
- Carry tablets for immediate use if necessary. Do not pack in luggage when travelling.
- Keep tablets in tightly-closed original container. Tablets need to be protected from exposure to light and moisture.
- Tablet should be stored in a cool dry place.
- Check expiry date on prescription. Tablet should be discarded after 6 months once the bottle has been opened. Plan for replacement of supply.

2. *Risk factor modification.*
   - Provide specific instruction on smoking cessation, daily exercise and diet modification.
   - Consider referral to a smoking cessation programme or outpatient cardiac rehabilitation program.
   - Encourage adherence to a diet low in calories saturated fats and cholesterol.
   - Discuss the benefits of stress management techniques in decreasing negative effect on oxygen demand. Refer to individual or group counselling as needed.
3. *Resumption of activities.*
   - Provide specific instructions on activities that are permissible and those that should be avoided.
   - Discuss resumption of driving and return to work.
   - Discuss guidelines for resuming sexual relations (e.g. 2 weeks for low risk patients to 4 weeks for Post-CABG patients) as given below:

   During sex, your heart beats should be about 117 items a minute.

Stages of sexual response

Arousal: Flushed, breathing and heart rate increase, BP goes up slightly.

Plateau: Increase in respiration, BP and heart rate.

Orgasm: (15 to 20 seconds): Pulse may reach 150 beats per min. BP reaches 160/90.

Resolution: Return to resting state within second; angina or palpations are most likely to occur during resolution.

General guidelines for sexual activity in MI

- Sexual foreplay at a relaxed pace allows your heart rate and BP to increase more slowly.
- Hugging, stroking, and touching are safe ways to get back in touch with your partner.
- Talk with your partner. Express your feelings.
- Extramarital affairs or sex with new partner may produce more stress.
- Avoid positions for sex that require you to support yourself on your arms for a long time.
- Have a sex in a pleasant, comfortable environment.
- Do not take very hot or cold baths or showers before or after sex.
- Be rested before sex.
- Do not have sex after a heavy meal or drinking alcohol.
- If you have any question about side effects of any drug, do not stop taking the drug, but talk to your health care provider.
- Masturbation and manual or oral stimulation are not harmful to your heart. Anal intercourse may lead to an irregular heartbeat. Avoid this choice unless you clear it with your health care professional.

Treatment of MI

The treatment of MI is aimed at the following.

- Protection of ischaemic and injured heart tissue to preserve muscle function.
- Reduce the infarct size and prevent death.
- Early restoration of coronary blood flow by innovation modalities, and
- Use of pharmocologic agents to improve oxygen supply and demand, reduce and/or prevent dysrhythmias, and inhibit the progression of coronary artery disease.
- Endogenous catecholamines release during pain imposes an increased workload on the heart muscle, thus causing an increase in oxygen demand.

Thus, the treatment modalities will include:

- The patient should be admitted in ICU of the hospital.
- The patient is given resuscitation if required and oxygen inhalation for respiratory distress. Good oxygen therapy improves oxygenation to ischaemic heart muscle.
- The patient is given analgesic to control pain. An opiate analgesic therapy includes:
  - Morphine is used to relieve pain, improve cardiac haemodynamics by reducing preload, and after load, and to provide anxiety relief. Those who are allergic to morphine- *meperdine* may be given to avoid respiratory depressions.
  - Nitroglycerin may be administered IV (severe cases) sublingual or paste, to promote venous (low-dose) and arterial (high-dose) relaxation as well as relaxation of coronary vessels and prevention of coronary spasm.
  - Benzodiazepinin (Diazapam) are also used with analgesics to reduce anxiety.

- In addition, following drugs will be used for MI:
  - Thrombolytic agents such as tissue plasminogen activator (Activase), Streptokinase (Streptase), and Urokinase (Abbokinase) are used to re-establish blood flow in coronary vessels by dissolving obstructing thrombus through IV or introcoronary.
  - Along with thrombolytic agents, anticoagulants are also useful for patients who are in situations like prolonged bedrest, pulmonary embolism, deep vein thrombosis, mural thrombi, cardiogenic shock and atrial fibrillation. Eg Heparine by subcutaneously and every 8 hours.
  - Beta-adrenergic blocking agents (eg. metaprolol as prescribed) are used for the purpose of limiting the extent of cardiac damage and to improve oxygen supply and demand, decrease sympathetic stimulation to the heart, promote blood flow in the small vessels of the heart, and antidysrhythmic effects.
  - For control of arrythmia, hypokalaemia if present, is corrected, and the patient is given lignocaine (xylocaine) as prescribed. Lignocaine decreases ventricular irritability, which commonly occurs in postmyocardial infarction.
  - Calcium channel blockers also may be used to improve the balance between oxygen supply and demand by decreasing heart rate, blood pressure and dilating coronary vessels.
  - In cases of sinus bradycardia, hypotension or syncope, the patient is given atropin sulphate 0.3 mg by IV and repeated if necessary.
  - If the hypotension is severe due to arrythmias, treatment is with direct current shock. In cases of ventricular fibrillation, treatment given with direct current shock. If it fails cardiac massage, alternating with direct mouth-to-mouth resuscitatiaon is given until defibrillator is available. The patient is also given IV infusion of 8.4 per cent solution of sodium bicarbonate, 50-100 ml. Thereafter, lignocain IV and follow-up as prescribed by the physician.

Nursing Management

- The patient is kept *in rest* with restriction of patients' physical activity and is advised to avoid alcohol and for abstinence from smoking (if they are in that habit). Once the acute phase is over, the patient can gradually increase physical activity and it is usually taking 6 weeks time to resume normal life.
- In *nursing assessment* the nurse should gather information regarding patient's chest pain, its nature, intensity, onset and duration, location and radiation and also precipitating and aggravating factors (any maneuvers and medications alleviating pain).
  - and also observe other symptoms experienced associated with pain i.e., diaphoresis, facial pallor, dyspnoea, guarding behaviours, rigid posture, weakness, and confusion.
  - and also previous health status- current medication, allergies, (opiate analgesics, iodine, Shellfish) recent trauma or surgery, aspirin ingestion, peptic ulcers, fainting spells, drug and alcohol use and also any significant ones.
- The probable *nursing diagnoses* will be:
  - Pain related to an imbalance in oxygen supply and demand.
  - Anxiety related to chest pain, fear of death, threatening environment.
  - Decreased cardiac output related to impaired contractility.
  - Activity intolerance related to insufficient oxygenation to perform ADL and deconditioning effects of bedrest.
  - Risk for injury (bleeding) related to dissolution of protective clot.
  - Altered tissue perfusion (Myocardial), R/T coronary restenosis and extension of infarction.

SHOCK

Shock is defined as a complex, life-threatening condition (or syndrome) characterised by inadequate blood flow to the tissues and cells of the body (Rice 1991). In other words, it is a failure of the circulatory system to maintain adequate perfusion of vital organs. Various disorders leading to inadequate tissue perfusion. This inadequate oxygenation results in anaerobic cellular metabolism and accumulated waste products in cells. If the condition is untreated, cell and organ death occurs.

Adequate blood flow to the cells and tissues require the following components.

- an adequate cardiac pump,
- an effective vasculature or circulatory system and
- adequate blood volume.

If one of these components is impaired, blood flow to the tissues will be threatened or compromised. Inadequate blood flow to the tissues results in inadequate oxygen and nutrients to the cells, cellular starvation, cell death, organ failure and eventual death if not treated. Thus, shock is a clinical syndrome resulting in decreased blood flow to body tissues, causing cellular dysfunction and eventual organ failure. Regardless of the cause of shock the end result is inadequate supply of oxygen and nutrients to body cells from impaired tissue perfusion.

Shock affects all body systems. It may develop rapidly or slowly depending on the underlying cause. During shock the body struggle to survive, calling on all its homeostatic mechanisms to restore blood flow and tissue perfusion. Shock may occur as a complication of many disorders and therefore all patients have the potential to develop shock.

(Text continue page no. 360)

Table 9.2: Nursing care plan for the patient with an acute myocardial infarction

Problem	*R*	*Objective*	*Nursing interventions*	*Rationales*
Nursing Diagnosis #1				
Tissue perfusion, alteration in, related to: 1. Coronary artery occlusion resulting in decreased myocardial tissue perfusion. 2. Ventricular dysfunction resulting in decreased perfusion to brain, kidneys, lungs and liver. 3. Thromboembolism resulting from deep venous thrombosis or mural thrombi.		Patient will: 1. Maintain haemodynamic stability: • BP within 10 mmHg of baseline. • HR 60-80/minute. • Absence of dysrhythmias. • Cardiac output 4-8 liters/minute. • Brisk capillary refill (within 2 sec). • Urine output > 30 ml/hr. • Mental status: alert, oriented. 2. Remain without thromboembolic events or, if they occur, thromboembolism will resolve without significant sequelae. • Extremities warm to touch; pulses palpable and equal bilaterally. • Absence of positive Homan's sign. • Circumference of extremities equal bilaterally.	• Initiate rest-promoting activities: Bedrest until haemodynamically stable, quiet environment; limit visitors if needed to ensure patient rest.	• Rest decreases myocardial oxygen consumption.
			• Allow bedside commode privileges if haemodynamically stable.	• Use of bedside commode is associated with less stress than use of a bedpan.
			• It MI is uncomplicated, patient should be allowed out of bed to the chair for periods of 1-2 hours and should be allowed to use the commode instead of a bedpan from the time of admission.	• Prolonged bedrest is associated with many complications (fluid shifting, orthostatic intolerance, increased heart rate, progressive decalcification resulting in osteoporosis and urolithiasis, and thromboembolism). Early ambu-lation is the most effective means to combat these.
			• For patient with complicated MI, initiate activities to counteract effects of bedrest. ◆ Elevate head of bed when possible. ◆ Have patient turn frequently in bed. ◆ Teach footboard exercises (limit contraction durations to less than 10 seconds when performing these). ◆ Apply anti-embolism stokings. ◆ Consult physician regarding initiation of mini-dose heparin (5,000 units subcutaneously q 8-12 hr).	• Footboard exercises may decrease venous stasis. Contractions less than 10 seconds in duration cause no significant detrimental cardiovascular response.
			Allow to feed self if able and if patient desires.	• Self-feeding is less stressful for most patients.
			• Assist with bathing the first day and as needed on subsequent days.	• Bed bathing is associated with insignficant cardiovascular responses in terms of blood pressure, ECG, heart sounds, oxygen uptake.
			• Monitor for factors that may cause an increase in myocardial oxygen consumption and institute measures to correct these.	• Hypotension, hypertension, increased heart rate, increased contractility, pain, fever, anaemia, volume depletion, and psychologic stress cause an increase in myocardial oxygen consumption and may increase infarct size.
			• Administer pharmacologic therapy as ordered (nitrates, nitroprusside, beta-blockers, calcium channel blockers) to increase myocardial oxygen supply or decrease MVO_2.	• Pharmacologic measures to increase myocardial oxygen supply or to decrease demand may help to limit infarct size.
			• Administer oxygen as prescribed. ◆ Monitor for possible negative effects of O_2 therapy including increased HR and systemic vascular resistance.	• Oxygen may have negative cardiovascular effects.
			• Monitor for signs and symptoms of pulmonary embolus including tachypnoea, tachycardia, shortness of breath anxiety, hypotension, deteriorating oxygenation, pulmonary artery pressure elevation, jugular venous distention.	• Early detection and treatment of thromboembolic events may aid in more successful recovery.
			• Monitor for signs of deep vein thrombosis: ◆ Positive Homan's sign. ◆ Change in colour, temperature, or girth of extremity. ◆ Presence of tenderness and/or cords.	• Early detection and treatment of thromboembolic events may aid in more successful recovery.

Contd...

Problem	*R*	*Objective*	*Nursing interventions*	*Rationales*
Nursing Diagnosis #2 Alteration in cardiac output, related to: 1. Dysrhythmias, conduction disturbances. 2. Left ventricular dysfunction. 3. Hypovolaemia.		Patient will: 1. Maintain electrophysiologic stability. • Absence of dysrhythmias. • 12-lead ECG return to baseline. 2. Maintain haemodynamic stability. • HR 60-80/min. • BP within 10 mm Hg of baseline. 3. Be normovolemic. • Cardiac output 4-8 liters/min. • Brisk capillary refill (2 seconds).	• Attach to cardiac monitor as soon as possible.	• Early detection of dysrhythmia allows for early treatment.
			• Select best lead to monitor based on type of MI patient is having type of conduction disturbance, and needs of monitor, especially if a computerized dysrhythmia detection system is used. Multiple lead monitoring is preferable.	• Appropriate lead monitoring allows ECG changes (i.e., ST segment, T wave, PR or QRS interval prolongation) to be seen and treated properly.
			• Treat lethal dysrhythmias immediately (V-tach, V-fib, asystole) per unit protocols. Notify physician.	• Prompt treatment of lethal dysrhythmias is more successful than delayed treatment.
			• Be aware of potential significance of warning dysrhythmias—VPBs > 6/minute, R-on-T VPBs, coupling.	• "Warning dysrhythmias" may precipitate episodes of V-tach, V-fib. These dysrhythmias may also occur without warning.
			• Notify physician and institute treatment of tachyarrhythmias and bradyarrhythmias as soon as possible.	• Bradyarrhythmias and tachyarrhythmias may compromise CO, and increase myocardial oxygen consumption.
			• Check vital signs (BP, HR, PAP, CVP, CO) with any change in rhythm or conduction.	• Rhythm or conduction changes may be associated with haemodynamic compromise, particularly in a patient with marginal left ventricular function.
			• Allow hot or cold beverages in small quantities if patient desires. Elevate head of bed during ingestion.	• Hot or cold beverages in small quantities (1 glass) consumed in a sitting position (at least semi-Fowler's) are not associated with dysrhythmias, ECG changes.58
			• Take oral temperature routinely; rectal temperature may be taken if necessary.	• Taking oral temperature is less stressful to the patient. • Rectal route is not associated with vagal stimulation and thus may be used if necessary.
			• Assess for signs and symptoms of left ventricular dysfunction. These include sinus tachycardia; dyspnoea, orthopnoea; pulmonary rales; S3 gallop, pulsus alternans; jugular venous pressure elevation, positive hepatojugular reflex, peripheral or sacral oedema; hypotension, elevated pulmonary capillary wedge pressure, elevated central venous pressure, decreased cardiac output and cardiac index.	• Myocardial ischaemia and/or infarct predisposes patient to left ventricular dysfunction. • Degree of LV dysfunction is a major determinant of post-MI mortality.
			• Assess for signs of ventricular septal defect (VSD) including a holosystolic murmur heard best at the lower left sternal border; left-to-right shunting; signs of heart failure as above with the degree dependent on the size of the VSD.	• Myocardial damage may result in a defect in the ventricular septal wall.
			• Assess patient for signs of hypovolaemia. These include hypotension (BP may be increased initially); decreased central venous pressure; decreased pulmonary capillary wedge pressure; tachycardia; oliguria; decreased cardiac output and cardiac index.	• Vomiting, severe diaphoresis, aggressive treatment with diuretics or nitrates may deplete intravascular volume.
Nursing Diagnosis #3 Alteration in comfort: Pain, related to: 1. Myocardial ischaemia, necrosis.		Patient will: 1. Be pain free. 2. Notify staff immediately of chest pain episodes.	• Have patient describe pain, including location, radiation, associated symptoms (nausea, vomiting, diaphoresis, shortness of breath,	• Description helps to determine aetiology of chest pain.

Contd...

Problem	*Objective*	*Nursing interventions*	*Rationales*
2. Extension of infarct. 3. Pericarditis. 4. Dressler's syndrome (late pericarditis).	3. Maintain haemodynamic stability: • BP with 10 mmHg of baseline. • HR at rest: 60-80/minute without dysrhythmias. • Mental status: Alert and oriented to person, place, and time. • Urinary output greater than 30 ml/hr.	palpitations), precipitating factors, quality, duration, relief mechanisms, association with movement, respiration or palpation.	
		• Administer nitrates and/or narcotic analgesia as needed and monitor response to therapy.	• Nitrates help to relieve pain by means of coronary vasodilatation and both preload and afterload reduction. Narcotics act centrally to relieve pain and also have some afterload reducing effects.
		• Monitor vital signs before and per unit protocol after medication administration. Assess for hypotension, tachycardia, and respiratory depression. Assess for relief of pain.	• Significant change in vital signs (BP decrease > 10 mmHg and/or HR increase >20 beats/minute and/or respiratory rate <10/minute) may necessitate discontinuation of medication.
		• Obtain 12-lead ECG prior to medication administration, particularly if this is undiagnosed or new-onset chest pain, or recurrence of chest pain in a patient who has been pain free for 24 hours.	• Documentation of changes on a 12-lead ECG helps to make the diagnosis of cardiac chest pain (vs. other types of chest discomfort), and also helps to diagnose infarct extension, Printzmetal's angina, or pericarditis.
		• Stay with patient until ischaemic chest pain is relieved.	• Presence of caring, supportive, knowledgeable nurse may reduce patient anxiety, which reduces stress response. This causes reduced circulating catecholamines (epinephrine), which help to increase the pain threshold, thereby reducing myocardial oxygen consumption.
		• Assess patient for pericarditis or Dressler's syndrome (depending on time interval after MI) if recurrent MI and infarct extension have been ruled out. Symptoms of pericarditis or Dressler's syndrome may include: ◆ Chest pain increased by deep inspiration. ◆ Chest pain alleviated by leaning forward. Presence of a pericardial friction rub. ◆ ECG changes associated with pericarditis (diffuse or localized ST segment elevation, with upward concavity). ◆ Atrial arrhythmias. ◆ Persistent fever > 101øF. (38.3°C). ◆ Symptoms of pleuritis, pericardial effusion, or tamponade. ◆ Response to aspirin or indomethacin. ◆ If patient is on anticoagulant medication, check with physician about continuation.	• Either condition may occur following myocardial infarction, particularly following transmural MIs. Symptoms are similar. Time courses are somewhat similar and overlap does occur, sometimes making it difficult to distinguish between these two syndromes. ◆ Anticoagulants may precipitate cardiac tamponade.
Nursing Diagnosis #4 Anxiety, related to: 1. Knowledge deficit regarding illness and its prognosis. 2. Pain. 3. Intensive care setting. 4. Disruption of daily life activities, role and self-image changes, family concerns.	Patient will: 1. Verbalize basic understanding of his/her illness. 2. Verbalize feeling less anxious. 3. Describe pain and verbalize when it is relieved. 4. Verbalize familiarity with ICU routines and practices.	• Assess level of understanding of disease process and readiness to learn. ◆ Provide patient with appropriate information on coronary artery disease and myocardial infarction when patient is ready. ◆ Reassure patient appropriately regarding prognosis. ◆ Initiate other anxiety-relieving measures; remain with patient during stressful periods or when patient needs to talk; encourage to verbalize fears and anxieties; listen attentively; explain all procedures and equipment	• Fear and anxiety initiate the stress response. This causes increased catecholamine release, which causes increased myocardial oxygen consumption (MVO_2), as well as decreasing the pain threshold, which further increases MVO_2.[60] ◆ Presence of a caring supportive individual may help to increase patient's ability to cope. ◆ Knowing what to expect help to reduce anxiety.

Contd...

Problem	*R*	*Objective*	*Nursing interventions*	*Rationales*
			involved in the patient's care; involve in decision-making whenever possible; instruct in relaxation techniques; limit nursing personnel caring for patient to increase continuity; orient patient and family to all ICU routines.	◆ Maintaining some sense of control helps to reduce anxiety. ◆ Use of relaxation techniques helps to promote a sense of control over situation.
			• Assess for signs and symptoms of anxiety: restlessness, agitation, tachycardia, tachypnoea, diaphoresis, crying, uncooperative or non-compliant behaviour, verbalization of fears, concerns, inability to concentrate.	• Underlying cause of anxiety must be determined in order to provide appropriate intervention. ◆ Some behaviours may be helpful during the acute phase of an MI, as for example, denial.
			• Administer nitrates and/or narcotic medications until pain is relieved or until significant decrease in BP occurs (<90-100 mmHg).	• Pain precipitates and/or aggravates anxiety. • Narcotics alleviate chest discomfort and also decrease anxiety and increase the patient's sense of well-being.
			◆ Administer sedatives as needed.	• Mild sedation helps to decrease anxiety and increase sense of well-being.
			• Manipulate ICU environment to promote as much rest for patient as possible.	• Physical rest reduces myocardial oxygen consumption, promotes a sense of well-being and reduces anxiety.
			• Assess family members' coping abilities. • Support family members in dealing with their own as well as patient's needs. • Encourage family members to avoid stressful and controversial issues at this time.	• Family coping behaviours influence patient's coping abilities and may positively or negatively affect patient's level of anxiety.[61]
			• Assess family members' level of knowledge and educate appropriately when they are ready. • Allow family members to verbalize fear, concerns.	• Family members' lack of knowledge may influence their level of anxiety and ultimately patient's anxiety level.[62]
			• Facilitate family visiting by individualizing visiting hours to patient and family needs.	• Short artificially terminated visiting hours are arousing to patient's cardiovascular system[63-64] and may increase anxiety and myocardial oxygen consumption.
			• Assess need for spiritual counselor.	• Spiritual support is helpful to some patients to decrease anxiety.
Nursing Diagnosis #5 Coping, potential inellective individual, related to: 1. Diagnosis and fear of death.	Patient will: 1. Verbalize feelings of fear and depression. 2. Use denial (if he/she chooses) as a defense mechanism to control fear and anxiety but not to interfere with ultimate acceptance of prognosis and rehabilitation program.		• Assess for symptoms of depression, including anorexia, insomnia, listlessness, crying, expression of feelings of hopelessness, lack of self-esteem. • Encourage to verbalize feelings.	• Depression may interfere with patient's ability to deal realistically with situation and may compromise patient's recovery.
			• Assess use of deniel as a defense mechanism; signs of this include explicit verbal denial, inappropriate cheerfulness, unrealistic non-compliance with medical regimen. • Support appropriate use of denial by the patient.	• Deniel is commonly used by patients after an MI to deal with theoverwhelming anxiety associated with having an MI. Survival rate during the first few days of CCU care is higher in patients who effectively deny their illness.[65,66]
			• Monitor physiologic parameters (HR + BP) closely during conversations that deal with potentially stressful topics.	• HR and rhythm changes may occur when patient engages in conversations about stressful topics[67] (pain, symptoms before admission, concerns

Contd...

Problem	*R*	*Objective*	*Nursing interventions*	*Rationales*
				about death, the consequences of death for their dependents, the consequences of continued survival, the life problems that await them after discharge, the difficulties they had with compliance, and guilt about noncompliance and its contribution to their present illness).
Nursing Diagnosis #6				
Sexual patterns, potentially altered, related to: 1. Fear and lack of knowledge about sexual activity after a myocardial infarction.		Patient and/or significant other will: 1. Feel comfortable expressing concerns about sexuality. 2. Verbalize that sexual activity is a form of exercise. 3. Be able to verbalize criteria for "safe sex" after an MI. 4. Be able to verbalize practices to be avoided.	• Answer patient's (or significant other's) questions regarding sex directly and honestly.	• Patient who brings this up during ICU stay is obviously anxious about it. Answering questions directly and honestly should decrease anxiety.
			• Describe the following guidelines to patient:	
			◆ Sex may be resumed when patient can climb 20 steps in 10 seconds without symptoms or when HR rises to 110-120 bpm without causing chest pain or shortness of breath.[68]	◆ These activities are the metabolic equivalent of sexual intercourse and can be used as guidelines for when the patient is physically ready to resume sexual activities.
			◆ Encourage foreplay before intercourse.	◆ Foreplay allows HR and BP to increase gradually.
			◆ Inform patient that intercourse in a familiar place, with a familiar partner, and in a familiar position has very little risk.	◆ Familiarity with place, partner, and position is associated with less anxiety.
			• Describe the things to avoid:	
			◆ Anal intercourse.	◆ Anal intercourse may precipitate vagal stimulation and bradycardia.68
			◆ Sex when fatigued or after a large meal or heavy alcohol intake.	◆ These increase metabolicm demands and workload on the heart.
			◆ Sex in very hot or cold environment.	◆ Same as above.

Shock is a complex clinical syndrome that may occur at any time and in any place. It is a life-threatening condition often requiring team action by many health care providers including nurses, physicians, laboratory technicians, etc.

Shock causes thousands of deaths and unknown number of permanent injuries every year. Because shock is potentially lethal, it is essential that nurses are able to identify clients at risk of developing shock, recognize the early assessment finding indicating shock, and initiate appropriate interventions before shock ensues. In order to recognize the development of shock, it is important for the nurses to understand the process taking place in the body.

Classification of Shock

There have been many attempts to classify shock, but none of these have been total satisfaction. Here, one classification suggested by many is that it is based on a consideration of defects in the three primary mechanisms responsible for adequate circulation:

i. Defect in vascular tone i.e., distributive shock.
ii. Defect in the ability of the heart to act as a pump i.e., cardiogenic shock.
iii. Defect in the intravascular volume i.e., hypovolaemic shock.

Distributive Shock

Distributive or vasogenic shock occurs when there is a maldistribution of the blood volume in the vasculature. It is due to changes in blood vessel tone, that increases the size of the vascular space without an increase in the circulating blood volume. This results in relative hypovolaemia (total fluid volume remains the same but is redistributed). Vasogenic shock is further divided into three types. i.e. anaphylactic, neurogenic and septic shock.

i. *Anaphylactic shock*

It is a severe hypersensitivity reaction resulting in massive systemic vasodilation. The precipitating factors of this anaphylactic shock will include drugs (penicillin), insect bites/stings, contrast media, blood transfusions, anaesthetic agents, foods and vaccine. Anaphylactic shock is an acute and potentially life-threatening allergic reaction. It is an immediate hypersensitive reaction characterized by dilatation of arterioles and capillaries and increased capillary permiability causing microvascular leakage throughout the body. anaphylactic shock can result in respiratory failure as a result of laryngeal oedema or severe bronchospasm and circulatory failure resulting from vasodilatation.

ii. *Neurogenic shock*

Neurogenic shock is an uncommon and often transitory disorder, is caused by massive vasodilatation as a result of loss of sympathetic vasoconstrictor tone in the vascular smooth muscle and impairment of autonomic function. The massive vasodilatation causes pooling of blood in the venous vasculature, decreased venous return to the heart, decreased cardiac output, and eventually inadequate tissue perfusion. Typically, the patient in neurogenic shock which develop hypotension, and bradycardia. There are several precipitating factors that can lead to neurogenic shock, which includes injury and disease to the spinal cord; spinal anaesthesia, deep general anaesthesia or epidural block; and vasomotor center depression due to severe pain, drugs, hypoglycaemia and emotional stress.

iii. *Septic shock*

Septic shock is due to a release of vasoactive substances. It is more commonly caused by gram-negative bacteria, although many patients with septic shock never have positive blood culture. Septic shock can also occur secondary to staphylococcal, streptococcal, fungal and protozoal infections. The causes of septic shock will include:

- Infections eg: urinary tract, respiratory tract, postabortion, postpartum, caused by invasive procedures, and indwelling lines and catheter.
- Compromised patients including older adults, patients with chronic diseases (Diabetes, Cancer and AIDS), patients receiving immonosuppressive therapy, and malnourished or debilitated patients.

Cardiogenic Shock

Cardiogenic shock often referred to as "Pump failure" occurs when heart can no longer pump blood efficiently to all parts of the body and when cardiac output is decreased. There is no decreased intravascular volume or vasodilatation of the vascular space. Cardiogenic shock is the usual result of left ventricular dysfunction. However, the right ventricle also may be involved. The ventricles are the pumping chambers of the heart and when either one fails, blood backs up into the systemic circulation. Left ventricular dysfunction causes blood to back up into pulmonary system causing pulmonary congestion and decreased cardiac output to the systemic circulation. A vicious cycle developes as the SVR increases in response to the decreased cardiac output. The failing heart has to pump harder against this higher systemic resistance.

Cardiogenic shock occurs when the heart has an impaired pumping ability, it may be of coronary or non-coronary origin. It is due to inadequate pumping action of the heart, because of primary cardiac muscle dysfunction or mechanical obstructions of blood flow caused by myocardial infarction (MI). Valvular insufficiency is due to disease or trauma, cardiac dysrythmias, or an obstructive condition such as pericardial temponade or pulmonary embolus, pericardial disease, tension pneumothorax, autovalvular damage and pulmonary embolism.

Hypovolaemic Shock

Hypovolaemic shock occurs when there is disease in the intravascular volume. It is due to inadequate circulating blood volume resulting from haemorrhage with actual blood loss, burns with a loss of plasma proteins and fluid shifts to dehydration with a loss of fluid volume. Hypovolaemic shock is the most common type of shock and develops when the intravascular volume decreases to the point where compensatory mechanisms are unable to maintain organ and tissue perfusion. The precipitatory factors of hypovolaemic shock as already stated above, to be specific, are given below:

- External fluid losses are due to:
  - Haemorrhage, (most common cause).
  - Burns.
  - Excessive use of diuretics.
  - Loss of GI Fluid (vomiting, diarrhoea, fistulas, nasogastric suctioning).
  - Diabetes insipidus.
  - Diabetic ketoacidosis.
  - Profound diaphoresis.
- Internal fluid shifts.
  - Pooling of blood in the interstitial spaces (ascitis, peritonitis and intestinal obstruction).
  - Internal bleeding (fracture of long bones, ruptured spleen, haemothorax, severe pancreatitis, femoral arterial puncture or catheters in patient on anticoagulant therapy).

Pathophysiology of Shock

Shock is a dynamic event in which several different processes may be occurring at the same time. In addition, patient may progress towards death or towards normal homeostatic functioning over widely varying time periods. The shock syndrome can be divided into four stages.

- Initial stage.
- Compensatory stage
- Progressive stage, and
- Irreversible or refractory stage.

Although there are no clear-cut divisions between the stages, in order to understand the pathophysiology of the shock syndrome, these stages are helpful.

1. *Initial stage*

During the initial stage, there will be no clinical sign or symptoms, however, changes are occurring at the cellular level. When body cells lack an adequate blood supply and an adequate supply of oxygen, the ability to metabolize energy is impaired. Energy metabolism occurs within the cell where nutrients are chemically broken down and stored in the form of adenosine triphosphate (ATP). Cells use this stored energy to perform necessary functions such as active transport, muscular contraction and biochemical synthesis as well as specialized cellular function such as the conduction of electrical impulses. ATP can be synthesized aerobically or anaerobically. Aerobic metabolism yields far greater amounts of ATP per mole of glucose than aerobic metabolism and therefore, is a more efficient and effective means of producing energy. Additionally, anaerobic metabolism results in the accumulation of the toxic and product, lactic acid which must be removed from the cell and transported to the liver for conversion into glucose and glycogen.

In shock, the cells lack adequate blood supply and are deprived of oxygen and nutrients, therefore, they must produce energy through anaerobic metabolism. This results in low energy yields from nutrients and an acidotic intracellular environment. The cell swells and its membrane becomes more permeable allowing electrolytes and fluids to seep from and into the cell. The sodium-potassium pump becomes impaired. Cell structures (mitochondria and lysosomes) are damaged and death of the cell results.

2. *Compensatory stage*

The compensatory stage is the reversible stage in which compensatory mechanisms are effective in maintaining adequate perfusion to the vital organs. In this stage, most of the metabolic needs of the body continue to be met. Here, regardless of the cause of shock, the body attempts to compensate for a decrease in tissue perfusion in a variety of ways. First, a decrease in arterial pressure causes a similar decrease in capillary hydrostatic pressure. When the hydrostatic pressure no longer exceeds the colloidal osmotic pressure, fluid moves from the interstitial space to the intravascular space. This process is sometimes called "auto-transfusion". It may add sufficient volume to the vascular space to maintain normal arterial pressure without the help of other compensatory mechanisms.

A reduction in mean arterial pressure will inhibit baroreceptor activity, resulting in stimulation of the vasomotor center in the medulla, causing activation of the sympathetic nervous system and release epinephrin. Stimulation of alpha adrenergic receptor causes selective peripheral vasoconstriction. Blood flow to the heart and brain is maintained, whereas the blood flow to the kidneys and skin is decreased. Beta-adrenergic receptors'stimulation causes a mild increase in heart rate and force of contraction, resulting in an increased cardiac output. This sympathetic stimulation causes dilatation of the coronary arteries, resulting in an increase in oxygen to the myocardium, which now has an increased oxygen demand as a result of increase in heart rate and contractability.

The decrease in the blood flow to the kidneys stimulates the release of rennin into the blood. In the blood-stream, renin activates angiotensinogen to produce angiotension I, which then circulates to the lungs where it is converted to angiotensin II. Angiotensin is a strong vasoconstrictor resulting in arterial and venous constriction. The net result is increased venous return to the heart and an increase in blood pressure. Angiotensin also simultaneously stimulates the adrenal cortex to release aldosterone, which results in sodium reabsorption by the kidneys. The increased reabsorption raises the serum osmolarity and stimulates the release of ADH. The action of ADH results in increased water reasorption by the kidneys, increased blood volume and increased venous return to the heart. Thus, venous return is increased by the combination of autotransfusion, vasoconstriction and hormonal changes. Increased venous return, as well as increased heart rate and myocardial contractility caused by beta-adrenergic receptor stimulation result in increased cardiac output, maintenance of blood pressure, and adequate tissue perfusion.

The clinical manifestation of the compensatory stage may be subtle and can be overlooked. One of the most reliable signs of this stage is the patient's level of consciousness. Subtle changes in sensorium, usually in the form of restlessness, irritability or apprehension are frequently observed and are primarily caused by hypoxia of brain cells. Sedation at this time is contraindicated because it will mask important neurologic signs. Pupil size may not be an accurate indicator of the degree of shock, because drugs such as atrophine and morphine will cause dilatation or constriction of the pupil.

During this stage, the resting supine, blood pressure may be slightly elevated, slightly decreased or normal for the patient. For this reason, blood pressure may not be useful indicator at this stage. Orthostatic hypotension (a decrease in at least 15 mm Hg. when a patient is raised from a flat position to an elevation of 90 degrees or standing) is significant and indicated absolute or relative volume depletion.

The heart rate in this stage is moderately increased. The pulse may be bounding or thready, depending on the stroke volume and the degree of peripheral vasoconstriction. Respirations increase in rate and depth in an attempt to compensate for tissue hypoxia, resulting in respiratory alkalosis. Urine output may begin to decrease because of reduced renal perfusion as a result of vasoconstriction. Because of extravascular volume, depletion, the patient complains thirst. In addition, thirst may be caused by decreased secretion of saliva secondary to peripheral vasoconstriction. Vasoconstriction in the skin will result in cool and pale extremities. An exception is septic shock, in which skin may be warm and dry. The body temperature at this stage will be slightly decreased except in septic shock, in which, it may be elevated. Bowel sounds will often be hypoactive because of decreased peristalisis as a result of reduced blood flow to the gastrointestinal system.

3. *Progressive stage*

In this stage of shock, compensating mechanisms are becoming ineffective and may even be detrimental to the patient. Aggressive management is necessary at this stage to reverse the shock stage.

When shock is not detected and the precipitating cause is not corrected during the earlier stages, a massive sympathetic nervous system occurs. Profound vasoconstriction of most vascular beds occurs with some peripheral vessels possibly becoming totally occluded. Renal ischaemia leads to activation of the renin-angiotensin mechanism, causing even more pronounced vasoconstriction. Despite the attempt of the body to increase cardiac output by increasing the heart rate and myocardial contractility, there is a net decrease in cardiac output. The decreased cardiac output and profound vasoconstriction leads to tissue hypoxia which causes the cells to undergo anaerobic metabolism. A by-product of anaerobic cellular metabolic is lactic acid production. Metabolic acidosis results from the accumulation of lactic acid and impaired renal excretion of acids. As the shock stage progresses, the rise in the lactic acid level will often correlate with the severity of the shock state. Acidosis has a direct depressant effect on cardiac function by impairing calcium metabolism within myocardial cells.

Associated with the sympathetic nervous system response is the secretion of large amounts of catecholamines from the adrenal medulla. Catecholamines enhance the cellular metabolism of the brain and heart. Catecholamines also stimulate the liver to undergo glycogenolysis, releasing its glycogen stores in the form of glucose. In addition, the pancreatic release of insulin is suppressed. Therefore, the brain, which does not require insulin for glucose utilization, has large quantities of glucose available for metabolism.

The clinical manifestation of progressive stage of shock includes the patient demonstrates listlessness, apathy and confusion. In addition a decreased response to painful stimuli may be observed. When the blood pressure begins to fall, the patient is no longer in compensatory shock. Regardless of the previous blood pressure, a systolic pressure below 80 mm Hg should be regarded as a danger signal. It is important to remember that a hypertensive patient does not often initially display a pressure this low. A guide for determining hypotension is a reduction in blood pressure greater than 25 per cent of the baseline for the patient. In addition to hypotension, a narrowed pulse pressure (difference between systolic and diastolic BP) is often present. This finding indicates decreased stroke volume from a decrease in systolic pressure and a normal or elevated diastolic pressure. Since cuff pressures are likely to be inaccurate during this stage of shock because of the severe peripheral vasoconstrictions, intra-arterial monitoring may be used to provide more reliable pressure readings.

Tachycardia is evident during this stage of shock, and the pulse is older adults and patients who are receiving beta-adrenergic blocking drugs may be an exception and show like heart rate change. Respirations increase in rate in an attempt to compensate for tissue hypoxi and metabolic acidosis. However, the respirations become more shallow as the patient begins to tire and weaken. Urine output decreases and fall below 0.5 ml/kg/hr. indicating inadequate renal perfusion, which can lead to renal failure. The lips and mucosa are dry, and the patient may continue to complain of thirst. The skin is cold, pale and clammy with slow capillary refill noted. There may be cyanosis caused by tissue hypoxia. Body temperature is usually subnormal.

4. *Irreversible or refractory stage*

Irreversible or refractory stage of shock is the stage during which compensatory mechanisms are either nonfunctioning or totally ineffective. Cellular necrosis and multiple organ dysfunction syndrome (MODS) may occur. Attempts to restore the blood pressure have failed and death is imminent.

As shock progresses, the sympathetic nervous system activity can no longer compensate to maintain homeostasis. Thus, one of the major compensatory mechanisms has failed. There is pooling and sludging of blood because of the lack of vasomotor tone. Thrombosis of small blood vessels also occurs. Tissue hypoxia resulting from peripheral vasoconstriction and decreased cardiac output makes it necessary for cells to metabolize anaerobically. The accumulation of lactic acid and other acid metabolities in the body's tissues contribute to cell death. The acid environment also causes increased capillary permeability, allows fluid and plasma proteins to leave the vascular space. Because the venous end of the capillaries remains constricted and the arterial end is dilated, blood pools in the capillary bed. This also causes further peripheral vasoconstrictions and a vicious cycle of decompensation ensues.

As shock progresses, hypotension and the resulting tachycardia decrease coronary blood flow leading to myocardial depression, which further decreases cardiac output. Cerebral ischaemia occurs. The body cannot maintain vasoconstriction for long with the vicious cycle repeating itself. Consequently, failure of the medullary vasomotor center occurs, which results in loss of sympathetic tone. The result is respiratory or cardiac arrest and death.

The clinical manifestation of this stage includes all body systems, especially the cardiovascular system, show evidence of decompensation. The patient is usually unconscious and may be unresponsive to all stimuli. The systolic blood pressure continues to fall and may not respond to therapeutic measures to raise it. The diastolic pressure blood pressure falls toward zero. The heart rate becomes progressively slower. The pulse is weak, and a pulse deficit may be present. Cardiac dysrythmias may develop because of an ischaemic myocardium and increased serum potassium levels from the release of potassium from the dead cells.

Because of the respiratory center depression, there are likely to be slow shallow respirations with an irregular rhythm and sometimes Cheyne-Stokes respirations. If the patient is in an ICU, intubation and mechanical ventilation will usually be used. Damage to the pulmonary endothelial cells increases capillary permeability and interstitial and alveola oedema and hemorahage an impaired gas exchange may occur. The resulting hypoxaemia and respiratory acidosis will further decrease tissue oxygen delivery.

Ischaemia of the intestinal mucosa also increases permeability, allowing bacteria and their toxins to enter the blood stream and causing sepsis. Renal ischaemia may result in acute tubular necrosis with altered fluid and other metabolic disturbances. Urine output is minimal, and there may be a considerable in serum creatinine and BUN level, indicating some degree of acute renal failure.

The skin is cold and clammy, with a significant decrease in temperature (except in septic shock). Cyanosis may be present and is usually observed in the lips, mucous membranes, and nail beds. However, it may be more obvious in the palms, soles and palpetral conjunctive (inside the eye lids) of dark-skinned patients.

Infection, acute tubular necrosis, acute respiratory distress and disseminated intravascular coagulation are the common complications of shock.

Management of Shock

It is difficult to know when shock actually exists and when therapy should begin. Treatment should generally be instituted for shock whenever at least two of the following three conditions occur.

- Systolic BP 80 mm Hg or less.
- Pulse pressure of 20 mm Hg or less.
- Pulse rate of 120 or more.

Pulse pressure is calculated by substracting diastolic BP from systolic BP. Normally pulse pressure is between 30 and 50 mm Hg.

Emergency Management

Emergency care of the patient in shock is important and may increase greatly the patient's chances of survival. For example, emergency management of *Hypovolaemic shock* is as follows:

The possible causes of hypovolaemic shock are major traumas resulting in multiple or serious injuries that are associated with blood or fluid loss, oesophageal varices, postoperative bleeding, etc.

The possible assessment findings are:

- Decreased level of consciousness.
- Restlessness, anxiety and weakness.
- Rapid, weak and thready pulse.
- Hypotension.
- Cool and clammy skin.
- Tachypnoea, dyspnoea or shallow irregular respirations.
- Extreme thirst.
- Nausea, vomiting.
- Chills.
- Feeling of impending doom.

Nursing intervention will be:

- Establish and maintain airway; anticipate need for intubation if respiratory distress is evident.
- Administer high flow humidified oxygen (100 per cent) by non-rebreather mask.
- Maintain cervical spine precautions if indicated.
- Monitor vital signs, level of consciousness and cardiac rhythm.
- Establish IV access with two large guage catheters and administer IV fluids.
- Assess for external bleeding sites and apply pressure dressings. Use of pneumatic antishock garment (PASG) to control bleeding if indicated.
- Assess for life-threatening injuries (ex. haemothorax, cardiac tamponade liver laceration and Pelvic fractures).
- Insert an indwelling cathetar and nasogastric tube if indicated.

Therapeutic Management

Whenever possible, the patient should be treated in an ICU and should receive continuous ECG monitoring. A general goal is to keep the mean arterial BP greater than 60 mm Hg.

- Establishment of patent airway:
- Management of shock begins by ensuring that the patient has an adequate airway. Maintaining clients' airway is vital to the treatment of shock. In all types of shock, supplemental oxygen is administered to protect against hypoxaemia. Oxygen can be delivered via nasal cannula, mask highflow nonrebreathing mask, endotracheal tube.
- Fluid Replacement:

In shock, various fluids are given to correct specific problems such as electrolyte or protein deficiencies or other defects of the blood, including acidosis and hyponatraemia. However, in treating hypovolaemic shock, the immediate result of therapy seems to depend less on the type of fluid administered for fluid replacement than on the amount of fluid administered. Because shock (except cardiogenic) almost always involves as a decreased effective circulating blood volume, the cornerstone of shock therapy is expansion of that volume by the IV administration of appropriate fluids either crystalloids, colloids or blood products or combinations. At least two large-guage IV catheters should be inserted immediately before severe vasoconstriction access and intravenous access becomes difficult.

Crystalloids are electrolyte solutions that are either hypotonic, hypertonic or isotonic relative to plasma. However, in the critically-ill patient, approximately two-thirds of the volume will diffuse out of the vascular space because of the increased permeability and reduced oncotic pressure. Therefore, large amount of crystalloids are needed for adequate volume replacement. Because of the expansion of the interstitial space following large amounts of crystalloid administration, the development of systemic oedema is common. The common crystalloids are 0.9 per cent Saline. Ringer's lactate (Isotonic); hypertonic saline 3 per cent i.e. D5 NS (Hypertonic) 45 per cent NS, 33 per cent NS D5W (hypotonic).

Colloids are primarily remaining in the intravascular space because of the size of the molecules. The osmotic pressure of these solutions draws fluid into the intravascular space expanding the intravascular volume. Colloids are extremely effective volume expanders. However, none is ideal. Each colloid has significant toxicities that must be considered. Colloids are used in the treatment of shock when plasma protein loss is excessive as in burn shock and peritonitis. If needed, packed cells are administered as soon as possible after they have been typed and crossmatched.

Pharmacologic Management

The primary purpose of drugs used in the treatment of shock is correction of the poor tissue perfusion. These drugs are administered intravenously. They are as follows:

1. *Sympathomimetic drugs* are drugs that mimic the action of the sympathetic nervous system. The effects of these drugs are mediated through action on the alpha-adrenergic, or beta-adrenergic receptors. The various drugs differ in their alpha and beta effects. Debutamine, dopaaine, epinephrine (adrenaline), isoproterenol, levarnenol, meteraminol, methaximine, and phenylephrine are examples of sympathomimetric drugs. Many of them (ephinephrine and norephinephrine) can cause peripheral. Vasoconstriction and are referred to as 'Vasopressor drugs'.
2. *Vasodilators* some patients in shock show evidence of excessive vasoconstriction and poor perfusion in spite of volume replacement and normal high systemic pressures. An excessive constriction can reduce blood flow. In such cases vasodilators are used. The common vasodilators are nitroglycerin, sodium nitroprusside, phentolamine and morphine sulphate.
3. *Corticosteroids* steroids have several effects that may assist the client in neurogenic shock after the spinal cord injury. IV corticoster roid therapy may be helpful in anaphylactic shock. Steroids may prevent the delayed symptoms that are thought to be caused by the release of chemical mediators. The common steroids used are dexamethesone, hydrocortisone and methylprednisolone. They inhibit inflammatory process, stabilizes lysosomal membranes, reduces capillary permeability, reduces release of chemical mediators in the septic process, and promotes sodium retention.
4. Antibiotics are essential when shock is due to infection. If septic shock, it is suspected that a blood specimen for culture and sensitivity is taken once and broad spectrum antibiotics are started even though the specific infections organism is not identified.

Nutritional Management

During the acute phase of shock syndrome, the patient receives nothing by mouth because of gastrointestinal tract is not adequately perfused. As recovery begins, nutrition plays an important role in limiting morbidity. Since anorexia is almost universally present, parenteral or enteral feeding is often used. Enteral tube feeding via a feeding pump is commonly the initial method of supplying nutrition. Parenteral feeding is generally adopted only if tube feeding is contraindicated or if they fail to meet the patient's caloric requirements.

Nursing Management

In shock, client's condition can change rapidly, frequent nursing assessment is essential. Documentations of progress and response to intervention needs to be concise, yet convey the client's status minute by minute.

The first step in assessing a person in shock via general overview, giving attention as necessary to the ABC's (airways breathing and circulation). Once the airway is patent, air exchange is adequate, a pulse is present and cervical spine is immobilized (if it is trauma....). Perform rapid cursory initial head-to-toe physical assessment. The initial assessment goal is to identify major problems and gross abnormalities. Give further detailed attention to specific injuries or problems after shock is stabilized with the use of physical assessment skills, the nurse has to make following observations.

- Airway patency: Presence of noisy respirations and obstructions.
- Breathing respiratory rate and efforts.
- Respiratory pattern: Chest wall expansion; Chest wall bulges or deflates. Tachypnoea, wheezing, crackles, absence of breath sounds, coughing (anaphylaxis) and choking.
- Circulation: Pulse, blood pressure, skin colour, and temperature. Tachycardia, hypotension, weak thready pulse, flat neck vein and fullness of jugular vein engorgment (JVE).
- Heart sounds: abnormal heart sounds and dysrythmias.
- Level of consciousness: Orientation X3 (Person, place, time)

ability to move extremities, sensation in all extremities, hand grasps, response to verbal and painful stimuli, pupil size and reaction to light; presence of abnormal posturing; restlessness, anxiety, altered orientation, lethargy, stupor, coma and so on to evaluate neurologic function.

- State of hydration and perfusion of skin: (eg. capillary refill time less than 3 seconds) condition of mucus membrane, sclera, and conjunctive presence of pallor cool, moist skins or warm, flushed skin (Septic and anaphylactic shock) cyanosis (Later shock) uriticaria, rash and angioedema (anaphylic shock).
- Position of trachea: tracheal deviation may indicate tension pneumothorax.
- Presence, location, intensity, duration of pain, what relieves the pain.
- Abdominal distension, rigidity, vomiting, hyperactive or diminished bowel sounds.
- Circumference of abdomen and or extremities.
- Peripheral pulses.
- Presence of incerations, contusions, ecchymoses, petechiae, purpura (also check bruising over flank area).
- Bone deformities.
- Presence of medical alert tags or bracelets.

Nursing Diagnoses

The possible potential nursing diagnoses for patient in shock are:

- Ineffective airway clearance.
- Ineffective breathing pattern.
- Impaired gas exchange.
- Altered tissue perfusion: cerebral, cardiopulmonary, renal, GI, peripheral.
- Decreased cardiac output.
- Fluid volume deficit.
- Altered nutrition: less than body requirement.
- Constipation.
- Activity intolerance.
- Impaired physical mobility.
- Sensory/perceptual alteration, visual, auditory, kinetic, olfactory, tactile gestating,
- Sleep patten disturbance.
- Impaired or risk for skin integrity.
- Self care deficit, bathing, grooming, dressing, toileting.
- Body image disturbance.
- Self esteem disturbance.
- Altered role performance.
- Personal identity disturbance.
- Anxiety, fears, pain and spiritual distress.
- Anticipatry grievance.

Planning

Nursing care of the client with shock is complex. Frequent reassessment of the client and nursing activities are essential because the client status often changes rapidly. Specific nursing and medical intervention vary according to individual needs and the setting in which care is delivered. However, these common objectives of the care of the client with shock are:

- Return of tissue perfusion and cellular function to normal.
- Meeting metabolic demands.
- Preventing further injury.
- Effective coping by the client and significant others.

Nursing Intervention

In terms of the patient's cardiovascular status, the recommended position for the treatment of shock (after the chest-X-Ray have ruled and neck and spine injury) is supine with the legs elevated to an angle of 45 degrees. The trunk should be horizontal, the head at the level of chest and the knees straight. This Trendelenburg (head down) position should be avoided in shock because it may:

- Initiate aortic and carotic sinus deflexes, causing impaired cerebral blood flow and decreased jugular venous flow.
- Cause the abdominal organs to press against diaphragm, thus limiting respiratory excursion and possibly contributing to respiratory distress.
- Decrease filling of the coronary arteries causing myocardia ischaemia.
- Cause an increase in intracranial pressure in the presence of head injury.

This modified Tredelenburg's position promotes increased venous return from the lower extremities without compressing abdominal organs against diaphragm.

(Further management refer *Nursing care plans)*

CARDIOGENIC SHOCK

Cardiogenic shock occurs when the heart muscle loses its contractile power. It is a grave condition resulting from sudden and complete loss of cardiac function.

Aetiology

Absence or inadequate contraction causing cardiac arrest occurs mainly due to: Ventricular fibrillations and occasionally due to ventricular aystole. The condition may also result from circulatory collapse with sudden hypotension as in syncope, vasomotor collapse, profound hyperthermia, CNS damage, hypovolaemic shock, severe haemorrhage, septicaemia, and accidents such as drowning and electrocution. It also occurs from drug or anaesthetic overdose and from cardiac catheterization. Extensive damage of the left ventricle due to myocardial infarction commonly initiates a perpetuating 'shock cycle'.

(Text continue on page no. 376)

Table 9.3: Nursing care plan for the patient with septic shock

Problem	*R*	*Objective*	*Nursing interventions*	*Rationales*
Nursing Diagnosis #1 Fluid volume deficit related to: 1. Distributional volume loss; shift to interstitial space. 2. Increased insensible loss with high fever.		Patient will: 1. Maintain adequate circulating blood volume and stable haemodynamic variables: • Heart rate 60-100/min when resting. • Systemic arterial blood pressure adequate for tissue perfusion. • Normal pulmonary capillary wedge pressure 8-12 mmHg. • Normal central venous pressure 0-8 mmHg. 2. Maintain normal body temperature. 3. Maintain adequate urine output > 30 ml/hour (ml/kg). 4. Maintain baseline and/or optimal neurological status. 5. Maintain fluid and electrolyte balance as demonstrated by laboratory data within normal limits: • Electrolytes. • Haemoglobin and haematocrit. • BUN and creatinine	• Assess for signs and symptoms of septic shock.	• Baseline assessment data is needed to establish the phase of septic shock: Early or late. Baseline data is useful in determining changes in patient status and evaluating response to therapy.
			• Assess for early signs of septic shock: Hyperthermia, warm, dry, flushed skin; chills; weakness; nausea, vomiting, diarrhoea.	• Early recognition of septic shock is important in order to institute prompt measures to prevent late or irreversible shock.
			• Assess neurological status: 1. Altered level of consciousness. 2. Anxiety.	• Neurologic assessment is a way to gauge cerebral perfusion. Orientation and anxiety are indicative of early septic shock, when cerebral perfusion is not as yet compromised. Confusion, disorientation, and coma may indicate decreased perfusion as seen in late septic shock.
			• Assess cardiovascular status: Hypotention; tachycardia; character of pulse. • Observe for ventricular dysrhythmias.	• Dysrhythmias may indicate decreased coronary perfusion, as seen in late septic shock.
			• Note colour and character of the skin: Cool, pale, diaphoretic.	• Cool, pale skin is a sign of decreased perfusion and peripheral vasoconstriction.
			• Assess renal function: Urine output; urine-specific gravity, urinary sodium.	• Reduced renal perfusion will reduce glomerular filtration, causing a decrease in urine output. A decrease in urinary sodium is indicative of hypovolaemia secondary to aldosterone release.
			• Obtain baseline laboratory data: Cultures: Urine, sputum; wound (if applicable).	• Determination of the portal of entry and focus of infection is crucial to successful treatment.
			• Blood cultures—two specimens from different sites by venipuncture.	• Bacteremia may be transient. Blood cultures should not be obtained through indwelling venous or arterial catheters, as they may be colonized with bacteria not responsible for the septicaemia.
			• Electrolytes. • Coagulation factors and clotting times; fibrin split products. • Haemoglobin and haematocrit. • White cell count with differential.	• These data will be helpful in monitoring fluid replacement therapy and in identifying complications such as DIC. • Eelvated leukocyte count with a left shift is frequently observed in septic shock; indicative of acute infection.
			• Assist with the insertion of haemodynamic monitoring devices. • Arterial catheters: Blood pressure; arterial blood gases.	• Haemodynamic variables (CVP, PCWP, CO, SVR, SvO_2, A-aDO_2, VO_2) are important in determining the effectiveness of fluid replacement therapy and in determining the phase of septic shock.

Contd...

Problem	*R*	*Objective*	*Nursing interventions*	*Rationales*
			♦ Pulmonary artery catheter: Central venous pressure; pulmonary artery pressure; cardiac output, SvO_2 (mixed venous gases).	♦ Reduction in oxygen tension (< 40 mmHg) in mixed venous gases (SvO_2) is indicative of compromised tissue perfusion.
			• Administer and monitor prescribed fluid replacement therapy: ♦ Monitor haemodynamic variables (as above).	♦ Higher than normal central venous pressure, pulmonary artery pressure, and wedge pressure may indicate a too rapid infusion of fluids and impending fluid overload.
			♦ Monitor hourly urine output.	♦ Urine output of greater than 30 cc/hour indicates adequate renal perfusion.
			♦ Assess respiratory status: Respiratory rate; rhythm of breathing; presence of adventitious breath sounds; crackles, wheezes.	♦ Tachypnoea and crackles may indicate fluid overload.
			• Institute measures to control body temperature.	• High body temperatrue increases the metabolic rate of the tissues and may exacerbate tissue ischaemia and hypoxia.
			♦ Monitor body temperature every 2 hours if the patient is febrile.	♦ Insensible fluid loss may increase when the patient is febrile.
			♦ Administer antipyretic drugs as ordered; evaluate response to therapy. ♦ Apply hypohyperthermia blanket as prescribed: – Manual mode. – Automatic cooling mode using rectal probe.	♦ Continuous measurement of temperature while the patient is on a cooling blanket will prevent excessive cooling and chills.
Nursing Diagnosis #2 'otential impaired gas exchange related to: 1. Hypovolaemia resulting in reduced pulmonary perfusion (ventilation/perfusion mismatch). 2. Altered alveolar-capillary membrane.		Patient will: 1. Maintain acceptable blood gas parameters: • pH 7.35-7.45 • pO_2 > 60 mmHg • pCO_2 ~ 35-45 mmHg 2. Maintain baseline and/or optimal neurological status.	• Assess respiratory status.	• Respiratory distress syndrome may occur in septic shock secondary to decreased perfusion and endotoxin damage to the pulmonary vasculature.
			♦ Respiratory rate and rhythm.	♦ Altered respiratory patterns such as hyperventilation and tachypnoea occur secondary to fever and sympathetic nervous system stimulation.
			♦ Breath sounds.	♦ Development of abnormal breath sounds such as crackles indicate fluid overload and pulmonary oedema.
Nursing Diagnosis #3 ineffective, related to: 1. Tachypnoea, hyperventilation.		Patient will: 1. Achieve effective alveolar minute ventilation (arterial blood gas values as above). 2. Verbalize ease of breathing.	♦ Monitor arterial blood gases and pH.	♦ Decreased PaO_2 creased $PaCO_2$ > 50 mmHg (room air) are signs of impending respiratory failure.
			• Maintain patent airway. • Administer and monitor oxygen and respiratory therapy. ♦ Monitor arterial blood gases.	• Patients with septic shock may require endotracheal intubation.

Contd...

Problem	*R*	*Objective*	*Nursing interventions*	*Rationales*
			◆ Observe for increase peak inspiratory pressures during mechanical ventilation.	◆ In the patient requiring mechanical ventilation, increased inspiratory pressures indicate decreased lung compliance observed in respiratory distress syndrome.
			• Assess neurological status.	• Changes in mental status may indicate cerebral hypoxia.
Nursing Diagnosis #4 Alteration in cardiac output: decreased, related to: 1. Decreased venous return (late septic shock).		Patient will: 1. Demonstrate stable haemodynamic variables: • Blood pressure > 90 mmHg systolic. • Pulmonary capillary wedge pressure 8-12 mmHg. • Cardiac output > 4 liters/min. • Systemic vascular resistance 800-1400 dyne-seconds/cm^5. 3. Maintain adequate urine output > 30 ml/hour (ml/kg). 4. Maintain adequate respiratory status: • Respiratory rate < 30/min. • Absence of adventitious breath sounds. • Arterial blood gases within acceptable limits. 5. Demonstrate adequate peripheral tissue perfusion: • Warm, dry skin. • Absence of cyanosis. • Absence of skin breakdown. 6. Maintain baseline/optimal neurological function: • Level of consciousness: Oriented to person, place, time. • Deep tendon reflexes brisk.	• Assess haemodynamic status. ◆ Cardiac output. ◆ Pulmonary capillary wedge pressure. ◆ Systemic vascular resistance. • Assess neurological status. • Assess respiratory status: ◆ Rate and rhythm of breathing. ◆ Adventitious breath sounds. • Administer and monitor the effects of prescribed medical interventions: Vasodilators; positive inotropes; antiarrhythmics.	• Increase cardiac output and decreased systemic vascular resistance are observed in early septic shock; however, in late septic shock, cardiac output is reduced and systemic vascular resistance is high. Monitoring these variables will determine the effectiveness of therapeutic interventions. • Changes in neurological status may indicate decreased cerebral perfusion, secondary to decreased cardiac output. • Acute respiratory failure may develop secondary to cardiac failure. Baseline data are needed in order to monitor the effectiveness of therapeutic interventions.
Nursing Diagnosis #5 Potential impairment of skin integrity, related to: 1. Immobility. 2. Decreased tissue perfusion.		Patient will: 1. Demonstrate skin integrity as evidenced by the absence of skin breakdown and pressure ulcers.	• Assess skin condition frequently. • Perform passive range of motion exercises. • Provide pressure relief device. • Teach the patient to shift position frequently. • Establish a turning schedule of every 1-2 hours depending on the patient's condition.	• To improve peripheral circulation. • Pressure ulcers may be prevented by reducing the amount and duration of pressure to a given area.

Contd...

Problem	*R*	*Objective*	*Nursing Interventions*	*Rationales*
Nursing Diagnosis #6 Potential for reinfection.		Patient will: 1. Re-establish and maintain normal body temperature. 2. Remain without new evidence of infection.	• For specific nursing interventions and rationales, refer similar, Nursing Diagnosis mentioned in earlier NCPs.	
Nursing Diagnosis #7 Anxiety related to: 1. Intensive care environment. 2. Septic shock.		Patient will: 1. State that he/she feels less anxious. 2. Verbalize feelings about illness and care in the intensive care unit. 3. Perform relaxation techniques.	• For specific nursing interventions and rationales, refer similar Nursing Diagnosis mentioned earlier NCPs.	
Nursing Diagnosis #8 Sleep pattern disturbance related to: 1. Intensive care environment. 2. Anxiety. 3. Assessments and treatments.		Patient will: 1. State that he/she feels rested. 2. Verbalize feelings about illness.	• Plan nursing care activities such as assessment, treatments, and tests to allow for rest periods. • Determine the patient's normal sleep pattern. • Assess the duration and quality of sleep as perceived by patient. • Administer prescribed sedatives and hypnotics. ◆ Monitor for signs of respiratory depression: Significantly decreased respiratory rate (< 8 spontaneous breaths/min); evidence of reduced alveolar hypoventilation.	• Longer periods of rest can be provided when nursing care is organized. • Knowledge of the patient's normal sleep pattern is useful to determine the timing and length of rest periods. ◆ Patients in ICU may sleep upto 50 per cent of their limited sleep time during the day; little or no sleep may occur at night due to frequent awakenings and anxiety.

Table 9.4: Sample care plan for the patient with anaphylactic shock

Problem	*R*	*Objective*	*Nursing Interventions*	*Rationales*
Nursing Diagnosis #1 Airway clearance, ineffective: actual or potential related to: 1. Bronchospasm, laryngospasm. 2. Increased pulmonary secretions in response to release of chemical mediators from degranulated mast cells.		Patient will: 1. Maintain adequate alveolar ventilation and oxygenation: • $PaCO_2$ ~ 35-45 mmHg (room air). • PaO_2 > 60 mmHg. • pH 7.35 - 7.45. 2. Verbalize ease of breathing; breath sounds clear on ausculation; absence of adventitions breath sounds. 3. Verbalize reduced perform relation exercises: demonstrate a relaxed demeanour.	• Assess respiratory function: ◆ Respiratory parameters: Respiratory rate, rhythm; diaphragmatic excursion; use of accessory muscles; ◆ Presence of abnormal or adventitious breath sounds on auscultation. ◆ Neurological parameters: Mental status: Orientation to person, place, and date. ◆ Cardiovascular parameters: Vital signs. ◆ Arterial blood pressure • Implement measures as to assure a patent air way:	• It is essential to establish baseline function to facilitate evaluating the patient's response to therapeutic measures. ◆ Adventitious sounds are noted with special emphasis placed on the pressure of stridor and wheezing. Inspiratory wheezes and stridor are ominous signs. ◆ A deterioration in the level of consciousness may be the first warning sign of inadequate oxygenation and tissue perfusion.

Contd...

Problem	*R*	*Objective*	*Nursing Interventions*	*Rationales*
			◆ Maintain upright position.	◆ Upright position allows for chest wall expansion and diaphragmatic excursion; accessory muscles can be utilized to the fullest.
			◆ Place suction and intubation equipment at the bedside.	◆ Suction equipment, etc., is needed for prophylactic readiness in case, laryngospasm or oedema compromises the airway.
			◆ Initiate oxygen therapy as prescribed (e.g., nasal cannula at 2 liters/min).	◆ Oxygen prevents hypoxia and consequent respiratory acidemia.
			◆ Obtain baseline arterial blood gases (room air) prior to initiating oxygen therapy. ◆ Monitor serial arterial blood gas parameters.	◆ Monitoring of arterial blood gasses provides a direct indication as to the effectiveness of therapeutic measures in assisting the patient to maintain adequate gas exchange.
			• Administer medication regimen as prescribed: ◆ Anticipate subcutaneous injection of epinephrine.	◆ Subcutaneous route may be safer because it is more slowly absorbed. There are fewer adrenergic side effects. Epinephrine will help to control bronchospasm, and improve ventilation.
			◆ Implement Alupent treatments in conjunction with the Respiratory Therapy department as per physician.	◆ Alupent, a frequently used adrenergic agent, stimulates beta receptors and thus exerts the following effects: Bronchodilation, positive inotropic and chronotropic cardiac activity, and decreased synthesis and release of chemical mediators by most cells.
			• Provide restful and calm environment to reduce tension and anxiety. ◆ Spend time at the patient's bedside. ◆ Keep abreast of progress. ◆ Instruct regarding relaxation exercises. ◆ Provide periods of uninterrupted rest and/ or sleep.	
Nursing Diagnosis #2 Fluid volume deficit, actual or potential, related to: 1. Vasodilation. 2. Increased capillary permeability with increased third- spacing (angioedema).		Patient will: 1. Maintain stable vital signs: • Blood pressure within 10 mmHg of baseline. – Heart rate < 100 beats/min.	• Monitor vital signs, particularly blood pressure and heart rate.	• An increase in blood pressure and decrease in heart rate may be indicative of restoring circulatory volume and cardiac output.
			• Monitor intake and output hourly.	• Renal function parallels normal cardiac output and normovolaemia. Urine output should be maintained at > 30 ml/hour.
		2. Remain without evidence of third-spacing. (e.g., no angioedema or pitting oedema).	• Implement prescribed fluid regimen.	• Initial fluid challenges must be monitored in relation to patient's clinical status.
			◆ Initiate intravenous therapy with lactated Ringer' solution (fluids may need to be infused wide open).	◆ Ringer's lactate is the most compatible physiologic (isotonic) solution and can be infused at a rapid rate in an attempt to stabilize intravascular volume.

Contd...

Problem	*R*	*Objective*	*Nursing Interventions*	*Rationales*
			♦ Anticipate repeated doses of SQ epinephrine, followed by intravenous administration if there is no clinical improvement.	♦ Epinephrine is an endogenous catecholamine that stimulates both alpha and beta receptors. It will increase the heart rate and myocardial contractility; it will increase systemic vascular resistance and thereby increase arterial blood pressure. It may be necessary to give epinephrine intravenously since peripheral perfusion may be inadequate for SQ or IM injection if the shock state progresses. The intravenous route is fast and efficacious, but when this route is unavailable, epinephrine may be instilled directly into the endotracheal tube after intubation (as prescribed).
Nursing Diagnosis #3 Anxiety related to: 1. Respiratory distress (hypoxia and dyspnoea stimulate flight/fight responses and emotional distress). 2. Hypotensive state.		Patient will: 1. Verbalize ways to reduce stress and avoid panicking. 2. Assume a relaxed demeanour.	• Implement measures to assist patient/family to maintain control and react appropriately in the event of an emergency.	
			♦ Assist patient to assume a position of comfort—may try orthoponea.	♦ Facilitates ease of breathing and may relieve respiratory distress.
			♦ Allow patient decision-making alternatives.	♦ Anxiety may be decreased when patients are permitted decision-making power. ♦ Choices facilitate autonomy and self-control.
			♦ Speak in a calm, soothing voice.	
			♦ Offer optimistic reassurances.	♦ There are positive psychological benefits derived from reassurances.
			♦ Do not leave patient unattended.	♦ Fear is perpetuated when patient is left alone. The patient's condition may deteriorate rapidly.
			♦ Keep patient/family informed of treatments and progress.	♦ Fear of the unknown is alleviated.
			♦ Consider the sedative effects of drugs such as Benadryl to assist in management anxiety.	♦ Benadryl can be used as an adjunct epinephrine therapy, after the acute symptoms are controlled.
Nursing Diagnosis #4 Skin integrity, impairment of, related to: 1. Severe urticaria with pruritus		Patient will: 1. Avoid scratching. 2. Demonstrate ways to avoid scratching (e.g., massaging with prescribed lotion). 3. Maintain intact skin, with absence of antioedema.	• Implement measures to relieve itching and maintain skin integrity:	
			♦ Apply cool compresses to affected areas, PRN.	♦ Cool temperatures reduce the discomfort that coincides with pruritus and angioedema.
			♦ Remove all unnecessary clothing/bedding.	♦ Removal of clothing sometimes relieves itching and feelings of constriction.
			♦ Instruct patient to avoid scratching: if all else fails, instruct patient to use fingertips rather than nails, and to use a massaging motion.	♦ Scratching disrupts skin integrity, the first line of defense against infection.
			♦ Administer Benadryl as prescribed.	♦ Benadryl competes with histamine for the histamine receptor sites. It effectively controls localized itching.

Contd...

Problem	*R*	*Objective*	*Nursing Interventions*	*Rationales*
			◆ A prescription may be given upon discharge that includes oral Benadryl and/or a topical cream.	◆ Since some chemical mediators (e.g., SRS-A) have slower and more prolonged action, an antihistamine and local, topical agents may be prescribed to counteract the annoying skin cryptions (urticaria).
Nursing Diagnosis #5 Knowledge deficit related to: 1. Inability to identify allergen (allergen was disguised as a preservative). 2. Delay in receiving treatment (driving to distant hospital rather than the one nearby; this may have exacerbated the shock-state).		Patient will: 1. Review sources of sulphur preparations. 2. Discuss cross-reactivity with allergens. 3. Verbalize need to expedite emergency treatment upon exposure to allergen(s).	• Assess patient/family knowledge regarding allergic status: Known allergens; precautions taken to avoid exposure to allergen(s); emergency care with onset of allergic reaction.	• Assessing patient/family knowledge base regarding anaphylaxis assists in determining essential information to include in patient/family instruction; it may also help to discern misunderstandings that might complicate the patient's care.
			• Assess readiness to learn. ◆ Identify support system in family.	• It is imperative that one or more family members be versed in emergency first-aid measures should the patient develop anaphylactic shock.
			• Implement patient/family education program: ◆ Teach the importance of reading all labels.	◆ Sulfiting agents (e.g., sulphur, sodium or potassium bisulphate or sodium sulphite) are commonly used as antioxidants and food preservatives. Potatoes, shellfish, and wines are just a few items that contain sulphites.
			◆ Reinforce responsibility to notify all health professionals of specific allergies.	◆ Patients are active participants as well as recipients of interdisciplinary health care.
			◆ Encourage patient to wear a "medic alert" tag/bracelet.	◆ Identification of the allergen or anaphylactoid reaction may be lifesaving, especially if only minutes can be spared.
			◆ Recommend an allergy referral.	◆ Clients who experience severe systemic reactions need a referral for further evaluation and care.
			◆ Inform patient/family that treatment must be sought immediately as subsequent reactions may be more severe.	◆ Phase two reactions cause chemical mediators to be released into the blood, since the patient is already sensitized (i.e., has preformed IgE antibody from initial exposure). Treatment must be solicited at nearest hospital, via ambulance if necessary.

Table 9.5: Nursing care plan for the patient with hypovolaemic shock

Problem	*R*	*Objective*	*Nursing Interventions*	*Rationales*
Nursing Diagnosis #1 Tissue perfusion, alteration in: Cerebral, renal, and peripheral, related to:		Patient will maintain adequate tissue perfusion:	• Assess for signs/symptoms of hypovolaemic shoc:	• A baseline assessment is necessary to establish stage of shock and to determine emergent measures

Contd...

Problem	*R*	*Objective*	*Nursing Interventions*	*Rationales*
1. Reduced circulating blood volume. 2. Fluid volume deficit.		1. Arterial blood pressure within 10 mmHg of baseline. 2. Heart rate less than 100 beats/minute. 3. Mental status: Alert; oriented to person, time, and place. 4. Skin warm, dry to touch; usual colour, good turgor, good capillary refill (<2 seconds). 5. Urinary output greater than 30 ml/hr. 6. Arterial blood gases within normal range: • PaO_2 > 80 mmHg • $PaCO_2$ 35-45 mmHg • HCO_3 22-26 mEq/liter • pH 7.35-7.45 7. SVO_2 about 75 per cent.		indicated; serves as a measure of the patient's response to therapy.
			◆ Assess cardiovascular function: ◆ Blood pressure (orthostatic).	◆ A drop in blood pressure of 10-15 mmHg from supine to sitting/standing position suggests blood loss of about 1 liter.
			◆ Heart rate, rhythm.	◆ Reflects effect of altered intravascular volume on cardiac function.
			◆ Resting peripheral pulses.	◆ Peripheral pulses, if palpable, may be weak and thready due to decrease in stroke volume and peripheral vasoconstriction.
			◆ Skin colour, moisture, temperature, and turgor.	◆ When tissue perfusion is decreased, skin becomes cool and clammy to the touch and pale in colour; cyanosis may occur if reduced haemoglobin concentration exceeds 5 g/100 ml.
			◆ Assess neurologic function: – Mental status. – Orientation.	◆ Appropriateness of patient's behaviour and responses reflects adequacy of cerebral tissue perfusion.
Nursing Diagnosis #2 Cardiac output, alteration in decreased, related to: 1. Decreased venous return (preload).		Patient will maintain stable haemodynamics: 1. Central venous pressure 0-8 mmHg. 2. Pulmonary artery pressure <25 mmHg (systolic). 3. Pulmonary capillary wedge pressrue 8-12 mmHg. 4. Cardiac output 4-8 liters/minute. 5. Systemic vascular resistance (SVR) 800-1200 dynes/sec/cm-5.	◆ Assess renal function: – Urine output. – Intake and output.	◆ Reduced circulating blood volume and hypotensive state compromise renal perfusion. Rine output is a reliable indicator of renal perfusion.
			◆ Assess gastrointestinal function: – Bowel sounds, abdominal distention, pain.	◆ Decrease in blood flow to fluids and fluid volume expanders and blood and blood products may be necessary to restore circulating blood volume.
			• Establish/maintain 1 or more large-gauge intravenous access sites.	• Rapid administration of fluids and fluid volume expanders and blood and blood products may be necessary to restore circulating blood volume.
			• Initiate timely and aggressive fluid replacement therapy and monitor response to therapy: ◆ Administer crystalloids, colloids. ◆ Transfuse blood/blood products.	
			• Initiate haemodynamic monitoring: Arterial, pulmonary artery, and pulmonary capillary wedge pressures.	• Insertion of systemic arterial and pulmonary artery catheters in the setting of massive haemorrhage and/or fluid loss with massive fluid volume replacement is essential to accurately follow trends and evaluate patient's response to therapy.
			◆ Initiate monitoring of mixed venous blood (SVO_2).	◆ Status of mixed venous blood reflects adequacy of peripheral tissue perfusion.
			• Monitor hydration status during fluid replacement therapy: ◆ Assess respiratory function:	◆ Detection of adventitious breath sounds (crackles, rhonchi) in

Contd...

Problem	*R*	*Objective*	*Nursing Interventions*	*Rationales*
			– Respiratory rate, rhythm, chest excursion, breath sounds, use of accessory muscles; status of neck veins.	previously clear lungs suggests overhydration.
			◆ Obtain daily weight. ◆ Monitor intake and output.	◆ Most accurate measure of hydration status.
			• Insert Folcy catheter to measure hourly urine output.	• Hourly urine outputs reflect status of renal perfusion and underlying haemodynamic status.
			• Insert nasogastric tube.	• Decompresses stomach to facilitate respiratory excursion and prevent aspirtion of stomach contents, and affords means to monitor for gastrointestinal bleeding.
			• Monitor haematology profile: ◆ Haematoacrit, haemoglobin, RBCs, platelets	• Reflects haemoglobin oxygen-carrying capacity; decrease in haemoglobin levels compromises oxygen delivery to tissues.
Nursing Diagnosis #3 Anxiety, related to: 1. Haemorrhage. 2. Transfusion therapy. 3. Inherent sympatho-adrenal activity (enhanced). 4. ICU setting.	Patient will: 1. Verbalize feeling less anxious. 2. Demonstrate relaxed demeanour. 3. Perform relaxation techniques with assistance. 4. Verbalize familiarity with ICU setting.		• Assess signs/symptoms of anxiety: ◆ Restlessness, agitation, diaphoresis; tachypnoea, tachycardia, palpitations; uncooperative or non-compliant behaviour; verbalization of fears and concerns.	• Thorough assessment assists in discerning underlying cause of anxiety and provides a basis for therapy. Patients with hypovo-laemic shock may experience anxiety associated with massive sympathoadrenal output.
			• Examine circumstances underlying anxiety.	• Removal of precipitating cause may reduce anxiety.
			◆ Manipulate ICU environment to provide calm, restful periods.	◆ Reduction instimuli is essential to assist patient to relax. This is especially important in the patient at risk of bleeding or rebleeding.
			• Assess patient coping behaviours and their effectiveness in dealing with current stressors.	• Experiencing a bleeding episode can be very distressing.
			◆ Provide positive reinforcement when desired outcome is achieved.	◆ Positive feedback and reassurance nurture self-confidence and confidence in health team.
			• Initiate interventions to reduce anxiety: ◆ Relieve pain or other discomfort. – Medication for pain; monitor response. – Comfort measures.	◆ Pain precipitates and/or aggravates anxiety.
			◆ Monitor effectiveness of ventilation and oxygenation. ◆ Serial arterial blood gases.	◆ Inadequate gas exchange, "air hunger," hypoxaemia, and/or hypercapnia may cause the patient to experience a "sense of doom."
			◆ Listen attentively, encourage verbalization, provide a caring touch.	◆ These nursing activities reassure the patient that he/she is not alone.
			◆ Let the patient know it's okay to feel anxious and afraid.	◆ Reassurance helps patient to focus on feelings and to work them through.
			◆ Remain with patient during periods of acute stress.	
			• Assess readiness to learn and implement the following when appropriate:	• Readiness to learn facilitates meaningful learning and a sense of accomplishment.
			◆ Orient patient to environment, ICU equipment and routines, and staff. – Explain all procedures and activities involving patient.	◆ Knowing what to expect helps to reduce anxiety.

Contd...

Problem	*R*	*Objective*	*Nursing Interventions*	*Rationales*
			♦ Involve patient in decision-making regarding care when possible and appropriate.	♦ Helps patient to maintain some degree of control of health management.
			♦ Assist in establishing short-term goals and desired patient outcomes.	♦ Builds and reinforces self-confidence.
			♦ Instruct patient in relaxation techniques when it is prudent to do so.	♦ Use of energy-release techniques allows an outlet for pentup feelings; enables patient to have some control over anxiety.
Nursing Diagnosis #4 Fluid volume, alteration in, related to: 1. Haemorrhage. 2. Fluid shifts associated with loss of plasma proteins (hypoprotenoaemia, hypoalbuminaemia).		Patient will: 1. Maintain body weight within 5 per cent of baseline. 2. Balance fluid intake and output. 3. Exhibit good skin turgor, absence of peripheral oedema, absence of jugular venous distention, absence of adventi-tious breath sounds. 4. Maintain serum electrolytes within normal limits.	• Maintain fluid and electrolyte balance. ♦ Administer prescribed fluid volume.	• Fluid therapy is the mainstay of treatment of hypovolaemic shock to restore/maintain tissue perfusion.
			♦ Document intake and output, urinezapecific gravity. ♦ Record daily weight.	♦ Close monitoring of urine output helps to evaluate renal perfusion and assess overall haemody-namics.
			♦ Monitor serum electrolytes.	♦ Rapid and massive fluid volume replacement therapy can dilute electrolytes and precipitate electrolyte imbalance.
			• Monitor haemodynamic parameters: ♦ Arterial blood pressure. ♦ Pulmonary artery pressure parameters. ♦ Central venous pressure. ♦ Cardiac output.	• These measures best reflect the patient's status and response to therapy. Rapid administration of crystalloids and colloids may precipitate fluid shift between extracellular and intracellular compartments.
			• Implement nursing measures to improve and/or maintain cardiac output: ♦ Assist patient into positions of comfort that facilitate breathing. – Head of bed elevated to 20-30 degrees.	♦ Placing patient with hypovolaemic shock into Trendelenburg's position (i.e., the legs higher than the head) may be of little value to haemodynamics or to improvement of cardiac output. Optimal ventilation/perfusion matching occurs in dependent areas of lungs.
			♦ Maximize patient activities in accordance with the acuity and limitations of the illness.	♦ Nursing interventions are implemented to maximize circulation, prevent pooling or stasis of blood, ensure adequate venous return, and promote comfort.
			♦ Provide special care to back and to skin over joints and pressure points. ♦ Assist with passive range-of-motion exercises.	♦ Compromised circulation in a patient with reduced tissue perfusion increases the risk of tissue ischaemia and stasis of blood predisposing to venous thrombosis, and reduces venous return and cardiac output.

Pathophysiology

Pathological changes occur according to predisposing factors. An impaired contractility causes a marked reduction in cardiac output. This decreased cardiac output results in a lack of blood and oxygen. The lack of blood and oxygen to the heart muscles results in continued damage to the heart muscle, a further decline in contractile power and a continued inability of the heart to provide blood and oxygen to the vital organs. At the end-stage, cardiomyopathy, severe valvular dysfunction, and ventricular aneurysm also precipitate cardiogenic shock.

Clinical manifestation

- Confusion, restlessness, mental lethargy due to poor perfusion of brain.
- Low systolic pressure (HP 80 mm Hg or dp mm Hg less than previous level).

- Oliguria-urine output less than 30 ml per hour for at least 2 hours - due to decreased perfusion of kidney - oliguria may lead to acute tubular necrosis.
- Cold, clammy skin- The onset is sudden or gradual, but it presents with pale, cold, sweaty skin (due to blood is shunted from the peripheral circulation to perfuse vital organs).
- This condition may give rise to hypotension, tachycardia and heart sound may be difficult to analyse as sinus tachycardia is more than 100 per minute.
- Weak thready, peripheral pulses, fatigue, hypotension are due to inadequate cardiac output.
- There may be peripheral vasoconstriction leading to peripheral cyanosis or gangrene.
- There will be dyspnoea, tachypnoea, cyanosis due to increased left ventricular pressures resulting in elevation of left atrial and pulmonary pressure, causing pulmonary congestion.
- There may be dysrythmias due to lack of oxygen to heart muscle and sinus tachycardia as a compensatory mechanism for decreased cardiac output.
  There may be Chenyes-stokes respiration, confusion, irritability and an impairment of continuousness.
- Chest pain due to lack of oxygen and blood to heart muscle.
- There may also be progressive acidosis, visual and cerebral impairment while the cardiac arrythmias may be intractable.
- If late, there may be permanent cerebral damage or loss of peripheral tissue even after recovery.
- Hypoxaemia is common particularly when there is pulminory oedema.
- Neurologic impairment, respiratory distress, renal failure, multiorgan dysfunction syndrome and death are the complications of cardiogenic shock.

Diagnosis

Diagnosis of the condition is made on clinical grounds PCWP, 18 mm Hg or greater, chest-x-ray (Pul. Vascular congestion) Abnormal laboratory value such as BUN, creatinine and liver enzymes.

Medical Measures

- Use of cardiac glycosides (Digoxin) and positive inotropic drugs (dopamir to stimulate cardiac contractility as prescribed).
- Use of vasodilators to decrease workload of heart and temporary cardiac output.
- Use of vasopressors (sometimes it requires).
- Use of diuretics to decrease total body fluid volume and to relieve systemic and pulmonary congestion.
- Introducing counterpulsation therapy.
- Cardiopulmonary bypass.
- Left ventricular assisting device.
- Emergency cardiac surgery.

Nursing Management

The nurses should make continuous nursing assessment which includes:

- Identify patients at risk for development of cardiogenic shock.
- Assess the early symptoms that are indicative to shock, restlessness, confusion, increasing heart rate, decreasing pulse pressure.
- Observe the presence of pulses alternansm (LHF), decreasing urine output, weakness, fatigue, etc.
- Observe the presence of central and peripheral cyanosis.
- Observe the development of oedema.
- Identify signs and symptoms indicative to myocardial infarctions.
- Identify patients' and significant others' reaction to crisis situation.

The probable nursing diagnosis may be:

- Decreased cardiac output related to impaired contractility due to extensive heart muscle damage.
- Impaired gas exchange related to pulmonary congestion due to elevated left ventricular pressure.
- Altered tissue perfusion (renal, cerebral, cardiopulmonary gastrointestinal, and peripheral) related to decreased blood flow.
- Anxiety related to ICU and threat to death.

Nursing intervention: The condition urgently calls for identification of the primary cause and immediate management. The patient is protected from unnecessary disturbance and is maintained adequate airway. The patient is also given oxygen inhalation and small doses of morphine (IV) for anxiety and pain. For further details please see nursing care plan.

HEART FAILURE

Heart failure occurs when the myocardium is unable to maintain a sufficient cardiac output to meet the metabolic needs of the body. This condition results from systolic dysfunction or diastolic dysfunction.

- Systolic dysfunction results from inadequate pumping of blood from the ventricle. The decrease in pumping power results in a decreased cardiac output. Any process that alters myocardial contractility can produce systolic dysfunction.
- Diastolic dysfunction (stiff heart syndrome) occurs when the ventricle does not fill adequately during diastole. Inadequate filling decreases the amount of blood in the ventricle for cardiac output. Systolic function is often normal or augmented.

(Text continue on page 379)

Table 9.6: Nursing care plan of cardiogenic shock

Problem	*Reason*	*Objective*	*Nursing Intervention*	*Evaluation*
1. Decreased cardiac output	(Write Subjective and Objective data)	Improved cardiac output.	• Position the patient properly as directed. • Establish continuous ECG monitoring. • Monitor haemodynamic parameters continually (PAP, PCWP, CO, CI,SVR) • Administer cautiously drugs as prescribed, i.e. digoxin, IV fluids, vasodilators, diuretics as prescribed. • Observe any side effects of drugs. • Monitor blood pressure and mean arterial pressure (MAP). • Maintain MAP less than 60 mm Hg. • Measure and record urine output every hour. • From indwelling catheter and fluid intake. • Obtain daily weight. • Evaluate serum electrolytes Na+, K+. • Be alert to chest pain and report immediately.	
2. Impaired gas exchange.	"	Improved gas exchange	• Monitor rate and rhythm of respiration every hour. • Ascultate lung sound for abnormal sounds. • Evaluate arterial blood gas (ABGs). • Administer oxygen therapy to increase O_2 tension and improve hypoxia. • Elevate the head of bed 20 to 30 degree as tolerated. • Reposition the patient to promote ventilation and maintain skin integrity. • Observe for frothy pink-tinged sputum & cough. • Report abnormality immediately.	
3. Altered tissue perfusion	"	Maintain tissue perfussion	• Perform a neurologic check every hour, using Glasgow coma scale. • Report changes immediately. • Obtain BUN and creatinine blood levels to evaluate renal function. Ausculate for bowel sounds every 2 hours. • Evaluate character, rate, rhythm and quality of arterial pulses every 2 hours. • Mention temperature every 2 to 4 hours. • Protect the skin breakdown.	
4. Anxiety	"	Reduce anxiety	As state in other NEP	
5. Knowledge deficit R/T cardiogenic management	"	Knows management of condition	• Teach the patient on degoxin the importance of medication is prescribed. • Teach how to take pulse before digoxin and after reporting any abnormality. • Teach the signs of impending heart failure. – increasing oedema, shortness of breath, decreasing urine output, increasing pulse and report immediately. – Teach specific measures as in MI.	

Aetiology

The incidence of heart failure increases with advancing age and coronary artery disease. An increase in the number of survivors of MI is in part responsible for the increasing number of patients with heart failure. Additional predictors of heart failure include diabetes, cigarette smoking, obesity and elevated total cholesterol-to-high density lipoprotein cholesterol ratio, and abnormally high or low haematocrit level and proticnuria.

The common causes for chronic and acute heart failure (CCF) are as follows:

Chronic	*Acute*
• Coronary artery disease	• Acute myocardial infarction.
• Hypertensive heart disease	• Arrhythmias
• Rheumatic heart disease	• Pulmonary emboli
• Cor pulmonale	• Thyrotoxicosis
• Cardiomyopathy	• Hypertensive crisis
• Anaemia	• Rupture of papillary muscle
• Bacterial endocarditis	• Ventricular sepral defect.

The common casues for systolic and diastolic dysfunctions are as follows:

Systolic	*Diastolic*
• Coronary artery disease	• Coronary artery disease
• Hypertension	• Hypertrophy
• Metabolic disorders	• Fibrosis of advanced age constrictive pericarditis
• Myocarditis	• Myocarditis
• Alcohol	• Hypertension
• Cocaine	• Aortic stenosis
• Cardiac valve diseases	• Ventricular remodelling
• Dilated cardiomyopathy	• Collagen diseases
	• Cardiomyopathy.

Congestive heart failure may be caused by any interference with normal mechanisms regulating cardiac output. Cardiac output depends on preload, afterload, myocardial contractility, heart rate and metabolic state of the individual. Any alteration in these factors can lead to decreased ventricular function and the resultant of manifestations of CCF; there are some precipitating causes for heart failure. The common precipitating causes for CCF and their mechanism are as follows:

- Anaemia : Decreases oxygen carrying capacity of the blood, stimulating increase in cardiac output to meet tissue demand.
- Infection : Increases oxygen demand of tissues stimulating increase in cardiac output.
- Thyrotoxicosis : Increases the tissue metabolic rate, accelerating heart rate and workload of the heart.
- Hypothyroidism : Indirectly predisposes to increase atherosclerosis, severe hypothyroidism decreases myocardial contractility.
- Arrhythmias : May decrease cardiac output and increase workload and oxygen requirement of myocardial tissue.
- Bacterial-endocarditis : Increases metabolic demands and oxygen requirements.
- Valvular dysfunction : Causes stenosis and regurgitation.
- Pulmonary embolism : Increases pulmonary pressure and exerts a pressure load on right ventricle, leading to right ventricle hypertrophy and failure.
- Pulmonary disease : Increases pulmonary pressure and exerts a pressure level on the right ventricle, leading to RVH failure.
- Paget's disease : Increases work load of the heart by increasing the vascular bed in skeletal muscle.
- Nutritional deficiencies : May decrease cardiac function by decreasing myocardial muscles mass and contractility.
- Hypovolaemia : Increases preload and causes volume load on Right Ventricle (RV).

Classification of Heart Failure

In addition to above types of heart failure, heart failure can be classified as follows.

1. *Left-sided V/S right-sided heart failure*
    - In left-sided heart failure, left ventricle cardiac output is less than volume received from the pulmonary circulation; blood accumulates in left ventricle, left atrium and pulmonary circulation.
    - In right-sided heart failure, right ventricle cardiac output is less than volume received from the peripheral venous circulation, blood accumulates in RA, RV and peripheral venous system.
2. *Forward v/s backward failure*
    - In forward failure, decreased cardiac output results in inadequate tissue perfusion.
    - In backward failure, blood remains in ventricle after systole, increasing atrial and venous pressure; rise in venous pressure forces fluid out of capillary membrane into extracellular spaces.
3. *High-output V/s low-output failure*
    - High output failure occurs in response to conditions that cause the heart to work harder to supply blood; the increased oxygen demand can be met only with an increase in cardiac output; systemic vascular resistance decreases to promote cardiac output.
    - Low output failure occurs in response to high blood pressure of hypovolaemia which, results in impaired peripheral circulation and peripheral vasoconstriction.

4. *Acute v/s chronic failure*
   - Acute failure occurs in response to a sudden decrease in cardiac output which results in rapid decrease in tissue perfusion.
   - So chronic failure, body adjusts to decrease in cardiac output through compensatory mechanisms which results in systemic congestion.

Recently New York Heart Association classified heart failure as follows:

- Class I : No symptoms tolerate ordinary physical activity.
- Class II : Comfortable at rest, ordinary physical activity results in symptoms.
- Class III : Comfortable at rest, less than ordinary physical activity results in symptoms.
- Class IV : Symptoms may be present at rest, symptoms with any physical activity.

Pathophysiology

In most cases heart failure begins with left ventricular systolic dysfunction. Ventricular failure can be described as:

- A defect in systolic functions that results in impaired ventricular emptying; or
- A defect in diastolic function that causes an impairment in ventricular filling.

It is now recognised that patients with heart failure actually comprise three distinct groups:

i. Those with failure of systolic ejection;
ii. Those with abnormal resistance to diastolic filling; and
iii. Those with mixed systolic and diastolic dysfunction.
   - Systolic failure is the most common cause of heart failure. It is a defect in the ability of the cardia myofibrils to shorten, which decreases the muscles' ability to generate enough pressure to eject blood forward through the high-pressure aorta. Inability to move blood forward through the aorta results in:
     - A decreased left ventricular ejection traction (LVET).
     - An acute increase in left ventricular endodiastolic pressure (LVEDP).
     - An increase in fluid accumulation in the pulmonary vascular bed (pulmonary congestion).

Systolic failure is due to impaired contractile function (MI), increased after local (HBP) or mechanical abnormalities (valvular disease).

- Diastolic failure is not a disorder of contractility, but of relaxation and ventricular filling. In fact, there is normal or hyperdynamic systolic function. Diastolic failure is characterized by high-filling pressure and the resultant venous engorgement in both the pulmonary and systemic systems. The diagnosis of diastolic failure is made on the basis of the presence of pulmonary congestion and pulmonary hypertension in the setting of a normal ejection pattern.
- Systolic and diastolic failure of mixed origin is seen in disease state such as dilated cardiomyopathy (DCM), a condition in which poor systolic function is further compromised by dilated left ventricular walls that are unable to relax. This patient often have extremely poor ejection tractions, high pulmonary pressures and biventricular failures.

Heart failures can have an abrupt onset as with acute MI or it can be an insidious process resulting from slow progressive changes. The overloaded heart resorts to certain compensatory mechanisms which include:

- Ventricular dilation.
- Ventricular hypertrophy.
- Increased sympathetic nervous system stimulation and
- Hormonal response.

Dilation is an enlargement of the chambers of the heart. It occurs where pressure in the heart chambers, usually, the left ventricle is elevated over time. The muscle fibres of the heart stretch and thereby increase that contractile force. Initially this increased contraction leads to increased cardiac output and maintenance of arterial blood pressue and perfusion. Therefore, dilation is an adaption mechanism to cope with increasing blood volume. Eventually this becomes inadequate because the elastic elements of the muscle fibres are overstretched and overstrained.

Hypertrophy is an increase in the muscle mass and cardiac wall thickness in response to overwork and strain. It occurs slowly because it takes time for this increased muscle tissue to develop. It generally follows persistent or chronic dilation and then further increases the contractile power of the muscle fibres. This will lead to an increase in cardiac output and maintenance of tissue perfusion. However, hypertrophic heart muscle has poor contractility.

Sympathetic nervous system activation is often the first mechanism triggered in low cardiac out put. It is a least effective compensatory mechanism, because there is inadequate stroke volume and CO. There is increased sympathetic nervous system activation resulting in the increased release of epinephrine and norepinephrine. This results in an increased heart rate. Myocardial contractility and peripheral vascular constrictions. This improves cardiac output (CO). However, later, it leads to worsening the ventricular performance with overlooked volume due to peripheral vascular conditions.

Hormonal responses—As the CO falls, blood flow to the kidneys decreases, causing decreased glomerular blood flow. This is interpreted by the juxtaglomerular apparatus in the kidney as decreased volume. The decrease in renal blood flow activates the renin-angiotensin system to correct a perceived hypovolaemia. Angiotension causes the adrenal cortex to release aldesterone which causes sodium retention and increased peripheral vasoconstriction, which increases asteral blood pressure. The posterior pituitary senses the increased osmotic pressure and it secretes ADH, which increases water absorption in renal tubules causing water retention and therefore increased blood volume. Therefore, the blood volume is increased in a person who is already volume overloaded.

Clinical Manifestations of Heart Failure

Classic symptoms of heart failure include dyspnoea with exertion, orthopnoea, nocturnal dyspnoea, a dry, hacking cough, and unexplained fatigue. When volume overload contributes to pathology, the following additional symptoms occur: rales, a third heart sound, peripheral oedema, unexplained weight gain, jugular venous distention, hepatic engorgements, ascitis and worsening dyspnoea. Compensatory mechanism accounts for many of the clinical signs and symptoms of heart failure.

The more common symptoms as well as symptoms encountered with progressive heart failure are as follows:

1. *Respiratory symptoms*
   - Dyspnoea.
   - Orthopnoea.
   - Paroxysmal noctural dyspnoea.
   - Persistent hacking cough.
   - Alternating periods of apnoea and hyperapnoea.
   - Rales (Crackles).
2. *Cardiovascular symptoms*
   - Angina.
   - Jugular venous distention.
   - Tachycardia.
   - Decrease in systolic blood pressure with increase in diastolic pressure.
   - S_3 and S_4 heart sounds.
3. *Gastrointestinal symptoms*
   - Enlargement and tenderness in the right upper quadrant of abdomen.
   - Ascitis.
   - Nausea.
   - Vomiting.
   - Bloating.
   - Anorexia.
   - Epigastric pain.
4. *Cerebral symptoms*
   - Altered mental status (confusion, restlessness).
5. *Generalized symptoms*
   - Fatigue.
   - Decrease in activity intolerance.
   - Oedema (Peripheral pitting).
   - Weight gain.
6. *Psychosocial*
   - Anxiety.

The clinical manifestations specific to right-sided and left-sided heart failure are as follows:

1. *Right-sided heart failure.*
   Signs
   - Right ventricle heaves.
   - Murmurs.
   - Peripheral oedema.
   - Weight gain.
   - Oedema of dependant body part (sacrum, anterior tibias, pedal oedema).
   - Ascitis.
   - Anasarea (Massive generalized body oedema).
   - Jugular venous distension.
   - Hepatomegaly (Liver engorgement).
   - Right-sided pleural effusion.

   Symptoms
   - Fatigue.
   - Dependent oedema.
   - Right upper quadrant pain.
   - Anorexia and GI bloating.
   - Nausea.
2. *Left-sided heart failure*
   Signs
   - Left ventricle heaves.
   - Cheyne-stokes respirations.
   - Pulsus alternans (alternating pulses: strong, weak).
   - Increased heart rate.
   - PMI displaced inferiorly and posteriorly (LV hypertrophy).
   - Decreased PaO_2, slight increased $PaCO_2$ (poor oxygen exchange).
   - Crackles (Pulmonary oedema).
   - S_3 and S_4 heart sounds.

   Symptoms
   - Fatigue.
   - Dyspnoea (Shallow respiration upto 32-40/m).
   - Orthopnoea (Shortness of breath in recumbent position).
   - Dry, hacking cough.
   - Pulmonary oedema.
   - Nocturia.
   - Paroxysmal nocturnal dyspnoea.

Management of Heart Failure

Along with other team members, nurses assess the health status of the patient with heart failure by identifying the clinical manifestations particularly paroxysmal nocturnal dyspnoea, orthopnoea, new-onset of dyspnoea on excretion, fatigue, lower extremity oedema, persistent cough and recent weight gain and records, and perform physical assessment which includes third heart sound, respiratory distress, pulmonary rales, elevated jugular venous pressure, increased in daily weight without increased intake, abdominal distension, cool extremities and decreased pulse, alteration in level of consciousness and decreased urine output.

In addition, nurses also assist in diagnostive test such as ABGs, serum chemistries, liver profile, chest X-ray, haemodynamic monitoring, Twelve-lead ECG and monitor echocardiogram, nuclear imaging studies and cardiac catheterization.

Nursing diagnosis are determined from analysis of patient's data. The possible nursing diagnosis will include:

- Decreased cardiac output R/T alteration in preload, afterload or inotropic changes in heart.
- Impaired gas exchange R/T alveololar-capillary membrane changes.
- Fluid volume excess R/T imbalance between O_2 supply and O_2 demand.
- Hopelessness R/T failing or deteriorating physiological changes.

The objectives of nursing intervention will be:

- Improving cardiac output.
- Improving gas exchange.
- Restoring fluid volume balance.
- Improving activity tolerance.
- Supporting the patient experiencing hopelessness and
- Educating the patient and family regarding care.

The guidelines for taking care of the person with heart failure are as follows:

1. *Support oxygenation*
   a. Administer oxygen by nasal cannula at 2 to 6L/min. for oxygen saturation greater than 90 per cent.
   b. Give oxygen as needed for dyspnoea.
   c. Patient should be well supported in a semi-Fowler's position.
   d. Encourage use of incentive spirometry fourth hourly.
2. *Balance rest and activity.*
   a. Reinforce importance of conservation of energy and planning for activities that avoid fatigue.
   b. Encourage activities within prescribed restriction; monitor for intolerance to activity (dyspnoea, fatigue, increased pulse rate doesn't stabilize).
   c. Assist with ADL as necessary; encourage independence within patient's limitations.
   d. Provide diversional activities that assist in conservation of energy.
   e. Provide calm and quiet environment.
3. Perform head-to-toe assessment in each shift, including assessment of lab. values, daily weight, and intake and output.
4. Provide skin care, particularly over oedematous areas; use prophylactic measures to prevent skin breakdown.
5. Assist in maintaining an adequate nutritional intake while observing prescribed dietary modifications (offer small meals with supplements).
6. Monitor constipation, give prescribed stool softners.
7. Give prescribed medications and monitor for adverse effects.
8. Provide patient and family with opportunities to discuss their concerns and time to learn about the diagnosis and plan of care.

Role of Nurses in Medication

Nurses are also responsible for educating the patient as well as family regarding the care of the person with heart failure which include:

1. Monitor for signs and symptoms of recurring heart failure and report these signs and symptoms to the primary provider.
   - Weight gain of 1 to 1.5 kg (2 to 3 lb).
   - Loss of appetite.
   - Shortness of breath.
   - Orthopnoea.
   - Swelling of ankles, feet or abdomen.
   - Persistent cough.
   - Frequent night-time urination.
2. Avoid fatigue and plan activity to allow for rest periods. Incorporate ADL, occupational activity and sexual activity into daily routine by pacing activities.
3. Plan and eat meals within sodium restrictions.
   - Avoid salty foods.
   - Avoid drugs with high sodium content (eg. some laxatives and antacids, Alee-seltser)- read the labels.
   - Eat several small meals rather than three large meals per day.
4. Take prescribed medications.
   - If several medications are prescribed, develop a method to facilitate accurate administration.
   - Digitalis: Check own pulse rate daily; report a rate of less than 50/min to primary provider and signs and symptoms of toxicity.
   - Diuretics:
     - Weigh self daily at same time of day.
     - Eat foods high in potassium and low in sodium (such as oranges, bananas) if on potassium-depleting diuretics.
   - Vasodilators:
     - Report signs of hypotension (light-headedness, rapid pulse, syncope) to physician.
     - Avoid alcohol when taking vasodilators.
5. Adopt healthy lifestyle choices; daily routines; develop support groups; smoking cessation; alcohol intake limited to not more than one drink per day and minimize risk of infections.
6. Comply with follow-up appointment.
   Thorough evaluation also needed for follow-up scheme.

Table 9.7: Nursing care plan for the patient with heart failure

Problem	*R*	*Objective*	*Nursing Interventions*	*Rationales*
Nursing Diagnosis #1				
Cardiac output, alteration in, decreased, related to: 1. Impaired myocardial contractile functioning. 2. Filling disorders. 3. Abnormal volume load. 4. Abnormal pressure load.		Patient will: 1. Demonstrate signs of haemodynamic stability: • Cardiac output 4-8 liters/minute. • Heart rate < 100 beats/minute. • Systolic blood pressure > 110 mmHg or within 10 mmHg of baseline. • Pulmonary capillary wedge pressure 8-12 mmHg (mean). • Absence of S3 and S_4. 2. Maintain electrophysiologic stability. • Absence of dysrhythmias. 3. Maintain state of normovolaemia. • Good skin turgor. • Absence of peripheral oedema. • Absence of jugular venous distention. • Absence of rales on auscultation. • Stable baseline body weight.	• Ongoing assessment of signs and symptoms of left ventricular failure:	• Provides a systematic approach to data collection to gauge the severity of the disease and the efficacy of therapeutic intervention.
			• Rales (crackles).	• Fluid in alveoli, the result of pressure increases in the pulmonary capillary bed.
			• Bronchial wheezing.	• Bronchiolar constriction from excess fluid.
			• Dyspnoea.	• Result of elevation in pulmonary interstitial oedema.
			• Paroxysmal nocturnal dyspnoea.	• Serum proteins are at lowest level in early morning; redistribution of volume secondary to recumbent position; nocturnal respiratory depression.
			• Nocturia.	• Increased renal perfusion secondary to postural redistribution of blood flow.
			• Orthopnoea.	• Result of increased venous return from postural redistribution of pulmonary blood flow.
			• Anxiety, restlessness, disorientation.	• Decreased cerebral perfusion and cerebral hypoxia.
			• Pulsus alternans (see Fig. 38-2).	• Secondary to variation in strength of ventricular contraction.
			• Gallop rhythms.	• S_3 associated with increased LVEDP, left atrial pressure, and PCWP. • S_4 related to decreased ventricular compliance.
			• Peripheral cyanosis.	• Secondary to decreased cardiac output and decreased peripheral circulation; blood stays in peripheral tissues longer to extract more oxygen, and when blood reaches distal vascular bed, it has a markedly diminished O_2 content.
			• Central cyanosis.	• Results when alveolar oedema impairs O_2 diffusion.
			• Blood-tinged sputum.	• Rupture of bronchiolar capillaries due to increased hydrostatic pressure in capillaries.
			• Cheyne-Stokes respirations.	• Decreased cardiac output causes prolonged circulation time, which in turn causes the respiratory center in the brain-stem to be underperfused and underoxygenated.
			• Ongoing assessment of the signs and symptoms of right ventricular failure:	
			• Jugular venous distention.	• Result of elevated venous pressures.
			• Peripheral oedema. • Weight gain. • Ascites.	• May gain as much as 10-15 lb of extracellular fluid before oedema is readily apparent.

Contd...

Problem	*R*	*Objective*	*Nursing Interventions*	*Rationales*
			◆ Hepatojugular reflux.	◆ Pressure on right upper quadrant compresses liver and acts as a temporary fluid challenge; dysfunctional right heart will show a visible increase in pressure in jugular veins; competent right heart will not show a visible increase in pressure.
			◆ Anorexia, nausea, vomiting.	◆ Increased pressure in capillaries of abdominal organs results in oedema; nausea is secondary to stretching of liver capsule secondary to oedema.
			• Identify and correct (if possible) precipitating factors of heart failure.	• Any factor that increases metabolic demand of body stresses the cardiovascular system, which can precipitate the development of heart failure in the patient with cardiac dysfunction. Identification fosters early, more effective intervention.
			• Monitor fluid balance: ◆ Measure weight daily. ◆ Document intake and output, urine specific gravity. ◆ Maintain fluid restriction as indicated. ◆ Use microdrip or infusion pump for fluid administration.	
			• Monitor haemodynamic parameters.	• Provide best indication of patient's response to therapy.
			◆ Arterial blood pressure.	◆ Decreased systolic pressure or narrowed arterial pulse pressure indicative of decreased cardiac output; increased diastolic blood pressure indicates increased peripheral vascular resistance.
			◆ Allow for frequent rest periods.	◆ Reduces ratigue, decreases myocardial oxygen consumption.
			◆ Administer oxygen as prescribed.	◆ Reduces workload of heart and supports cellular energy requirements. ◆ Correction of hypoxia related to pulmonary congestion. ◆ Myocardial tissue hypoxia predisposes to dysrhythmias and further decreases myocardial contractility.
			• Institute measures to allay anxiety (see Nursing Diagnosis #4).	
			• Administer prescribed medication regimen to maximize effects of preload, afterload, and myocardial contractility.	
			◆ Cardiac glycosides.	◆ Positive inotropic and negative chronotronic agent - improved cardiac output.
			◆ Diuretics: – Monitor I and O; daily weight. – Monitor for side effects of diuretic therapy (hypokalaemia, hyponatra-emia, fatigue, muscle cramps, hypotension, tachycardia).	◆ Decrease intravascular volume by their direct action on the kidney and by reducing sodium reabsorption; increase venous capacitance, reduce preload to maximize Frank-Starling mechanism.

Contd...

Problem	*R*	*Objective*	*Nursing Interventions*	*Rationales*
				• Increased venous capacitance provides beneficial effect in patients with left heart failure and pulmonary oedema; in patients with right heart failure with vigorous diuresis, this may be detrimental as it contributes to systemic venous pooling, thereby limiting venous return and right ventricular filling and further contributing to a decreased cardiac output.
			• Vasodilators: – Monitor for side effects and efficacy of therapy (headache, dizziness, hypotension, postural hypotension, muscle weakness, syncope; $\downarrow$ SVR, $\downarrow$ PCWP, $\downarrow$ RA pressure, diuresis, increased exercise tolerance, resolution of heart failure symptoms).	• Vasodilators increase cardiac output by decreasing SVR and/or reducing LVEDP by decreasing vascular tone. Vasodilators reduce myocardial oxygen demand, which may help minimize ischaemia and infarction size.
			• Pulmonary capillary wedge pressure.	• Pulmonary oedema develops when PCWP exceeds plasma osmotic pressure (> 28 mmHg). • Measure of LVEDP preload; optimal PCWP maximizes contractility via Frank-Starling mechanism. Elevated in aortic stenosis and regurgitation, mitral stenosis and regurgitation, cardiogenic shock, dilated cardiomyopathy, hypertropic cardiomyopathy, and restrictive cardiomyopathy.
			• Cardiac output and cardiac intake.	
			• Systemic vascular resistance.	• Determinant of afterload; increased impedance to left ventricular ejection increases intramyocardial wall tension; result of sympathoadrenergic stimulation; increased SVR increases myocardial oxygen requirements and decreases myocardial contractility.
			• Right atrial pressure.	• Elevated in pulmonary hypertension, tricuspid and pulmonic stenosis, tricuspid regurgitation right heart failure, and hypervolaemia.
			• Monitor laboratory/diagnostic data.	
			• Arterial blood gases.	• Increased work of breathing secondary to pulmonary congestion leads to hypoxia and hypercapnia, which further depress myocardial contractility.
			• Electrolytes.	• BUN, Na—reflect hydration status; hypokalaemia—diuresis-induced; hyperglycaemia—secondary to stress-related catecholamines.
			• ECG.	• May reveal evidence of ischaemia, LVH, RVH, dysrhythmias.

Contd...

Problem	*R*	*Objective*	*Nursing Interventions*	*Rationales*
			◆ Chest x-ray.	◆ Presence of pleural effusion, usually right-sided or bilateral (rarely on the left); interstitial pulmonary oedema; enlarged cardiac silhouette.
			◆ Circulation time.	◆ Prolonged secondary to decreased contractility of ventricles leading to decreased cardiac output.
			◆ Elevated bilirubin, SGOT, and LDH.	◆ Result of hepatic congestion in right heart failure.
			◆ Protenuria, increased specific gravity, increased BUN and creatinine.	◆ Indicate renal dysfunction as a result of decreased cardiac output and decreased glomerular filtration rate.
			• Implement measures to reduce cardiac workload:	
			◆ Place patient in semi-Fowler's position if blood pressure tolerates.	◆ Diminishes venous return and promotes adequate lung expansion.
			◆ Sympathomimetics.	◆ Positive inotropic agents that increase cardiac output by increasing stroke volume and contractility; myocardium becomes dependent on circulating catecholamines in heart failure, and sympathomimetic administration provides an exogenous source of catecholamines to support myocardial contractility.
			• Assess the effects of systemic congestion and decreased cardiac output on drug therapy.	• Hepatic congestion and renal dysfunction may alter drug metabolism and excretion, predisposing the patient to toxic side effects.
			• Assess medication regimen for drugs with negative inotropic effects; discuss with physician before discontinuing.	• Such drugs may cause further compromise of cardiac function but may be controlling dysrhythmias, which may also precipitate a deterioration in patient's condition and in cardiac output.
			• Monitor for dysrhythmias.	
			◆ Maintain continuous ECG monitoring.	
			◆ Monitor conditions that precipitate dysrhythmias (hypoxia, acidosis, alkalosis, digoxin toxicity, electrolyte imbalcne) and implement corrective action.	◆ Increased irritability of myocardium predisposes to dysrhythmias.
			◆ Document rhythm changes and assess for haemodynamic compromise; notify physician of patient response.	◆ Bradyarrhythmias may decrease cardiac output secondary to decreased stroke volume. ◆ Tachyarrhythmias reduce diastolic filling time and increase myocardial oxygen consumption. Loss of atrial kick contributes to a decreased cardiac output.
			◆ Administer treatment to correct dysrhythmias (may include pacing, antiarrhythmics, and/or cardioversion).	
			• Identify factors that exacerbate structural abnormalities of cardiac function and institute appropriate therapy.	
			◆ Hypertrophic cardiomyopathy: Avoid conditions that increase the degree of	◆ Digitalis, exercise, beta-agonists, and Valsalva maneuvers increase

Contd...

Problem	*Objective*	*Nursing Interventions*	*Rationales*
		obstruction and/or decrease ventricular volume (digitalis, diuretics, nitrates, exercise, sudden postural changes, Valsalva maneuvers, beta-antagonists). ◆ Encourage factors that increase cardiac output (alpha-stimulants, supine or squatting position). • Prepare for insertion of mechanical circulatory assist devices. • Maintain properly functioning emergency equipment and ensure its availability on each shift.	contractility and the degree of obstruction should be avoided. Diuretics, nitrates, sudden postural changes decrease ventricular volume.
Nursing Diagnosis #2 Tissue perfusion alteration in, related to: 1. Severely impaired myocardial contractility.	Patient will: 1. Demonstrate signs of haemodynamic stability: • Systolic BP > 90 mmHg. • Diastolic BP 60-90 mmHg. • PCWP 8-12 mmHg (mean). • Cardiac output 4-8 liters/minute. • Heart rate < 100 beats/minute. • SVR 800-1200 dynes/sec/cm-5. 2. Maintain adequate tissue perfusion. • Patient awake, alert, oriented. • Urine output > 30 ml/hr. • Skin warm and dry. • Absence of peripheral oedema. • Absence of rales (crackles) on auscultation. 3. Maintain electrophysiologic stability. • Absence of dysrhythmias. 4. Maintain arterial blood gases within normal limits. 5. Verbalize anxieties and concerns.	• Identify patients at risk of developing cardiogenic shock.	• Early recognition and intervention are crucial determinants to patient survival.
		• Assess signs of inadequate tissue perfusion. ◆ Coronary: ◆ Blood pressure.	◆ Decreased pulse pressure, increased diastolic blood pressure, systolic pressure less than 90 mmHg: Indicative of increased SVR and decreased cardiac output.
		◆ Heart rate.	◆ Compensatory tachycardia.
		◆ Cardiac output/cardiac index.	◆ Decreased in heart failure; indicator of tissue perfusion.
		◆ SVR.	◆ Measurement of afterload; increased secondary to sympathetic nervous system stimulation.
		◆ MAP.	◆ Decreased MAP and increased LVEDP (PCWP) result in decreased coronary artery perfusion potentially resulting in myocardial ischaemia and necrosis.
		◆ Right atrial pressure.	◆ Measurement of adequacy of central venous return.
		◆ PAP, PCWP.	◆ Increased secondary to impaired myocardial contractility; maintained slightly higher than normal to maximize Frank-Starling mechanism; serial measure-ments to evaluate left ventricular function and response to therapy.
		◆ Monitor for signs of left or right ventricular failure and dysrhythmias.	◆ See Nursing Diagnosis #1.
		◆ Evaluate medication regimen for any treatments that may cause myocardial depression.	◆ See Nursing Diagnosis #1.
		◆ Assess for signs and symptoms indicative of myocardial ischaemia and necrosis.	◆ Refer to discussion of myocardial infarction.
		◆ Renal: ◆ Measure urine output hourly; notify physician <30 ml/hr. ◆ Measure intake and output. ◆ Monitor BUN and creatinine. ◆ Assess for increased tolerance to diuretic therapy.	◆ Decreased cardiac output results in decreased renal perfusion and function; the afferent arterioles vasoconstrict and glomerular filtration decreases, which results in a decreased ability of the kidneys to filter, excrete, and reabsorb.

Contd...

Problem	*R*	*Objective*	*Nursing Interventions*	*Rationales*
			• Cerebral:	
			• Assess neurologic status: LOC; restlessness, agitation, confusion, and somnolence; response to verbal and tactile stimuli; EOMs and pupillary responses.	• Decreased cardiac output causes diminished carotid and vertebral artery blood flow. Blood flow to medulla remains normal until late in the stages of shock; midbrain, cerebellum, and cerebral cortex are under-perfused.
			• Respiratory.	• For respiratory assessment, interventions, and rationales see Nursing Diagnosis #3, below.
			• Cutaneous:	
			• Assess capillary refill.	
			• Assess warmth, colour, and moistness of skin.	• Cool, moist skin indicates decreased perfusion secondary to redistribution of blood flow to central circulation.
			• Assess quality of peripheral pulses.	• Weak, thready peripheral pulses are indicative of vasoconstriction.
			• Visceral:	
			• Monitor bowel sounds.	
			• Assess for abdominal discomfort.	• Indicative of decreased perfusion and ischaemia to splanchnic area secondary to a profound decrease in cardiac output.
			• Laboratory data (see Nursing Diagnosis #1):	
			• Arterial blood gases.	• Acidosis depresses myocardial contractility; acidosis indicates inadequate tissue perfusion and accumulation of lactic acid.
			• Venous blood saturations.	• Increased arterial-venous O_2 difference indicates increased O_2 extraction by tissues in response to a decreased cardiac output.
			• Electrolytes.	• Hyponatraemia and hyperkalaemia are myocardial depressants.
			• Serum lactate level.	• Elevated secondary to anaerobic metabolism.
			• Assess for hypovolaemia (hydration status).	
			• Intake and output including extrarenal (insensible) losses; urine output; PCWP; and weight changes.	
			• Keep physician informed of patient's status.	
			• Monitor effects of fluid challenge if ordered.	• Contraindicated for PCWP > 20 mmHg; CVP > 12 cmH_2O.
			• Administer fluid challenge (0.9 per cent normal saline) rapidly: 100 ml every 5-10 minutes.	• Ensures intravascular expansion.
			• Determine CVP or PCWP after each bolus.	• End points of challenge are hypotension; PCWP at 20 mmHg; CVP increase by 2 cmH_2O. • PCWP > 20 mmHg increases likelihood of precipitating pulmonary oedema.
			• Administer medications as prescribed.	

Contd...

Problem	*R*	*Objective*	*Nursing Interventions*	*Rationales*
			• Monitor medications for efficacy and toxicity.	• Hypotension, redistribution of blood volume, impaired renal and hepatic perfusion may impair absorption and metabolism.
			• Monitor haemodynamic parameters to assess efficacy of pharmacologic therapy.	• Best indices to LV function and systemic perfusion.
			• Monitor arterial pH.	• Most vasoactive therapy has decreased efficacy in an acidotic or alkalotic environment.
			• Prepare for use of mechanical circulatory assistance if above measures are ineffective in restoring tissue perfusion.	• Decreases after load during systole and increases perfusion by increasing aortic pressure during diastole.
			• Institute measures to allay anxiety.	• See Nursing Diagnosis #4, below).
Nursing Diagnosis #3 Gas exchange, impaired, related to: 1. Pulmonary congestion with increased ventilation/ perfusion mismatching, and shunting.		Patient will: 1. Demonistrate signs of adequate cerebral oxygenation: Alert mental status; oriented to person, time, and place.	• Perform ongoing mental status assessment: Confusion, restlessness, anxiety, stupor, loss of consciousness.	• Hypoxaemia may predispose to cerebral tissue hypoxia.
			• Monitor respiratory function on ongoing basis.	
		2. Demonstrate normal respiratory effort: • Rate < 25/minute; pattern—eupneic.	• Respiratory rate and rhythm.	• Reflects work of breathing: Increased work of breathing increases oxygen consumption and myocardial oxygen demand.
			• Dyspnoea.	• Secondary to increased pulmonary interstitial oedema.
		3. Maintain optimal arterial blood gases: • pH 7.35-7.45. • PaO_2 > 60 mmHg. • $PaCO_2$ 35-45 mmHg.	• Orthopnoea.	• Increased venous return secondary to postural redistribution of pulmonary blood flow.
			• Cough.	• Usually nonproductive, periodic, and nocturnal.
		4. Maintain breath sounds clear to auscultation. 5. Demonstrate clear lung fields on chest x-ray.	• Status of weakness and fatigue.	• Secondary to decreased perfusion to skeletal muscles; increased work of breathing further fatigues the patient and predisposes to alveolar hypoventilation with hypercapnia and respiratory acidemia.
		6. Maintain effective cardiovascular function: • HR 60-80/minute. • Cardiac output 4-8 liters/minute.	• Secretions: Quality, quantity, presence of blood (frequently pink and frothy secretions).	• Result of capillary hydrostatic pressure exceeding pulmonary capillary oncotic pressure, which allows fluid to leak into pulmonary interstitium; when this cannot be reabsorbed via the pulmonary lymphatic system, fluid fills the alveoli.
			• Cyanosis, pallor.	
			• Auscultation of lungs for presence of adventitious sounds: Rales, bronchial and wheezing.	• Frequent assessments allow for early intervention, minimizing deleterious effects of respiratory compromise.
			• Monitor diagnostic tests and studies:	
			• Arterial blood gases.	• Reflect effectiveness of gas exchange; decreased PaO_2 result of alveolar flooding; $PaCO_2$ initially decreases secondary to hyperventilation; then it elevates secondary to patient fatigue.
			• Chest x-ray.	• Butterfly distribution of pulmonary infiltrates; may take 24

Contd...

Problem	*R*	*Objective*	*Nursing Interventions*	*Rationales*
				hours after symptoms develop to become apparent on chest x-ray.
			◆ ECG.	◆ May reflect signs of myocardial ischaemia.
			• Assess cardiovascular function frequently:	
			◆ Heart rate.	◆ Initial tachycardia is the result of sympathetic nervous system stimulation; return of heart rate to baseline may be indicative of resolving pulmonary oedema.
			◆ Haemodynamic parameters: ◆ Systemic blood pressure.	◆ May become hypertensive from sympathetic stimulation.
			◆ Cardiac output.	◆ Reflects tissue perfusion.
			◆ PCWP.	◆ Increased LVEDP reflected back to pulmonary capillary bed, increasing pulmonary intravascular hydrostatic pressure; PCWP > 20 mmHg.
			◆ Jugular venous distention; peripheral oedema, sacraloedema; presence of S_3, S_4; gallop rhythm; pulsus alternans; palpitation, chest pain.	◆ Affords noninvasive evaluation of changes in venous pressure (see Nursing Diagnosis #1).
			• Implement measures to allay patient anxiety.	• Anxiety causes patient to become tachypneic, which causes him/her to consume more oxygen.
			◆ Assess patient's anxiety. ◆ Explain treatment plan and procedures. ◆ Maintain calm, reassuring approach to care.	
			• Implement measures to increase gas exchange.	
			◆ Administer oxygen as prescribed and monitor response to therapy.	◆ O_2 is given to raise PaO_2 above 60 mmHg when there is hypoxaemia without hypercapnia. ◆ Hypoxia enhances likelihood of dysrhythmia development, depresses myocardial contractility, and causes pulmonary vasoconstriction, which increases the workload of the right side of the heart; elevating the PaO_2 will minimize and/or reverse these processes.
			◆ Reassure patient of the need for oxygen and its temporary nature. ◆ Administer positive pressure as needed.	◆ Most patients tolerate administration of oxygen by mask poorly and frequently fear suffocation. ◆ Increases mean lung volume (functional lung capacity), allowing more alveoli to participate in gas exchange.
			◆ Assess haemodynamic parameters meticulously during positive pressure therapy (PEEP).	◆ Positive pressure can impede venous return, thereby decreasing cardiac output.
			◆ Initiate intubation and mechanical ventilation as necessary.	
			• Implement measures to decrease preload and afterload.	
			◆ Place patient in high Fowler's position with dependent lower extremities if blood pressure allows.	◆ Dilates peripheral arteries and veins and causes venous pooling, thereby decreasing venous congestion.

Contd...

Problem	*R*	*Objective*	*Nursing Interventions*	*Rationales*
			◆ Administer morphine sulphate IV. ◆ Monitor for respiratory depressant effects; have morphine antagonist at bedside.	◆ Reduces patient's anxiety, decreases tachypnoea, causes peripheral pooling of blood, decreases preload and afterload. ◆ Respiratory depression occurs in approximately 7 minutes.
			◆ Monitor blood pressure for hypotension.	◆ Hypotension, the result of baroreceptors' vasoconstrictive reflexes, is inhibited by morphine.
			◆ Administer intravenous vasodilators such as nitroprusside and nitroglycerin. Carefully monitor arterial blood pressure while administering these drugs.	◆ Reduce vascular hydrostatic pressure and reduce PCWP; these drugs have systemic venous and arterial vasodilatory properties.
			◆ Administer intravenous diuretics as ordered (usually potent loop diuretics such as furosemide and ethacrynic acid). Carefully monitor for hypotension and tachycardia, and check for signs of hypokalaemia.	◆ Reduce total blood volume and increase venous capacitance. ◆ Cause reduction in sodium reabsorption in loop of Henle; direct effect on arterial and venous dilatation. ◆ Evidence of circulatory intolerance and potassium wasting is associated with use of these diuretics.
			◆ Apply rotating tourniquets as ordered (automatic tourniquet machine) following appropriate procedure: ◆ Connect to upper portion of arms and legs; only 3 cuffs should be inflated simultaneously.	
			◆ Inflate blood pressure cuffs to 10 mmHg below the diastolic pressure.	◆ Higher pressures will cause fluid loss into the patient's peripheral extravascular spaces. ◆ Should not occlude arterial blood flow.
			◆ Check for presence of peripheral pulses, warmth, and colour of extremities.	◆ Pulse should be palpable with cuff inflated.
			◆ Make certain tourniquets rotate every 15 minutes.	
			◆ When discontinuing tourniquets, remove one by one in a counterclockwise direction every 15 minutes.	◆ Avoids excessive increase in venous return.
			◆ Assess patient's tolerance to discontinuance of treatment.	
			• Implement measures to improve left ventricular contractility.	• Increased myocardial contractility leads to increased cardiac output with a reduction in LVEDP and PCWP.
			◆ Administer cardiac glycosides as prescribed.	
			◆ Administer dopamine, dobutamine in low doses as prescribed.	◆ Stimulate myocardial beta-receptors to enhance contractility.
			◆ Administer aminophylline as prescribed (observe for hypotension, dysrhythmias).	◆ Bronchodilator; also increases myocardial contractility and enhances diuresis.
Nursing Diagnosis #4 Anxiety, related to: 1. Potential for life-style modification. 2. Powerlessness. 3. Intensive care setting.		Patient will: 1. Verbalize anxieties and fears. 2. Verbalize feeling and less anxious. 3. Demonstrate a relaxed demeanour.	• Obtain baseline assessment of anxiety level and coping patterns from patient, family members, or significant others. • Assess level of anxiety; include heart rate, blood pressure, increased muscle tension,	• Baseline data are essential in evaluating the effectiveness of therapeutic interventions and the patient's ability to cope. ◆ Assists in determining the underlying cause of anxiety and provides a basis for intervention.

Contd...

Problem	*R*	*Objective*	*Nursing Interventions*	*Rationales*
4. Uncertainty related to illness and diagnosis.			increased startle response, a change in sleeping patterns, nightmares, irritability, diaphoresis, nausea, diarrhoea, repetitive behaviours.	
			• Ascertain what the patient or family member is experiencing; eliminate a physiologic basis of symptoms.	• Hypoxaemia, hypercarbia, decreased cardiac output, and pain precipitate and intensify feelings of apprehension and anxiety.
			• Determine what the individual's needs are and what resources can be mobilized to decrease feelings of anxiety; provide positive reinforcement when appropriate.	• Positive feedback helps nurture confidence.
			• Implement therapeutic measures to decrease anxiety.	
			◆ Encourage the patient and/or family to verbalize anxieties and concerns; encourage them to ask questions; listen attentively; provide a caring environment.	◆ Helps to create a trusting relationship; reassures patient he/she is not alone.
			◆ Explain procedures and limitations to patient/family. Relate to nature of heart disease.	◆ See Nursing Diagnosis #7, below.
			◆ Familiarize patient with ICU staff, routines, equipment.	◆ Knowing what to expect will help to reduce anxiety.
			◆ Mobilize appropriate resources: ◆ Consult social services, chaplaincy program, financial advisor, or other such services, as appropriate. ◆ Modify the environment to decrease anxiety; modify the policy regarding visitors; increase or decrease environmental stimuli as indicated; increase frequency of nurse/patient contacts.	◆ Removed of multification of precipitating factors may reduce anxiety; social interaction helps modify feelings of depersonalization that accompany hospitalization.
			◆ Involve patients in their own care within physical limitations.	◆ Will decrease anxiety by reestablishing sense of control and purpose.
Nursing Diagnosis #5 Infection, potential for, related to: 1. Decreased mobility. 2. Invasive lines. 3. Pulmonary congestion. 4. Valvular heart disease.		Patient will: 1. Demonstrate absence or resolution of infection as indicated by: • White blood cell count within normal limits. • Normal body temperature (37°C, 98.6°F). 2. Demonstrate understanding of importance of antibiotic prophylaxis (as patient's condition warrants). 3. Remain without complications of infectious process (e.g., embolization associated with infective.	• Identify patients at high risk of developing an infection: Elderly; rheumatic heart disease; prosthetic heart valves; valvular lesions; intravenous drug abuse; hypertrophic cardiomyopathy; multiple invasive lines; immunocompromised; chronic debilitating diseases.	• Patients with heart disease are at high risk due to alterations in endothelial integrity on cardiac valves secondary to surgical, congenital, or rheumatic causes. Early detection and treatment may improve prognosis.
			• Maintain strict aseptic technique during insertion and changing of haemodynamic monitoring lines; strict adherence to handwashing protocols.	• Minimises likelihood of airborne and contact organisms entering sterile field.
			◆ Maintain closed system; use sterile stopcocks with caps.	◆ Stopcocks that are not maintained as a closed system contribute to 5-10 per cent of the infections associated with intravascular catheters.
			◆ Change pressure tubing and flush solutions every 48 hours or as per unit protocol.	◆ Has proven sufficient for minimizing incidence of line-related septicaemia.
			◆ Change dressings and observe for signs of infection, as per unit protocol.	
			◆ Record date of insertion of each line; arterial, CVP and PA lines should be changed every 3-4 days, or as per unit protocol.	◆ Irritation of vessel or endocardium predisposes to thrombophlebitis and infective endocarditis.
			◆ Culture tips of catheters when removed, if indicated.	
			• Monitor for signs of infection.	

Contd...

Problem	*R*	*Objective*	*Nursing Interventions*	*Rationales*
			◆ Monitor temperature every 4 hr; report elevation to physician. ◆ Monitor WBC count. ◆ Observe for tachycardia, chills, or diaphoresis. Keep patient warm and dry.	◆ Fever increases basal metabolic rate and causes tachycardia and increase in cardiac output to meet tissue metabolic demands. This hyperdynamic response is likely to precipitate severe heart failure by markedly elevating myocardial oxygen demand and reducing the time for diastolic filling. ◆ Early detection of an inflammatory or infectious process encourages prompt intervention to minimize deleterious effects of the causative organism on the heart and other body processes.
			• Administer antibiotics and antipyretics as prescribed and monitor response to therapy.	
			• Turn every 2 hr while on bedrest. • Initiate measures to prevent atelectasis.	• To maintain skin integrity and mobilize pulmonary secretions.
			◆ Encourage hourly deep breathing while awake and during periods of immobility. ◆ Teach use of incentive spirometer if appropriate. ◆ Progress activity as tolerated.	◆ Maximizes alveolar inflation and minimizes atelectasis and hypoventilation.
			◆ Note colour, quantity, character of secretions (pulmonary).	◆ Pulmonaryoedema results in frothy, blood-tinged sputum; pneumonia results in thick, purulent sputum.
			◆ Auscultate breath sounds every 4 hr and record.	◆ Assessment for atelectasis, increasing left heart failure, or pneumonia.
			• Assess for potential source of infection: ◆ Urine: Haematuria, cloudy, flank pain. ◆ Sputum, character, colour, quantity. ◆ Monitor cultures and sensitivities.	◆ Assists in assessing response to therapy.
			• Assess for signs and symptoms of infective endocarditis:	• Infective endocarditis can precipitate the development of heart failure.
			◆ Change in murmur.	◆ Murmurs are usually absent in patients with right-sided endocarditis, particularly with tricuspid valve involvement. ◆ Murmurs that develop with endocarditis are usually regurgitant; vegetative lesion (if large enough) can cause stenotic murmur. ◆ New or changing murmur may indicate crosive complications of valve.
			◆ Fever	◆ Siaphylococcus is usually associated with acute infectious process and causes temperature elevations with high fever spikes and rigours; Streptococcus usually produces a subacute process with moderate temperature elevations.
			◆ Haematuria	◆ Result of renal emboli and infarction.
			◆ Petechiae	◆ One of the most frequent signs

Contd...

Problem	*R*	*Objective*	*Nursing Interventions*	*Rationales*
				noted in neck, conjunctivae, clavicles, wrists, ankles, and mucous membranes.
			◆ Osler's nodes	◆ Painful, red subcutaneous nodules noted in the pads of the fingers or toes.
			◆ Roth's spots	◆ Retinal haemorrhages with white or pale center, located near optic disc.
			◆ Janeway nodes	◆ Non-tender haemorrhagic lesions 1-5 mm in diameter; occur on arms, legs, palms, and soles; intensify when extremity is elevated.
			◆ Nailbed splinter haemorrhages.	◆ In distal one-third of nail; thought to be result of an allergic vas-culities of the arterioles.
			• Assess for complications of embolization:	
			◆ Change in level of consciousness, visual disturbances, headache.	◆ CNS embolization from left heart endocarditis.
			◆ SOB, chest pain, haemoptysis.	◆ Result of right-sided endocarditis causing pulmonary infarction.
			◆ Haematuria, decreased urine output, increased BUN and creatinine.	◆ Embolization to renal vasculature.
			◆ Dysrhythmias, pericardial friction rub, sudden haemodynamic compromise.	◆ Left heart endocarditis; result of erosive vegetations. Can cause VSD, fistulas, pericarditis, cardiac tamponade, or myocardial infarction.
			◆ Left upper quadrant pain radiating to left shoulder.	◆ Spleen is most common site of embolic infarction in bacterial endocarditis.
			• Instruct patient with valvular heart disease regarding importance of antibiotic prophylaxis.	• See Nursing Diagnosis #7, below.
Nursing Diagnosis #6 Potential for activity intolerance, related to compromised cardiac reserve.		Patient will: 1. Maintain normal muscle tone. 2. Maintain highest level of activity that does not produce symptoms of myocardial dysfunction. 3. Identify end-points of activity tolerance.	• Perform assessment of activity and exercise tolerance.	• Initial assessment provides pertinent data that will guide individualized activity prescription from acute to rehabilitative phase.
			◆ Age	◆ Physical endurance decreases with age; older patients will tolerate less activity.
			◆ Weight	◆ Obesity increases myocardial burden.
			◆ Gender	◆ Females have more endurance; men can tolerate workload of higher intensity secondary to the increased ratio of muscle mass: total body weight.
			◆ Cardiovascular disorder	◆ Cardiovascular history may influence the attitude of the patient to activity (i.e., if angina or palpitations developed on exertion, this may influence the patient's attitude towards exercise).
			◆ Previous activity and motivation.	◆ Identifies patients who may need encouragement to exercise.
			• Initiate gradual activity progression in the critical care setting.	• Minimizes the deleterious effects of deconditioning, which include a decreased work capacity, tachycardia,

Contd...

Problem	*R*	*Objective*	*Nursing Interventions*	*Rationales*
				orthostatic hypotension, venous thrombosis, and feelings of hopelessness and dependency.
			• Encourage to participate in ADL (feed self, wash hands, shave, active ROM).	• Such activities improve circulation and help to prevent phlebitis or thromboembolism.
			• Maintain bedrest with commode privileges during acute phase of heart failure. • Prevent complications of immobility.	• Physical activity redistributes blood from viscera and kidneys to the skeletal muscle and skin. Bedrest allows for a limited cardiac output and decreases myocardial oxygen demand. However, myocardial oxygen consumption is greater when a patient uses bedpan than during commode use.
			• Assist with frequent position changes. • Provide frequent back care and skin care.	• Maintenance of skin integrity and muscle tone.
			• Encourage hourly deep breathing while awake.	• Minimizes development of atelectasis.
			• Maintain in semi-Fowler's position.	• Reduces venous return to the heart; increases ability to expand lungs during deep breathing exercises.
			• Assess tolerance to activity progression by checking blood pressure, heart rate, and respiratory rate 1 minute and 4 minutes after the activity. Indicators of poor tolerance include dyspnoea, syncope, angina, diaphoresis, cyanosis, fatigue, weakness, dysrhythmias; heart rate should return to baseline within 4 minutes. Heart rate should not exceed 20 beats/minute above resting heart rate and it should not exceed 110 beats/minute.	• Physical activity increases venous return to the heart, increases myocardial workload, and increases metabolic heat production, i.e., one- fifth of cardiac output is shunted to skin in thermoregulation and the patient with impaired myocardial function cannot compensate for this with a tachycardia or increased contractile force; symptoms of pulmonary venous congestion and decreased cardiac output intensify.
			• Monitor systolic blood pressure.	• Fall of 20 mmHg below resting level and failure of systolic blood pressure to increase above the resting level suggest poor exercise tolerance.
			• Assess readiness to learn and instruct regarding indicators of activity intolerance, as noted above.	• Readiness to learn facilitates meaningful learning.
			• Teach patient how to take own pulse.	
			• Isometric exercises should be discouraged.	• Result in increased blood pressure and cardiac workload; do not improve cardiovascular conditioning.
			• Encourage gradual resumption of aerobic activity when free of heart failure.	• Increases functional capacity and cardiovascular conditioning.
			• Re-emphasize to patient that activity will be progressed gradually and will be supervised during the initial stages; provide positive reinforcement when appropriate; gradually transfer supervision of tolerance from health care personnel to patient and family.	• Builds and reinforces self-confidence; helps minimize deleterious effects of phychophysiologic responses to stress (increased myocardial oxygen consumption).

Contd...

Problem	R	Objective	Nursing Interventions	Rationales
Nursing Diagnosis #7 Knowledge deficit, related to: 1. Underlying heart disease, treatment, and follow-up.		Patient will: 1. Describe underlying disease process and relationship to heart failure. 2. Identify own risk factors or precipitating conditions that require modification. 3. Identify importance of follow-up care and symptoms requiring medical intervention. 4. Describe the importance of medications, diet, and activity to the overall treatment plan. 5. Identify signs and symptoms of activity intolerance. 6. Identify indications for endocarditis prophylaxis (if patient is in high-risk profile.)	• Assess knowledge of heart failure, underlying disease process, and expectations of disease progression.	• Readiness to learn varies because of differences in general education background, intellectual ability, and motivation. Assessment establishes baseline data from which to build or determine need to alter misconceptions.
			• Encourage verbalization of patient/family concerns and their learning needs.	• Fosters establishment of open, trusting relationship. Learning is enhanced when patient participates in goal setting. Heart failure affects patient and his/her lifestyle and impacts on the entire family to varying degrees.
			• Assess readiness to learn.	• Readiness facilitates more effective learning.
			• Implement teaching plan, which should include: ◆ Explanation of normal heart function, heart failure, and underlying disease process. ◆ Explanation of signs and symptoms and appropriate action regarding their development. ◆ Explanation of risk factors and factors that will aggravate the symptoms of heart failure and methods to modify these factors. ◆ Explanation of medication regimen (including name, dosage, frequency, action, and side effects). ◆ Explanation of diet modification if indicated. ◆ Activity prescription and signs and symptoms of activity intolerance.	• Patient and family have a right to receive information about the disease, treatment, and prognosis; understanding enhances compliance; knowledge allays anxieties and the adverse effects associated with psychophysiologic stress.
			• Assist patient/family in identifying family strengths and resources.	• Engenders self-confidence.
			• Initiate referral to appropriate resources if indicated (social services; community resources).	• It is reassuring to have support services available.

ARRHYTHMIAS/CARDIAC DYSRHYTHMIAS

Arrhythmias are abnormal cardiac rhythms also called as dysrhythmias. The ability to recognize arrhythmias is an essential skill for the nurse. Cardiac monitoring is now used in a wide range of hospital and clinical settings. Prompt assessment of an abnormal cardiac rhythm and patient response to the rhythm is critical.

Cardiac tissue has those properties which enable the conduction system to initiate an electrical impulse that is transmitted through the cardiac tissue stimulating muscle contraction. The four properties are:

- Automaticity i.e. ability to initiate an impulse spontaneously and continuously.
- Contractility i.e. ability to respond mechanically to an impulse.
- Conductivity i.e. ability to transmit an impulse along a membrane in an orderly manner.
- Excitability i.e. ability to be electrically stimulated.

The conduction system of the heart is made up of specialized neuromuscular tissues located throughout the heart. A normal cardiac impulse begins in the sinoatrial (SA) node in the upper right atrium. It is transmitted over the atrial myocardium via Bachman's bundle and internodal pathways to the atrioventricular (AV) node. From the AV node, the impulse spreads through the bundle of his and down the left and right bundle branches, emerging in the purkinje's fibres, which transmit the impulse to the ventricles. A rhythm is classified as 'normal' when it meets the following criteria in ECG.

- Presence of one upright and consistent-appearing P wave before each QRS complex, all PR intervals between 0.12 and 0.20 seconds.
- The PR intervals are consistent and the heart rate is between 60 and 100 beats per minute.

Conduction to the point just before the impulse leaves the Purkinje's fibres take place within the time of the PR intervals of the ECG. When the impulse emerges from the Purkinje's fibers, ventricular depolarization occurs, producing mechanical contraction of the ventricles and ....QRS complex on the ECG. Rates of conduction system are:

- SA node 60-100 times/min.
- AV junction 40-60 times/min.
- Purkinje's fibres 20-40 times/min.

The autonomic nervous system plays an important role in the rate of impulse formation, the speed of conduction, and the strength of cardiac contraction. The components of the autonomic nervous system that affect the heart are this right and left vagus nerve fibres of the parasympathetic nervous system and fibers of the sympathetic nervous system. Stimulation of the vagus nerve causes a decreased rate of firing of the SA node, slaved impulse condition of the AV node and decreased force of cardiac muscle contraction. Stimulation of the sympathetic nerves that supply the heart has essentially the opposite effect on the heart.

Aetiology

Cardiac arrhythymias are the result of alterations in impulse formation or propagation. Arrhythmias are often classified by the anatomical site of the dysfunction. For example, sinus dysrhythmias and atrial dysrhythmias. Common causes of arrhythmias include underlying cardiac disease, sympathetic stimulation, vagal stimulation, electrolyte imbalances and hypoxia, which are due to:

- Drug effects of toxicity.
- Myocardial cell degeneration.
- Hypertrophy of cardiac muscle.
- Emotional crisis.
- Connective tissue disorders.
- Alcohol.
- Metabolic conditions (eg. thyroid dysfunction)
- Coffee, tea, tobacco.
- Electrolyte imbalances.
- Cellular hypoxia.
- Oedema.
- Acid-base imbalance.
- Myocardial ischaemia.
- Degeneration of conduction system.

Pathophysiology

Alterations in impulse formation and propagation arise from one of the three pathophysiological processes: altered automaticities, altered conduction resulting in delays or blocks and re-entry mechanisms.

i. *Altered automaticity*

Automaticity is the ability to depolarize spontaneously without external stimulation, it is a property that normally confineds to the cells of the *SA node*. The SA node usually depolarizes at a faster rate than other potential pacemaker cells because of the steep slope of phase 4, allowing sinus cells to reach threshold at faster rate. A variety of conditions can alter the automaticity of SA node and produce faster or slower than usual heart rates. Vagal stimulation will decrease this slope, resulting in a slower heart rate. Sympathetic stimulation and hypoxia will steepen phase 4 resulting in faster heart rates. If the phase-4 depolarization is found, the *AV node* or ventricular condition system increases, enhanced automaticity is said to exist. Some causes for enhanced automaticity are hypoxia, catecholamines, hypokalaemia, hypocalcaemia, atrophine, trauma and digital toxicity.

Even cells that do not normally have automaticity may develop abnormal automaticity if the resting membranes potential or threshold potential is altered, increasing the threshold slows the heart rate because it then takes longer to reach threshold. If the resting membrane potential is made, less negative automaticity will increase because it is easier to reach threshold. Altered automaticity may be a consequence of ischaemia, infarction, hypokalaemia, hypocalcaemia or cardiomypathy. This abnormality is not easily impressed by the activity of the faster pace makers.

ii. *Altered conductivity*

When the rate of amplitude of depolarization decreases, conduction also decreases. Electrolyte imbalances affect the rate of depolarization by altering the resting membrane potential. Hypokalaemia causes the resting membrane potential to be positive, decreasing the rate of depolarization and slowing conduction. Any condition decreases the amplitude of the action potential such as ischaemia, hypercalaemia, or calcification of the conducting figures can cause cardiac conduction disturbances. Abnormality in conduction occur anywhere in the conduction system, including the SA node, the AV node, and the bundle branches. The severity of impaired conduction ranges from a slight delay to complete cessation or block of impulse transmission.

iii. *Re-entry*

Re-entry occurs when an impulse is delayed within a pathway of slow conduction, long enough that the impulse is still viable when the remaining myocardium repolarizes. The impulse then re-enters surrounding tissue and produces another impulse. This typically occurs when two different pathways share an initial and final segment. The first impulse travels down the faster pathway, leaving behind its refractory trail. Should a second, early impulse follow, it will be blocked because that path is refractory. The second impulse then enters the slow pathway and can return retrograde through the fast path, initiating a circuitous pattern.

Clinical Manifestation

In most cases with arrhythmias are asymptomatic as long as cardiac output meets the body's metabolic demands. The clinical manifestations associated with most arrhythmias directly relate to decrease in cardiac output from slow or fast heart rates. Significant changes in heart rate may not allow adequate time for the ventricles to fill and empty. The clinical manifestation includes:

i. *General*
- Palpitations (racing heart, skipped beats)
- Anxiety.
- Fatigue.

ii. *Altered cardiac output*
- Pallor
- Cool and clammy skin
- Cyanotic
- Shortness of breath
- Rales
- Decreased blood pressure
- Confusion
- Dizziness
- Weakness
- Presyncope
- Syncope with loss of consciousness
- Chest pain
- Atrial thrombi (may dislodge to causes systemic emboli).

Management

The diagnosis of arrhythmias begins with the 12-lead ECG. Each arrhythmia exhibits characteristic changes in the ECG tracing. A systematic approach to analyzing the ECG rhythm helps distinguish the different dysrhythnias. The systematic interpretation of ECG tracing are:

- Rale (atrial and ventricular).
- Rhythm (atrial and ventricular).
- Presence or absence of P waves.
- PR inteval 0.12-0.20 seconds.
- QRS complex 0.06-0.12 seconds
- QT internal less than 0.55 seconds.
- Interpretation.

Please note that normal sinus rhythm has an atrial (P) and ventricular (QRS) rate of 60 to 100 beats per minute, a regular rhythm (consistent PP and RR intervals) and a P wave before every QRS.

The other diagnostic tests used in the assessment of arrhythmias include signal-averaged electrocardiomyography, ambulatory holter monitoring and electrophysiological studies.

Medical and nursing management of arrhythmias focuses on alleviating symptoms from altered cardiac output and eliminating or reversing the aetiology. Arrhythmia occurring in out-of-hospital setting and present problems of management. Determination of the rhythm by cardiac monitoring is a high priority. Emergency management of arrhythmias indicated where arrhythmias may be due to hypoxia, shock, poisoning, drug ingestion, myocardial infarction, CCF, conduction defects, pulmonary disorders near-drowning, electrolyte imbalances, metabolic imbalances, and electric shock.

During this assessment findings will be:

- Irregular rate and rhythm, palpitations.
- Chest, neck, shoulder or arm pain.
- Dizziness, syncope.
- Dyspnoea.
- Extreme restlessness.
- Decreased level of consciousness.
- Feeling of impending doom.
- Numbness, tingling of arms.
- Weakness and fatigue.
- Cold and clammy skin.
- Diaphoresis.
- Pallor.
- Nausea and vomiting.
- Decreased blood pressure.
- Decreased oxygen saturations.

The nursing intervention will include initially:

- Ensure patient airway.
- Administer O_2 via nasal cannula or non-breather mask.
- Establish IV access.
- Apply cardiac electrodes.
- Identify underlying rhythm.
- Identify ectopic beats.

and ongoing monitoring includes:

- Monitor vital signs, level of consciousness, O_2 saturation and cardiac rhythm.
- Anticipate need for intubation if respiratory distress is evident.
- Prepare to initiate CPR, defibrillation or both.

Management of specific arrhythmias according to their types are as follows with their descriptions.

i. *Sinus bradycardia*

Sinus bradycardia is characterized by atrial and ventricular rates less than 60 beats per minute. It is a normal sinus rhythm in aerobically trained athlets and in other individuals during sleep. It occurs in response to carotid sinus massage Valsalva's maneuver, hypothermia, increased intraocular pressure, increased vagal tone, and administration of parasympathomimetic drugs. It can be associated with hypothyroidum, increased intracranial pressure, obstructive jaundice and inferior wall MI.

ECG shows the P wave precedes each QRS complex and has normal encounter and a fixed interval. The clinical significance of sinus bradycardia depends on how the patient tolerates haemodynamically. Hypotension with decrease CO (cardiac output) may occur in some circumstances. An acute MI may predispose the heart to escape arrhythmias and premature beats.

Treatment consists of administration of atrophane (Anticholenergic) or isoproterenol is usually effective in increasing HR.

ii. *Sinus tachycardia*

Sinus tachycardia is characterized by an atrial and ventricular rate of 100 beats per minute or more (upper limit 150/m). It is associated with physiologic stressors such as exercise, fever, pain, hypotension, hypovelaemia, anxiety, anaemia, hypoxia, hypoglycaemia, myocardial ischaemia, CCF and hyperthyroidism. It can also be an occur by using of drugs such as epinephrine, non-epinephrine, caffeine, atropine theophylline, nifedripine, hydralozine and ingestion of alcohol, caffeine and tobacco.

ECG shows P wave is normal, precedes each QRS complex

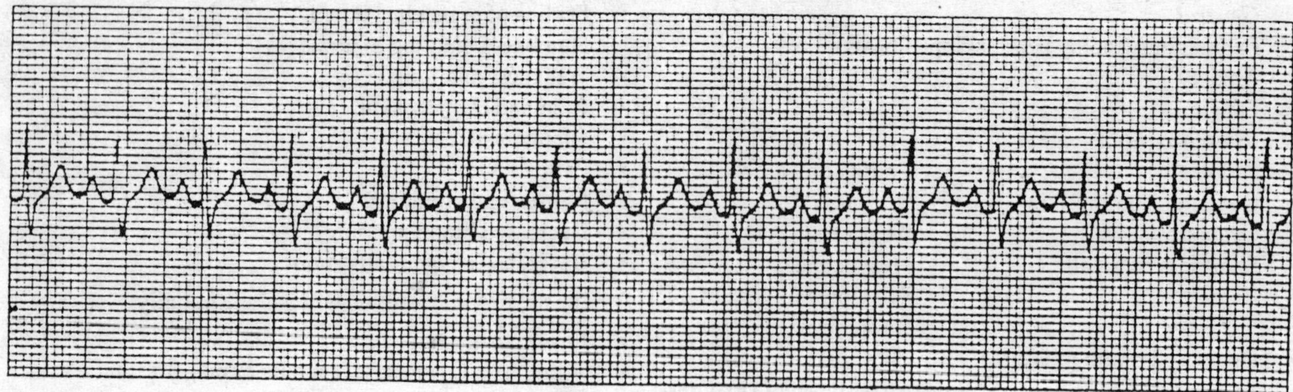

Fig. 9.5: (A) Sinus tachycardia

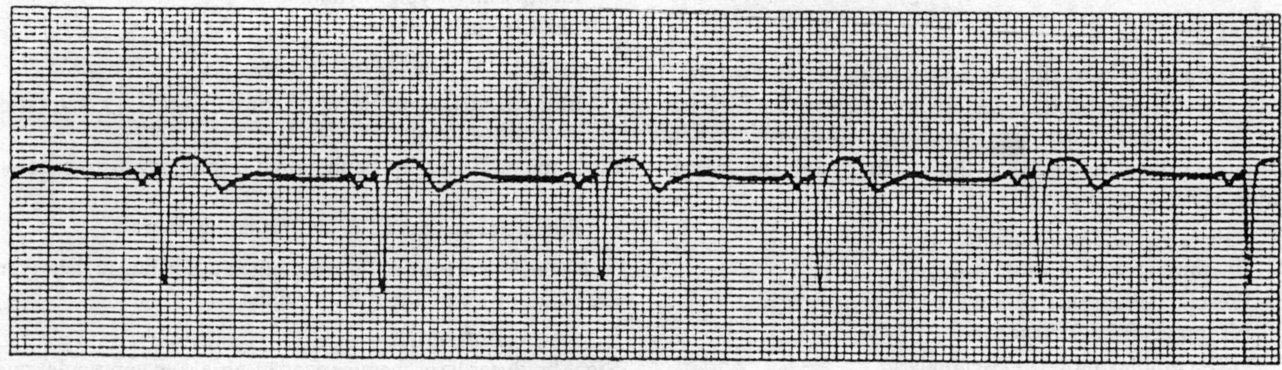

Fig. 9.5: (B) Sinus bradycardia

and has a normal contour and a fixed interval. It is normal, but HR greater than 100 beat/minute. The clinical significance depends on the patient tolerance on increased heart beat. The patient may complain of palpitations of has no symptoms or has symptoms and dizziness and hypotension. In the patient with compromised myocardium, and tachycardia may cause decrease in CO with resultant lightheadedness, chest pain and heart failure.

Treatment is determined by underlying causes. Sinus tachycardia can usually be slowed with digoxin, beta blockers if necessary.

iii. *Sinus dysrythmia*

Sinus dysrhythmia is the most common arrhythmia. It is typically found in young adults and elderly persons. It is an irregular rhythm in which PP intervals are accompanied by changes in RR intervals. The cyclic pattern of changing PP or RR intervals correlates with the pattern of inspiration and expiration. During inspiration, the intervals shorten as the heart rate increases. Conversely, intervals lengthen during expiration. This condition cannot be treated unless the bradycardia phase is marked, causing symptoms that can be treated with administration of atropine.

iv. *Sick sinus syndrome (SSS)*

SSS is one type of tachycardia—bradycardia syndrome, which is characterized by the presence of bradycardia with intermittant episodes of tachydysrythmias. The episode of tachy-dysrythmia often is followed by a long pause before returning to sinus bradycardia. Complication of this inefficient rhythm includes heart failure and CVA resulting from thromboembolism. This condition is associated with ischaemia degeneration of SA node, in which (SSS) some patient remian free of symptoms or complain only palpitations. For the patient with severe symptoms, the heart rhythm is stabilized with a permanent implantable pace maker for the slow phase and administration of digoxin or beta blockers to control the ventricular rate of the tachycardia phase.

v. *Sinus exit block and sinus arrest*

Sinus exit block occurs when an impulse originates in the SA node but is blocked immediately. No P wave or QRS complex is generated resulting in a long pause. The next impulse occurs in a time interval representing the normal PP interval. Sinus arrest infers that the SA node never fired; therefore, there is no P or QRS complex. The next impulse is asynchronous to the normal PP interval.

This condition may occur as a result of medication such as degoxin hypoxin, myocardial ischaemia and damage or injury to the SA node. The patient is symptomatic from a decrease in cardiac output the pauses or long or frequent. The patient may feel palpitations from the strong stroke volume that accompanies the next beat after the pause. When the patient is symptomatic, atropine may be administered to increase the HR and CO. Definitive therapy includes the insertion of permanent pacemaker.

vi. *Premature atrial contraction or beat (PAC or PAB)*

PAC or PAB is a contraction originating from an ectopic focus on the atrium in a location other than the sinus node. It originates in the left or right atrium and travel across the atria by abnormal pathway creating a distorted P wave. In normal heart, PAC can result from emotional stress or the use of caffeine, tobacco or alcohol. PAC also occurs in disease state such as infection, inflammation, hyperthyrodism COPD, heart disease (AHD), valvular diseases and others.

ECG shows HR variation with the underlying rate and frequency of PAC and the rhythm is irregular. The P wave has a different contour from that of a normal P wave. It may be notched to have negative deflection or it may be hidden in the preceding T wave. The PR interval may be shroter or stronger than a normal PR interval originating from the sinus node. But it is within normal limits. The QRS complex is usually normal. A PAC may be a prelude to supraventricular tachycardia.

Treatment depends on the patient's symptoms, withdrawal of sources of stimulation warranted. Drugs such as digoxin, quinidine, procainmide, flecanamide and betablocker are used.

vii. *Wantering atrial pacemaker (WAP)*

WAP occurs when at least three ectopic sites create the impulse for the cardiac rhythm. ECG shows P waves of different shapes and PR intervals of different lengths. The impulse can originate from the area around the AV node creating inverted P waves from retrograde conduction. Impulses from this lower area may also cause stimulation of the atria at the same time or after the ventricles. The P wave that appear buried in the QRS or occur inverted after the QRS.

WAP usually signify underlying heart disease or drug toxicity. The patients are asymptomatic unless the HR increases or decreases enough to affect cardiac output. The nurse mentions for changes in the rhythm and in the patient's symptoms. Then treat accordingly.

viii. *Atrial tachycardia or paraxysmal suppraventricular tachycardia (PSVT or PAT)*

PSVT or PAT in an arrhythmia originating in an ectopic focus anywhere above the bifurcation of the bundle of HIS. Paroxysmal refers to an abrupt onset and termination. Termination is sometimes followed by a brief period of asystole. Some degree of AV block may be present.

In the normal heart, paraxysmal atrial tachycardia (PAT) or PSVT is associated with overexertion, emotional stress, changes

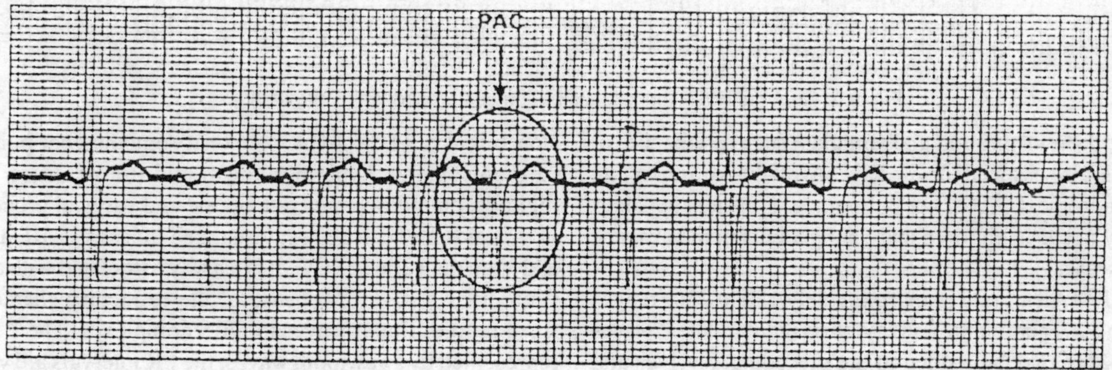

Fig. 9.6: (A) Normal sinus rhythm with premature atrial contraction.

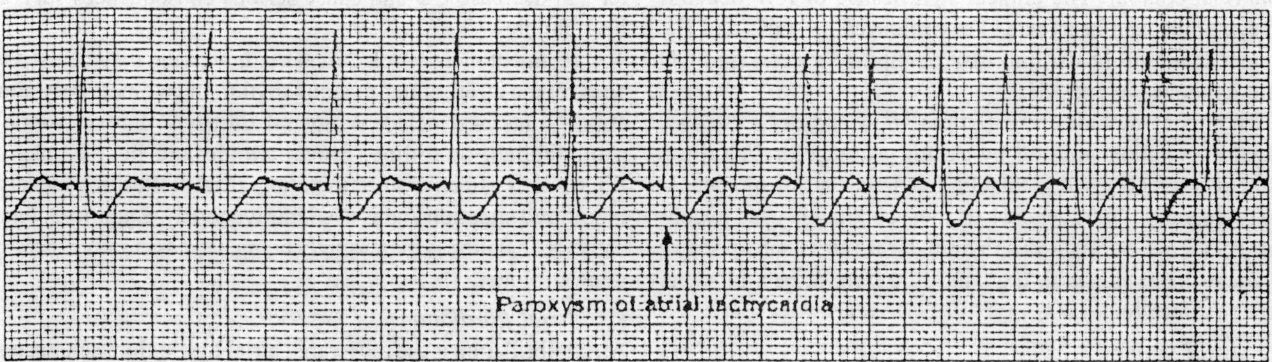

Fig. 9.6: (B) Paroxysmal atrial tachycardia.

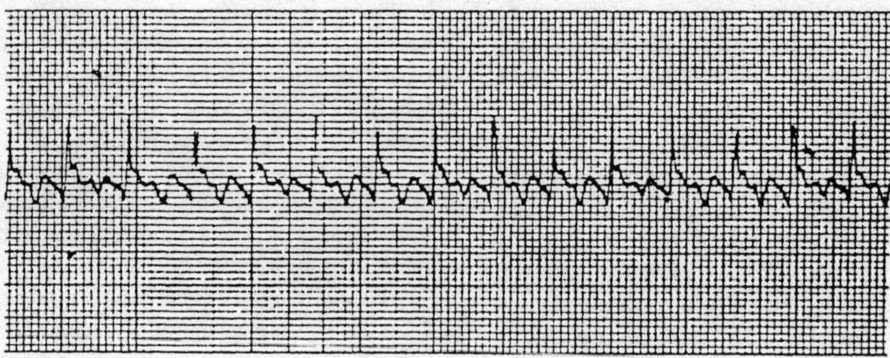

Fig. 9.6: (C) Atrial flutter

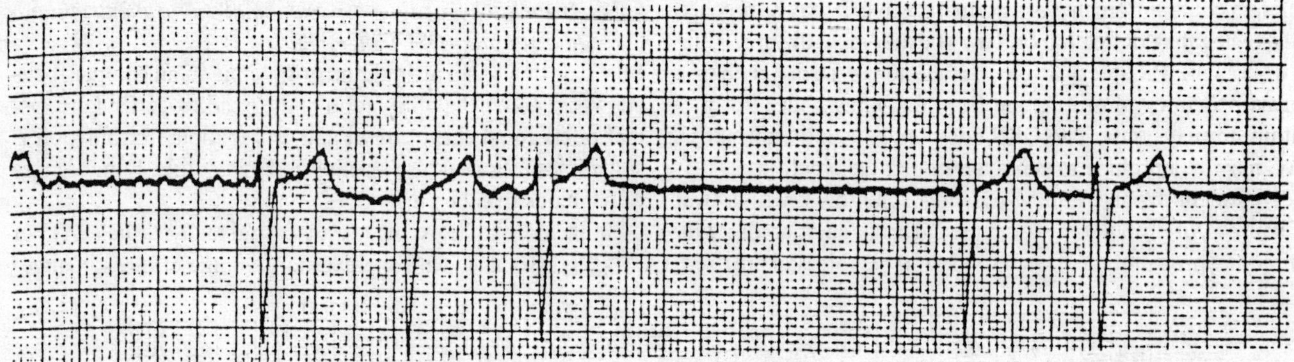

Fig. 9.6: (D) Atrial fibrillation with slow ventricular response (controlled).

in position, deep inspiration and stimulant such as tobacco, or caffeine. It is also associated with RHD, Woff-Parkinson-White (WPW) syndrome, CAD or cor pulmonale. Transient episodes of PAT may occur in children and young adults in the absence of heart disease.

ECG in PAT, heart rate is approximately 150 to 250 (ranges from 100 to 300) per minute and rhythm is regular. The P waves are present, but may be hidden in the preceding T waves and has an abnormal contour. The PR interval may be prolonged, shortened or normal and QRS complex may have a normal or abnormal contour. The clinical significance of PAT depends on symptoms and heart rate. The prolonged episodes and HR greater than 180 beats/ mib may precipitate a decreased CO with hypotension and MI.

Treatment includes vagal stimulation and drug therapy. Vagal stimulation induced by carotid massage or Valsalva's maneuver may be used to treat PAT. Administration of adenosine (Adenocard) intravenously is most commonly used to convert PSVT to a normal sinus rhythm. If the rate is unresponsive to adenosine, verapamil, digoxin, dilitrazen, or beta blockers may be effective.

ix. *Atrial flutter*

Atrial flutter is an atrial tachyarrhythmia identified by recurring regular, sawtooth-shaped flutter waves. It rarely occurs in normal heart. In disease state, it is associated with CAD, hypertension, mitral valve disorders, pulmonary embolus, cor pulmonale, cardiomyopathy, hyperthyroidism and use of drugs such as digitalis, quinidine, and epinephrine and surgical procedures.

Atrial flutter can be best visualized in leads II, III, and AVF and V on the 12-lead ECG. It is usually associated with a slower ventricular response, because of the refractory characteristic fixed ratio of flutter waves to QRS complexes. The P wave is represented by swawtooth waves, the PR intervals are variable, and QRS complex is normal in contour. Atrial rate is 250 to 350 beats/minute. High ventricular rates associated with atrial flutter can decrease CO and cause serious consequences such as heart failure.

Treatment includes electrical cardioversion may be used to convert the atrial flutter to sinus rhythm in an emergency situation. Drugs used include verapamil, dilitizem, digoxin, soralol, propafenone, quinidine, procainamide and beta blockers. Ilbutilide is effective at terminating atrial flutter in a closely-monitored situation and is used intravenously. Radiofrequency catheter abalation is increasingly being used as curative therapy of atrial flutter.

x. *Atrial fibrillation*

Atrial fibrillation is the most rapid atrial dysrhythmia characterized by a total disorganization of atrial electrical activity without effective atrial contraction. Atrial fibrillation may be paroxysmal and transient or chronic. Generally associated with underlying heart disease and typically with pericarditis, thyrotoxicosis, cardiomyopathy, CAD, HHD, Rh. mitral valve disease, cardiac surgery, heart failure and excessive alcohol intake (holiday heart), gastroenteritis and stress.

The ECG demonstrates baseline fibrillatory wave or undulations of variable contour at a rate of 300 to 600 per minute. Atria depolarizes chaotically at rates of 350 to 600 per minute. The baseline is composed of irregular undulations without definable P waves. The QRS complex is usually normal, but the ventricular rhythm is irregularly irregular.

Because of ventricular rhythm irregularity and the loss of synchronous atrial contractions (atrial kick), CO is decreased. Symptoms include fatigue, dyspnoea and dizziness. Thrombi may form in the atria and cause emboli, which may lodge in the pulmonary or peripheral blood vessels. The goal of treatment is to prevent complications through control of the ventricular rate and restoration of normal sinus rhythm (NSR). The risk of emboli may necessitate long-term anticoagulation in some patients. Drugs used to control fast ventricular rates include dililtazem, digoxin and beta blockers.

xi. *Premature junctional beat (PJB)*

PJB arises from an ectopic focus either (a) at the junction of atrial and AV nodal tissue or (2) at the junction of AV nodal tissue and bundle of HIS. If the PJBs arise from the first junction, the P wave will be inverted and premature and will precede the QRS complex. In the second case, the P wave is either hidden in the QRS or is inverted and follows the QRS. The abnormal timing and the inversion of the P wave are caused by depolarization of the atria in a retrograde fashion. The QRS is normal, but the PR interval is less than 0.12 second.

PJB mainly occurs in normal heart. They also may result from digitalis toxicity, ischaemia, hypoxia, pain, fever, anxiety, nicotine, caffeine, or electrolyte imbalance. Treatment when needed is directed towards correcting the underlying cause.

xii. *Junctional arrhythmias*

Junctional arrhythmias refer to an arrhythmia which originates in the area of AV node. The PJB is one among junctional arrhythmia. Other junctional arrhythmia include junctional escape rhythm (JER), accelerated junctional rhythm (AJR) and junctional tachycardia (JT). JER is often associated with the aerobically trained person who has sinus bradycardia, which may occur with acute MI and dysfunction of SA node. AJR and JT is observed with acute MI digital toxicity and acute Rh, fever during open heart surgery.

Treatment according to the patient tolerance of the rhythm and the patient's clinical condition. Inderol, cardizem and phenytoin are used.

xiii. *Premature ventricular contraction/beat (PVC/PVB)*

PVC or PVB is contraction originating in an ectopic focus in the ventricles. They are associated with stimulants such as caffeine, alcohol aminophylline, epinephrine, isoproterenol and digoxin. They are also associated with hypokalaemia, hypoxia, fever, exercise and emotional stress diseases associated are MI, CHF, CAD and mitral valve prolapse (MVP).

PVC is the premature occurrence of a QRS complex, which is wide and distorted in shape compared with a QRS complex initiated from the supraventricular tissue. The QRS complex is usually wider than 0.12 seconds, and the T wave is generally large and opposite in direction to the major deflection of the QRS complex. Retrograde conduction may occur and the P wave may be seen following the ectopic beat. PVC that are initiated form different foci appear different on contour from each other called multifocal PVCs. When every other beat is a PVC, it is called "VENTRICULAR BIGEMING". When every third beat is PVC, it is called "VENTRICULAR TRIGEMING" two consecutive PVCs are "Couplets". Three consecutive PVCs are called "TRIPLETS". Ventricular tachycardia occurs when there are three or more consecutive PVCs. When a PVC falls on the T wave of preceding beat, the R on T phenomenon occurs and is considered to be dangerous because it may precipitate ventricular tachycardia or ventricular fibrillation.

ECG finding shows HR variation according to intrinsic rate and a number of PVCs rhythm is irregular because of premature beat. A retrograde P wave is possible. The P wave is rarely visible and is usually lost in the QRS complex of PVC. The PR interval is not measurable. The QRS complex is wide and distorted in shape, more than 0.12 second.

PVCs are usually a benign finding in the patient with a normal heart PVCs may reduce the CO and precipitate angina and heart failure. PVCs in ischaemic heart disease or acute MI represents ventricular irritability. They may also occur as "reperfusion arrhythmias after lysis of a coronary artery clot with thrombolytic therapy in acute MI or following plaque reduction from percutaneous transluminal coronary angioplasty (PTCA).

For treating PVCs, lidocaine is the drug of choice, with an initial IV bolus of 1 to 1.5 mg/kg following by a second bolus of 0.5 to 1.5 mg/kg and continuous lidocaine infusion of 2 to 4 mg/minute.

Procainamide in the second drug of choice if lidocaine is ineffective.

xiv. *Ventricular tachycardia*

If the SA node and AV junction fail to initiate impulses, a ventricular pacemaking cell will automatically begin to initiate impulses at a rate of 20 to 40 beats per minute. This is known as "idioventricular rhythm". P-waves when seen are not associated with the ventricular rhythm. The QRS complex is greater than 0.12 wide and bizzarre. If the rate of ventricular initiated rhythm increases, to 40 to 100 beats per minute, it is known as an "accelerated idioventricular rhythm (AIVR). AIVR may be seen in hypoxin, in digital toxicity, as complication of acute MI and as reperfusions dysrhythmia after thrombolytic therapy.

Ventricular tachycardia (VT) may be sustained (lasting longer than 30 seconds) or non-sustained (lasting 30 seconds or less). VT is associated with acute MI, CAD, significant electrolyte imbalance (Eg. K) cardiomyopathy MVP, long QT syndrome, and coronary reperfusion after therapy.

ECG shown ventricular rate 110 to 250 beats per minute. Rhythm may be regular or irregular. ECG may be taken when a run of three or more PVCs occur. The QRS complex distorted in appearance, with a duration exceeding 0.12 seconds and with the ST-T direction pointing opposite to the major QRS deflection. It occurs when an ectopic focus or foci fire repetitively and the ventricle takes control as the pacemaker. The ventricular rate is 110 to 250; the RR interval may be regular or irregular. AVdissociation may be present, with P waves occurring independently of the QRS complex. VT may cause a severe decrease in CO as a result of ventricular diastolic filling times and loss of atrial contraction. The result may be pulmonary oedema, shock and decreased blood flow to the brain. It should be treated immediately.

Treatment includes, if the patient is haemodynamically stable lidocaine bolus administration. If lidocaine is ineffective, IV procainamide may be tried. The third drug of choice is bretylium IV at a dose of 5 mg/kg for several minutes and increased to 10 mg/kg at 15 to 30 minutes (not to exceed 30 to 35 mg/kg). A continuous infusion of bretylium (1 to 2 mg/min) may be started.

xv. *Torsades de pointe's*

Torsades de pointes, a variation of ventricular tachycardia, can also progress a ventricular fibrillation if not managed appropriately. It is otherwise known as polymorphic ventricular tachycardia. It is a type of VT characterised by a QRS contour that gradually changes into polarity over a series of beats. It usually occurs when QT prolongation is present.

Magnesium sulphate infusion is the drug of choice for torsade de pointes. Other drugs can be used, are isoproterenol or lido-caine infusion if haemodynamic state is stable. If the patient is unconscious or haemodynamically unstable, immediate cardioversion starting initially with 50 Joules. A defibrillator is used in the synchronized mode of cardioversion.

xvi. *Ventricular fibrillation (VF)*

VF is a severe derangement of the heart rhythm characterized on the ECG by irregular undulations of varying contour and amplitude. This represents the firing of multiple ectopic foci in the ventricle. Mechanically, the ventricle is simply "quivering" and no effective contraction or CO occurs. VF occurs in acute MI, CAD, myocardial ischmia and cadiomyopathy. It also occurs during cardiac pacing or cardiac catheterization procedure.

ECG shows HR is not measurable. Rhythm is irregular and chaotic. The P wave is not visible and the PR interval and QRS interval are not measurable. VF may result in unconsciousness, absence of pulse, apnoea, and seizures, if not intervened, death may occur.

Treatment consists of immediate initiation of CPR and initiation of advanced cardiac life support (ACLS) measures with the use of defibrillation and definitive drug therapy.

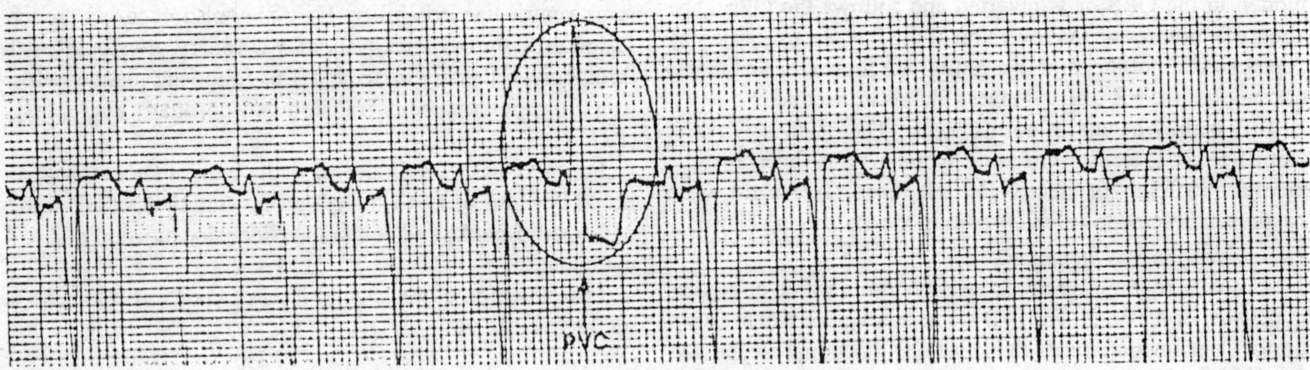

Fig.9.7: (A) Normal sinus rhythm with premature ventricular contraction

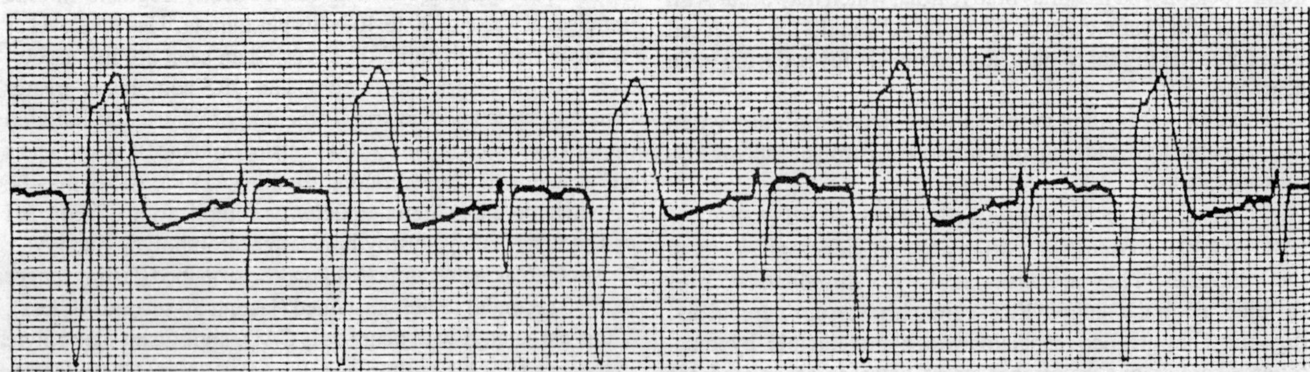

Fig.9.7: (B) Ventricular bigeminy

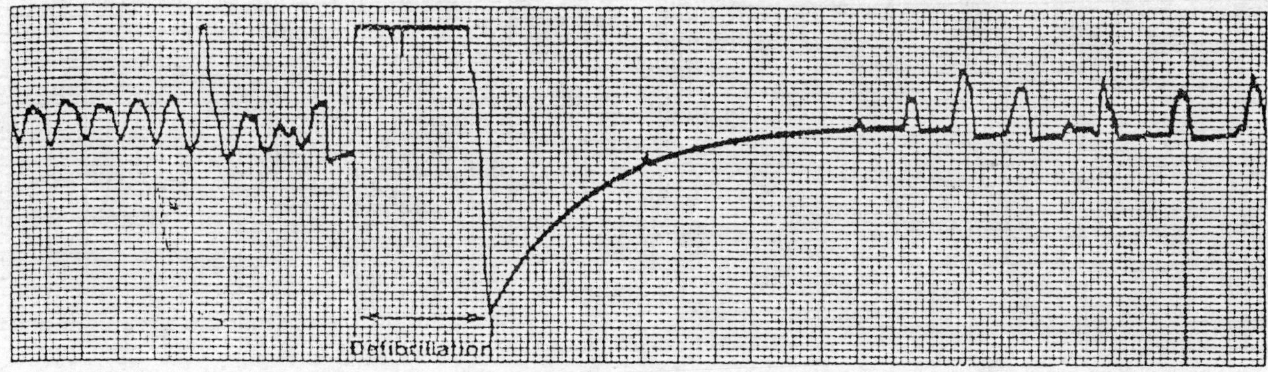

Fig.9.7: (C) Ventricular fibrillation with defibrillation

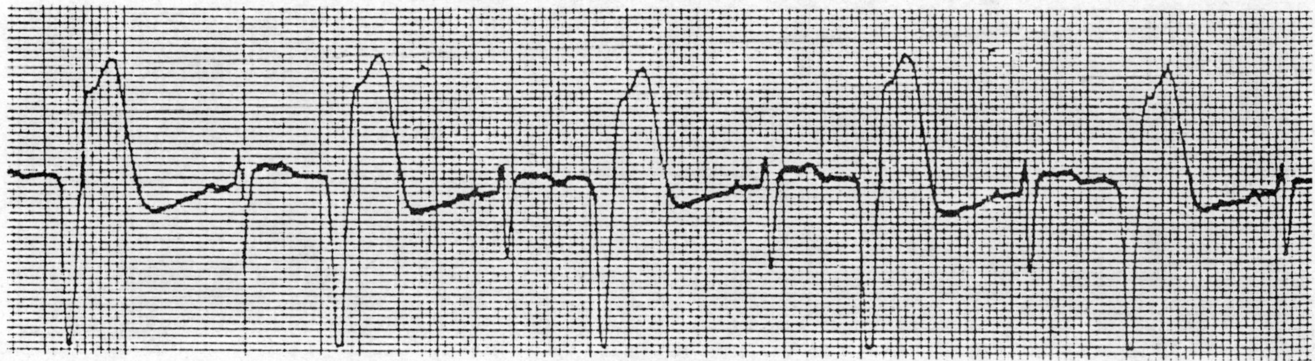

Fig.9.7: (D) Ventricular tachycardia

xvii. *Asystole*

Asystole represents the total absence of ventricular electrical activity. Occasionally P waves can be seen. No ventricular contraction occurs because of depolarization does not occur. This is a lethal arrhythmia that requires immediate treatment. Asystole is usually a result of advanced cardiac disease. Treatment consists of CPR with initiation of ACLS measures which includes itubation and IV therapy with epinephrine and atrophine.

xviii. *Atrio-ventricular block (AV block)*

A block to conduction of an impulse may occur at any point along the conduction pathways. One common area in the AV junction. The severity of the block is identified by degrees i.e., first, second, and third degree AV blocks.

- First degree AV block is present when the PR interval is prolonged to greater than 0.20 second, indicating a conduction delay in the AV node. It is usually found in association with rheumatic fever, digitalis toxicity, acute inferior MI and increased vagal tone. When this occurs in isolation, the patient is asymptomatic and no treatment is needed.
- Second-degree AV block may be devided into two categories. Type I (Mobitz I or Wenckabach phenoma) and Type II (Mobitz II)

Type I AV block may result from use of digoxin or beta blockers, and may be associated with cardiac and other diseases that can slow AV conduction. In this atrial rate is normal, but

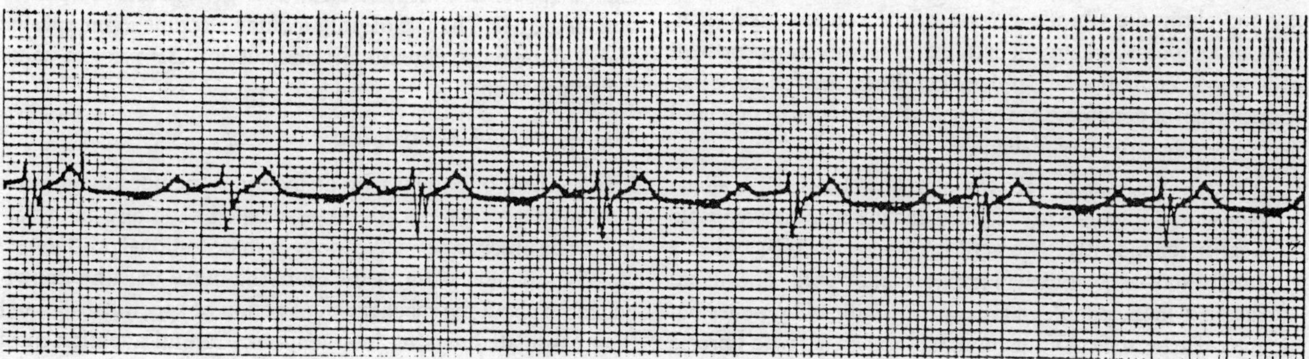

Fig.9.8: (A) First-degree AV block

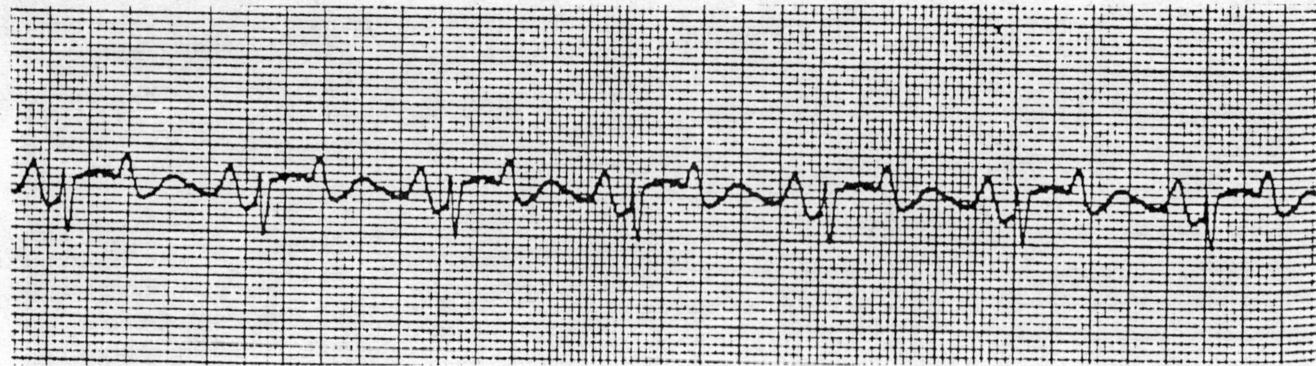

Fig.9.8: (B) Second-degree AV block (Mobitz 1)

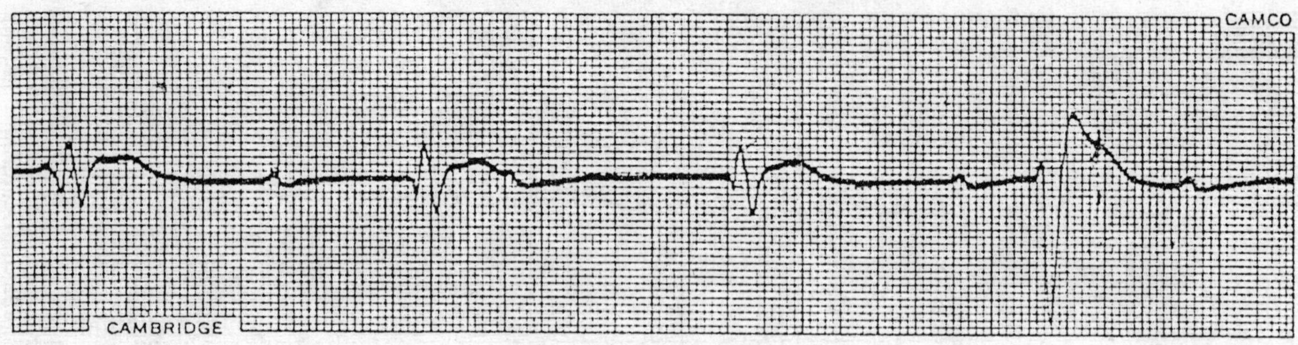

Fig.9.8: (C) Third-degree AV block

ventricular rate may be slower as a result of dropped QRS complexes. Ventricular rhythm is irregular. The PR interval progressively lengthens before the non-conducted P wave occurs. The P wave has a normal contour. The PR interval lengthens progressively until a P wave is nonconducted and a QRS complex is dropped. The QRS complex has a normal contour of the patient in symptomatic atropine it is used to increase heart rate or temporary pacemaker may be needed (for MI).

Type II AV block is less common but more serious. It is characterized by non-conducted sinus impulses despite constant PR intervals for the conducted P waves. The nonconducted P waves may occur at random or in patterned ratio (2:1, 3:1). The QRS complexes are widened unless the block is within the bundle of HIS type II blocks may occur in CAD, MI, RHD, cardiomyopathy and chroronic fibrotic disease of the conduction system. For this temporary treatment before the insertion of permanent pacemaker, i.e. temporary pacemaker drugs such as atropine, epinephrine, or dopamine can be tried to increase heart rate until pacemaker therapy is available.

- Third degree AV block is a complete heart block. Here all the sinus atrial impulses are blocked and the atria and ventricle beat independently. The ventricles are driven by either a junctional or a ventricular pacemaker cell. The usual lesion is in the bundle of HIS or the bundle of branches but may also be at the AV junction. It is associated with fibrosis or calcification of the cardiac conduction system, CAD myocarditis, cardiomyopathy, open heart surgery and some systemic diseases such as amyloidosis and scleroderma.

ECG shows the atrial rate usually a sinus rate which is usually a sinus rate of 60 to 100 beats/min artery. The ventricular rate depends on the site of block. The P wave has normal contour. The PR interval is variable and there is no relationship between the P wave and the QRS complex. The QRS complex is normal if escape rhythm is initiated in the bundle of his or above. The third-degree AV block almost always results in reduced CO with subsequent ischaemia and heart failure. Syncope from this block may result from severe bradycardia or even episodes of asystole.

Treatment includes insertion of temporary pacemaker or an external pacemaker applied on an emergency basis in a patient with acute MI. The use of drug include atropine, epinerphrine and dopamine to increase HR and support BP prior to pacemaker insertion.

Management of Arrhythmias

Management of patient with arrhythmias includes diagnosing the specific arrhythnia and its associated aetiology and treating the disorders with medications or interventional procedures.

When patient is on medication, the nurse must be knowledgeable about the mechanism of action of specific drugs and their associated nursing interventions. Careful attention must be given to potential drug interactions and synergetic effects when combination of therapy is used. The metabolism and excretion of medications may be impaired in the elderly and in patients with decreased perfusion to the kidney and liver. The nurse must be aware of new agents approved for the management of cardiac arrhythmian and how to monitor their safe use.

Nursing management of the patient experiencing arrhythmia include interventions to decrease oxygen demand. The nurse spaces activities and encourages frequent rest periods. While medication therapy is being adjusted, patients are on continuous monitoring (telemetry). Rhythms are documented every 4 to 8 hours and as needed. Skin care is provided to minimize the irritation of monitoring electrodes.

The nurse must be alert to changes in a patient's rhythm. Assessment for changes in the cardiac output are documented. Emergency drugs should be available and intravenous access should be ensured. Ancillary equipment such as defibrillators, oxygen suction and temporary pacemaker should be readily available and in good working condition.

Interventions such as cardioversion defibrillation, coronary ablation, pacemaker therapy, automatic implantabel cardioverter-defibrillators, and CPR are also part of the managements of patients with arrhythmias.

INFLAMMATORY HEART DISEASE

Pericarditis

Pericarditis is an inflammatory process of the visceral or parietal pericordium (inflammations of the pericardial sac). It can be acute or chronic and can spread from or to the myocardium.

Aetiology

Pericarditis can occur as a result of bacterial, viral or fungal infection. The causes of pericarditis are as follows:

i. *Infections*
   - Viral causes including Coxsakie virus B, Coxsakie virus A, adeno virus, mumps, epstein-barr, varicella Zoster and hepatitis B.
   - Bacterial causes including pneumococci, staphylococci, streptococci septicemia from gram-negative organisms and tuberculosis.
   - Fungal causes including histoplasma, candida species, infections such as toxoplasmosis and lyme disease.

ii. *Non-infections*
   - Uraemia.
   - Acute MI.
   - Neaplasms such as lung cancer, breast cancer, Hodgkin's disease and lymphoma.
   - Trauma after thoracic surgery, pacemaker insertion and cardial diagnostic procedures.
   - Radiation.
   - Dissecting aortic aneurysm.
   - Myxedema

iii. *Hypertensive or autoimmune*
   - Delayed post-myocardial-pericardial injury.
   - Post-myocardial infarction syndrome (Dresslers).
   - Post-pericardiotomy syndrome.
   - Rheumatic fever.
   - Drug reactions (eg. Procainamide and hydralazine).

Pathophysiology

In acute pericarditis, the membranes surrounding the heart become inflammed. The inflammed membrane rub against each other and produces the classic pericardial friction rub of percarditis. The friction rub sounds scratching and harsh on the auscultation and lasts throughout systole and diastole. The patient complains of severe precordial chest pain, which may closely resemble that of acute MI. The pain intensifies when the person is lying supien and decreases with sitting. The pain also intensifies when the patient breathes deeply. Patient shows other signs and symptoms (See clinical manifestation.)

Chronic pericarditis can be constrictive or adhesive. It usually begins with an initial episode of acute pericarditis (often secondary to neoplasia, radiation, previous surgery, or ideopathic causes) and is characterized by fibrin deposition with clinically undetected pericardial effusion. Organization and resorption of the effusion slowly follows with progression towards the chronic stage of fibrous scarring, thickening of the pericardium from calcium deposition, and eventual obliteration of the pericardial space. The fibrositic, thickened and adherent pericardium encases the heart, thereby, impairing the ability of the atria and ventricles to stretch sufficiently during diastolic filling.

Clinical Manifestations

In acute pericarditis, patient may complain chest pain, dyspnoea and a pericardial friction rub. The intense, plueretic chest pain is generally sharpest over the left precardium or retrosternally but may radiate to the trapezius ridge and neck (mimicking angina) or sometimes to the epigastrium or abdomen (mimicking abdominal or other non-cardiac pathologic condition). The pain is aggravated by lying supine, deep breathing, coughing, swallowing and moving the trunk and is eased by sitting up and leaning forward. The dyspnoea accompanying acute pericarditis is related to the patients' need to breathe in, rapid, shallow breaths to avoid chest pain and may be aggravated by fever and anxiety. The pericardial rub is a scratching, grating, high-pitched sound believed to arise from friction between the roughened pericardial and epicardial surface. It is best heart with stethoscope.

The two major complications of acute pericarditis induced are pericardial effusion and cardiac tamponade. The accumulation of fluid within the pericardial sac is called "Pericardial effusion". The fluid may be serous, purulent, or haemorrhagic. Serous effusion usually accompany heart failure. Purulent effusions indicate underlying disorders such as tuberculosis or neoplasm. Haemorrhagic effusions most often occur from trauma, aneurysm, rupture, coagulation abnormalities. Large effusions may compress adjoining structures. Pulmonary tissue compression can cause cough dyspnoea and tachypnoea. Phrenic nerve compression can induce hiccups and compression of the laryngeal nerve may result in hoarseness. Heart sounds are generally distant and muffled, although BP is maintained by compensatory meçhanism.

The cardiac tamponade develops as the pericardial effusion increases in size compensatory mechanism ultimately fail to adjust to the decreased cardiac output. This can lead to cardiac failure, shock and death. The signs and symptoms of cardiac temponade include

- Decrease in systolic BP.
- Narrowing pulse pressure.
- Pulses Paradoxus (Greater than 10 mm Hg).
- Increase in venous pressure and distention fo neck veins.
- Tachycardia.
- Tachypnoea.
- Possible friction rub.
- Muffled heart sounds.
- Low voltage EGG.
- Rapid enlargement of cardiac heart on chest X-Ray.
- Peripheral cyanosis.
- Anxiety.
- Chestpain.

The chronic pericarditis patient may complain of dyspnoea and fatigue and exhibits symptom of heart failure as a result of diminished ability of the heart pump.

Management of Ac. pericarditis

To diagnose, careful history and physical examination are needed. In addition, auscultation of chest, EGG, Chest X-Ray, echocardiography, pericardiocentesis, CT scan, nuclear scan of the heart are useful. The management includes.

- Treatment of underlying disease.
- Bedrest.
- Aspirin.
- NSAIDs (Non-steroid anti-inflammation drug)
- Corticosteroids.
- Pericardiocentesis (for large pericardial effusion or cardiac temponade)

In chronic pericarditis, removal of the pericardium may be necessary to restore cardiac function.

The management of the patient's pain and anxiety during acute pericarditis are primary nursing considerations. Assessment and careful observation of pain and attending to it are important and also monitor the anxiety level and take anxiety-reducing measures in addition to regular treatment including care of surgical patients.

In addition, the nurse teaches the patient and their significant others about the nature of the disease and the purposes and correct use of all medications. She teaches measures to decrease fatigue and provides information on how to minimize the risk of complications. The nurse also provides an overview of the signs and symptoms of recurrent pericarditis that would need to be promptly reported to the health care provider.

MYOCARDITIS

Myocarditis, a focal or diffuse inflammation of the myocardium that causes an infiltrate in the myocardial interstitium and injury to an adjacent myocardial cells.

Aetiology

Myocarditis may be primary with an unknown aetiology or secondary from an identifiable cause such as drug sensitivity or toxicity, connective tissue disease, sarcoidosis, or infection. The inflammation process often develops secondary to infective endocarditis. Myocarditis may be acute or chronic. It has been associated with variety of a etiologic agents including viruses, bacteria, rickettsia, fungi, parasites, radiation and pharmacological and chemical factors. Viral infection is the most common cause. It includes viruses like coxsackievirus B, coxsackievirus A, echovirus, poliovirus, influenza A and B, rubella, mumps, rabies, Epstein-Barrs, lepatitis and HIV.

The pathophysiologic mechanisms of myocarditis are poorly understood because there is usually a period of several weeks after the initial infection before the development of manifestations of myocorditis. Immunologic mechanisms may play a role in the development of myocarditis. The majority of infections are benign, self-limiting, and sub-clinical although viral myocordium in infants and pregnant women may be virulent.

Clinical Manifestation

During the acute viral phase, symptoms are flu-like and include fever, lymphadenopathy, pharyngitis, myalgia and gastrointestinal complaints. Hepatitis, encephalitis, nephritis and orchitis also can occur. The clinical manifestations for patient with myocarditis are variable ranging from a benign course without any overt manifestations to severe heart involvement of sudden death:

Usually early cardiac manifestations appear 7 to 10 days after viral infection and include pericardial chest pain with an associated friction rub because pericarditis often accompanies myocarditis. Cardiac signs (S_3 Crackles, jugular venous distention and peripheral oedema) may progress to CHF including pericardial effusion, syncope, and possibly ischaemic pain. ECG changes include ST segments, elevation and QT interval prolongation.

Management

Diagnosis can be made through as in pericarditis. In addition, histologic confirmation of myocarditis through endomyocardial biopsy (EMB). The patient with myocarditis are treated with bedrest and digitalis to prevent heart failure and cardiogenic shock. Immunosuppression may be beneficial in reducing inflammation and preventing irreversible myocardial damage. Medical therapy also includes treatment of underlying disease with antibiotics, conventional therapy for CHF and management of arrhythmias.

Nursing care includes ongoing monitoring of the patients, physiological status. Patients are commonly anxious about the sudden onset of heart disease and its implications for the future. The nurse provides emotional support and encourages verbalizations of feelings. If EMB is performed, postbiopsy nursing care focuses on the potential for injury that can occur, such as haematoma or bleeding at the connulation site, cardiac tamponade or pneumothorax. Any alteration should be referred to the physician concerned immediately. Vital signs are monitored closely to assess for continual haemodynamic stability. Monitoring for heart failure is an important consideration. Measure to decrease cardiac workload include frequent rest periods, provisions for a quiet environment, and the use of semi-Fowler's position. The patients and their family members/significant and others were educated regarding the disease. The nurse encoruages slow progression of activities with frequent rest periods and the use of medication with instructions.

INFECTIVE ENDOCARDITIS

Infective endocarditis previously known as bacterial endocarditis is an infection of the endorcordial surface with micro-organism, present in the lesion. The endocardium, the inner layer of the heart, is contagious with the valves of the heart. Therefore, inflammation from infective endocarditis usually affects the cardiac valves.

Infective endocarditis classified as subacute and acute. The subacute form has a longer clincial course of more insidious onset with less toxicity, and the causative organisms usually of low virulence. In contrast, the acute form has a shorter clinical course with more rapid onset, increased toxicity and more pathogenic causative organism.

Aetiolocy

Aetiologic organisms associated with infective endocarditis includes:

- Streptococci
  - Alpha and haemolytic streptococci
  - Enterococci
  - Streptococcus bovis and
  - Streptococcus pneumoniae.
- Staphylococci
  - Staphylococcus aureus
  - Staphylococcus epidermidia.
- Gram-negative bacteria;
  - Escherichia coli
  - Klebsialla and
  - Pseudomonas.
- Polymicrobic endocarditis.
  - Staphylococcus agalaective and methicillin susceptible Staphylococcus areus.
  - Pseudomonas aeruginosa, a-hemolytic streptococci and micrococcus.
- Haemophilus
- Actinobacilus
- Cardiobacterium
- Eikenella and
- Kingella.

The predisposing conditions to the development of infective endocarditis are as follows:

- Cardiac conditions:
  - Rheumatic heart disease.
  - Aortic valve leaflet abnormalities.
  - Mitral valve prolapse with murmur.
  - Cyanotic congenital heart disease.
  - Prosthetic valve.
  - Degenerative valvular lesions.
  - Prior endocarditis.
  - Morjan's syndrome.
  - Asymmetric septal hypertrophy.
  - Idiopathic hypertrophic subs-lesions.
- Non-cardiac diseases:
  - Associate risks.
  - Intravascular devices (leading) bacteraemia.
- Procedure
  - Associated risks.
  - Intravascular devices (leading to nosocomial bacteraemia.
  - Procedures that require endocarditis antibiotic prophylaxis.

The patient populations at risk for infective endocarditis are:

High risk

- Prosthetic heart valves.
- Previous history of endocarditis.
- Complex congenital cyanotic heart disease.
- Surgically constructed systemic pulmonary shunts or conduits.

Moderate risk

- Patent ductus arteriosus.
- Ventricular septal defect.
- Primum atrial septal defect.
- Coarctation of aorta.
- Acquired valvular dysfunction.
- Hypertrophic cardiomyopathy.
- Some clinical presentation of mitral valve prolapse.

Pathophysiology

A damaged cardiac valve or a ventricular septal defect produces turbulent blood flow, which allows bacteria to settle on the low pressure side of the valve or defect. The hallmark of endocarditis is the "Platletfibrin-bacteria mass" on the value called a vegetation. The organism-surround the heart valve become embedded on the valve matrix, and result in vegetative, the primary lesions of the infective endocarditis consist of fibrin, leukocytes, platelets, and microbes that adhere to the valve surface or endocardium. The loss of portions of these friable types of vegetation into the circulation results in embolization. Systemic embolization occurs from left-sided heart vegetation, progressing to organ (particularly brain, kidneys and spleen) and limb infarction. Right-sided heart lesions embolize to the lungs. If the vegetative emboli enter organs, abscesses may form.

The infection may spread locally to cause damage to the valves or to their supporting structures. The resulting valvular incompetence and eventual invasion of the myocardium in the infectious disease result in CHF, generalized myocardial dysfunction and sepsis.

Clinical Manifestations

The onset of SBE (Subacute Bacterial Endocarditis) is gradual and the patient reports malaise and general achiness. Low grade fever is usually present, although a high fever usually occurs with S. aureus, infection. The other non-specific manifestations that may accompany fever include chills, weakness, malaise, fatigue, and anorexia. Arthrelgia, myalgia, backpain, abdominal discomfort, weight loss and headache, clubbing of fingers may occur in SBE.

Vascular manifestation's infective endocarditis include splinter haemorrhages (black longitudinal streaks) that may occur in nail beds. Petechiae may occur as a result of fragmentation and microembolization of vegetative lesions and are common in the conjunctiva, the lips, the buccal mucosa, the palate, and over the ankles, the feet and the antecubital and popl, eteal areas oslers nodes (painful, tender, red or purple pea-size lesions) may be found in figertips or toes. Janeway lesions (flat painless, small red spots) may be found on the palms and soles. Funduscopic examination may reveal haemorrhagic retinal lesions called Rohith's spots.

Auscultation reveals murmurs over the affected area and clinical manifestations secondary to embolizations in various body organs may also be present, if embolization of organs and cardinal symptom are as follows:

- Spleen – Sharp left upper quadrant pain and splenomegally, local tenderness and abdominal rigidity.
- Kidney – Pain in the flank, haematuria and azotaemia.
- Peripheral – Blood vessel of arms and legs may cause gangrene.
- Brain – Hemiplegia, ataxia, aphasia, visual changes. LOC changes.
- Pulmonary emboli, occurs in right-sided endocarditis.

Management

For diagnosis obtaining the patient's recent health history is very important particularly inquiry regarding any recent dental urologic, surgical or gynaecologic including normal or abnormal obstetric delivery, heart disease diagnostic procedures, infection of skin and respiration or urinary origin are helpful.

In addition to thorough physical examination and routine diagnostic procedures, useful are blood culture and sensitivity, WBC count with differential rheuma old factor, urin analysis, chest X-Ray, ECG, echocardioraphy and cardiac catheterization.

The major aim of the therapy is to eliminate all micro organisms from the vegetative grown and prevent complications. The therapy includes:

- Appropriate antibiotic therapy.
- Antipyretics.
- Rest.
- Repetitions of blood cultures and sensitivity tests.
- Surgical valvular repair or replacement (for severe valvular damage).

The nurse teaches the patient to avoid excessive fatigue and to stop activity immediately if chest pain, dyspnoea, lightheadedness, or faintness occurs. Patients should avoid others with infections. The nurse instructs the patient to inform all primary care providers including physicians, and dentists about history of infective endocarditis, so that appropriate antibiotic therapy can be administered prior to intrusive procedure. American Heart Association recommended following antibiotic prophylaxis of infective endocarditis.

1. For dental, oral, respiratory tract or oesophageal procedure, if streptococcus viscidan is a pathogen, the antibiotic choice will be:
   - Amoxicillin 2g 1 hr before procedure, alternative if unable to take oral or if allergic to penicillin.
   - Ampicillin IV.
   - Clindamycin, oral or IV.
   - First-generation Cephalosperins - Cefazin. IV Azithromycin or Clatithromycin.
2. For genitourinary and nonesophageal GI, procedures if pathogens is entered coccus faecalis, antibiotic choice will be parenteral Ampicillin or Amoxicillin, IV/IM Gentamycin IV Nafcillin, IV Vancomycin (for Staphylococcus).

In addition, the patient should brush with soft-bristled toothbrush and floss regularly to protect the gums and or event caries. Good dental hygiene is of utmost importance in decreasing the risk of recurrent infective endocarditis.

Problems

- Activity intolerance related to imbalance between oxygen supply and demand.
- Ineffective management, R/T Therapy.
- Pain related to arthralgia. Myalgia and embolization.
- Altered health maintenance.
- Emboli R/T dislodging vegetation and immobility.
- Anxiety R/T Critical illness.

RHEUMATIC HEART DISEASE

Rheumatic heart disease is an acute inflammatory reaction involving all layers. The resulting damage to the heart from Rh fever is termed "Rheumatic heart disease" a chronic condition characterized by scarring and deformity of heart valves.

Aetiology

Rheumatic fever almost always occurs as a delayed sequela (usually after 2 to 3 weeks) of a group A-beta-haemolytic streptococcal infection of the upper respiratory system. In addition socio-economic factors, familial factors and presence of an altered immune response have a predisposing role in the development of rheumatic fever.

Pathophysiology

The inflammation of rheumatic heart disease may involve:

- The lining of the heart or endocardium (endocarditis) including the valves, resulting scarring, distortion and stenosis of the valves.
- The heart muscle (myocarditis) or
- The outer covering of the heart (Pericarditis), where it may cause adhesions of surrounding tissues.

Clinical Manifestations

The development of symptoms of chronic rheumatic heart disease depends on the involvement of the particular part of the heart.

Management

Careful history and physical examination are needed to diagnoses rheumatic heart disease. In addition, ASO titre (Antistreptolysin Otiter) ESR, C-reactine protein, throat culture, WBC count, RBC parameter, chest-X-Ray, ecocardiography and ECG are useful to identify RHD.

Prophylactic penicillin is prescribed during acute episodes of rheumatic fever and for several years thereafter lifelong antibiotic prophylaxis may be necessary for persons with significant rheumatic heart disease. Corticosteroids may be prescribed during acute rheumatic fever to decrease the cardiac inflammation. If congestive heart failure occurs, bedrest, sodium and fluid restrictions, diuretics, and inotrope usually are prescribed. Antipyretics are also used cautiously.

The nurse emphasizes to the patient and family the importance of rest and adequate nutrition. Additional education to be given as in cardiac diseases.

VALVULAR HEART DISEASE

The heart contains two atro-ventricular valves, the mitral and tricuspid, and two semilunar valves, the aortic and the pulmonic which are located in four strategic locations to control unidirectional blood flow. Types of valvular heart diseases are defined according to the valve or valves affected and the two types of functional alterations, stenosis and regurgitation.

1. Mitral Stenosis

Mitral stenosis occurs when the blood flow from the left atrium to the left ventricle during ventricular diastole (Ventricular filling) is impeded due to thickening or fibritic changes in the mitral valve.

Aetiology

The primary cause is rheumatic fever and carditis, which causes an inflammatory process of the mitral valves chordaectendineae or commissures (leaflets). Less common causes include bacterial vegetation, thrombus formation, calcification of the mitral annulus and atrial myexaema (tumour).

Pathophysiology

In mitral stenosis, the mitral valve leaflets become thickened and fibrotic from scar tissue formation and calcification. As the valve leaflets become stiff and fosed, the valve lumen progressively narrows and becomes immobile. In addition, the chorda tendinea may shorten and thicken. The mitral value of orifice may decrease in size from its normal 4 to 6 cm to less than one cm. With progressive mitral stenosis, left atrial pressure elevates as a result of incomplete emptying of the left atrium. Sustained elevated left atrial pressure causes the myocardium to compensate with left atrial dilation and hypertrophy. In addition, high pressures in the left atrium lead to elevated pulmonary venous capillary and arterial pressures. Eventually sustained elevation of the left atrial pressure can produce pulmonary hypertension and subsequent right ventricular hypertrophy. With the increased pressure in the pulmonary vasculature, leakage of fluid across the pulmonary pillary membrane into the lung enterstitium can be produced pulmonar oedema. Persons with mitral stenosis also have reduced cardiac output and increases cardiac arrhythmias - (atrial fibrillation), later this may allow thrombus formation and arterial embolization to vital organs.

Clinical Manifestations

The most common cause rheumatic fever. In addition there will be fatigue, weakness. The primary symptoms include dyspnoea, an exertion orthopnoea, paraxysmal nocturnal dyspnoea, predisposing causes to respiratory infections, haemoptysis, pulmonary hypertension and oedema. These symptoms may be precipitated by emotional stress, respiratory infections, sexual intercourse or atrial fibrillation. Later neural deficits only associated with emboli (haemiparasis) CVA, ascitis, hepatic angina with hepatomegaly, chest pain, palpitations (AF) diastolic murmurs accentuated first heart sound, opening snap. If not treated and right ventricular failrue occurs leads to jugular vein distentions, pitting oedema and hepatomegaly.

Management

Diagnosis of mitral stenosis is established by the clinical symptoms such as an opening snap (best heard at the apex with stethoscope diaphragm) and a low-pitched, rumbling diastolic murmur (best heard at the apex with the stethoscope bell) results from increased velocity of blood flow. If valve calcified no murmr, heard. ECG echocardiagram and cardiac catheterization are also helpful in diagnosis of mitral stenosis.

Mildly symptomatic patient with mitral stenosis are treated with diuretics, and digitalis is used to control heart rate in the event of atrial fibrillations. Anticoagulation therapy is used to prevent embolization. Medical therapy includes antibiotic prophylaxis before dental and surgical procedures to reduce the risk of bacterial endocarditis. Mechanical enlargement of the mitral valve is indicated when the disease causes either loss of exercise capacity or pulmonary hypertension.

- Percutaneous valvuloplasty using baloon dilation provides a non-surgical alternative to repair of mitral stenosis.
- Surgical commissurotomy can also be performed while the valve leaflets remain mobile.
- Mitral valve replacement using open heart surgery.
- Cardiopulmonary bypass is performed when the valve is severely calcified.

Patient who experiences symptoms related to mitral stenosis are prescribed sodium-restricted diet to help prevent fluid retention, and progressive heart failure. Nursing interventions are taken accordingly.

2. Mitral Regurgitation

Mitral regurgitation (mitral insufficiency) occurs when the mitral valve fails to completely close during ventricular systole, and consequently some blood flows backward into the left atrium. Mitral regurgitation can be acute or chronic.

Aetiology

The causes of mitral regurgitations are numerous and may be inflammatory, degenerative, infective, structural, or congenital in nature. The majority of cases may be attributed to chronic rheumatic heart disease, isolated rupture of chordae tendineae, mitral valve prolapse, ischeni papillary muscle dysfunction and infective endocarditis.

Pathophysiology

The regurgitant mitral orifice is parallel with aortic valve, so that burden imposed on the left ventricle and the left atrium are determined by the aetiology, severity and duration of mitral regurgitation. In chronic regurgitation, volume overload on the left ventricle, the left atrium, and the pulmonary bed is created by the backward flow of blood from the left ventricle into the left atrium during ventricular systole, resulting in varying degrees of left atrial enlargement and left ventricular dilation. Acute mitral regurgitation does not result in dilation of the left atrium or left ventricle. Without dilation to accommodate the regurgant volume, pulmonary vascular pressure rise ultimately, causing pulmonary oedema.

Clinical Manifestation

The resultant clinical picture in acute M. regurgitation is that of pulmonary oedema and shock. Patient will have thready, peripheral pulses and cool, clammy extremities. Auscultation findings of a new systolic murmur may be obscured by a low cardiac output.

Patient with chronic mitral regurgitation may remain asymptomatic for many years until the development of some degree of LVF. Initial symptoms include weakness, fatigue and dyspnoea that gradually progress to orthopnoea, paraxysmal nocturnal dyspnoea, and peripheraloedema, and brisk carotid pulse. Auscultatory findings reflect accentuated left ventricular filling leading to an audible third heart sound (S_3) even in the absence of left ventricular dysfunction. The murmur is a loud pansystolic or holosystolic murmur at the apex radiating to the left axilla.

Management

The diagnosis of mitral regurgitation is made by auscultatory findings. Chest-X-ray reveals left atrial enlargement need occassional left ventricular dilation. ECG echocardiogram also is used for diagnosis. Definitive diagnosis is made through cardiac catheterization, which assess left ventricular function and the degree of regurgitation.

Patient with mild mitral regurgitation are generally managed medically. Acute mitral regurgitation need hospitalization and haemodynamic stabilization. As with other cardiac cases, management of heart failure, arrhythmias, and others by antibiotic prophylaxis, diuretics and digitalis are useful accordingly. The nursing care is also designed accordingly.

3. Mitral Valve Prolapse (MVP)

Mitral valve prolapse occurs when abnormalities in the mitral valve leaflets, cordae tindinea or papillary muscles allow prolapse of the mitral valve leaflets backward into the left atrium during ventricular systole. It is also known as Barlow's syndrome as well as a "floppy or billowing" mitral valve.

Aetiology

The cause of MVP is unknown but related to pathogenic mechanisms of mitral valve apparatus. If incidence is possibly linked to an autosomal dominant inherited trait, and is associated with other inherited connective tissue disorders such as Marfan syndroma, Ehlers-Danlos syndrome and oestrogenisis imperfecta. Other causes include endocarditis, CAD, myocarditis, cardiomyopathy, cardiac trauma and hyperthyroidism.

Pathophysiology

In mitral valve prolapse, the leaflets of mitral valve become enlarged or thickened, and the chordae tindineae may become elongated. These changes permit the valve leaflets to billow upward into the left atrium during ventricular systole. Depending on the degree of prolapse and integrity of the valve leaflets mitral regurgitation may occur. The subsequent pathophysiology parallels that of mitral regurgitation.

Clinical Manifestation

Many cases of MVP are symptomatic. Persons with symptomatic complain of palpitations secondary to arrhythmias and tachycardia, other systems include light-headedness, syncope, fatigue, lethargy, weakness, dyspnoea, and chest tightness. In addition, hyperventilation, anxiety, depression, panic attacks and atypical chest pain may occur. Many symptoms are vague, and puzzling and are not necessarily degree of prolapse.

Management

MVP is diagnosed principally by echocardiography, although cardiac angiography may be used to confirm diagnosis. Individuals who experience palpitations require 24 hours ambulatory ECG monitoring to determine severity of arrhythmias.

Asymptomatic persons with MVP usually do not require treatment. Symptomatic persons may require medications for the arrhythmias. Beta blockers are the treatemnt of choice for managing palpitations and chest pain. The drug of choice is atenolol or propranolol. Antibiotic prophylaxis are used to prevent endocarditis. All persons with MVP need regular follow-up and should have an echocardiogram every few years to monitor disease, severity and progression.

Persons with MVP are encouraged to avoid caffeine which may exacerbate the incidence of tachycardia and atrial dysrhythmias.

4. Aortic Stenosis (AS)

Aortic stenosis occurs when the aortic valve leaflets become stiff, fused or calcified and impede blood flow from the left ventricle into the aorta during ventricular systole.

Aetiology

Aortic stenosis is caused by congenital malformation of the aortic valve inflammatory heart disease (endocarditis) or degenerative disease (calcification). Hypertrophic cardiomyopathy leads to subvalvular lesion that may mimic aortic stenosis.

Pathophysiology

Aortic stenosis results in obstruction of flow from the left ventricle to the aorta during systole. The effect is concentric for left ventricular hypertrophy and increased myocardial oxygen consumption because of the increased myocardial mass. As the disease course progresses and compensatory mechanisms fail, reduced cardiac output leads to pulmonary hypertension.

Clinical Manifestation

The general symptoms is fatigue, dyspnoea on exertions, syncope (especially on exertion), pain resembles angina pectoris, bradycardia, dysrhythmias (with heart failure). Systolic murmurs normal or soft S_1, Prominent S_4 Crescendo-decrescendo murmur.

Management

A diagnosis of aortic valve stenosis is made by clinical symptoms, clinical findings and diagnostic test. Test that help are ECG, Chest X-ray echocardiogram, and cardiac catheterization. Percutaneous balloon valvuloplasty may be used to alleviate aorta stenosis. The definitive therapy for patients with aortic stenosis is valve replacement with a prosthetic aortic valve. In addition, measures to be taken to manage arrhythmias and heart failure. Nursing care is designed accordingly.

The diet of persons with aortic stenosis is unrestricted, unless heart failure is present, in which case the nurse instructs patient to restrict their daily intake of sodium and fluid. Activity level must be carefully monitored because patients are at risk for sudden cardiac death. Patients are cautioned against undue physical exertion or stress, which may precipitate heart failure or arrhythmias. Patients and families need ongoing teaching, and support effectively to manage this ongoing challange in their daily lives. The nurse also reminds patient of the seeking prophylactic antibiotic treatment against endocarditis before any invasive dental procedure or surgery.

Aortic Regurgitation

Aortic regurgitation occurs when an incompetent aortic valve allows blood to flow backward from the aorta into the left ventricle during diastole.

Aetiology

Aortic regurgitation may result in a primary disease of the aortic valve leaflets, the aortic root, or both acute aortic regurgitation may be the result of a primary disease of the aortic valve leaflets, the aortic root, or both. Acute aortic regurgitation is caused by bacterial endocarditis, trauma or aortic dissection and constitute a life-threatening emergency. Chronic aortic regurgitation is generally the syphillis, or chronic rheumatic conditions such as ankylosing spondylitis, or Reiter's syndrome.

Pathophysiology

The basic physiologic consequence of aortic regurgitation is retrograde blood flow from the ascending aorta into the left ventricle resulting in volume overload. The left ventricle initially compensates for chronic aortic regurgitation by dilation and hypertrophy. Myocardial contractility eventually declines and blood volume increases in the left atrium and pulmonary vasculature. Ultimately, pulmonary hypertension and right ventricular failure develops.

Clinical Manifestation

Patients with acute aortic regurgitation have sudden clinical manifestations of cardiovascular collapse. Abrupt onset of profound dyspnoea, transient chest pain, progression to shock which need immediate medical attention.

Patient with chronic aortic regurgitation have pulses that are of the "water-hammer" or collapsing type with abrupt distension during systole and quick collapse during diastole

(Corrigan's pulse). Pistol-shot pulse sounds can be auscultated over the femoral arteries, and some persons demonstrate a typical head bobbing with each heart beat. Auscultaty findings include a soft or absent S_1, presence of S_3 or S_4 and a soft decrescendo and high-pitched diastolic murmur. A systolic murmur also can be heard i.e., systolic ejection click.

In chronic aortic regurgitation it appear symptomatic for many years and seen with external dyspnoea, orthopnoea, paraxysmal nocturnal dyspnoea only after considerable myocardial dysfunction. Nocturnal angina with diaphoresis and abdominal discomfort may be present.

Management

The diagnosts of aortic regurgitation made by auscultative finding, regular chest X-ray, ECG, and echocardiogram digitalis and diuretic are helpful to persons with heart failure. Aortic valve replacement is indicated for symptomatic persons, after thorough diagnosis. The other measure as in other valvular diseases.

6. Tricuspid Valve Disease

Tricuspid stenosis is a restriction of the tricuspid valve orifice that impedes blood flow from the right atrium to the right ventricle during right ventricular diastole (filling). Conversely, tricuspid regurgitation involves an imcompetent tricuspid valve that allows blood to flow backward from the right ventricle to the right atrium during ventricular systole.

Aetiology

Tricuspid stenosis is extremely uncommon and occurs almost exclusively in patient with rheumatic mitral stenosis. It is also seen in IV drugs users. Tricuspid regurgitation is usually the result of pulmonary hypertension or right ventricular dysfunction.

Pathophysiology

In tricuspid stenosis, right atrial outflow is obstructed, resulting in right atrial enlargement and elevated systemic venous pressures. Volume overload of the right atrium and ventricle occur in tricuspid regurgitation.

Clinical Manifestation

Tricuspid stenosis and regurgitation result in the backward flow of blood into the systemic circulation. Common manifesta tions are peripheral oedema, ascitis, and hepatomegaly. The murmur of ste-nosis is presystolic (Sinus rhythm) or midsystolic (AF) and pan-systolic murmur may be heard in regurgitation. Both types of murmurs dramatically increased in intensity with inspiration.

Management

As in other valvular disease are according to underlying cause.

7. Pulmonic Valve Disease

Tricuspid and pulmonary valve disease all cause similar consequences to cardiac function. Pulmonic valve disease is an uncommon entity and in the case of pulmonary stenosis, it is always congenital. Pulmonary regurgitation as an isolated abnormality has a benign course but it generally is associated with disease of other valves.

To sum up, the management of valvular heart disease includes following measures.

1. *Diagnostic measures*
   - History and physical examination.
   - Chest X-ray.
   - ECG.
   - Echocardiography.
   - Cardiac catheterization.
2. *Nonsurgical measures*
   - Prophylactic antibiotic therapy to prevent- Rh fever, Inf. endocarditis.
   - Digitalis.
   - Diuretics.
   - Sodium restriction.
   - Anticoagulant agents-warfarin-dipyramidole.
   - Aspirin.
   - Antiarrhythmic drugs.
   - Oral nitrates.
   - Beta-adrenergic blockers.
   - Percutaneous transluminal balloon valvulopathy.
3. *Surgical measures*
   - Valvuloplasty-Repair of valve and suturing of tornleaflets.
   - Closed commissurotomy (Valvulotomy-dilation of valve; repair of leaflet or commissure, fibrous band or ring).
   - Annuloplasty- Repair of ring or annulus of incompetent or diseased valve.
   - Valve replacement.

CARDIAC SURGERY

Numerous diseases and conditions may create the need for cardiac surgery. The most common reason for an adult to undergo cardiac surgery is myocardial revascularization (CABG). In addition, patients undergo cardiac surgery for valve repair or replacement, repair of structural defects (acquired or congenital) implantation of devices and cardiac transplantation. The indication for cardiac surgery includes:

- Aneurysm of sinus of valsalve.
- Constrictive pericarditis.
- Congenital heart defects.
- Coronary artery disease.
- Dissecting aortic aneurysm.
- Valvular insufficiency or stenosis.
- Ventricular aneurysm.
- Ventricular spetal defect.
- Ventricular arrhythmias.

The indications for cardiac surgery and associated procedures are:

- Ischaemic heart disease- Coronary artery bypass graft. (CABP)

- Repair of structural abnormalities
  - Valve repair
  - Atrial septal defect repair
  - Ventricular septal defect repair
  - Atrial tumour resection
  - Aortic aneurysm (Thoracic) repair
- Implantation of devices
  - Automatic implantable cardioverter-defibrillator.
  - Ventricular assist device.
  - Artificial heart chamber.
- Transplantation- Replacement of diseased heart with healthy heart.

Cardiac surgery is classified either as an open heart surgery or closed heart surgery, depending on whether the heart is "Opened" during the course of the surgery. Cardiac surgery involving the repair of internal structural defects is open heart, whereas revascularization is a closed heart procedure.

Cardiac surgery today provides pain relief, improvement in lifestyle, and improved survival and for the patient undergoing open heart surgical treatment.

Nursing Management

Care of the person undergoing cardiac surgery involves multidisciplinary team approach utilizing the skills of a variety of health care professionals including nurses, physicians, nutritionists and others.

The nurse caring for the cardiac surgery patient provides individualized care that is appropriate for the patient's medical condition, health history and psychosocial history. Important goals for the preoperative period include obtaining an accurate and complete patient history, providing preoperative teaching to the patient and family about the planned surgery and preparation of patients physiologically and psychologically for surgery. The nurse has to take active part in or collect information by required preoperative diagnostic test such as Chest X-ray, cardiac catheterization, coronary angiography, cardiography, stress testing and serum blood analysis as appropriate. A complet-baseline database is documented before surgery. Baseline vital signs including apical and radial heart rates and bilateral arm blood pressure integrity of all pulses (both proximal and distal), neurological status, height, weight, nutritional status, elimination pattern and psychological status are assessed and recorded in the immediate preoperation period. Before surgery, patient continues their normal medical and activity routines. With the exceptions of the withholding aspirin for 1 to 3 days before the day of surgery. Patients remain NPO after midnight before surgery.

Nurse has the main responsibility to perform preoperative teaching to patient undergoing cardiac surgery, which includes the following.

1. General information.
   - Places of care during hospitalization
     - CCU or ICU after surgery.
     - Return to general patient care unit in 2 to 3 days.
     - Visiting hours and location of waiting rooms.
2. Description of surgery.
   - Simple explanation of anatomy of heart and effect of the patient's cardiovascular disorder (eg. incompetent valve, CAD).
   - Explanation of surgical procedure including planned incision.
   - Definition of any unfamiliar terms: Bypass, extracorporeal.
   - Length of time and surgery: 2 to 4 hours.
   - Length of time until able to see family (1-1/2 to 2 hours after surgery).
3. Preparation for surgery.
   - Shower or bath at night before surgery with special antimicrobial soap.
   - Surgical shave: Shaving the entire chest and abdomen, neck to groin and left mid-axillary line to right.
   - Legs shaved in saphenous vein grafts will be used.
   - Preoperative medication.
4. Explanation of monitors.
   - Round patches on chest connected to cardiac monitor that record patient's heart beats.
   - Monitor makes beeping sound all the time.
5. Explanation of lines.
   - Intravenous routes for fluid and medications.
   - Central venous line in neck or chest to monitor fluid status.
   - Pulmonary artery catheter in chest or neck to measure pulmonary pressure and mobitor fluid status.
   - Plastic connector line to obtain blood samples without needle stick.
6. Explanation of drainage tube.
   - Indwelling urinary catheter.
   - Chest tube: bloody drainage expected.
7. Explanation of breathing tube.
   - Tube in windpipe connected to machine called ventilator.
   - Unable to speak with tube in place but can mouth words and communicate in writing.
   - Tube is removed when patient is awake and stable.
   - Secretions in lungs or tube removed by nurse using a suction catheter.
   - Food and oral fluids are not permitted until breathing tube is removed.
8. Explanation and demonstration of activities and exercises.
   - Purpose of activity is to promote circulation, keep lungs clear, and prevent infection.
   - Activities include turning from side to side in bed; sitting on edge of bed. Sitting on chair at the night or morning after surgery.
   - Range of motion exercises.

- Deep breathing using sustained maximal inspiration.
- Tubes and lines will restrict movement to a certain extent but nurse assists.

9. Releif of pain.
   - Some pain will be experienced, but it will not be excruciating.
   - Frequent pain medication will be given to relieve pain but patient should inform always when there is pain.

And following guidelines for care of the person who has undergone cardiac surgery.

1. Monitoring of:
   i. Cardiovascular
      - Blood pressure and pulse (rate, pulse devidit).
      - Pulmonary artery pressure (PAP). Pulmonary capillary wedge pressure. (PCWD), cardiac output (CO), central venous pressure (CVP) and left atrial-pressure (LAP).
      - ECG for signs of arrhythmias.
      - Body temperature.
      - Skin colour, temperature and capillary filling.
      - Signs of hypovolemic shock (decreased CVP, decreased LAP and decreased CO).
      - Signs of cardiac temponadle (cessation of chest drainage) restlessness, increased CVP, PAP and LAP, tachycardial paradioxical pulse, narrowed pulse pressure, diminished or absent point of maximal impulse, diminished heart sound, distended neckvein (CVP).

   ii. Respiratory:
      - Respirations : rate, depth, quality
      - Breach sounds
      - Chest tubes for patency and drainage
      - Autotransfuse chest tube drainage.

   iii. Neurological.
      - Level of consciousness
      - Pupillary size and reaction
      - Orientation
      - Movement and sensation of extremities.

   iv. Gastrointestinal - •nausea, •anorexia.

   v. Urinary output (amount)-colour, pH and specific gravity.

   vi. Fluid and electrolytes balance.
      - intake/output balance
      - Daily weight
      - Serum potassium and calcium levels

   vii. Presence of discomfort-pain, fatigue.

   viii. Ability to sleep

   ix. Behaviour: Repression, fear, disorientation and hallucinations.

2. Promoting oxygen/carbon dioxide exchange.
   - Preoxygenation and suction during intubation: suction as necessary after extubation.
   - Position with head only slightly elevated; turn side to side.
   - Encourage breathing exercises; incentive spirometry.
   - Encoruage range of motion exercises and progressive activity.
3. Promoting fluid and electrolytie balance.
   - Record accurate intake and output.
   - Maintain prescribed flow rates of parenteral fluid.
   - Give prescribed supplemental IV potassium chloride.
4. Promoting comfort.
   - Give narcotic analgesia every 3 hours during first 24 hours then as needed.
   - Give frequent mouth care.
   - Control environment for comfort.
   - Change bedlinens when diaphoresis presents (assure patient it is common).
   - Plan activities to permit periods of sleep.
   - Provide backrubs for backache.
   - Splint incision during coughing.
   - Encourage patient to share feelings and experiences.
   - Support family visits.
5. Promote activity.
   - Provide for passive than active range of motion exercises.
   - Encourage ambulation when permitted.
6. Teaching.
   - Piogressive return to physical activity as recommended by the physician.
   - Rehabilitation exercise programme.
   - Sexual activity usually permitted in 3 to 4 weeks.
   - Signs of overexertion include fatigue, dyspnoea and pain.
   - Eat a balanced diet with prescribed modifications (Low Na+, low fat).
   - Medications:
     Name, dosage, schedule action and side effects of prescribed drugs use prescribed education as needed.
   - Signs that may persist: dyspnoea, pain and night sweats.
   - Signs requiring medical attention fever, increasing dyspnoea or chestpain with minimal exertion.
   - Need for ongoing medical care.

The nurse has to provide discharge instruction for the patient who undergoes cardiac surgery includes:

1. Incision care:
   - Clean twice a day.
   - Care of sterile stips staples, sutures.
   - Incision massage with cocoa butter after 10 days.
2. Showering:
   - Wash with soap that is unscented, gentle, bactericidal
   - No tube bath until incision is completely healed.

3. Activity:
   - No lifting greater than 10 pounds.
   - No driving for 6 weeks.
   - No prolonged sitting.
   - Activity as tolerated, cardiac rehabilitation if ordered.
   - May resume sexual activity when comfort level allows.
4. Nutrition:
   - Low sodium, low-fat and heart-healthy diet
   - Increase protein intake for 4 to 6 weeks.
5. Medications:
   - Pain medications, do not drive or operate machine if taking narcotics.
6. Miscellaneous:
   - Women should wear a bra to help support chest TED stockings.
   - Daily weights - notify physician for gain of 6 pounds in 2 days.
   - Incentive spirometer three times a day.
   - Prevent constipation with fiber, fluids and stool softners.
   - Instruct any adverse symptoms should be reported to physician concerned.

VASCULAR PROBLEMS

ARTERIAL DISORDERS

1. Aneurysms

Aneurysms are outpouchings or dilation of the arterial wall and are a common problem involving aorta. Aneurysm is a Greek word meaning "widening". Aneurysms are points of weakness, dilation of outpouching of arteries to at least 1.5 times their normal size. Aneurysm occurs most commonly on the aorta but they can occur in any artery of the body. The other common sites include the femoral and popliteal artery.

Aetiology

The exact cause of aneurysm is unknown. The several factors are associated with developments of aneurysm, including hypertension, smoking, atherosclerosis, trauma, syphilis, congenital abnormalities of the vessel infection, (TB) and connective tissue disorders that cause weakness on the wall of the vessel.

Pathophysiology

Most aneurysms are found in the abdominal aorta below the level of renal arteries. The aortic wall weakens and dilates with the turbulent blood flow. The growth rate of aneurysm is unpredictable, but the larger the aneurysm, the greater the risk of rupture. Thrombi are deposited on the aortic wall and can embolize. There are three types of aneurysm.

- A *fusiform* aneurysm involves a circumferential dilation of the vessel well and is relatively uniform in shape.
- A succular aneurysm is pouch-like with a narrow neck connecting the bulge to one side of the arterial wall.
- A *dissecting* aneurysm develops from a tear in the time of the artery that causes an accumulation of blood in the newly formed cavity between the intima and the media. They further classified according to type of tear and degree of haematoma.

A cause of aortic aneurysm is atherosclerosis with plaques composed of lipids, cholesterol, fibrin, and other debris deposited beneath the intima or lining of the artery. This plaque formation causes degerative changes in the media (middle layer of arterial wall), leading to loss of elasticity, weakening and eventual dilation of aorta.

Clinical Manifestation

Patients with aneurysm are commonly asymptomatic. Abdominal aneurysm may be felt as a palpable mass and a systolic bruit may be heard. The patient may complain of abdominal or back pain. If the aneurysm leaks or ruptures, the patient will develop severe pain signs of shock, decreased RBCs count, and increased WBCs count.

Symptoms of thoracic aneurysm vary and depend on the size and placement of the aneursysm and its effect on the surrounding structures. Most patients may experience anterior chest wall, back, flank or abdominal pain or may develop signs of shock if the aneurysm leaks. Symptoms such as dyspnoea, cough, wheezing may develop if the aneurysm puts pressure on the trachea or bronchi.

Management

Most aneurysms are found on routine physical or X-ray examinations (chest and abdomen), ECG, CT scan, and MRI may also be used to diagnose and assess the severity of aneurysms.

Examples

Aortography: Anatomic mapping of the aortic system by contrast imaging is not a reliable method, but it helps the surgeon with accurate information about the visceral, renal or distal vessels.

The goal of management is to prevent rupture of the aneurysm. Therefore, early detection and prompt treatment of the patient are imperative. Once an aneurysm is suspected, studies are performed to determine its exact size and location. A careful review of all body systems is necessary to identify and coexisting disorders, especially of the lungs, heart or kidney because they may influence the patient's risk of surgery.

The choice of treatment is surgery. The surgical technique involves:

i. Incising the diseased segment of the aorta.
ii. Removing intraluminal thrombus or plaque;
iii. Inserting a synthetic arterial graft (Dacron or Polytetra fluroethylene) which is sutured to the normal aorta proximal or distal to the aneurysm; and
iv. Suturing the native aortic wall around the graft so that it will act as a protective cover.

(Text continue on page 425)

Table 9.8: Nursing care plan for preoperative care of the cardiac surgical patient

Problem	*R*	*Objective*	*Nursing Interventions*	*Rationales*
Nursing Diagnosis #1				
Anxiety, related to: 1. Opening cardiac surgery.		The patient will demonstrate decreased anxiety by indicating willingness to discuss the following: 1. Normal function of the heart. 2. Disease process, including: a. Risk factors. b. Surgical procedure. c. Expected outcomes of the surgery.	• Teach the patient about the normal function of the heart; underlying disease process including risk factors; the surgical procedure; and the expected outcomes of the surgery.	• Teaching provides a basic understanding of the problem, the solution, and what to exepct, thereby decreasing the patient's anxiety. However, not all patients experience a decreased level of anxiety when bombarded with new informations.
			• Use simple terms or explain medical terms used.	• Using simple terms or explaining medical terms enhances learning because the patient can understand the explanations. Using medical terms sometimes confuses and overwhelms the patient.
			• Utilize posters, models, and handouts/pamphlets.	• Visualization aids learning.
			• Teach in short blocks if time allows.	• Allows assimilation of information before more is added, and thus enhances learning.
			• Observe patient's nonverbal cues.	• Enables the nurse to evaluate patient's understanding and anxiety level. The nurse can determine whether to proceed, reiterate, or stop.
			• Allow time for questions.	• Relieves anxiety, clarifies information, and prevents misconceptions.
			• Answer questions honestly.	• Establishes a trusting relationship and attains patient cooperation.
			• Maintain a calm, relaxed, nonrushed atmosphere with little or no interruptions.	• Enhances the learning experience.
			• Have the patient discuss the information in his/her own words.	• Assists in evaluating what has been learned.
			• Correct any misconceptions.	• Patient knows what to expect, thereby reducing some of his/her anxiety.
Nursing Diagnosis #2				
Knowledge deficit regarding preoperative and postoperative expectations.		Patient will verbalize an understanding of the preoperative routine: 1. Tests, procedures. 2. Medications. 3. The night before the surgery. 4. The day of the surgery. 5. The immediate postoperative care.	• Provide information regarding the following: ◆ Tests and procedures that will be performed before surgery.	◆ This is a time when the patient needs and wants to be with family but is frequently interrupted, causing frustration and sometimes anger. Knowing about these studies ahead of time will help in coping with the interruptions.
			◆ Blood studies: CBC, serum electrolytes, BUN, creatinine, cardiac enzymes, clotting time, prothrombin time, fibrinogen levels, platelets, type and cross-match of blood, arterial blood gases.	◆ To evaluate baseline values. If any abnormal values are present, treatment can be initiated so as to prevent complications intraoperatively and postoperatively. Patient is typed/cross-matched to ensure, blood is available if needed.
			◆ ECG.	◆ Provides a baseline for comparison.
			◆ Chest x-ray.	◆ To examine for abnormalities; provides a baseline for comparison. ◆ To evaluate for signs of infection.

Contd...

Problem	*R*	*Objective*	*Nursing Interventions*	*Rationales*
			• Urine analysis. • Pulmonary function tests (PFTs).	• To evaluate patient's pulmonary status.
			• Changes in medication regimen and necessary preoperative medication:	• Changes in medication regimen can cause anxiety. Understanding of what the changes will help decrease anxiety and enhance patient cooperation.
			• Sedation the evening before/prior to surgery.	• Decreases anxiety, allows a good night's sleep.
			• All aspirin, anticoagulants, and anti-inflammatory drugs should be discontinued at least 2 days prior to surgery.	• Prevents bleeding due to altered coagulation studies.
			• Digitalis is usually held 1-2 days prior to the surgery unless the patient is in uncontrolled atrial fibrillation.	• Digitalis toxicity is a common complication postoperatively, related to low potassium levels. If given to control atrial fibrillation, the patient must be monitored closely for signs of toxicity postoperatively, especially in the immediate postoperative phase.
			• Propranolol is tapered 24 hr-2 weeks prior to surgery.	• Negative chronotropic and inotropic action postoperatively further decreases the cardiac output. If needed early in the postoperative period, dopamine, epinephrine, isoproterenol, and/or glucagon can be given.
			• Diuretics are discontinued 24-48 hours prior to the surgery if congestive heart failure is controlled.	• Diuretics increase the loss of fluids and potassium, which could cause adverse reactions postoperatively (i.e., hypovolaemia, acidaemia, hyponatraemia, digoxin toxicity).
			• Nitroglycerin is kept at the bedside and can be taken for chest pain (as per protocol).	• Relieves chest pain associated with anxiety.
			• Long-acting insulin is changed to regular insulin and patient is placed on a sliding-scale coverage 24 hours prior to the surgery.	• Insulin requirements change due to the stress of the surgery and NPO status. Administration of insulin on a sliding scale provides a more precise dosage to meet the patient's needs, thereby preventing hyperglycaemia/hypoglycaemia.
			• Potassium supplements are given to maintain the patient's potassium level at 4.0 mEq/liter.	• To prevent intraoperative and postoperative complications (i.e., acidemia, digoxin toxielty, dys-rhythmias).
			• Norpace may be discontinued 24 hours prior to the surgery.	• Norpace may cause heart failure in the postoperative phase.
			• Antidysrhythmics are maintained to control the dysrhythmias.	• Prevent further decrease in the cardiac output related to the dysrhythmias; help to prevent serious or life-threatening dysrhythmias.
			• Antihypertensive medications are maintained.	• Maintain the patient's blood pressure. Nitrofrusside (Nipride) can be given intraoperatively.
				• Prevents infection.

Contd...

Problem	*R*	*Objective*	*Nursing Interventions*	*Rationales*
			◆ Prophylactic antibiotics are given prior to the surgery and continued for 2 days post-operatively.	
			◆ Check the patient for allergies to any medications, especially antibiotics, iodine preparations, or fish.	◆ Prevents anaphylaxis.
			• The night before the surgery, the patient will:	
			◆ Receive a light dinner, then nothing to eat or drink after midnight.	◆ Prevents aspiration of the stomach contents.
			◆ Be shaved from the chin to the toes (CABG) or chin to shins (valve replacement).	◆ Decreases the possibility of infection since skin and hair har-bour bacteria.
			◆ Shower with an antibacterial agent (i.e., Betadine).	◆ Decreases the possibility of infection by decreasing the bacteria on the skin.
			• The morning of the surgery, the patient will:	
			◆ Shower again with the antibacterial agent.	
			◆ Put on a hospital gown.	
			◆ Receive a preoperative sedative.	◆ Decreases anxiety and helps the patient to relax.
			◆ Receive family for a brief visit (according to hospital policy).	◆ Allays anxiety of patient and family.
			◆ Give valuables to the family to take home.	◆ There is little room in the ICU for the patient's personal effects. Family will be told what to bring in when it is needed.
			◆ Be transferred to a stretcher and transported to the OR.	
			• Explain the immediate postoperative care: Inform the patient of the ICU routine:	• Knowing what to expect decreases the patient's anxiety and enhances cooperation.
			◆ Patients remain in the ICU for 2-3 days if no complications occur.	
			◆ The unit may be noisy and the lights left on.	◆ The patient should understand that frequent assessments are part of usual ICU protocols.It does not mean that anything is wrong.
			◆ Patients are checked frequently for vital signs and assessments.	
			◆ Visiting hours are restricted to brief periods.	◆ Awareness of the unit's environment will decrease the anxiety level for some patients. The patient will not become alarmed in response to the noise, frequency of vital signs, and absence of family except during brief visits.
			◆ A tour of the unit is offered to those who want it. Patient may be able to meet the nurse who will be taking care of her/him in the ICU.	
			• Explain expectations of postoperative period (e.g., equipment/routines). Patient will:	• Knowledge regarding expectations of care enables the patient to be co-operative and participate in care (e.g., not trying to pull the tubes out, fighting procedures, afraid of moving). The patient needs to know that needs will be anticipated and a method of communication worked out. This serves to redcue anxiety.
			◆ Have an endotracheal tube connected to a ventilator that will help with breathing.	◆ The endotracheal tube is usually left in place for 8-24 hrs.
			◆ Be unable to talk.	◆ An alternate means of communication should be set up (i.e., mou-thing words, finger writing, sign language).
			◆ Experience breathlessness when suctioned.	◆ The patient should know that the feeling of breathlessness, should it occur, will last only for a few seconds.
				◆ The patient should be encouraged

Contd...

Problem	*R*	*Objective*	*Nursing Interventions*	*Rationales*
				to breathe with the ventilator and not to "fight" the ventilator.
			• The patient will:	
			◆ Have a Foley catheter postoperatively.	◆ Allows for an accurate measurement of urine output.
			◆ Have peripheral, jugular, and subclavian IVs.	◆ Access for emergency medications, fluids, blood and blood products, and plasma expanders as needed. Once stabilized postoperatively, all but one will be discontinued while in the ICU.
			◆ Have an arterial line for approximately 1 day.	◆ Access for arterial blood gases and other blood specimens. Allows for continuous monitoring of arterial blood pressure.
			◆ Be connected to a cardiac monitor.	◆ To monitor heart rhythm and rate.
			◆ Have a rectal temperature probe in place postoperatively until temperature stabilizes (usually 8 hr).	◆ Allows frequent monitoring of the patient's temperature. In the absence of a temperature probe, rectal temperatures can be taken hourly until stabilized.
			◆ Have chest tubes in place for approximately 2 days.	◆ Allows evaluation of bleeding in the chest, which may indicate improper closure of a graft, cardiac tamponade, or coagulation abnormality. ◆ The drainage will be bloody initially and then gradually become serous.
			• Explain the various suture lines.	Patient will have a midline chest incision (medial sternotomy) that will be dressed initially. The dressing is usually removed 24 hours postoperatively. Patient may have some chest discomfort related to the sternum being opened; this pain differs from the chest pain experienced previously. Pain medication will be available. • Patient will have an incision in one or both legs. It may extend from the thigh to the knee, the thigh to the ankle, or the knee to the ankle, depending on the amount of graft needed, the surgeon's preference, and the condition of the vein. *Note*: When a mammary artery is used as bypass graft, incisions in lower extremities are unnecessary.
			◆ Advise that postoperatively Ace bandages or elastic stockings are applied.	◆ Ace bandages/elastic stockings aid in the venous return from the legs; they are also used to prevent thrombi.
		Patient will demonstrate activities expected to be performed in the postoperative period: 1. Coughing and deep breathing.	• Demonstrate, and have the patient return the demonstration, activities to be performed postoperatively:	• Enhances cooperation in the postoperative activities needed to prevent complications. Ensures that the patient knows what must be done, why, and how it is to be done.

Contd...

Problem	*R*	*Objective*	*Nursing Interventions*	*Rationales*
		2. Splinting the chest incision. 3. Use of the incentive spirometer. 4. Arm and leg exercises. 5. Turning side to side. 6. Getting out of bed the day after the surgery.	• Coughing and deep breathing: Take 4-5 deep breaths, then cough. • Pain medication will be given prior to the exercises (as indicated). • Splinting the chest incision. • Arm exercises—range of motion and walking up the wall. • Leg exercises—ankle range of motion, "ankle pump," and dorsiflexion. • Turning side to side every 2 hrs. • Getting out of bed—splint chest. • Inch legs over the side of the bed. Sit up straight on the edge of the bed, then ease the feet down to the floor. Nurses will be present for support and guidance of tubings.	• Prevent atelectasis and pneumonia. • Deep breaths loosen the secretions so they can be mobilized. • Decreases the amount of pain so the exercises can be done effectively. • Decreases the amount of pain. • Prevent frozen shoulder. • Increase circulation in the lower extremities and prevent stasis and thrombosis. Range of motion also prevents foot drop. • Early ambulation helps prevent many complications, especially pneumonia and thrombosis. It is not as simple a task postoperatively as patients may believe.

Table 9.9: Nursing care plan for early postoperative care of the cardiac surgical patient

Problem	*R*	*Objective*	*Nursing Interventions*	*Rationales*
Nursing Diagnosis #1 Cardiac output, alteration in: Decreased, patient in: 1. Cardiopulmonary bypass. 2. Low cardiac output syndrome.		Patient will demonstrate stabilization of body functions monitoring and life-supportive systems: 1. Arterial blood pressure within 10 mmHg of patient's baseline. 2. Stable pulmonary artery pressures: • PAP < 25 mmHg. • PCWP 8-12 mmHg. • CVP 0-8 mmHg. 3. Cardiac output ~5 liters/minute. • Heart rate > 60 < 100 beats/minute. 4. Urine output > 30 ml/hour. 5. Alert mental status; oriented to person, place, time. 6. Electrolyte balance. 7. Acid-base balance: • pH 7.35-7.45. • PaO_2 > 80 mmHg. • $PaCO_2$ 35-45 mmHg. 8. Stable haematology profile: • Hct: male, 45-52 per cent; female, 37-48 per cent.	• Monitor vital signs (BP, heart rate, respiratory rate, and temperature) q 5 minutes within lim-its stable, then q 1 hr × 12. • Assess the patient q 1 hr until stable, including heart sounds; ECG changes; cardiac rhythm; neck veins; lung sounds; peripheral pulses; capillary refill; skin turgour, colour and temperature; movement and sensation. • Monitor haemodynamic parameters: Mean arterial pressure (MAP), pulmonary artery pressure (PAP), pulmonary capillary wedge pressure (PCWP), central venous pressure (CVP), or right atrial pressure (RAP), and left atrial pressure (LAP). • Assess the pacemaker concerning type (fixed or demand), the rate it is set at, the milliamperes (mA), and whether it is functioning properly. (Pacing wires are commonly used in valve replacement surgery.) • Keep exposed wires wrapped in gauze and place in a plastic covering.	• Frequent monitoring of the vital signs allows early detection of abnorma-lities, and treatment for provable complications. • Changes may indicate haemodynamic decompensation or complications. Signs of low cardiac output syndrome include a decrease in arterial pressure, urine output below 30 ml/hr, signs of vasoconstriction cool, pale, or cyanotic skin and mucous membranes), tachycardia, dysrhythmias, tachypnoea, narrow pulse pressure, weak peripheral pulses, decrease in level of consciousness, restlessness. • Parameters will reflect left ventricular function, fluid status, and arterial perfusion. • Need to be familiar with equipment in order to use it properly, identify if it is functioning properly, and how to trouble-shoot problems. Pacemaker is usually kept on standby to keep the patient's heart rate above 60 beats/minute and to treat other dysrhythmias. • Prevents the possibility of electrical shock or short circuit.

Contd...

Problem	*R*	*Objective*	*Nursing Interventions*	*Rationales*
		• Hgb: male, 13-18 g/100 ml; female, 12-16 g/100 ml. • Platelet count: 150,000-350,000/mm3.	• Report any abnormalities in vital parameters to physician immediately:	• Immediate intervention can be ordered to prevent further deterioration/complications.
			◆ BP: Systolic < 80, > 180. Diastolic > 100. ◆ MAP: < 60, > 100.	◆ Pressures below 80 mmHg could cause graft closure or indicate shock; pressures above 180 mmHg could cause the graft to "blow," or could cause a CVA.
			◆ CVP: < 5, > 15.	◆ CVP readings below 5 cmH_2O indicate inadequate intravascular fluid; readings above 15 cmH_2O indicate fluid overload.
			◆ Heart rate: < 60, > 100.	◆ Heart rates below 60 could cause graft closure; rates above 100 will decrease the oxygenation to the myocardium and increase the workload of the heart.
			◆ Temperature: Remains hypothermic or rises above 101°F.	◆ Hypothermia prolongs vasoconstriction, adding to low cardiac output syndrome. Temperatures above 101°F may indicate infection.
			◆ Excessive or bloody chest tube drainage > 100 ml/hr.	◆ Excessive and/or bloody drainage suggests bleeding at surgical site.
			◆ Urine output < 30 ml/hr.	◆ Reduced urine output warns of prerenal failure.
			◆ Extremities: Cool, moist, mottled, with sluggish capillary refill and poor or absent peripheral pulses.	◆ Signs of decreased peripheral perfusion related to emboli or decreased cardiac output. If accompanied by pain, arterial occlusion of the extremity may have occurred.
			◆ A decrease in movement or sensation.	◆ May indicate possible neurologic involvement or may be due to the effect of the anaesthesia.
			◆ Presence of anginal pain or ECG changes: ST segment elevation ro depression; T wave peaked/inverted.	◆ Indicative of myocardial ischaemia.
Nursing Diagnosis #2 Breathing pattern, ineffective, related to: 1. General anaesthesia. 2. Incisional pain with splinting.		The patient will maintain: 1. A patent airway. 2. Respiratory rate <25-30/minute; eupneic rhythm. 3. ABGs within normal range: • pH 7.35-7.45. • PaO_2 > 80 mmHg. • $PaCO_2$ 35-45 mmHg. • HCO_3 22-26 mEq/liter.	• Assess respiratory function: Rate, rhythm, pattern, chest excursion, use of accessory muscles; breath sounds; presence of adventitious sounds.	• It is essential to establish baseline function with which to compare subsequent findings; assists in following trends.
			• Maintain patient on ventilator at prescribed settings.	• Maintains patient's respirations when the respiratory center is depressed due to the anaesthesia and narcotics. Provides adequate oxygenation. Decreases the work-load of the heart.
			◆ Check the endotracheal cuff for adequate inflation.	◆ Improper cuff inflation reduces tidal volume and may compromise ventilation.
			• Administer pain medications to decrease pain and prevent "fighting" the ventilator.	• Pain and "fighting" the ventilator can lead to hyperventilation, which may predispose to respiratory alkalosis. Acid-base imbalances can cause dysrhythmias.

Contd...

Problem	R	Objective	Nursing Interventions	Rationales
				◆ Tachycardia related to pain can increase workload of the heart.
			• Suction prn. Sigh the patient before and after suctioning. (Sigh is a deeper than normal breath with 100 per cent oxygen.) ◆ Use hand resuscitator to ventilate and preoxygenate prior to and following each suction pass (some mechanical ventilators have "sigh" capability.)	• Remove secretions for adequate oxygenation and gas exchange. Sighing the patient before and after expands the alveoli, mobilizes the secretions, and prevents drastic drops in the patient's oxygen levels.
			• Monitor ABGs q 1-4 hr as the patient's condition warrants; or continuously monitor mixed venous gases (SvO_2) as prescribed.	• Respiratory and metabolic alterations are reflected in the ABGs. Adjustment in the ventilator settings or pharmacologic interventions can be initiated to prevent severe imbalances.
			• Wean patient off the ventilator as prescribed, when alert, breathing spontaneously, and demonstrating adequate ABGs and appropriate ventilatory parameters (i.e., inspiratory pressure, expiratory pressure, tidal volume, minute volume, and vital capacity).	• The patient must be able to breathe spontaneously with adequate respiratory excursion, tidal volume, minute ventilation, and peak inspiratory pressure.
			• Administer oxygen through a heated humidified face mask or tent after weaning.	• Provides oxygenation with humidification to assist in thinning the secretions and thereby facilitating deep breathing and coughing.
			• Encourage patient to cough and deep breathe hourly; administer chest percussion; encourage the use of the incentive spirometer q 1-2 hr while awake. ◆ Have respiratory therapist administer IPPB and nebulizer treatments as ordered.	• Loosens and mobilizes the secretions, thereby preventing atelectasis and pneumonia. Incentive spirometer provides patients with a visual feedback as to how well they are breathing.
			• Assess breath sounds q 2 hr and/or when indicated.	• Decreased breath sounds may indicate atelectasis, pneumonia, or poor breathing technique due to splinting. Absence of breath sounds on one side suggests atelectasis or malpositioning of the endotracheal tube. Endotracheal tube may have slipped down into right bronchus. Pneumothorax, if present, is usually accompanied by unequal chest excursion and shifting of trachea to opposite side.
			• Notify the physician of any significant abnormalities in respiratory parameters.	• Interventions may be taken expeditiously to prevent complications.
Nursing Diagnosis #3 Fluid volume deficit, actual and potential, related to: 1. Surgery-related blood loss or haemorrhage. 2. NPO status. 3. Peripheral vasodilation associated with rewarming (dis proportion between size of vascular bed and intravascular blood volume).		Patient will: 1. Maintain stable haemodynamic parameters: • BP, pulses, CVP, PAP, PCWP (see Nursing Diagnosis #1, above). 2. Demonstrate adequate peripheral perfusion; peripheral pulses 2+ bilaterally; brisk capillary refill; skin warm, no cyanosis of nailbeds or mucous membranes. 3. Be alert and oriented.	• Monitor vital signs q 15 minutes while the patient is rewarming.	• The vascular bed increases during rewarming, causing a disproportion in the vascular volume and the vascular bed size. If the disproportion is great enough the patient will become hypotensive, predisposing to shock. Under these circumstances, there is a risk that the grafts may close off. In response to the hypotension the patient may develop myocardial ischaemia with dysrhythmias, prerenal failure, or DIC.
			• Administer fluids as ordered. (Usually less than 100 ml/hr total volume unless the patient is hypovolaemic).	• Adequate fluids are necessary to prevent hypovolaemia; overhydration can cause the patient to develop pulmonary oedema.

Contd...

Problem	*R*	*Objective*	*Nursing Interventions*	*Rationales*
		4. Maintain urinary output above 30 ml/ hour with no haematuria. 5. Show no sign of haemorrhage (stable vital signs). 6. Maintain a haematocrit above 30 per cent.	• Monitor the patient's intake and output carefully. Weigh daily.	• Patient may be retaining fluid if fluid intake is greater than output plus the insensible losses. Daily weighing is a reliable indicator of hydration status (2.2 1b is equal to 1 liter of fluid).
			• Monitor urine output q 1 hr; specific gravity q 2 hr.	• Urine output less than 30 ml/hr may, indicate decreased cardiac output, hypovolaemia, or renal failure. A decrease in specific gravty indicates hypovolaemia.
			• Monitor BUN and creatinine.	• The BUN is an indicator of renal function and fluid status, the creatinine is an indicator of renal function. The physician should be notified of an increase in either, or of any change in BUN/creatinine ratio.
			• Assess skin turgour and mucous membranes for hydration status.	• Tenting of the skin when pinched indicates dehydration. Oedema indicates fluid excess or decreased cardiac output. Dry mucous membranes indicate dehydration; moist mucous membranes indicate adequate hydration.
			• Monitor haemodynamic parameters especially when rehydrating the patient.	• PAP, LAP, and CVP will be decreased in volume depletion. As fluids are administered the pressures also will increase. Pressures will be elevated in fluid overload.
				• Low Hgb and Hct are indicative of blood loss or haemodilution; an elevated Hct is indicative of haemo concentration.
			• Monitor serum electrolytes and haemoglobin and haematocrit (Hgb and Hct). Administer potassium to maintain level within 3.5-5.5 mEq/liter.	• Elevation of potassium may be related to renal failure, cardiopulmonary bypass, or acid-base imbalance. Abnormal potassium levels can cause dysrhythmias.
			• Monitor amount and colour of chest tube drainage.	• Chest tube drainage greater than 100 ml/hr for the first 4 hr is indicative of abnormal bleeding, which could be related to platelet destruction, inadequate reversal of the heparin, inadequate suturing of arteries during the surgery, or diffuse intrathoracic ooze.
			◆ Observe the dressings and bedding for signs of haemorrhage.	◆ Bleeding may occur at the suture line. Excessive bleeding may ooze down the patient's side and pool under him.
			• Monitor coagulation studies.	• Abnormal coagulation caused by anticoagulants or DIC can cause haemorrhage related to oozing at injection sites, suture lines, insertion sites of IVs.
			• Administer blood, plasma expanders, and clotting factors as prescribed.	• Blood and plasma expanders are given to maintain the intravascular volume. Fresh-frozen plasma and cryoprecipitate may be administered to bolster concentration of clotting factors to ensure appropriate blood coagulation and prevent haemorrhaging.

Contd...

Problem	*R*	*Objective*	*Nursing Interventions*	*Rationales*
Nursing Diagnosis #4				
Tissue perfusion, alteration in peripheral, related to: 1. Low cardiac output syndrome.		Patient will: 1. Demonstrate normotension (MAP within 10 mmHg of patient's baseline). 2. Demonstrate normothermia (98.6°F, 37.0°C). 3. Maintain palpable peripheral pulses and brisk capillary refill. 4. Exhibit warm, dry skin, pink in colour with good turgour. 5. Maintain heart rate >60, <100. 6. Maintain urine output > 30 ml/hr.	• Assess peripheral pulses. Compare right with left. Note characteristics: Rate, rhythm, quality (bounding, weak, and thready), and equality. ◆ Mark sites of pulses if difficult to palpate. • Assess the skin for temperature, colour, capillary refill, breakdown, and sensation. • Have patient perform leg and arm exercises as taught in the preoperative phase. • Apply elastic stockings or Ace bandages to lower extremities as prescribed. ◆ Check size of elastic stockings and apply properly; check pulses q 4 hr, administer skin care. Remove stockings once each shift. • Assess the patient for calf tenderness, swelling, and a positive Homan's sign. • Measure girth of calves and thighs bilaterally. • Do not gatch the bed or use pillows under the knee. Discourage the patient from crossing knees and/or ankles.	• Peripheral pulses are indicators of the arterial flow through the extremity. An absence or decrease in the pulse may indicate occulusion of the vessel due to emboli. ◆ Marking the sites makes it easier to find the pulse, especially if the pulse is weak. • Indicators of peripheral perfusion. A decrease may be indicative of poor perfusion. • Exercises increase circulation. • Properly applied elastic stockings and Ace bandages assist in venous return, reducing risk of venous stasis. • Signs of thrombophlebitis. • Often the means of detecting that a deep venous thrombosis is pre-sent is by monitoring the circumference. • Applies pressure under the knee, thereby decreasing circulation to the lower leg.
Nursing Diagnosis #5				
Tissue perfusion, alteration in cerebral, related to: 1. Anaesthesia. 2. Cardiopulmonary bypass. 3. Narcotics. 4. Postcardiotomy delirium (PCD).		Patient will: 1. Demonstrate an intact, direct, and consensual pupillary light reflex bilaterally. 2. Demonstrate an intact gag reflex. 3. Be alert and oriented to person, place, and time. 4. Follow commands/behaviour appropriately. 5. Speak clearly and understandably. 6. Demonstrate movement in all extremities equal to preoperative state.	• Assess neurologic status at least every 2-4 hr, or when indicated: Pupils—size and equality, reaction to light; level of consciousness; orientation; speech, obeys commands; movement of all extremities. • Assess the patient's behaviour every shift. Orient to person, place, and time. Provide frequent explanations. Allow family to visit. Reinforce normality of the disorientation (if no other signs of neurologic deficit are present).	• Abnormal neurologic findings may be indicative of permanent or temporary alterations related to the anaesthesia, intraoperative stroke, cardiopulmonary bypass machine, hypothermia, decreased cardiac output. Abnormal findings may occur in the immediate postoperative phase but they should gradually return to baseline within the initial 4-8 hr postoperatively. • Confusion and disorientation may be indicative of postcardiotomy delirium (PCD). Frequent explanations, reorientation, and visits from family help the patient cope with PCD. Postcardiotomy delirium is associated with cardiopulmonary bypass and is manifested in some patients post-bypass by changes in behaviour, confusion, and frank psychosis.
Nursing Diagnosis #6				
Infection, potential for, related to: 1. Interruption in integrity of skin barrier (surgical incision). 2. Invasive monitoring. 3. Chest tubes, Foley catheter.		The patient will remain infection free: 1. Temperature at baseline (98.6°F, 37.0°C). 2. WBC at baseline. 3. Incisional area clean, dry, and healing.	• Assess incision, IV sites, intravascular lines for signs of infection (warmth, redness, swelling). • Change IV lines and haemodynamic lines per hospital protocol. Maintain sterility of the lines. • Change dressings daily or according to hospital protocol.	• The skin is the first line of defense against infection. Any break in the skin's integrity is prone to infection. • These are access sites through which bacteria enter. • Dressing changes permit visualization of the surgical site. Redness, warmth, and swelling suggest infection.

Contd...

Problem	*R*	*Objective*	*Nursing Interventions*	*Rationales*
			• Administer antibiotics as prescribed.	• Timely and accurate administration of antibiotics helps to maintain therapeutic blood levels.
			• Culture any draining wound.	• Detection of the causative organism is necessary so that appropriate antibiotic therapy can be prescribed.
			• Assess breath sounds and appearance of sputum.	• Presence of adventitious sounds and sputum production can signal possible onset of pneumonia.
			• Maintain the Foley catheter as a closed system. Discontinue as soon as possible.	• Foley catheters are a common source of infection and can lead to gram-negative sepsis.
			• Assess the patient for signs of systemic infection (sepsis): Change in behaviour, hyperthermia/hypothermia, chils, diaphoresis.	• The first sign of sepsis is a change in behaviour. Timely and aggressive intervention is necessary to prevent septic shock and multisystem organ dysfunction.
			• Practice good handwashing technique.	• Good handwashing technique is the main way to prevent inspection or its spread.
Nursing Diagnosis #7 Anxiety, related to: 1. Outcome of surgery. 2. Recuperative period. 3. Lack of sleep/rest. 4. Noisy ICU environment.		Patient will verbalize: 1. Feelingless anxious. 2. Ability to rest and to sleep. 3. Progress made in recuperation. 4. Willingness to cooperate in care. 5. Desire to make decisions concerning care.	• Familiarize with ICU environment: Equipment, procedures, and protocols.	• Appropriate explanation decreases anxiety.
			• Explain condition and treatments. Stress the patient's progress.	• Reassures the patient. Gives positive reinforcement.
			• Administer pain medication as needed. Withhold if the patient is hypotensive, is being weaned off the ventilator, or has neurologic changes.	• Decreasing the pain will decrease the patient's anxiety by breaking the pain-fear-anxiety triangle. Narcotics are not given if they will interfere with assessment or stabilization of the patient.
			• Provide rest periods. Administer sedatives/ pain medication to enhance sleep at night.	• Sleep and rest deprivation causes irritability, which increases anxiety.
			• Allow the patient to take an active part in care; allow patient to make decisions concerning care.	• Decision-making and active participation in care give positive feedback to the patient that he/she is making progress, as well as giving the patient a sense of self-worth.
			• Allow the family to visit as much as possible according to unit/hospital policy.	• The family is a support system that the patient depends on. Family interaction helps prevent social isolation and gives the patient a sense of being needed.

Prior to surgery, every effort is made to bring the patient into best possible state of hydration and electrolyte balance. Any abnormalities in coagulation and blood cell count are corrected. The patients may receive antibiotics and baths with antiseptics before surgery. If aneurysm has ruptured immediate, surgical intervention is needed. All aneurysm resections require cross-clamping of the aorta proximal or distal to aneurysm. When aneurysms are repaired electively, the patient is systematically anticoagulated with IV heparin before cross clamping aorta. This prevents clotting of pooled blood distal to the aneurysm. If surgery is emergent, no anticoagulative is indicated.

All patients undergoing aneurysmectomy should be placed in an intensive care unit with appropriate support services and equipment. The nursing role during the preoperative period should include teaching, providing support for the patient and family, and carefully assessing all body systems. It is imperative that problems be identified early and proper intervention instituted. In addition to maintaining adequate respiratory function, fluid and electrolyte balance, and pain control in the post-operative period, the nurse must monitor graft patency and renal perfusion. The nurse can also assist in preventing ventricular arrhythmias, infections and neurologic complications.

2. Aortic Dissection

Aortic dissection, occurring most commonly in the thoracic aorta, is a longitudinal splitting of the medial layer of the artery by a column of blood.

Aetiology

Exact cause is unknown; but most people with aortic dissection problem have hypertension, or Marfan's syndrome.

Pathophysiology

Aortic dissection results from a small tear in the intimal lining of the artery, allowing blood to "track" between the intima and media and creating a false lumen of blood flow. As the heart contracts each systolic pulsation causes increased pressure on the damaged area, which further increases dissection. As it extends proximally, distally, it may occlude major branches of the aorta, cutting of blood supply to the areas such as the brain, abdominal organs, kidneys, spinal cord, and extremities. Occasionally a small tear develops distally and the blood flow reenters the true vested lumen. Aortic dissection differes from an aortic aneurysm. Aortic dissections are usually classified as Type I, II, and III.

- Type I involves the ascending aorta and descending thoracic aorta.
- Type II involves the ascending aorta only and
- Type III invovles the aorta distal to the subclavian artery.

Clinical Manifestation

The patient with acute aorta dissection usually has sudden severe pain in the back, chest, or abdomen. The pain is described as "tearing" or "ripping". The severe pain resembles MI. As the dissection progresses pain may be located both above and below the diaphragm. Dyspnoea may also be present.

- If the arch of aorta is involved, the patient may exhibit neurologic deficiencies, including altered LOC, dizziness, and weakened or absent carotid and temporal pulse.
- An ascending aorta dissection usually produces some degree of aorta valvular isufficiency and a murmur audible on auscultation. Severe insufficiency may produce left ventricular failure with development of dyspnoea and orthopnoea caused by pulmonary oedema.
- When either subclavian artery is involved, pulse quality and readings may vary between the left and right arms. As the dissection progresses down the aorta, the abdominal organs and lower extremities may begin to demonstrate evidence of altered tissue perfusion and ischaemia. The complications of aortic dissection are cardiac tamponade and haemorrhage in the mediestinal, pleural or abdominal cavities, Ischaemia of concerned organs, spinal cord, abdoman and kidneys.

Management

The diagnostic studies used to assess dissecton of aortas are history and physical examination, ECG, Chest X-Ray, CT Scan, transesophageal echocardiography, MRI, and aortography. The goal fo therapy for aortic dissections without complications is to lower the BP and myocardial contractility to diminish the pulsatile forces within the aorta. The use of trimethapan and nitroprusside IV reduces BP and IV beta blockers may be used. Propranolol is used to decrease the force of myocardial contractility. Supportive treatment directed towards pain relief, blood transfusion and management of heart failure is indicated. Surgery is indicated when drug therapy is ineffective or when complications are present. Surgery invovles resection of the aortic segment containing intimal tear and replacement with synthetic graft material.

The nursing intervention includes:

- Bedrest—keep patient in semi-Fowler's position and maintain quiet environment.
- Administrate narcotic or transquilizers as ordered to reduce anxiety.
- Continuous IV administration of anti-hypertensives.
- ECG monitoring.
- Monitoring of vital signs, level of consciousness (LOC).
- Preoperative care.
- Postoperative care.

ACUTE ARTERIAL OCCLUSIVE DISORDERS

The arteries are thick-walled vessels that transport blood and oxygen from the heart to the tissues. Arterial disease can affect any artery of the body and can manifest itself as an acute or chronic condition. Disruption of the arterial blood flow can be caused by narrowing or complete obstruction of the wall of the vessels.

Acute arterial occlusion occurs suddenly without warning signs.

Aetiology

Acute arterial occlusion caused by embolism, thrombosis of the already narrowed artery, or trauma, embolization of a thrombus from the heart or an atherosclerotic aneurysm is the most frequent cause of acute arterial occlusion. Heart condition in which thrombi are prone to develop include infective endocarditis, MI, mitral valve disease, chronic atrial fibrillation, cardiomyopathic and prosthetic heart valves.

Pathophysiology

The thrombi becomes dislodged and may travel to the lungs if they originate in the right side of the heart or to anywhere in the systematic circulation if they originate in the left side of the heart. Arterial emboli tend to lodge at sites of arterial branching or in areas of atherosclerotic narrowing. An acute arterial occlusion causes the blood supply distal to the embolus to decrease. The degree and extent of symptoms depend on the size and location of the obstruction, the occurrence of clots fragmentation with embolism to smaller vessels, and the degree of peripheral vascular disease already present. Sudden local thrombosis may occur at the location of an atherosclerotic plaque. Traumatic injury to the extremity itself may produce partial or total occlusion of a vessel from compression and shearing or laceration.

Clinical Manifestation

Signs and symptoms of an acute arterial occlusion usually have an abrupt onset. Clinical manifestation of it includes the six "Ps". Pain, pallor, pulselessness, paresthesia, paralysis and poikilotherma (adaptation of ischaemic limb to its environmental temperature, most often cool). Without immediate intervention, ischaemia may progress to tissue necrossis and gangrene within hours. Paralysis is a late sign.

The nurse should note the symptoms that occur suddenly and are severe as follows:

Pain	:	When the obstruction is complete, the pain is severe and constant and is not relieved by rest.
Pallor	:	The limb typically appears pale and mottled.
Pulselessness	:	Numbness, tingling and burning in the extremity are common when ischaemia is severe.
Poikilotheremia	:	The limb is typically cool, if not frankly cold to the touch.
Paralysis	:	Mobility of the part in limited. The development of frank paralysis is an ominous sign because it may indicate the ischaemic death of nerves in the extremity.

If perfusion is not rapidly restored, the limb will develop signs of necrosis and gangrene often is a matter of hours.

Management

Diagnosis of acute occlusion is primarily established through physical assessment of affected limb, Doppler Ultrasonic studies, ABI measurement, MRI and angiographing if indicated.

Drug therapy by immediate initiation of anticoagulant through continuous IV Hepatin. A few long-term measures i.e. procedure used and treatment includes:

- Percutaneous balloon angioplasty.
- Intravascular ultrasound.
- Laser-assisted balloon angioplasty (LABA).
- Peripheral atheroctomy.
- Intravascular stents.

The options for surgical repairs of acute arterial occlusion are:

- Endarterectomy - A direct opening is made into the artery to remove the obstruction.
- Embolectomy - Removal of embolus from artery.
- Femoral-Femoral bypass - A graft from one femoral artery to other.
- Axilla-femoral bypass - A graft from axilla artery to femoral.
- Femoral-paplital bypass.
- Aorta iliac bypsss.

The patient may be undergoing varieties of emergency tests and procedures and will have extensive needs of teaching and support. Preoperative care focuses on the physical, emotional and psychosocial preparation of severely-stressed patient. The nurse is an important mediator between the patient and the rest of the treatment team and attempts to keep the channel of communication open while taking care of the person with acute arterial occlusion are as follows:

- Monitor the patient for any change in circulatory status to the affected limb. Monitor temperature, colour, sensation and pain. A change in these parameters may indicate worsening occlusion.
- Monitor peripheral pulses bilaterally for presence, strength, quality and symmetry.
- Keeping the extremity warm, but do not apply direct heat or heat lamps.
- Avoid chilling.
- Maintain bedrest unless activity is specifically ordered.
- Keep the extremity flat or in a slightly dependent position to promote perfusion.
- Use an overbed cradle to protect a painful extremity from the pressure of linens.
- Use sheepskin and 4-inch forum mattress beneath the extremity.
- Do not use the knee gatch on the bed; instruct the patient not to cross the legs at the knee or ankle.
- Do not apply any restraint to the affected limb.
- Keep the head of the bed low to support circulation to the lower extremities.
- Monitor the effects of anticoagulant and thrombolytic therapy.
- Monitor prothrombin time, partial thromboplastin time, platelets and other studies.
- Assess for local and systematic bleeding.

The patient receives meticulous general surgical care. The complications of vascular surgery can affect virtually any organ system. The more invasion procedure, the greater the risk of complication. Potential complications include bleeding, infection at graft site, cardiac failure, myocardial injury to the adjacent organs and tissues (eg. ureters and nerves). The nurse is responsible for meticulous postoperative monitoring of all the body systems and supporting circulation and perfusion, preventing respiratory complication, supposing fluid balance, and promote wound healing and providing discharge instruction to the patient. The discharge instructions after bypass graft surgery includes:

- Shower daily, clearing the incision gently with a mild or antibacterial soap without lotion of perfume added. Pat dry. Use a shower chair or stool to prevent falling if any instability. Avoid tube baths until healing is complete.
- Monitor the incision daily for signs of infections-redness, swelling, increased pain, discharge of suture or staple separation. Report any of these symptoms to surgeon promptly.
- Advance activity gradually as tolerated initiate a daily walking regime. Expect to feel fatigued and plan for rest periods throughout the day. Avoid lifting anything heavier than 10 pounds until approved by the surgeon.
- Resume a low-fat, low-cholesterol diet as tolerated. Use supplements as needed to ensure adequate calories, proteins and vitamin C during the healing period. Four to six small meals a day are often better tolerated than three large ones.
- Avoid constipation and straining at stool. Eat a high-fiber diet with plenty of fluids to avoid constipation. Remain active. Take a stool softener daily plus a bulk-forming laxative if constipation cannot be managed through diets and fluids.
- Use prescribed pain medication as needed to ensure adequate rest and activity. Take oral medication with food to prevent gastric irritation.

CHRONIC ARTERIAL OCCLUSIVE DISEASE

Chronic peripheral arterial occlusive disease involves progressive narrowing and degeneration and eventual obstruction of the arteries to the extremities occurring predominantly in the legs. It may effect the aortoiliac, femoral, popliteal, tibial, peroneal vessels or any combinations of these areas. Arteriosclerosis obliterans is the most common form of chronic arterial occlusive disease.

Aetiology

The leading cause of chronic arterial occlusion is the atherosclerosis a gradual thickening of the intima and media, which leads to narrowing of the vessel of lumen. Atherosclerosis primarily affects large arteries. The involvement is generally segmental with normal segments, interspersed between involved ones. The femoral-politeal area is the site most commonly affects in the non-diabetic persons. The patient with diabetes tend to develop disease in the arteries below the knee (specifically the anterior tibial, posterior tibial, and peroneal arteries). In advanced stages, multiple level of occlusions are seen.

The risk factors of peripheral vascular disease (PVD) include-increased age, smoking, hypertension, atherosclerosis, obesity, diabetes mellitus, stress, family history of PVD or atherosclerosis, sedantary life style, hyperlipidaemia.

Pathophysiology

Atherosclerosis, the build-up of cholesterol and triglyceride plaque within the arteries, combines with process of diffuse arteriosclerosis is calcification produced widespread, slowly progressive and narrowing of the arteries. Chronic arterial obstruction leads to progressively inadequate oxygenation of the tissues supplied by the obstructed arteries. The pain attributable to ischaemia is produced by end products of anaerobic cellular metabolism, such as lactic acid. This usually occurs in the larger muscle groups of the legs (buttocks, thighs and calves) during exercise. Once the patient stops exercising the metabolites are and pain subsides. As disease process becomes advanced, pain develops at rest. "Restpain" most often occurs in the feet or toes and indicates insufficient blood flow to the nerve supplying the distal extremity. The patient may notice rest pain more often at night and achieve partial relief by lowering the limb below heart level (eg. dangling the leg over the side of the bed). The clinical manifestations depend on the site and extent of the obstruction and the extent and the amount of collateral circulation.

Clinical Manifestation

- Intermittent claudication in:
  - Buttocks and upper thigh due to occlusion of aortoiline arteries.
  - Calves due to occlusion of femoral or popletal artery.
  - If disease extends internal iliac artery results impotence and sexual dysfunction occurs in aortoiliac artery occlusion.
- Rest pain in advanced diseases-precipitated by a predictable amount of exercise, relieved by resting and reproducible (Rest ischaemia).
- Diminished hair growth on affected extremities.
- Thick, brittle and slow-growing nails.
- Shiny, thin, fragile, taut skin, dry and scaly.
- Cool temperature.
- Diminished or absent pulses.
- Palees blanched appearance with extremity elevation.
- Reddish discolorition: rubor with extremity in dependent position.
- Reactive hyperaemia.
- Decreased motor function.
- Ulcer formation with advanced disease.
- ABI (Ankle-Bracheal Index) of 0.5-0.95.

The complication of chronic occlusion disorder is that ischaemia leads to atrophy of the skin and underlying structure which in turn leads to decreased ability to heal, infection and necrosis and may result from even minor trauma (eg. diabetes).

Ischaemic ulcer and gangrene are the most serious complications, may result in lower extremity amputation if blood flow is not restored.

Management

Various tests have been used to diagnose arterial occlusive disorder. Non-invasive tests include ultrasonography, segmental limb pressure, pulse volume recordings and exercise testing. In addition, Doppler ultrasound studies, duplex imaging, angiography, magnetic resonance angiography are also used.

The conservative therapy includes projecting the extremity from trauma, slowing the progression of atherosclerosis, decreasing vasospasm, preventing and controling infection, and improving collateral circulation. The patient's risk factors should be assessed and proper intervention should be begun regarding cessation of smoking, weight reduction (if indicated) and control of lipid disorders. Hypertension should also be properly managed. The nurse should assist in teaching diet modification to reduce the intake of animal fat and refined sugars, proper care of the feet, and the avoidance of injury to the extremities. The patient with family history of cardiac, diabetes and vascular disease should be encouraged to obtain regular follow-up case.

The common drugs used for arterial occlusive diseases include antiplatelets (aspirin, ticlopidine, dipyridamale) Xanthine derivative (Pentoxifylline) bihydrophridine (Nifedipine), israldipine, (Felodipine) and vasodilators (hydralazine, minoridil). The nurse should know the action of drugs and monitor the effects and side effects of the drugs.. and monitor the effect of claudication and exercise tolerace. Monitor BP and Pulse.

The patient with atherosclerosis should be taught and encouraged to do the following:

- Adjust calorie intake so that optimum weight can be achieved and maintained.
- Decrease dietary cholesterol to less than 200 mg/day.
- Substantially reduce saturated dietary fat.
- Restrict sodium to 2 g per day if oedema is present.

The procedure/therapy used for acute care of the person with chronic arterial occlusive disease including:

- Percutaneous transluminal angioplasty with or without stent.
- Atherectomy.
- Arterial bypass.
- Patchgraft angioplasty, often in conjunction with bypass.
- Thrombolytic therapy/Anticoagulation.
- Endarterectomy (done rarely, with localized stenosis).
- Amputation required, if gangrene is extensive.

BUERGER'S DISEASE

Buerger's disease is an obstructive vascular disorder caused by segmental inflammation in the arteries and veins of the upper or lower extremities. It is also known as thromboanginitis obliterans (TAO).

Aetiology

It typically occurs in men between the ages of 20 and 40 years but rare in women. The basic cause is unknown. But incidences are strongly associated with cigarette smoking—the disease does not occur in non-smokers.

Pathophysiology

Buerger's diseas causes an inflammatory response in the arteries, veins and nerves. There is infiltration of white cells and the area becomes fibroitic as healing occurs, which can result in vessel occlusion. Occlusion of the vessel occurs when development of collateral circulation around areas of obstruction. Necrotic lesions form at the tips of fingers and toes and recurrent superficial thrombophlebitis commonly occurs in both upper and lower extremities.

Clinical Manifestation

Symptoms include slowly developing claudication, cyanosis and coldness which can progress necrosis and gangrene. Rest pain is common. The risk of gangrene increases with the presence of collagen disease or atherosclerosis and in response to cold weather. The other symtoms may include colour and temperature changes in the affected limb or limbs, parasthesia thrombophlebitis, and cold sensitivity, painful ulceration and gangrene.

Management

Buerger's disease is difficult to treat and management is focussed on assisting the patient to quit smoking and avoidance of trauma to the extremity. Patients are often told that they have choice between their cigarettes/Beedis and their legs. They cannot have both. In addition to cessation of smoking efforts, the patient has to avoid exposure to cold and protect the extremities from injury and trauma. Supportive psychotherapy and pharmacologic treatment of underlying anxiety disorders are sometimes helpful in assisting the patient to stop smoking. Although this disorder is difficult to treat, anticoagulants and vasodilator therapy have been used. A sympathectomy may help to eliminate vasospasm, but it must be performed early in the disease process. Amputation generally below the knee may be necessary in advanced cases.

RAYNAUD'S DISEASE

Raynaud's disease (arteriospastic disease is an episodic vasopastic disorder of the small cutaneous arteries, usually involving the fingers and toes. First described by Maurice Raynaud (1802).

Aetiology

The exact cause is not known. Associated disorder includes

systemic sclerosis, systemic lupus erythematosus, rheumatid arthritis, haematological disorders, trauma, and arterial obstruction, other contributing factors includeoccupation-related trauma and pressure to the fingertips (eg. typists-pianists and workers who use handheld vibrating equipments). Symptoms are commonly precipitated by exposure to cold, emotional upset, caffeine ingestion and tobacco use.

Pathophysiology

Vasoconstriction is regulated by alpha-2 receptors. Sympathetic stimulation or cold exposure causes the release of noradrenaline which activate the alpha-2 receptors and cause vasoconstriction and vasospasm. Persons with Raynaud's disease may have increased number of alpha-2 receptors. They may also have a decreased is betareceptors and calcitonin which are responsible for vasodilation. The pathological sequence is not completely understood.

Clinical Manifestation

The symptoms are symmetrical and bilateral. The vasospasm confined to the ditits and does not usually thumb. Only the tip of the finger distal to the metacarpophalangeal joint is typically affected. Toes may also be affected in same pattern. The disorder is characterised by three colour changes (white, red and blue). Initially the vasoconstrictive effect produces pallor (white), followed by cyanosis (bluish purple). These changes are subsequently followed by rubor (Red) or hyperemia. The patient usually describes cold and numbness in the vasoconst rictive phase and throbbing aching pain; tingling and swelling in the hypermic phase. This type of episode usually lasts only for minutes but in severe cases, may persist for several hours. Complications include punctuate (small hole) lesions of the fingertips and superficial gangrenous ulcers in advanced cases.

Management

Mild cases do not require any treatment. Patients are advised to have protection from cold by wearing loose, warm clothing or gloves when handling refrigerator, extreme should also be avoided and advised to stop smoking, avoid caffeine. Advise to immerse hands in warm water to decrease spasm. The drugs used are calcium channel blockers and beta-adrenergic blocking agents may help to some extent. Sympathectomy is considered only in advanced cases.

AMPUTATION AND ITS MANAGEMENT

Amputation is a surgical intervention commonly used in the treatment of peripheral vascular disease. It is the last resort of treatment when other medical and surgical measures have failed to save the limb. Amputation, although radical and traumatic for the patient, it can provide relief of chronic pain, the potential to walk against with the use of prosthesis and an improved quality of life.

The possible causes for indications or factors responsible for amputation are diabetes with pathology, peripheral vascular disease, birth defects, trauma and malignancy. Chronic tissue ischaemia that results in necrosis and then gangrene is the most common pathological sequence that results in amputation.

The goal of amputations is to preserve as much of the functional length of the extremity as possible while removing all infected of ischaemic tissue. Lower extremity amputations are roughly classified as follows:

1. Below-the-knee amputation (BKA).
2. Above-the-knee amputation (AKA).
3. Amputation of the foot and ankle (Symes).
4. Amputation of the foot between metatarsus and tarsus (Hey's or Lisfracs).
5. Hip diarticulation - Removal of the limb from the hip joint.
6. Hemicorporectomy - Removal of half of the body from pelvis and lumbar areas.

Preoperative Care

The preoperative period focuses on the careful evaluation and preparation for surgery include carrying out routine diagnostic measure as indicated according to the underlying disease. Stabilization of patient from infection, diabetes and others. The nurse focuses on teaching and patient support in the preoperative period. Amputation can have tremendous psychological implication. This radical change in body image can evoke feelings of loss, anger, fear, shock and denial, so that psychological preparation of the patients in very essential preoperative teaching emphasizes care that will be provided in the postoperative period, pain management strategies, plans for prosthesis fitting, and a basic introduction to stump care routines. The patient should be told to anticipate the occurrence of phantom limb sensation, a sensation of aching, tingling or simple awareness of the amputated part. In addition, other routine for surgery performed by the nurses.

The nursing care of the person after amputation includes:

1. Assess stump and monitor drainage for colour and amount, report signs of increased drainage.
2. Position of the patient with no flexion at hip or knee to avoid contractures and encourage prone position.
3. Maintain patient in low-Fowler's or flat position after AK.
4. Support stump with pillow for first 24-hours (according to physician or Surgeon's preference and avoiding flexion); place rolled bath blanket.
5. Encourage exercises to prevent thromboembolism:
   - Active ROM of unaffected leg, ankle rotations and pumps.
   - Use of overhead trapeze when moving in bed.
   - Push-ups from sitting position in bed.
   - Quadriceps sets.

- Lifting stump and buttocks off bed while lying flat on back to strengthen abdominal muscles.

6. Teach care of stump:
   - Inspect for redness, blister and abrasions.
   - Wash stump with mild soap, rinse with water, and pat dry.
   - Avoid use of alcohol, oils and creams.
   - Remove stump bandage or stump sock and reapply as needed; use firm smooth figure of -8 Ace wrapping to reduce swelling and shape stump (if rigid dressing not used).
7. Encourage patient to ambulate using correct crutch walking-techniques.
   - Keep elbows extended, limit elbow flexion to 30 degrees or less.
   - Avoid pressure on axilla.
   - Bear weight on palms of hands, not on axilla.
   - Maintaining upright posture (head up, chest up, abdomen in, pelvis in foot straight).
8. Monitor patient's ability to use a prosthesis.

VENOUS DISORDERS/DISORDERS OF VEINS

DEEP VEIN THROMBOSIS/THROMBOPHLEBITIS (DVT)

The most common venous disorder, results from incompetent valves in the veins and obstruction of venous return to the heart usually results in a thrombus. The formation of thrombus (clot) in association with inflammation of the veins is called "Thrombophlebitis".

Aetiology

Venous thrombosis typically results from at least one element of virchows traid: Venous stasis, damage to the endothelial lining of the vein, and hypercoagulopathy. The patients at risk for the development of thrombophlebotis usually has predisposing conditions to these three disorders. Risk factors for deep vein thrombosis are as follows:

- Advanced age - the elderly typically have a number of risk factors.
- Gender-DVT occurs more often in women.
- Positive history of thromboses.
- Immobility/stasis
  - Surgery, bedrest, paralysis, fractured hip, spinal cord injury.
  - Prolonged sitting (automobile or air travel).
  - Obesity and pregnancy.
- Increased viscosity (Hypecoagulatable stumps)
  - Dehydration, fever and malneutrition.
  - Polycythaemia vera and Severe anaemias.
- Intimal damage.
  - Central and peripheral IV catheters, pacemaker wires, IV therapy.
  - IV drug abuse.
- Associated conditions/disorders.
  - Malignancy.
  - Varicose veins.
  - Inherited coagulation disorder.
  - Haemolytic anaemia (Sickle cell anaemia).
- Trauma
  - Fractures especially involving the pelvis and long bones.
  - Burns.
- Use of oral contraceptives (risk primarily related to oestrogen content).
- Chronic lung and heart disease (CHF, cerebrovascular disease).
- Cigarette smoking.
- Venous cannulation or catheterization).

Pathophysiology

Thrombi develop from platelets, fibrin and both red and white cells. They typically form in areas where the blood flow is slow or turbulent. The major elements of stasis increased coagulability, and intimal damage dramatically accelerate the process. Muscle spasm and changes in the intravascular pressure can cause the developing thrombus to dislodge and move towards the heart and lungs. The lungs are rich in heparin and plasmin activators and can effectively dissolve some thrombi. However, if the thrombus is not successfully dissolved, it can lodge in an artery and obstruct perfusion to the lung segment causing problems.

Clinical Manifestation

Clinical manifestation of the thrombophlebitis varies according to the size and location of the thrombus and the adequacy of collateral circulation. The patient with superficial thrombophlebitis may have a palpable firm, subcutaneous cord-like vein. The area surrounding the vein may be tender to the touch, reddened, and warm. A mild systemic temperature elevation and leukocytoses may be present. Oedema of the extremity may occur or may not occur.

The patient with deep thrombophlebitis may have no symptoms or have unilateral leg oedema, pain, warm skin, and temperature greater than 38°C. If the calf is involved, tenderness may be present on palpation. Homan's sign, pain on dorsiflexon of the foot when the leg is raised is a classic but unreliable sign because it is not specific for DVT. If the inferior vena cava involved, the lower extremities may be oedematous and cyanotic. If the superior venacava is involved, the upper extremities, neck, back and face may be oedematous and cyanotic.

The most serious complication of DVT are pulmonary embolism, chronic venous insufficiency and phlegmasia cerulea-dolens.

Management

Various diagnostic studies are used to determine the site or location and extent of the thrombus or embolic which includes chest X-ray, APTT (activated partial thromboplastin time), PT (Prothrombin time) venous studies, venogram of the affected limb (Rarely), Lung scan and pulmonary angiogram.

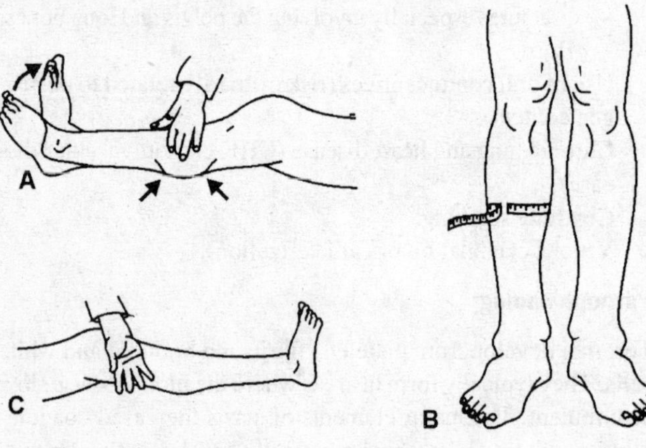

Fig.9.9: Nursing assessment for deep vein thrombosis. (A) Pain and tenderness in the calf of the affected extremity, especially on dorsiflexion of the foot (Homan's sign). (B) The affected extremity may have a larger circumference than the unaffected extremity caused by oedema. (C) The affected extremity will be warm to touch compared to the unaffected extremity.

The patients with DVT are treated with complete bedrest, because the patient on traditional heparian therapy will be on bedrest for 5 to 7 days. Patient on low-molecular-weight heparian can be out of bed after 24 hours if pain level permits. Patient can be treated with the use of local heat to extremity when inflammation is acute, fit the patient carefully for graduated compression stockings and teach correct use.

Patients are on anticoagulant therapy should be taught the action, dosage and side effects of medication, and they are advised to eat dark green and yellow leafy vegetables moderately because these are rich in vitamin K, which can counteract the effect of Coumadin (Warfran) and advise them to use alcohol only in moderation because it increases the anticoagulant effect.

In addition, patient should be taught the following.

- Risks and complications of DVT, signs and symptoms of complication.
- Risk, complications of heparin administration, signs and symptoms and complications.
- Bleeding precautions.
- Need for ongoing laboratory follow-up of anticoagulation levels after discharge.

The conservative treatment includes:

- Continuous IV heparin.
- Bedrest with bathroom privileges.
- Elevation of legs above the heart level.
- Anticoagulant therapy and heparin, warfarin.
- Elastic compression stockings.
- Measurement and charting of size of both thighs and calves every morning.
- Mild oral analgesics such as aspirin and codiene.
- NSAIDS

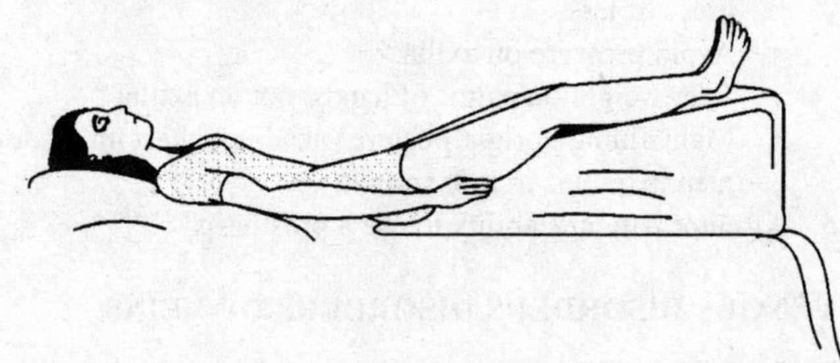

Fig.9.10: This leg elevator is of foam construction with a removable cotton cover t'iat may be machinc washed. It is clamped to the lower end of the mattress. This position is anatomically correct and provides adequate support to all parts of the leg oedema and stasis of the lower extremities can be controlled.

Surgical procedure if indicated incl:'de.

- Intracaval filter insertion.
- Venous thrombectomy (rarely done)

The primary option is transvenous filteration device placed in the vena cava to trap embolie before they reach the heart and pulmonary vessels. Two types are currently in use; the Greenfield filter and bird's nest filter. Both filters are permanently implanted and rarely become dislodged or occluded. The nursing care of the patient with a venacaval filter includes:

- Assess venipuncture site for signs of bleeding or infection. Maintain an adhesive covering over the insertion site.
- Immobilize the extremity after the procedure per institution protocol or physician's order.
- Assess peripheral pulses, temperature, colour and sensation in affected extremity per protocol. Assess for pain and presence of positive Homan's sign.
- Assess respiratory status and monitor pulse oximetry or blood gases as indicated. Position is partial or high-Fowler's position.

- Implement bleeding precautions and associated safety measures if systemic anticoagulation is to be continued. Monitor appropriate laboratory test results (PTT, HB, HctINR).
- Teach the patient to monitor for signs of infection at insertion site. Signs of systemic bleeding (eg. blood in stool, urine, gums, nosebleed easy bruises); bleeding precaution for home use, if anticoagulation is continued (eg. use of soft toothbrush, electric razor, stool softener), symptoms to report to the health care provider (bleeding and infection) DVT. Pulmonary embolism-swelling and warmth in extremity, sudden chest pain, dyspnoea, tachypnoea, restlessness, filter occlusion.
- Localized pain, venous stasis, or swelling and unusual symptoms.

VARICOSE VEINS

Varicose veins or varcosites are prominent, abnormally dilated, tortous subcutaneous veins most frequently occur in saphenous system, most oftenly in the lower extremities because of the effects of gravity on venous presence.

Aetiology

The aetiology of varicose veins is unknown. The increased venous pressure may result from congenital weakness of the vein structure, obesity, pregnancy, venous obstruction resulting from thrombosis or extrinsic pressure by tumours or occupations that require prolonged standing (eg. police constable, OT. nurse, etc). It may be hereditory and effects chronic diseases such as cirrhosis or CHF.

Pathophysiology

As the veins enlarge, the valves are stretched and become incompetent allowing blood flow to be reversed. As back pressure increases and the calf muscle pump (muscle movement that squeezes venous blood back towards heart) fails. Further venous distention results. The increased venous pressure is transmitted to the capillary bed and oedema develops.

Clincial Manifestation

Discomfort from varicose veins varies dramatically among people and tends to be worsened by superficial thrombophlebitis. In addition, many patients voice concern about cosmetic disfigurement. The most common symptom of varicose veins is an ache or pain after prolonged standing, which is relieved by walking or by elevating the limb. Some patients feel pressure or a cramp-like sensation. Swelling may accompany discomfort nocturnal leg cramps, especially in calf area occurs. The common complication is superficial thrombophlebitis. Ulceration may develop as a result of skin infections or trauma.

Management

A duplex ultrasound can detect obstruction and reflux in the vertease system with considerable accuracy. Treatment is not indicated if varicose veins are only a cosmetic problem. If incompetency of venous system develops, the care involves rest with the affected limb elevated, compression stocking and exercise such as walking. Sclerotherapy is a technique used in the treatment of unsightly superficial varicosites. Direct IV injection of a sclerosing agent such as sodium tetradecyl induces inflammation and results in eventual thrombosis of vein. After procedure leg is wrapped with an elastic bandage for 24 to 72 hours to maintain persons over the vein- local tenderness subsides within 2 to 3 weeks and eventually thrombosed vein disappears. After this patients are advised to wear compression stockings to prevent further varicosites.

The nurse should instruct patients to avoid sitting or standing for long time, maintain ideal body weight, take precautions against injury to the extremities and avoid wearing constrictive clothing. After vein ligation, the nurse should encourage deep breathing for promoting venous return. The extremities should be checked regularly for colour, movement, sensation, temperature presence of oedema and padal pulses. Postoperatively the extremities are elevated at a 15 degree angle to prevent development of verious stasis and oedema. Following measures are also to be taken.

VENOUS STASIS ULCER

Chronic venous insufficiency can lead to venous stasis ulceration, which may occur as a resultt of previous DVT.

Aetiology

Leg ulcers can be caused by many conditions including venous hypertension, infection, diabetes mellitus, malignancy, connective tissue disorders, rheumatid arthritis and damage through DVT or VS, external injuries such as trauma, pressure, and insect bites.

Pathophysiology

The basic dysfunction is imcompetent valves of the deep veins. As capillaries rupture, RBCs breakdown and release haemosiderin causing a brownish discoloration of the skin due to the deposition of melanin, and hemosiderin. The venous stasis ulcers usually develop around the ankles, especially in the area of the medial malleoli. Loss of epidermis occurs, and portions of the dermis may also be involved, depending on the degree of venous stasis.

Clinical Manifestation

The skin of the lower leg is leathery, with a characteristic brownish or "brawny" appearance. Oedema has usually been present for a prolonged period. The ulcer is concave lesion below the margin of skin surface. Pain may occur when the limb is in a dependent position or during ambulation. Pain is usually relieved by elevation of the foot. If the ulcer is not treated, infection may occur. Scar tissue is formed around the rim of the ulcer. Poor hygiene, debilitation, and inadequate nutritional status contribute to severity of ulcer.

Management

- Elevation of affected limb to reduce venous stasis and V. hypertension and oedema.
- Extrinsic compression methods- Stocking's elastic bandages and hydrocolloid dressings.
- Routine prophylactic antibiotic therapy (Culture and Sensitivity if needed).
- Protein- Vitamin supplementation.
- Calorie limitation for weight reduction.
- Surgery- Excision of ulcer.

PULMONARY EMBOLISM

Pulmonary embolism is the most common complication in hospitalized patients.

Aetiology

Thrombi in the deep veins can dislodge spontaneously. However, more common mechanism is jarring of the thrombus by mechanical forces, such as sudden standing, and changes in the rate of blood flow such as those that occur with Valsalvas manoeuvre. In addition, less common causes include fat emboli, (from fractured long bones), air emboli (from improper IV therapy) and amniotic fluids and tumours.

Pathophysiology

Most pulmonary embolies arise from thrombi in the deep veins of the legs. Other sites of origin include right side of the heart, upper extremities (rarely) and the pelvic veins (after surgery or childbirth). Lethal pulmonary embolie originate most commonly in the femoral or iliac veins. Emboli are mobile clots that generally do not stop moving until they lodge at a narrowed part of the circulatory system. The lungs are an ideal location for emboli to lodge because of their extensive arterial and capillary network. The lower lobes are more frequently affected because they have higher blood flow than the other lobes. Occasionally, the presence of deep vein thrombosis is unsuspected until pulmonary embolism occurs.

Clinical Manifestation

The severity of clinical manifestation depends on the size of the emboli and the size and number of blood vessels occluded. Most common are the sudden onset of unexplained dyspnoea, tachypnoea, or tachycardia. Other manifestations are cough, chest pain, haemoptysis, crackles, fever accentuation of the pulmonic heart sound, and sudden change in mental status as a result of hypoxaemia. Massive emboli may produce sudden collapse of the patient with shock, pallor, severe dyspnoea, and crushing chest pain. Some patients may have no pain. The complications of pulmonary embolism are pulmonary infarction and pulmonary hypertension.

Management

Diagnosis measures of pulmonary emboli include in addition to routin history need physical assent; venous studies, chest X-Ray, continuous ECG monitoring, ABGs, CBC, lung scan, and pulmonary angiography treatment measures includes:

- Oxygen by mask on Cannula.
- Establishment of IV route for drugs and fluids.
- Continuous IV heparin.
- Bedrest.
- Narcotics for pain relief.
- Thrombolytic agents in certain patients.
- Vena cava filter.
- Pulmonary embolectomy in life-threatening situation.

PROCEDURE 9.1: **CENTRAL VENOUS PRESSURE (CVP) MONITORING*

Equipment		
	Venous pressure tray	Arm board (for antecubital inserton).
	Cutdown tray	Sterile dressing tape.
	Infusion solution/infusion set with CVP manometer	Gowns, masks, caps and sterile gloves.
	Heparin flush system/ pressure bag (if transducer to be used)	ECG monitoring
		Carpenter's level (for establishing zero point).
	IV Pole	

STEPS OF PROCEDURE

Nursing Action	*Rationale*
Preparatory Phase	1. Evaluate patient's PT, PTT, and CBC.
1. Assemble equipment according to manufacture's directions.	
2. Explain the procedure to the patient and obtain informed consent.	2. Procedure is similar to an IV, and the patient may move in bed as desired after passage of catheter.
a. Explain to the patient how to perform the valsalva's maneuver.	a. The Valsalva's maneuver performed during catheter insertion and removal decreases chance of air emboli.
b. NPO 6 hours before insertion.	
3. Position patient appropriately.	3. Provides for maximum visibility of veins.
a. Place in supine position.	
i. Arm vein—extend arm and secure on armboard.	Trendelenburg's position prevents chance of air emboli.
ii. Neck veins—place patient in Trendelenburg's position, place a small rolled towel under shoulders (Subclavian approach).	Anatomic access and clinical status of the patient are considered in site selection.

Contd...

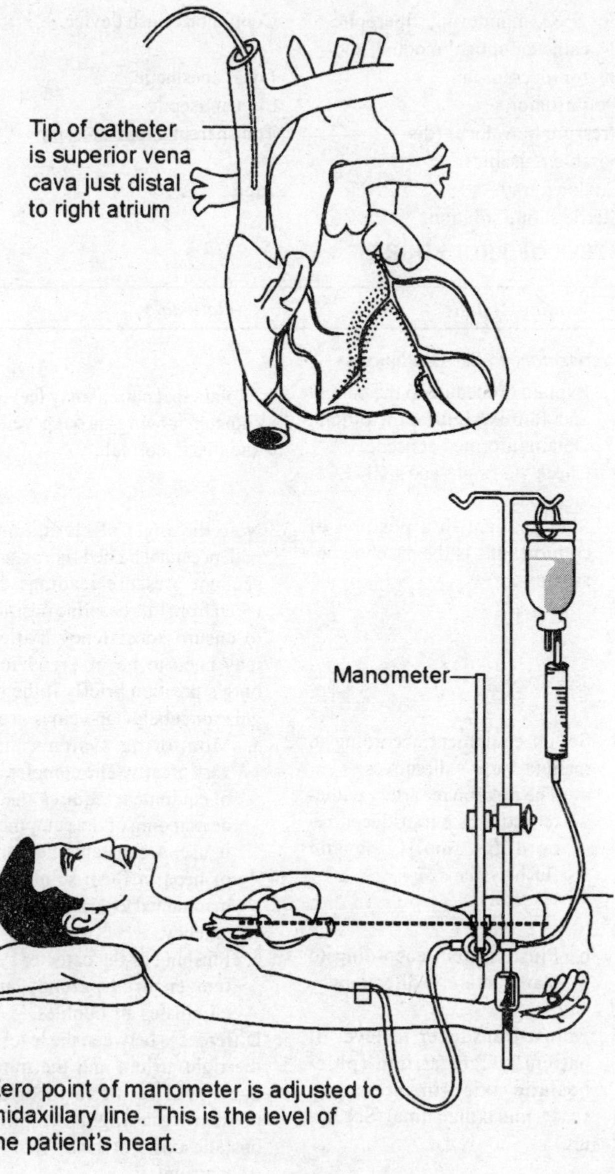
Tip of catheter
is superior vena
cava just distal
to right atrium
Manometer
Zero point of manometer is adjusted to
midaxillary line. This is the level of
the patient's heart.

Fig.9.11: Central venous pressure

Nursing action	*Rationale*
4. Flush IV infusion set and manometer (measuring device) or, prepare heparin flush for use with transducer.	4. Secure all connections to prevent air emboli and bleeding.
a. Attach manometer to IV pole. The Zero point of the manometer should be on a level with the patient's right atrium.	a. The level of the right atrium is at the 4th intercostal space midaxillary line.
b. Calibrate/Zero transducer and level port with patient's right atrium.	b. Mark midaxillary line with indelible ink for subsequent readings.
5. Place patient on ECG monitor.	5. Dysrhythmias may be noted during insertion as catheter is advanced.

Contd...

Nursing action	*Rationale*
Insertion phase (By Physician)	
1. Physician dons gown, cap, and mask.	1. VP insertion is a sterile procedure.
2. The CVP site is surgically cleansed. The physician introduces the CVP catheter percutaneously or by direct venous cutdown.	2. Patient may be asked to perform Valsalva's maneuver to protect against chance of air embolus.
3. Assist patient to remain motionless during insertion.	
4. Monitor for dysrhythmias as catheter is threaded to great vein or right atrium.	
5. Connect primed IV tubing/heparin flush system to catheter and allow IV solution to flow at a minimm rate to keep vein open (25 ml. maximum).	5. Catheter placement must be verified before hypertonic or blood products can be administered.
6. The catheter should be sutured in place.	6. Prevents inadvertent catheter advancement or dislodgement.
7. Place a sterile occlusive dressing over site.	
8. Obtain a chest X-ray.	8. Verify correct catheter position.
To Measure the VP	
1. Place the patient in a position of comfort. This is the baseline position used for subsequent readings.	
2. Position the zero point of the manometer at the level of the right atrium (See accompanying figure). Central venous pressure.	2. The zero point of baseline for the manometer should be on a level with the patient's right atrium. The middle of the right atrium is the midaxillary line in the 4th intercostal space.
3. Turn the stopcock so the IV solution flows into the manometer, filling to about the 20 to 25cm level. Then turn stopcock to solution in manometer flows into patient.	
4. Observe the fall in the height of the column of fluid in manometer. Record the level at which the solution stabilizes or stops moving downward. This is the central venous pressure. Record CVP and the position of the patient.	4. The column of fluid will fail until it meets an equal pressure (ie, the patient's central venous pressure). The CVP reading is reflected by the height of a column of fluid in the manometer when there is open communication between the catheter and the manometer. The fluid in the manometer will fluctuate slightly with the patient's respirations. This confirms that the CVP line is not obstructed by clotted blood.
5. The CVP catheter may be connected to a transducer and an electrical monitor with either digital or calibrated CVP wave readout.	
6. The CVP may range from 5 to 12cm H_2O (Absolute numerical values have not been agreed on) or 2 to 6mm Hg.	6. The change in CVP is a more useful indication of adequacy of venous blood volume and alterations of cardiovascular function. The management of the patient is not based on one

Contd...

Nursing action	*Rationale*
	reading, but on repeated serial readings in correlation with patient's clinical status.
7. Assess the patient's clinical condition. Frequent changes in measurements (interpreted within the context of the clinical situation) will serve as a guide to defect whether the heart can handle its fluid load and whether hypovolaemia or hypervolaemia is present.	7. CVP is interpreted by considering the patient's entire clinical picture hourly urine output, heart rate, blood pressure, cardiac output measurements. a. A CVP near zero indicates that the patient is hypovolaemic (verified if rapid IV infusion causes patient to improve). b. A CVP above 15 to 20 cm H_2O may be due to either hypervolaemia or poor cardiac contractility.
8. Turn the stopcock again to allow IV solution to flow from solution bottle into the patient's veins.	8. When readings are not being made, flow is fromed a very slow microdrip to the catheter, bypassing the manometer.
Follow-up Phase:	
1. Observe for complications.	1. Patient's complaints of new of different pain must be assessed closely.
a. From catheter insertion, pneumothorax, haemothorax, air embolism, haematoma, and cardiac tamponade.	a. Signs/symptoms of air embolism include; severe shortness of breath hypotension, hypoxia, rembling murmur, cardiac arrest.
b. From indwelling catheter infection, and air embolism.	b. If air embolism is suspected, immediately place patient in left lateral Trendelenburg's position and administer oxygen. Air bubbles will be prevented from moving into the lungs and will be absorbed in 10 to 15 minutes in the right ventricular outflow tract.
2. Carry out ongoing nursing surveillance of the insertion site and maintain a septic technique. a. Inspect entry site twice daily for signs of local inflammation/phlebitis. Remove immediately if there are any signs of infection. b. Change dressings as prescribed. c. Label to show date/time of change. d. Send the catheter tip for bacteriologic culture when it is removed.	*Nursing focus* A CVP line is a potential source of septicemia.

PROCEDURE 9.2: **MEASURING PULMONARY ARTERY PRESSURE BY FLOW-DIRECTED BALLOON-TIPPED CATHETER* (SWAN-GANZ CATHETER).

Equipment:

Swan-Ganz catheter, set

ECG, monitor and display unit with paper recorder.

Pressurized bag.

Heparin infusion in plastic bag.

For SVO_2 monitoring, fiberoptic PA catheter, optical module, and microprocessor unit.

Defibrillator

Pressure transducer (disposable/reusable)

Cutdown tray

Sterile saline solution.

Continuous flush device.

Local anesthetic.

Skin antiseptic

Transparent/gauze dressing

Tape.

STEPS OF PROCEDURE

Nursing Action	*Rationale*
Preparatory Phase (By Nurses)	
1. Explain procedure to the patient and family/significant others. Obtain informed consent.	1. Explain that patient may feel the catheter moving through veins, and this is normal.
2. Check vital signs and apply ECG electrodes.	
3. Place patient in a position of comfort, this is the baseline position.	3. Note the angle of elevation of patient cannot be lied flat, as subsequent pressure readings are taken from this baseline position to ensure consistency. Patient may need to be in Trendelenburg's position briefly if the jugular or subclavian vein is used.
4. Set up equipment according to manufacturer's directives. a. The pulmonary artery catheter requires a transducer, recording, amplifying and flush systems.	4. a. Monitoring systems may vary greatly. The complexity of equipment requires an understanding of the equipment in use. A constant microdrip of heparin flush solution is maintained to ensure catheter patency.
b. Flush system according to manufacturer's directions.	b. Flushing of the catheter system ensures patency and eliminates air bubbles.
5. Adjust transducer to level of patient's right atrium (phlebostatic axis 4th intercostal space, midaxillary line) (See figure).	5. Differences between the level of the right atrium and the transducer will result in incorrect pressure readings, the phlebostatic axis is at the level of the right atrium.
6. Calibrate pressure equipment (especially important when reusable transducers are employed).	6. A known quantity of pressure is applied to the transducer (usually by mercury manometer) to ensure accurate monitoring of pressure readings.
7. Clip excess hair prepare skin over insertion site.	7. The Catheter is inserted percutaneously under sterile conditions.
Performance Phase (By the physician)	
1. Physician dons sterile gown and gloves, and places sterile drapes over patient.	1. Sterile field is established to prevent chance of infection.
2. The balloon is inflated with air understerile water or saline to test for leakage (bubbles). The catheter may be flushed with saline at this time.	2. To ensure that the balloon is intact and to remove air from catheter.

Contd...

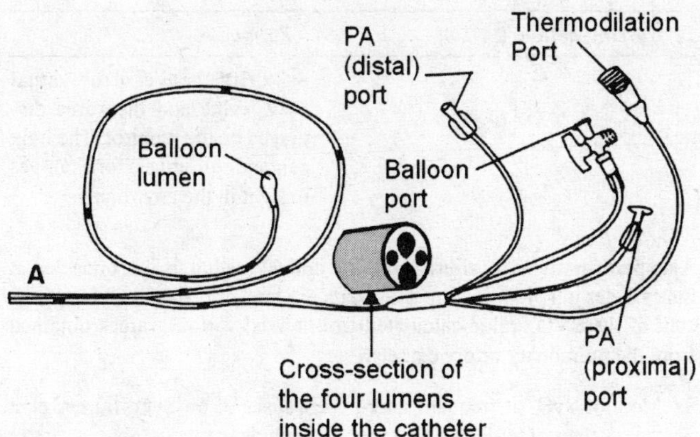

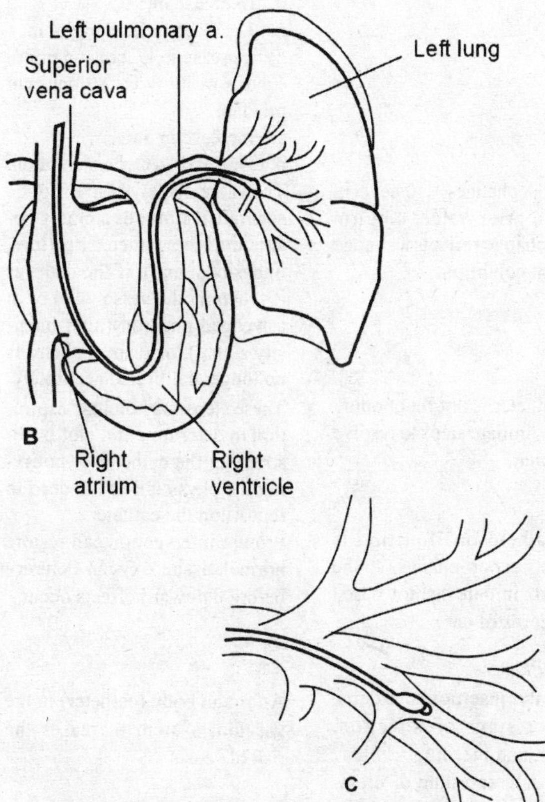

Fig.9.12: (A) Swan-Ganz catheter. (B) Location of the Swan-Ganz catheter within the heart. The catheter enters the right atrium via the superior vena cava. The balloon is then inflated, allowing the catheter to follow the blood flow through the tricuspid valve, through the right ventricle, through the pulmonic valve, and into the main pulmonary artery. Wave form and pressure readings are noted during insertion to identify location of the catheter with the heart. The balloon is deflated once the catheter is in the pulmonary artery and properly secured. (C) Pulmonary capillary wedge pressure (PCWP). The catheter floats into a distal branch of the pulmonary artery when the balloon is inflated, and becomes "wedged." The wedged catheter occludes blood flow from behind, and the tip of the lumen records pressures in front of the catheter. The balloon is then deflated, allowing the catheter to float back into the main pulmonary artery.

Nursing action	*Rationale*
3. The Swan-Ganz catheter is inserted through the internal jugular, Subclavian, or any easily accessible vein by either percutaneous puncture or venotomy.	3. The internal jugular vein establishes a short route into the central venous system.
4. The catheter is advanced to the superior vena cava. Oscillations of the pressure wave forms will indicate when the tip of the catheter is within the thoracic cavity. The patient may be asked to cough.	4. Catheter placement may be determined by characteristic wave forms and changes. Coughing will produce deflections in the pressure tracing when the catheter tip is in the thorax.
5. The Catheter is then advanced gently into the right atrium and the balloon inflated with air.	5. The amount of air to be used is indicated on the catheter.
6. The inflated balloon at the tip of the catheter will be guided by thc flowing stream of blood through the right atrium and tricuspid valve into the right ventricle. From this position, if finds its way into the main pulmonary artery. The catheter tip pressures are recorded continuously by specific pressure wave forms as the catheter advances through the various chambers of the heart.	6. Watch ECG monitor for signs of ventricular irritability as catheter enters the right ventricle. Report any signs of dysrhythmia to the physician.
7. The flowing blood will continue to direct the catheter more distally into the pulmonary tree. When the catheter reaches a pulmonary vessel that is approximately the same size or slightly smaller in diameter than the inflated balloon, it cannot be advanced any further. This is the wedge position, called palmonary capillary wedge pressure (PAWP).	7. With the catheter in the wedge position, the balloon blocks the flow of blood from the right side of the heart towards the lungs. The sensor at the tip of the balloon detects pressures distally, which results in the sensing of retrograde left a trial pressures. The PCWP is thus equal to left atrial pressures. a. Normal PCWP is 8-12 mmHg. Optimal LV function appears to be at a wedge between 14-18 mmHg. b. Wedge pressure is a valuable parameter of cardiac function. Filling pressures less than 8-10 mm Hg may indicate hypovolaemia and in an actuely injured heart are often associated with reduction in cardiac, output, hypotension, and tachycardia. Filling pressures greater than 20mm Hg are associated with left ventricular failure, pulmonary congestion, and hypervolaemia.
8. The balloon is diflated, causing the catheter to retract spontaneously into a larger pulmonary artery. This gives a continuous pulmonary artery systolic, diastolic, and mean pressure.	8. The normal systolic pulmonary pressure rangers are 20-30 mm Hg, and the diastolic pulmonary artery pressure (average pressure in pulmonary artery throu-ghout the entire cardiac cycle) is 15-20 mm Hg.

Contd...

Nursing action	*Rationale*
9. The catheter is then attached to a continuous heparin flush and transducer.	9. A low-flow continuous irrigation ensures that the catheter remains patient. The transducer converts the pressure wave into an electronic wave that is displayed on the oscilioscope.
10. The catheter is sutured in place and covered with a sterile dressing.	10.
11. A chest x-ray is obtained after. Swan-Ganz insertion if fluoroscopy was not used to guide insertion.	11. To confirm catheter position and to provide a baseline for future reference.
To obtain a wedge pressure reading	
1. Note amount of air to be injected into balloon, usually 1ml. Do not introduce more air into balloon than specified.	
2. Inflate the balloon slowly until the contour of the pulmonary arterial pressure changes to that of pulmonary wedge pressure. As soon as a wedge pattern is observed, no more air is introduced.	2. The transducer converts the pressure wave into an electronic wave that is displayed on a screen.
a. Note the digital pressure recordings on the monitor (an average of pressure waves is displayed, but these waves are not taken at end expiration).	a. PCWP should be determined at end expiration because respiratory variation of the wave form occurs due to changes in intrathoracic pressures.
b. Obtain a strip of the pressure tracing.	b. A calibrated osciloscope or graph paper is needed to read pressures at end expiration.
c. Determine PCWP from strip at end expiration.	
3. Deflate the balloon as soon as the pressure reading is obtained. Do not draw back with force on the syringe because too forceful a deflation may damage the balloon.	3. Segmental lung infarction may occur if the catheter balloon is left inflated for long periods. Pulmonary, capilary wedge pressures are only measured intermittently. Do not allow catheter to remain in wedge position when patient is unattended or when not directly making the measurement.
4. Record PCWP reading and amount of air needed to obtain wedge reading. Document recorded wave form is placing a strip of the waveform in patient's chart showing wedge tracing reverting to pulmonary artery waveform.	4. Overinflation of the balloon may cause a "Superwedge" wave form and data obtained will be inaccurate. Overinflation of balloon may cause balloon to lose elastic properties and rupture. The strip provides documentation that catheter was not left in wedge position.
To obtain a SVO$_2$ reading:	
1. Before insertion, perform a preinsertion calibration of the catheter.	1. This calibrates the catheter to light intensity in the environment.
2. After insertion, perform a calibration for light intensity and an in vivo calibration every 8 hours.	2. The in vivo calibration ensures that there is minimal difference, or "drift" between the actual SvO$_2$ value and the value displayed on the monitor. The light calibaration adjusts for changes in light in the environment.

Nursing focus

Also perform in vivo calibration if the optical module is disconnected at the catheter junction, if calibration data are lost, or if the SVO$_2$ is + 4 per cent of the SVO$_2$ value calculated from mixed various values obtained from the pulmonary artery catheter.

Nursing action	*Rationale*
3. Monitor SvO$_2$ at frequent intervals. Values of 60-80 per cent are normal.	3. Causes of an SvO$_2$ 60 per cent include. a. Decrease in cardiac output. b. Decrease in SaO$_2$. c. Decrease in Haemoglobin. d. Increase in Q$_2$ consumption. Causes of an SvO$_2$ 80 per cent include; a. Increase in SaO$_2$. b. Decrease in O$_2$ consumption.
4. If the SvO$_2$ changes + 10 per cent from the prior value, confirm that the change reflects a change in patient condition.	4. The value displayed may not be accurate if fibrin or a clot is obstructing the catheter tip (low-intensity signal), if the catheter is touching the vessel wall or in a wedged position (high intensity signal), or if the catheter is no longer calibrated accurately.
5. If the catheter is not functioning properly, initiate steps to resolve the problem.	5. These steps may include aspiration to determine if a clot is obstructing the catheter or notifying the physician of the need to reposition the catheter.
6. If no catheter malfunction is identified, report changes to the physician, initiate therapy based on standards of care.	6. Prompt intervention can restore normal tissue oxygen delivery before untoward effects occur.
Follow-up Phase	
1. Inspect the insertion site daily. Look for signs of infection, swelling, and bleeding.	1. A foreign body (catheter) in the vascular system increases the risk of sepsis.
2. Record date and time of dressing change and IV, tubing change.	
3. Assess contour of waveform, frequently and compare with previous documented waveforms.	3. Catheter may move forward and become lodged in wedge position or drift back into right ventricle. Turn patient to left side and ask him to cough (may dislodge catheter from wedge position). If not dislodged notify physician.
4. Assess for conplications, pulmonary embolism, dysrhythmias, heart block, damage to tricuspid valve, intracardiac knotting of	4. Blood coming back into syringe indicates balloon rupture. Notify physician immediately.

Contd...

Contd...

Nursing action	Rationale
catheter, thrombophlebitis, infection, balloon rupture and rupture of pulmonary artery.	
5. When indicated, the catheter is removed without excessive force or traction, pressure dressing is applied over the site.	5. The site should be checked periodically for bleeding.

PROCEDURE 9.3: **MEASUREMENT OF CARDIAC OUTPUT (CO) BY THERMODILUTION METHOD.*

Equipment:

Flow directed thermodilution Catheter in place.
CO Set, which includes IV tubing 10ml Syringe and three-way stopcock.
Normal saline or D5W solution bag.
Cardiac monitor with CO computation capability or stand-alone CO computer.
Temperature sensor cable.

STEPS OF PROCEDURE

Nursing Action	Rationale
1. Explain procedure to patient.	
2. Connect IV solution bag and CO set maintaining aseptic teachnique.	2. Solution will be injected directly into the heart and must be sterile.
3. If you do not have a prepackaged CO set, attach IV solution bag to IV tubing connect a three-way stopcock to the end of the tubing, connect a 10 ml syringe to the middle part of the three-way stopcock.	
4. Attach the three-way stopcock to the proximal injectate port of the thermodilution catheter. This port should be reserved solely for determination of CO. No medications.	4. The Proximal injectate port should have its distal end in the right atrium. If medications are infusing in this port, they will be flushed through in bolus form when CO measurements are taken.
5. Another three-way stopcock may be used to allow for IV solution to run at a keep open rte.	5. Once the CO set is connected, the system should remain closed.
6. Connect temperature sensor cable to the thermistor port of the thermodilution catheter.	6. When solution is injected through catheter, it mixes with the blood in the right side of the heart and flows to the pulmonary artery where blood temperature is detected by the thermistor.
7. Set cardiac monitor to CO computation format. If using a standalone CO computer, enter the temperature of the injectable solution and the code number for the size of thermodilution catheter in use (Code will be located on the thermodilution catheter packaging).	7. The injectate solution should be 15-20 degrees cooler than the patient's body temperature. Room temperature injectate is usually adequate.
8. Fill 10-ml syringe with injectate solution by turning stopcock off to patient and open to syringe and solution.	

Contd...

Nursing action	Rationale
9. Turn off IV keep open solution if present.	9. Need closed system from syringe to catheter.
10. Turn stopcock off to injectate solution and open to patient and syringe.	
11. Press inject button on the CO computer or monitor and inject 10ml, rapidly (within 4 seconds) and smoothly into the proximal port).	11. Delay will interfere with results.
12. Wait for computation to be complete. Repeat the procedure two or three times to obtain an average.	12. Same monitors display a waveform for the injectate dispersal to evaluate the adequacy of dispersal and temperature sensing.
13. Turn stopcock off to the syringe and injectate and allow keep open IV fluid to infuse through the proximal port.	

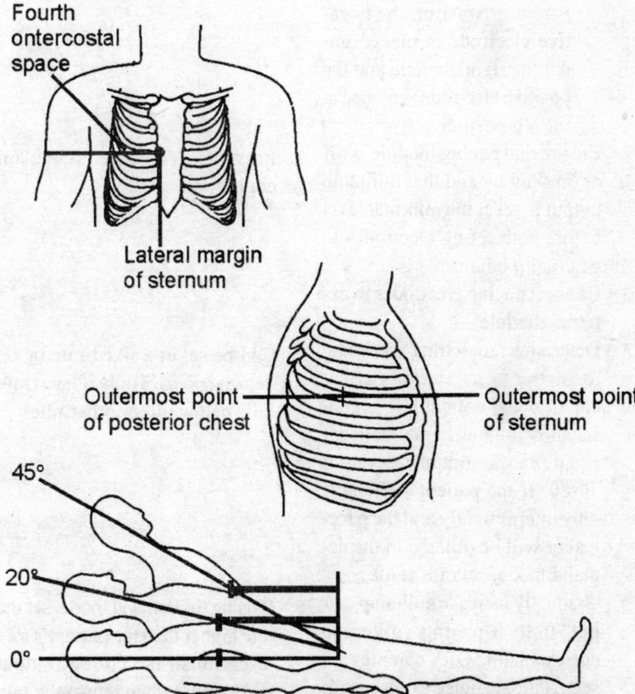

Fig.9.13: The phlebostatic axis and the phlebostatic level. (A) The phlebostatic axis is the crossing of two reference lines: (1) a line from the fourth intercostal space at the point where it joins the sternum, drawn out to the side of the body beneath the axilla; (2) a line midpoint between the anterior and posterior surfaces of the chest. (B) The phlebostatic level is a horizontal line through the phlebostatic axis. The transducer or the zero mark on the manometer must be level with this axis for accurate measurements. As the patient moves from the flat to erect positions, the chest moves and therefore the reference level; the phlebostatic level stays horizontal through the same reference point.

PROCEDURE 9.4: **TRANSCUTANEOUS CARDIAC PACING.*

Equipment

Disposable electrode pads
External pacing module
Resuscitative equipment.

STEPS OF PROCEDURE

Nursing Action	*Rationale*
Preparatory Phase	
1. Explain procedure to patient.	1. Allays anxiety.
2. Explain sensation of discomfort with external pacing.	2. Discomfort is felt with each firing, but can be relieved with analgesics.
Performance Phase	
1. Place electrodes as follows. a. Anterior/posterior. The negative electrode is placed on the anterior chest at the V3-V1 position, the positive electrode is placed on the back to the left of the spine. b. Anterior/Anterior, the negative electrode is placed under the right clavicle and the positive electrode is placed at the V6 position.	1. Electrodes must be placed so the current passes through as much of the myocardium as possible with the least distance between the pads.
2. Ensure that pacing module is off or on standby and that milliamp output is set at the minimal level before connecting electrodes to external module.	2. Prevents accidental shock on connection.
3. Connect pacing electrodes to external module.	
4. Determine rate setting according to instructions and/or patient condition. If patient HR is consistently too low to maintain adequate cardiac output, set rate at 70-80, If the patient's HR falls only intermittently and the pacemaker will be utilized in the demand mode, set rate at 60.	4. Can be set at a fixed rate or on demand, to pace only if heart rate falls below 60 (or other rate).
5. Gradually increase milliamp output, until a pacing spike and corresponding QRS complex are seen. Palpate pulse to ensure adequate response to electrical event.	5. If using the demand mode, set the rate higher than the patient's rate to establish the correct output and capture, then return the rate to 60.
6. Check pad placement frequently.	6. Patient perspiration may cause pads to loosen or slip.
Follow-up Phase	
1. Check vital signs at least every 15 minute, while continuous pacing is employed.	1. To determine if cardiac output is adequate.
2. Monitor ECG continuously for pacer functioning.	2. To detect malfunction (may occur due to electrodes loosening).

Contd...

Nursing action	*Rationale*
3. Assure patient that treatment is temporary.	3. Should only be used continuously for 2 hours.
4. Prepare patient for transvenous or permanent pacemaker insertion as indicated.	

PROCEDURE 9.5: **DIRECT CURRENT DEFIBRILLATION FOR VENTRICULAR FIBRILLATION.*

Equipment:

DC defibrillator with paddles.
Interface material (disposable conductive get pads, electrode gets and pastes).
Resuscitative equipment.

STEPS OF PROCEDURE

Nursing Action	*Rationale*
Performance Phase	
1. Monitored patient—if Ventricular fibrillation recognized with 2 minutes, give precordial thump, assess rhythm and carotid pulse, and expose anterior chest. Unmonitored patient-expose anterior chest.	
2. Unmonitored patient—Start cardiopulmonary resuscitation Immediately. Monitored patient—if within 2 minutes of detection of ventricular fibrillation, defibrillate before initiating cardiopulmonary resuscitation. Beyond 2 minutes, start resuscitation efforts immediately.	2. This procedure should be carried out immediately after ventricular fibrillation is detected to minimize cerebrial and circulatory deterioration. Cardiopulmonary resuscitation, is essential before and after defibrillation to ensure blood supply to the cerebrial and coronary arteries.
3. Apply interface material to the patient (gel pads) or to the paddles (gel, paste). The electrode paddies should be in firm contact with the patient's skin.	3. The interface material helps provide better conduction and prevents skin burns. Do not allow any paste on the skin between the electrodues. If the paste areas touch, the current may short circuit (Severely burning the patient and may not penetrate the heart. Saline pads are not recommended because the saline can easily drip, forming a path for the current.
4. Remove oxygen from immediate area.	4. Prevents danger of fire or explosion.
5. A second person should turn on the defibrillator to the prescribed setting. The American Heart Association recommends that initial defibrillation should be 200-300 watt-seconds of delivered energy. A second attempt at same level should be given if first attempt unsuccessful. A third attempt within increase of energy	5. The shock is measured in joules or Watt-seconds (the dose is 2 joules kg in paediatric, patients based on estimated body weight). The ideal energy dose for defibrillation remains controversial.

Contd...

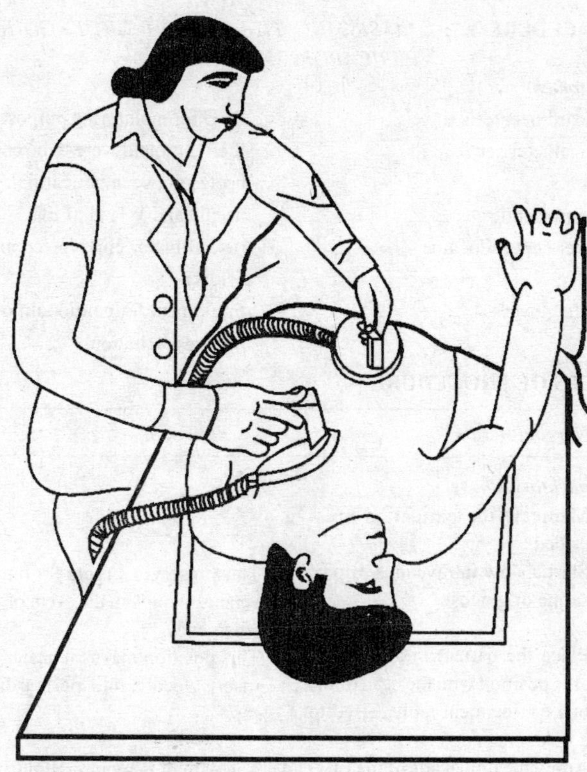

Fig.9.14: Paddle placement in ventricular defibrillation

Nursing action	Rationale
level to 360 watt-seconds should be attempted. Allow only approximately 5 seconds between the successive attempts to assess rhythm and pulse.	
6. Apply one electrode just to the right of the upper sternum below the clavicle and the other electrode just to the left of the cardiac apex or left nipple (See figure). About 20-21 1b of pressure is applied to paddles to ensure good contact with the patient's skin.	6. The paddies are placed so that the electrical discharge flows through as much myocardial mass as possible. If anteropastenor paddies are used, the anterior paddle is held with pressure on the middle sternum while the .patient lies on the posterior paddle under the left infrascapular region. In this method the countershock more directly traverses the heart.
7. Grasp the paddles only by the insulated handles.	
8. Charge the paddles, once paddles are charged. Give the command for personnel to stand clear of the patient and the bed. Look quickly to make sure all are away from the patient and bed.	8. If a person touches the bed, he or she may act as a ground for the current and receive a shock, especially if there are electrolyte solutions on the floor.
9. Push the discharge buttons in both paddles simultaneously.	
10. Remove the paddles from the patient immediately after the shock is administered (Unless monitoring leads are in the paddles).	

Contd...

Nursing action	Rationale
11. Resume cardiopulmonary resuscitation efforts until stable rhythm, spontaneous respirations, pulse, and blood pressure return.	11. After the third attempt to countershock, CPR efforts should be resumed, total delay should be no more than 5 seconds to oxygenate the patient and restore circulation.
12. Look at the ECG monitor to determine the specific therapy for the resultant electrical mechanism. Further high energy countershocks may be necessary.	

Paddle placement in ventricular defibrilatillation.

Follow-up Phase

1. After the patient is defibrillated and rhythm is restored, indocaine is usually given to prevent recurrent episodes.	1. Any resultant dysrhythmia may require appropriate drug intervention.

PROCEDURE 9.6: ***SYNCHRONIZED CARDIOVERSION.***

Equipment:

Cardioverter and ECG machine.

Conduction jelly or gel pads and cardiac medications.

Resuscitative equipment.

STEPS OF PROCEDURE

Nursing Action	Rationale
1. If the procedure is electrive. It is advisable to have the patient "NPO" 12 hours before the cardioversion.	1. During sedation or the procedure the patient may vomit and aspirate if the stomach is full.
a. Reassure the patient and see that informed consent has been obtained.	a. Do not use word "shock" because this will increase the patient's apprehension.
b. Make sure the patient has not been taking digitalis and that the serum potassium is normal.	b. Low potassium may precipitate postshock dysrhythimias.
2. Make sure IV line is secure.	2. An IV line may be necessary for administration of emmergency medications.
3. Obtain a 12-lead ECG before and after cardioversion with the ECG machine. The ECG machine wires are best left on the patient, because the ECG printout is of much better quality than that of the monitor. This fact is especially important when one is trying to dissect complicated dysrhythmias.	3. An ECG is taken to ensure that the patient has not had a recent myocardial infarction (either just before or after the cardioversion).
4. a. Allow the patient to receive oxygen before and after cardioversion.	4. a. Oxygen will help prevent unwanted dysrhythmias after cardioversion.
b. Do not give oxygen during the procedure.	b. An explosion could occur if a spark from the paddles should ignite the oxygen during the procedure.
5. Place the paddles in one of the following two positions:	
a. Anterior posterior position. One paddle-left infrascapular area. Other paddle-upper sternum at 3rd interspace.	

Contd...

Nursing action	Rationale
b. Anterior position. One paddle-just to right of sternum at 2nd interspace. Other paddle-just under left nipple.	
6. Determine if the machine's synchronization mechanism is working before applying the paddles.	
a. The discharge should hit near the peak of the R wave.	a. If the electrical discharge hits the T wave. Ventricular fibrillation may occur.
b. The R wave usually must be of substantial height. If it is not, adjust the gain (sensitivity) or change in the lead. On many machines the R wave must be upright before there is synchronization.	b. Synchronization is not used for ventricular fibrillation if the synchronization mode is on.
7. If using paste, apply to all of the paddle surface, but make sure there is no excess around the edges of the paddles.	7. If there is excess paste around the paddles, the discharge may run onto the skin, causing a burn. If there is not firm contact between the paddle and skin, a burn may occur, also electricity is lost from the heart.
a. The paste should be rubbed on the skin very thoroughly; this allwos more electricity to penetrate the body surface.	
b. Make sure paddles are clean because surface material will interfere with the flow of electricity.	
c. Apply firm pressure to the paddle.	
8. If using gel pads, place pads where paddles are to be positioned.	8. Excessive energies may cause unnecessary discomfort to the patient.
9. Set dial for lowest level of electrical energy that can be expected to convert the dysrhythmia. Some dysrhythmias (such as atrial flutter) can be converted with very low energies, such as 25 watt-seconds (joules).	9. This helps, produce amnesia concerning the cardioversion.
10. A short acting sedative such as midazolan (versed) should be given if the patient is conscious.	
11. After the patient is in a light sleep from the IV medication and when no one is touching the bed of patient, discharge the cardioverter. If cardioversion does not occur, proceed to a higher energy level.	11. The patient may revert to previous dysrhythmias after conversion.
12. Monitor the ECG after conversion occurs, blood pressures should be recorded about every 15 minutes until the preshock blood pressure is reached.	

PROCEDURE 9.7: **ASSISTING THE PATIENT UNDERGOING PERICARDIOCENTESIS.*

Equipment:

Pericardiocentesis tray	ECG for monitoring purposes.
Intracatheter set	Sterile ground were to be connected between pericardial.
Skin antiseptic	needle and V lead of ECG
1-2 per cent Lidocaine	(use alligator clip type connectors).
Sterile gloves.	Equipment for cardiopulmonary resuscitation.

STEPS OF PROCEDURE

Nursing Action	Rationale
Preparatory Phase	
1. Medicate the patient as prescribed.	
2. Start a slow intravenous drip of saline or glucose.	2. This preserves a route for intravenous therapy in the event of an emergency.
3. Place the patient in a comfortable position with the head of the bed or treatment table raised to a 45 degree angle.	3. This position makes it easier to insert weedle into pericardial sac.
4. Apply the limb leads of the ECG to the patient.	4. The patient is monitored during the procedure by ECG.
5. Have defibrillator available for immediate use.	5. In case the procedure has severe adverse effect.
6. Have pacemaker available.	
7. Open the tray using aseptic technique.	
Performance Phase (By physician)	
1. The site is prepared with skin antiseptic, the area is draped with sterile towels and injected with anaesthetic.	
2. The pericardial aspiration needle is attached to a 50-ml, syringe by a three-way stopcock. The V lead (precordial lead wire) of the ECG is attached to the hub of the aspirating needle by a sterile wire and alligator clips or clamp.	2. There is danger of laceration of myocardium/coronary artery and of cardiac dysrhythmias.
3. The needle is advanced slowly until fluid is obtained.	3. Fluid is generally aspirated at a depth of 25-4cm (+ to 1-1/2 inches).
4. When the pericardial sac has been entered, a haemostat is clamped to the needle at the chest wall just where it penetrates the skin. Pericardial fluid is aspirated slowly.	4. This prevents movement of the needle and further penetration while fluid is being removed. Aspirated fluid may be cloudy, clear or bloody.
5. Monitor the patient's ECG blood pressure, and venous pressure constantly.	5. a. The ST segment rises if the point of the needle contacts the ventricle, there may be ventricular ectopic beats.

Contd...

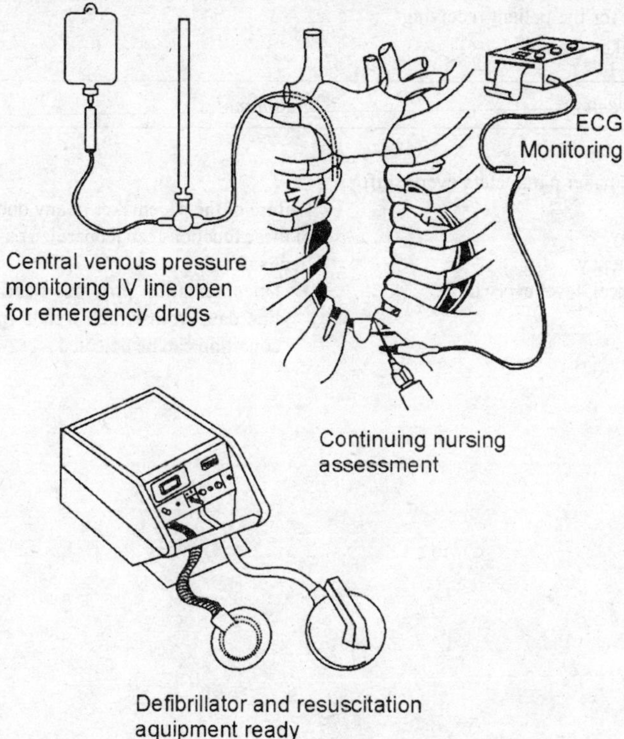

Fig.9.15: Nursing support of the patient undergoing pericardiocentesis. (Small circles indicate sites for pericardial aspiration.)

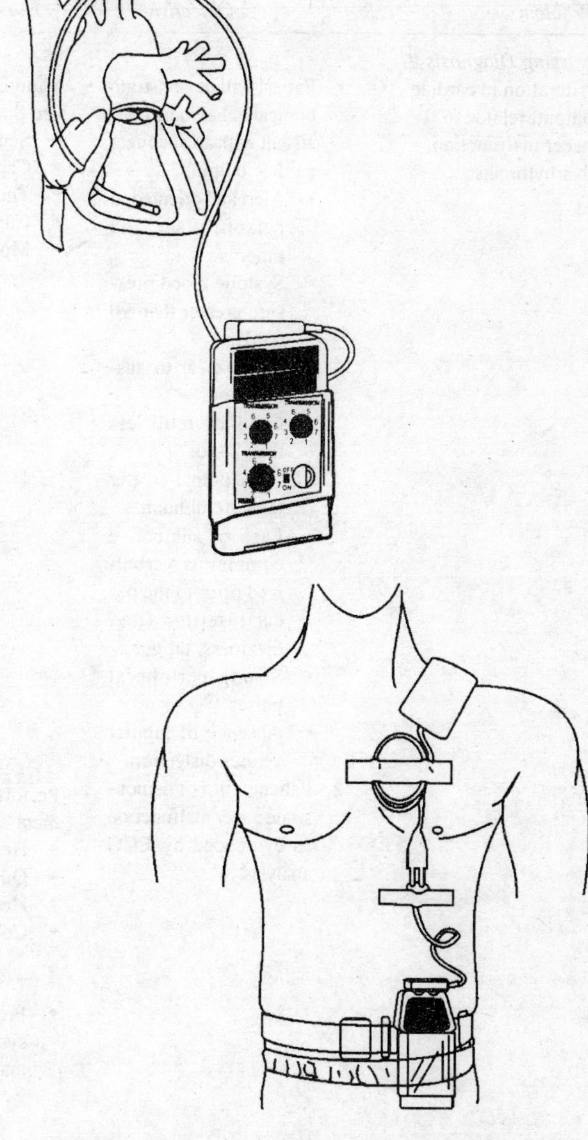

Fig.9.16: Temporary transvenous pacer wire with external pulse generator.

Nursing action	*Rationale*
	b. The PR segment is elevated when the enedle touches the atrium. c. Large, erratic QRS complexes indicate penetration of the myocardium.
6. If a large amount of fluid is present, a polyethylene catheter may be inserted through a needle (an intracath) and left in the pericardial sac.	6. An indwelling catheter left in the pericardial space permits further slow drainage of fluid and prevents recurrence of cardiac tamponade.
7. Watch for presence of bloody fluid. If blood accumulates rapidly, an immediate thoracotomy and cardiorrhaphy (Suturing of heart muscle) may be indicated.	7. Bloody pericardial fluid may be due to trauma. Bloody pericardial effusion fluid does not clot readily, where as blood obtained from inadivertant puncture of one of the heart chambers does clot.
Follow-up Phase	
1. Monitor patient closely. a. Watch for rising venous pressure and falling arterial pressure. b. Auscultate the area over the heart.	1. After pericardiocentesis, careful monitoring of blood pressure, and heart sounds will be necessary to indicate possible recurrence of tamponade, repeated aspiration is then necessary.
2. Prepare for surgical drainage of pericardium if. a. Pericardial fluid repeatedly accumulates, or b. The aspiration is unsuccessful, or c. Complications develop.	2. In the presence of these sign the patient is probably experiencing cardiac temponade.
3. Assess for complications. Inadvertent puncture of heart chamber. Dysrhythmias, Puncture of lung, stomach or liver. Laveration of coronary artery or myocardium.	3. Listen for decrease in intensity of heart sounds indicating recurring cardiac tamponade.

Contd...

Table 9.10: Nursing care plan for the patient receiving temporary pacemaker therapy

Problem	*R*	*Objective*	*Nursing Interventions*	*Rationales*
Nursing Diagnosis #1 Alteration in cardiac output, related to pacer malfunction, dysrhythmias.		1. Patient will demonstrate clinical behaviours consistent with an adequate cardiac output: • Alert and oriented to person, place and time. • Systolic blood pressure greater than 90 mmHg. • Lungs clear to auscultation. • Capillary refill less than 2 sec. • Urine output greater than 30 ml/hour. • Lack of subjective complaints verbalized prior to the pacer insertion (i.e., dizziness, fatigue). • Strong peripheral pulses. • Absence of jugular venous distention.	• Monitor the pacemaker parameters every shift and document: ◆ Sensing ability. ◆ Capture frequency. ◆ Threshold (check level every day). ◆ Current setting. ◆ Mode.	• Failure of the pacemaker in any one of these functions can jeopardize patient safety.' ◆ Documentation provides baseline data from which trends in condition can be detected.
		2. Patient will not demonstrate pacer malfunction as evidenced by ECG analysis.	• Perform comprehensive cardiovascular assessment at least once per shift. Include: ◆ Heart rate, rhythm. ◆ Quality of peripheral pulses. ◆ Heart sounds. ◆ Colour, temperature of skin. ◆ Presence of pulsus paradoxus (a drop of the systolic blood pressure more than the normal 10 mmHg during inspiration). – Blood pressure. – Quantity of urine output. – Presence of JVD. – Subjective comments. – Level of consciousness. – ECG strip interpretation.	• Baseline assessment will provide data from which comparisons can be made. ◆ Development of additional heart sounds may reflect decreased myocardial compliance or incompetence fo valves. ◆ Decreased or muffled heart sounds, jugular venous distention, and the presence of pulsus paradoxus may reflect tamponade. – Quality of pulses, urine output, temperature, colour of skin reflect tissue perfusion. – Jugular venous distention reflects elevation of rightsided heart pressures, which can be associated with tamponade. – First symptom of decreased cardiac output may be a change in mentation.
		3. Patient will be free of haemodynamically significant dysrhythmias.	• Check pacemaker system every shift including: ◆ Integrity of lead connections. ◆ Battery. ◆ Pacer generator.	• Pacemaker function may be closely assessed through strip analysis.

Contd...

Problem	*R*	*Objective*	*Nursing Interventions*	*Rationales*
			◆ Pacer settings.	◆ Ensure all components of system are functioning appropriately.
			• Monitor patient for presence of dysrhythmias and document type, patient's response, any associated activity, pacer activity (i.e., inability to sense).	• Dysrhythmias may or may not be haemodynamically significant or related to pacer activity. The pacemaker may need to be adjusted.
			• Notify physician at onset of any dysrhythmias. Keep Lidocaine at bedside. Ensure patent IV line is present.	• Physician may want to reposition pacing wire or initiate antiarrhythmic therapy.
Nursing Diagnosis #2 Potential for injury from microshock.	1. 2.	Patient's environment will be free of microshock hazards. Patient will not receive microshock.	• Cover any exposed lead wires with rubber gloves, finger cots, or scotch tape. • Wear rubber gloves if handling exposed wires. • Use only properly-grounded equipment, including the electric bed. • Inspect all electric equipment in room for signs of cord fraying. • Do not touch patient while handling electrical equipment.	• Insulating the lead wires will decrease the risk of conduction. • Improperly grounded equipment poses serious threat to patient safety. • It is possible for energy to travel through you from the equipment to the patient.
Nursing Diagnosis #3 Anxiety, related to invasive procedure, "heart failure."	1.	Patient will demonstrate decreased anxiety as evidenced by: • Subjective comments. • Decreased restlessness. • Facial expressions. • Nonverbal behaviour. • Ability to concentrate.	• Assess patient's understanding of situation, reasons for anxiety. • Provide information in supportive manner. • Assess patient's understanding of information provided. o Observe patient's response. • Assess past coping. ◆ Establish calm, quiet environment. • Provide sedation if needed.	• Pattern interventions to patient's level of comprehension. • Establishing calm rapport will reassure patient. • Patient's level of anxiety may prevent integration of information. • Assessing past coping skills will help you develop a more effective plan of care. • Sedation may be appropriate if nonpharmacologic interventions are ineffective.
Nursing Diagnosis #4 Knowledge deficit, related to need for pacemaker, procedure for insertion.	1.	Patient/family will verbalize understanding of: • Need for pacemaker. • How pacemaker is helping the heart. • Procedure for insertion.	• Assess patient/family's level of knowledge with pacemakers. • Establish teaching plan, including: ◆ Need for pacemaker. ◆ How the pacemaker will help. ◆ How long the procedure will take. ◆ Sensations of events expected during insertion. ◆ Post insertion events. • Provide only necessary information. • Encourage questions.	• Assessing prior level of knowledge will help in developing a more effective teaching plan. ◆ Including family will help their understanding of events. • Clarification of questions improves understanding.
Nursing Diagnosis #5 Potential for infection: Invasive line placement.	1.	Patient will be infection-free, as evidenced by: • Normal temperature. • Lack of redness, heat, swelling, discharge at insertion site.	• Monitor insertion site every day and document findings. • Monitor patient's temperature every 8 hours; every 4 hours if an elevation is noted. • Change dressing using sterile procedure every 24 hours or per unit protocol. • Change IV solution every 24 hours if a central line is present.	• Signs/symptoms of infection often begin at local level. • Temperature elevation is a clinical sign of the immune system's activity in combating pyrogens. • Frequent sterile dressing changes can prevent infections by providing an aseptic barrier once the skin integrity has become impaired. • Changes in IV solution will decrease medium for bacterial growth.

Contd...

Problem	*R*	*Objective*	*Nursing Interventions*	*Rationales*
			◆ Culture any drainage from site, and notify the physician.	
			• Culture all catheter tips if spike in temperature is noted (i.e., central line, pacing catheter).	• Identification of organism involved in the infectious process is vital for determining course of treatment.
			• Do not administer antipyretics for pain.	• Antipyretics may mask temperature elevation and signs of infection.
Nursing Diagnosis #6 Alteration in comfort, related to invasive line insertion.		1. Patient will verbalize statements of comfort.	• Assess patient's level of comfort (verbal and nonverbal cues).	• Patient may not openly admit discomfort.
			• Reposition patient frequently using pillows for support.	• Repositioning will prevent development of pressure areas and fatigue of dependent sites.
			• Rub areas of discomfort with lotion.	• Rubbing areas of discomfort promotes relaxation of sore muscle groups and enhances circulation to the area.
			• Provide medication for pain as needed.	• Medication can provide analgesia necessary to improve the patient's level of comfort.

Table 9.11: Nursing care plan for the patient with a permanent pacemaker

Problem	*R*	*Objective*	*Nursing Interventions*	*Rationales*
Nursing Diagnosis #1 Alteration in cardiac output, related to: 1. Pacemaker malfunction. 2. Pacemaker-induced dysrhythmias. 3. Electromagnetic interference.		1. Patient will demonstrate clinical behaviours consistent with an adequate cardiac output: • Alert and oriented to person, place, and time. • Systolic blood pressure greater than 90 mmHg. • Lungs clear on auscultation.	• Monitor ECG continuously for 24-48 hrs after pacemaker insertion for: ◆ Sensing ability. ◆ Ability to capture. ◆ Firing rate that is consistent with settings. ◆ Frequency of pace-assist. ◆ Presence of dysrhythmias.	• The pacemaker may "oversense" (i.e., become inhibited by other electrical potential in the body) or it may "undersense" and not recognize intrinsic cardiac activity. • Conditions may develop that can increase the threshold and decrease the pacemaker's ability to capture (i.e., fibrosis at the pacing catheter tip, hypoxia, dislodgement of pacing catheter, concurrent drug therapy, electrolyte imbalance).
		• Capillary refill less than 2 sec. • Urine output greater than 30 ml/hr.	• Confirm that the pacemaker is firing at the present rate.	• Determining how frequently the patient's rhythm requires pacemaker assistance will provide you with pertinent clinical information.
		• Lack of the subjective complaints that might have been verbalized before the pacemaker insertion, indicative of low cardiac output (i.e., dizziness, fatigue, nausea). 2. Patient will not demonstrate pacemaker malfunction as evidenced by ECG analysis.	• CV assessment same as temporary pacer.	◆ Foreign object in ventricle can irritate the myocardium and cause dysrhythmias.
		3. Patient will be free of haemodynamically significant dysrhythmias.	• Assess patient's response to dysrhythmias and communciate with physician for appropriate treatment regimen.	• The pacemaker-induced dysrhythmias may be self-limiting and haemodynamically insignificant, or they might be life-threatening. The physician should be made aware of their

Contd...

Problem	*R*	*Objective*	*Nursing Interventions*	*Rationales*
				occurrence to determine if therapeutic intervention is warranted.
			• Rule out any other potential cause of dysrhythmias (i.e., electrolyte imbalance, ischaemia and hypoxia).	• Other variables in the patient's clinical picture may be causing the dysrhythmias and should be excluded before the pacing catheter is implicated.
			• If cardioversion/defibrillation is required, do not place sternal paddle directly over pulse generator. Keep current approximately 10 cm away from pulse generator at all times. Anteroposterior paddle placement is strongly recommended if possible.	• Discharge of high amounts of energy over the electrical circuitry can damage the pacemaker and cause malfunction.
			• Do not expose patient to any conditions known to cause interference: ◆ Nuclear magnetic resonance. ◆ Cautery. ◆ Electroconvulsive therapy. ◆ Electric razors.	• Electrical and magnetic fields can alter pacer function.
Nursing Diagnosis #2 Potential for infection, related to the surgical procedure.		1. Patient will be infection-free as evidenced by: • Approximation of surgical incision. • Lack of elevation of temperature. • Lack of redness, swelling, discharge, heat at site of incision.	• Monitor incision site and document findings.	• Signs/symptoms of infection often begin at local level.
			• Cleanse incision with Betadine daily; keep open to air after 24 hr.	• Washing the wound with antibacterial solution will prevent infection. Keeping the incision open to air will promote granulation of tissue.
			• Monitor patient's temperature every 8 hours, every 4 hours if elevation noted.	• Temperature elevation is an accurate clinical sign of the immune system's activity in combating pyrogens.
			• Do not administer antipyretics for pain.	• Antipyretics may mask temperature elevation and signs of infection.
Nursing Diagnosis #3 Alteration in mobility, related to the surgical procedure.		1. Patient will be able to demonstrate full range of motion in affected extremity.	• Encourage patient to perform ROM exercises 24-48 hours after the insertion to prevent stiffness of shoulder; provide passive ROM if unable.	• Stiffness in affected shoulder occurs because of surgical manipulation of large supportive muscle groups.
Nursing Diagnosis #4 Anxiety, related to surgical procedure.		1. Patient will demonstrate decreased levels of anxiety as evidenced by: • Subjective comments. • Decreased restlessness. • Facial expressions. • Non-verbal behaviour. • Ability to concentrate.	• Assess patient's understanding of situation, reasons for anxiety.	• Pattern interventions to patient's level of comprehension.
			• Provide information in calm, supportive manner. ◆ Assess patient's understanding of information provided. – Observe patient's response.	• Establishing calming rapport will reassure patient. ◆ Patient's level of anxiety may prevent integration of information.
			• Assess past-coping behaviours. • Establish calm, quiet environment.	• Assessing patient's coping skills will help you develop a more effective plan of care.
			• Provide sedation if needed.	• Sedation may be appropriate if nonpharmacologic interventions are ineffective.
Nursing Diagnosis #5 Potential disturbance in self-concept after dependence on the pacemaker, disfigurement.		1. Patient will verbalize acceptance of the pacemaker as integral part of body.	• Assess patient's level of comfort with the pacemaker. Note comments related to: ◆ Dependence on "a machine." ◆ Fear of malfunction. ◆ Insecurity, embarrassment about cosmetic appearance. ◆ Loss of self-control and independence.	• Patients often have difficulty accepting the pacemaker because it is a continual reminder that they have a cardiac condition and because of its limited lifespan.

Contd...

Problem	*R*	*Objective*	*Nursing Interventions*	*Rationales*
			• Encourage patient to ventilate concerns; reassure and counsel to dispel misconceptions.	• Many patients have misunderstandings that promote disturbances.
			• Assess past coping mechanisms and apply if pertinent. ◆ Consult psychiatry if necessary.	• Past-coping mechanisms will indicate adaptive/maladaptive behaviour.
			• Have patient speak with another recipient of permanent pacemaker. • Refer to support group (if applicable).	• Recognition that problems are not unique provides comfort and strength for recovery.
Nursing Diagnosis #6 Knowledge deficit, related to: 1. Indication for permanent pacer. 2. How it will function. 3. Monitoring pacer function. 4. Signs and symptoms of malfunction. 5. Return to prior lifestyle. 6. Changes in lifestyle. 7. Medical alert information. 8. Electrical precautions. 9. Follow-up care.		1. Patient/family will verbalize understanding of: • Indication for permanent pacer. • How it will function. • Signs and symptoms of malfunction. • Monitoring pacer function. • Return to prior lifestyle. Changes in lifestyle. • Medical alert information. • Electrical precautions. • Follow-up care. 2. Patient and/or family member will demonstrate how to measure pulse rate with 100 per cent accuracy.	• Assess patient/family level of knowledge regarding pertinent information. • Develop teaching plan specific to their learning needs.	
			• Provide written information for reference of the material covered.	• Written materials are helpful referecnes when at home.
			• Explain in layman's terms: ◆ Purpose of conduction system. ◆ Why patient needs pacer.	• Understanding will improve patient's ability to care for self. ◆ A common misperception is that the pacer is replacing patient's own heart function.
			◆ How it will work to supplement the patient's cardiac activity – Signs and symptoms of malfunction (relate to signs/symptoms patient presented with if applicable). – Changes in lifestyle required. – Need to carry Medic-Alert card with pacer information at all times—use of bracelet or necklace. – Follow-up care.	◆ Must be able to identify specifics about pacemaker should it malfunction.
			◆ Electrical precautions: – Magnetic fields (i.e., store theft devices, some microwaves and radar). – Electrical fields (i.e., electric razors and cautery).	◆ Magnetic/electrical fields may cause interference with electrical circuitry; ability of pacemaker to function.
			• Demonstrate to patient/family how to check pulse. ◆ Have patient/family do return demonstration with 100 per cent accuracy.	• Patient needs to monitor appropriate functioning of the pacemaker.

Table 9.12: Nursing care plan for the patient requiring intra-aortic balloon pumping

Problem	*R*	*Objective*	*Nursing Interventions*	*Rationales*
Nursing Diagnosis #1 Potential alteration in tissue perfusion, related to myocardial ischaemia, peripheral vascular disease and embolic phenomena.		1. The patient will demonstrate adequate tissue perfusion as evidenced by: • Absence of angina. • Capillary refill of less than 2 seconds. • Warm extremities. • No change in baseline peripheral pulse quality. • Normal respiratory effort. • Sensorium alert and oriented.	• Check peripheral pulse quality, compare with baseline every hour, and document findings.	• Peripheral ischaemia or occlusion may occur due to embolization or diminished flow distal to the catheter.
			• Place patient in vascular position (reverse Trendelenburg).	• Vascular position promotes blood flow to the peripheral bed.
			• Monitor patient for complaints of chest pain, shortness of breath and peripheral pain.	• Complaints of pain can be indicative of ischaemia or embolization. ◆ Sudden onset of shortness of breath can indicate development of pulmonary oedema or pulonary embolism.
			• Assess colour and temperature of extremities with peripheral pulse checks, and compare bilaterally.	• The circulation distal to the IABP catheter is most at risk for compromised flow.

Contd...

Problem	*R*	*Objective*	*Nursing Interventions*	*Rationales*
			• Avoid flexion of patient at hips.	• This may cause migration of balloon catheter upward in the aorta. ◆ If the balloon catheter migrates forward it will occlude the left subclavian or carotid artery, causing diminished flow to the areas they service.
			• Monitor left radial pulse quality (or arterial pulse, complaints of dizziness.	
			• Place a sheet over the leg in which the but loca is inserted for restraint of movement.	• This will minimize the possibility of catheler migration cephaled.
Nursing Diagnosis #2 Impaired physical mobility related to cannulation of femoral artery.		1. Patient will maintain range of motion in all extremities except cannulated leg.	• Position patient with head of bed at 30-degree angle.	• This will permit swallowing and performance of some self-care activities. Elevation of head of bed greater than 30 degrees will cause hip flexion and may encourage migration of the IABP catheter.
			• Encourage patient to perform ROM exercises in all extremities except the cannulated leg.	• Maintenance of muscular tone.
			• Reposition patient frequently, log-rolling from side to side.	• Repositioning of patient will maintain use of muscle groups. The patient must be log-rolled to maintain alignment of the cannulated extremity.
			• Have patient continue ankle and foot exercises in affected leg.	• Ankle and foot exercises will help maintain full ROM of these areas without jeopardizing the catheter placement.
Nursing Diagnosis #3 Potential alteration in cardiac output, related to left ventricular dysfunction, dysrhythmias.		1. Adequate cardiac output will be maintained as evidenced by: • MAP 70-90 mmHg. • Urine output > 30 ml/hour. • Cardiac index > 2.0 liters/minute/m2. • PCWP < 20 mmHg. • SVR 800-1200 dyne-seconds/cm^{-5}.	• Monitor the following haemodynamic parameters every 15-30 minutes: ◆ Systolic and diastolic blood pressure, mean arterial pressure, diastolic blood pressure, mean arterial pressure, diastolic augmentation. ◆ Heart rate. ◆ Pulmonary artery systolic, diastolic, and mean pressures. ◆ Urine output every hour. ◆ CVP, PCWP. ◆ CO/CI, SVR.	• Ongoing assessment of clinical data is necessary to detect changes in left ventricular function.
			• Check balloon timing every hour or more frequently with changes in heart rate + 10 per cent.	• Timing must be precise to optimize effects IABP.
			• Monitor for dysrhythmias. Note patient's haemodynamic response.	• Dysrhythmias may or may not affect cardiac output.
			• If patient is tachycardic (HR greater than 150 bpm) it may be necessary to change IABP frequency to 1:2.	• At high heart rate, shuttling of gas and ability of IABP to inflate and deflate may be compromised.
			• If CPR is required, turn balloon to 1:3 frequency and decrease the volume to minimal level.	• It is impossible to coordinate IABP with resuscitative efforts, but the balloon should never remain still in the aorta because of the risk of thrombus formation.
Nursing Diagnosis #4 Anxiety (patient/family).		1. Patient/family will verbalize feelings of anxiety. 2. Patient/family will demonstrate relaxed demeanour as evidenced by	• Explain all aspects of treatment or care to patient/family.	• Understanding of patient care activities minimizes misconceptions and fears.
			• Explain/describe all expected equipment, sounds before they occur.	• Anticipation of sights and sounds helps prepare the patient.

Contd...

Problem	*R*	*Objective*	*Nursing Interventions*	*Rationales*
		verbal and nonverbal clues.	• Maintain interpersonal contact throughout performance of technical care. • Approach patient and family with confident, calm and professional behaviour.	• Recognition of human factor amidst technology is vital. • Patient/family must have confidence in care givers.
Nursing Diagnosis #5 Potential alteration in sensory perception, related to sensory overload.	1.	Patient will demonstrate lucid mentation as evidenced by: • Appropriate conversation. • Orientation to person, place, and time.	• Maintain quiet, soothing environment. • Attempt to preserve day/night sleep cycle. • Ensure patient has adequate sleep periods. • Restrict traffic around patient's bed; coordinate care to minimize disruptions. • Assess patient's mentation. • Reorient as necessary.	• Interventions are designed to minimize overstimulation, which can contriabute to disorientation.
Nursing Diagnosis #6 Potential for infection, related to indwelling catheters.	1.	Patient will be free of infection as evidenced by: • Lack of temperatre elevation. • Lack of redness, heat, swelling, or discharge at catheter insertion site.	• Maintain meticulous handwashing. • Change femoral dressing with aseptic technique. ◆ Observe insertion site for signs and symptoms of infection. • Monitor temperature every 4-8 hrs. ◆ Do not administer antipyretics for pain. • Meticulous perineal and Foley care.	• Handwashing decreases incidence of nosocomial infections. • Sterile dressings protect site from organisms. • Temperature elevation is an accurate clinical sign of the immune system's activity in combating pyro-gens. ◆ Antipyretics may mask temperature elevation and signs of infection. ◆ Signs and symptoms of infection often begin at a local site. • Maintain area free of contamination.
Nursing Diagnosis #7 Potential for physiologic injury: Bleeding, related to: 1. Indwelling arterial catheter. 2. Concomitant anticoagulation.	1.	Patient will not have active bleeding as evidenced by: • Stable haematocrit, haemoglobin levels. • Cuaiac-free stools. • Absence of haematoma, bruising, or ecchymosis. • Stable blood pressure and heart rate.	• Monitor laboratory values indicative of bleeding status (PTT, haematocrit, haemoglobin). • Monitor all stools for presence of occult blood. • Inspect the patient for oozing and haematoma formation at the catheter insertion site. ◆ Inspect the flank area for retroperitoneal ecchymosis. Generally inspect the skin for evidence of bleeding. • Apply pressure dressing, direct pressure manually or with a C-clamp if bleeding is noted at the insertion site. • Monitor the patient's blood pressure and heart rate for evidence of diminished intravascular volume.	• PTT will identify the ability of patient's blood to form clots. The haematocrit and haemoglobin will identify the level of circulating red blood cells. • Anticoagulation can promote internal bleeding. • Most common site of bleeding is the catheter insertion site. ◆ Retroperitoneal ecchymosis may indicate dissection of the iliac artery upon insertion. • Stasis of blood can be achieved by application of pressure of the site of bleeding. • Unexplained drop in systolic pressure with concurrent rise in heart rate may indicate active bleeding.

Table 9.13: Nursing care plan for the patient with percutaneous transluminal coronary angioplasty

Problem	*R*	*Objective*	*Nursing Interventions*	*Rationales*
Nursing Diagnosis #1 Anxiety, related to upcoming procedure.	1.	Patient will demonstrate decreased anxiety as evidenced by:	• Assess patient's understanding of the procedure, any past experiences or misconceptios, and reasons for anxiety.	• Identifying patient's level of comprehension and contributing factors to anxiety will allow for clarification

Contd...

Problem	*Objective*	*Nursing Interventions*	*Rationales*
	• Subjective comments. • Decreased restlessness. • Facial expressions. • Nonverbal behaviour. • Ability to concentrate.		through provisions of meaningful information.
		• Provide information based on assessment in a calm, concise manner.	• Information will be integrated if it is perceived as meaningful.
		• Assess the patient's understanding of the information provided, noting nonverbal cues.	• Patient's anxiety level may prevent integration of information.
		• Assess patient's past coping behaviours.	• Assessing patient's coping skills will help you develop a more effective plan of care.
		• Establish calm, quiet environment.	• Environmental stimuli can add to anxiety level.
		• Provide sedation if needed.	• Sedation may be appropriate to decrease catecholamine release and minimize myocardial oxygen demand if nonpharmacologic interventions are ineffective.
Nursing Diagnosis #2 Potential alteration in comfort, related to: Myocardial ischaemia, immobility.	1. Patient will remain pain-free as evidenced by lack of verbalization of symptoms of angina. 2. Patient will promptly report any symptoms of angina and will verbalize rapid relief after intervention. 3. Patient will verbalize comfort during period of immobility.	• Instruct patient to report immediately any discomfort. Emphasize the importance of this responsibility.	• Many patients are afraid or do not understand the implications of chest pain after the procedure.
		• Assess the patient for signs and symptoms of angina.	• Manifestations of angina may mimic gastric distress.
		• Assess type of discomfort along with associated symptoms and compare with presenting symptoms.	• It is important to differentiate pain of cardiac angina.
		• Perform stat ECG; note ST segment changes.	• ECG will reflect changes consistent with ischaemia.
		• Notify physician immediately of any complaints of chest pain or changes in condition.	◆ May need to repeat procedure.
		• Administer sublingual nitroglycerin, procardia, or IV nitroglycerin as per protocol.	• Vasodilation with nitrates and antispasmodic medication is needed to improve coronary perfusion.
		• Instruct patient that although he/she must lie flat during the time interval that the introducer sheaths remain in and for 6 hours after sheaths are removed, there are measures that can be taken to improve his/her comfort level.	• Reassurance that this immobility is limited promotes compliance and tolerance.
		◆ Place eggcrate or air mattress on bed. ◆ Elevate head of bed 30 degrees. ◆ Reposition patient on side with pillows. Place rolled towel under small of back. ◆ Medicate as necessary. ◆ Provide diversional activities.	◆ Interventions are patterned to minimize time lying flat on back.
Nursing Diagnosis #3 Potential alteration in tissue perfusion, related to cannulation of femoral artery.	1. Patient will demonstrate adequate tissue perfusion of extremities as evidenced by: • No change in peripheral pulse quality from baseline. • No change in colour sensitivity, or movement from baseline. • Brisk capillary refill (less than 2 seconds).	• Check bilateral pedal pulse quality every 15-30 minutes until sheaths are pulled. ◆ After sheaths are pulled, check pulse quality every 30 minutes for four hours then every hour for 6 hours. Mark location of pulse with pen. ◆ Compare findings with baseline.	• The circulation of the extremity distal to the sheath insertion is at high risk for compromise of flow during the period of time that the sheaths remain in and immediately after their removal.
		• Place patient in mild vascular position (reverse Trendelenburg).	• Vascular position promotes flow to lower extremities.
		• Remind patient not to bend at waist.	• Bending at waist could cause puncture of cannulated artery.
		• Instruct patient to report any pain, tingling, or numbness immediately.	• Pain, tingling, or numbness of the cannulated extremity can indicate vascular compromise and decreased tissue perfusion.
Nursing Diagnosis #4 Potential for physiologic injury: Bleeding, related to:	1. Patient will evidence no bleeding at site of sheath	• Check femoral insertion site every 15-30 minutes with pulse checks.	• Bleeding frequently occurs at the sheath insertion site.

Contd...

Problem	*R*	*Objective*	*Nursing Interventions*	*Rationales*
1. Cannulation of an artery. 2. Concomitant anti-coagulation.	insertion or retroperitoneal area.		• Assess the integrity of the sheaths. Ensure that the dilator remains within the arterial cannula.	• The dilator prevents blood from flowing out of the arterial cannula. If the dilator is not in completely, blood loss can occur.
			• Assess for oozing, haematoma formation.	• Frank oozing can occur around the cannulae, or haematomas can occur within the subcutaneous tissue.
			• Place 5-1b sandbag over site of insertion.	• Sandbag promotes haemostasis at insertion site by providing direct pressure.
			• Instruct patient to report any warmth in groin or leg area or sharp flank pain.	• Warmth may indicate unintentional blood flow from the cannulae. Flank pain may indicate iliac dissection, peritoneal bleeding.
			• Monitor PTT levels.	• PTT is indicative of clotting ability and will help direct therapy with heparin. The goal of treatment is to prevent reocclusion of the artery that was dilated.
			• Assess patient for retroperitoneal ecchymosis. Notify physician immediately if present.	• May indicate femoral or iliac dissection, internal bleeding.
			• Place direct pressure over site for 20 minutes, or until bleeding stops.	• Direct pressure prevents blood loss and promotes haemostasis.
Nursing Diagnosis #5 Potential alteration in cardiac output, related to: 1. Left ventricular dysfunction. 2. Sheath removal. 3. Dysrhythmias. 4. Orthostatic hypotension.		1. Patient will exhibit cardiac output adequate for tissue perfusion as evidenced by: • Systolic blood pressure greater than 90 mmHg. • No change in mentation. • Brisk capillary refill time less than 2 seconds. • Urinary output greater than 30 ml/hour.	• Assess vital signs, rhythm, mentation, capillary refill every 15-30 minutes until sheath removal, then every 30 minutes for 6 hours. Notify physician with status changes.	• Frequent assessment of patient status promotes detection of subtle changes in condition.
			• Assess urinary output every hour.	• Urinary output is a consistent noninvasive measure of cardiac output, renal perfusion.
			• Assess peripheral circulation with vital signs.	• Vasoconstriction is a compensatory mechanism for decreased CO.
			• Assess patient's mentation along with vital signs. Assess patient's mentation along with vital signs.	• Mentation is one of the most sensitive indicators of altered tissue perfusion.
			• Encourage fluid intake after procedure.	• Fluids are important in maintaining intravascular volume.
			• Monitor patient's response to sheath removal, direct groin pressure. Observe for bradycardia, hypotension, complaints of dizziness. Administer normal saline or other rapid volume replacement; place patient in Trendelenburg position and administer atropine, 1 mg IVP, as per protocol.	• It is common to observe a vasovagal reaction to the removal of femoral arterial sheaths.
			• Check blood pressures in lying and sitting positions once patient is able to get out of bed, and note decrease in systolic blood pressure greater than 20 mmHg or complaints of dizziness. Return patient to lying position if this occurs.	• Orthostatic changes are common after PTCA due to prolonged bedrest, venodilation with nitrates.
Nursing Diagnosis #6 Knowledge deficit, related to coronary artery disease post-PTCA expectations.		1. Patient/family will be able to verbalize an understanding of: • What CAD is. • Why this is a problem for the patient. • Purpose of PTCA. • Immediate post-PTCA care.	• Determine patient/family understanding of coronary artery disease, and how it affects them.	• Identification of baseline level of knowledge is necessary in providing individualized teaching.
			• Develop comprehensive teaching plan in conjunction with patient and family, based onlearning needs. ◆ Utilize diagrams and audiovisuals to enhance understanding of CAD.	• Mutual agreement on what information is needed is helpful in meeting perceived needs and providing meaningful information.

Contd...

Problem	*R*	*Objective*	*Nursing Interventions*	*Rationales*
		• Risk factors of CAD that the patient can modify. • Name, dosage, and purpose of homegoing medications. • Follow-up care (appointments). • What to do in an emergency.	◆ Supply patient with written instructions for information pertaining to medications, risk factors, expected behavioural changes, and emergent care.	◆ Levels of anxiety during hospitalization as well as quantity of information communicated necessitate written instructions for clarity.
			• Reinforce teaching during care and evaluate level of understanding. • Encourage questions and verbalization of feelings.	• It is important to assess patient's understanding after any teaching to identify any misconceptions.

Table 9.14: Nursing care plan for the patient with disseminated intravascular coagulation

Problem	*R*	*Objective*	*Nursing Interventions*	*Rationales*
Nursing Diagnosis #1 Tissue perfusion, alteration in: Decreased cerebral, peripheral, renal, gastrointestinal, related to: 1. Intravascular coagulation with thrombosis in the microcirculation. 2. Hypotension.		Patient will: 1. Remain alert, and oriented to person, place and date. 2. Maintain peripheral pulses that are strong proximally and distally; skin normal pink in colour, warm and dry to touch. 3. Maintain urine output > 30 ml/hour. 4. Maintain negative values for occult blood in body secretions and drainage.	• Assess neurologic status. ◆ General cerebral functions: Mental status; level of consciousness; monitor for confusion, lethargy, obtundation, coma, seizures, behavioural changes, headache, dizziness.	• Ongoing assessment of neurologic status is essential because of risk of possible cerebral emboli/thrombi, intracranial bleeding, cerebral anoxia related to cerebral oedema, hypoxaemia.
			◆ Cranial nerve function:	◆ Alterations in cranial nerve function reflect brainstem involvement.
			– Assess pupillary reaction to light and accommodation; drooping upper eyelid.	– Signals occulomotor nerve involvement.
			– Assess for drooping lower eyelid and facial drooping.	– Signals facial nerve involvement.
			– Ability of patient to talk; presence of protective reflexes: cough and gag.	– Reflect function of cranial nerves IX, X. Airway must be protected especially in the compromised patient.
			◆ Sensorimotor function: Assess movement and strength of all extremities.	◆ Peripheral thrombosis compromises systemic circulation.
			– Assess for the presence of paresthesias, numbness and tingling.	– Deep retroperitoneal bleed may cause pressure on lumbar nerve roots.
Nursing Diagnosis #2 Cardiac output, alteration in: Decreased, related to: 1. Fluid volume deficit. 2. Myocardial infarction. 3. Dysrhythmias		Patient will: 1. Maintain stable haemodynamics: • BP within 10 mmHg of baseline. • Heart rate < 100/ beats/min. • Central venous pressure ~0-8 mmHg. • PAP ~25 mmHg. • PCWP ~8-12 mmHg. • Cardiae output 4-8 liters/min.	• Assess cardiovasculae status. ◆ Assess vital signs: BP and heart rate; heart sounds: gallop rhythms, murmur; CVP, PAP, PCWP, CO; monitor for dysrhythmias.	• Ongoing assessment assists in identifying potential underlying bleeding, and helps to evaluate the patient's response to fluid and blood replacement therapy.
			◆ Assess for chest pain.	◆ Sluggish circulation predisposes to cardiac ischaemia.
			◆ Assess peripheral vascular status: – Degree of peripheral or dependent oedema; peripheral pulses; capillary refill.	– Oedema may occur with altered capillary permeability and osmotic pressure dynamics. Note quality of peripheral pulses both proximally and distally; monitor refill time.
			◆ Monitor skin colour and temperature of arms and legs. Monitor for signs of thromboemboli: Homan's sign.	◆ Presence of acrocyanosis reflects microthrombi within peripheral vasculature.

Contd...

Problem	*R*	*Objective*	*Nursing Interventions*	*Rationales*
Nursing Diagnosis #3 Fluid volume deficit, related to: 1. Bleeding/haemorrhaging.		Patient will: 1. Remain without signs of re-bleeding: • Without haematemesis, melena. • Without haematuria. • Without oozing around invasive lines and wounds. 2. Maintain balanced intake and output. • Skin turgour good; warm to touch. 3. Maintain stable laboratory parameters: • RBC and WBC counts. • Hgb: 12-18 g/100 ml. • Hct: 37-54 per cent. • BUN, creatinine, electrolytes, calcium, and glucose all within acceptable levels. 4. Maintain normovolaemia. • Body weight within 5 per cent of baseline. 5. Achieve resolution of impaired coagulation. 6. Achieve resolution of underlying cause.	• Initiate activities to detect the presence of occult bleeding.	
			◆ Assess skin and mucosal membranes for pallor, cyanosis, jaundice, petechiae: observe sclera and conjunctiva; gingival bleeding? epistaxis? ecchymosis? purpura?	◆ Acrocyanosis reflects microemboli within peripheral circulation; presence of jaundice suggests extensive hemolysis associated with underlying coagulopathy.
			◆ Determine overall status: presence of fatigue, weakness, malaise. – Myalgia, haemarthrosis (i.e., bloody effusion into joint cavity).	◆ Bleeding into joint cavities may underlie joint/bone pain.
			– Presence of visual disturbances.	◆ Retinal hemorrhages may underlie vision disturbances.
			◆ Measurement of blood loss: All body fluids and secretions: Stool (especially if diarrheal), haematochezia (i.e., stool containing red blood); urine; emesis, nasogastric drainage; sputum and/or haemoptysis; diaphoresis, wound drainage, drains. – Bandages and lines should be weighed; sanitary napkins counted.	◆ Multi-organ system involvement in some patients with DIC requires a delicate balance between hypovolaemic shock on the one hand, and overhydration from overly aggressive fluid/blood replacement therapy on the other. The key to therapy is accurate measure of all fluid and blood losses.
			◆ Sequential measurement of extremity circumference as well as abdominal girth. – Observe arterial and venipuncture sites for oozing of frank blood.	◆ Persistent oozing or increase in bloody drainage may indicate a developing/increasing coagulopathy.
			◆ Monitor laboratory parameters: Haemoglobin and haematocrit.	◆ These parameters are chief indicators as to the presence of bleeding; however, the patient's hydration status must be considered when evaluating these values; blood administration may also alter these values. ◆ Early identification of bleeding enables timely initiation of therapy to minimize and/or prevent bleeding.
			• Administer prescribed fluid/blood replacement therapy.	• Adequate tissue perfusion requires an adequate intravascular blood volume.
			◆ Administer lactated Ringer's/saline solutions; albumin and other plasma expanders.	◆ Massive fluid resuscitation is frequently necessary to maintain intravascular volume at levels to maintain intravascular volume at levels to maintain opti-mal cardiac output and blood pressure to meet the oxygen and nutrient needs of body tissues.
			◆ Blood/blood products replacement therapy. – Whole blood, platelets and fresh, frozen plasma may be given for severe depletion of platelets and coagulation factors. – Cryoprecipitate is given for depletion of factors V and VIII.	◆ Blood replacement therapy remains controversial. When utilized, it should be initiated after heparin therapy has been administered to prevent rapid consumption of blood products through the underlying disease process.
			◆ Nursing care considerations: Monitor vital signs before, during, and after administrational double-check product with patient's identification, and with donor's type and cross-match.	◆ For nursing care considerations and precautions to be taken when administering blood/blood products.

Contd...

Problem	*Objective*	*Nursing Interventions*	*Rationales*
		◆ Monitor patient for transfusion reaction. Note: Hives, chills, fever, facial flushing, headache, palpitations, tachycardia, chest pain, dyspnoea.	◆ Patient should be closely monitored for the initial 30 minutes.
		◆ Use blood administration set with a filter and large gauge needle (19 gauge). Infuse blood products with normal saline.	◆ Helps to remove injured cells and other debris in blood that may be antigenic. Minimizes injury to red blood cells. Dextrose solutions will cause RBCs to clump.
		◆ Allow blood products (e.g., platelets) to warm to room temperature before administering.	◆ Infusion of chilled blood/blood products may induce hypothermia. However, blood/blood products should be administered within 15 minutes of arrival on unit to minimize bacterial contamination/colonization.
		• Initiate actions to prevent further bleeding.	
		◆ Gentleness is the rule of thumb when caring for the patient with DIC. Use an electric razor.	◆ Gentle care minimizes injury to fragile tisseus, which may predispose to further bleeding.
		◆ Gentle tooth brushing; cleansing of mouth with cotton swabs.	◆ Use of mild saline solution, bicarbonate, and peroxide as a rinse are recommended instead of a mouthwash; if a mouthwash is used, dilute it 1 : 1.
		◆ Skin protection through gentle handling; special attention to skin and mucous membranes especially around catheters, endotracheal tubes, and other invasive lines and catheters.	
		– Orotracheal suctioning should be performed only when absolutely essential, and with meticulous aseptic technique.	◆ Careful and timely suctioning minimizes injury to mucosal lining, reducing the risk of bleeding and infection.
		– Blood pressure cuffs should be used as infrequently as possible.	◆ To avoid rupture of superficial capillaries with further bleeding. While an arterial line is invasive, it may be preferred to monitor vital signs and to obtain blood samples.
		• Administer prescribed medications and monitor response: Oral medications should be given whenever possible; parenteral medications should be administered using the smallest gauge needle and applying pressure to the puncture site for a 5 to 10 minute period.	
		◆ Stool softeners should be given.	◆ Help to prevent constipation with straining at stool.
		◆ Aspirin preparations contraindicated:	◆ Aspirin inteferes with platelet aggregation thus inhibiting coagulation.
		◆ Heparin therapy via continuous infusion pump or intermittently (via minidose protocol).	◆ Controversy regarding use of heparin in treatment of DIC. – Heparin is most effective when given early in the course of DIC. – Heparin is most effective when given early in the course of DIC. – Preferred route of administration is continuous intravenous drip. Doses are adjusted according to patient's overall status.

Contd...

Problem	*R*	*Objective*	*Nursing Interventions*	*Rationales*
				– Heparin therapy is usually continued until clinical and laboratory data indicate patient's condition is stabilizing.
			♦ Vasopressors (e.g., dopamine).	♦ Vasopressors may be indicated if blood pressure does not stabilize with full hydration.
			• Monitor haematopoietic function. ♦ Asses the following: Bleeding—estimate loss; presence of petechiae, ecchymosis, purpura, baematoma; note size and location. ♦ Monitor haemoglobin, haematocrit, coagulation studies especially platelets, prothrombin time, partial thromboplastin time, fibrin degradation products, and bleeding time.	• Changes in laboratory values are indicative of the patient's status and response to therapy; they afford the capability of following trends in the patient's condition that enable timely and appropriate therapy to be instituted.
			♦ Monitor for exacerbation of bleeding.	♦ Exacerbation of bleeding in patients receiving heparin therapy longer than eight days may be indicative of antiplatelet antibody formation.
Nursing Diagnosis #4 Gas exchange, impaired, related to: 1. Increased pulmonary capillary permeability, pulmonary embolism, ARDS, with increased pulmonary shunting.		Patient will: 1. Maintain respiratory rate < 30/min. 2. Maintain adequate ventilation as gauged by the work of breathing and arterial blood gases: • $PaO_2 > 60$ mmHg (room air). • PaCO2 ~ 35-45 mmHg. • pH 7.35-7.45. 3. Maintain breath sounds clear to auscultation.	• Assess pulmonary function. ♦ Respiratory rate and breathing pattern. ♦ Breath sounds. ♦ Adventitious sounds: Rales, rhonchi, stridor. ♦ Chest pain: pleuritic causes. ♦ Sputum production; haemoptysis.	• Onset of respiratory distress suggests intravascular clotting and/or bleeding into pulmonary tissues. ♦ Tachypnoea, orthopnoea, tachycardia reflect effort to maintain tissue oxygenation. ♦ Haemoptysis suggests possible pulmonary emboli.
			♦ Monitor arterial blood gases.	♦ Altered pulmonary vascular dynamles predisposes to pulmonary shunting with compromised gas exchange and consequent hypoxaemia.
			• Initiate precautionary/supportive therapy. ♦ Teach patient to cough, sneeze, and blow nose gently. ♦ Avoid sudden Valsalva's maneuver.	♦ Reduce risk of dislodging clots and causing rebleeding.
			♦ Provide humidified supplemental oxygen. ♦ Encourage to breathe deeply at regular intervals.	♦ Humidification helps to keep secretions moist and easier to mobilize and remove; helps avoid infection.
			– Encourage use of incentive spirometer.	– Helps to expand the lungs and prevent areas of atelectasis.
Nursing Diagnosis #5 Urinary climination, alteration in, related to; 1. Haematuria. 2. Hypovolaemia. 3. Renal dysfunction associated with microemboli. 4. Haemoglobinopathy.		Patient will: 1. Maintain urinary output > 30 ml/hour. 2. Maintain urine without red blood cells/haemoglobin/protein. 3. Maintain renal function studies at baseline. • BUN, creatinine.	• Assess renal status. ♦ Hydration: Intake and output; urine specific gravity; body weight. ♦ Haematuria.	• Urine output less than 30 ml/hour suggests dehydration, hypovolaemic state, or possible microemboli within the kidneys. ♦ Oliguria may be associated with renal insufficiency or acute tubular necrosis. ♦ Massive fluid resuscitation may be necessary to maintain intravascular volume.

Contd...

Problem	*Objective*	*Nursing Interventions*	*Rationales*
		◆ Monitor renal function studies: BUN, creatinine; urine glucose, acetone; renal calculi, if bedrest is prolonged. • Monitor urinary function. ◆ Assess for haematuria, burning on urination, urgency, frequency. ◆ Maintain sterility of closed urinary system if Foley catheter is in place. ◆ Use leg strap to secure teh tubing to the leg to prevent pulling. ◆ Maintain hydration.	◆ Major complication is urinary infection. ◆ Tugging on the catheter can cause injury to the urinary meatus and urinary tract.
Nursing Diagnosis #6 Bowel elimination, alteration in, related to: 1. Bleeding potential.	Patient will: 1. Remain without signs of intra-abdominal bleeding: • Without abdominal distention and pain. • Stable abdominal girth. • Without nausea and vomiting. • Negative for occult blood in nasogastric drainage, emesis, stools. • Bowel sounds appropriate. • Vital signs stable.	• Assess gastrointestinal function. ◆ Assess for signs of distention and increasing abdominal girth; abdominal cramps or pain; nausea/vomiting. ◆ Assess bowel sounds. – Presence of paralytic ileus. ◆ Haematest for occult blood: Nasogastric secretions; emesis, stools. • Implement precautionary/supportive measures. ◆ Maintain good oral hygiene. ◆ Avoid loose fitting dentures. Keep lips lubricated. ◆ Monitor patient's response to antacid protocol: cimetidine; ranitidine; maalox. – Avoid use of rectal temperatures. – Avoid use of suppositories. – Avoid use of aspirin and steroids. Administer stool softeners as prescribed.	◆ Bleeding into peritoneal cavity should be suspected in the presence of increasing abdominal girth. – Presence of microthromboemboli within splanchnic circulation may underlie mesenteric ischaemia and/or necrosis. ◆ Helps patient to feel good and reduces the risk of infection. ◆ Potential for injury to oral mucosa causing bleeding. ◆ Reduce secretion and deleterious effects of HCl acid (gastric). ◆ May irritate friable rectal tissues, resulting in bleeding. ◆ These drugs compromise haematologic and immunologic functions leading to potential bleeding and infection.
Nursing Diagnosis #7 Nutrition, alteration in: Less than body requirement, related to: 1. NPO status in the presence of potential bleeding. 2. Anorexia, fatigue.	Patient will: 1. Maintain body weight within 5 per cent of baseline. 2. Maintain plasma protein levels 6-8 gm/100 ml. 3. Maintain triceps skinfold and midarm circumference measurements within acceptable range. 4. Maintain blood chemistries within acceptable range. • BUN, creatinine. • Serum glucose. • Serum electrolytes including calcium, phosphorus, magnesium, sodium, potassium, chloride.	• Collaborate with nutritionist in assessing nutrition status. ◆ Implement prescribed dietary feeding or hyperalimentation. – Maintain strict intake and output. ◆ Encourage liquids and soft foods as tolerated. – Avoid use of hot, spicy foods/fluids. ◆ Encourage carbonated beverages as tolerated.	• Dietary regimen must meet tissue protein needs to promote healing. ◆ Avoids oral mucosal irritation and gingival bleeding. ◆ Carbonated beverages help to loosen crusts around mouth and oral cavity without bleeding.

Contd...

Problem	*R*	*Objective*	*Nursing Interventions*	*Rationales*
Nursing Diagnosis #8 Mobility, impaired, related to: 1. Pain caused by bleeding into muscle and joints. 2. Debilitated state. 3. Increased risk of rebleeding.		Patient will: 1. Be able to resume pre-illness activity.	• Assess mobility. ◆ Assess movement of all extremities. ◆ Assess for the presence of joint/muscle pain; haemarthrosis. Assess extremities and joints for swelling and tenderness. • Institute precautionary measures: ◆ Utilize a bed cradle. ◆ Immobilize affected areas. ◆ Treat bone/joint pain with hot or cold compresses as prescribed. ◆ Maintain proper body alignment. ◆ Provide gentle passive range of motion. ◆ Utilize extra assistance when moving patient; use draw sheet to lift patient. • Monitor all peripheral pulses, colour of skin, and temperature of skin.	◆ Thrombosis/bleeding into muscle and joints may necessitate restriction of movement to minimize further trauma. • Goal is to protect the patient from further trauma; minor injury/stress may potentiate bleeding. ◆ This avoids dragging the patient, as for example, when moving the patient up in bed; such action could cause skin abrasions and other trauma increasing potential for bleeding.
Nursing Diagnosis #9 Skin integrity, impaired, related to: 1. Capillary fragility, bleeding sites. 2. Inadequate dietary intake. 3. Immobility.		Patient will: 1. Maintain skin intact, no breaks, lesions, irritations, or signs of infection; good skin turgour. 2. Without signs of acrocyanosis or tissue necrosis.	• Assess integrity of skin and mucous membranes. • Institute precautionary measures. ◆ Avoid unnecessary intramuscular and subcutaneous injections; if necessary, use small-gauge needle, rotate sites, and apply steady pressure for 5-10 minutes. ◆ Implement use of pressure relief device (e.g., air mattress).	◆ Reduces the risk of bleeding. ◆ Reduces pressure points which can predispose to skin breakdown especially in the compromised patient.
Nursing Diagnosis#10 Oral mucous membranes, alteration in.		Patient will: 1. Maintain integrity of mucous membranes. • Mucous membranes moist. • Lips without cracking/fissuring. • No evidence of bleeding. • No evidence of infection (stomatitis).	◆ Implement turning and postitoning schedule. ◆ Identify pressure areas: include stage and depth of ulcer if present. – Review patient's nutritional status. ◆ Keep skin well lubricated. – Provide meticulous skin and wound care. – Be gentle with patients. Discourage scratching; removing scabs; keep nails trimmed.	◆ Helps to maximize tissue perfusion. ◆ Dietary intake should ensure adequate sources of protein for tissue repair. ◆ To avoid dryness and cracking which can predispose to skin breakdown and infection. – To prevent infection. – To avoid trauma.
Nursing Diagnosis #11 Anxiety, fear, related to: 1. Knowledge deficit regarding bleeding and status of condition. 2. Altered level of body function and capability for carrying out self-care activities.		Patient will: 1. Verbalize fear about bleeding. 2. Exhibit relaxed facial expression and overall demeanour. 3. Heart rate at baseline for patient.	• Assess level of anxiety/discomfort. ◆ Sigsn and symptoms: Verbalization of fear and anxiety; body posture: Clenched fists, restlessness, irritability, insomnia; evaluate pain. • Provide comfort measures. • Monitor response to pain medication. • Promote rest and sleep periods. • Offer necessary explanations regarding condition and therapy.	• Relaxation affords comfort. • Assist in conserving strength. • Prevents unnecessary anxiety and concern on the part of patient and family.

Contd...

Problem	*R Objective*	*Nursing Interventions*	*Rationales*
Nursing Diagnosis#12 Coping, ineffective: Individual/family.	Patient/family will: 1. Verbalize feelings regarding underlying disease and prognosis. 2. Identify strengths and coping mechanisms. 3. Make decision of importance to the patient/family. 4. Identify familial and community resources.	• Assess patient/family's prior coping methods. ◆ Identify family/community resources. • Evaluate patient/family's understanding of illness: Anticipate needs; be accessible; make necessary explanations. • Provide emotional and psychological support. • Assist in self-care activities.	• Identifying past coping capabilities may assist patient/family in dealing with current illness; familiarity breeds self-confidence. • Knowledge of underlying problem may be especially helpful in coping with a bleeding disorder. The sight of even a little blood can be frightening. • Encourages patient/family to assume responsibility for their own health. This is especially important in those instances where the bleeding problem is a chronic problem.
Nursing Diagnosis#13 Potential for infection, related to: 1. Debilitated state. 2. Stagnation of blood. 3. Open wounds. 4. Impaired skin integrity.	Patient will remain without signs and symptoms of infection. 1. Body temperature at baseline. 2. Haematology profile within acceptable limits.	• Assess patient for signs and symptoms of possible infection: Monitor temperatures; productive cough with rust-coloured or purulent sputum; purulent drainage from open wounds, incisions; redness, swelling, and pain at catheter sites. • Implement protocols in the event of infection: Cultures/sensitivity of body secretions and excretions—sputum, blood, urine, wounds and catheter tips.	• Patients in a compromised, debilitated state are at increased risk of developing infection and sepsis. • Sepsis may be the underlying cause of DIC. • See for nursing care considerations in the patient with or at risk of infection.

Orthopaedic Nursing

INTRODUCTION

The word "orthopaedic" was invented by French Surgeon NICHOLAS ANDRY (1743). It is derived from two greek words: 'orthos' meaning straight or correct and 'paedios meaning' of a child, and so can be taken to mean the rearing of straight childrens. Modern orthopaedics, however, means much more than that and indeed the word no longer does justice to the vast field of practice in which medicine, surgery, nursing, physiotherapy and many other skills meets and merge in the treatment of disorders of nerves, muscles and skeleton.

Now 'orthopaedics' emerged as a branch of surgery dealing with correction of deformities of bone and muscles. 'Orthopaedic Nursing' refers to nursing management of disorders of bones and muscles i.e. diseases and deformities of the muscles and skeleton for thick correction. It can also be called as "musculoskeletal nursing".

Individuals often show the ability to move about freely in the environment. The ability to perform complex and precise movements permits human beings to interact and adapt to environment. Proper functioning of the musculoskeletal system makes such movements possible. The musculoskeletal system consists of bones, muscles, joints, cartilage, ligaments, tendons, fascial and bursal. All the components of the system work together to produce movement and to supply structure. The musculoskeletal system is particularly vulnerable to external forces. Any disturbance in this well-integrated system results in musculoskeletal dysfunction. Problems can arise as a result of disease affecting the nerves, bones, muscles or joints or as a result of trauma to these or surrounding structures. Problems arising outside the musculoskeletal system such as endocrine, or neurological diseases may also directly affect the system resulting in some form of disability. The consequences may be deformity, alteration of body image, alteration in mobility, pain or permanent disability. These problems may produce long-term health problem that interfere with activities of daily living and quality of life.

Individuals with alterations in musculoskeletal functioning requires planning for appropriate interventions. This requires a careful and thorough assessment, based on the nurses' knowledge and understanding of the anatomy and physiology of the musculoskeletal system. Text Plans for the care of any person with a musculoskeletal system disorders are based on the systemic assessment of needs, capabilities and resources.

Assessment of the Musculoskeletal System

Correct diagnosis depends on an accurate patient history and a thorough examination. A musculoskeletal assessment can be made on a specific body part, as a part of general physical examination in itself. Decision should be used on the basis of patients' problems in selecting all or part of the components of the musculoskeletal history and physical examination. Accidents often result in trauma to the musculoskeletal system and require a thorough assessment. If the injury is serious or life-threatening, only pertinent information related to the accident is obtained and complete assessment is deferred. A thorough assessment includes subjective data gathered from the patient and family interviews, which includes past health history, medications and other treatment and functional health patterns.

Health History

Symptomatic health information to be obtained are poor health history i.e. certain illnesses are known to affect musculoskeletal system either directly or indirectly which include tuberculosis, diabetes mellitus, gout, inflammatory or degenerative arthritis, haemopillia, parathyroid problems, rickets, oesteomalacia, scurvy, oesteomyelitis or soft tissue infection, fungal infection of the bones or joints, and neuromuscular disabilities. If the patient has history of any of these, detailed account of illness should be obtained. In addition, sources of secondary bacterial infections can be obtained.

And obtaining information about medication used by the patient for musculoskeletal problems also are very important. i.e., reason for taking the drug, its name, dose, frequency and length of time it was taken, its effect and side effects. Because some drugs may lead to adverse effects on patient, which incldue anti-seizures (osteomalacia), phenothiozines (gait disturbances), corticosteroids (abnormal fat distribution) avascular necrosis, and decreased bone and muscle mass), and potassium-depleting diuretics (muscle cramps and weakness), amphetamines and caffein intake can cause increase in motor activity. And any previous surgery or other treatments, musculoskeletal are also obtained.

In addition to medical and surgical history, family history of genetic disorders/abnormalities, congenital abnormalities, also should be obtained. And general history of patients which include patients' age, sex, height and weight, nutritional pattern, occupation, exercise regimen, elimination pattern, ADL, habits like smoking, alcohol, recreational drug use, etc. are also important, for assessment of musculoskeletal system.

Physical Examination

The primary methods used in the physical examination of the musculoskeletal system incldue inspection and palpation. The data gathered from careful health history will provide the nurse with clues about areas on which to concentrate for examination. The nurse should observe the following.

1. *Behaviour*
   - Mental status
     - Orientation to time, place and person.
     - Ability to understand direction.
     - Capacity to retain information.
     - Attention span.
     - Ability to relate to others (is the person's attitude, quiet, talkative, tense, guarded, negative appropriate and inappropriate).
2. *General Appearance*
   - *Age, sex* may relate to a specific disorder or attitude towards disorder (eg. elderly susceptible for fall, old women risk for oesteoporosis, etc.).
   - *Posture* may be characteristic of a specific problem (e.g. Scoliosis, Kyphotic posture in ankylosing spondylitis, etc.)
   - *Nutritional status*
     - Overweight may indicate diminished ability to perform regular exercise or activity. Excess weight causes increased stress on joints.
     - Underweight may indicate inability to secure or prepare nutritional meals or to carry out feeding activities adequately; may relate to specific systemic conditions causing anorexia, nausea vomiting or malabsorption of food.
3. *Skin*
   - Turgor (fullness). This papery skin may indicate aging, systemic connective tissue disease, or long-term steroid use. Skin is easily broken.
   - Texture (feel). Thick leathery patches over forearms, hands, chest, face, indicate scleroderma; ulcerates easily, especially over joints.
   - Integrity.
     - Breaks in skin, ulcerations reddened areas-
     - Impaired circulation to extremities-Breakdown of distal parts.
   - Temperature- Warmth over the painful joints indicative of presence of inflammation or infection.
   - Erythema over joints—indicates inflammation of joint-need for joint to keep rest.
   - Colour change on exposure to cold-white (resulting from anterior spasms), blue (cyanosis caused by stagnation of blood), red (warming and reactive vasodilation).
   - Bruising often present in following trauma.
   - Swelling of extremities denote prolonged dependent position, lack of activity, circulatory or renal impairment.
   - May indicate presence of effusion (serous, purulent or blood).
   - Rony enlargement- indicative of disease process.
     Eg. Hyberden nodes in oesteoarthritis (hard, irregular swellings over the distal interphalangeal joints of the fingers) or Bouchard's nodes (Cartilaginous or bony enlargement of proximal interphalangeal joint of fingers).
   - Subcutaneous nodules- indicative of rheumatid arthritis, hard mobile swellings commonly found in subolecranon area.
   - Bursal swellings indicative of bursal inflammation, palpated as soft swelling over the bursae.
   - Synovial cyst - indicative of hypertrophy of synovial tissue (for eg. Baker's Cyst - swelling of the popliteal area often extending to calf).
   - Tophaceous deposits—indicative of gout, hard translucent swelling over joints as in cartilage such as that of the ear.
   - Tenderness may be elevated by direct pressure and graded by amount of pressure required to produce discomfort. Degree of tenderness is visually in direct proportion to severity of imflammation or trauma. For eg. in joint inflammation or injured soft tissue or overlying fracture.
   - General hygiene - Evidence of uncleanliness of body, clothing, may indicate inability to adequately carry out hygiening requirements.
4. *Nails and Hairs*
   - Poorly kept or diseased nails may indicate lack of strength or inability to reach nails to care of nails, change in nail structure may indicate presence of connective tissue disease.
   - Poorly kept hair may indicate inability to lift arms to comb hair.
   - Alopecia, scaling of scalp may indicate connective disease and medications.

Inspection begins during the nurse's initial contact with the patient. The nurse should observe the patient for any apparent symmetry and for sitting and standing posture, gout, general body build, and configuration of the muscles and signs of any abnormalities of behaviour in general appearance, skin, nails, hairs as stated above. And in a head to toe fashion palpate all bones, joints, and soft tissue for temperature, swelling, tenderness, pain or masses. Palpate the spinous processes and intervertebral spaces for tenderness. In addition, assess the sensory function, deep tendon reflex activities, and range of motion. The most common movement that occur at synovial joint includes.

- Flexion – Bending of joint that decreases angle between two bones, shortening muscle strength.
- Extension – Bending of joint that increases angle between two bones.
- Hyperextension – Extension which angle exceeds 180 degrees.
- Abduction – Movement of part away from midline.
- Pronation – Turning of palm downwards or sole outwards.
- Supination – Turning of palm upwards or sole inwards.
- Circumduction – Combination of flexion, extension, abduction and adduction resulting in circular motion of body part.
- Rotation – Movement about longitudinal axis.
- Inversion – Turning of sole inwards towards midline.
- Eversion – Turning of sole outward away from midline.

In addition to above, limb length and circumferential measurement of muscle mass are often obtained when subjective problems or length discrepancies are noted and muscle-strength testings performed to know the strength of individual muscles or grasps of muscles is graded in performance of movements during contraction against applied resistance. The muscle strength scale is as follows:

0. No, detection of muscular contraction.
1. A barely detectable flicker or trace of contraction.
2. Active movement of body part with elimination of gravity.
3. Active movement against gravity.
4. Active movement against gravity and some resistance.
5. Active movement against full resistance without evidence of fatigue (normal).

The normal physical assessments of the musculoskeletal system are:

- Full range of motions of all joints.
- No joint swelling, deformity or crepitation.
- Normal spinal curvatures.
- No tenderness on palpitation of spine.
- No muscle atrophy or asymmetry.
- Muscle strength of 5.

Assess the person's ability to discern light, touch, gentle pressure, pain and temperature which will evaluate sensory innervation. Perform each test bilaterally and compare results. Check sensation in the dermatomes, which will show abnormalities in spinal nerve innervation. Also evaluate the person's sense of proprioception (position sense) in the extremities.

Absence of reflexes may indicate neuropathy or a lower motor neuron lesion, whereas brisk reflexes indicate an upper motor neuron lesion. Again be sure to compare bilateral responses. The grading of responses of deep tendon reflex activity are as follows (Scale of responses to score DTRA).

0. No response.
1. Sluggish or diminisher.
2. Active or expected response.
3. More brisk than expected, slightly hyperactive.
4. Brisk, hyperactive with intermittent or transient clonus.

The nurse assesses gait by having the patient walk across the room and back. The normal gait cycle will be:

- Stance phase - Begins with heel strike and ends with toe-off.
- Swing phase - Begins with toe off and continues through heel strike.
- Double support - Brief period when both feet are on ground.

Musculoskeletal and neurologic problems can result in gait abnormalities.

In addition, the special assessment techniques for musculoskeletal system are as follows followed by abnormality detected.

i. *Limb measurement*: Measurement in centimeters of extremities from a major landmark. Asymmetrical limb length may indicate pelvic obliquity of hip deformities; discrepancies in circumference may indicate atrophy or paresis of muscle groups, less than 1 cm discrepancy is normal in most people.
ii. *Ballottement*: Compression of the suprapatellar pouch, which is normally snug against the femur. Fluid wave indicates excess fluid in the knee (effusion).
iii. *Bulge sign*: Stroke the medial aspect of the knee, then tap the lateral side of the patell; a fluid wane or if fluid is present.
iv. *McMurray's test:* External rotation and valgus stress applied to the knee while the leg is held flexed at the knee and hip (patient is lying supine), normally there is no pain or sound. "Click" or pain indicates meniscal tear.
v. *Drawer test* (Anteroposterior or mediolateral): With the patient supine and knee flexed, push forwards and backward on tibia at the joint line; with the patient supine with knee extended, stabilize the femur and ankle while attempting to abduct and adduct the knee; normally there is little or no movement, assess symmetry of responses. Laxity or movement suggests instability of the anterior or posterior cruciates ligaments or the medial or lateral collateral ligaments of the knee.
vi. *Straight leg raising (LaSegue) test*: With the patient supine raise the leg straight with the knee extended; normally there is no pain. If the maneuver reproduces sciatic pain, it is considered positive and suggest a herniated disk.
vii. *Trendelenburg's test*: While the patient stands on one foot and then the other, both iliac crests should appear symmetrical. Asymmetry suggests hip dislocation.

viii. *Thomas test*: With the patient lying supine and one leg fully extended and other flexed on the chest, observe the ability of the patient to keep extended leg flat on the table. Inability to keep the leg extended suggest a hip flexion contracture in the extended leg that may be masked by increased lumbar lordoses.

ix. *Phalen's test:* Flex both wrists together at 90 degrees and hold for 60 seconds; normally this produces no symptoms, numbers, tingling or burning in the median nerve distribution suggests carpal tunnel syndrome.

x. *Tinel's sign:* Tap over the median nerve where it passes through the carpal tunnel in the wrist; nomally this does not produce any symptom. Tingling along the median nerve distribution is associated with carpal tunnel syndrome.

xi. *Drop arm test:* Raise the affected arm to - 90 degree of flexion, then have the patient slowly adduct the arm to the side. Inability to lower the arm slowly or smoothly is associated with disruption of the rotator cuff mechanism of the shoulder.

xii. *Scoliasis Screening:* "Forward bend" test, observe symmetry and height of scapulae, shoulders, iliac crests and rib-cage. A symmetry of scapulae or shoulder height, "winged" iliac crests, demonstrable curve of the spine and rib hump indicates scoliasis.

COMMON ABNORMALITIES OF MUSCULOSKELETAL SYSTEM

1. *Ankylosis:* Scarring within a joint leading to stiffness or fixation. Eg. Chronic joint inflammation.
2. *Atrophy:* Reduction in size of an extremity or body part. Wasting of muscle, characterized by decrease in circumference and flab by appearance and resulting decrease in function and muscle tone. Example: Wasting of muscles to that they appear to be lacking the bulk of normal muscle, can result from lack of use or disease process. For example: Polymyelitis. It may be due to prolonged disuse, con tracture, ligament structure, tightness of soft tissue, immobilization or muscle innervation.
3. *Contracture:* Resistance to movement of muscle or joint as a result of fibrosis of supporting soft tissues. It may be due to shortening of muscle or ligaments structure, tightness of soft tissue, immobilization and incorrect positioning.
4. *Crepitation:* Cracking sound or grating sensation as a result of friction between bones. May be due to fracture, chronic inflammation and dislocation.
5. *Effusion:* Fluid in joint possibly with swelling and pain. It occurs in trauma especially in knee.
6. *Felon:* Abscess occurring in pulp space (tissue mass) of distal phalax of finger as a result of infection due to hand injury, puncture, wound and laceration.
7. *Ganglion:* Small, fluid-filled synovial cyst usually on dorsal surface of wrist and foot. It is due to degeneration of connective tissue close to tendens and joints leading to formation of small cysts.
8. *Hypertrophy:* Increase in size of muscle as a result of abnor-mal enlargement of existing cells or organ or body part. Limitation of function is associated with enlargement. It may be due to exercise, increased andeogens and increased stimulation or use.
9. *Kyphosis* (round back): Anteroposterior i.e., forward bending of spine with convexity of curve in posterior direction; common at thoracic and sacreal levels. It may be due to poor posture, tuberculosis, chronic arthritis, growth disturbance of vertebral epiphysis and osteoporesis.
10. *Lordosis:* Deformity of spine resulting in anteroposterior curvature with concavity in posterior direction; common in lumbar spine. It may be secondary to other deformities of spine, muscular dystrophy, obesity, flexion contracture of hip, congenital dislocation of hip.
11. *Pes Planus:* Flat foot, may be due to congenital condition, muscle paralysis, mild cerebral palsy and early muscular dystrophy.
12. *Per Cavus:* High in step.
13. *Scoliasis:* Deforming resulting in lateral curvature of spine. It is idiopathic or congenital condition or due to fracture or dislocation, osteomalacia and functional condition.
14. *Subluxation:* Partial dislocation of joint. It is instability of joint capsule and supporting ligaments (eg. from trauma or arthritis).
15. *Swan neck deformity:* Flexion contracture of the metacarphalangeal joint, hyperextention of the proximal interphalangeal joint, and flexion of the distal interphalangeal joint of the fingers found in the advanced rheumatoid arthritis.
16. *Ulnar deviation or drift*: Fingers deviate at the metacorpophalangeal joints towards the ulnar aspect of the hand.
17. *Valgus deformities:* Angulation of bone away from midline. Distal arm of the angle of the joint points away from midline of the body.
    - Hallux valgus - Great toe turns towards the other toes.
    - Genuvalgum - Knock knees.
    - Talipes valgus - Eversion of the foot.

This may lead to alteration in gait, pain and abnormal erosion of articular cartilage.

DIAGNOSTIC STUDIES OF THE MUSCULOSKELETAL SYSTEM

Diagnostic studies provide important information to the nurse in monitoring the patient's condition and planning appropriate intervention. The common diagnostic studies performed and used are as follows:

1. Radiological Studies

i. *Standard x-ray:* An X-ray is taken to determine density of bone. Study evaluates structural or functional changes of bones and joints. In an interoposterior view, X-ray beam passes from front to back, allowing one-dimensional view; Lateral position provides two-dimensional view. Nursing responsibility here is to avoid excessive exposure of patient and self; Before procedure, remove any radio-opaque objects that can interfere with results and explain procedure to the patients.

ii. *Arthrogram:* This study involves injection of contrast medium or air into joint cavity, which permits visualization of joint structures. Joint movement is followed with series of X-rays. Here nurse has to assess patient for possible allergy to contrast medium including iodine or seafood. Explain the procedure to patient and prepare the area to be injected aseptically.

iii. *Diskogram:* An X-ray of cervical or lumbar intervertebral disk is done after injection of contrast dye into nucleus purposes. Study permits visualization of intervertebral disk abnormalities. Preparation of the patient as in arthrogram may be performed in surgery.

iv. *Sinogram:* An X-ray is taken after injection of contrast dye into sinus tract (deep-draining wound). Study visualizes course of sinus and tissues involved. Preparation is as in arthrogram.

v. *Tomogram:* Multiple X-ray views of body region are focussed at successively deeper layers of tissue lying in predetermined planes. Study focuses on certain tissues, eliminating or blurring surrounding structures. Technique is useful in locating bone destruction, small body cavities, foreign bodies and lesions overshadowed by opaque structures. Usual preparation includes informing the patient in this procedure is painless.

vi. *Computed Tomography SCAN*: An X-ray beam is used with a computer to provide a three-dimensional picture. It is used to identify soft tissue abnormalities, and various musculoskeletal trauma. Usual preparation plus informing the patient that it is painless, and importance of remaining still during procedure.

vii. *MRI:* Radio waves and magnetic field are used to view soft tissues. Study is especially useful in the diagnosis of a vascular necrosis, disk disease, tumours, osteomyelitis, ligament tears, and cartilage tears. Patient is placed inside scanning chamber. Gadolinium may be injected into a vein to enhance visualization of the structures. Open MRI does not require the patient to be placed inside a chamber. The nurse's responsibilities here include:
- Inform that it is painless procedure.
- Be aware that it is contraindicated in patients with aneurysm clip metaling implants, pacemakers, electronic devices, hearing aids, sharpner and extreme obesity.
- Ensure that patient has no metal on clothing (eg. snaps, zippers, jewellery and credit cards).
- Convert IV to heparin lock.
- Inform patient about importance of remaining still throughout examination.
- Inform patients who are claustrophobic that may experience symptoms during examination.
- Administer anti-anxiety agent (if indicated or ordered).
- Open MRI may be indicated for obese patient or patient with large chest and abnormal girth or severe claustrophobia.
- Open MRI may not be available at all facilities.

2. Bone Mass Measurement

- Radiogrammetry, radiodensitometry- study evaluation bone mass of metacarpals. A very low dose of radiation is used.
- Single-photon absorptiometry (SPA): Low dose radiation scanner measures mostly peripheral cortical bone at distal radius or midradius. This study is not useful for follow-up because of slow changes in cortical bone.
- Dual-photon absorptionetry (DPA) - Technique measures mixed trabecular and cortical bones at sites such as hip and lumbar spine. It can be used to calculate total body calcium concentration.
- Dual-energy X-ray absorptiometry (DEXA)-Technique measures bone mass of spine, femur, forearm, and total body. Considered to be fast and precise with low dose of radiation.

In these procedures, nurse explains the procedure to patient and inform that the procedures are painless.

3. Radioisotope Studies

- *Bone Scan* - Technique involves injection of radioisotopes, usually sodium pertechnate) that is taken up by bone. Camera scans entire body (front and back) and recording is made on paper. Degree of uptake is related to blood flow to bone. Increased uptake is seen in osteomyelities. Osteoporosis, primary and metastatic malignant lesions of bone, and with certain fracture. Decreased uptake is seen in areas of avascular necrosis.

The nurse's reponsibility includes:
- Give calculated dose of radioistope 2 hours before procedure.
- Ensure the bladder emptied before scan.
- Inform patient that procedure requires 1 hour while patient lies supine and no pain or harm will result from isotope. Be aware that no follow-up scans are required.

4. Endoscopy

1. *Arthroscopy*- The study involves insertion of arthroscope into joint usually knee for visualization of structure and contents. It can be used for exploratory surgery (removal of loose

bodies and biopsy) and for diagnosis of abnormalities of meniscus, articular cartilage ligaments of joint capsule. Other structures that can be visualized through the arthroscope include the shoulder, elbow, wrist and ankle. The nurse has to:

- Inform patient that procedure performed in opening room with strict asepsis and that either local or general anaesthesia is used.
- After procedure, cover wound with sterile dressing.
- Wrap leg from midthigh to midcalf with compression dressing for 24 hours for knee arthroscopy.
- Instruct patient to limit activity for few days.

2. *Serological studies*

For all the serological studies, nurses have to obtain blood samples by venipuncture and send the sample, to concerned laboratories at right time. Prior to procedure, inform the patient that procedure does not require fasting to some and some need fasting. After procedure, observe the venipuncture site for bleeding or haematoma formation.

i. *Mineral metabolism test*

- *Alkaline phosphatase:* This enzyme produced by osteoblast of bone, is needed for mineralization of organic bone matrix. Elevated levels are found in healing fractures, bone cancers, osteoporosis, osteomalacia rickets, and Paget's disease (normal 20-90 UL).
- *Calcium:* Bone is primary organ for calcium storage. Calcium provides bone with rigid consistency. Decreased serum levels are found in osteomalacia, renal disease and hypothyroidism rickets. Increase in serum level is immobility and bone demineralization bone cancer, multiple myeloma (Normal 3-4.6 mg/dl).
- *Phosphorus:* Together with calcium K+ plays vital role in bone metabolism. Decreased level is found in osteomalacia; increased level is found in chronic renal disease, healing fractures, osteolytic metastatic tumour (Normal 2.8-4.5 mg/dl).

ii. *Serum test*

- Rheumatoid Factor (RF)-Study assesses presence of autoantibody (RF) in serum. Factor is not specific for rheumatoid arthritis and seen in other connective tissue diseases, as well as in a small percentage of normal population (Normal : negative or less than 1.20).
- *Erythrocyte Sedimentation Rate (ESR):* This study is nonspecific index of inflammation. Study measures rapidity with which RBCs settle out of unclotted blood in 1 hour. Results are influenced by physiologic factors as well as diseases. Elevated levels are seen with any inflammatory process especially rheumatoid arthritis, rheumatic fever, oesteomyeltis, and respiratory infections. (Normal less than 20mm/hr. general variation 1-3m/hr (M), 4-7 mm/hr (P).
- *Lupus Erythrematosus* (LE) cells: Used in the diagnosis and treatment of systemic lupus aerythrematosus (SLE). Obtain blood from patient and smear made on slide. Normally no LE cells ore present.
- *Antinuclear Antibody (ANA):* Study assesses presence of antibodies capable of destroying nucleus of body's tissue cells, positive in 95 per cent SLE cases and may be positive in cases of scleroderma and Rh arthritis.
- *Anti-DNA Antibody.* Study detects serum antibodies that react with DNA. It is the most specific test for SLE cases.
- *Serum complement:* Complement, a normal body protein is essential to both immune and inflammatory reactions, complement components used in these reactions are depleted. Subsequent tests applied to serum yields little or no serum complement components. Complement depletion may be found in patients with Rh. arthritis or SLE.
- *Serological Test for Syphilis (STS):* False-positive STS results occur in 10-15 per cent of persons with connective tissue diseases. So test may help in diagnosis. FTA-ABS (Fluorescent treponemal antibody absorption) excludes the presence of syphylis.
- *C-reactive Protein* (CRP) - Study used to diagnose inflammatory diseases, infections, and active widespread malignancy. CRP is synthesized by the liver and is present in large amounts in serum 18-24 hours after onset of tissue damage (Normal negative).
- *Human Leukocyte Antigen (HLA-B27).* Antigen present in disorders such as ankylosing spondylitis and variants of rheumatoid arthritis.
- *Serum muscle enzyme test.*

  AST (Serum aspartate aminotransferase transaminase).
  SGOT (Serum-gutamic-oxaloacetic transminase).
  Alolase.
  CPK (Creatinine phosphokinase) isoenzymes MM.MB.

Enzymes can be elevated in the presence of primary myopathic (muscle) disease. Elevated levels may result from muscle degeneration or from diffusion., through a muscle membrane that has increased permeability. Enzyme levels are an index of both progress of the myopathic disorder and effectiveness of treatment.

- Higher concentration of CPK is found in skeletal muscle. Increased values are found in progressive muscular dystrophy, polymyositis and traumatic injuries (Normal: 5.5 u/L (M), 5.35u/L (F)).
- Aldolase study is useful in monitoring muscular dystrophy and dermatomyosites (Normal 1.0-7.5u/L).
- AST or SGOT enzyme is found in skeletal muscle but primary and enzyme of cardiac and hepatic cell (Normal 1-4.5 u/L. (SGOT), AST 8.204/L).

3. *Urinary tests*

- 24 hour urine for creatine-creatinine ratio.

In the presence of muscle disease, the ability of the muscle to convert creatines decreased; the amount of creatine excreted by the kidneys increases, and the ratio of creatine to creatinine increases. Periodic studies are helpful in diagnosis and evaluation of progress of treatment of primary myopathies.

- Urinary uric acid level (24 hrs. collection); End product of purine metabolism is normally excreted in urine. Helpful in diagnosis and decisions regarding treatment modalities for gout. (Normal value should not exceed 900-mg uric acid excretion per day).
- Urine for deoxypyridineline (Dpd) - first or second morning void. Routine collection - Dpd cross links assay provides a quantitative measurement of Dpd. which is excreted unmetabolized in the urine during bone resorption.

4. *Invasive procedures*
   - Arthrocentesis is incision or puncture of joint capsule is done to obtain samples of synovial fluid from within joint cavity or to remove excess fluid. Local anaesthesia and aseptic preparation are used before needle is inserted into joint and fluid aspirated. Study is useful in diagnosis of joint inflammation.

In this, nurse has to inform patient that procedure is usually done at bedside or in examination room. Send sample of synovial fluid to lab examination (if indicated). After procedure, apply compression dressing and have patient rest joint 8-24 hours. Observe for leakage of blood or fluid on dressing.

- *Electromyogram* (EMG) study evaluates electrical potential associated with skeletal muscle contraction. Long, small-guage needles are inserted into certain muscles. Needle probes are attached to leads that feed information to electromyogram machine. Recordings of electrical activity of muscles are traced on audiotransmitter, as well as oscilloscope and recording paper. Study is useful in providing information related to lower motor neuron dysfunction and primary muscle diseases. In this procedure, the nurse must inform the patient that the procedure is usually done in electromyogram laboratory while the patients lie supine on special table. Keep patient awake to cooperate with voluntary movement. Inform patient that the procedure involves some discomfort from needle insertion. Avoid administration of stimulants and sedatives 24 hours prior to procedure.

In addition to this, other procedures are thermography, plethysmography, and somatosensory evoked potential (SSEP).

- *Thermography* is a technique (noninvasive) uses infrared detector, which measures degrees of heat radiating from skin surface. Study is useful in investigation of cause of inflammed joints and in following up patient's response to anti-inflammatory drug therapy.
- *Plethysmography* study (noninvasive) records variation in volume and pressure of blood passing through tissues. Test is nonspecific and quantitative.
- *SSEP* is invasive procedure, it evaluates evoked potential of muscle contractions. Electrodes are placed on muscle and provide recordings of electrical activity of muscle. Study useful in identifying subtle dysfunction of lower motor neuron and primary muscle disease. SSEPT measures nerve conduction along pathways not accessible to EMG. Transcutaneous or percutaneous electrodes are applied to the skin and help identify neutropathy and myopathy. Here, nurse informs the patient that the procedure is similar to EMG, but does not involve needles. Electrodes are applied to the skin.

In addition, biopsies of tissues from a variety of organs are helpful in the diagnosis of disease or disorders affecting the musculoskeletal system.

- Skin biopsy (Punch biopsy).
- Muscle biopsy (Operative procedure).
- Synovium biopsy (closed performed with needle, open performed in surgery).
- Buccal mucosa (Punch biopsy).
- Bone biopsy (operative procedure).

The nurse should prepare the patient according to procedure.

SOFT-TISSUE INJURIES

Soft-tissue injuries include sprains, strains, dislocations and subluxation. These common injuries are usually caused by trauma.

Sprains and Strains

A sprain is an injury to ligamentous structures surrounding a joint, usually caused by a wrenching or twisting motion. A sprain is classified according to the amount of ligament fibres torn.

- A first degree involves tears only a few fibres resulting in mild tenderness and slight swelling.
- A second degree sprain is partial disruption of the involved tissue with more swelling and tenderness.
- A third degree sprain is a complex tearing of the ligament. A gap in the muscle may be apparent or felt through the skin of the muscle is torn. Because these areas are nerve endings, the injury is extremely painful.
- The most common areas of sprain occurs in the ankle and wrist.

A *strain* is a stretching of muscles and its fascial sheath.

Aetiology

Acute soft injuries caused by falls, direct blows, crust injury, motor vehicle collisions and sport injuries. The common sport-related injuries are:

- Impingement syndrome: Entrapment of soft-tissue structures under coracoa cromial arch of the shoulder.

- Rotator cuff tear: Tear within muscle or ligaments of shoulder.
- Skin splints: Inflammation along tibial shaft from tearing away of tendons caused by improper shoes, overuse, or running on hard pavement.
- Tendenitis: Inflammation of tendon in upper or lower extremities as a result of overuse or incorrect use.
- Ligament injury: Tearing or stretching of ligament: usually, as a result of direct blow: characterized by sudden pain, swelling and instability.
- Meniscal injury: Injury to fibrocartilage of the knee characterized by popping, clicking or tearing sensation and swelling.

Clinical Manifestation

The clinical manifestation of sprains and strains are similar and include pain, oedema, decrease in function and bruising. Usually the patient will recount a history of traumatic injury. Possibly of a twisting nature, or recent exercise activity. Minor sprains and strains are usually self-limiting with full function returning within 3 to 6 weeks. A severe sprain can result in an avulsion fracture, in which, ligaments pull loose a fragment of bone. Alternatively the joint structure may become unstable and result in subluxation or dislocation. At the time of injury haemarthorosis (bleeding into a joint space or cavity) or disruption of the lining may occur. An acute strain may involve partial or complete rupture of muscle.

Management

X-rays of the affected part are usually taken to rule out a fracture or widening of the joint structure. Surgical repair may be necessary if the injury is significant enough to produce severe disruption of ligamentous or muscle structures, fracture or dislocation.

To reduce sprains and strains, individuals are encouraged to stretching and warm-up exercises before vigorous activity. Preconditioning exercises protect an inherently weak joint, because slow stretching is tolerated better by biological tissues than quick stretching. Warm-up exercises "prelengthen" potentially-strained tissues by avoiding the quick stretch often encountered in sports. Warm-up exercise also increases the temperature of muscle, which increases the speed of cell metabolism and the speed of nerve impulse transmission. The increased metabolism contributes to better oxygenation of muscle fiber during work. Stretching also is thought to improve kinesthetic awareness, thus lessening the chance of uncoordinated movement.

In acute soft-injury, nurse should assess the patients.

The assessments finding may include:

- Oedema.
- Ecchymosis.
- Pain, tenderness.
- Decreased pulse, coolness and capillary refill.
- Decreased sensation with severe oedema.
- Decreased movements.
- Pallor.
- Shortening or rotation of extremity.
- Inability to bear weight when lower extremity is involved.
- Decreased function with upper extremity involvement.
- Muscle spasms.

An initial nursing intervention includes:

- Ensure airways, breathing and circulation.
- Assess neurovascular status of involved limb.
- Rest and limitation of movement.
- Application of ice to the injured area.
- Compression of the involved extremity.
- Elevation of the extremity and to prevent oedema.
- Analgesia as necessary to relieve pain (Mild analgesic, aspirin, ibuprofen.
- Administer tetanus prophylaxis of skin integrity is broken.

Cold in several forms can be used to produce hypothermia to the involved part. Physiological changes that occur in soft tissue as a result of the use of cold include vasoconstriction, reduction in transmission of nerve impulses, and reduction in conduction velocity. These changes result in analgesia and anaesthesia, reduction of muscle spasm without changes in muscular strength or endurance, reduction of local oedema and inflammation and reduction of local metabolic requirements. Few unwanted side effects accompany the use of cold to treat a soft tissue injury. Cold is most useful when applied immediately after the injury had occurred. Ice application should not exceed 20 to 30 minutes per application, allowing a warm-down time for 10 to 15 minutes between applications.

Compression also helps in limit swelling, which, if left uncontrolled could lengthen healing time. The elastic compression bandage can be wrapped around the injured part, but it should not be too tight or too loose.

After the acute phase (usually lasting 24 to 48 hours), warm, moist heat can be applied to the affected part to reduce swelling and provide comfort. NSAIDS may be recommended to decrease oedema and pain. The patient is encouraged to use the limb provided that the joint is protected by means of casting, taping or splinting. Movement of the joints maintains nutrition to the cartilage, and muscle contraction speeds circulation and resolution of the haematoma.

DISLOCATION AND SUBLUXATION

Dislocation is a severe injury of the ligamentous structures that surround a joint. It results in the complete displacement or separation of the articular surfaces of the joint.

A Subluxation is a partial or incomplete displacement of joint surface. The aetiology of both are associated with accidents.

Clinical Manifestation

The clinical manifestations of dislocation and subluxation are similar. The most obvious clinical manifestation of the dislocation is asymmetry of the musculoskeletal contour. For example, if a hip is dislocated, the limb is shorter on the affected side. Additional manifestation includes local pain tenderness, loss of function of the injured part and swelling of the soft tissues in the region of that joint. The major complications of a dislocated joint are open joint injuries, intra-articular fractions, fracture dislocation, avascular necrosis and damage to adjacent neurovascular tissues.

Management

X-ray studies are performed to determine the extent and shifting of the involved structures. The joint may also be aspirated to determine the presence of blood (haemarthorosis) or fat cells. Fat cells from the synovial fluid indicate probable intra-articular fracture.

The dislocation requires prompt attention. The longer the joints remain unreduced, the greater the possibility of avascular necrosis (bone cell death due to inadequate blood supply, eg. hip joint dislocation). The first goal of management is to realign the dislocated portion of the joint in its original anatomic position. This can be accomplished by a close reduction, which may be performed under local or general anaesthesia. Anaesthesia is often necessary to produce muscle relaxation so that the bones can be manipulated. In some situation surgical open reduction may be necessary. After reduction the extremity is usually immobilized by taping or using a sling to allow the torn ligaments and capsular tissue time to heal. Observation is indicated for the patient with a posterior sternoclavicular dislocation because delayed intrathoracic complications such as pneumothorax or subclavian vessel injury may occur.

Nursing management of subluxation or dislocation is directed towards relief of pain and support and protection of the injured joint. After joint has been reduced and immobilized, motion usually is restricted. A carefully-regulated rehabilitation programme can prevent formation of contractures.

CARPAL TUNNEL SYNDROME (CTS)

Carpal tunnel syndrome is a condition caused by compression of the median nerve beneath the transferse carpal ligament within the narrow confines of the carpal tunnel location at wrist.

Aetiology

This condition frequently is due to pressure from trauma or oedema caused by inflammation of a tendon (tenosynovitis) neoplasm, rheumatoid synovial disease or soft tissue masses such as ganglia. CTS occurs in mostly middle-aged or post-menopausal women. This syndrome is associated with occupations that require continuous wrist movement (eg. butchers, musicians, hair-stylists, secretaries, typists, carpenters and computer operators).

The clinical manifestation of carpal tunnel syndrome are weakness (especially of the thumb, pain and numbness or impaired sensation in the distribution of the median nerve and clumsiness in performing hand movements. Numbness and tingling may be present that awaken the patient at night. Holding the wrist in acute flexion for 60 seconds will produce tingling and numbness over the distribution of the median nerve, the palmar surface of the thumb, the index finger, the middle finger, and part of the ring finger. This is known as positive *phalen sign*. Tapping gently over the area of the inflammed median nerve may reproduce the paresthesia. This is known as a positive Tinel's sign. In late stages there is atrophy of the thenar muscle around the base of the thumb. This syndrome can result in recurrent pain and eventual dysfunction of the hand.

Management

Prevention of carpal tunnel syndrome involves educating employees and employer to identify risk factors. Adaptive devices such as wrist splints may be worn to hold the wrist in slight dorsiflextion to relieve pressure on the median nerve. Special keyboard pads that help prevent repetitive pressure on the median nerve are available for computer operators to help reduce CTS by decreasing tension on the carpal tunnel.

Care of patient with CTS is directed towards relieving the underlying cause of the nerve compression. The early symptoms associated with CTS can usually be relieved by stopping of the aggrevating action and by placing the hand and wrist at rest by immobilizing them in a handsling. If the cause is inflammation, injection of hydrocortisone should be given directly in carpal tunnel. If the problem continues the median nerve may have to be surgically decompressed by longitudinal division of the transferse ligament under regional anaesthesia. Endoscopic carpal tunnel release is new procedure used for decompression.

REPETITIVE STRAIN INJURY (RSI)

Repetitive strain injury is defined as a comulative trauma disorder resulting from prolonged, forceful or awkward movements. Repeated movements strain tendens, ligaments, and muscles causing tiny tears that become inflammed. If the tissues are not given time to heal properly, scarring can occur. Blood vessels of the arms and hands may become constricted, depriving tissues of vital nutrients and causing an accumulation of factors such as lactic acid. Without intervention, tendons and muscles can deteriorate and nerves become hypersensitive. At this point, even the slightest movement can cause pain.

In addition to the repetitive movements, other factors related to RSI include poor posture and positioning, ill-fitting furniture, a badly designed keyboard, and a heavy workload. The result in damage to the muscles, tendons and nerves of the neck, shoulder, forearm and hand. Symptoms of RSI include pain, weakness, numbness or impairment of motor function. Persons most often affected with RSI are as stated in CTS.

RSI can be prevented through education, ergonomics (consideration of the interaction of humans and their work environment) and appropriate job design. Once diagnosed, the treatment of RSI consists of avoidance of the participating activity, physical therapy, and careful use of analgesia. In most cases, the muscle and tendon damage associated with RSI cannot be surgically repaired.

ROTATOR CUFF INJURIES

The rotator cuff is a complex of four muscles in the shoulder: Supraspinatus, infraspinatus, teres minor and subscapularis. These muscles act to stabilize the humeral head in the glenoid fossa and rotate the humerus.

A tear in the rotator cuff may occur as a gradual degenerative process resulting from aging, poor posture, repulsive stress (especially overhead arm motions) or using arm to break or fall. Young adults are more prone to experience a tear as a result of trauma such as fall, lifting heavy objects or throwing a ball.

Patient with a rotator cuff injury will complain of shoulder pain and cannot initiate or maintain abduction of the areas or shoulder. An X-ray alone cannot benefit in diagnosis, so a tear can be confirmed by arthogram or MRI.

The patient may be treated conservatively with rest, ice and heat, NSAIDS, periodic corticosteroid injections into joint, and physical therapy. If the patient does not respond to conservative treatment or if a complete tear is present, surgical repair may be necessary. This can be performed through arthroscope. If extensive tear or pressure, open repair is indicated. An immobilization device such as sling or more commonly a shoulder immobilizer may be used for several weeks after surgery. Exercises and physical therapy begin within few days of surgery.

MENISCUS INJURY

The meniscus is the fibrous cartilage in the knee and other joints. Meniscus injuries are closely associated with ligament sprains, commonly occurring in athletes engaged in sports such as basket ball, rugby, foot ball, soccer and hockey. These activities produce a rotational stress when the knee is in a flexed position and the foot is fixed. A blow to the knee can cause the menscus to be trapped between the femoral condyles and the plateau of the tibia, resulting in a torn meniscus. A causal relationship exists between occupations that require working in squatting or kneeling position and meniscus injury.

Meniscus injuries alone do not usually cause chronic oedema because cartilage is avascular and aneural. However, a torn meniscus may be suspected when local tenderness or pain is reported. Pain is elicited by abduction or adduction of the leg at the knee. The usual clinical picture is feeling by the patient that knee may click and lock periodically. Quadriceps atrophy is evident if the injury has been present for some time. Degenerative joint disease can occur if a damaged roughened meniscus is not surgically removed.

Management

An arthrogram or arthroscopy or both can diagnose knee problems. MRI also is beneficial before arthroscopy. Because meniscal injuries are commonly caused by sports-related activity, athletes should be educated about warm-up activities. Proper stretching may make the person less prone to meniscal injury when a fall or twisting occurs.

Examinations of the acutely injured knee should occur within 24 hours of injury. Initial care of this type of injury involves application of ice,, immobilization, and partial weight bearing with crutches. Most meniscal injuries are treated in an outpatient setting. The patient should be allowed to ambulate as tolerated. Crutches may be necessary. Use of an immobilizer during first few days protects the knees.

After acute pain has decreased, gradual increase in flexion and strengthening help return the patient to full functioning. Physical therapy may be needed to help the patient strengthen muscles before returning to sport activities. Surgical repair or excision of part of meniscus (menisectomy) may be necessary. Frequently this can be done by arthroscopy. Use of the laser for arthroscopy is undergoing clinical research.

BURSITIS

Bursaes are closed sacs that are lined with synovial membrane and contain small amount of synovial fluid. They are located as sites of friction such as between tendons, bones and overlying joints. A bursac may become inflammed (bursitis) from repeated or excessive trauma or friction, gout, rh, arthritis or infection.

The primary clinical manifestations of bursitis are warmth, pain and swelling and limited range of motion in the affected part. Since parts of the body at which it occurs include the hand, knee, trochanter, shoulder and elbow.

Management

Attempts are made to determine and correct the cause of the bursitis. Rest is often only the treatment needed. Icing the area will decrease pain and may reduce inflammations. The affected part may be immobilized in a compression dressing or plaster splint. NSAIDS may be used to reduce pain and inflammation. Aspiration and bursal fluid and injection of hydrocortisone may be necessary. If the burn has become thickened and continued to interfering joints' function, require surgical excision (bursectomy).

MUSCLE SPASMS

Local muscle spasms are common conditions often associated with excessive everyday activities and sports activities. Injury to a muscle results in inflammation and oedema, which stimulates free nerve endings, resulting in muscle excitation and spasm. The spasms produce additional pain, creating a repetitive cycle.

The clinical manifestation of muscle spasm include pain.

Palpable muscle mass in spasm, tenderness, diminished range of motions of affected site, and limitations of the daily activities.

Management

A careful history should be taken and physical examination should be performed to relevant CNS problems. Muscle spasms can be managed with drug therapy (Mild analgesics, NSAIDS, skeletal muscle relaxants), physical therapy or both. The physical therapy program might include the use of heat or ice, supervised exercises, massage hydrotherapy, local heat-producing application (Oil of Wintergreen) ultrasound (deep heat) manipulation and bracing.

FRACTURES

Aetiology

Fractures are disruptions or break in the continuity of the structure of bone. Fractures of bone usually occur as a result of blow to the body, a fall, or another accident. Traumatic injuries account for the majority of the fractures, although some fractures are secondary to a disease (pathological fractures).

The highest incidence of fractures is in males 15-24 years old and in elderly persons especially women aged 65 years or more. Osteoporosis is the most common cause of bone fractures. Neuromuscular instability is an important contributory factor to risk falls, which commonly proceeds a fracture in the elderly ones. Wrist, hip, and vertebral fractures are most common in elderly persons. Persons in high-risk occupations (steel-workers and race car drivers and persons with chronic degenerative or neoplastic diseases are also at higher risk for injury.

Pathophysiology

A fracture is a complete or partial interruption of osteous tissue. Fractures can be described and classified according to type, communication or non-communication with external environment and location of the fracture. Fractures are also described

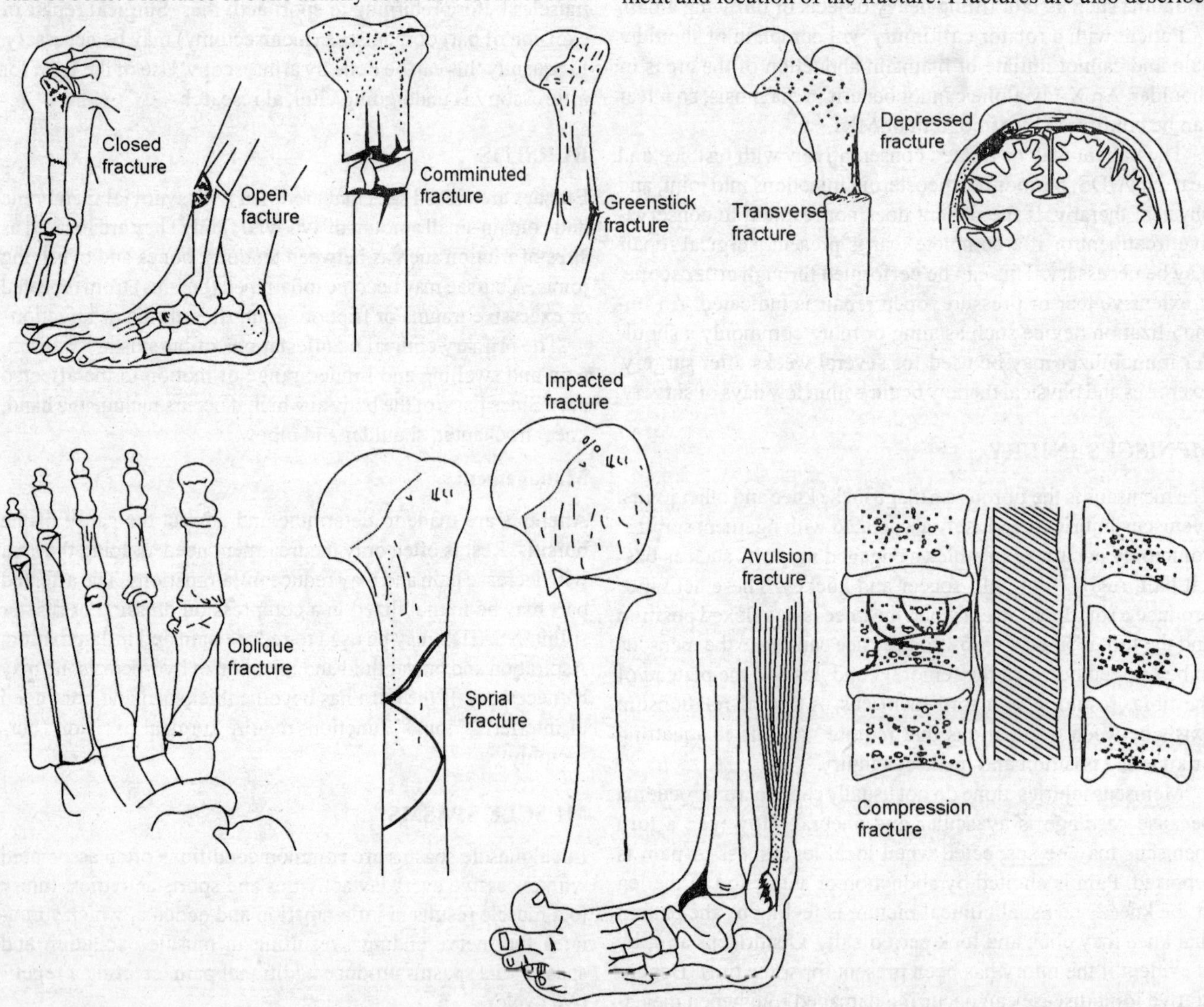

Fig. 10.1: Types of fractures

as stable or unstable. A *stable* fracture occurs when some of the perioesteum is intact across the fracture either external or internal fixation has rendered the fragments stationary. Stable fractures are usually transverse, spiral, greenstick. An *unstable* fracture is grossly displaced during injury and in a site of poor fixation. Unstable fractures are usually comminuted or oblique.

Fracture can be described as complete or incomplete. *Complete* fractures penetrate both cortexes, producing two bone fragments, by only one cortex is broken in *incomplete* fracture. A typical complete fracture and incomplete fracture are as follows:

1. Typical complete fractures.
   - Closed (simple) fracture - Noncommunicating wound between bone and skin.
   - Open (compound) fracture - communicating would be between bone and skin-high risk for contamination.
   - Comminuted fracture - It is a fracture with more than two fragments. These smaller fragments appear to be floating.
   - Linear fracture - Fracture line parallel to the long axis of the bone. The periesteum is not torn away from the bone (Longitudinal fracture).
   - Oblique fracture - is a fracture in which the line of the fracture extends in an oblique direction. Fracture line is 45 degree angle to the long axis bone.
   - Spiral fracture - Fracture line encircling bone, in which the line of the fracture extends in a spiral direction along the shaft of the bone.
   - Transverse fracture - Fracture line is perpendicular to long axis of bone, in which line of the fracture extends across the bone shaft at a right angle to the longitudinal axis.
   - Impacted fracture - Fracture fragments are pushed into each other. It is displaced (overriding) fracture which involves a displaced fracture fragment that is overriding the other bone fragments. The periosteum is disrupted on both sides.
   - Pathological fracture - Fracture occurs at a point in the bone weakened by a disease. For e.g. tumour or oesteoporosis.
   - Avulsion: It is a fracture of bone resulting from the strong pulling effect of tendons or ligaments at the bone attachment. A fragment of bone connected to a ligament breaks off from the main bone.
   - Extracapsular- Fracture is close to the joint but remains outside the joint capsule.
   - Intracapsular- Fractures within the joint capsule.
2. Typical incomplete fractures.
   - Greenstick fracture- Break on one cortex of bone with splintering of inner bone surface.
   - Torus fracture- Buckling of cortex.
   - Bowing fracture- Bending of the bone.
   - Stress fracture- Microfracture - Normal or abnormal, subject to repeated stress such as from jogging or running.
   - Transochondrial fracture- Separation of cartilagenous joint surface (articular cartilage) from main shaft bone.

Clinical Manifestation

The clinical manifestation of fractures differ depending on the location and type of fracture and associated with soft-tissue injuries. The common signs and symptoms include the following.

- *Oedema and swelling*: Disruption of the soft tissues or bleeding into surrounding tissues. Unchecked oedema in closed space can occlude circulation and damage nerves (i.e. there is risk of acute compartment syndrome).
- *Pain and tenderness*: Muscle spasm as a result of involuntary reflex action of muscle, direct tissue trauma, increased pressure on sensory nerve, movement of the fracture parts. Pain caused by swelling at the site, muscle spasm, damage to periosteum. It may be immediate, severe and aggravated by pressure at the site of injury and attempted motion.
- *Loss of normal function*: Due to disruption of bone, preventing functional use, the injured part is incapable of voluntary movement. Fracture must be managed properly to ensure restoration of function.
- *Deformity*: Obvious deformity resulting from loss of bone continuity. Abnormal position of bone as a result of original forces of injury and action of muscles pulling fragment into abnormal position seen as a loss of normal bony contours. Deformity is cardinal sign of fracture. If incorrected, it may result in problems with bony union and restoration of function of injured part.
- *Excessive motion at site*: i.e., motion when motion does not usually occur.
- *Crepitation*: Crepitus or grating sound occurs if limb is moved gently. Grating or crunching together of bony fragments, producing palpable or audible crunching sensation. Examination of crepitation may increase chance for nonunion and bone ends are allowed to move excessively.
- *Soft tissue* oedema in area of injury resulting from extravasation of blood and tissue fluid.
- *Warmth* over injured area resulting from increased blood flow to the area.
- *Ecchymosis*: of skin surrounding injured area (may not be apparent for several days). This is discoloration of skin as a result of extravasation of blood in subcutaneous tissue. It usually appears several days after injury and may appear distal to injury. The nurse should reassure patient that process is normal.
- *Impairment* or loss of sensation or paralysis distal to injury is resulting from nerve entrapment or damage.
- Signs of shock related to severe tissue injury, blood loss or intense pain.
- Evidence of fracture on X-ray film.

Healing of Fracture

It is important to understand the principles of fracture healing to provide appropriate therapeutic interventions. Bone goes through a remarkable reparative process of self-healing (termed union) that occurs in following stages:

1. *Fracture haematoma*: When fracture occurs, bleeding and oedema create a haematoma, which surrounds the ends of fragments. The haematoma is extravasated blood that changes from a liquid to a semi-solid clot.
2. *Granulation tissue*: During this stage, active phagocytosis absorbs the products of local necrosiš. The haematoma converts to granulation tissue. Granulation tissue (consisting of young blood vessels, fibro-blasts and oesteoblasts) produces the basis for a new bone substance called 'osteoid'.
3. *Callus formation*: As minerals (Calcium, Phosphorous and magnesium) are deposited in the osteoid, it forms an unorganized network of bone that is woven about the fracture parts. Callus is primarily composed of cartilage, osteoblasts, and end of the first week of injury. Evidence of callus formation can be verified by X-ray.
4. *Ossification*: Ossification of the callus begins within 2 to 3 weeks after the fracture and continues until the fracture has healed. This stage is marked by ossification of callus that is sufficient to prevent movement at the fracture site when the bones are gently stressed. However, the fracture is still evident on X-ray. During this stage, of clinical union, this patient can be converted from skeletal traction to a cast or the cast can be removed to allow limited mobility.
5. *Consolidation*: As callus continues to develop, the distance between bone fragments diminishes and eventually closes. This stage is called "Consolidation" and ossification continues. It can be equated with radiograph union.
6. *Remodelling*: Excess tissue absorbed in the final stage of bone healing, and union is completed. Gradual return of the injured bone to its preinjury structural strength and shape occurs. Remodelling of bone is enhanced as it responds to physical stress. Initially, stress is provided through exercise. Weight-bearing is gradually introduced. New bone is deposited in sites subjected to stress and resorbed at areas where there is little stress. Radiographic union occurs when there is X-ray evidence of complete bony union.

Many factors, such as age, initial displacement of the fracture, site of the fracture and blood supply to the area, influence the time required for fracture. Fracture healing may not occur in the expected time (delayed union) or may not occur at all (nonunion). The ossification process is arrested by causes such as inadequate immobilization and reduction, excess movement, infection and poor nutrition. Healing time for fractions increases with age. For example, an uncomplicate midshaft fracture of the femur heals in 3 weeks in a new born and requires 20 weeks in an adult. Electrical stimulation is used successfully to stimulate bone healing in some situation of nonunion or delayed union. The complication of fracture healing are delayed union, nonunion, malunion, angulation pseudoarthrosis, posttraumatic osteoporosis, refracture and myositis ossificants.

The major factors that impede bone healing are as follows:

- Excess motion of fracture fragments -
  Inadequate immobilization resulting in movement of fragments.
- Poor approximation of fracture fragments.
  - Inaccurate reduction or malalignment of fracture fragments.
  - Excessive bone loss at time of fracture, preventing sufficient bridging of broken ends.
  - Excessive fragmentation of bone, allowing soft tissue to be interposed between bone ends.
  - Inability of patient to comply with restrictions imposed by immobilization, fixation device(s) resulting in movement of fragmentation.
- Compromised blood supply.
  - Damage to nutrient vessels.
  - Periosteal or muscular injury.
  - Severe comminution.
  - Avascularity (type of fracture and result of internal fixation device).
- Excessive oedema at fracture.
  - Tissue swelling impedes supply of nutrients to area of fracture.
- Bone necrosis.
  - Injury to blood vessels impedes supply of nutrients to involved bone.
- Infection at fracture side.
  - Infection disrupts normal callus formation.
- Metabolic disorders or diseases (cancer, diabetes, malnutrition, immunodeficiencies- Paget's disease).
  - Retard osteogenesis.
- Soft tissue injury.
  - Disruption of blood supply.
- Medication use, (e.g. steroids, anticoagulants).
  - Steroids can cause osteoporosis, avascular necrosis, long-term use of heparin may cause osteoporosis.

Management of Fracture

Diagnosis of fracture is confirmed by X-ray. Other studies may be indicated if multiple injuries have been sustained. The goals of fracture treatment are:

- Anatomic realignment of bone fragments known as reduction.
- Immobilization to maintain realignment, and
- Restoration of functions of the injured part.

Immediate treatment principles implemented at the time of injury include the following:

- Maintain airway and assess signs of shock.
- Splinting the fracture to prevent movement of the fracture fragments, and further injury to the soft tissues by bony fragments. Splinting and immobilization will also decrease pain.
- Preserve correct body alignment.
- Elevate the injured part to decrease oedema.
- Apply cold packs (during first 24 hours) to reduce haemorrhage, oedema, and pain.
- Observe for changes in colour, sensation, circulation, movement, or temperature of injured part.

Secondary management goals include the following.

1. For simple fracture:
   a. Optimal reduction (replacing bone fragments in their correct anatomical position).
      - Manual manipulation or closed reduction (moving bone fragments into by applying traction and pressure to distal fragment).
      - Traction.
      - Open reduction (Surgical involvement that may incorporate use of internal fixation device).

   b. Immobilization.
      - External fixation cast, splint, external fixator device (wires, external frame).
      - Traction.
      - Internal fixation-pins, plates, screws, wires and prosthesis.
      - Combination of the above.
2. For compound fracture:
   a. Surgical debridement and irrigation of wound to remove dust, foreign material, devitalized tissue and necrotic bone.
   b. Wound culture.
   c. Pack the wound.
   d. Observe for signs of osteomyelitis, tetanus, and gangrene.
   e. Wound closure when there is no sign of infection.
   f. Reduce fracture.
   g. Immobilize fracture.
3. Use of bone-growth stimulators that use low-voltage electrical impulses to enhance healing in cases of nonunion.

Fracture Reduction

1. *Closed reduction* (manipulation): Manipulation is a nonsurgical manual realignment of bone fragments to their previous anatomic position. Traction and counter-tractions are manually applied to the bone fragments to restore position, length and alignment. Closed reduction or manipulations, the injured part is immobilized by traction, casting, external fixation, splints or orthoses (braces) to maintain alignment until healing occurs.
2. *Open reductions*: Open reduction is the correction of bone alignment through a surgical incision. It frequently includes internal fixation of the fracture with the use of wire, screws, pins, plates, intramedullary rods or nails. The type and location of the fractures, age of patient and concurrent disease as well as the result of attempted closed reduction by means of traction, may influence the decision to use open reduction. The main disadvantages of this form of treatment are the possibility of infection, and the complications associated with anaesthesia. If open reduction with internal fixation (ORIF) is used, for intra-articular fractures involving joint surfaces, early initiations of ROM of the joint is indicated. Machines that provide continuous passive motion (CPM) to various joints are now available, which help so many ways to prevent certain associated problems.

TRACTION

Traction is the mechanism by which a steady pull is exerted on a part or parts of the body. Traction may be used to accomplish the following:

- Reduce a fracture.
- Maintain correct alignment of bone fragments during healing.
- Immobilize a limb while soft tissue healing takes place.
- Overcome muscle spasm.
- Stretch adhesions.
- Correct deformities.

Types of Traction

Two types of traction are used: Skin traction and skeletal traction.

- *Skin traction* is achieved by applying wide bands of moleskin, adhesive or commercially available devices directly to the skin and attaching weights to them. The pull of the weights is transmitted indirectly to the involved bone or other connective tissues. Skin traction is generally used for short-term treatment (48 to 72 hours) until skeletal traction or surgery is possible. Tape, boots or splints are applied directly to the skin to maintain alignment, assist in reduction and help diminish muscle spasm in the injured part. The traction weight is usually limited to 5 to 10 1bs (2.3 to 4.5 kg). Commonly in skin traction are as follows with nursing implications.
- *Buck's extension* is used for condition affecting hip, femur, knee, or back. It can be unilateral or bilateral may also be used to correct knee and hip joint contracture while taking care of these patients, nurse has to make all assessments at least on 4th hourly. Assess for altered neurovascular status caused by original injury to or the application of the bandages used. Injury in Buck's traction especially note decreased peripheral vascular flow and peroneal nerve deficit by assessing for ability to dorsiflex toes and foot and for changes in sensation in the first website between the great and second toes. Pressure from the elastic wrap may result in pressure necrosis, especially over the boney prominence and areas prone to pressure. (Anterior tibial border, fibular head, both malleoli, achilles tendon, calcaneous, and dorsum of the foot). In addition, assess for an allergic reaction to the adhesive material, rotation of the extremity, and constant traction and counter-traction forces.
- *Russel's traction* used for fracture of femur or hip. Nursing implications are as in Buck's. An additional area prone to

pressure necrosis in the area over the hamstring tendons in the popliteal space.

- *Bryant's traction* used for fracture of the femur, fracture in small children and immobilization of hip joints in children and 2 years of 30 1b (14) kg in weight. Nurses should be aware that with traction in place, buttocks just clear the mattress. Check for undue pressure over the outer-head and neck of fibula, dorsum of foot. Achilles tenden, scapulae, and shoulders. Check that bandages or boot has not slipped. Be aware that traction are usually removed for skin care and assessment every 4th hourly.
- *Pelvic belt* (or girdle) used for sciatica, muscle spasm (low back), and minor fractions of the lower spine. Nursing implication include
  - Check for security of the pelvic belt.
  - Check frequently for skin irritation over iliac crests and in the intergluteal fold.
  - Use measures to prevent skin breakdown.
  - Check and adjust pelvic belt straps so that they are unrestricted and equal in length. Secure the straps with adhesive tape.
  - Use a foot board to prevent foot drop.
  - Maintain correct angle of pull of the traction.
  - Be aware that the physician orders the type fo counter-traction.
- *Pelvic sling traction* used for pelvic fractures to provide compression for separated pelvic girdle. Here the sling should keep the pelvis just above the surface of bed. Nurses should assess for pressure necrosis and skin irritation every 4th hourly especially pressure over the iliac crests, intergluteal fold and greater trochanter. Monitor for soiling of the sling and change is needed. Use a fracture bedpan for toileting. Limit use of trapese since it will reduce compressive force from the sling. Use alternating air pressure mattress or other pressure dispersing devices and provide frequent back care.
- *Circumferential* Head halter used for soft tissue disorders and degenerative disk disease of the cervical spine. It is not commonly used for unstable fractures of the cervical spine. Nursing implications include assessment for alignment with trunk, areas of local pressure over the ears, and mandibular joints and under the chin and occipital area and pain or dysfunction in the temperomandibular joint. Patients may be permitted to remove traction for meals, if not provide a liquid or mechanical soft diet to reduce the temperomandibular joint pain. Since this traction is commonly used in the adults ensure patient can demonstrate safe and effective set up, application and use of the traction before discharge.
- *Skeletal traction* is a traction applied directly to bone. It is generally in place for longer period of time is used to align injured bones and joints or to treat joint contractures and congenital hip dysplasia. It provides long-term pull that keeps the injured bones and joints aligned. To establish skeletal traction the physician inserts a pin or wire into the bone, either partially or completely to align and immobilize the injured part. Weight for skeletal traction ranges from 5 to 45 1b. (2.3 to 20.4 kg). The commonly used are:
  - *Overhead arm* (90°–96°). Commonly used for immobilization for traction and dislocation of the upper arm and shoulder. Here, be aware that the shoulder and elbow joint are maintained at 90° angles. Assess for pressure necrois beneath the sling, especially over the bony prominences, assesses distal neurovascular status because of the exposure, skin temperature may be indicative of decreased perfusion. Perform assessment 4th hourly. Inspect the pin sites and perform pin site care according to hospital policies.

    Later arm Commonly used in immobilization of the fracture and dislocation of the upper arm and shoulder. Here, inspect the pin site and perform skin care according to hospital policy assess neurovascular status.
  - *Balanced suspension traction*: Used for fr injury or fracture of the femoral shaft of the femur, acetabulum, hip, tibia, or any combination of these. In this traction, nurses should be aware that this traction uses half ring Thomas splint (1) and Pearson attachment (2) and then suspension of the extremities and direct skeletal traction are applied. This allows raising of the buttocks off the bed for bedpan use and skin care without altering the line of traction. Use nursing assessment so that counter-traction is maintained (e.g. position patient high in bed so that feet do not press on foot of bed; do not elevate the head of bed more than 25°, if it causes continual movement toward foot of the bed). Encourage self-help in patients' performances of activities of daily living, movement in bed with help of trapeze, and flexion and extension of affected foot to prevent foot drop. Assess for pressure necrosis, in areas contacted by traction, especially greater trachanter, ischial tuberosity, hamstring tendons, fibular head and both mallioli. Assess distal neurovascular status 4th hourly and inspect pin site and give pin site care accordingly.

The signs and symptoms of neurovascular impairment include pallor, cyanosis, prolonged capillary refill, oedema, tissue cold or cool to touch. Patient is unable to move part distal to injury. Patient reports severe pain, decreased sensation or paresthesia in part distal to injury and diminished of absent pulses.

The following guidelines will help to take care of person with traction.

a. Patient education

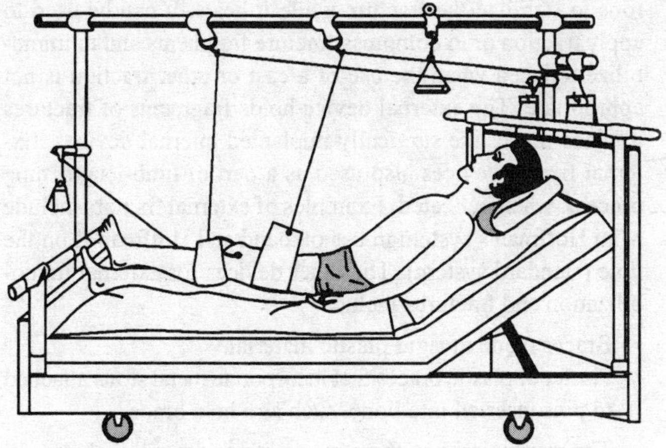

Fig.10.2: Balanced skeletal traction using slings for support and suspension.

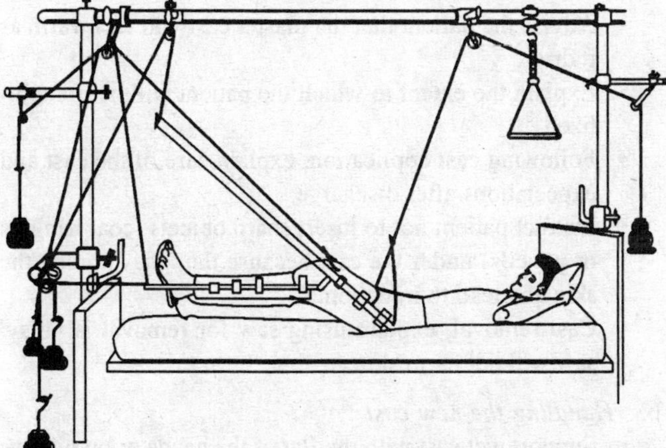

Fig.10.3: Balanced skeletal traction using Thomas leg splint and Pearson attachment.

- Explain traction in relation to fracture and surgeon's plans of treatment.
- Explain amount of movement permitted and how to achieve it (e.g. how trapeze can be used to assist with movement).
- Explain correct body positioning. Maintain proper body alignment.

b. Maintain continuous traction, unless indicated otherwise.
   - Inspect traction apparatus frequently to ensure that ropes are running straight and through the middle of the pulleys; that weights are hanging free that bed clothes, the bed or the frame and bars on the bed are not impinging on any part of the traction apparatus.
   - Check ropes frequently to be sure, they are not frayed.
   - Avoid releasing weights or altering the line of pull of the traction.
   - Avoid adding weight to the traction.
   - Check the position of the Thomas splint frequently; if the ring slides away from the groin, read just the splint to its proper position without releasing traction.
   - Avoid bumping into or jarring the bed or traction equipment.
   - Be sure weights are securely fastened to their ropes.
   - Avoid manipulation of pins.

c. Maintain countertractions.

d. Skin care.
   - Encourage the patient to turn slightly from side-to-side and to lift up on the trapeze to relieve pressure on the skin of the sacrum and scapulae, have the patient lift up for routine skin care to prevent friction and shearing forces.
   - Avoid padding the ring of the Thomas splint, because this will create dampness next to the skin. Bathe the skin beneath the ring, dry it thoroughly and powder the skin lightly.
   - Inspect the skin frequently to be sure it is not being rubbed, contused, or macerated by traction equipment, readjust splints or the extremity in the splint to free the skin from pressure.
   - Keep the skin areas aound pin sites clean and dry; direct care to pin sites (e.g. cleansing with cotton applicators and hydrogen peroxide, povidone iodine, or alcohol) is controversial check with the surgeon regarding method of pin site care.

e. Toileting.
   - Use a fracture pan with blanket roll or padding as support under the small of the back.
   - Protect the ring of the Thomas splint with water proof material when female patients are using the bed pan.

FRACTURE IMMOBILISATION

External fixation of fracture is achieved by a cast or an external fixator.

Casts

The most common external fixation device is the cast. Casting is a common treatment often closed reductions has been performed. It allows the patient to perform many normal activities of daily living. While providing sufficient immobilization to ensure stability. Major cast materials include fiberglass, plaster of paris, polyurethane, thermoplastic resins and thermolabile plastic.

- Plaster of paris, after immersion in water, is wrapped and moulded around the affected part. It is anhydrous calcium sulphate embedded in gauze roll. The strength of the cast is determined by the number of layers of plaster bandage and the technique of application. As the cast dries, it recrystalises and hardens. Heat is generated during the drying process. Increased oedema as a result of the increased circulation may occur as a result of heat produced by the drying cast. After the cast is completely dry, it is strong and firm and can withstand stresses. The plaster is hard within 15 minutes, so the patient can move around without problems. However, it is not strong enough for weight bearing until it is dry (after about 24 to 48 hours).

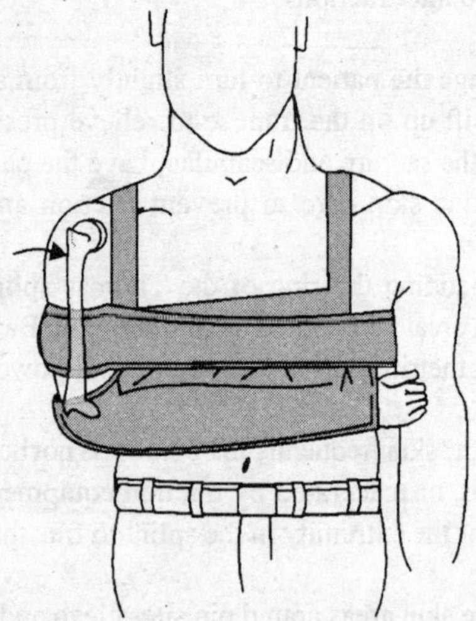

Fig. 10.4: Immobilization of fracture of upper humerus can be achieved with conventional sling and swathe.

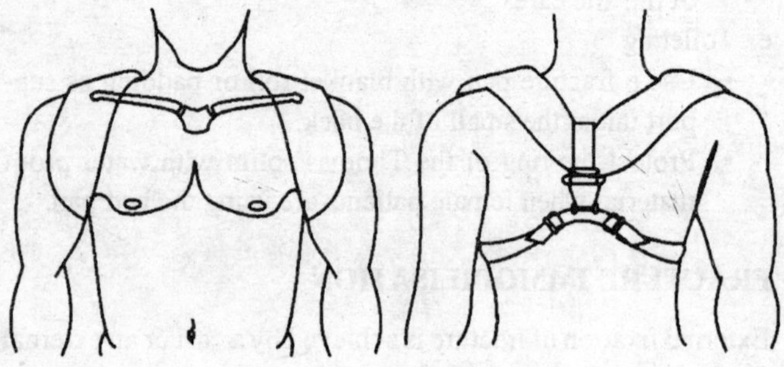

Fig. 10.5: Method for immobilizing a clavicular fracture with a clavicular strap.

Thermolabile plastic (orthoplast) and thermoplastic resin (Hexcelite) are moulded to fit the torso extremities after being heated in warm water. Polyurethane, which is formed for polyester and cotton fabric impregnated with a chemical in water activated by immersing in cool water to start chemical process. Casts made by this fiber glass tape are frequently used because they are light weight and relatively waterproof and support earlier mobilization. They are appropriate in cases in which severe oedema is not present or when multiple cast changes are not anticipated.

An external fixator is a metallic device composed of metal pins that are inserted into the bone and attached to external rods to stabilize the fracture while it heals. It can be used to apply traction or to compress fracture fragments and to immobilize reduced when the use of a cast or other traction is not appropriate. The external device holds fragments of fractures in place much like surgically implanted internal devices. External fixator devices also used as a part of limb-lengthening process, when indicated. Examples of external fixators include Mini Hoffman's system in use on hand and Hoffman II on the tible (standard system). The other devices for external immobilization and fractures include:

- Braces made of rigid plastic material.
- Plaster or plastic braces that incorporate metal struts attached to pins inserted into bone, such as a helo brace.

The nursing care of the person with a cast will include:

a. *Patient education*
   - Before cast application, explain why and how the cast will be applied.
   - Advise the patient that the plaster cast will feel warm as it dries.
   - Explain the extent to which the patient will be immobilized.
   - Following cast application, explain care of the cast and expectations after discharge.
   - Instruct patient not to insert sharp objects (coat hangers or pencils) under the cast because they may abrade the skin and lead to infection.
   - Cast removal, explain using saw for removal is noisy; saw will not harm skin.

b. *Handling the new cast*
   - Support wet cast with the flat of the hands or on pillows to avoid indentations that will cause pressure on underlying skin.
   - Place cotton blankets or other absorbent material under the cast to aid the drying process.
   - Turn the patient frequently to aid the drying process.
   - Use a fan to circulate air over the cast.
   - Do not apply paint varnish, or shellac to the cast; plaster is porous material that allows air to circulate the skin.

c. *Skin care*
   - Inspect skin at edges of cast and underlying cast for redness or irritation; apply petal-shaped strips of adhesive type or moleskin around rough edges of cast.
   - Remove plaster crumbs from skin with a wash cloth moistered with warm water.
   - Use cream and lotion sparingly, because they may soften the skin and cause the cast to stick to the skin.
   - Apply waterproof material around perineal area to prevent skin irritation and soiling of and damage to cast.
   - Attend to patients report of pain under the cast, particularly over bony prominences, because this may indicate

pressure on the skin. If discomfort is not relieved by repositioning, report to physician. Cast pressure may need to be relieved by windowing or bivalving (cutting cast into two halves).

- Following cast removal, skin care to remove built-up exudate to secretions and dead skin. Mineral oil and warm water soaks are helpful.

d. *Turning*
- Turning to any position is generally permitted, as long as the integrity of the cast is not compromised and the patient is comfortable.

e. *Toileting (For a long leg or hip spica cast)*
- Use a fracture pan with blanket role or padding as support under the small of the back.
- Elevate the head of the bed if permitted, or place the bed in reverse Trendenburg position.

f. *Abdominal discomfort*
- Spice cast may be "windowed" (cut an opening into cast) to provide relief of abdominal distention or as a port for checking bladder distention.

g. *Mobilization*
- Weight-bearing is at the discretion of the surgeon/physician who will prescribe specific limitations.
- A cast shoe or a walking heel incorporated into a lower extremity cast will permit weight-bearing without damaging the cast.

h. *Prevention of neurovascular problems*
- Perform neurovascular checks every hour for at least 24 hours after cast application to detect difficulty from swelling or pressure of cast on nerves or vessels. Notify physician of colour changes, alterations sensation, or motion unrelieved by position change, cast may need to be bivalved to relieve pressure.
- Elevate affected extremity on pillows until danger of swelling is over (usually 24 to 48 hours).
- After mobilization of patient with lower-extremity or upper-extremity cast, avoid keeping extremity in dependant position for prolonged periods.
- After lower extremity cast is removed, encourage patient to wear elastic stocking and elevate affected leg at rest until full mobility is regained.

INTERNAL FIXATION

Internal fixation devices are surgically inserted at the time of realignment. Internal fixation is carried out under the most vigorous aseptic conditions, and patients may receive a course of perioporative prophylactic intravenous antibiotics. Example of internal fixation devices include pins, plates and screws. They are biologically inert metal devices such as stainless steel, vitallium or titanium that are used to realign and maintain bony fragments. Proper alignment is evaluated by X-ray studies at regular intervals. A variety of internal fixation devices are also available include:

- Plates and nails.
- Intramedullary rods (ex-Kuntsher nail-Old shaft femur fracture) and Neufeld nail and screw for intrastrachenter fracture).
- Transfixation screws (Eg. Richard's intramedullary hipscrew, for femur. Richard's compression crew and plate for hip frature).
- Prosthetic implants-used particularly fracture is jeopardized, for example fracture through or immediately below the femoral head (e.g. Bipolar modular prosthasis for femurs, and bipolar (left) and unipolar (right) hip prosthesis for hip fracture).

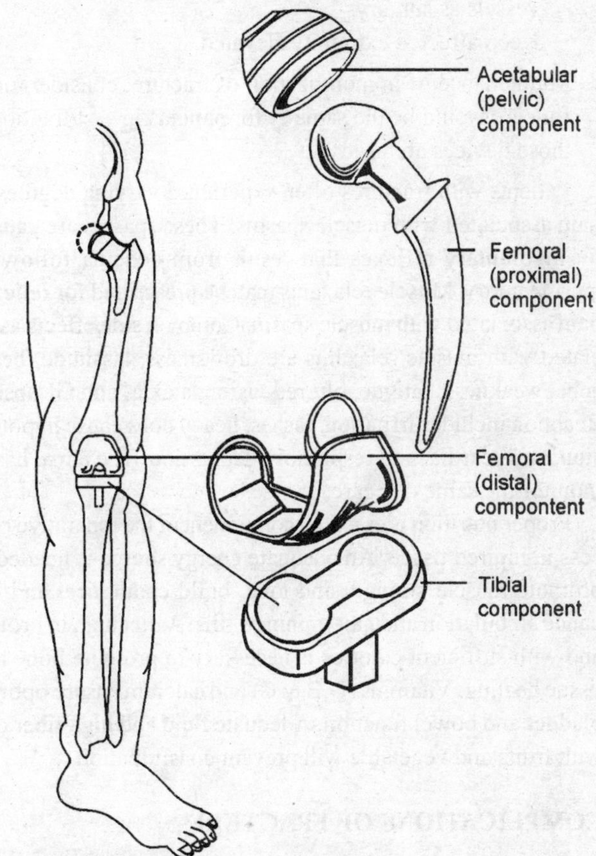

Fig.10.6: Hip and knee replacement.

The nursing care of the person with an internal fixation device are as follows:

a. Patient Education
- Prepare the patient for anaesthesia.
- Explain the surgical procedure and general nursing care after surgery.
- Postoperatively, explain the limits of motion and weight bearing to the affected parts.

b. Promoting Mobility

- Determine in consultation with the physician, the limits of motion and weight bearing is permitted.
- Instruct and assist the patients to turn, transfer and ambulate within the prescribed limits (mobilization may begin as early as the day of surgery).
- Instruct and assist the patients to use an appropriate ambulatory aid if the fracture is of a lower extremity.

c. Prevention of Neurovascular Problems

- Perform neurovascular checks every hour for the first 24 to 48 hours, notify the physician if any change from preoperative status, because this may indicate pressure from swelling, constricting bandages, or damage to nerves or vessels as surgery.
- Keep affected extremity elevated.

d. Maintenance of immobilization of fracture; considerations for care would be the same as for patients in cast/traction if those devices are used.

Patients with fractures often experience varying degrees of pain associated with muscle spasms. These spasms are caused by involuntary reflexes that result from oedema following muscle injury. Muscle relaxants may be prescribed for relief of pain associated with muscle spasm. Common side effects associated with muscle relaxants are drowsiness, lassitude, headache, weakness, fatigue, blurred vision, ataxia, and GI upsets. Reaction includes irritation, rashes, heavy does cause hypotension, tachycardia, and respiratory depression. The nurse has to monitor the same day care.

Proper nutrition is essential component of the reparative process in injured tissue. An adequate energy source is needed to promote muscle strength and tone, build endurance, and enhance ambulation and gait training skills. A diet high in protein and with sufficient calories is necessary to promote bone and tissue healing. Vitamins (D,B & C) and calcium ensure optimal bladder and bowel function. Adequate fluid and high fiber diet with fruits and vegetable will prevent constitipation.

COMPLICATIONS OF FRACTURE

The majority of fractures heal without complications. If death occurs after a fracture, it is usually the result of damage to underlying organs and soft tissue or from complications of the fracture or immobility complication include problems with bone union, avascular necrosis and bone infections. Indirect complications of fractures associated with blood vessel and nerve damage resulting in conditions such as compartment syndrome, venous thrombosis, fat embolism, and traumatic or hydrovolium, fatembolism and traumatic or hypovolumic shock. Although most musculoskeletal injuries are not life-threatening, open fractures or fracture accompanied by severe blood loss and fractures that damage vital organs (such as the lung and bladder) are medical emergencies requiring immediate attention).

Proper nursing interventions help to prevent complication in appropriate management of fracture are as follows:

1. Preventing Trauma and Injury/Promoting Self-Care

As health progresses and pain diminishes, patient should be advised to follow the following instructions for preventing trauma and injury and promoting self-care.

- How to move comfortably in bed.
- Safe transfer technique.
- Duration and extent of weight-bearing restriction.
- Type of activity restrictions.
- Proper use of ambulatory or other ADL assistive devices.
- Use and care of immobilization devices (slings, casts, pins)
- Proper positioning of the affected extremity.
- Pain and discomfort relief measures.
- Exercises to maintain strength and enhance circulation.

2. Maintaining Strength and Mobility/Promoting Activity

The nurse can use the following intervention to assist the patient to maintain mobility, muscle tone and strength.

- Allow and encourage the patient to move about to the greater extent possible within the restrictions of the fracture reduction and the immobilizing devices.
- Allow and encourage the patient to accomplish as much self-care as possible.
- Encourage the patient to perform muscle toning (isometric) exercises on a regular basis. For example quadriceps, sitting and glutal sitting.
- Encourage and assist the patient to follow through with exercise program (including ambulation) prescribed by the physician and taught by the physiotherapist and nurse).
- Encourage and assist patient to resume normal functioning of all ADL within limits of immobilization or fixation device) as soon as possible for example using bedside commode or toilet instead of bedpan.

3. Promoting Comforts

The person with a fracture will often have severe pain in the fracture site, pressure from oedema and damage of soft tissues adjacent to the fracture and spasm of the muscles in the fracture area. Measures the nurse can take to help reduce pain include the following.

- During initial stages of treatment, administer prescribed narcotic and non-narcotic analgesics in appropriate doses at timely intervals.
- Instruct the patient about principles of pain management and use of patient-controlled analgesia, if prescribed.

- Administer prescribed agents such as diazepam to reduce muscle spasm.
- Apply ice compress, as ordered to the affected part to reduce swelling and decrease pain.
- Reposition patient frequently with prescribed position or activity limitation to avoid prolonged pressure over bony prominences and to prevent stiffness.
- Instruct patient how to use relaxation techniques (deep-breathing, imagery).
- As pain subsides, negotiate with the patient a reduction in the strength or frequency of analgesic administration.

In addition, positioning is a measure that promotes comfort, provides for adequate ventilation and mobilization of pulmonary secretions, enhance circulation, and relieves pressure on vulnerable skin areas. Before positioning, the nurse should know the location and type of traction, reduction technique, and special activity or positioning restriction according to type of traction, cast, fixation as described earlier.

4. Maintaining Intact Neurovascular Status and Tissue Perfusion

To maintain an intact neurovascular status and tissue perfusion the nurse has to monitor the neurovascular status of the injured part includes:

- Palpating for warmth.
- Observing colour.
- Assessing length of capillary-filling time.
- Questioning patient about pain and paresthesias in injured part.
- Assessing patient's ability to discriminate sensation.
- Observing patient's ability to voluntarily move body part distal to fracture.
- Institute measures to promote venous blood flow:
  - Elevate extremities to level slightly above the heart.
  - Apply elastic stockings or intermittent pneumatic copression devices.
  - Use proper positioning techniques.
  - Avoid external compression on pressure sites.
  - Encourage ROM and isometric exercises.
- Assessing for presence of positive Homan's sign (although not always released).
- Encourage ambulation if possible.
- Obtaining baseline and ongoing measurements of circumferences of both calves for compression.

5. Preventing Infection

Nursing intervention to promote wound healing include:

- Carefully attending to aseptic technique during dressing changes to prevent infections; assessing wound for signs of healing or presence of infection.
- Monitoring drains for correct placement.
- Assessing pin sites regularly: perform pin site care as specified to prevent infection.
- Providing and encouraging patient to eat a well-balanced diet to provide the nutritional elements necessary for tissue healing.
- Assessing patient for any systemic signs of infection.
- Monitoring laboratory data (e.g. WBCs, C and S, ESR).
- Assessing patient for therapeutic response to antibiotics if prescribed.

6. Maintaining Skin Integrity

To prevent skin breakdown, and to promote wound healing, nurse has to take measures to maintain skin integrity which includes:

- Identifying skin areas at risk, particularly areas over bony prominence. Eg. heels, sacrum, elbows, scapulae, ischial tuberosities).
- Inspecting the skin (at least every 8 hrly) for signs of pressure (erythema or induration, nonblandible areas).
- Turning at least every 2 hours, while maintaining fracture immobilization using a turning sheet.
- Moving patient from one surface to another with a pull sheet or roller board.
- Rolling patient on to side or lifting patient to place him or her on bedpan rather than sliding pan under the patients.
- For patient who cannot be fully turned because of traction apparatus or other limiting factor, possibly using one or more of the following pressure-relieving devices.
  - Sheep skin pads,
  - Flotation pads.
  - Alternating air pressure mattress or alternating air pressure system.
  - Foam mattress.
  - Foam heal or elbow pads.
  - Special bed such as the clinitron, mediscus, or bidyne.
  - Turning frames such as the Foster or Stry Ker frames.
- Regularly inspecting the skin areas in contact with cast edges or traction apparatus and taking appropriate measure to eliminate chafing or rubbing these areas.
- Assisting patient to keep skin clean and dry, especially under casts, slings and traction apparatus.

7. Promoting Nutrition/Stabilizing Weights

The essentials of nutritions diet including fruits, vegetables, proteins and vitamins are especially important for the persons after a fracture. Nursing intervention to ensure adequate nutrition of the patient include:

- Encourage the patient to eat regular meals.
- Allow the patient adequate time to eat.

- Encoruage self-feeding but help the patient whenever needed.
- Attend to patient's need for roughage and fluids and protein.
- Position the patient to facilitate comfortable intake of food and fluids.

8. Promoting Autonomy and Sense of Control

To promote autonomy the following actions will be helpful.

- Assess and incorporate patient's locus of control (internal or external) into plan of care.
- Explain course of treatment to patient and family.
- Provide opportunities for decision making.
- Incorporate patient preferences into daily plan of care.
- Allow the patient to manipulate the environment wherever needed.
- Involve family and significant others in patient's care.
- Assist patient to set realistic goals.

INFLAMMATORY AND DEGENERATIVE DISORDER-MUSCULOSKELETAL SYSTEM

RHEUMATOID ARTHRITIS (RA)

Arthritis, an inflammation of the joint is a common disorder of the musculoskeletal system that causes pain and stiffness in the joint. Rheumatoid arthritis (RA) is a chronic, systemic disease characterized by recurrent inflammation of the diarthrodial joints and related structures and surrounding tissues. The disease process is characterized by recurrent inflammations of the connective tissue throughout the body. Systemic manifestation includes pulmonary, cardiac, vascular, opthalmological, dermatological, and haematological involvement, showing extra-articular manifestation such as rheumatoid nodules, arteritis neuropathy, scleritis, paricarditis, lymphadenopathy and splenomegaly.

Aetiology

The cause of rheumatoid arthritis is unknown. Whether a single causative factor is responsible or multiple factors are involved, several theories have been postulated regarding its pathogenicity.

- *Infection*: Studies continue to probe the possibility of specific infections pathogens, such as Epstein-Barr virus, Parvovirus and mycobacteria, which may trigger the process.
- *Auto-immunity*: Although no virus particles have been identified, it is likely that an antigenic stimulus such as a virus leads to the formation of an abnormal immunoglobulin G (IgG). RA is characterised by the presence of autobodies against this abnormal IgG. The antibodies to this altered IgG termed as "Rheumatoid Factors" and they combine with IgG to form immune complexes that deposits in the joints, blood vessels and pluera. Complement is activated and an inflammatory response occurs.

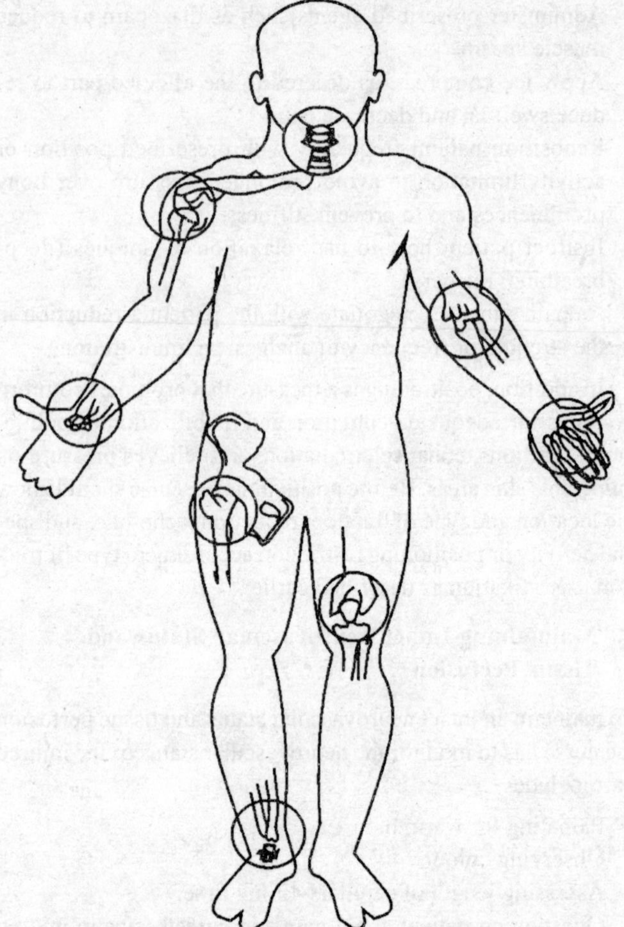

Fig.10.7: Rheumatoid arthritis characteristically involves the joints of the hands, wrists, feet, ankles, knees, elbows, and the glenohumeral and acromioclavicular joints and the hips. The articulations of the cervical spine are also affected.

- *Genetic factors*: A genetic predisposition has also been identified related to certain human leukocyte antigen (HLA) known as the HLA-DR4.
- *Other factors*: Metabolic and biochemical abnormalities, nutritional and environmental factors and occupational and psychosocial influences may play a part in the cause or expression of the disease but their contribution is entirely speculative. RA occurs in young and middle-aged females more often than male.

Pathophysiology

The disease progresses through four stages which include:

- *First State*: The unknown aetiologic factor initiates joints imflammation synovitis, with swelling of the synovial lining membrane and production of excess synovial fluid.
- *Second Stage*: Pannel (Inflammatory granular tissue) is formed at the juncture of the synovium and cartilage. This extends over the surface of the articular cartilage and eventually invades the joint capsule and subchondria bone.

- *Third Stage*: Tough fibrous connective tissue replaces pannus, occluding the joint space. Fibrous ankylosis results in decreased joint motion malalignment and deformity.
- *Fourth Stage*: As fibrous tissue calcifies, bony ankylosis may result in total joint immobilization.

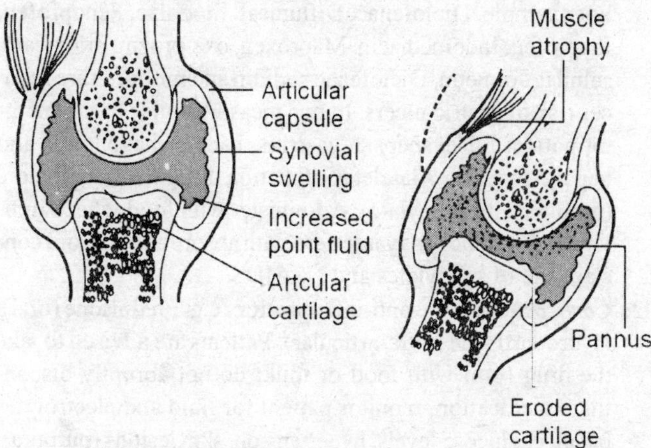

Fig.10.8: Pathophysiology of rheumatoid arthritis. (A) Joint structure with synovial swelling and fluid accumulation in joint. (B) Pannus, eroded articular cartilage with joint space narrowing, muscle atrophy, and ankylosis.

Actually disease begins in the synovial membrane within the joint, oedema, vascular congestion, fibrin exudate, and cellular infiltrate occur as a result of the inflammatory process. Joint changes are characterized by chronic inflammation with the presence of inflammatory cells and mediators. The infiltrating macrophages are activated and released a variety of cytokines, including interlukin-1 and interlukin-6 tumour necrosis factor (TNF), and colony-stimulating factor. The activity of these cytokines accounts for many of the features of rheumatoid synovity including synovial tissue inflammation, synovial proliferation, cartilage and bone damage and systemic manifestation of rheumatoid arthritis.

Normally synovial tissue secretes synovial fluid that both lubricate the joint and is the medium through which nutrients are supplied to the articular cartilage. Inflammation causes oedema, vascular congestion, fibrins exudate and cellular infiltrate to build up around synovium. WBCs move into the synovium, releasing superoxide radicals, H_2O_2, prostaglanding Leukopneou, and callagenases, which manifest synovium thickens particularly at articular junctions. Symptoms of inflammations occur within and overlying the joint (pain, swelling, erythaema, warmth). Joint mobility is limited by pain.

Generally articular cartilage covers the ends of articulating bones to provide a smooth surface for movement. When pannus forms at junctions of synovial tissue and articular cartilage, covers the ends of articulating bones to provide a smooth surface for movement. When pannus forms at junctions of synovial tissue and articular cartilage, interfering with nutrition cartilage. Articular cartilage becomes necrotic. Pannus invades subchondrial bone and supporting soft tissue structure (ligaments, tendon destroying them. This leads to joint pain increases at rest and with movement. Destruction of soft tissue structure (ligaments tenden) causes joint to sublux or dislocate. Depending on the amount of articular cartilage destroyed adhesions can develop and the joints can fuse, prohibiting joint motion.

Clinical Manifestations

Rheumotoid arthritis typically develops insidiously. Non-specific manifestations such as fatigue, anorexia, weight loss, fever, malaise, morning stiffness. Pain at rest and with movement, night pain, oedematous, erythematous, "boggy" joint. The stiffness becomes more localized after weeks to months. Some patients report a history of precipitating stressful event such as infection, work stress, physical exertion, childbirth, surgery, or emotional upset.

Specific articular involvement is manifested clinically by pain, stiffness, limitation of motion, and signs of inflammation (heat, swelling and tenderness). Joint symptoms are generally, bilaterally symmetric and frequently affect small joints of the hands (proximal interphalangeal) and feet (metatorsophalangeal) as well as larger peripheral joints, including wrists, elbows, shoulders, knees, hips, ankles and jaw. The cervical spine may be affected but axial spine is generally spared. The patient characteristically has joint stiffness on arising in the morning and after periods of inactivity. This morning stiffness may last for 30 minutes to several hours or more depending on disease activity.

Later symptoms of rheumatoid arthritis include;

- Pallor.
- Anaemia.
- Colour changes of digits (bluish, rubor, pallor).
- Muscle weakness, atrophy.
- Joint deformities.
- Paresthesias.
- Decreased joint mobility.
- Contractures (usually flexion).
- Subluxation.
- Dislocation.
- Increasing pain.

Rheumatoid arthritis may also affect other body systems and rheumatoid nodules takes form in the heart, lungs spleen. The systemic manifestations of RA are as follows:

- Cardiovascular : Pericarditis, valvular lesions, myocarditis, vasculitis, Raynaud's phenomenon.
- Pulmonary : Pleurisy; rheumatoid nodules in lungs, pneumoconiosis, (Caplan syndrome), interstitial pneumonitis, pulmonary fibrosis, pulmonary hypertension.

- Neurological : Compression neuropathy, peripheral neuropathy, cervical myelopathy.
- Haematological : Anaemia, leukopoenia (Felty's syndrome) when accompanied by hepatosplenomegally).
- Renal : Rheumatoid nodules in kidneys.
- Dermatological : Rheumatoid nodules, brown lesions, on skin, due to ischemia, ulcers and draining fistulae.
- Ophthalmological : Scleritis, Sicca syndrome (Keratoconjunctivitis) Sjögren's syndrome (Kerato conjunctivitis, xerostomia, dryness), glaucoma, scleromalacia.
- Others : Fever, malaise and weakness.

Management

Several findings are helpful in diagnosing rheumatoid arthritis in conjunctions with the history and physical examination. The diagnostic criteria for RA includes:

- Morning stiffness: 1 hour and at least 6 weeks duration.
- Symmetric joint swelling.
- Swelling of wrist metacorpophalangeal (MCP) and proximal intraphalangeal (PIP) joints.
- Rheumatoid nodules.
- Positive serum rheumatoid factor test.

According to American Rheumatoid Association, the following presence of four of the seven/nine criteria in nursing for diagnosis of RA i.e., the diagnostic tests result usually include:

- An elevated erythrocyte sedimentation rate (ESR).
- Positive creactive protein test during acute phases.
- Positive antinuclear antibody test.
- Mild leucocytosis.
- Anaemia (hypochromic, nomocytic).
- Positive rheumatoid factor or latex fixation test.
- Narrowing of the joint spaces and erosion of articular surfaces on roentgenographic examination, subluxation and dislocation.
- Inflammatory charges in synovial tissue obtained by biopsy.
- Increased turbidity and decreased viscosity of synovial fluid obtained by arthrocentesis, immune complexes and WBCs present.

Care of the patient with RA begins with a comprehensive program of drug therapy and education. Physical comfort is promoted by NSAIDS and rest. The patient and family are educated about the disease process and have management strategies. Compliance with medications, includes correct administration, reporting of side effects and lab. follow up visits. Physical therapy maintains joint motion and muscle strength. Occupational therapy develops upper extremity function and encourages joint inspection through the use of splinting packing techniques and assistive devices.

The purpose of drug therapy is to control inflammation and prevent bone erosion. The common medications used for RA are as follows:

1. *NSAIDS*, Salicylate: modify inflammatory process by inhibiting prostaglandin synthetase, analgesics and antipyrotic. For example, Diclofenac, Diflunisal, Etodolac, Fenoprofen, Ibuprofen, Indomethacin. Maproxen, oxa-prozin, prioxicam, sulinlac Jolmetin, Diclofenac sodium and misopros are reduces risk of gastric ulcers. In this measure, nurse has to monitor patient for dyspepsia, gastritis, haemorrhage, renal and hepatic function, platelet dysfunction, headache, confusion, (tinnitus with salicylate). Administer with food (check individual drug, food may interfere with absorption). Avoid constant use of salicylates and NSAIDS.
2. *Corticosteroids* are anti-inflammatory e.g. Prednisone (oral), Hydrocortisone (intra-articular). Patients are advised to take the drug (oral with food or milk; do not abruptly discontinue medication, monitor patient for fluid and electrolytes balance, glucose levels, hypertension, skin lesions (purpura); decreased healing potential, cataract formation; encourage adequate calcium and vitamin D intake to retard osteoporosis; teach patient to avoid sources of infection. The systemic effects are rate with intra-articular use; avoid more than three injections per joint per year.
3. *DMARD*. (Disease-modifying anti-rheumatic Drugs).
   - Methotrexate (oral or I.M.) 3 hr
   - Rhematrex.

Rapid onset of action inhibits degradation of folic acid, which inhibits DNA synthesis of inflammatory cell. In this, before starting therapy renal function should be evaluated. Then monitor patient for hepatic and pulmonary toxicity, leukopoenia, anaemia, explain to patient that nausea, diarrhoea and stomatitis are common. Advise patient to use birth control while taking medication; check for drug interactions that may increase toxicity risk.

- Hydroxychloroquine (Naqenil); mechanism of this is unclear; acts on DNA synthesis, anti-inflammation. In this, inform patient of need for eye examination before therapy and every 6 months thereafter (Retinal oedema may result in blindness); monitor patient for haematological toxicity, gastrointestinal irritation, and hypertension, evaluate renal function.
- Sulfagalazine (Azylfidine) - action is unknown. But anti-inflammatory. Here monitor patient for neurological and gastrointestinal toxicity. Leukopoenia, anaemia and Stevens-Johnson syndrome; educate patient about need for CBC and liver function test throughout therapy.
- Gold salts (Myochrysine, Ridaura, Joganal). It may be given oral or IM anti-inflammatory mechanism of these drugs is unclear, effect not noted until several months of therapy. Here nurse monitors patient's renal and hepatic damage,

dramatitis and mouth ulcerations. Inform patient of need for CBC and urinalysis before and at intervals throughout therapy, stress the need for oral hygiene, therapy, may cause metallic taste in mouth. Oral gold has fewer side effects.

- Azathioprine (Smuran): Action is unknown. It is immune suppressant. In the nursing intervention include monitor patient for blood dyscrasiasis, hepatitis and pancreatitis. CBC necessary as baseline & throughout course of treatment.
- D-Penicillamine (Depon, Cuprimine), action is unknown. In this treatment nurse monitors patients for fever, rash, GI upset, blood dyscrasiasis, and delayed wound healing; assess for penicillin allergy; Inform patient of potential for dysgeusia (taste alteration. For interferes with absorption. Rare side effects include polymyositis and Good pasture's syndrome. Urinalysis and CBC counts are needed.
- *Antineoplastics*: (Cyclophosphamide-Cytotoxin) suppresses synovitis; retards bony erosions. Here monitor patient for toxic effects including GI distress, bone marrow suppression, alopecia and haemorrhagic cystitis. Inform patients of need for monitoring CBC and urin analysis during therapy; teach patients to increase fluid intake to ensure frequent bladder emptying.

The goal of therapy for persons with RA to relieve symptoms prevent joint destruction, maintain joint functions, and promote independence, and quality of life. In addition to medication, occupation therapy and physical therapy are mainstays of treatment to preserve joint mobility and promote independence, which splints and orthoses (braces) are prescribed by the physician. The purposes of *splints* and *braces* are as follows:

- Stabilize or support the joints.
- Protect a joint or body part from external trauma.
- Mechanically correct dysfunction such as foot drop by supporting the joint in its functional position.
- Assists patients to exercise specific joints.

Splints and braces are designed to be as light weight and cosmetically acceptable as possible. The type and function of splints and braces include.

- Spring-loaded braces - Oppose the action of unparalyzed muscles and act as partial functional substitue for paralyzed muscles.
- Resting-splints - Maintain a limb or joint in a functional position while permitting the muscles around the joint to relax.
- Functional splints - Maintain the joint or limb in a usable position to enable the body part to be used correctly.
- Dynamic splints - Permit assisted exercises to joints, particularly following surgery of finger joints.

Many assistive devices are available for persons who have impaired upper and/or lower extremity function, which include:

- Utensil with built-up handle
- Long-handled shoe horn.
- Utensil with cuffed handle
- Long-handled reacher.
- Combination knife-fork
- Stocking guide.
- Mug with special handle.

In addition supportive devices or ambulatory aids (walkers, canes and crutches) are usually recommended for-persons who cannot bear weight on one or more joints of the lower extremities. Nurses are expected to supervise patient in their use of these devices and encourage patients to use their walking aids correctly.

Other treatment modalities for person with RA include the application of hot and cold packs at the affected joints. It can be achieved by the following:

- Hydrocollator packs (packs containing chemical filter that expands in water and retains heat; may be heated in pot of water or special machines that maintain a constant temperature of 80°C (174°F).
- Paraffin baths.
- Electric heating pads that are approved for use with moist towels.
- Electric heating pads that produce moisture.
- Warm soaks, tub soaks or showers.

The application of cold or ice packs helpful in reducing or preventing swelling (especially after injury) reducing pain, and relieving stiffness.

When conservative therapies are ineffective, surgery is indicated for correction of deformity, relief of pain or restoration of function. The objectives of surgical itervention are as follows:

- Restoration or maintenance of a body part.
- Prevention of deformity.
- Correction of deformity if not already exists.
- Development of the patient's powers of compensation and adaptation of loss of function or permanent deformity is not preventable.

Prior to surgery, the orthopaedician considers the procedure best suited to achieve the desired objective for individual clients.

The commonly-performed surgical procedures are as follows:

1. *Arthroscopy* - Is endoscopic examination of joint, indicated for diagnosis, synovectomy, chondroplasty, removal of bone spurs, osteophytes, and joint mice.
2. *Arthrotomy* - Opening of a joint indicated for exploration of joint-drainage of joint and removal of damaged tissue.
3. *Arthroplasty* - Reconstruction of a joint, indicated for restore motion, relieve pain, correct deformity and avascular necrosis.

- Interposition-Replacement of part of a joint with a prosthesis or with soft tissue.
- Hemiarthroplasty - Replacement of one articulating surface.
- Replacement (total joint) - Replacement of both articulating surfaces of a joint with prosthetic implants.

4. *Synovectomy* - Removal of part or all of the synovial membrane, indicated when delay the progress of RA.
5. *Osteotomy* - Cutting a bone to change its alignment indicated in correct deformity (varus or valgus) alters the weight-bearing surface of diseased joint to relieve pain.
6. *Arthodesis* - Surgical fusion of a joint by removal of articular hyaline cartilage, introduction of bone grafts, and stabilization with internal or external friction devices. Indicated for stabilizing a joint and relieve pain.
7. *Tendon Transplants* - i.e. moving tendon from its anatomical position, indicated for substitute one tendon for another that is not working or realign tendon function for example for stability.

In addition to the above, diet, rest, exercises are important in treatment of RA.

Diet. There is no special diet for RA. However, balanced nutrition is important. There is evidence to suggest that ingestion of fish oil (a type of n-3 poly unsaturated fat) as dietary fat is beneficial to persons with RA. A diet containing adequate calories and balanced nutrition is necessary to prevent fatigue and increase energy. If the patient is overweight, a weight reduction diet, combined with exercises, is recommended to decrease the strain on weight-bearing joints.

Rest is a therapy often used with RA. There are two forms of rest viz. Absolute rest or no activity and potential rest of limited activity. This should be decided on the basis of part affected, devices used and so on.

Exercises are advised to accomplish the following.

- Preserve joint mobility (active and passive ROM).
- Maintain muscles tone (active ROM and isometrics).
- Strengthen selected muscle groups (Resistive exercises performed against resistance provided by another person or by weights).

Exercises may be facilitated by the application of heat or cold or the administration of analgesics before exercise period. Exercises are contraindicated in the presence of acute joint or muscle inflammation until it subsides. Exercises may be tailored to the patient's specific needs and capabilities.

Patient and Family Education

As for any chronic illness, patient teaching is perhaps the most important aspect of nursing care and the patient with rheumatoid arthritis. Patient teaching should include the following information.

- Proper balance of rest and activity, assisting the patient in determining his/her activity tolerance.
- Joint protection and energy conservation techniques.
- Proper use of medication (i.e. names of drugs dosages, precautions in administration and side effects or toxic effects).
- Plans for implementation of the exercise program prescribed by the physician and physical therapist.
- Proper application of heat and/or cold packs.
- Proper use of walking aids and other assistive devices.
- Safety measures to prevent injury.
- Application, appropriate use and care of splints and braces.
- a. Inspect patient's skin after the orthosis has been applied for short time, to be certain it has caused no skin irritation.
  b. Notify orthotist if adjustment needs to be made in orthosis to make it more comfortable or to relieve chafing.
  c. Instruct patient in the proper application and care of the orthosis
     - Metal braces should be stored upright.
     - Leather materials should be treated occasionally with meets foot compound or other leather preservative to prevent cracking and drying.
     - Orthoses fabricated of moulded material should be stored away from sources of heat.
     - If patients fitted with moulded orthoses are braces gain or lose weight, the brace may have to be adjusted or replaced.

  d. Assist patient to make the psychological adjustment to wearing the orthoses.
- Basics of good nutrition and the importance of avoiding weight gain.
- Importance of regular following with physician.
- Risks of following programs that promises "cure".
- Joint protection and energy conservative is advised through
  - Maintaining good posture and proper body mechanism.
  - Maintain normal weight.
  - Use assistive devices if indicated.
  - Avoid positions of deviation and stress.
  - Find less stressful ways to perform tasks.
  - Avoid task that causes pain.
  - Develop organising and pacing techniques.
  - Avoid forceful repetitive movements.

Osteoarthritis (OA)

Osteoarthritis also known as degenerative joint disease (DJD) is a slowly progressive disorder of articulating joints, particularly weight-bearing joints, and is characterized by degeneration of articular cartilage. The damage from osteoarthritis is compared to the joints and surrounding tissues.

Aetiology

Osteoarthritis (OA) may occur as a primary OA is unknown.

After both primary and secondary OA are influenced by multiple factors (i.e. metabolic mechanical, genetic and chemical). Secondary OA has an identifiable precipitating event, such as previous trauma, fractures, infection or congenital deformities, that is believed to predispose the person to later degenerative changes. Although symptomatic OA is usually seen in the 50-70 years (45-55 years) age-group, it has been observed as early as 20 eyars of age. The other factors that influence the development of OA include congenital structural defects (e.g. Legg-Calve-Perthes disease i.e. osteochondritis of head of femur in children) metabolic disturbances (e.g. Diabetes Mellitus, Acromegaly), repeated intra-articular haemorrhage (haemophilia) neuropathic arthropathies (e.g. Charcots joints) and inflammatory and septic arthritis.

Specific predisposing factors such as excessive use of stress on joints have been identified as accelerating osteoarthritic changes (eg. on the knees of football players and the feet and ankle in ballet dancers). Genetic factors influence the development of Heberdensnodes, which involve a single autosomal gene, dominant in women and recessive in men.

Pathophysiology

Although oestoarthritis is generally termed "noninflammatory", a small amount of low-grade inflammation is observed, and mechanical abnormalities in the joints irritate surrounding soft tissue and bone cause inflammation. Both primary OA and secondary OA affect the articular cartilage. Characteristic of pathological changes include:

- Erosion of articular cartilage.
- Thickening of subchondral bone.
- Formation of osteophytes or bone spurs.

Degenerative changes over time cause the normally smooth, white, translucent joint cartilage to become yellow and opaque with rough surfaces and areas of malacia (softening). As the layers of cartilage become thinner, bony surfaces are drawn closer together. As the cartilage breaks down, fissures may appear and fragments of cartilage becomes loose. Inflammations of the synovial membrane secondary to cartilage causes break down. As the articular surface becomes totally denuded of cartilage, subchondrial bone increases in density and becomes sclerotic (eburnated). New bone outgrowth (osteophytes) are formed at joint margins and at the attachment sites of ligaments and tendens. These may break off and appear in the joint cavity as "joint mice".

There are several possible causes for cartilage deterioration, which is an active process. The enzyme hyaluronidase, which is normally found in the synovial fluid, may be responsible for digestion of proteoglycans via cracks in the surface layer of articular cartilage. Another possible cause is that the inadequate nutrition of cartilage may result in cartilage degeneration. Because cartilage is avascular, nutrients are provided by the synovial fluid. DNA synthesis, which is normally absent in the adult articular cartilage is active in OA tissue and appears to be directly proportional to disease severity.

Clinical Manifestation

Clinical manifestation include, joint pain, stiffness and limited range of motions (ROM). Persons generally seek medical help because of pain i.e., deep aching in the joints. Weather changes and increased activity tend to increase the pain loss of joint motion may be caused by the loss of articular cartilage, muscle spasms, shortening ligaments and osteophytes. Loss of articular cartilage and subchondrial bone can lead to joint subluxation and deformity. As the joint degenerates, the person may report decreased mobility and the sensation of grinding and catching.

Arthritis of the hand is more common in women between 65 to 74 years. Hip involvement more common in men; women are more likely to have knee involvement. Arthritic changes in hip cause antalgic gait, and pain usually felt on the aspect of the hip, in the groin, buttocks, inner thigh and knee. OA of the knee are most likely to report pain with motion, stiffness after inactivity and decreased flexion. Neurological symptoms may be caused by osteophytes, foraminal stenosis, disc protrusion and subluxation.

To sum up, clinical manifestation of OA includes:

- Joint enlargements - may be from inflammatory exudate, or blood entering in capsule, increasing synovial fluid or fragment of osteophytes in synovium.
- Crepitus- may be present on movement.
- Pain increased with weight bearing relieved with rest.
- Limitation of joint motion depends on amount of destroyed cartilage.
- Non-inflammatory effusion.
- Morning stiffness less than 1 hour.

And the characteristic changes or symptoms in certain joints include:

- Knee involvement- Varus valgus (knocked knees), flexion deformity crepitus and limited ROM.
- Heberden's nodes—Bony portuberences occurring on the dorsal surface of the distal interphalangeal joints of the fingers.
- Bouchard's nodes—Bony portuberances occurring on proximal interphalangeal joints of the fingers.
- Coxarthrosis (degenerative joint disease of the hip)-Pain in the hip on weight bearings, with pain progressing to include groin and medial knee pain and limited ROM.

Management

Diagnosis is made on evaluation of history and physical examination and the results of radiological studies. X-ray of the involved joints. ESR and synovial fluid analysis are also helpful in diagnosis of OA.

There is no specific treatment for OA. Therapy is aimed at

symptomatic relief and control of pain, prevention of progression and disability and restoration of joint function. First line of therapy starts with acetaminophen 1 g and upto four times daily. Typical agents, such as Capsaican cream may be used alone or in conjunction with acetaminophen. This cream made from chilli peppers, causes depletion of substance P from nerve endings, thus blocking pain signals to the brain. Low dose of ibuprofen. 400 mg upto Qds may be used.

If acetominophen is contraindicated (Liver and renal diseases) NSAIDS are the next choice of therapy.

Intra-articular injection of corticosteroids are used to treat a symptomatic care of OA. No use of this is restricted, because it may accelerate disease process. A newly approved treatment for OA of knee uses intra-articular injection of synthetic and naturally occurring hyaluronic acid derivatives (orthovise, synvise, and Hyalgan). This is viscosupplementation. Although exact mechanism is unknown but it is beneficial.

Appropriate nutritional intake is encouraged to maintain ideal body weight and avoid weight gain. Weight gain places an unnecessary stress on joints, particularly the hip and knees. Emphasis is placed on the following activities.

- Unloading the stress on painful weight-bearing joints through the use of canes, walkers or crutches.
- ROM exercises to prevent deformities and contractares, muscle strengthening exercises to icrease or maintain muscle, muscle tone and strength.

Aerobic exercise should be included in the regimen to increase endurance and increase overall conditioning. Exercise also is beneficial in reducing fatigue a common complaint of chronic diseased persons.

Surgical Management

When medications and physical therapy have failed, surgery is performed. Surgical management of person with OA is indicated to relieve pain. Improve function, or correct deformity. Surgical procedures include those that preserve or restore articular cartilage and thsoe that realign, fuse or replace joints. Surgical management usually provides the patient with excellent results. However, the patient is at risk for developing surgical complications including infection, nerve and blood vessel injury, deep vein thrombosis and pulmonary fat embolism. The common surgical procedures performed for OA are:

- Abrasion chondroplasty (to stimulate growth of cartilage).
- Osteotomy (to realign joint or to redistribute cartilage).
- Arthrodesis (to relieve pain, to restore stability and alignment).
- Arthroplasty (Joint replacement).

Praperatively nurse has to carry out routine assessment procedure collaboratively with other team members as in other surgical procedure with special emphasis on elective surgery. In addition, nursing intervention include preoperative teaching which should focus on assessed risk factors, then may influence his or her case intraoperatively or postoperatively. Major concerns identified by patients with total joint replacement including fear of the unknown, pain, performance, altered body image, dependency depression and fatigue.

Postoperative care of joint replacement surgery includes monitoring vital signs and level of consciousness, coughing and deep breathing, monitoring and recording intake and output, providing adequate nutrition and hydration, managing pain, assessing the surgical site for drainage, and signs of infection, maintaining the position of the operative extremity to prevent dislocation of prosthesis, performing neurovascular checks, providing skin care, encouraging progressive ambulation, preventing infection, teaching and monitoring signs of complication and attending accordingly.

Postoperative Care of the Person with Total Hip Replacement

1. *Positioning*
   - Positioning will depend on the design of the prosthesis and the method of insertion. Restriction designed to avoid dislocation of the prosthesis usually include the following.
     - Flexion is limited to 60 degrees for 6 to 7 days, then 90 degrees for 2 to 3 months.
     - No adduction is permitted beyond midline for 2 to 3 months. Therefore, no sidelying on operative side unless ordered by the surgeon. Leg is maintained in abduction when lying supine or on non-operative side.
     - No extreme internal or external rotation is permitted.
2. *Wound care*
   - Drains are inserted in wound to prevent formation of haematoma and left in place for 24 to 48 horus.
   - Maintain constant suction through self-contained suction device.
   - Note amount and types of drainage.
   - Use aseptic technique.
   - Following initial dressing change, change dressing once daily and prn, using a septic technique. Observe the incision line for signs of infection. The wound may be left open to air if there is no drainage. Staples are removed 7 to 10 days postoperatively.
3. *Activity*
   - Observe flexion restriction when elevating head of bed.
   - Encourage periodic elevation and lowering of head of bed to provide motion at hip.
   - Instruct patient in use of overhead trapeze to shift weight and lift for bedpan and change of linen.

- Encourage active dorsiplantar flexion exercise of ankles and quadriceps and gluteal setting exercises to promote venous return, prevent thrombus formation, and maintain muscle tone.
- Patient may be turned to unoperative side with operative leg maintained in abduction and extension.
- Begin ambulation as early as possible as the first postoperative day, if tolerated.
  - Observe flexion and adduction restrictions.
  - Observe weight-bearing restrictions prescribed by surgeon (usually partial weight bearing assisted with walker or crutcher).
  - Increase amount of walking each day according to patient tolerance.
- Begin sitting when patient demonstrates sufficient control of leg to sit within flexion restrictions (usually requires elevation of sitting surfaces, including use of raised toilet seat).

4. *Medications*
   - Prophylactic anticoagulant drug may be prescribed to decrease risk of thrombus formation.
   - Initially control pain with positioning and narcotics, gradually tapered to non-narcotic analgesia according to patient tolerance.
5. *Discharge instructions*
   - Patient must use ambulatory aid, avoid adduction, and limit hip flexion to 90 degree for about 2 to 3 months.
   - A raised toilet seat is to be obtained and used at home until flexation restrictions are removed.
   - Patient may need a long-handled shoehorn and reacher to facilitate ADL within flextion restriction.
   - Patient must be made aware of the life-long need for antibiotic prophylaxis when undergoing invasive procedures or dental work to protect prosthesis from bacteremic infection.

Postoperative Care of the Person with Total Knee Replacement

1. *Positioning*
   - The operative leg(s) is elevated in pillows to enhance venous return for the first 48 hours. Pillows are placed with caution not to flex the knee (s). It is becoming more common for patients who have bilateral total knee replacements at one surgery.
   - The patient may be turned from side to back to side.
2. *Wound care*
   - Care of drains is as for total hip replacement.
   - Patient is assessed for systemic evidence of loss of blood, (hypotension, tachycardia) if bulky compression dressing is used, since it may hold large quantities of drainage before drainage is visible.
   - Bulky dressings are removed before the patient begins active flexion.
   - Assess wound for heal in and signs of infection. Perform dry sterile dressing change once bulky dressing is discontinued. Leave incision open to air if there is no drainage.
3. *Activity*
   - Passive flexion in a CPM machine within prescribed flexion-extension limits. Patient's leg may remain in machines as much as tolerated (upto 22 hours per day) to facilitate even healing of tissue.
   - Patient is encouraged to perform active dorsiplantar flexion of the ankles, quadriceps setting and after the drain is removed, straight leg-raising exercises.
   - Patient begins active flexion exercises three to four times per day on about the third postoperative day. The time when active flexion is permitted varies.
   - Partial weight bearing with an assistive device may be started as early as the first postoperative day and increased as the patient tolerates.
   - Sitting in a chair with leg(s) elevated may be started on the first postoperative day.
   - Patient may be encouraged to wear a resting knee extension spling (immobilizer) on the operative extremity untilable to demonstrate quadriceps control (independent straight leg raising)
4. *Pain control*
   - Initial control of pain is with narcotics (PCA) and positioning medication is gradually decreased to non-narcotic analgesics as patient tolerates.
   - Ice is usually prescribed to be applied to the knee to reduce swelling and pain.
   - Patient is encouraged to apply ice to knee (1) for 20 to 30 minutes before and after active flexion exercise.
5. *Discharge instructions*
   - Patient must observe partial weight-bearing restriction and use ambulatory aid for approximately 2 months after discharge.
   - Patient should continue active flexion and straight leg-raising exercises at home.
   - Patient must be made aware of the life-long need for antibiotic prophylaxis before invasive procedure or dental work.

In surgery, total replacement of shoulder, elbow and ankle also performed. Position and other care should be taken accordingly. The complications of total joint arthroplasty are as follows:

1. *Hip*
   - Dislocation.
   - Infection.
   - DVT.
   - Pulmonary embolus.
   - Leg length discrepancy.
   - Pat embolus.
   - Altered gait.
   - Pneumonia.
   - Foot drop.

2. *Knee*
   - Infection.
   - DVT.
   - Pulmonary embolus.
   - Acute compartment syndrome.
   - Instability.
   - Loosening of prosthesis.
   - Pattellar fracture.
   - Poor patellar tracking.
   - Vascular injury and haemorrhage.
   - Reflex sympathetic dystrophy.
   - Nerve damage.

3. *Shoulder*
   - Infection.
   - Loosening of prosthesis.
   - Gleno-humeral instability.
   - Dislocation, subluxation.
   - Intraoperative fracture.
   - Rotation cuff tears.
   - Deltoid dysfunction.
   - Nerve damage.
   - Impingement syndrome
   - Pulmonary embolus.

4. *Elbow*
   - Infection.
   - Loosening of prosthesis.
   - Glenohumer 1 instability.
   - Dislocation, subluxation.
   - Intraoperative fracture.
   - Rotator cuff.

5. *Elbow*
   - Infection.
   - Dislocation.
   - DVT.
   - Pulmonary embolus.
   - Loosening prosthesis.
   - Delayed healing of wound.

6. *Ankle*
   - Infection.
   - Residual pain.
   - Impingement.
   - Loosening prosthesis.

Juvenile Rheumatoid Arthritis (JRA)

JRA is a major rheumatoid disease of youth and is defined as RA beginning before 16 years of age. It may be classified on the basis of the type of onset. Systemic, pauciarticular or polyarticular. Polyarticular resemble adult RA systemic JRA with onset during childhood.

JRA may occur with arthritis confined to one joint (Pauciarticular) or several (Polyarticular). Children, most often, do not complain of joint pain, but may assume a position of flexion to minimize pain, carefully limit movement or refuse to walk at all. A more constitutional variant known as stills disease (systemic onset) causes high-spiking fever, vague arthralgins, generalized rash, hepatosplenomegally, lymphadenopathy and pleuritis or pericarditis. Complication of JRA includes retarded growth and development, and chronic asymptomatic eye inflammation.

The criterion diagnosis of JRA is persistent athritis of one or more joints for at least 6 consecutive weeks, provided certain other similar disorders are ruled out. High-spiking fever, generalized lymphadenopathy and splenomegaly are more common in children. Leucocytosis is common. JRA can be treated with NSAIDS, if no resposne to NSAIDS use chrystotherapy (treatment with gold sales).

Nursing intervention includes the education of parents and significant ones about the course and prognosis of their child's arthritis according to the onset of classification. Daily participation in planned physical training progress encourages full ROM and muscle strengthening and does not strain affected joints. Swimming, bicycling and dance therapy are better than running, jumping and kicking and routine ophtholmological examinations are advised.

GOUT/GOUTY ARTHRITIS

Gout is characterized by recurrent attacks of acute arthritis in association with increased levels of serum uric acid. It may be classified as primary or secondary.

Aetiology

Primary gout occurs predominantly in middle-aged men, with almost no incidence in premenopausal women. Gout was considered a disease of the wealthy, associated with rich food and wine. Uric acid is the major end product of the catabolism of purines and primarily excreted by the kidneys. Thus, hyperurecaemia may be result of increased purine synthesis, decreased renal excretion or both. There are folklores associated with excess of food and drink with acute attacks of gouty arthritis. Although high dietary intake of purine alone has relatively little effect on uric acid levels, it is clear that hyperurecaemia may result from prolonged fasting or excessive alcohol drinking because of increased production of keto acids, which then inhibit normal excretion of uric acid.

The causes of secondary gout include:

Overproduction of uric acid

- Paget's disease.
- Cancer
- Polycythemia vera.
- Multiple myeloma.
- Chronic myelocytic and lymphonytic leukaemia.
- Haemolytic anaemia
- Cytotoxic drugs.

Under-excretion of uric acid

- Chronic renal insufficiency.

- Ketoacidosis.
- Lactic acidosis.
- Drug ingestion (diuretics, cyclosporine, lovadopa, pyrazinamide. Low-dose salicylism.

Unknown aetiology

- Hyperparathyroidism.
- Hypoparathyroidism.
- Hypothyroidism.
- Adrenal insufficiency.

Associated condition leading to hyperuricaema are acidosis and ketosis, alcoholism, atherosclerosis, cytotoxic drugs, diabetes mellitus, drug-induced renal impairment, hyperlipidaemia, hypertension, intrinsic renal disease, malignant disease, myeloproliferation disorder, obesity and sickle cell anaemia.

Pathophysiology

Uric acid levels are controlled by diet, purine metabolism and renal clearance. Persons with chronically-elevated uric acid levels will develop gouty arthritis. As stated earlier, gout is classified primary and/or secondary. Undersecretion of uric acid is caused by decreased tubular secretion, increased tubular resorption, or a combination of both. Seventy-five per cent cases of primary gout as a result of undersecretion of uric acid, twenty-five per cent of primary gout are oversecretion of uric acid. Primary gout is idiopathic, affected persons also tend to have hypertension and obesity.

Secondary gout results from an overproduction of uric acid secondary to increased purine catabolism or impaired excretions of uric acid. Secondary gout usually occurs in the acute care setting. Urate crystals form in the synovial tissue causing severe inflammation.

Chemical Manifestation

In acute phase, gouty arthritis may occur in one or more joints but usually less than four. Affected joint may appear dusky or cyanotic and are extremely tender. Inflammation of the great toe (Podagra) is most commonly the initial involvement. Other joints affected are midtarsal, ankle, knee and wrist joints and olecranon bursa. Acute gouty arthritis is usually precipitated by events such as trauma, surgery, alcohol, ingestion or systemic infection. Onset of symptoms usually are rapid with swelling and pain peaking within several hours. Often accompanied by low grade fever. Individual attacks usually subsides, treated or untreated in 2 to 10 days. They affect joint returns entirely to normal and patients are often free of symptoms between attacks.

Chronic gout is characterized by multiple joint involved and deposits of sodium urate crystals called tophi. These are typically seen in the synovium subchondral done, olecronon burns, and vertebrae; along tendens, and in the skin and cartilage. Tophi are rarely present at the time of the initial attack and generally noted only many years after the onset of disease. Chronic inflammation may result in joint deformity. Destructing the cartilage may predispose the joint to secondary osteoarthritis. Excessive uric acid excretion leads to kidney or urinary tract stone formation.

Management

The diagnosis can be established by finding monosodium urate, monohydrate crystals in the synovial fluid of an inflammed joint or tophus in addition to history and physical examination. Family history of gout, elevated serum uric acid levels, and elevated 24-hour urine for uric acid levels.

Acute gouty arthritis is treated with one of three types of anti-inflammatory agents such as colchicine, NSAIDS, or cortiocosteroids. Corticosteroids should be reserved for cases in the cochicine and NSAIDS are contraindicated or ineffective. Colchicine and NSAIDS are also used as prophylaxis to prevent further attacks of gout.

Acute gouty arthritis may be prevented by maintenance of the serum uric acid at normal levels, Nursing interventions is directed at supportive care of the inflammed joints—Bedrest may be appropriate, with affected joint properly immobilized. The limitation of motion and degree of pain should be assessed. Treatment effectiveness should be documented. Special care is taken to avoid causing pain so the inflammed joint by careless handling. Involvement of a lower extremity may require use of cradle or footboard to protect the painful area from the weight of bed clothes. In addition, nursing management includes the following.

1. *Patient teaching*
   - Instruct patient on nature of disease.
   - Instruct patient on proper use of prescribed medication.
   - Encourage patient to lose weight gradually if overweight.
   - Encourage lifestyle modification to control hypertension or adherence to pharmocological regimen (medication).
   - Encourage patient to take in sufficient fluid to assure daily output of 2000 ml to 3000 ml.
   - Advise the patient to avoid excessive intake of purine (sweet bread yeast, heart, herring, herring roe and sardines and excessive alcohol intake).
   - Explain to patient that severe dietary purine restriction is not necessary as long as his or her hyperuricaemia is well controlled by daily-drug tehrapy.
2. *Promoting comfort*
   - Provide absolute rest until the pain of an acute attack subsides.
   - Avoid touching the joint or moving the affected extremity until the acute pain subsides.

Thorough explanation should be given concerning importance of drug therapy and the need for periodic determination of blood and uric acid levels. The patient should be able to demonstrate knowledge of precipitating factors that may cause an attack, including overindulgence in the intake of calories, purines, and alcohol, starvation (fasting), medication use (aspirin, diuretics) and major medical events (eg. surgery, MI).

SEPTIC ARTHRITIS

Septic arthritis (Infection or Bacterial Arthritis) is caused by invasion of the joint cavity with micro-organism.

Aetiology

Various bacteria are commonly responsible including

- Neisseria gonorrhoeas (children).
- Meningococci.
- Streptococcus haemolyticus.
- Staphylococcus aureus.
- Coliform bacteria.
- Salm nella.
- Haemophilus influenzae.

Haematogenous infection is the most common cause of bacterial arthritis. Persons with an underlying medical illness are at greatest risk. Immunodeficiency, chronic disease intravenous drug abuse, local joint surgery or trauma, intra-articular injections and theumatoid arthritis also place the person at risk.

Pathophysiology

A site of active infection is often responsible for bacteraemia (micro-organism reaching the blood stream). Leading to haematogenous seeding joints. Synovial tissue respond to bacterial invasion by becoming

- Signs and symptoms of septic arthritis.
- Importance of diagnosis and treatment.
- Importance of antibiotic therapy.
- Instructing in care of cast or other immobilizing device.
- Encouraging active joint motion when motion is permitted.
- Instructing about use of crutches or assistive devices.
- Instruct on proper administration of antibiotics if it is continued after discharge.
- Ensuring that patient should be aware of plans for follow-up with physician.

inflammed. The joint cavity may become involved and pus will be present, in the synovial membrane and the synovial fluid. If allowed to progress, the infection will cause abscesses in the synovium and subchondral done; eventually destroying cartilage. Ankylosis of the joints may result. The patient will report pain, swelling and tenderness of the joint.

Clinical Manifestation

Inflammation of the joint cavity causes severe pain, erythaema, and swelling of one or several joints. Large joints, such as the knee and the hip are most frequently involved. Fever or shaking chills often accompany particular symptoms because bacterial entry into a joint is usually by the haematogenous route from a primary site of infection.

Management

Process diagnosis is made by aspiration of the joint and culture of the synovial fluid. Blood cultures for aerobic and anaerobic organism, should be obtained. Strict aseptic technique must be followed to avoid introducing additional bacteria into the joint. WBC counts will be high, and X-ray of joint reveals loss of joint space and lythic changes in bones.

Septic arthritis is a medical emergency that requires prompt diagnosis and treatment to prevent joint destructions. Parenteral antibiotic administration is maintained until there are no clinical signs of active synovitis or inflammation in the joint fluid. The treatment of septic arthritis includes.

- Appropriate antibiotic therapy.
- Rest or immobilization of the joint.
- Surgical drainage by needle aspiration arthroscopy, arthrotomy, or a system of irrigation and drainage if injection does not respond to antibiotic therapy or if osteomyelitis, required daily until drainage ceases. Infection of the hip joints must be drained immediately to prevent necrosis of the femoral head.
- Resumption of active range of motion when infection subsides and motion can be tolerated.

Nursing management includes the following.

- Promoting rest of the affected joints.
- Assessment and monitoring of joint inflammation, pain and fever.
- Immobilization of affected joint to control pain is often by resting splints or traction.
- Administering antibiotics on time and as prescribed to maintain blood level.
- Administering prescribed pain medication as necessary.
- Strict aseptic technique should be used during assistance with joint aspiration procedure.
- Support should be offered to the patient requiring repeated arthrocentesis or operative drainage.
- Gentle ROM exercise should be done.
- Patient teaching should be done regarding.

LYME'S DISEASE (LD)

Lyme's disease is tick borne spirochetal infection caused by the "Borrelia Burgeloferi" and transmitted by the bite of an infected tick. It was first identified in 1975 in Lyme, Connecticut (US) after an unusual clustering of arthritis in children.

Aetiology

Lyme's disease is caused by the spirachete (Borrelia-Burgeloferi). This disease is transmitted by ticks, present most commonly on deer, dogs, cats, raccons, cows and horses. Birds help spread infected ticks by their migratory flights.

Pathophysiology

Lyme's disease has been called "great imitator" because it resembles, mimics other diseases such as influenza, RA multiple sclerosis, chronic fatigue syndrome, and others. Infection with B. Burgelorferi stimulates inflammatory cytokines, and autoimmune mechanisms which result in Lyme arthritis. Primarily an extracellular organism B. Burgelorferi is thought to invade some cells and cross the blood-brain barrier, resulting in the neurological manifestation of Lyme disease. Infection with this spirochate can be divided into three stages (I, II, III). Not all patients develop all states (See clinical manifestations).

Clinical Manifestation

Stage I (Early localized infection)

- Symptoms appear days to 16 weeks after tick bite.
- Erythaema, migraine appear in 50-70% of patients, resolve spontaneously in a few weeks.
- Fatigue.
- Headache.
- Lethargy.
- Myalgia, arthalgia.
- Lymphadenopathy.

Stage II (Early disseminated infection):

- Symptoms occur weeks to months after tick bite.
- Cardiac Symptoms—Carditis, dysrhythmias, hear failure, pericarditis, palpitation, dyspnoea.
- Neurological symptom—Meningitis, encephalitis, cranial and peripheral neuorpathy and myelitis.
- Musculoskeletal—Arthralgia, myalgia, fibromyalgia.
- Other symptoms-Conjunctivitis, optieneuropathy, Hepatomegaly, hepatitis, generalized lymphadenopathy.

Stage III (Late infection)

Symptoms occur months to years after tickbite.

- Monoarticular or dioarticular arthritis.
- Chronic arthritis.
- Aerodermatitis chronic atrophicans (bluish, red, doughy lesions).
- Ataxia.
- Spastic paresis.
- Periventricular lesions.
- Memory loss.
- Behavioural changes.

Management

Diagnosis is made on the basis of clinical manifestation, history of exposure in an endemic area and a positive serological test for B. Bureldorferi. Differential diagnoses also should be made. Serological test includes ELISA (Enzyme linked immu-noabsorbent assay, Western blot, and indirect immunofluorence assay.

Patients in Stage I disease should be treated with tetracycline or deoxycycline to prevent development of further symptoms. During Stage II and III, intravenous therapy is indicated, usually cefiaxone (crosses the blood-brain barrier), cefotaxime or penicillin. The patient should be monitored for development of cardiac and neurological sequalae. Persons with musculoskeletal symtoms resulting in impaired mobility require physical therapy and occupational therapy. Nursing interventions are as in RA. Education is the best way to prevent Lyme disease in endemic areas, which include:

- Avoid walking through tall grasses and low bush.
- Avoid tick-infested areas and sitting directly on the ground, stay on paths while hiking.
- Mow grass and remove brush along paths, buildings and camp sites.
- When outdoors in high risk areas, wear long sleeves and long pants and pants into shoes or sockes.
- Wear closed shoes when hiking.
- Use EPA approved tick repellants on skin and clothing. Wash off repellant thoroughly when returning inside.
  Avoid spraying repllants directly on skin of small children.
- Check frequently for ticks crawling from legs to open skin.
- Have pets wear collars, inspect them often, and do not allow them on furniture or beds.
- If a tick is found, use a fine-pointed tweezer to grasp the tick, at the point of attachment, gently pull the tick straight out, place the tick in a sealed jar and have it tested by a local veterinarian or health department. Don't squeeze the tick, doing so may release infected fluid.
- Dispose off tick in alcohol or flush down toilet. Do not crush with fingers.
- Wash the tick site thoroughly with soap and warm water, apply antiseptic and disinfect the tweezers. Wash hands and clothes properly.
- Ticks are susceptible to dehydration. Reduce humidity by pruning trees, clearing brush, and mowing the lawn on your property.
- Do not have bird feeders or birdbaths in your yard, these attract animals that may have ticks.
- Keep woodpiles away from the house- Move woodpiles and bird-feeders away from house.
- Keep children's play areas away from wooded areas.
- See a doctor or nurse practitioner immediately if flu-like symptoms or bull's-eye rash develop, within a few weeks after removal of tick.

SERONEGETIVE ARTHROPATHIES

Seronegetive arthropathies is a term used to describe a group of disease characterized by arthritis (arthropathy) in which the rheumatoid factor is not present in the serum. Diseases included in this category are Ankylosing spondalitis, Psoriatic arthritis, enteropathic arthritis and Reifer's syndrome. These diseases also are known as the 'Spondyle arthritis, and have several characteristics other than a negative rheumatoid factors which include.

- Frequent bouts of spondylitis (inflammation of the vertebrae characterized by stiffness and pain).
- Presence of the cell marker HLA-B_{27}-strong association with H antigen B_{27}.
- Common extra-articular manifestation (eye, heart, skin, mucus membrane).
- Predilection for involvement of sacroiliac joint and spine.
- Oligoarticular asymmetric arthritis.
- Absence enthesitis (inflammation at tendon attachment sites to bone).
- Enthesopathy (plantor facitis and Achilles tendenitis).
- Absence of rheumatoid factor and anti-antibiotics.
- Male predominance.

1. Ankylosing Spondylitis (AS)

Ankylosing spondylitis is a chronic inflammatory disease that primarily affects the sacroiliac joints, apophysical and costovertebral joints of the spine and adjacent soft tissues.

Aetiology

The cause of AS is unknown. The course of disease is marked by remissions and exacerbations. The disease in both sexes, with progressive disease more common in men. Genetic predisposition appears to play an important role in the disease pathogenesis, but the precise mechanisms are unknown. Environmental factors and infection agents are also suspected.

Pathophysiology

Inflammation in joint and adjacent tissue causes the formation of granulation tissue and eroding vertebral margins, resulting spondylitis. Calcification tends to follow the inflammation process, leading to bony ankylosis. Spondylitis means inflammation of the spine. As a result of inflammation, the bones of the spine grow together and ankylose (fuse). The primary site of pathological findings is in the enthesis where ligament tendens and joint capsule insert into bone. In ankylosing, spondylitis, fibrous ossification and eventually fusion of the joint occur. The joint capsule articular cartilage, and periosteum are invaded by inflammatory cells that trigger the development of fibrous scar tissue and growth of new bone. The bony growth changes the contour of the vertebrae and form a new enthesis called a "syndesmophyte" on top of the old one. As the spinal ligaments continue to undergo progressive calcification, the vertebral bodies lose their original contour and appear square, which gives the spine the classic "bamboo" appearance of ankylosing spondylitis. Inflammation usually begins around the sacroiliac joints and progresses up the spine, eventually resulting in fusion of the entire spine. As the inflammatory process involves the costosternal and costovertebral cartilage, it causes the chest pain, which is worse on inspiration.

Clinical Manifestation

The patient typically has lower back pain, stiffness and limitation of motion that is worse during the night and in the morning, but improves with mild activity. General constitutional feature, such as fever, fatigue, anorexia and weight loss are rarely present. Other symptoms depend on the stage of the disease and include arthritis of the shoulders, hips and knees and occasionally ocular inflammation (iritis). Involvement of the costovertebral joints leads to a decrease in chest expansion. Advancing kyphosis leads to a bent-over postage and compensating hipflexion contractures may occur. There is pronounced impairment of neckmotion in all direction. Extraskeletal involvement may include iritis, aortitis, valvular regurgitation and apical pulmonary fibrosis.

Management

Diagnosis is made by history and physical examination and the following findings.

- X-ray films shows that the presence of syndesmophytes and bamboo spine ankylosis of peripheral joints seen. CT and MRI show changes.
- ESR elevated.
- Test by RF is negative.
- HLA-B_{27} present in the serum.

The objectives of the treatment are to relieve pain, achieve and maintain the best possible alignment of the spine, strengthening the paraspinal muscles and maximal breathing capacity. For which:

- Administration fo salicylates, NSAIDS (phenybutazone effective but may cause bone marrow toxicity).
- Sulfasalazine and systemic steroids are avoided except for patients with severe eye disease.
- Exercise is an important component of treatment. Swimming in a warm pool is a good choice for exercise. Rest should be discouraged unless a fracture is present.
- Physical therapy to maintain mobility and reduce severties of deformity. For example ROM exercises and lying prone (extension) 3 to 4 times per day for 15 to 30 minutes and deep-breathing exercises to promote maximum chest expansion (rib cage mobility) is decreased.
- Heat.
- Use of thoracic lumbar sacral orthosis (TLSO).
- Cervical head halter traction to decrease muscle spasms and distractive spine.

- Spinal osteotomy and fusion are usually cervical.
- Hip arthroplasty.
- Value replacement of pace maker insertion if cardiac involvement is present.

Patient teaching is essential. It should focus on the following:

- Facilitating learning.
  - Nature and cause of disease.
  - Prescribed exercises.
  - Appropriate use of prescribed medication.
  - Methods of applying heat to back and hips.
- Promoting maximum ability and reducing severity of deformity.
  - Maintain proper posture and walk erect.
  - Provide firm mattresses and bed board.
  - Encourage patient to sleep without pillow under the head to maintain extension of spine, lying prone or supine is recommended; avoid sidelying.
  - Supervise and encourage regular exercises; assist as necessary.
  - Regular deep-breathing exercises are important to optimize respiratory function. Persons with ankylosing spondylitis should not smoke.
  - Encourage participation in ADL and usual activities to the fullest extent possible.
  - Refer to an occupation therapist for adaptive or supportive devices. Recommend use of long-handled reachers, sponges, and shoe horn, for patient with hip involvement.
- Promoting comfort and relieving pain.
  - Provide heat applications/hydrotherapy and especially prior to exercises.
  - Administer prescribed medications on time.
  - Assess effectiveness of pain relief measures.
  - Promoting acceptance of body image.

PSORIATIC ARTHRITIS

Psoriatic arthritis can be defined as an association of clinically-apparent psoriasis with inflammatory polyarthritis. Psoriatic skin changes may precede or follow articular symptoms. It affects few joints of peripheral-i.e. distalphalanges of hands, feet and metatorsal bones. X-ray findings show asymmetric distribution and resorption of tufts at joints. These patients get spondylitis, Hypauricaemia, at present of HLA-B_{27}. Forms of treatment include splinting, joint protection, and physicial tehrapy. Treating the cases with drug methotrexate is most effective.

REITER'S SYNDROME

Reiter's syndrome is a self-limiting disease associated with arthritis, urethritis, conjunctivitis, and mucocutaneous lesions. The cause of disease is unknown, but it appears to be a reactive arthritis after certain enteric (eg Shigella) or veneral (eg Chlamydia trachomatis) infections. This disease usually affects in males, shows HLA-B27 positive, which provides evidence of genetic predisposition.

Diagnosis measures as in ankylosy spondylitis. The arthritis of Reiter's syndrome tends to be asymmetric, frequently involving weight-bearing joints of the lower extremities and sometimes lower parts of the back. Arthralgia usually begins 1 to 3 weeks after the appearance of initial infection. The full attack accompanied by fever and other constitutional complaints including anorexia with considerable weight loss and may prove highly debilitating. Soft tissue manifestations cause induced Achilles tendinitis. Treatment is symptomatic and joint inflammation is treated with NSAIDS. Autoimmune is connected two diseases.

SYSTEMIC LUPUS ERYTHMATOSUS

Systemic lupus erythmatosus (SLE) is a chronic multisystem inflammatory disease of connective tissue that often involves the skin, joints, serous membrane (Pleura, Pericardium)-kidneys, haematological system and central nervous system.

Aetiology

The cause of SLE is unknown. However, factors implicate in the aetiology of SLE include genetic predisposition, sex hormones, race, environmental factors (Eg. ultraviolet, radiation, drugs, chemical) viruse and infections, stress and immunologic abnormalities, SLE is a disorder of immunoregulation.

- Genetic factors may contribute to the development of the disease. Family members of persons with SLE have an increased chance of developing disease.
- Environmental factors associated with cases of SLE. For example, exposure for ultraviolet light is a known cause of execerbations. Drugs-including procainamide (Pronestyl), isonicosonic acid hydrazial (INH) hydralazine anticonvulsants and chloropromozin are known to induce lupus-like syndromes. Persons with drug-induced lupus do not develop renal and neurological disease. The symptoms usually resolve after the drug is discontinued. Other areas being considered include viral-origin and disturbance is aestrogen metabolism (menses and pregnancy).
- Alterations in the immune response may cause immune complexes containing antibodies to be deposited in tissue causing tissue damage.

Pathophysiology

The exact mechanism of is not known. However, several alterations in the immune system are associated with SLE. Numerous cellular antibodies have been identified with it. Antinuclear antibodies, antibodies to DNA, antihistones, and antibodies to ribonucleoprotein (Smith antigen) are strongly associated with SLE.

Abnormalities in both B cells and T cells have been exempted in the persons with SLE. The appearance of B cells is thought to cause an increase in production of antibodies to self and non-self antigen. These antibodies are responsible for the tissue injury seen in SLE. Most visceral lesions are mediated by type III hypersensitivity and antibodies against red blood cells are mediated by type II hypersensitivity. An acute necrotizing vasculitis can occur in any tissue. Most lesions are found in the blood vessels, kidney, connective tissue and skin.

Clinical Manifestation

The clinical manifestation of SLE can be overwhelming. The criteria for classification are remissions and ommissions Fixed erythaema, flat or raised, over the molar eminences tending to spare the nasolabial fold.

- *Discord rash*: Erythematus raised patches with adherent keratotic scaling and follicular plugging, atrophic scarring may occur in older lesions.
- *Photosensitivity*: Skin rash as a result of unusual reaction to sunlight by patient history or physician observation.
- *Oral ulcers*: Oral or nasopharyngeal ulceration, usually painless observed by care taken.
- *Arthritis*: Non-erosive arthritis involving two or more peripheral joint characterized by tenderness, swelling of effusion.
- *Serositis*: Pleuritis- Pleuritic pain or rub hears.
  : Pericarditis- document by ECG or rub.
- Renal Disorders.
  - Persistent orotienuria greater than 0.5 g/dl.
  - Cellular casts - may be RBCs haemoglobin-granular, tubular or medial.
- Neurological disorder.
  - Seizures: in the absence of offencing drugs and known metabolic derangements eg. anaemia, ketoacidosis, or electrolyte imbalances.
  - Psychoses - " -
- Haematological disorders.
  - Haemolytic anaemias - with reticulosis or
  - Leukopoenia-less than 4.0 × 109/L total on two or more occasions.
  - Lymphopoenia-less than 1.5 × 109/L. total on two or more occasions or
  - Thrombocytopoenia less than 100 × 109/L in the absence of offending drug.
- Immunological disorder
  - Positive lupus erythematous cell preparation or
  - Anti-DNA antibody to negative DNA is abnormal or
  - Anti-Sm - Presence of antibody to Sm nuclear antigen or
  - False positive STS known to be positive for at least 6 months and confirmed by negative. Trepenoma palladium immobilization.
- Antinuclear antibody
  - An abnormal titer of antinuclear antibody by immunofluorescence of an equivalent assay at any point in time and in the absence of drugs known to be associated with drug-induced lupus syndrome, and general constitutional complaints include fever, weight loss, arthralgia, and excessive fatigue and may precede an exacerbation of disease activity.

Management Diagnosis is made after evaluation of the history and physical examination and results of the laboratory test-lupus cell preparation, Antibodies, CBC count, urinalysis, X-ray of the joints, Chest X-ray, complement level CH 50, C3) and ECG.

The following medications are given for SLE:

- NSAIDs to control arthritic symptoms; diclofenic, naproxen, and oxaprozine are effective in treating lupus. Renal function are monitored carefully.
  - Antimalarial drugs, particularly if rasin is extensive.
- Corticosteroids for severe neurological and renal involvement or if NSAIDS or are ineffective.
- Cystotoxic agents if other drugs fail (Cyclophosphamide).
- Ointments or skin creams for rash.

Nursing care will depend upon the symptoms manifested. Nursing intervention to maintain musculoskeletal functioning are similar to those for caring for persons with rheumatoid arthritis. Nursing intervention must emphasize health teaching and home management which includes the following.

- Education on the disease process.
- Names of medications and actions, side effects, dosage and administration.
- Energy-conservation and pacing techniques.
- Daily heat and exercise program (for Anthralgia).
- Avoidance of physical and emotional stress, overexposure to ultraviolet light and unnecessary exposure to infection.
- Regular medical and laboratory follow-up.
- Marital counselling if necessary.
- Referral resources to community and health care agency.

All nursing intervention can assist the patient in accepting changes and coping with a chronic disease.

The other autoimmune connective diseases are:

- Scleroderma (Systemic sclerosis).
- CREST syndrome (Limited Cutaneous Scleroderma).
- Sjogren's syndrome.

The brief description of these diseases are as follows.

SYSTEMIC SCLEROSIS

Systemic sclerosis (SS) or scleroderm is a disorder of connective tissue characterized by fibrositic, degenerative and occasionally inflammatory changes in the skin, blood vessels, synovium, skeletal muscle, and internal organ.

It is most common in middle-aged women, causes microvascular damage and fibrous degeneration of tissues in the skin, GI tract, lungs and kidneys. The exact cause is unknown but possible links include environmental toxin, exposure to vinyl chloride, epoxy resins and trichloroethylene. Occupational silica dust exposure increases insidious scleroderma.

Clinical Manifestation

- Raynaud's phenomenon (Paraxysmal vosospasm of the digits).
- GI: dysphagia, diarrhoea and malabsorption.
- Renal: haematuria, protienuria, renal crisisa and hypertension.
- Cardiopulmonary: Pericarditis, dysrhythmias, pulmonary hypertension, fibrosis.
- Dermatologeal: hardening, thickening and tightening of the skin, oedema,

Management

- Routine diagnostic measures.
- Avoidance of cold; protective clothing.
- Skin care for ulcers.
- Thoracic sympathectomy for Raynaud's phenomenon.
- Metoclopramide, is apride, H_2 blockers and oesophageal dilation for gastrointestinal symptoms.
- NSAIDS, Calcium channel blockers, prednisone, bronchial lavage, for cardiopulmonary symptoms.
- Splints for contractures and deformities.
- Heat and cold application is needed.
- D-penacillamine and colchicine used to decrease collagen with some success.

CREST SYNDROME

This is variant of scleroderma classified by the extent of skin thickening. It has more favouruable prognosis and less organ involvement. Sclerosis may range from a diffuse cutaneous thickening with rapidly progressive and fatal visceral involvement to more benign variant called CREST SYNDROME (Calcinosis, Raynaud's phenomenon, oesophagial hyperomotility Sclerodactyly) Skin changes of the (fingers) and Telangiectasia (macule-like angioma on the skin).

Clinical Manifestation

- Calcinosis (result of chronic vascular insufficiency):
  - Intracutaneous or subcutaneous calcification on digital pads, particular tissues, extensor surfaces of forearms, olecranon and prepatellar bursae.
- Raynaud's phenomenon.
- Oesophageal dysmotility.
- Sclerodactyl.
- Telegrectasia.
- Pulmonary involvement in many patients.

Management

Treatment as for scleroderma. Surgical removal of calcium deposits.

SJÖGREN'S SYNDROME

Sjögren's syndrome is characterizedly autoantibodies to two protein-RNA complexes termed SS-A/Ro and SS-B/La. The clinical manifestations are caused by inflammation and dysfunction of the exocrine glands particularly the salivary and lacrimal glands, which result in dryness of the mouth, eyes and mucus membrane. Lymph nodes, bone marrow and organ involvement is present. RA is 50 per cent of patients.

The clinical manifestations include xerostomia, dyspareunia, decreased tearing, gritty sensation in eyes, dysphagia, dental caries, cough, enlarged parotid glands, rheumatoid and antinuclear antibody factor, positive in most patients and anaemia.

Ophthalmalogical examination (Schimer's Test) salivary flow rates and lower lip biopsy of minor salivary glands confirm the diagnosis. The treatment is symptomatic including:

- Instillation of artificial tears as often as necessary to maintain adequate hydration and lubrication.
- Vaginal lubrication with a water soluble product such as K-Y jelly may increase comfort during intercourse.
- Surgical punctal acclusion.
- Increased fluid intake, especially with meals.
- Good dental and oral hygiene especially after meals.
- Avoidance of respiratory infections.
- Increased humidity in home and work environment.
- Carticosteroids and immunosuppressive drugs are indicated for treatment of Pseodolymphoma.

POLYMYOSITIS/DERMATOMYOSITIS

Polymyositis (PM) is a chronic acquired inflammatory disorder of skeletal muscle. When a characteristic skin rash is present, this disorder is called "dermatomyositis" (DM). Both are diffuse inflammatory myopathies of straited muscle, producing symmetric weakness usually most severe in the proximal muscle (e.g. trunk, shoulder and hip).

Aetiology

The aetiology of both disorders is unknown, but abnormal reaction of the immune system have been implicated, perhaps triggered by Virus. Autoantibodies are found in the serum of affected muscle. These disorders occur twice as frequently in women as in men; usually occurs in the fifth and sixth decades of life.

Pathophysiology

Both polymyositis and dermato polymyosits are characterised by inflammation of muscle fibres and connective tissues, resulting in extensive tissue necrosis and destruction of muscle fibers. Both cell-mediated and humoral immune mechanisms are associated with the diseases. Inflammatory cells found at the perimysical and perivascular sites contain B cell and helper T cells in dermatomyositis. Less vascular involvement occurs in polymyosites and B and T cells are found in surrounding the muscle fibers and foscicles.

Clinical Manifestation

The initial symptoms of both disorders are similar to those associated with any inflammatory response: fever, swelling, malaise and fatigue. The diseases which run a course of exacerbations and remissions are usually first noted in proximal muscles in particular, the pelvic and shoulder girdles. The weakness is symmetric. Climbing stairs, raising from a chair and other activities that involve lifting the body becomes increasingly difficult or impossible. Lifting the arm becomes progressively more difficult, and hair combing may be impossible. Other muscles such as the neck flexors and the muscles of swallowing may also be involved. Muscle pain or tenderness is present in some instances in early stages.

Clinical manifestations of both disorders include dysphagia, dyspnoea, decreased oesophegeal motility, cardiomyopathy and Raynaud's phenomenon. A dusky red lesions may be found in the preorbital region (heliotype) along with preorbital oedema in persons with dermatomyositis. This dusky red rash may extend over the face, forehead, neck, upper shoulders, chest and upper back. Scaly lesions on the arms and legs commonly affect the exterior surfaces. Erythema occurs over the metacarpophalangeal and proximal phalangeal joints. Calcinosis can also occur in dermatomyosisis. The weakness of myositis, if it persits, can lead to contractures and atrophy.

Management

Diagnosis is based on the following.

- History and physical examination including manual muscle test to delineate weakness in specific muscles.
- Electromyogram to delineate a specific pattern of findings to differentiate polymyositis from other types of muscle disease.
- Muscle biopsy to define specific pathological changes in muscle.
- Serum enzyme levels (creatine phosphokinase, lactate dehydrogenase, aldolase) which are elevated in the presence of active disease.
- 24-hour urine test to determine abnormal creatine/creatinine ratio.

Treatment includes high dose corticosteroid therapy (Prednisone upto 60 mg. daily). If steroid therapy contraindicated, or ineffective, an immunosuppressant such as methotrexate is prescribed. Cyclophosphamide has been used effectively in some patients and hydroxychloquine may improve rash in persons with dermatomyositis.

Nursing responsibilities include the following.

a. *Promoting comfort*
   - During acute episodes, assist with frequent changes of position.
   - Administer prescribed analgesics.
   - Assist with ADL.
   - Provide adequate rest.

b. *Promoting mobility*
   - Elevate sitting surfaces to facilitate transfer.
   - Provide appropriate ambulatory device to facilitate comfortable walking.
   - Provide for frequent changes of positive and ROM to prevent contraction.
   - Encourage patient to gradually resume independent ADL as symptoms subside.
   - Refer patient to physical therapy for exercise program.

c. *Preventing skin breakdown*
   - Reposition patient frequently.
   - Assess skin for integrity.
   - Topical steroids may be prescribed for the rash in persons with dermatomyositis.

In addition, patient should have a thorough understanding of the chronic nature of the disorders, the usefulness and the side effects of all prescribed medications and the importance of regular medical care and serial laboratory testing.

FIBROMYALGIA SYNDROME (FMS)

Fibromyalgia is a musculoskeletal chronic pain syndrome, is characterized by fatigue, stiffness, myalgias, arthralgias, headache, irritable bowel syndrome and sleep disturbance. It has association with arthritis and other rheumatic disorder as discussed earlier. Other generalized pain syndrome affecting musculoskeletal system include polymyalgia rheumatica which often occurs with giant cell arteritis.

Aetiology

The aetiology is unknown; but there is an association between sleep disturbance and fibromyalgia. Muscle microtrauma and imbalance of neurotransmitters have also been implicated as possible causative factors. Trauma or infection may trigger the onset of symptoms. Symptoms typically occur between the ages of 20-40 years, mainly in women (80%).

Pathophysiology

FMS may appear with RA or SLE or other pain syndrome like polymyalgia rheumatica. Several abnormalities in muscles have been documented in persons with FMS, including lower ATP and ADP levels, higher levels of AMP and changes in the number of capillaries and fiber area. Increased muscle tenderness may be the result of generalized pain intolerance perhaps as a result of CNS abnormalities.

Clinical Manifestations

The characteristic symptom of fibromyalgia is a generalized chronic pain, which may be described as "burning or gnawing". Chronic aching, nonrestorative sleep, morning stiffness and fatigue are commonly reported patients with FMS demonstrate loss of functional abilities similar to patient with RA. Yet no radiographic changes in articular structures are found in FMS. Temperomandibular joint dysfunction, premenstrual symptoms, and mitral valve prolapse may also accompany the disorder. Cognitive disturbances such as memory problems (brain fog) or difficulty in concent rating are common. Depression, anxiety and feelings of hopelessness often result because of the nature of chronic nature of FMS. There is no visible signs of FMS. Headaches, sensitivity to extreme temperature, abdominal pain, paresthesias, menstrual irregularities, irritable bowel and difficulty in concentration may be reported.

Management of FMS

The diagnosis of FMS is made by the presence of typical symptoms and the location of tender points. Eighteen points, tender in normal persons have been identified than one hypersensitive in persons with FM. The diagnostic criterion for FM is a history of widespread pain and the presence of at least pain in 11 of 18 specific tender points sites when palpated (digital palpations) is significant for diagnosis. Bilateral tender point sites are:

- Occiput-Suboccipital muscle insertion.
- Cervical-low cervical-anterior aspects of the intratrans-verse spaces C_5-C_7.
- Trapezius-Midpoint of the upper border.
- Scapular-Supraspinatus-above the medial border of the scapular spine.
- Epicondyle-lateral epicondyle 2 cm distal to the epicondyles.
- Gluteal-upper outer quadrants of buttocks.
- Trocanter-greater tochanter-posterior to the trochantic prominence.
- Medial knee-Medial fat pad proximal to the joint line.
- Second rib-Second costochondrial junctions.

FMS may be localized to a specific region of the body (often termed "myofascial pain) or generalized with migratory tender points. Myofascial pain most often involves the posterior neck, lowback, shoulder and chest.

Treatment of FM is symptomatic and requires a high level of patient motivation. The nurse can play a key role in educating the patient to be an active participant in the therapeutic regimen. Pain, aching, and tenderness can be helped by rest and NSAIDS are effective for some patients. Stress, fatigue, and sleep disturbance can be helped by low-dose tricyclin antidepressants (eg. anaitriptyline, imipramine, or trazodone, muscle relaxants, stress management and stress reduction techniques, deep relaxation and a healthful diet. One of the most beneficial approaches to reducing symptom, FM is to encourage patient participation in safe, moderate and exercise programme (eg. Swimming, walking). In addition, gentle stretching exercises, yoga, massage therapy, or taichai may be helpful. Other treatments that may be effective include heat in the form of whirlpools. Moist packs, or hot shower, acupuncture and acupressure.

INFECTIOUS BONE DISEASES

Osteomyelitis

Osteomyelitis is an infection of bone by direct or indirect invasion of an organism. The two types of osteomyelitis are classified by the mode of entry of the pathogen i.e., exogenous and haematogenous osteomyelitis.

Aetiology

1. *Exogenous osteomyelitis* or as described by the Waldragel system as secondary to a contagious source of infection, is caused by a pathogen from outside the body. Examples include pathogens from an open fracture or surgical procedure, involving instrumentation. The infection is also caused by human and animal bites and fist blows to the mouth. The most common organism found in human bite is "Staphylococcus aureas" and in animal bites is "Pasteurella multicida. The infection spreads from the soft tissues to the bone. Risk factors for developing exogenous osteomyelitis are chronic illness, diabetes, alcohol or drug abuse, and immunosuppression. In diabetes or vascular disease, osteomyletis occur in the feet.
2. *Haematogenous Osteomyelitis* is caused by blood-borne pathogen originating from infectious site within the body. Examples include sinus, ear, dental, respiratory and genitourinary infections. In haematogenous osteomyletis the infection spreads from the bone to the soft tissues and can even break through the skin, becoming a draining fistula. This type of oesteomyelitis is common in infants, children and elderly persons. The most common organism is S. Areus and other organisms are streptococcus B. haemophilus influenza, salmonella and gram-negative bacteria.

Pathophysiology

In haematogenous osteomyelitis the organisms reach the bone through the circulatory and lympatic systems. The bacteria lodged in the small vessels of the bone, triggering an inflammatory response. Blockage of the vessels causes thrombosis, ischaemia and necrosis of the bone. The femur, tibia, humerus and radius are commonly affected. Infections of the pelvic organs frequently spread to the pelvic and vertebrae. Bone inflammation marked by oedema, increased vasculature, and leucocytes activity exudate seals the bone canaliculi, extends into the metaphysics and marrow cavity and finally reaches the cortex. New bone laid down over the infected bone by osteoblasts is termed "involucrum". Opening in the involucrum allows infected material to escape into soft-tissues. The infectious process weakens the cortex, thereby increasing risk of pathological fracture. `Bordies abscesses' are characteristics of chronic osteomyelitis. These are isolated encapsulated pockets of micro-organisms surrounded by bone matrix, usually found in long bones. These pockets of virulent organisms are capable of reinfections at any time. The microscopic channels found in bone allow bacteria to proliferate without being affected by body defences. In patient with osteomyelitis the infection begins in the soft tissues disrupting muscles and connective tissues and eventually forming absciss. Acute osteomyelitis left untreated or unresolved after 10 days is termed Chronicosteomyelitis.

Clinical Manifestation

Acute oesteomyelitis refers to the initial infection or an infection of less than one month in duration. The clinical manifestation of acute osteomyelitis are both systemic and local. Systemic manifestations include fever, night sweats, chills, restlessness, nausea and malaise. Local manifestation includes severe bone pain that is unrelieved by rest and worse with activity; swelling, tenderness, and warmth at infection site; and restricted movement of affected part. Later signs include drainage from sinus tracts to the skin and fracture site.

Chronic oesteomy elitis refers to a bone infection that persists for longer than 4 weeks or an infection that has failed to respond to the initial course of antibiotic therapy. Chronic type can represent either a continuous, persistent problem or a process of exacerbations and aquiescence. It results from inadequately treated acute osteomyletis. Pus accumulation causing ischaemia of the bone. Over time, granulation tissue turns to scar tissue. This avascular scar tissue provides an ideal site for bacterial grown and is impenetrable to antibiotics.

Management

Diagnosis based on the following:

- A culture and sensitivity test of the drainage (wound) will reveal the causative organisms and identify appropriate antibiotics.
- Blood tests reveal an increase in WBCs, ESR, C-reactive probe levels.
- Blood cultures will determine the presence or absence of septicaemia.
- Radiological signs suggestive of osteomyelitis, after the appearance of clinical symptoms.
- MRI, CT scan, Gallium scan are also given usefully to confirm diagnosis.

The goals of treatment of osteomyelitis are:

- Complete removal of dead bone and affected soft tissue.
- Control of infection.
- Elimination of dead space (after removal of necrotic bone).

Many modes of treatment are available. Use of treatment modality is used depends on the area of bone involved. Causative organism, ability to maintain a functional limb, duration of treatment and expected outcomes. Treatment options include:

- Antibiotic therapy: Intravenous antibiotics may be prescribed for upto 6 weeks and oral antibiotic therapy may continue for upto 6 months eg. ciprofloxacin and ofloxacin.
- Irrigation and drainage systems: This involves a surgical procedure in which holes are drilled into the cortex of the bone, allowing continuous infusion of antibiotic solution and drainage of inflammatory exudate. Drains are usually removed after a few days to prevent secondary infection.
- Analgesics and antipyretics as necessary.
- Hyperbaric oxygen therapy may be used as an adjunctive therapy.

When conservative modalities fail to control the infection, surgical intervention is indicated. Many types of surgery are possible from simple debridements to amputation.

Nursing management of patient with osteomyelitis includes the following:

- Using aseptic technique during dressing changes.
- Observing the patient for signs and symptoms of systemic infection.
- Encouraging range of motion exercises to prevent contrctures and flexion deformities.
- Administering antibiotics on time and as prescribed.
- Administering analgesics and/or antipyretics as prescribed and monitoring patient for effectiveness.
- Promoting rest of affected joint or limb. The affected limb should be handled carefully to avoid pathological fracure. Splints are often used for immobilization.
- Encouraging participation in ADL to fullest extent.
- Instructing the patient in correct use of assistive devices as needed.

In addition, patient/family education is to be given by the nurse regarding follow-up measures of treatment modalities.

LOW BACK PAIN

Low back pain (LBP) is one of the most common conditions a nurse will encounter in practical setting. Although a common disorder, LBP is also a challenge to health care professionals as the problem is worldwide.

Aetiology
Several risk factors are associated with low back pain, including lack of muscle tone and excess weight, poor posture, smoking and stress. Jobs that require repetitive heavy lifting, vibration (e.g. Jachammer operator) and prolonged period of sitting are also associated with LBP. Pain in the lumbar region is common problem because this area:

- bears most of the weight of the body.
- is the most flexible region of the spinal column.
- contains nerve roots that are vulnerable to injury or disease and
- has an inherently-poor biochemical structure.

Low back pain is most often due to musculoskeletal problem. However, other causes such as metabolic, circulatory, gynaecologic, urologic, or psychologic problems, which may refer pain to the lower back, must not be overlooked. The causes for low back pain of musculoskeletal origin include:

- Acute lumbosacral strain.
- Instability of lumbosacral bony mechanism.
- Osteoarthritis of the lumbosacral vertebrae.
- Intervertebral disk degeneration and
- Herniation of the intervertebral disk.

There are two varieties of low-back pain, i.e., acute low back pain and chronic low back pain.

Acute Low Back Pain

Acute low back pain is usually associated with some type of activity that causes undue stress on the tissues of the lower back. Often symptoms do not appear at that time of injury but develop later because of gradual increase in paravertebral muscle spasms. Few definitive diagnostic abnormalities are present with paravertebral muscle strain. The straight leg raise test may produce pain in the lumbar area without radiation along the sciatic nerve. If muscle spasms are not severe, the patient may be treated on outpatient basis with a combination of the following:

- Analgesics.
- NSAIDS.
- Muscle relaxants (cyclobenzaprine) and
- Use of corset. A corset prevents rotative, flexion and extension of lower back.

If spasms and pain are severe, a brief period of rest at home may be necessary. Since paravertebral muscle spasms are worse when the patient is upright, bed rest is the prime treatment for severe acute low back pain. Bathroom previliges are usually allowed. Bedrest is maintained until patient can move and turn from side to side with minimal discomfort. At this time, gradually increasing activity is initiated. When the patient is comfortable on oral pain medication, a progressive therapy program is begun to regain mobility and strength in lower back structures. If conservative treatment is ineffective, the cause of the pain is nerve root irritation, and epidural corticosteroid infection may be performed.

The nurse should assess the patient' use of body mechanics and offer advice when activities could produce back strains are used. Some 'Do nots' 'Dos' for low back problem are as follows:

Do nots

- Lean forward without bending knees.
- Lift anything above level of elbow.
- Stand in one position for prolonged time.
- Sleep on abdomen or on back or side with legs outstraight.
- Exceed prescribed amount and type of exercise without consulting health care provider.

Do

- Prevent lower back from straining forward by placing a foot on step or stool during prolonged standing.
- Sleep in a side-lying position, knees and hips bent.
- Sleep on back with a lift under knees.
- Sit on a chair with knees higher than hips and support arms on chair or knees.
- Exercise 15 minutes in the morning and 15 minutes in the evening regularly, begin exercises with a 2-or 3-minutes warm-up period by moving arms and legs, by alternately relaxing and tightening muscles, exercise slowly with smooth movements as directed by the physical therapist.
- Avoid chilling during and after exercising.
- Maintain appropriate body weight.
- Use a lumbar role or pillow for sitting.

Some exercises to strengthen the back as follows:

1. *Knee-to-chest lift* (to stretch hip, buttocks, lower back muscles).
   - Lie on back on the floor with knees bent and feet flat on floor.
   - Draw both knees upto chest.
   - Place both hands around knees and pull them firmly against chest. Hold for 30 seconds.
   - Lower legs and return to starting position.
   - Repeat 5-10 times.
2. *Simple leg lift*
   - Lie flat on back on floor with left knee bent and left foot flat on floor.
   - Raise right leg as high as comfortably as possible.
   - Hold for counting upto 5.
   - Slowly return leg to floor.
   - Bend right knee and put right foot flat on floor.
   - Raise left leg and hold for 5 counts.
   - Repeat 5-10 times for each leg.
3. *Double leg lift*
   Lie flat on back.
   - Slowly lift legs until feet are 12 inches from the floor.

- Keep legs straight and hold this position for counting upto 10.
- Lower legs to floor.
- Repeat five times.

4. *Pelvic tilt*
   - Lie flat on back on floor with knees bent and feet on the floor.
   - Firmly tighten your buttock muscles.
   - Hold for counting upto 5.
   - Relax buttocks.
   - Repeat 5-10 times.
   - Be sure to keep lower back flat against floor.
5. *Half sit-ups* (to strengthem abdominal muscles)
   - Lie flat on floor on back with knees bent, feet flat on floor and hand on chest.
   - Slowly raise head and neck to top of chest.
   - Reach both hands forward and place them on knees.
   - Hold for counting upto 5.
   - Return to starting position.
   - Repeat 5-10 times.
6. *Elbow Props* (to extend lower back)
   - Lie face down with your arms beside your body and your head turned to one side.
   - Stay in this position for 2-5 minutes, making sure that you relax completely.
   - Remain face down and prop yourself on your elbows.
   - Hold this position for 2-3 minutes.
   - Return to starting position and relax for one minute.
   - Repeat 5-10 times.
7. *Hip tilts*
   - Lie flat on back with knees bent.
   - Slowly bend legs and hips to one-side as far as possible.
   - Bend to other side.
   - Repeat five times.
8. *Toe touches*
   - Stand straight and relaxed.
   - Lower head and body and try to touch floor with finger tips.
   - Keep knees straight.
   - Do not jerk or lunge towards floor.
   - Bend only as far as you can.
   - Repeat the some for 5 times.

Chronic Low Back Pain

The causes of chronic low back pain include degenerative disk disease, lack of physical exercise, prior injury, obesity, structural and postural abnormalities, and systemic disease.

Pathophysiology

The pathophysiology includes common causes of back pain, such as herniated disc, spinal stenosis, and spondylolisthesis. If disk-herniation is the cause of back pain, the pain comes from the irritated dura and spinal nerves as the nucleus purposes lacks intrinsic innervation can arise from the joint capsule, ligaments, or muscles in the lumb spine. The ligamentous structures of the lumbar spine are richly supplied with pain receptors and are susceptible to tears, sprains and fracture. Muscle sprains and strains are also common causes of backpain.

Clinical Management

The most common feature of a lumbar herniated intervertebral disk in backpain with associated buttock and leg pain along with distribution of the sciatic nerve (radiculopathy). Specific manifestations based on the level of lumbar disk herniation which include:

- L3-L4- Subjective pain. Back to buttock to posterier thigh to inner calf.
- L4-L5- Subjective back to buttock to dorsum of foot and beg toe.
- L5-S1- Subjective back to buttock to sole of foot and heel.

Straight leg raise test may be positive. Back or leg pain may be reproduced by raising the leg and flexing the foot at 90 degrees. Reflex may be depressed or absent, depending on the spinal nerve root involved. Paresthesia or muscle weakness in the legs, feet, or toes may be reported by the patient. If the disk ruptures in the cervical area, the clinical manifestations are stiff neck, shoulder pain radiating to hand, and parasthesias and sensory disturbances of the hand.

Management of CLBP

Diagnosis made on the basis of the following:

- History and physical examination with emphasis on neurologic deficits and straight leg raising.
- CT Scan-MRI, myelogram, diskogram, EMG. Somatosensory evoked potential.

Degenerative disk disease is managed by conservatively with rest, limitation of spinal involvement (corset) local heat or ice, ultrasound, transcutaneous electrical nerve stimulation (TENS) and NSAIDS, analgesic muscle relaxants diathermy, thermotherapy, physical therapy. If conservative treatment is unsuccessful, radiculopathy becomes progressively worse, or there is documented loss of bowel or bladder control (Cauda equina), surgery may be indicated. The common surgical procedure includes:

- Laminectomy with or without spinal fusion.
- Diskectomy.
- Percutaneous lateral diskectomy.
- Spinal fusion with or without instrumentation.

Patients who have undergone spinal surgery require vigilant postoperative care. Nursing intervention is aimed at maintaining proper alignment of the spine at all times until healing has occurred.

- Flat bedrest may be maintained for 1 to 2 days depending on the extent of surgery.
- Logrolling patients when turning is essential to maintain proper body alignment.
- Pillows can be used under the thighs of each leg when supine and between the legs when in sidelying position to provide comfort and ensure alignment.
- Severe muscle spasms in the surgical area can be managed with medication and with correct turning and positioning.
- The nurse must offer reassurance to the patient that proper technique is being used to maintain body alignment.
- Watch for severe headache or leakage of CSF if it is so reported.
- Frequent monitoring of peripheral neurologic signs of the extremities is a routine postoperative nursing responsibility after spinal surgery. Movements of arms and legs and assessment of sensation be unchanged when compared with preoperative status.

The patient should be instructed to avoid sitting or standing for prolonged periods. Activities that should be encouraged include walking, lying down, and shifting weight from one foot to the other, when standing. The patient should learn to think through an activity before starting any potentially injurious task such as bending, lifting, or stopping. Any twisting movement of spine is contraindicated. A firm mattress or bedboard is essential.

Degenerative Disorders of Spine

Degenerative disease of the spine is a common but difficult problem. The spine has been intervertebral disk joints and 46 posterior facets joints. The intervertebral disks are composed of an outer layer of cartilage called the anulus fibrosus and an inner layer of the cartilage called "nucleus pulposure. Several common problems arise with the structures in degenerative disease of the spine. These include degenerative disc disease, herniated vertebral disk, spinal stenosis, spondylolisthesis and spondylosis.

Aetiology

Degenerative disc disease develops as a result of biochemical and biomechanical changes in the intervertebral discs. The gelationous mucoid material of the nucleus pulosus is replaced with fibrocartilage as a result of aging. Spinal stenosis, occurs as a result of aging, degenerative disc disease, spondylosis, oesteophyte formation or a congenial condition. The disc space is narrowed, losing its resiliency, and may be unstable at the affected levels. Smoking is a risk factor for the development of disc degeneration and herniation. Other risk factors include sedantary life style and extensive motor vehicle driving. Heredity plays a role in spondylosis, occurring more frequently in conjunction with other congenital spine defects.

Pathophysiology

Pathophysiological changes associated with degenerative disc disease include spinal stenosis (narrowing of the spinal canal), spondylosis (degeneraton and stiffness of the vertebral joints), subluxation and vertebral degeneration. Initial disc changes are followed by facet arthropathy, osteophyte formation and ligamentous instability, myelopathy osteophyte formation and ligamentous instability. Myelopathy and radiculospathy (disease involving a spinal nerve root) may follow. The degenerative process usually involves synovitis, which causes cartilage erosion, leading to the formation of osetophytes.

Herniated intervertebral disk is a protrusion of the nucleus purpose through a tear or rupture in the anulus. Herniation occurs anterior, posterior or laterally. Extrusion of the disk material may impinge on a nerve root or on the spinal cord. Herniation occurs in cervical spine (C-5-6, C-6-7), (C4-5), lumbar spine (L5-S1 and L-4-5) levels. It may be the result of trauma, sudden or sharp material or degeneration.

Spinal stenosis is narrowing of the spinal cord or intervertebral foramine at any level, creating pressure on the involved nerve root (s) resulting in neurological symptoms.

Spondyl olisthesis is a forward slipping of one vertebra on another. It can be a congenital abnormality or be caused by degenerative changes trauma or bone disease.

Clinical Manifestation

a. Herniated intervertebral disk shows following possible signs and symptoms.

Cervical

- Decreased range of motions of cervical spine.
- Paresthesia of upper extremities, depending on nerve root involved.
- Weakness or atrophy of upper extremity musculature, depending on level involved.
- Pain in affected nerve root distribution.
- Abdominal reflex activity.
- May have motor or sensory disturbances in lower extremities.

Lumbar

- Sciatica.
- Tenderness or pain with palpation of disk spaces and sciatic notch.
- Painful and/or decreased range of motion of lumbar spine.
- Motor and sensory impairment in affected nerve root distribution (may note discrepancies in calf circumference, weakness in lower extremity, muscle groups, pain and numbness in dermatomal distribution).
- Decreased or absent reflexes.
- Bowel or bladder impairment.
- Positive straight leg raising (Laseques test): Straight leg raising with opposite leg flat will produce a leg pain or radicular symptoms).

- Pain radiating down by in dermatomal distribution.
- Pain relieved by lying down.

Spinal stenosis resulting neurological symptoms. In spondylolisthesis, pain weakness and/or bowel and bladder involvement are seen. The slip may be detected when the spinous processes are palpated.

Management

Diagnostic tests to determine defects in the spine include X-Ray films, myelography, CT scanning, and MRI, Conservative management degenerative disorders of spine includes NSAIDS, avoidance of alcohol or aspirins (Leads to GI irritation and bleeding) and prolonged use of narcotic analgesics Risk of depending oral corticosteroids helps to relieve pain and skeletal muscle relaxants may be used if necessary.

SURGICAL MANAGEMENT

1. Postoperative Care of the Patient with Lumbar Spinal Surgery

a. Positioning
   - Head of the bed is kept flat.
   - Patient is encouraged to legroll to change position from side to back to side.
   - Use of turning sheet is advised until patient can assist with turning.

b. Neurological checks to assess motor and sensory functions.

c. Wound care (drain placed in wound to prevent haematoma formation SOS).
   - Maintain constant suction through drain as required.
   - Maintain drain free of contamination.
   - Monitor excessive output from drains. Output ranges from 20 to 250 ml/8 hours for the first 24 hours, tapers for 12 hours postoperatively and usually is removed 24 to 36 hours postoperatively. Drains that allow reinfusion of serous drainage may be used.
   - Inspect surgical area frequently for evidence of excess drainage or formation of haematoma (bulging of tissues surrounding surgical site).
   - If a spinal fusion has been done, inspect donor site (usually iliac crest) for drainage, haematoma.

d. Promoting comfort.
   - Reposition patient frequently.
   - Administer narcotic medications as needed; gradually reduce to non-narcotic analgesics as patient tolerates.
   - Monitor use and effectiveness of PCA pump if ordered.
   - Use fractured bedpan.

e. Promoting mobility.
   - Activity out of bed varies. Patient with fusion may need bedrest for 1 to 2 days.
   - Transfer patient out of bed with a little time spent in the sitting position as possible.
     - Start transfer with patient in a side-lying position at the edge of the bed.
     - Have the patient push off the bed with the uppermost hand and the lowermost elbow.
     - One person assists by guiding the patient's trunk and another assists the patient's leg, over the side of the bed.
     - Reverse process for return to bed.
   - The patient may be permitted to walk as much as tolerated with an assistive aid if necessary.
   - Braces or corsets, if prescribed, and applied before the patient gets out of bed.
   - Encourage patient to participate in ADL within prescribed limits of mobility.

f. Discharge instructions.
   - Do not lift or carry anything heavier than 2.25 kg (5 lb).
   - Do not drive a car until permitted by surgeon.
   - Avoid twisting motions of the trunk.

2. Postoperative Care of the Person with Cervical Surgery

a. Positioning
   - Keep head of bed elevated 30 to 45 degrees, particularly if anterior surgical approach was used, to decrease swelling in throat and facilitates respirtions.
   - If patient is cervical brace, position is not restricted except by patients tolerance.
   - If patient is in cervical traction, patient may be turned side to back to side to patient's tolerance.

b. Promoting safety
   - Assess airway and respiratory function frequently. Airway may be compromised by swelling.
   - Provide suction equipment and tracheotomy set in patient's room until swelling in throat subsides and patient is swallowing and breathing normally.
   - Check adjustment screws and straps frequently to ensure there is no loosening of the brace.
   - Advise physician or orthotist of loosening of the brace consequent to decrease in oedema, so brace can be readjusted.

c. Wound care
   - Inspect surgical areas, including iliac crest donor site, frequently for evidence of excess drainage or formation of haematoma. Use icebag to donor site for comfort.
   - If tong or halo traction is being used, pin care may be required.

d. Promoting comfort and reducing pain.
   - Provide ice chips to soothe sore throat.

- Make progressive diet changes slowly; patient will have difficulty in swallowing and will be afraid of smoking. Full liquids or semi-solids (ice cream, custards, jello, nectars) are often better tolerated than clear juice or broth; however, milk products may increase mucous production.
- Administer analgesics as for any patient having spine surgery. Donor sites often cause more discomfort than does neck incision.
- Patient may require aerosol treatment or humidifications of air to loosen mucus scretions or make breathing more comfortable.

e. Promoting mobility.
- If a patient is in traction, encourage patient to perform ankle dorsiplanar flexion exercises and quadriceps settign on a regular basis to promote circulation and maintain leg strength.
- If patient is in brace, out of bed activity, inducting walking, it may begin as soon as patient tolerates.
- Provide temporary use of walker if donor site pain restricts mobility.
- Encourage patient to participate in ADL to greatest extent possible.
- Report any difficulty with brace to physician immediately.
- Do not drive a car during period that brace must be worn.
- Report symptoms of graft dislodgingment (dysphagia and a feeling of "fulness" in the throat).

3. Postoperative Care of the Person with Thoracic Spinal Surgery

Same as for lumbar surgery with the following additions and exceptions.

a. Positioning
- Head of bed may often be elevated to 30 degrees.

b. Wound care
- If pleural cavity entered, a chest tube will be inserted and must be managed postoperatively.

c. Promoting comfort.
- Assist patient to splint chest while coughing.

d. Promoting mobility.
- Encourage and assist patient in vigorous pulmonary hygiene measures.
- Discourage patient from vigorous pulling or pushing with the arms because weight bearing through the arms poses a threat to the integrity of the graft.
- Brace is routinely prescribed and must be applied before patient is allowed out of bed.
- Permit patient to perform whatever activities are comfortable within the limitation of the brace.
- Encourage patient to participate in ADL within prescribed limits of mobility.

e. Discharge instructions.
- Apply and remove the brace before getting out of bed.
- Wear the brace whenever out of bed, assess skin under brace.

Complications associated with general anaesthesia and important consideration after surgery. These include complications such as atelectorsis, paralytic ileus, and urinary retention. Infection is a complication associated with the operative procedure. When instrumentation is used, the risk for infection increases. There is also a risk for hardware failures. Complication of the procedure, postoperative include dural tear, CSF leakage, blood loss, hypovolaemia, decreased cardiac output haematoma formation, infection, instruments or graft failure, pseudoarthosis loss of correction deformity, persistent pain, neurological problem, DVT pulmunary embolism, fluid volume overload, and fat embolism.

SCOLIOSIS

There were two types of scoliosis viz. nonstructural and structural.

1. *Nonstructural scoliosis* is also termed postural or functional and is caused by posture pain, leg length inequality and other factors. This form of scoliosis is usually easily corrected either by exercise or by removing the underlying causes. An important distinction is the absence of vertebral rotation. However, untreated nonstructural scoliosis can progress to structural scoliosis.
2. *Structural scoliosis* involves a rotational deformity of the vertebrae. It is further divided into three major categories.
   - Congenital scoliosis (Present at birth) occurs as a result of vertelbral malformation in foetal life (accounts for 15 per cent).
   - Neuromuscular scoliosis result as a consequence of several diseases.
   - Idiopathic scoliosis has an unknown cause but genetic factors have been lined to the development of disease.

Aetiology

i. Congenital

ii. Neuromuscular
- Cerebral palsy.
- Charcot-Marie - Tooth disease.
- Syringomyelia.
- Spinal cord injury.
- Poliomyelitis.
- Myelomenigocele.
- Muscular dystrophy.
- Neurofibromatosis.
- Marfan's syndrome.

iii. Idiopathic
- Infantile : 0 to 3 years of age.
- Juvenile : 3 to 10 years of age.
- Adolescent : older than 10 eyars of age.

Pathophysiology

Scoliosis may develop in localized areas of the spinal column or involve the whole spinal column. Curvatures may be 'S' Shaped or 'C' shaped. The earliest pathological changes begin in the soft tissues. Muscles and ligaments shorten on the concave side of the curve, progressing to deformities of the vertebrae and ribs. In skeletally immature persons, vertebral formations occur as asymmetrical forces are applied to the epiphysis by the shortened and tight soft tissues structures on the concave side of the curve.

Deformities are classified by magnitude, direction, location and aetiology. Curve direction is designated by the convex side or the curve. The degree of rotation of the curve is important, because, it determines the amount of impingement on the rib cage. The amount of compression and twisting depends on the position of the vertebrae in the curve. The force of compression is greatest on the apical vertebrae, which becomes the most deformed. Deformity progresses quickly-during skeletal growth and slows later in life, but the greater increase in the curfacture may occur in adult life. Gravity and increase in upper body weight may increase in the deformity in adulthood.

Clinical Manifestation

The person can initially have slight, mild, or severe deformity. Early deformity may not be obvious except on specific examination. In the early stages, the person may note that clothing does not fit correctly or hand evenly, because the height of shoulders is uneven. Pain is not usually an accompanying factor. Persons affected with structural scoliosis may exhibit asymmetry of hip height, pelvic obliquity (tilting of the pelvis from the normal horizontal positions; inequalities of shoulder height, scapular prominence; rib prominence; and rip humps which are posterior, unilateral humpings of rib cages visible on forward bending.

In severe cases, cardiopulmonary and digestive functions may be affected because of compression or displacement of internal organs. Total lung capacity, vival capacity and maximum voluntary ventilation are decreased in persons with scoliosis. Cardiac output may be compromised. Significant deviations in the balance of the curve may also affect gait patterns. Right thoracic, right thoracic and lumbar, and right thoracolumbar curves are most common or idiopathic scoliosis. A compensatory durve may develop, allowing the head to be centered over the pelvis. In general, compensatory curves are of less degree, more flexible and less rotated.

Management of Scoliosis

A complete radiological examination of the spine is performed, curve angles, flexibility and degree of vertebal rotation are calculated. Radiographs also help to determine skeletal maturity. In severe case, pulmonary function studies also indicated. Treatment of scoliosis depends on the individual patient and the degree of lateral curvature:

i. Early or postural scoliosis may be amenable to postural exercises or exercise combined with traction. Cotrelis traction which is a combination of a cervical head halter with 5 to 7 1b and pelvic traction with 10 to 20 1b may be used.
ii. When the curve is flexible (less than 40°) and the patient is cooperative, bracing in combinatioan with exercise may be sufficient to correct the deformity (e.g., Milwaukee brace, Rissar Caster, halofemoral or halopelvic traction). Maintaining the ideal weight is consideration in reducing the stress on the spine. The patient should be advised against weight gain, especially if bracing is prescribed, because the brace is specifically fitted and contoured to the individual. The brace can usually accomodate a 10 1b gain or loss.
iii. Transcutarean electrical muscle stimulation may be used to stimulate the muscle on the convex side of the curve. Repeated stimulation strengthens the muscle and pulls the spine into alignment. The patient usually uses the stimulator at night.

Surgery is indicated for patients when conservative treatment has failed to halt curve progression for those with severe progressing curves, intractible pain, or compromised pulmonary function or for cosmesis. Many individuals with neuromuscular scoliosis are unable to walk. Surgical corection sometiems performed in these patients to facilitate the ability to transfer or to increase sitting ability or tolerance. Surgical correction is usually involves a posterior approach to the spine with instrumentation and bony fusion. The complication of scoliosis fusion are similar to spinal surgery discussed earlier. Nursing management of the patient with scoliosis correction is similar to spinal surgery discussed earlier.

COMMON HAND AND FOOT PROBLEMS

Hand's Problem

Dupuytren's Contracture

Dupuytren's contracture is a progressive condition maked by hypertrophic hyperplasia of the Palmar fascia that results in a flexion of the distal palm and fingers.

The causes of this contracture is not known. A familar tendency has been noted. And it is associated with diabetes, epilepsy, alcoholism, penile lesions (Peyrobie's disease), and hyperplasia of the plantar fascia (Lederhoses disease). Pathophysiology of this is not completely understood the contracture may take upto 20 years to reach maximum deformity. Depends upon the severity of the deformity and hand dominance, the patient may experience difficulty in gasping objects. Burning pain may accompany attempts at grasping. Usually main complaints are deformity and mild interference with hand function.

Surgery is the preferred method of treatment. Persons with fixed flexion contractures of 30° or more at the metacorpophalangeal or proximal interphalangeal joints are persons for surgery. Surgical repair involves regional faciectomy or subtotal palmar fasciectomy to allow the patient full motion. Surgical repairs is performed as in outpatient procedure. The most common complication is haematoma and inadequate skin closure. The nursing intervention focuses on postoperative care which includes:

- Elevating hand to control swelling.
- Checking fingers for circulation, sensation and movement of every 1 to 2 hours.
- Administering prescribed analgesics as necessary to maintain comfort.
- Encouraging active extension of fingers.
- Encouraging patient to use hand in self-care activities after 2 to 3 days.

Foot Problem

The foot is the platform that provides support for the weight of the body and absorbs considerable shock in ambulations. It is a complex structure composed of bony structures, muscles, tendons and ligaments. It can be affected by congenital conditions; structural weakness; traumatic injuries; and systemic conditions Diabetes Mellitul, (D.M.), Rheumatid Arthritis (R.A.).

Forefoot

1. *Hallux valgus (Bunion)*

Hallux Valgus is the lateral angulation of the proximal phalanx on the metatarsal head of the great toe. It is a painful deformity of great toe consisting of great toe towards second toe, bony enlargement depending upon the degree of angulation, prominence of the medial eminence may occur resulting bunion deformity.

- Conservative treatment includes wearing shoes with wide forefeet or bunion pocket and use of bunion pads to relieve pressure on bursal sac and NSAIDS for pain relief.
- Surgical treatment is removal of bursal sac and bony enlargement and correction of lateral angulation of great toe may include temporary or permanent internal fixation.

2. *Hallux Rigidus* is a painful stiffness of first metatorso-phalangeal joint caused by osteoarthritis or local trauma.
   - Conservmative treatment includes intra-articular corticosteroids and passive manual stretching of first metatorsophalangeal joint. A shoe with a stiff sole decreases pain in the joint during walking.
   - Surgical treatment is joint fusion or arthoplasty with silicone rubber implant.

3. *Hammer toe*

It is the deformity of second through fifth toes including dorsiflexion of metatarsophalangeal joint, plantar flexion of proximal interphalangeal joint, and callu on dorsum of proximal interphalangeal joint and end of involved toe complaints related to hammer toe include burning of the bottom of foot and pain and difficulty in walking when wearing shoes.

- Conservative treatment consists of passive manual stretching of proximal interphalangeal joint and use of metatorsal arch support.
- Surgical correction consists of resection of base of middle phalanx and head of proximal phalanx and bring raw bone and together. Kirschner wire maintains straight position.

4. *Mortons neuroma (Mortons toe or plantar neuroma)*

It is neuroma in webspace between third and fourth metatorsal heads causing sharp, sudden attacks of pain and burning sensation. Surgical excision is usual treatment.

Midfoot

1. *Pes Planus* (flat foot) is a loss of metatarsal arch causing pain in foot or leg. Symptoms are relieved by use of resilient longitudinal arch supports. Surgical treatment consists of triple arthrodesis or fusion of subtular joint.
2. *Pes Cavus* is the elevation of the longitudinal arch of foot of arch. Treatment is manipulation and casting (in patients of younger than 6 years of age); Surgical correction is necessary if it interferes with ambulation (in patient older than 6 years of age).

Hindfoot

1. *Painful Heels* complaint of heel pain with weight bearing. Common cause plantar bursitis or calcaneal spur in adult. Treatment includes:
   - Cortecosteroids are injected locally into inflammed bursa and sponge rubber heel cushion is used.
   - Surgical excision of bursa or spur is performed.

Local problems

1. *Corn* is a localized thickening of skin caused by continual pressure over bones prominences, especially metatarsal head, frequently causing localized pain. Treatment incldues:
   - Corn is softened with warm water or preparation containing salicyl acid and trimmed with razor blade or scalpal. Pressure on bony prominences caused by shoes is relieved.
2. *Soft corn* is painful lesion caused by bony prominences of one toe pressing against adjacent toe; usual location in web space between toes, softness caused by secretions keeping web space relatively moist. Here pain is relieved by placing cotton between toes to separate them. Surgical treatment is excision of projecting bone spur (if present).

3. *Callus:* A similar formation to corn but covering of wider area and usual location on weight-bearing part of foot. Treatment is as for corn.
4. *Plantar Wart:* A painful papillomatus growth caused by virus that may occur on any part of the skin or sole of foot. Treatment is excision with electrocoagulation or surgical removal is done. Ultrasound may also be used.

Nursing management of common foot problems

Much of the pain, deformity and disability associated with foot disorders can be directly attributed to or accentuated by improperly fitting shoes. Which causes . . . . . . an angulation of the toes., and inhibition of the normal movement of foot muscles. The purposes of footwear are to:

- Provide support, foot stability, protection, shock absorptions and a foundation for orthosis.
- Increase friction with the walking surface and
- Treat foot abnormalities.

For which well-constructed and properly-fitted shoes are essential for healthy, pain-free, feet. Fashion styles especially for women often influence selection of footwear instead of consideration of comfort and support. Patient education should stress the importance of having shoe that comforms to the foot rather than to current fashion trends. To prevent feet problems good foot care is essential. Then education should be given to patient and family by the nurse concerned as follows;

In addition to recognizing common problems, there are many that the person can do to promote healthy feet and prevent feet problems; Nurse has to advise the person, that measures as follows:

- Walk regularly. This will improve circulation. Increase flexibility and encourage bone and muscle development. Walking is very important for maintaining over all foot health.
- Always wear comfortable shoes that provide proper support. The shoes should be sufficiently wide and have low enough heels so that person feels no leg fatigue, leg or foot cramps or pain.
- Advise to massage their (persons) feet to improve circulation and promote relaxation of the feet at least daily.
- If person (Patient) have bunions, wear shoes that are extra-long and wide, this will help ease pressure on thick toes. In addition, used donut-shaped bunion cushions, or (mole skin) to take pressure off of the joints.
- Wear heel pads or cushions in the bottom of their (affected persons) shoes to provide theri heels if they walk on hard surfaces for long times.
- Advise to wash their feet every day in warm water. Dry them by blotting with a towel, rather than rubbing.
- If their (affected persons) feet perspire a lot, ask them to dust their feet with talcum or hygienic foot powder. They may also sprinkle some powder into their shoes. Do not use cornscratch powder because it may lead to fungal infection.
- Advise them to trim their nails shortly after they have taken a bath or shower, while they are soft, cut the nail across with a toenail cliper.
- Advise them that they do not go barefoot outdoors especially in area that is not theirs own or a yard. A foreign body may cut or puncture their feet.
- Inspect themselves their feet every day against dust, blisters, and scratches. Provide care as needed and observe for proper heeling.

Many foot problems require surgery. When surgery is performed, the foot is usually immobilized by a bulky dressing shortly cast, slipper (plaster) cast, or a platform shoe that fits over the dressing and has a rigid sole (bunion foot). The foot should be elevated with the head off the bed to help reduce discomfort and prevent oedema. Neurovascular status should be assessed postoperatively and routine nursing intervention to be performed accordingly as in other similar surgery.

MUSCULOSKELETAL TUMOURS

Tumours may arise from any of the structures of the musculoskeletal system. The type of tumour is determined and classified by the tissue of origin. Tumours can be benign or malignant and can affect both adults and children. The common tumours of musculoskeletal system are:

1. *Bone*: Osteoma (benign), osteosarcoma (Malignant).
2. *Cartilage*: Osteochondroma, enchondroma, periosteal chondroblastomas are benign and chondrosarcomas malignant.
3. *Fibrous*: Fibroma (benign) fibrosarcoma (malignant).
4. *Bone Marrow*: Giant cell (benign). Ewing's sarcoma and myeloma are malignant.
5. *Uncertain cell*: Unicameral bone cyst, and aneurysmal bone cyst. Brief description of the common tumours are as follows:

   1. *Osteosarcoma* exhibits a moth-eaten pattern of bone destruction with poorly-defind margins. Osteoid and callus produced by the tumour invades and resorbs normal cortical bone. The tumour erodes through the cortex and periosteum and eventually invades soft tissue. Metastasis to the lungs is common. It mostly affects the long bones of the extremities and pelvis.

The clinical manifestation of oesteosarcoma are usually associated with a past history of minor injury and gradual onset of pain and selling especially line around the (knee of femur) initial complaint is often described as dull, aching, and intermittent, but the pain rapidly increases in intensity and duration. Night pain is common. Other frequent complaints include generalized malaise, anorexia and weight loss.

The diagnosis confirmed from biopsies, tissue specimen, elevation of serum alkaline, phosphates calcium levels, X-ray, CT Scan and MRI findings.

Treatment of surgical excision. Preoperative chemotherapy is used to decrease tumour size. Surgical excision (amputation) is the procedure, necessary depending on the size and location of the tumour.

2. *Osteochondroma* is characterized by
   - Compromise of cancellous bone with cartilaginous cap.
   - Develops during growth periods at metaphysis of bone.
   - Also appears in tendens.
   - May limit joint motion and may recur.

   Surgical excision is choice of treatment.
3. *Enchondroma* is characterized by
   - Destruction of cancellous bone.
   - Usually occurs in humerous or fingers.
   - Can cause pathological fracture.
   - May become malignant, especially in long bones or pelvis.

   Surgical excision with wide margin, if not amputation is the treatment.
4. *Chondrosarcoma.* The characteristics of chondrosarcomas include:
   - Usually affects persons 50-70 years of old.
   - Comprises 20 per cent of all bone tumours.
   - Affects males more than females.
   - Slow growing, insidious onset.
   - Most common in humerouses femur and pelvis.
   - Local pain, swelling.
   - May have palpable mass.
   - Serene persistent pain.
   - May infiltrate joint space and soft tissue.
   - May metastatize to lung tissue and may recur.

   Treatment: Surgical excision; amputation.
5. *Fibrosarcoma*
   - Usually affects persons 30-50 years old.
   - Affects females more than males.
   - Occurs in bony fibrous tissue of femur and tibia.
   - Comprises 4 per cent of primary malignant bone tumour.
   - May result from radiation therapy, paget's disease or chronic.

   -osteomyelitis.
   - Night pain, swelling possible palpable mass.
   - May cause pathological fracture.
   - May metastaxises to lungs.

   Treatment: wide surgical excision, amputation.
6. *Gaint Cell Tumour* (osteoclastoma)
   - Usually affects ages 20-40 years.
   - Affects females more than males.
   - Comprises 4-5 per cent of all benign bone tumours.
   - Appears in epiphysical area, destroys bone matrix and can invade soft tissues.
   - Commonly found in femur, tibia or humerus.
   - Dull aching night pain.
   - Limitation of motions.
   - Swelling.
   - High incidence of recurrence.

   Treatment: Wide excision; May require bone graft and amputation.
7. *Myeloma, Multiple Myeloma (Multifocal)*
   - Poor prognosis
   - Common in persons 40 years above.
   - Affects males more than females.
   - Comprises 27-1 bone tumours.
   - Neoplastic proliferation of plasma cells.
   - Causes cortical and medullary bone lysis and infiltrates bone marrow.
   - Aching, intermittent pain in spine, pelvis, ribs, or sternum.
   - Pain increased with weight-bearing.
   - May complain of weight loss, malaise, anorexia.
   - Causes pathological fracture.

   Treatment: Palliative treatment. Radiation, Chemotherapy.
8. *Osteoma*
   - Usually affects persons of 10-20 years old.
   - Comprises 20 per cent of benign tumour of bone.
   - Slow growth.

   Treatment is only symptomatic and then excision.

MUSCLE TUMOURS

1. *Leiomyoma*
   - Affects smooth muscles, usually uterus, there will be palpable mass and tenderness. Treated by surgical excision.
2. *Rhabdomyoma* is rare, affects straightened muscle, cause tenderness. Usually treated by surgical excision.
3. *Leomyosarcoma* affects smooth muscle, usually uterus, stomach and small bowel. This radical growth treated by surgical excision with wide margin and radiation and chemotherapy are also used.
4. *Rhabdosarcoma* affects straightened muscle, usually inguinal, popliteal or gluteal areas. There is slow-growing mass and tenderness, treated with radiation, surgical excision and chemotherapy.

NURSING MANAGEMENT OF BONE TUMOUR

The patient with bone tumour should be assessed for the location and severity of pain. Weakness caused by anaemea and increased debility may be noted. Swelling at the involved site and decreased joint function depending on the tumour site should also be monitored. The possible nursing diagnosis for these patients include:

- Pain related to the disease process, inadequate pain medication or comfort measures.
- Impaired physical mobility related to disease process, pain, weakness and debility.
- Body image disturbance, related to possible amputation, deformity, swelling and effects of chemotherapy.
- Anticipatory grieving related to poor prognosis of the disease.
- Risk for injury (Pathological fracture) related to diseased process and inadequate handling or positioning of the effected body parts.

Nursing care planning and implementation are taken accordingly on the basis of nursing diagnosis in addition to routine preparation and assistance.

(Please refer to Oncological Nursing Chapter).

METABOLIC BONE DISEASES

Normal bone metabolism is dependent on adequate intake, absorption and use of calcium, phosphorous, protein, and vitamins. When there is dysfunction in any of these critical factors, generalized reduction of bone marrow may result. Metabolic bone diseases affect the normal haemeostatic functioning of the skeletal system. The aetiology of metabolic bone diseases include hormonal, genetic and dietary factors. Common metabolic bone diseases include rickets, osteomalacia, osteoporosis, oesteitis, deforman (Paget's disease).

Osteomalacia

Osteomalacia is an uncommon disorder of adult bone associated with vitamin D deficiency, resulting in decalcification and softening of bone. This disease is the same as rickets in children, except that epiphysical growth plates are closed in the adult. Vitamin is required for the absorption of calcium from the intestines. Insufficient vitamin D intake can interfere with the normal minimalization of the bone causing failure or insufficient calcification of bone, which results in softening of bone pain and deformities.

Aetiology

Aetiological factors development of oesteomalacia include lack of exposure to ultraviolet rays, gastrointestinal malabsorption, extensive burns, chronic diarrhoea, pregnancy, kidney disease, medication such as phenytoin (Dilantin).

Clinical Manifestation

- Persistent skeletal pain, especially while bearing weight.
- Low back pain.
- Progressive muscular weakness.
- Weight loss.
- Progressive deformities of the spine (kyphosis) or extremities.
- Fractures are common and demonstrate delayed healing when they occur.
- Decreased serum calcium or phosphorus.
- Elevated serum alkaline phosphates.
- X-rays demonstrate the effects of generalized bone demineralization especially calcium in the bone of thc pelvis and pressure associated with bone deformity.
- Looser's transformation zones (ribbons of recalcification in bone found on X-ray.

Management

Collaborative care for osteomalacia is directed towards corrections of the underlying cause. Vitamin D (Cholecalciferol) is usually supplemented, and the patient often shows a dramatic response, calcium or phosphorus intake may also be supplemented.

Paget's Disease (Osteitis Deformans)

Sir James Paget, an English surgeon first described this disorder also called 'osteitis deformans. It is skeletal bone disorder in which there is excessive bone resorption followed by replacement of normal marrow by vascular, fibrous connective tissue, and new bone that is larger, disorganized and weaker.

Aetiology

The aetiology of Paget's disease is unknown. But genetic predisposition is identified in 15 to 30 per cent. Probably a autosomal dominant pattern of inheritance. And other causative theories include autoimmune dysfunction vascular disorder, vitamin D deficiency in childhood, and mechanical stressors to bone. It may be due to viral infection. The Average age (50 to 60 years). It occurs most often after the fourth decade of life and most commonly in men.

Pathophysiology

The axial skeleton is usually affected by Paget's disease, particularly the vertebrae and skull, although the pelvis, femur and tibia are the common sites of disease. Initial changes in this disorder involve an increase in osteoclast-mediated resorption of cancellous bone, in addition to an increase in osteoblast-mediated bone formation. Bone resorption and formation are increased, resulting in mosaic-like mix of abnormal women and normal lamellar bone. Mineralization may encroach into the marrow and excessive bone formation usually occurs around partially resorbed trabeculae, causing thickening and hypertrophy. Vascularity is increased at affected portions of the skeleton.

Lesions may occur in one or more bones, but the disease does not spread bone to bone. Deformities and bony enlargements often occur. Deformities of bone caused by unexplained abnormal focal remodelling with structurally uneven bone. As stated earlier, the region of the skeleton commonly affected are the pelvis, long bones, spine, ribs, sternum and cranium. Bowing of the limbs and spinal curvature may occur in persons with advanced disease.

Clinical Manifestation

In milder forms of Paget's disease, patients may remain free of symptoms and the disease may be discovered incidentally on X-ray or serum chemistry.

The initial clinical manifestations are usually insidious development of skeletal pain (which may progress to severe intractible pain), complaints of fatigue, and progressive development of a waddling pain. Patients may complain that they are becoming shorter or that their heads are becoming larger.

Bone pain is the most common symptom. Degenerative arthritis may occur at adjacent joints. Microfractures, cortical swelling, and lytic bone lesions contribute to the pain. Pain is usually worse with ambulation or activity, but may also occur at rest. Involved bones may feel spongy and warm due to the increased vascularity. Weight-bearing bones such as tubia and femur may become deformed and pressing gait will be affected.

Skull pains usually accompanied by headache, warmth tenderness and enlargement of the head. Flattening of the base of the skull or platybasia may result in serious complication of the obstructive hydrocephalus or brain stem compression. Facial bone involvement may cause deformity or less frequently affect the airway. Conductive and/or sensori-neural hearing loss may develop due to otosclerosis or neurological abnormalities.

Pathological fractures are a problem, because of the increased vascularity of invovled bone, bleeding is potential danger. Lytic lesions of the long bones are the most susceptible to fracture.

Long-standing disease may lead to malignate transformation usually osteosarcoma, fibrosarcoma, and benign giant cell tumour. Most common sites for malignancy are the pelvis, femur and humerous.

Features of Paget's Disease and the Bone

Musculoskeletal Manifestation:

- Bone and joint pain (may be in a single bone) that is aching, poorly described, and aggraved by walking.
- Low back and sciatic nerve pain.
- Loss of normal spinal curvature.
- Enlarged, thick skull.
- Pathological fracture.
- Osteogenic sacroma.

Skin Manifestation:

- Flushed, warm skin.

Other manifestation.

- Apathy, lethargy and fatigue.
- Hyperparathyroidism.
- Chronic calcium deficiency
- Urinary or renal stones.
- Heart failure from fluid overload.

Laboratory Finding

- Elevated levels of alkaline phosphates due to osteoblastic activity
- Serum calcium usually normal except with generalized disease immediately.

Management of Paget's Disease

Radiography of individual with Paget's disease will reveal radio-lucent areas in the knee, typical fo increased bone resorption. Deformities and fractures may also be present. A bone scan is indicated at diagnosis to determine the extent of disease.

Management of Paget's disease is usually limited to sympatomatic and supportive care and correction of secondary deformities by either surgical implementation or braces. The goals of treatment are to relieve pain and prevent fractures and deformity. Asymptomatic patient generally does not require treatment.

Bone resorption, relief of actute symptoms, and lowering the serum alkaline phosphatase levels may be significantly influenced by administration of *calcitonin*, which inhibits the osteoclastic activity. Biphosphonates such as alendronates (Posamax) tiludronate (Skelid), risedronate (Actonel), and pamidronate (aredia) are nonhormonal agents are effective in reducing the bone resorption. The biphosphonates and calcitonin are effective agents and effective in reducing the bone resorption. The biphosphonates and calcitonin are effective agents to decrease bone pain and bone warmth, and may analgesic and NSAIDs also be in practice.

Radiation therapy and local surgical procedures such as periosteal stripping may be used for the control of the patient's pain.

A firm mattress should be used to provide back support and to releive pan. The patient may be required to wear a corset or light brace to relieve back pain and provide support when in the upright position. The patients should be proficient in the correct application of such devices knowhow to regularly examine areas of the skin for friction damage. Activities such as lifiting and twisting should be discouraged. Good body mechanics are essential. Analgesics and muscle relaxants may be administered to relieve pain. A properly-balanced nutritional program is important in the management of metabolic disorders of bone, especially pertaining to vitamin D, calcium and protein, which are necessary to ensure the availability of the components for bone formation. Preventive measures such as patient education, use of assistive device, and environmental changes should be actively pursued to prevent falls and subsequent fractures.

OSTEOPOROSIS

Osteoporosis or porous bone is a condition characterized by low bone mass and structural deterioration of bone tissue, leading to increased bone fragility. This metabolic bone disease is the major cause of fractures (especially hip, spine and wrist) in postmenopausal women and older adults in general.

Aetiology

The exact aetiology of osteoporosis is unknown, several risk factors have been identified as follows.

i. Aging: Osteoporosis is increasing in incidence, because more people are getting into an older age, usually occurs at over 65 years of age in both sex.
ii. Sex: Osteoporosis is eight times more common in women than men for several reasons:
   - Women tend to have lower calcium intake than men throughout their lives.
   - Women have less bone mass because of their generally smaller frame.
   - Resorption begins at an earlier age in women and is accelerated at menopause.
   - Pregnancy and breastfeeding depletes a woman's skeletal reserve unless calcium intake is adequate and
   - Longevity increases the likelihood of osteoporosis and women live lower than men.
iii. White race: Caucasian or Asian-American.
iv. Family history of osteoporosis.
v. Nulliparity.
vi. Diet low in calcium: Chronic calcium deficiency and vitamine D deficiency.
vii. Sedentary lifestyle: An inactive lifestyle.
viii. Small frame, low body weight. Thin and small-framed.
ix. Diet high in protein and fat.
x. Excessive use of alcohol: Chronic alcohol use.
xi. Excessive caffeine intake.
xii. Excessive cigarette smoking.
xiii. Postmenopausal including early or surgically-induced menopause.
xiv. History of anorexia, nervosa or bulimia, chronic liver disease or malabsorption.
xv. Long-term use of corticosteroids, thyroid replacement and antiseizure medications.

Osteoporosis is redefined as Type I (Postmenopausal) and Type II and further classified as primary or secondary. *Primary*, osteoporosis is the more common form; has no underlying pathological condition. *Secondary* osteoporosis results from another cause or medical condition. The causes of secondary osteoporosis are as follows:

i. Endocrine disorder: Diabetes, Cushing syndrome, hyperparathyroidism, parathyroidism, hypogonadism, prolactinoma.
ii. Rh. Arthritis drug-induced: Glucocorticoids, heparin, chronic use of phosphate binding antacids, loop diuretics, anticonvulsants, barbiturates, lithium and chemotherapy.
iii. Disuse: Prolonged immobilization (Prolonged bedrest, immobilization of limb by casting or splinting), paraplegia, Quadriplegia and lower motor neuron disease.
iv. Chronic illness: Sarcoidosis, cirrhosis, renal tubular acidosis.
v. Cancer: Multiple myeloma, lymphoma, leukaemia.
vi. Malabsorption syndrome.
vii. Anorexia nervosa.
viii. Prolonged parenteral nutrition.
ix. Alteration in gastrointestinal and hepatobiliary functions.

Pathophysiology

Bone is continually being deposited by osteoblasts and resorbed by osteoclasis, a process called remodelling. Normally, the rate of bone deposition and resorption are equal to each other. So, the total bone mass remains constant. i.e., in the process of normal bone remodelling, bone formation equals bone resorption. An osteoporotic state develops if bone resorption exceeds bone formation (bone deposition). Age-related bone loss begins in both sexes approximately at the age 40 years. Women experience a 35 to 40 per cent loss in trabecular bone and upto 60 per cent of cancellous bone stores, in contrast; men lose only about two-third of that amount throughout life. By the time a person reaches the age of 75 years, the skeletal mass is reduced 50 per cent. From age 30 level, the skeleton continues to lose bone mass at the hip and appendicular skeleton, even after the age of 80 years. Although resorption affects entire skeletal system, osteoporosis occurs most commonly in the bones of the spine, hips and wrists.

Overtime, wedging and fractures of the vertabrae produce gradual loss of height and a humped back known as dowager's hump or khyposis. The usual first signs are back pain or spontaneous fractures. The loss of bone substance causes the bone to become mechanically weakened and prone to either spontaneous fractures from minimal traumas.

Clinical Manifestation

Osteoporosis is often called the "silent thief" and the silent disease, because bone loss occurs without symptoms. People may not know they have osteoporosis until their bones become so weak that a sudden strain, bump, or fall causes a hip, vertebral or waist fracture.

Many fractures related to osteoporosis occur without the patient's knowledge, although some are associated with excrutiating pain. The earliest manifestation of oesteoporosis may be an acute onset of back pain in the mid to low thoracic region as a result of vertebral fracture, occurring at rest with minimal activity. Vertebral fracture can involve the entire vertebrae (compression) or portion, usually the anterior section (wedge). Anterior compression fracture of thoracic vertebrae may cause "dowager's hump" or thoracic khyphosis. Loss of height and protruding abdomen (due to pressure on abdominal viscera) are associated with conditions. Eventually lower rib cage may rest on iliac crest, paravertebral muscle spasm often occurs, but neurological deficits are rare with spontaneous vertebral compression. These postural changes may affect exercise tolerance and food tolerance. The patient will report early satiety and bloatedness. The patient's body image may also be affected as a result of the spinal deformity and collapsed vertebrae may initially be manifested back pain, loss of height, or spinal deformation such as kyphosis or severely stooped posture. Later on, distal radial fractures (Colles' fracture), fracture of the proximal femur and osteoporotic hip fracture occur.

Management

The risk for fracture can be assessed by the patient's risk factors and history and measured precisely with non-invasive diagnostic tools. Measurements of bone mineral deficiency (BMD) and biochemical markers of bone resorption are the basic tools for diagnosis of oesteoporosis.

The goal of pharmacological therapy for persons with osteoporosis is to prevent further bone loss and to decrease risk of fractures which includes:

- Calcium supplements.
- Vitamin D supplements
- Diet high in calcium.
- Exercise program. All four arm/leg lifts, the elbow prop. prone press-ups with deep breathing, standing back band, Isometric posture corrections. Standing and pelvic tilt.
- Oestrogen replacement therapy.
- Calcitonin.
- Biphosphonates-Etidonate (Didronel), Alendronate (Fosamax).
- Raloxifene (Evista).

Surgical intervention is necessary to repair some fractures.

Table 10.1: Nursing care plan for the patient with multisystems trauma: thoracic, abdominal and long bone (orthopaedic)

Problem	*R*	*Objective*	*Nursing Interventions*	*Rationales*
Nursing Diagnosis #1				
Alteration in tissue perfusion related to: 1. Hypovolaemia, 2. Impaired blood supply, and/or 3. Vascular compromise from fracture.		Patient will maintain: 1. Skin temperature, colour, and moisture—pink, warm, and dry. 2. Capillary refill of more than two seconds. 3. Normal neurovascular assessment of extremities: Sensorimotor function intact. 4. Urinary output of 30-50 ml per hour.	• Perform patient assessment and monitoring (includes ABCs with C-spine, and haemorrhage control). • Perform "mini" neuro exam (Glasgow Coma Score, and pupils). • Note vital signs (including temperature) at frequent intervals (every 15 minutes unless patient condition dictates more frequent vitals, than every 1-5 minutes). • Perform capillary refill checks with vital signs. • Assess neurovascular function of immobilized extremity (pain, pulse, pallor, puffiness, paralysis, paresthesias).	• Complete patient assessment and monitoring aids the nurse in discovering overt/covert changes in patient status at frequent intervals in those with multisystem trauma. • Early recognition of these changes results in timely care and the appropriate interventions to decrease trauma patient morbidity and mortality. • Reflects status of tissue perfusion.
Nursing Diagnosis #2				
Impaired gas exchange related to: 1. Disruption of alveolar-capillary membrane. 2. Decreased tissue perfusion, and/or		Patient will maintain: 1. Arterial blood gases: • $PaO_2 > 80$ mmHg (room air) • $PaCO_2$ 35-45 mmHg; pH 7.35-7.45.	• Ensure patent airway via appropriate route (chin lift, jaw thrust, without neck hyperextension). • Provide high flow oxygen at 6-10 liters/minute (use mask or cannula, or oral or nasal adjuncts).	• Establishing a patent airway provides the initial route for adequate intake of oxygen. • Oxygen delivery in the proper amount via the appropriate method assists in the maintenance of adequate tissue oxygenation.

Contd...

Problem	*R*	*Objective*	*Nursing Interventions*	*Rationales*
3. Other complication (e.g., fat emboli).		2. Minimum pulmonary function: • Tidal volume > 7-10 ml/kg • Vital capacity > 15 ml/kg 3. Cardiac output of 4-8 liters/minute. 4. Respiratory rate of 12-20/minute, eupnete. 5. SvO_2 within normal limits.	• Give ventilatory support as needed FIO_2 of 100 per cent (endotracheal or nasotracheal intubation; cricothyrotomy or tracheotomy, if indicated, for obstructed airway).	
			• Monitor serial arterial blood gases (ABGs) per physician.	• Serial blood gas measurements accurately reflect gas exchange requirements in impaired patients with decreased tissue perfusion.
			• Obtain serial chest x-rays per physician.	• Serial chest x-rays provide for ongoing monitoring for potential or missed lung injury (i.e., pulmonary contusion).
			• Cover suckling or open cheat wounds.	• Covering sucking or open wounds provides for more effective gas exchange until the defect can be repaired.
			• Observe for tension pneumothorax.	
Nursing Diagnosis #3 Fluid volume deficit related to: 1. Blood loss.		Patient will maintain: 1. Wedge pressure (PCWP) of 8-12 mmHg. 2. Systolic B/P of > 100 mmHg (including orthostatic B/P). 3. Pulse pressure of > 30 mmHg. 4. Strong, palpable peripheral pulses of 2+ bilaterally. 5. No external bleeding noted. 6. Normal skin turgour. 7. Level of consciousness: Alert, awake, and oriented × 3. 8. Absence of signs of internal bleeding (haematochezia, perlumbilical ecchymoses).	• Control external bleeding with direct pressure.	• Controlling external bleeding prevents exsanguinating haemorrhage—direct pressure is the best method.
			• Position patient in Trendelenburg if not contraindicated.	• Trendelenburg aids in venous return to augment B/P. Contraindicated in possible head injury, impedes blood flow from cranium.
			• Assess for signs of occult bleeding frequently (i.e., rigid abdomen, stools for guaiac).	• Assessment for occult bleeding is necessary to prevent missed injuries and to note the changing status of the patient.
			• Start IVs with large bore 14-16 gauge needles; crystalloids, colloids, and blood may be administered. ♦ Fluid replacement therapy: – Crystalloids: 3 ml/1 ml blood loss. – Blood: 1 ml/1 ml blood loss.	• Large bore IVs with crystalloids, colloids, and/or blood help replace fluid volume deficit.
			• Assist with cutdowns or central lines as needed.	• Cutdowns or central venous lines provide quick fluid access to central circulation.
			• Prepare for autotransfusion if indicated with chest injuries.	• Autotransfusion provides an immediate autologous blood transfusion to the patient.
			• Consider use of antishock garment (controversial). Monitor response: Blood pressure in hypotension; assess trouser pressure in bleeding: monitor ventilatory response as pressure over abdomen can compromise chest excursion.	• Antishock trousers enhance peripheral resistance, perform arterial tamponade, promote shunting of blood to vital organs, and splint fractures to decrease blood loss.
			• Splint and immobilize extremities, prevent gross movement.	• Immobilization of fractures prevents further haemorrhage; reduces risk of fat emboli.
			• Provide haemodynamic monitoring for critical patients.	• Haemodynamic pressure monitoring assists in determining fluid requirements in patients with fluid volume deficit.
			• Monitor serial haematocrits (as physician).	• Serial Hets determines the amount of packed red cells found in the blood.
Nursing Diagnosis #4 Alteration in cardiac output (decreased) related to:		Patient will maintain: 1. Normal electrocardiogram.	• Obtain 12-lead electrocardiogram (per physician).	• 12 lead-ECG provides baseline electrocardiographic data.

Contd...

Problem	R	Objective	Nursing Interventions	Rationales
1. Haemorrhage shock. 2. Cardiac injury.		2. Heart sounds S1 and S2 normal without extra sounds. 3. Cardiac output of 4-8 liters/minute. 4. Normal skin temperature, colour, and moisture (as noted above). 5. Pulse rate of 60-100 beats/minute. 6. Signs of adequate tissue perfusion (e.g., brisk capillary refill).	• Perform continuous ECG monitoring. • Consider antishock garment (controversial) • Monitor haemodynamic status to titrate fluids (see Nursing Diagnosis #3, above). • Obtain serial labwork (Hgb, Hct, chemistrics, and enzymes).	• Continuous EKG monitoring is performed to note potential cardiac dysrhythmias since they are a complication of impaired gas exchange and alteration in cardiac output. • Antishock garment enhances peripheral resistance (see Nursing diagnosis #3, above). • Haemodynamic monitoring defects status of cardiopulmonary function and measures cardiac output. • Maintaining haematocrit within normal range assures tissue oxygenation.
Nursing Diagnosis #5 Impaired skin integrity related to: 1. Open wounds from fractures. 2. Penetrating trauma. 3. Abrasions, contusions, lacerations, oedema, or 4. Eurovascular compromise.		Patient will maintain: 1. Absence of bacterial infection and secondary infections. 2. Intact skin surfaces. 3. Proper wound healing and reduced inflammatory response. 4. Absence of sepsis or other systemic reactions. 5. Body temperature at baseline: 98.6°F (37°C).	• Stabilize all impaled objects prior to operative removal. • Cleanse and irrigate all open wounds with solution of choice. • Cover all open wounds with sterile dressings. Perform sterile dressing changes as needed. Note amount, colour, and consistency fo drainage from wounds. • Cover "sucking" wounds with impregnated (petroleum jelly) gauze. • Provide antibiotic therapy as ordered (IV, IM, or oral). ◆ Obtain specimens for culture and sensitivity (as appropriate). • Give tetanus toxoid or tetanus immunoglobulin (per physician). • Turn and position q2hr; range of motion exercises (as indicated).	• Stabilization of impaled objects prevents further injury. • Cleansing and irrigation of open wounds removes debris and decreases bacteria, which cause infection. • Covering wounds maintains sterile environment. • Covering sucking wounds with impregnated gauze temporarily restores skin integrity and may reduce chest wall defect. • Antibiotic therapy inhibits and/or kills microorganisms and the growth of anaerobic gram-positive and gram-negative organisms. • Tetanus toxoid and tetanus immune globulin prevent tetanus. • Maximizes perfusion, reduces risk of thrombophlebitis and pressure ulcer in immobilized patient.
Nursing Diagnosis #6 Impaired physical mobility related to: 1. Chest, abdominal, and/or long bone trauma.		Patient will: 1. Demonstrate mobility to pre-injury capacity, or to optimal level of restored function.	• Remove all constrictive clothing and jewelry. • Splint and immobilize all extremities above and below joints. • Provide gait training and crutches during limited mobility. • Assist with cast, traction, pin, and/or fixator application if indicated. • Encourage early ambulation in multisystem trauma patients.	• Removing constrictive clothing and jewellery provides for enhanced mobility and increased circulation to promote healing. • Immobilization and splinting allow for increased mobility and the prevention of further injury. • Proper gait training prevents injury, a nd crutch-walking provides a method of early ambulation in patients with long bone trauma. • Casting, pin insertion, external and/or internal fixators, and/or traction promote alignment of bone, restore tissue function, and increase circulation to the affected area to promote healing. • Early ambulation prevents other complications (i.e., pulmonary).

Contd...

Problem	*R Objective*	*Nursing Interventions*	*Rationales*
Nursing Diagnosis #7 Alteration in comfort (pain) related to: 1. Tissue, nerve, or vessel disruption from penetrating, blunt, or extremity trauma.	Patient will: 1. Verbalize that pain is diminished or that pain relief has occurred (if conscious). 2. Display relaxed musculature, no facial grimace, and minimal signs of combativeness.	• Provide position of comfort for patient as permitted by patient's clinical status. • Provide pain medication via proper route and monitor response. • Use other pain reduction techniques if alternative therapy indicated (biofeedback, TENS, distraction and guided imagery). • Splint and immobilize all injured extremities. • Cover all wounds.	• Providing position of comfort for patients in pain may alleviate or reduce discomfort. • Pain medication binds to receptor sites, which function to reduce perception of pain. • Pain reduction techniques alter pain perception and/or sensation. • Splinting of injured extremities brings about immobilization, which reduces oedema, restores circulation and therefore tissue perfusion, to reduce or eliminate pain. • Dressings to wounds decrease pain to the injured site and reduce risk of infection.
ursing Diagnosis #8 Alteration in elimination (bowel or urinary) related to: 1. Decreased circulating volume. 2. Associated hyperfusion from multisystem organ failure, gastrointestinal injury, or renal trauma.	Patient will maintain: 1. Urinary output of 30-50 ml/hour (ml/kg). 2. Urine specific gravity of 1.010-1.025. 3. Normal colour, amount, consistency of urine. 4. Decreased gastric distention. 5. Expected nasogastric drainage (if NG tube is in place). 6. Abdomen, soft and nontender. 7. Normal bowel sounds, bowel movement if appropriate.	• Insert continuous urinary drainage catheter. Monitor urinary output. Note colour, amount, consistency, and specific gravity. • Insert nasogastric or orogastric tube. • Monitor gastric drainage (to suction if indicated). • Note colour, amount, and consistency of drainage.	• Continuous urinary drainage allows for monitoring of potential alterations in urinary and/or renal function. • Continuous gastric drainage allows for monitoring of gastrointestinal function and potential bleeding; decompressed stomach allows for full chest excursion and lung expansion; minimizes risk of aspiration in patients with an altered level of consciousness.
Nursing Diagnosis #9 Knowledge deficit related to: 1. Lack of information regarding injury or illness.	Patient/family comprehends treatment regimen through verbalization and resultant compliance in self-care.	• Assess for readiness of the learner(s). • Provide for patient and family education. • Give one-to-one teaching regarding specific aspects of care. • Teach to level of patient/family.	• Assessing for learner readiness provides information as to the patient/family level of comprehension. • Patient/family education may promote an understanding of the injury and therefore greater acceptance and compliance with treatment regimens. • One-to-one teaching may result in enhancing absorption of information and reinforcement. • Teaching to the level of the patient allows for greater retention and understanding.
Nursing Diagnosis#10 Ineffective coping patterns (patient and/or family or significant others) to stress of trauma.	Patient/family will: 1. Exhibit effective coping mechanisms. 2. Verbalize feelings. 3. Identify/access support systems (persons, institutions, associations).	• Assess for life-threatening injury or illness and/or patient and family perceptions of such illness. • Communicate and develop trusting relationship with patient/family.	• Assessing for life-threatening injuries may assist in relating patient prognosis information to patient/family, and clarifying patient's overall clinical status. • Development of a trusting relationship increases communication thereby giving clear messages to the client.

Contd...

Problem	*R*	*Objective*	*Nursing Interventions*	*Rationales*
		4. Identify past coping mechanisms that have been successful. 5. Be able to set short-term goals and objectives. 6. Eventually be able to set long-term goals, and a plan of action for the future. Anxiety reaction, if present, will be appropriate to crisis or event.	• Act as patient/family advocate. • Encourage patient/family to verbalize feelings. • Assist patient/family to identify past-coping mechanisms. • Help patient/family define immediate areas where decision-making is involved. • Provide emotional and verbal support during crisis. • Involve patient/family in as many decisions as possible (includes care activities, short and long-term decisions). • Encourage the development of new coping mechanisms where past mechanisms have proven ineffective for problem-solving. • Initiate referral system as needed.	• Acting as patient/family advocate may assist in patient support. • Verbalization of feelings encourages dealing with perceptions about the injury, and known/unknown fears. • Identifying past coping mechanisms may help in knowing which techniques were helpful. • Patient/family participation is imperative for future well-being and overall health care management. • Providing emotional support during crisis may decrease anxiety. • Involving patient/family in decisions about care allow them to assume responsibility for actions and promotes dignity and patient self-esteem. • Encouraging the use of new coping methods may strengthen patient/family and assist them in identifying effective coping mechanisms. • Utilization of a referral system (social service, pastoral care, psychological counseling) will be of significance in planning total, comprehensive, holistic patient care during acute phase, and rehabilitation.
Nursing Diagnosis#11 Alteration in nutritional status, decreased from multisystem trauma.		Patient will maintain: 1. Adequate nutritional intake via oral, IV, and/or parenteral or enteral route (reguular diet or diet to tolerance). 2. Positive nitrogen balance will be achieved. 3. Normal serum electrolytes: • Potassium 3.5-5.0 mEq/liter • Sodium 135-145 mEq/liter • Chloride 100-106 mE/q liter • CO_2 content 24-30 mEq/liter • Glucose 70-110 mg/100 ml • Creatinine 0.6-1.5 mg/100 ml • BUN 8-25 mg/100 ml 4. Normal skin turgor present.	• Provide nutritional support via appropriate route (oral, parenteral or enteral route as indicated). • Obtain serial electrolytes per physician. • Assess skin turgour and mucous membranes during complete patient assessment. • Monitor nitrogen balance in critically-injured patients.	• Nutritional support is necessary for the repair of injured tissue and the promotion of health. • Serial electrolytes provide baseline data for the monitoring of the patient's nutritional and overall status. • Skin turgour assessment detects dehydration or overhydration status of the patient. • Positive nitrogen balance is imperative for the multisystems trauma patient in a compromised, catabolic state due to injury.
Nursing Diagnosis#12 Alteration in body image related to:		Patient will: 1. Be able to discuss body image disturbance if present and verbalize	• Assess patient-coping style.	• Assessment of patient coping styles assists in discovering successful methods of dealing with body image crises.

Contd...

Problem	*R*	*Objective*	*Nursing Interventions*	*Rationales*
1. Traumatic incident. 2. Disfigurement, or 3. Perceived body image disturbance.		feelings about self, including positive comments. 2. Demonstrate signs of acceptance of self in actions like dress and performance of the ADL.	• Discuss with patient body image perceptions. • Offer praise and accomplishment when appropriate. • Establish open lines of communication. • Make appropriate referrals as needed.	• Verbalizing feelings regarding body perceptions may reduce anxiety and fears and help patients overcome disturbances. • Offering praise and support when appropriate creates feelings of enhanced human dignity, self-worth, and self-esteem. • Open lines of communication allows for verbalization of body image concerns. • Making appropriate referrals will assist in patient well-being.

Neurological Nursing

ASSESSMENT OF THE NERVOUS SYSTEM

The human nervous system is a highly-specialized system responsible for the control and integration of the body's activities. The ability to conduct an accurate neurological assessment depends on the nurse's knowledge of neuroanatomy and neurophysiology and skill in recognizing and interpreting subtle deviations from normal. (Refer to Standard anatomy and Physiology Text on). Although neurological assessment usually is complete in phases and depends on the condition of the person and the urgency of the situation, assessment of mental status, level of consciousness, language and speech, perceptual status and sensory status.

History

A careful history i.e. a skillfully taken history often holds the key to diagnosis. The person is asked to give a time-to-time account of the illness including the onset and progression as well as the nature of the symptoms. It is particularly important to note the speed of onset, frequency of remissions, (if any), and any diurnal patterns or intensity changes in symptoms. Symptoms that require further assessment are complaints of pain, headache, seizures, vertigo, numbness, visual changes, and weakness. Identification of specific patterns of symptoms may provide pertinent diagnostic information about the pathological process.

When eliciting data about health history, the nurse should ask the patient specific questions about diabetes mellitus, pernicious anaemia, cancer, infections, thyroid disease, substance abuse, and hypertention, because these conditions can affect the nervous system. Any hospitalization, injuries, or surgeries related to nervous system and use of medications, especially sedatives, narcotics, tranquilizers, mood-elevating drugs and their side effects should also be asked about.

In addition, information is collected about family members and their relationships and interactions, ethnic background, housing, recreational interests, occupation, education, coping mechanisms, dependence-independence characteristics, and how the person manages usual activities of daily living. Particular attention should be paid to reports of any recent changes in the patient's usual behaviours such as increased irritability or memory loss. A family health history and developmental history also are included.

Mental Status

While determining the presence of organic brain disease, specific abnormalities of higher cerebral functions are very significant for which clinical observation of mental function is important change in the level of consciousness (LOC) it can be most sensitive indicator of neurological function. The functional components of consciousness are aroused (alertness) and awareness (consent) of self and environment. *Arousal* is mainly controlled by brainstem activity including the reticular activating system (RAS). Awareness requires an intact cerebral cortex and association fibers. Thus, the state of consciousness depends on the interaction between the brainstem and cerebral hemisphere.

Arousal is determined by eye opening. A spontaneous opening of the eyes occurs where a person is spoken to by the examiner. A painful stimulus may be applied to determine whether the arousal mechanism is intact if eye opening does not occur with verbal and auditory stimulus.

Awareness is assessed by determining the patient's orientation to self and environment, which includes assessment of person, place, and time (day, month, year) is the most effective method.

Assessment of mood and behaviour also includes in the mental examination, because of a particular mood may be associated with a specific disease. For example:

- Emotional liability is often seen in bilateral (diffuse) brain disease where the mood shifts easily and quickly from one extreme to the other.
- Euphoria is a superficial elevation of mood accompanied by unconcern even in the presence of threatening events. It needs to be determined whether the persons mood is appropriate to the topic of conversation.
- Personality change with the appearance of violent temper and aggressive behaviour may occur with destructive lesions of the inferior frontal parts of the limbic system.

.... should assess mental status. The components of the mental status examination will include:

- General appearance; which includes motor activities, body posture, dress and hygiene, facial expression, and speech.
- State of consciousness: which includes orientation to place, person, and situation, as well as memory, general knowledge, insight, judgement, problem-solving and calculation.

- Mood and affect which includes noting agitation, anger, depression, euphoria and the appropriateness of these states. Questions should be directed to bring out the feelings of the patient.
- Thought content: which includes noting illusions, hallucinations, delusions or paronia.
- *Intellectual capacity*: i.e., noting retardation, dementia, and intelligence.

Language and Speech

Language ability is concentrated on a cortical field includes parts of the temporal lobe, the temporoparietaleoccipital junction, the frontal lobe of the dominant (usually left) hemisphere and occipital lobe. Lesion in any of these areas will produce some impairment in language ability aphasia or dysarthria.

- Aphasia is the impairment of language functions. There were different types of aphasias what had been identified as follows:
  - Motor expression aphasia is the impairment of ability to speak and write. Patient can understand written and spoken words. This may be due to lesions in the insular and surrounding region including Broca's motor area.

In the anomic, fluent, and non-fluent aphasia are as follows:

- Anomic refers to inability to name objects, qualities, and conditions although speech is fluent due to lesion in area of angular gyrus.
- Fluent refers to speech in well-articulated and grammatically correct but lacking in content and meaning.
- Non-fluent aphasia refers to problems in selecting, organizing and initiating speech patterns, may also affect writing. It is due to lesion and motor cortex at Broca's area.
  - i. Sensory (Receptive) aphasia refers to impairment of ability to understand written or spoken language, is due to disease of auditory and visual word centers. Wernick's aphasia is also the same as sensory aphasia due to lesion lying in Wernick's area of left hemisphere.
  - ii. Mixed aphasia refers to combined expressive and receptive aphasia deficits due to damage to various speech and language areas.
  - iii. Global aphasia refers to total aphasia involving all functions that make up speech and communication. Few if any imbibe language skills. This is due to severe damage to speech area.
  - iv. Dysarthria is an indistinctness in word articulation or enunication resulting from interference with the peripheral speech mechanisms (e.g. the muscles of the tongue, palate, pharynx or lips).

Dysarthria may be manifested by a single alteration or a variety of alterations and there are characteristic changes in particular diseases. For example in crebellar disease, speech is often thick with prolongation of speech sounds occurring at intervals. In Parkinsonism, speech is characterized by a decrease in loudness and a change in vocal emphasis patterns that makes sound seem monotonous.

Perception

Sensation is integrated and interpreted in the sensory cortex, especially in the parietal lobe. It is important for the nurse to recognise perceptual problems, because they can be more difficult to deal with the changes in the patient's ability to move or sense. Disorders of perceptions commonly involve spatial-temporal relationships or the perception of self.

The ability to recognize objects through any of the special senses is known as "gnosia". Lesions involving a specific association area of the cortex produces a specific type of agnosia (absence of the ability). One type of ability often tested is stereognosis, the ability to perceive—an object's nature and form by touch. This is assessed by asking the person to identify familar objects placed in the hand at a time, while keeping his eyes closed.

Apraxia is another perceptual problem, refers to the inability to perform skilled, purposeful movements in the absence of motor, sensory or coordination losses. The different types, of apraxia are as follows:

i. Constructional apraxia is an impairment in producing designs in two or three dimensions, involves copying, drawing, or constructing. This is due to lesion in occipitoparietal lobe of either hemisphere.
ii. Dressing apraxia is an inability to dress oneself accurately. Makes mistakes as putting clothes on backwards, upside down, inside out, or putting both legs in the same pantleg. This is due to lesion in occipetal or parietal lobe usually in nondominant hemisphere.
iii. Kinesthetic apraxia is a loss of kinesthetic memory pattern, which result in patient inability to perform a purposeful motor task although it is understood. This is due to lesion in frontal lobe of either hemisphere or precentral gyrus.
iv. Idiomotor apraxia is an inability to imitate gestures or perform a purposeful motor task on command. May be able to do spontaneous. This is due to lesions in parietal lobe of dominant hemisphere and supramarginal gyrus.
v. Ideational apraxia is an inability to carry out activities automatically or on command, because of inability to understand the concepts of the act. This is due to lesion in parietal lobe of dominant hemisphere or diffuse brain damage as in arteriosclerosis.

Sensory Status

Accurate assessment of sensory function depends on the person's cooperation, alertness, and responsiveness. The person should be relaxed and have the eyes closed during all portions of the sensory examination to avoid recovering visual clues. Also, sensation should be tested side by side and distally to proximity. Both superficial and deep sensations are tested on trunk and extremities. Areas of sensory loss or abnormality are mapped out on a body diagram according to the distribution of the spinal dermatomes and peripheral nerves.

PAIN

- Superficial pain perception is assessed by stimulating an area by pinprick and asking the person to report discomfort. Sharp and dull objects can be alternated for increased discrimination.
- Deep pain can be assessed by multiple means, some of which have the potential of causing tissue injury. It is necessary to assess deep pain only when the person has a decreased level of consciousness. Deep pain can be assessed by applying pressure over the nail beds or supraorbitally. Pressure may also be applied over bony areas, such as sternum. Nailbed pressure is applied by placing a pin or similar object on the nail bed and squeezing it between the examiner's thumb and forefinger. Deep pain may also be elicited by squeezing the trapezius muscle. Pinching and pricking may damage tissues and are avoided wherever possible.
- Crude touch may be assessed by touching area with cotton and requesting that the person indicate when the touch is felt.
- Temperature is tested by touching particular areas with warm to hot and cold to cold object and asking the person to state the sensations felt.

Motion and Position

Proprioceptive fibers transmit sensory impulses from muscles, tender ligaments, and joints. This results in an awareness of the position of one's limbs in space (Kinesthetic sense). Proprioception is tested by the examiner's grasping the sides of the person's distal phalax and moving it up and down. If proprioception is intact, the person reports correctly the direction in which the joint is being moved. Proprioceptive ability can also be assessed by the Remberg test, in which the person is asked to stand erect with the feet together and the eyes closed. A positive test occurs where the person loses balance which indicates a pathological condition.

Vibration is tested by placing a low frequency tuning fork on a bony prominence of each extremity and assessing the person's ability to feel it.

Neurological Examination

Generally neurological examination assesses six categories of functions and reflex function. The primary purpose of the nursing neurologic examination is to determine the effects of the neurologic dysfunction on daily living in relation to the patients and the family's ability to cope with the neurologic deficits, for which the medical model of examination also used for nursing purposes. The mental status examination already discussed. The nurse has to use or keep ready following equipment needed to perform a neurological examination which include:

- Compass.
- Cotton applicators.
- Dermatomes.
- Dynomemeter.
- Flash light.
- Miscellanous items of varied shape and size (coin, key, marble).
- Ophthalmoscope.
- Otoscope.
- Coloured pencil.
- Pins with sharp and blunt ends.
- Printed page.
- Reflex hammer.
- Tape measure.
- Tongue depressor.
- Tuning fork.
- Snellen chart.
- Stoppered vials containing:
  - Peppermint, oil of cloves, coffee and soap (small).
  - Sugar, salt, vinegar and quinine (taste).
  - Cold and hot water (temperatures).
- Watch with second hand.

Cranial Nerves

Testing of each cranial nerve (CN) is an essential component of the neurological examination. The 12 cranial nerves may be tested in numbered sequence. Some nurses prefer to test at the same time with those cranial nerves with similar function such as voluntary motor function visceral motor function, and special sensory or general sensory functions. However, some cranial nerves have both motor and sensory functions. Prior to the test the CN, it is better to review.

The cranial nerves and their functions are as follows:

i.	Olfactory	- Sensory :	Smell reception and interpretation.
ii.	Optic	- Sensory :	Visual acuity and visual fields.
iii.	Oculomotor	- Motor :	Raise eyelids, most extraocular movements.
iv.	Trochlear	- Motor :	downward, inward eye movements.
v.	Trigeminal	- Motor :	Jaw opening and clenching, chewing and mastication.
		- Sensory :	Sensation to cornea, iris, lacrimal glands, conjunctiva, eyelids, forehead, nose, nasal and mouth mucosa, teeth, tongue, ear facial skin.

vi. Abducens - Motor : Lateral eye movement.

vii. Facial - Motor : Movement of facial expression of muscles except jaw, close eyes, labial speech sounds (b.m.w. and rounded vowels).

- Sensory : Taste-anterior two-thirds of tongue-sensation of pharynx.

- Parasympathetic-secretion of salivary glands and carotid reflex.

x. Vagus - Motor : voluntary muscles of phonation (guttural speech sounds) and swallowing.

- Sensory : Sensation behind ear and parts of external ear canal.

xi. Spinal accessory - Motor - turn-head. shrug shoulders, some action for phonation.

xii. Hypoglossal - Motor-tongue movement for speech sound articulation (l, t, n.) and swallowing.

Testing cranial nerves.

i. *Olfactory Nerve*: Special receptors located within the superior or uppermost part of each nasal chamber transmit neural impulse over the olfactory bulbs to the olfactory nerves in the area of central cortex concerned with olfaction. When testing thus CN, the nurse asks the patient to close one nostril, close both eyes and sniff from a bottle containing coffee, spice, soup, or some other readily-recognised odour. If yes, the patient is asked to name the odour. Awareness of an odour must be differentiated from the ability to name a specific substance. The same may be repeated in other nostril. Anosmia (absence of smell) or hypotmia (decreased sensitivity of the sense of smell) is often associated with complaints of lack of taste, even though test may demonstrate sense to be intact. Anosmia caused by varied lesion involving any part of the olfactory pathways.

ii. *Optic Nerve*: When retina is stimulated, nerve impulses are transmitted over the optic nerves (extending from the optic disc to the chiasm) and the optic tracts with radiation terminating in the visual cortex of the occipital lobes. Optic nerve function is assessed in relation to visual acuity, visual fields and the appearance of fundus. Each eye is tested separately.

Visual acuity is mediated by the cones of the retina. Central vision is grossly tested by reading newspaper print. Distance visual activity is assessed through the use of the 'Snellen Chart'. Individuals with vision impairment are tested to determine light perception (LP), hand movement (Hm), and finger count (fc).

Visual fields are assessed grossly by confrontation techniques. The examiner, positioned directly opposite to the patient asks the patient to close one eye, look directly at the bridge of the examiner's nose and indicate when an object (finger, pencil tip, head of pins) presented from periphery of the four visual quadrants. The same test is repeated for the other eye. Visual field defects may arise from lesions of the optic nerve, optic chiasma, or tracts that extend through the temporal, parectal or occipital lobe. Visual charges resulting from brain lesion are hemianopsia (one-half of the field affected) a quadrantanopsia (one-fourth of visual field affected) or monocular.

The ocular fundus is defined as that portion of the interior of the eyeball, that lies posterior to the lens. It includes optic disc, blood vessels, retina and macula. Funduscopy reveals the physical condition of the optic disc (head of the optic nerve) as well as the retina and blood vessels.

iii. *Oculomotor, trochlear and abducens nerves*: Cranial nerves III, IV and VI are motor nerves that arise from the brainstem and innervate the six extraocular muscle attached to the eyeball. These muscles function as a group in the coordinated movement of each eyeball is the six cardinal fields of gaze, giving the eye both straight and rotary movement. The four straight or rectus, muscles are the superior, inferior, lateral and medial rectus muscles. The two slanting or oblique muscles are the superior and inferior. Since these three cranial nerves all help move the eye, they are tested together. The patient is asked to follow the examiner's finger as it moves horizontally and vertically (making cross) and diagnoally (making an X). If there is weakness or paralyses in one of the eye muscles, the eyes do not move together, and the patient has a disconjugate gaze. The presence and direction of nystagmus (fine, rapid, jerking movements of the eyes) is observed at this time even though it is most often indicated to vestibula cerebellar problems.

Double vision (diplopia) squint (strabismus) and involuntary rhythmic movement of the eye balls (nystagmus) may indicate weakness of some of the extraoccular muscles because of deficits of these motor nerves. Ptosis or drooping of the upper eyelid over the globe may be caused by damage to the oculomotor nerve. Other functions of the oculomotor nerve are tested by checking for pupillary constriction and for convergence (eye turning inward) and accommodation (Pupils constricting with near vision).

iv. *Trigeminal Nerve*: Cranial nerve V is a mixed nerve with motor and sensory components. It is the largest cranial nerve. The motor part innervates the temporal and masseter muscles, the sensory part supplies the cornea, face, head, and mucus membranes of the nose and mouth.

The sensory component of the trigeminal nerve is tested by having the patient identify light touch (cotton) and pinprick in each of the three divisions (ophthalmic maxillary and mandibular) of the nerve on both sides of the face. The patient's eyes should be closed during this part of the examination.

The corneal reflex test evaluates trigeminal nerves and facial simultaneously. It involves applying a cotton wisp strand to the cornea. The sensory components of this reflex (corneal sensation) is innervated by the ophthalmic division of VCN. The motor component (eye blink) of thin reflex is innervated by facial nerve. Normally, the person blanks laterally. This is especially important reflex to assess in persons with decreased level of consciousness because the absence of the blink reflex can result in corneal damage.

v. *Facial Nerve*: It is a mixed nerve that is concerned with facial movement and sensation of taste. It innervates the muscles of facial expression. The inability to smile, close both eyes slightly look upward wrinkle the forehead, show the teeth, purse the lips, and blow out the cheeks constitutes weaknesses or paralysis of the facial muscle innervated by this nerve. Its function is tested by asking the patient to raise the eyebrows, close the eyes tightly, purse the lips, draw back the corners of the mouth in an exaggerated smile, and frown. The examiner should note any asymmetry in the facial movements, because they can indicate damage to the facial nerve. The sensation of taste is tested by placing salty sweet, bitter and sour substances, in turn on the side of the protruded tongue for identification. A loss of task over the anterior two-third of the tongue is present when this nerve is diseased, as occurs in mastoid canal lesions.
vi. *Acoustic Nerve*: (VIII) is composed of a cochlear division related to hearing and a vestibular division related to equilibrium. The conchlear portion of this nerve is tested by having the patient close the eyes and indicate when a ticking watch or the rustling of the examiner's finger tips is heard as the stimulus is brought closer to the ear. Each ear rested individually and the distance from the patient's ear to sound source when first hand is retarded. A more complete examination, including bone and air conduction of sound involves assessment with a tuning fork and audiometric testing.

The vestibular portion of this nerve is not routinely tested unless the patient complains of dizziness, vertigo, or unsteadiness or has auditory dysfunctioning. There are variety of ways in testing this portion of the nerve. In the past-pointing test, the person is asked to raise the arms and bring the index fingers down on the examiner's finger with the arm outstretched, first with the eyes open and then with the eyes closed. Normally, the person's fingers touch the examiner's without difficulty. In vertibular disease, the finger points to one side or the other consistently. The person is also assessed for nystagmus.

vii. *Glossopharyngeal and Vagus nerves*: These two cranial nerves are tested together because both innervate the pharynx. Both nerves supply the posterior pharyngeal wall and normally when the wall is touched, there is contraction of these muscles on both sides, with or without gagging. This test is unreliable for either nerve alone, because the vagus nerve is chief motor nerve and the soft palatal, pharyngeal and laryngeal muscles assessment includes testing voice and cough sounds. In unilateral movement of the motor portion of the vagus nerve the voice is harsh and nasal. Bilateral involvement produces more severe speech problems, swallowing difficulty and fluid regurgitation through nose. Sensory function of the vagus is usually not tested.
viii. *Spinal accessory nerve* is motor nerve that supplies the sternocleido mastoid and the upper part of the trapezius muscles. This nerve tested by asking the patient to shrug the shoulders against resistance and to turn the head to either side against resistance. There shall be smooth contraction of the above-said muscles. Symmetry, atrophy or fasciculation of the muscle should be noted.
ix. *Hypoglossal nerve* is purely motor nerve. The person's tongue is first inspected at rest. Any asymmetry unilaterally decreased bulk, deviations, or fasciculation (fine twitching) are noted. When the nerve is involved, the tongue deviates towards the side of the lesion. In an upper motor neuron lesion, the tonge is affected on the side opposite the lesion (contralateral). Atrophy of the tongue shown through wrinkling and loss of substance on the affected side.

Motor Status

Function of the nerve system assessed through gait and stance, muscle strength, muscle tonus, coordination, involuntary movement and muscle stretch reflexes.

- Gait and stance are compelx activities that require muscle strength, coordination balance, proprioception, and vision. Ataxia is general term meaning lack of coordination in performing planned, purposeful motion such as walking or gait. It is caused by disturbance of position sense or by cerebellar or other diseases. To evaluate the gait, the person is asked to walk freely and naturally and then walk heel to toe in a straight line, tandem walk, because this exaggerates abnormality. To evaluate stance, the person is asked to perform the Romberg standing with the feet close together, first with eyes open and then with eyes closed. Patients with problem and proprioception have difficulty in maintaining balance with their eyes closed. Patients with cerebellar disease have difficulty even with their eyes open. A variety of distinctive gait characterizes specific neurological disorder (e.g. Parkinsonism).
- Muscle strength or power is assessed systematically-including trunk and extremity muscles. One common assessment of muscle strength is asking the patient to grasp both hands of the nurse or doctor and squeeze them simultaneously. The nurse or doctor compares the squeezing ability of one hand to another. Assessment of muscular strength of the feet can be performed by plantar flexion and dorsiflexion.
- To test muscle tonus, the nurse passively moves the person's

limbs through a full range of motion. A skilled examiner can differentiate hypertonic from hypotonic muscles, Hypertonic extremities are in fixed positions and feel firm; hypotonic extremities assume a position governed by gravity over extension and overflexion found in hypertonic.

- Coordination can be tested in several ways. The finger to nose test involves having the patient alternately touch the nose with index finger then touch the examiner's finger. Other tests include asking the patient to pronate and supinate both hands rapidly and to do a shallow knee bend, first on one leg and then on another. Dysarthria—a sign of uncoordination of speech muscles.

Involuntary movement: It is important to observe the location of muscle involved amplitude of movement, speed of onset, duration of contraction and relaxation and rhythm. The effects of posture, rest, sleep, distraction, voluntary movement and emotional stress on involuntary movement are determined. Emotional stress usually increases involuntary movement and they may subside during sleep. Abnormal movement may be the result of organic disease or psychosomatic in origin. Example: involuntary movements are tremor, chorea and arthecosis.

Reflexes

The reflex is a predictable response that results from a nerve input over a reflex arc. Tendons attached to skeletal muscles have receptors that are sensitive to stretch. A reflex contraction of the skeletal muscles occurs when the tendon is stretched. A simple muscle stretch reflex is initiated by briskly tapping the tendons of a stretched muscle, usually with reflex hammer. Assessment of reflexes requires an experienced examiner, a reflex hammer and a relaxed patient. The reflex is elicited by striking the hammer onto the muscle insertion tendon. Comparison of right and left sides should reveal equal responses. The reflex response graded as subjective, four-point scale that requires clinical practice to use accurately (as follow).

0 = Absent	0 =	Areflexia
1 = Weak response	1+ =	Hyporeflexia
2 = Normal response	2+ =	Normal
3 = Exaggerated response	3+ =	Brisker than normal
4 = Hyper reflexia with clonus	4+ =	Hyper-reflexia

Clonus, an abnormal response, is a continued rhythmic contraction of the muscle after the stimulus has been applied. In general the biceps, triceps, brachioradialis and patellar and Achilles tendon reflex are tested. Some common diagnostic reflexes of the CNS are as follows:

1. *Abdominal reflex* is an anterior stroking of the sides of lower torso causes contraction of the abdominal muscles. Absence of reflex indicates lesions of peripheral nerves or in reflex centers in lower thoracic segments of spinal cord; may also indicate multiple sclerosis.
2. *Achilles* reflex (ankle jerk) refers to tapping of calcaneal (Achilles) tendon of soleous and gastroenemius muscle cause both muscles to contract, producing plantar flexion of food. Absence of reflex may indicate damage to nerves innervating posterior leg muscles or to lumbosacral neurons; may also indicate chronic diabetes, alcoholism syphilis, subarachnoid haemorrhage.
3. *Biceps reflex* refers to tapping of biceps tendon in elbow produces contracton of brachialis and biceps muscle, producing flexion at elbow. Absence of reflex may indicate damage at the C5 or C6 vertebral level.
4. *Brudzinskis* reflex refers to forceful flexion of neck produces flexion of legs, thighs. This indicates irritation of meninges.
5. *Kernig's reflex* refers to flexion of hip, with knee straight and patient lying on back, produces flexion of knee. This reflex indicates irritation of meninges or herniated intervertebral disc.
6. *Patellar reflex* (knee jerk) refers to tapping of patellar tendon-causes contraction of quadriceps femoris muscle, producing upward jerk of leg. Absence of this reflex may indicate damage at the L2, L3, or L4 vertebral level; may also indicate chronic diabetes and syphilis.
7. *Plantar reflex* refers to stroking of the lateral part of sole-causes toes to curl down. If corticospinal damage, great toe flexes upward and other toes fan out (Babinskie's sign). This reflex indicates damage to upper motor neuron. Normal in children less than 1-year old.
8. *Triceps reflex* refers to tapping of triceps tendon at elbow-causes contraction of triceps muscle, producing extension at elbow. Absence of reflex may indicate damage at C6, C7 or C8 vertebral level.

DIAGNOSTIC STUDIES OF THE NERVOUS SYSTEM

Diagnostic studies provide important information to the nurse in monitoring the patient's condition and planning appropriate interventions. The common diagnostic studies and the nurse's responsibility in particular diagnostic studies of the nervous system are as follows:

1. Cerebrospinal Fluid (CSF) Analysis

CSF is a clear fluid that is formed in the third, fourth and lateral ventricles of the brain. Samples are obtained through either a lumbar puncture or cisternal puncture and examined for any increase or decrease in its normal constituents and foreign substances such as pathogenic organism and blood. The normal CSF values are as given below.

- Specific gravity .. 1.007
- pH .. 7.35
- Apearance .. Clear, colourless

- RBCs .. None
- WBCs 0-8/μl (0.0.008/L)
- Opening pressure with LP 60-150 mm H_2O
- Pressure 75 to 180 mm H_2O
- Protein - Lumbar 15-45 mg/dl
  - Cisternal 15-25 mg/dl
  - Ventricular 5-15 mg/dl
- Glucose 45-75 mg/dl.
- Microorganisms none.

Generaliy CSF is aspirated by needle insertions in L3-4 or L4-5 interspace to assess many CNS diseases. Nurse's responsibility while obtaining specimen through LP includes-

- Assist patient to assume and maintain lateral recumbent position with knees flexed.
- Ensure maintenance of strict aseptic technique.
- Ensure labelling of CSF specimen in proper sequence.
- Keep patient flat for at least a few hours depending on physician's preference.
- Encourage fludis.
- Monitor neurologic and vital signs.
- Administer analgesia as needed.

2. Radiological Tests

i. Skull and spine X-rays of the skull and spinal column is done to detect fractures, bone erosion, calcification and abnormal vascularity. Here nurse has to explain that procedure is non-invasive. Explain position to be assumed during X-ray.

ii. *Cerebral angiography* involves the injection of contrast medium into the cerebral arterial circulation which assists in determining aetiology of strokes, seizures, headaches and motor weakness. A catheter is inserted into the femoral artery (the most common entry site) and advanced to the carotid and cerebral vessels. Serial films are taken as the dye circulates through the cerebral circulation.

The nurse informs the patient that the procedure takes one to two hours.

- Keep patient withhold preceding meal 6 to 10 hours prior to procedure.
- Explain that patient will have hot flush of head when dye is injected.
- Administer premedication as ordered.
- Explain need to be absolutely still during procedure.
- Monitor neurologic and vital signs every 15-30 minutes for first hours.
- Maintain pressure dressing and ice to injection site.
- Maintain bedrest until patient is alert and vital signs are stable.
- Report any sign of change in neurologic status.

iii. *Computed tomograph (CT) Scan*. Computer assisted X-ray of several levels of thin cross sections of body parts are done to detect problems such as haemorrhage, tumour, cyst, oedema, infarction, brain atrophy and hydrocephalus. In this procedure, the nurse:

- Explains the procedure is noninvasive (if no dye is used).
- Observe for allergic reactions and note puncture site (if dye is used).
- Explain appearance of scanner.
- Instruct the patient on need to remain absolutely still during procedure.

iv. *Myelography* refers to X-ray of spinal cord and vertebral column after injection of dye into subarchnoid space is used to detect spinal lesions (e.g.) ruptured disk, tumour). In this, the nurse's responsibilities are to:

- Administer pre-procedure sedation as ordered.
- Instruct patient to empty bladder.
- Inform patient that test is performed with patient on tilt in table that is moved during test.
- Encourage fluids.
- Monitor neurologic and vital signs.

v. *MRI*- In MRI internal body parts are visualized by means of magnetic energy. No invasive procedures are required unless contrast material is used. Here, there is need for nurse to screen patient for metal parts and pace maker in the body. Instruct patient to be on knee to lie very still for upto 1 hour. Sedation may be necessary if patient is claustophobic.

vi. Positron Emission Tomography (PET) measures metabolic activity of brain regions to assess cell death or damage by using radioactive compounds. In this procedure, nurse:

- Explains procedure to patient.
- Explains that two IV Line will be inserted.
- Instruct patient not to take sedatives or tranquilizers.
- Empty bladder before procedure.
- May be asked to perform different activities during test.

3. Electrographic Studies

i. *Electroencephalography* (EEG): In this, electrical activity of brain is recorded by scalp electrodes to evaluate cerebral disease, CNS effects of systemic diseases and brain death. In this procedure, the nurse:

- Informs patient that procedure is painless and without danger of electric shock.
- Withhold stimulants.
- Informs that patient may be asked to perform various activities such as hyperventilation during test.
- Determines whether any medication (e.g. tranquilizer, antiseizures) should be withheld.

- Resume medications after test.
- Assist patient to wash electrode paste out of hair.

ii. *Electromyography* Nerve conduction is an electrical activity associated with nerve and skeletal muscles is recorded by insertion of needle electrodes to detect muscle and peripheral nerve disease. Here inform patient of slight discomfort associated with insertion of needle.

iii. *Evoked potentials* refer to electrical activity associated with nerve conduction along sensory pathways is recorded by electrodes placed on skin and scalp. Stimulus generates the impulse. Procedure is used to diagnose disease, locate nerve damage, and monitor function intraoperatively. This needs explaining procedure to patients.

iv. *Visual evoked potentials* refer to electrical activity in visual pathway is recorded with rapidly reverting checkerboard pattern on television screen. One eye is tested at time. Needs explaining the procedure to patients.

v. *Braunstem auditory evoked potentials* refer to electrical activity in auditory pathway is recorded with earphones that produce clicking sounds. One ear is tested at time.

vi. *Somatosensory evoked potentials* refer to electrical activity in certain nerve pathways is recorded with mild electrical pulse (several per second). This procedure needs to inform patient that stimulus may cause mild discomfort or muscle switch.

4. Ultrasound

i. *Carotid duplex studies*: in which sound waves determine blood flow velocity, which indicates presence of occlusive vascular disease.

ii. *Transcranial doppler*: Same technology as carotid duplex, but evaluates intracranial vessels. In these procedures, the nurse needs to explain the procedure to the patient.

INTRACRANIAL PROBLEMS

Altered Level of Consciousness (LOC)

Consciousness and coma (unconsciousness) exist as opposite ends of a spectrum. Full consciousness is a state of awareness and ability to respond optimally to one's environment. Coma is the opposite, a state of total abscence of awareness and ability to respond, even when stimulated. Unconsciousness is an abnormal state in which the patient is unknown of self or environment. It can range from brief episode, such as the prolonged unconsciousness of coma from which the person cannot be roused, even with vigorous external stimuli. Between these two extremes are degrees of unconsciousness varying in length and severity. A wide range of awareness and responsiveness exists between these extremes are shown as follows: (figure)

Alert→confused→lethargic→obtunded→stuporous→comatase.

The terminology used in this figure (continum of consciousness).

- Alert : attends to environment, responds appropriately to commands and questions with minimal stimulation.
- Confused : disoriented to surroundings, may have impaired judgement, may need cues to respond to commands.
- Lethargic : drowsy, needs gentle verbal or touch stimulation to initiate response.
- Obtunded : responds slowly to external stimulation, needs repeated stimulation to maintain attention and response to the environment.
- Stuporous : responds only minimally with vigorous stimulation may only mutter or moan as a verbal response.
- Comatose : no observable response to any external stimuli.

The labels used to identify the various points along the continuum are arbitrary and do not reflect any universal agreement as to the nature of consciousness. Consciousness has two primary components—arousal and content.

i. Arousal is a function of the brainstem pathways that govern wakefulness, particularly the reticular activating system (RAS) i.e., a network of nerve fibers and cell bodies that is located in the reticular formation in the central part of the nervous system. An intact RAS can maintain a state of wakefulness, even in the absence of a functioning of cortex.

ii. Content refers to the ability to reason, think and feel and to react to stimuli with purpose and awareness. Content is the sum of multiple interconnected cerebral hemisphere functions, including thought, behaviour, language and expression. These activities are mediated by the higher centres. Intellect and emotional functions are also controlled by these centers.

Disruptions in arousal, content or both can alter the individual level of consciousness (LOC). Interruptions of impulses from the RAS or alterations of the functioning of the cerebral hemisphere can cause unconsciousness. Any condition that markedly alters the functions of the hemispheres or that depresses or destroys the upper brainstem results in impaired consciousness.

Aetiology

The two general causes for altered LOC are structural and metabolic as follows:

1. *Structural causes*
   a. Trauma: Concussion, contusion, traumatic intracranial

haemorrhage subdural haematoma, epidural haematoma, cerebral oedema intracerebral haematoma.

b. Vascular disease: Cerebral infarction, intracerebral haemorrhage, subarachnoid haemorrhage, brainstem infarction, brainstem haemorrhage, cerebellar haemorrhage.
c. Infections: meningitis, encephalitis, brain abscess, cerebellar abscess.
d. Neoplasms: Primary brain tumours, metastatic tumours, brainstem tumours.

2. *Metabolic causes*
   a. Systemic metabolic derrangements: hypoglycaemia, diabetic ketoacidosis, hyperglycaemic nonketonic hyperosmalar states, uraemia, hepatic encephalopathy, hyponatraemia, myxedaema.
   b. Hypoxic or anoxic encephalopathies: Severe congestive heart failure, chronic obstructive pulmonary disease with execerbation, severe anaemia, prolonged hypertension, postictal states and concussions.
   c. Toxicity: Exogenous toxins- Drug overdose (opiates, barbiturates and alcohol)
      - Alcohol intoxication.
      - Lead poisoning.
      - Heavy metals.
      - Carbon monoxide.
      - Endogenous toxins - Hypoglycaemia, uraemia, Hepatic encephalitis, thiamine deficiency.
   d. Extremes of body temperature- Heat stroke, hypothermia.
   e. Deficiency states: Wernick's encephalopathy.
   f. Seizures.

Pathophysiology

Full consciousness is a product of many delicate interactions within the nervous system. Arousal is a function of the RAS. Fibres from the upper brainstem, thalamus, and hypothalamus receive input from sensory pathways in the brain and peripheral nervous system. The RAS fibres supply stimulation to the cerebral haemispheres to initiate and maintain arousal. When a person is aroused, or awake, he or she is ready to respond to the environment. The cerebral cortex also provides feedback to the RAS to modulate and regulate the information sent to the cortex. The ability to consciously respond to the environment is a function of cerebral hemispheres. The cerebral cortex, diencephalon, and upper brain stem act together to control voluntary motor function, language, memory and emotion. These higher level cognitive functions represent the content portion of consciousness. A person needs both arousal, or wakefulness, content to be considered fully conscious.

Many specific aetiologic events can result in unconsciousness. Above-stated causes can be grouped according to the pathophysiologic mechanisms such as supratentorial mass lesions, subtentorial mass lesions, destructive lesions, or metabolic and diffuse cerebral disorders. Psychic disorders such as depression, catotonia and schizophrenia can result in failure to respond to the environment.

Supratentorial mass lesions generally interfere with consciousness by compressing and shifting the cerebral contents and causing pressure on the upper brainstem containing the RAS. These lesions, occuring above the tentorium may include those resulting from trauma, subarachnoid haemorrhage, intracerebral haemorrhage or infarction, tumours, and abscesses. The most serious consequence of supratentorial mass lesion is herniation of the cerebral hemisphere through the tentorial notch, causing compression of the brainstem. Another form of herniation occurs if the brain shifts laterally, forcing the cingulate gyrus under the falx and compressing the blood vessels and brain tissue of the opposite hemisphere. The end result herniation is ischaemia and irreversible infarction.

Subtentorial masses or destructive lesions that occur below the tentorium interfere with consciousness by compressing or destroying the RAS above the midpons. Pontine or cerebellar haemorrhage, infarction, tumour, or abscess can affect the subtentorial area of the brain through direct brain compression, upward herniation into the foramen magnum.

Metabolic or diffuse cerebral disorders of either intracranial or extracranial origin can cause alterations in the conscious state. These disorders can disturb cerebral metabolism and thus alter the regulation of cellular nutrition, electrolyte balance, oxygen and carbon dioxide regulation, and enzymatic functions. Specific metabolic problems that can cause unconsciousness include uraemia, diabetic mellitus, hypoglycaemia alcohol intoxication, drug overdose, and lead poisoning. Regardless of the cause of the unconscious state, two pathophysiologic processes that affect cerebral metabolism generally occur which include, cerebral ischaemia, anoxia and cerebral oedema. In which cerebral ischaemia-anoxia managed by instituting measures to ensure adequate systemic circulation and cerebral oedema treated by hyperosmotic drugs and cortico-steroids Eg. 50 per cent dextrose IV with cortisone.

Clinical Manifestation

The clinical manifestation associated with altered LOC are as follows:

- Decreased wakefulness.
- Decreased attention to surrounding environment.
- Confusion.
- Hallucinations.
- Illusions.
- Disorientation.
- Agitation
- Poor memory.
- Decreased ability to carry out activities of daily living.
- Decreased mobility.
- Incontinence.

Management

Diagnostic tests.Diagnostic evaluation of altered LOC include searching for the structural or metabolic aetiology of the changes. The work-up includes a detailed history, extensive neurological examination, radiological examination and laboratory testing, which include the following.

Structural tests	*Metabolic test*
• Skull X-Rays	• Complete blood count
• Electroencephalography	• Urinalysis
• Computorized tomography of Head	• Electrolytes (glucose, bun, Creatinine)
• Cerebral angiogram	• Calcium
• Magnetic Resonance Imaging	• Liver function studies
• Evoked potential	• Cardiac enzymes
	• Serum osmolarity
	• Lumbar puncture
	• Arterial blood pressure
	• Toxicology serum for drug abuse.

While diagnostic test results are pending, or tests are being scheduled, a detailed history is obtained from the patient, when possible and also from family, significant others and physical examination. The detailed neurological examination provides the foundation for assessment of the patient with altered LOC, but health care providers including nurses use a variety of scales to standardize the ongoing evaluation of a patient's functioning. Example includes Glasgow Coma scale (GCS), the Rancho Los Amigo Scale (RLAS) and mini-mental state examination.

- Glasgow coma Scale (GCS): The GCS was developed to evaluate head injured patients but can be used with a wide variety of neurological patients. GCS does not take place comprehensive neurological examination, but the results (scores) can be graphed and used to identify trends in the patient's overall function and predict outcomes. The GCS is as given below:

1. *Glasgow coma scale*

Category and Response	*Score*
• *Eye opening*	
Spontaneously open	4
Open to verbal request	3
Open with painful stimuli	2
No opening	1
• *Best verbal Response*	
Oriented to time, place, person, converse appropriately.	5
Converse, but confused.	4
Words spoken, but conversation not sustained.	3
Sounds made, no intellible words.	2
No response.	1
• *Best Motor Response*	
Obeys commands.	6
Localizes to painful stimuli	5
Withdraws to painful stimuli	4
Abnormal flexion to pain (decorticates posturing)	3
Abnormal extension to pain (decerebrate posturing)	2
No response.	1

2. *Rancho los amigos scale (RLAS)*

RLAS was developed as a behavioural rating scale to aid in the assessment and treatment of brain injured patients. It assesses the progressive recovery of cognitive abilities as demonstrated through behavioural changes and is most commonly used in subacute and rehabiliative setting.

RLAS is used to know the level of cognitive functioning as follows:

i. No response	:	Patient is completely unresponsible to any stimuli.
ii. Generalized response	:	Patient reacts inconsistently and nonpurposefully to stimuli in non-specific manner.
iii. Localized Response	:	Patient reacts specifically but inconsistant.
iv. Confused-Agitated	:	Patient is heightened state of activity with severely decreased ability to process information.
v. Confused-Inappropriate	:	Patient appears alert and is able to respond to simple commands fairly consistently.
vi. Confused-Appropriate	:	Patient shows goal-directed behaviour but depends on external input for direction.
vii. Automatic-Appropriate	:	Patient appears appropriate and oriented within hospital and homesetting, goes through daily routine automatically with minimal to absent confusion and has shallow recall of actions.
viii. Purposeful-Appropriate	:	Patient is alert and oriented, is able to recall and integrate past and recent events, and is aware of end responsive to culture.

Nursing Assessment

Nursing assessment begins with patient's detailed history and the specific factors to assess in a patient experiencing altered LOC are subjective data which include:

- When the change in LOC was not noticed.
- Onset-sudden or slowly progressive.

- Patient and family awareness and understanding of the symptoms.
- Ability to think, think abstractly, calculate and make everyday decisions.
- Recent history of falls, infection or other trauma.
- Medication in use—Prescription and over-the-counter drugs, alcoholism.
- Visual changes.
- Other symptoms, pain, fever, nausea, headache and objective data which includes:
- Motor status, presence of posturing.
- Sensory status.
- Cranial nerve assessment, protective reflexes.
- Breathing pattern.
- Oxygen status.
- Laboratory results (electrolytes, HB per cent blood glucose, BUN, creatinine.
- Drug level.

Nursing Diagnosis

The possible nursing diagnosis is altered LOC will be:

- Ineffective breathing pattern R/T neuromuscular impairment, cognition.
- Altered tissue perfusion, cerebral R/o decreased or altered blood flow.
- Altered thought process R/T structural or metabolic imbalance.
- Ineffective thermoregulation R/T impaired regulatory function.
- Risk for injury R/T Sensory/motor deficits, loss or integrative function.
- Impaired physical mobility R/T neuromuscular impairment.
- Altered nutrition (body requirement R/T decreased alertness, chewing/swallowing difficulty.
- Bowel incontinence R/T perceptual or cognitive impairment.
- Altered urinary elimination R/T perceptual or cognitive impairment.
- Altered urinary elimination R/T neuromuscular impairment.
- Impaired health maintenance R/T perceptual or cognitive impairment.
- Risk for impaired skin integrity R/T impairment mobility, nutrition pressure.
- Ineffective family company R/T temporary family disorganisation.
- Knowledge deficit. R/O disorder, plans of treatment, etc.

Objectives

Patient with altered LOC should achieve the following:

- Maintain effective breathing pattern.
- Maintain adequate systematic blood pressure to perfuse the brain.
- Maintain coherent thought process, is not confused.
- Maintain body temperature within normal limits.
- Safety precautions in place does not experience injury.
- Maintains highest possible mobility with use of assistive devices and assistance of others.
- Consume adequate balanced nutrients to maintain stable body weight.
- Maintain regular pattern of bowel elimination without constipation, diarrhoea or incontinence.
- Maintain urinary incontinence with or without external continence device.
- Participate in self-care to the maximum degree possible.
- Skin integrity maintained, no evidence of redness or injury.
- Family activity participates in all decision-making and planning for patient care, use coping strategies to adapt family role changes.
- Patients and family indicate understanding of diagnosis of LOC.

Nursing Intervention

The following measures to be taken to achieve the above objectives of the patient with altered LOC.

1. Protect the airway and promote gas exchanges.
   - Turn side to side 4th hourly.
   - Encourage coughing and deep breathing every hour while awake.
   - Suctions oral and pharyngeal airway promptly if necessary.
   - Monitor oxygen saturation and blood gases.
2. Promote cerebral tissue perfusion.
   - Maintain hydration, prevent hypovolaemia.
   - Monitor effects of antihypertensive, other medication and promote adequate cardiac output and systemic blood pressure.
3. Promote tissue perfusion.
   - Turn patient 4th hourly.
   - Perform passive or active range of motion to enhance circulation at least once per shift.
   - Apply elastic stockings or intermittent compression devices to prevent deep vein thrombosis.
4. Promote sensory-perceptual function.
   - Provide meaningful stimuli.
   - Speak to patient before touching.
   - Orient patient to surroundings.
   - Provide adequate lighting.
   - Have calender and clock within patient's view.
   - Have familiar objects in patient's view.
5. Maintain normal body temperature.
   - Hyperthermia – Remove excess bed coverings.
     – Maintain a cool room temperature.
     – Administer antipyretic medication.

– Provide tepid bath.

- Hypothermia – Apply warmed blankets.
  – Use heat lamps with caution
  – Increase room temperature.

6. Prevent Injury.
   - Keep a call bell within the reach of patient.
   - Implement seizure precautions as needed.
   - Provide eye care to prevent corneal damage at least once per shift.
   - Apply restraints only as last resort at physician's order.
7. Promote mobility.
   - Perform active or passive range of motion every shift.
   - Assist patients with ambulation at position changes.
8. Maintain nutrition.
   - Record intake to assess quantity and quality.
   - Assist patient with feeding and swallowing safely with instruction to take small bites and chew carefully.
   - Administer enteral feedings at recommended rate for needs.
   - Weigh patient daily or weekly to assess gain or loss.
9. Maintain regular bowel function.
   - Provide adequate hydration.
   - Ensure adequate fiber in diet or tube feedings.
   - Administer stool softener as needed.
10. Maintain bladder continence.
    - Remove indwelling catheters as soon as possible.
    - Provide, regular toileting to prevent incontinence.
11. Maintain hygiene.
    - Assist patient with ADL as needed.
    - If patient is unable to care for self, provide bath, mouth, eye and skin care regularly.
    - Shampoo patient's hairs as needed.
12. Maintain skin integrity.
    - Reposition patient at least at every 2 hours' interval.
    - Use lotion or other skin moisturizers to prevent dry skin.
    - Keep sheets dry, free of wrinkles.
    - If skin breakdown is present or if patient is at high risk use pressure-relief device.
    - Avoid shearing and friction when moving patient.
13. Supporting family coping.
    - Assess family for usual coping skills and resources used.
    - Introduce family to new resources available for support.
    - Listen and address family concerns and provide needed information.
    - Teach patient care skills needed for home care to family.

In addition, the patient with confusion or disorientation may be taken care by using following measures.

1. Promote communication.
   - Touch may be useful to establish communication.
   - Use calm, quiet and unhurried voice to talk to patient.
   - Talk slowly and distinctly and use short sentences.
   - Face patient when talking and stay with conversational range.
2. Promote orientation.
   - Explain procedure in advance.
   - Environment should be well-lighted.
   - Keep large calender and clock in view.
   - Introduce self when caring for patient.
   - Keep sensory stimulation to a minimum.
   - Provide consistency in staff caring for patient.
   - Keep decision making to a minimum.
3. Support family.

Increased Intracranial Pressure (IICP)

Normal intracranial pressure (ICP) is the pressure exerted by the total volume from the three components within the skull: brain tissue, blood and CSF. ICP can be measured in the ventricles, subarachnoid space, subdural space, epidural space, or brain paranchymal tissue using a water manometer or a pressure transducer. With the patient in the lateral recumbent position, the pressure is generally recorded at 60 to 150 mm H_2O with the use of the water manometer. When the patient is lying with a 30-degree elevation of the head and the pressure is measured intracranially, it is 0 to 15 mm Hg with the use of the pressure transducer. A sustained pressure above the upper limit is considered abnormal.

Increased ICP is a life-threatening situation that results from an increase in any or all of the three components i.e. brain tissue, blood and CSF. It is a pathological process common to many neurological conditions. The intracranial volume composed of brain tissue (85 per cent) intracranial blood volume (5 per cent) and cerebrospinal fluid (10 per cent). Any increase in the volume of any of these contents singly in combinations, results in an increase in ICP, because the cranial vault is rigid and nonexpandable.

Aetiology

Any lesion that increases one or more of the intracranial content is called a space-occupying lesion. Cerebral oedema is the important factor contributing to increased ICP. Conditions associated with cerebral oedema are as follows:

i. Mass lesions
   - Neoplasms (Primary and materialistic).
   - Abscess Hydrocephalus.
   - Haemorrhage (intracerebral and extracerebral haematoma).

ii. Head injuries (Haemorrhage, contusion, Posttraumatic brain swelling.

iii. Brain surgery.

iv. Brain infections.

v. Vascular insult.
   - Infarction (thrombolic and embolic).

- Venous thrombosis.
- Anoxic and ischaemic episodes.

vi. Toxic or metabolic encephalophatic conditions.
Lead and arsenic intoxication.
Renal failure and liver failure.
Reye's syndrome.

Contributory factors are increased ICP will include

- Hypercapnia ($PaCO_2$ 45 mm Hg)
- Hypoxaemia (PaO_2 60 mm Hg)
- Cerebral vasodialatory agents (e.g. alothane, Antihistamine)
- Valsalva manuoever.
- Body positioning (Prone, flexion of neck, extreme hip flexion).
- Isometric muscle contractions
- Coughing or sneezing
- Rapid eye movement sleep
- Emotional upsets
- Noxious stimuli
- Arousal from sleep
- Clustering of actions.

Pathophysiology

The cranial vault is a rigid, closed compartments. The intracranial contents of the brain, blood and CSF occupy the skull fully and exists in a dynamic equilibrium under normal conditions. The Monro-Kellie hypothesis states that conditions that increase one or more of the intercranial conent must cause a reciprocal change in the remaining contents or an increase in ICP will occur. As the intercranial volume increases, compensatory mechanisms take place. CSF-filled spaces can be compressed and CSF redistributed to the lumbar cistern to reduce intracranial CSF volume. Intracranial blood vessels, especially the veins can be compressed by surrounding brain tissue and displace intracranial blood volume. These compensatory mechanisms initially are able to accommodate a growing intracranial volume without significant increases in ICP, but these mechanisms are quickly exhausted if the intracranial volume continues to increase. When the volume within the skull overwhelms, the compensatory mechanisms and intracranial pressure begins to rise. Small increase in pressure occurs in response to initial increase in volume. As compensatory mechanisms fail, additional increase in volume causes dramatic increase in ICP. Normal ICP between 0 to 15 mm Hg. pressure over 20 mm Hg are considered to be increased ICP.

As pressure within the skull increases, the cerebral blood vessels may be compressed, causing a reduction in cerebral blood flow (CBF). CBF is the amount of blood in millilitres passing through 100 gms of brain tissue in 1 minute. The global CBF is approximately 50 ml per minute per 100 gram of brain tissue. There is a difference in flow between the white and gray matter of the brain. The white matter has a slower blood flow (25 ml/m/100 g brain tissue) and the gray matter has a faster blood flow (75 ml/minute/100 g. brain tissue). The maintenance of blood flow to the brain is critical because the brain requires a constant supply of oxygen and glucose. The brain uses 20 per cent of the body's oxygen and 25 per cent of its glucose. Inadequate perfusion initiates a vicious cycle, causing the partial carbon dioxide pressure (PCO_2) to increase and the partial oxygen pressure (PO_2) and pH to decrease cerebral arterioles have the ability to autoregulate, which allows them to dilate or constrict to maintain a constant blood supply to the brain. Changes such as an increasing PCO_2 or decreasing pH cause vasodilatation of the cerebral blood vessels and an increase in ICP. Autoregulation works when the mean arterial pressure (MAP) is between 50mm Hg and 150 mm Hg and when the metabolic environment of the brain is normal. Severe anoxia and hypotensive state cause autoregulation to fail, subjecting the brain blood supply to the wide variations of systolic blood pressure (SBP).

Cerebral perfusion pressure (CPP) is a parameter used to monitor the adequacy of blood flow to the brain in the face of increased ICP. As ICP increases, blood vessels may be compressed, reducing blood flow to the brain in the face of increased ICP. As ICP increases, blood vessels may be unpressed, reducing blood flow to the brain. SBP needs to be high enough to overcome the ICP and deliver sufficient oxygen and glucose to brain tissues. The CPP measured by subtracting ICP from MAP. The formula is

$$CPP = MAP - ICP$$

$$MAP = DBP + 1/3\,(SBP - DBP) \text{ or } \frac{SBP + 2\,(DBP)}{3}$$

(DBP = Diastolic Blood Pressure.)

For example, SBP = 122/84
MAP = 97, ICP = 12 mmHg. CPP = 85 mm Hg.

The actual brain structure can also be affected by increased ICP. The brain is surrounded and divided into compartments within the skull by the dura matter. The presence of oedema or space-occupying lesions may cause brain tissue to shift or herniate. Subfalcial or cingulate herniation occurs when the brain is forced under the falx-cerebri that separates the cerebral hemispheres. Uncal herniation occurs when the uncal portion of the temporal lobes shift over the edge of the tentorium cerebelli. Transformental herniation occurs when the brainstem is forced downward through the foramen magnum.

Clinical Manifestations

The clinical manifestations of increased ICP can take many forms, depending on the cause, location and rate at which the pressure increase occurs. The common clinical manifestation of increased ICP are as follows:

Early Signs

- Decreasing level of consciousness in the earlier and most sensitive sign.

- Headache that increases in intensity with coughing and straining.
- Pupillary changes
  - Dilation with slowed constrictions.
  - Visual disturbances such as diplopia and ptosis.
- Contralateral motor or sensory losses
  - Decrease in motor function.

Late Signs

- Further decrease in level of consciousness.
- Changes in vital signs
  - Rise in systolic blood pressure.
  - Decrease in distolic blood pressure.
  - Widened pulse pressure.
  - Slow pulse.
- Respiratory dysrhythmias
  - shallow, slowed respirations.
  - Irregular patterns or periods of apnoea.
  - Hiccups.
- Fever without clear source of infection.
- Vomitting (more common in children).
- Decerebrate (Extensor or decorticate (flexor) posturing).

It is often difficult to identify increased ICP as the cause of coma-loss of consciousness also confuses the interpretation of clinical signs making it difficult to follow the progression of the increasing ICP.

Diagnostic Studies

- History and physical examination.
- Vital signs, neurologic checks, ICP measurements (via intraventricular catheter, subdural bolt or epidural transducer) every hour.
- Skull, chest and spinal x-rays.
- MRI, CT scan, EEG, angiography.
- Cerebral blood flow and velocity studies, PET.
- Lubricating studies including CBC, coagulation profile, electrolytes creatinine, ammonia level, general drug and toxicology screen, CSF protein, cells and glucose. ABGS.
- ECG.

The nurse has to assist in carrying out these diagnostic studies.

Management

- The goals of management are to identify and treat the underlying cause of increased ICP and to support brain function. A careful history is an important diagnostic aid that can direct the search for the underlying cause. The possible causes of unconsciousness may be:
- Trauma: Head and neck trauma.
- Infection, Meningitis and encephalitis.
- Poison: Drug overdose, toxic exposure and carbon monoxide.
- Metabolic : Diabetic coma, insulin shock, liver failure, uraemia, cardiac arrest and CVA.

An assessment finding (possible) over dose of drug and others elicited are:

- Unresponsive to voice and pain.
- Dilated or pinpoint pupils may be unreactive.
- Involuntary movements.
- Flaccidity or rigidity of muscles.
- Depressed or hyperactive reflexes.
- Decerebrated or decorticate posturing.
- Diaphoresis.
- Hyperthermia.
- Flushed dry skin.
- Glasgow coma scale score < 12.
- Abnormal vital signs.
- Arrythmias.
- Odour of alcohol, acetone on breath.
- Track marks.
- Signs of trauma.
- Petechae or rash.

An intervention included in emergency management of unconscious patient will indicate:

In initial stages:

- Ensure patent airway
- Administer oxygen via nasal cannula or nonrebreather mask
- Establish IV access with one large-bore catheter and normal saline.
- Administer IV naloxine if narcotic overdose suspected.
- Administer thiamine to malnourished or known alcoholic patient to prevent Wernick's encephalopathy.
- Administer one vial 50% dextrose if blood glucose < 60 mg/dl (3.3 mm 01/L).
- Prepare for IV insulin administration of glucose > 400 mg/dl (22.2 mm 01/L).
- Elevate head of bed or position on side to prevent aspiration (unless trauma involved).

And ongoing monitoring instituted to:

- Monitor vital signs, level of consciousness, oxygen saturation, cardiac rhythm, glasgow coma score, pupil size and reactivity, respiratory status.
- Anticipate need for intubation if gag reflex is absent.
- Anticipate gastric lavage if drug overdose is suspected.

The nursing intervention to be continued along with collaboration management of patient with increased ICP are:

- Elevation of head of bed to 30 degrees with head in a neutral position to facilitate reduction of cerebral oedema.
- Intubation and controlled ventilation to $PaCO_2$ of 30 to 35 mmHg because CO_2 is a potent cerebral vasodilator and hyperventilation reduces $PaCO_2$.

- Good pulmonary toilet to improve ventilation and prevent pulmonary complication by removing accumulated secretions, which helps to reduce risk of aspiration and ensure patent airway.
- Maintenance of fluid and electrolyte balance and assessment of osmalality.
- Maintenance of systolic arterial pressure between 100 and 160 mm Hg.
- Maintenance of CPP > 70 mmHg.
- Maintenance of PaO_2 at 100 mm Hg or greater.
- Maintenance of normothermia.
- Adequate sedation.
- Drug therapy as prescribed.
  - Osmotic diuretics (mannitol).
  - Loop diuretics fursomide (lasix), ethacrynic and (Edecrin).
  - Corticosteroids (methylprednisone, demamethosone (Decadran).
  - GI ulcer prophylactic (H_2^- Receptor antagoinst e.g. Cimetedine).
- ICP monitoring.

Table 11.1: Nursing care plan for the patient with increased intracranial pressure

Problem	*R*	*Objective*	*Nursing Interventions*	*Rationales*
Nursing Diagnosis #1				
Alteration in cerebral tissue perfusion, related to: 1. Increased intracranial pressure associated with cranial and/or cere bral insult (head injury, haematoma formation, cerebral haemorrhage, cerebral oedema).		Patient will: 1. Maintain cerebral perfusion pressure (CCP) > 60 mmHg. • Intracranial pressure (ICP) <15 mmHg. • Mean arterial blood pressure (MAP) ~80-100 mmHg or baseline (for patient).	• Monitor continuously for signs and symptoms of increasing ICP.	• Continuous monitoring is necessary as patient responses related to intracranial pressure can change rapidly from moment to moment.
			• Establish baseline parameters.	• Baseline measurements can be used to compare subsequent responses.
			• Determine arousability and assess for changes in level of consciousness and mentation: restlessnss, agitation, irritability: disorientation, inattentiveness; disturbed thought processes, loss of memory; inability to answer questions or follow commands.	• Arousability reflects functioning of reticular activating system within brainstem. • Level of consciousness provides earliest clinical evidence of a change in intracranial volume/ pressure dynamics. It reflects the status of cerebral hemispheres and diencephalon.
			• Assess for sensory function: – Special senses: visual acuity and visual fields; hearing. – Somatic senses: touch, pressure, pain, temperature, proprioception, vibration.	• Assessment of sensory function affords an evaluation of sensory pathways and functioning of primary sensory center (post-central gyrus, parietal lobe).
			• Assess for motor function (somatic): appropriate or inappropriate responses (decorticate or decerebrate posturing, flaccidity); muscle strength, tone, deep tendon reflexes.	• Appropriate motor responses and deep tendon reflexes reflect intact sensory pathways and total or partial intact motor pathways and neuromuscular junctions.
			• Assess for motor function (autonomic): respiratory rate and pattern; pupillary size and reactivity; ocular movements; dysconjugate gaze, nystagmus; oculocephalic and oculovestibular reflexes (doll's eyes phenomenon and caloric tests).	• Pupillary responses reflect status of midbrain and pons. In the patient with an altered state of consciousness who has fixed, moderately dilated pupils, ocular reflexes may provide the only clinical data reflective of the level of brainstem function.
			• Assess cranial nerves and status of protective reflexes.	• Increasing ICP causes pressure on brainstem, disrupting cranial nerve function (IX and X) and compromising protective reflexes (gag, cough, epiglottal closure). This places airway in great danger.

Contd...

Problem	*R*	*Objective*	*Nursing Interventions*	*Rationales*
			• Assess for headache, nausea, vomiting, papilledaema, diplopia, blurred vision, seizures.	• Many signs/symptoms of early rise in ICP tend to be nonspecific.
			• Assess vital signs: mean arterial blood pressure, pulse pressure, heart rate.	• A rise in blood pressure, widening pulse pressure, and slow, bounding heart rate are classic, late-occurring signs of increasing ICP.
			• Maintain intracranial pressure monitoring (ICPM) system.	• ICPM is a highly invasive technique with a high risk of infection.
			• Take measures to reduce risk of infection: wash hands meticulously, use aseptic technique at all times.	
			• Maintain integrity of ICPM system: – Check for leaks of air and ensure all stopcocks are in their appropriate positions.	• Maintaining a closed system and avoiding disconnections reduce the risk of infection.
			• Flush system as per protocol if appropriate for method in use. – Turn off stopcock to patient if it is absolutely necessary to disconnect the system.	• Introduction of any fluid into the system for whatever reason can be very dangerous in the compromised patient. If done, it should only be done with continuous ICPM. Such activities are usually the responsibility of the patient's physician; nurses do not routinely inject fluid into the ICPM sustem.
			• Avoid rapid or prolonged drainage of cerebrospinal fluid (CSF); follow unit protocol.	• Aspiration of CSF is a critical procedure, which can markedly reduce ICP, especially when intracranial volume is increased and compliance is significantly reduced. Risk of infection is a major disadvantage of this pressure-reducing measure. It can also precipitate a collapse of the ventricle or cause brain tissue to be sucked into the monitoring catheter or other device (subarachnoid screw). – Excessive loss of CSF in the presence of increased ICP can alter intracranial pressure dynamics and precipitate herniation.
			– Protect ICPM system when moving or positioning patient, or if patient is restless or agitated.	
			• Perform insertion site care as per unit protocol.	• Reduce risk of infection.
			• Obtain the record pressure measurements:	• Avoid treatment of increased ICP without accurate pressure measurements.
			– Confirm accurate placement of transducer; use carpenter's level for accuracy.	– The venting port of transducer should always be at pressure source, the foramen of Monro. Use edge of eyebrow and tragus of ear as guidelines.
			– Balance and recalibrate system if appropriate for method in use.	– For every inch that the measurement is off, approximately 2 mmHg is added or

Contd...

Problem	*R*	*Objective*	*Nursing Interventions*	*Rationales*
				subtracted from the digital readout. This is significant in a low pressure system and must be avoided.
			◆ Observe for fluctuation of CSF column.	◆ Reflects cardiovascular dynamics and indicates proper placement of catheter or screw.
			◆ Obtain baseline wave form configuration and digital readout.	◆ Establishes measure with which to compare subsequent data.
			◆ Monitor pressure waveform and digital readouts continuously.	◆ Waveform configuration and amplitude can reflect patency of system, rise in ICP, and status of intracranial compliance.
			– Be consistent in taking ICP readings. – Calculate and record cerebral perfusion pressure hourly.	
			◆ Analyze waveforms and pressure readings and identify trends.	◆ *Trends* are more significant in determining status of ICP and intracranial compliance.
			◆ Troubleshoot the system if unable to obtain a waveform, or if the waveform is dampened.	
			• Implement measures to prevent rise in and/or reduce ICP.	
			◆ Maintain proper positioning: elevate head of bed 30 to 45 degrees; avoid using pillows.	◆ Allow for optimal venous drainage from cranium via gravity; prevents compromise of cerebral blood flow.
			– Maintain body alignment in midline, and avoid neck flexion or head rotation.	– Prevents jugular vein compression or obstruction.
			– Avoid hip flexion. – Maintain head-neck alignment when turning.	– May increase intra-abdominal pressure and impede cerebral drainage via jugular veins and vena cavae.
			◆ Prevent increase in cerebral blood flow.	◆ Increase in cerebral blood volume may compromise compensation and compliance in the patient with increased ICP.
			– Initiate controlled hyperventilation: – Maintain $PaCO_2$ 25-35 mmHg, $PaO_2 > 80$ mmHg. – Monitor arterial blood gas.	– Reduced $PaCO_2$ (hypocapnia) causes cerebral vasoconstriction and thus lowers cerebral blood volume. A reduction in cerebral blood volume augments compensatory mechanisms or compliance.
			◆ Minimize cellular metabolism: – Relieve pain and anxiety.	◆ Reduction in cellular metabolism decreases need for metabolic substrates (e.g., carbon dioxide and hydrogen ions). The end result is a decrease in cerebral blood flow and intracranial pressure.
			◆ Pain nursing care activities so as to avoid a *cumulative* increase in ICP.	◆ A potential increase in ICP can occur when nursing care activities are implemented in close succession.
			– Identify activities that cause a change in ICP (e.g., coughing, suctioning, positioning)	– Provides a guide for planning nursing care.

Contd...

Problem	*Objective*	*Nursing Interventions*	*Rationales*
		– Incorporate planned rest periods into daily nursing care spaced between those procedures known to increase ICP.	
		♦ Administer prescribed sedatives or analgesics prior to procedures that may cause an increase in ICP.	♦ These measures may prevent an inordinate increase in ICP.
		♦ Avoid discussing patient's condition at the bedside or within earshot of the patient.	♦ Such conversations, if overheard, could be upsetting to the patient and may predispose to an increase in ICP.
		♦ Teach the responsive patient to avoid excessive coughing. Valsalva's manoeuver (straining), isometric exercises, or pushing against bed rails; avoid use of foot-board or restraints.	♦ These activities increase intrathoracic and intra-abdominal pressures, which can impede outflow of blood from cranium.
		♦ Assess for bladder distention, paralytic ileus, constipation. – Maintain quiet environment with a minimum of stimuli; gently stroke the patient and speak with a soothing tone of voice.	♦ These conditions may cause abdominal distention, thus increasing intra-abdominal pressures and limiting diaphragmatic excursion.
Nursing Diagnosis #2 Airway clearance ineffective, related to: 1. Compromised cough, 2. Immobility with pooling of secretions.	Patient will: 1. Maintain intact airway and protective reflexes. 2. Demonstrate secretion-clearing cough. 3. Have breath sounds clear on auscultation.	• Prevent accumulation of tracheobronchial secretions.	• Accumulation of secretions reduces alveolar ventilation; a consequent hypercapnia causes an increase in cerebral blood flow, which increases ICP.
		♦ Perform suctioning only when indicated by auscultation of breath sounds or excessive coughing. • Suction only breifly (<10 seconds).	♦ Suctioning stimulates cough reflex and Valsalva's manoeuver; a consequent increase in intrathoracic pressure reduces venous outflow from the brain via jugular veins and vena cava.
		♦ Pre-oxygenate and hyperventilate with 100 per cent oxygen before suctioning; repeat after suctioning.	♦ Proper suctioning technique minimizes the risk of hypoxaemia.
Nursing Diagnosis #3 potential for fluid and electrolyte imbalance, related to: 1. Osmotic diuretic therapy. 2. Diabetes insipidus.	Patient will: 1. Maintain baseline body weight. 2. Balance fluid intake with output. 3. Maintain baseline laboratory values. • Serum electrolytes, BUN, creatinine, serum protein, serum osmolality. • Urine-specific gravity—0.010 to 0.025.	• Limit or decrease cerebral oedema: ♦ Administer diuretic (furosemide) and hyperosmolar agents (Mannitol, urea) as prescribed. Monitor response to therapy.	• Fluid restriction coupled with pharmacologic therapy helps to decrease extracellular fluid volume that may contribute to oedema formation. A mild dehydrated state is usually maintained.
		♦ Administer prescribed corticosteroid therapy (dexamethasone or methylprednisolone). – Monitor response to therapy.	♦ Corticosteroids are thought to amellorate cerebral oedema, which occurs secondarily to the primary craniocerebral insult.
		♦ Restrict fluid intake (usually 1200-1500 ml/day).	♦ Intake/output includes intravenous medications (IV piggybacks) and CSF.
		♦ Meticulously record intake and output (hourly). – Weigh patient daily if not contraindicated.	♦ A Foley catheter is usually inserted to reduce patient activity and to monitor urine output. Physician should be notified if urine output is <30 or >200 ml/hr for 2 consecutive hours.
		♦ Monitor urine-specific gravity.	♦ Craniocerebral insults frequently predispose to diabetes insipidus.

Contd...

Problem	*R*	*Objective*	*Nursing Interventions*	*Rationales*
			◆ Monitor serum electrolytes and replace as prescribed. ◆ Monitor serum osmolality and maintain at 305-315 mOsm/kg.	◆ Increased serum osmolality helps to draw fluid from brain interstitium and reduce cerebral oedema.
Nursing Diagnosis #4 Potential for physiologic injury, related to seizures.		Patient will remain seizure free on anticonvulsant medications.	• Prevent seizure activity by administering prescribed anticonvulsant therapy. – Monitor patient's response to anticonvulsant therapy. ◆ Maintain normothermia and prevent shivering.	• Seizure activity greatly increases the demand for oxygen and glucose and, thus, cerebral blood flow. ◆ Pyrexia causes cerebral vasodilation with increased blood flow. For every 1øF increase in-body temperature, metabolic rate increases by 10 per cent.
Nursing Diagnosis #5 Potential for physiologic injury, related to gastrointestinal bleeding associated with stress, and possibly corticosteroid therapy.		Patient will: 1. Remain without gestrointestinal bleeding: • Absence of blood in gastric contents and stool. • Stable haematocrit, haemoglobin, and RBC values. 2. Maintain gastric pH >4.5.	• Initiate therapy to reduce the risk of gastrointestinal bleeding. – Administer prescribed histamine receptor antagonists: ranitidine (Zantac)2 is used most commonly. – Initiate antacid prophylaxis therapy as prescribed. ◆ Monitor acidity of gastric pH every 1 to 2 hr.	• Patients under extreme stress who receive corticosteroids seem to be at higher risk of developing gastrointestinal bleeding. ◆ Ideal gastric pH is greater than 4.5.
Nursing Diagnosis #6 Potential for infection, related to: 1. Invasive monitoring technique. 2. Compromised proprotective reflexes (gag, cough, epiglottal closure). 3. Compromised immune response (stress, corticosteroid therapy). 4. Altered nutrition.		Patient will: 1. Maintain normal body temperature ~ 98.6°F (37°C). 2. Maintain white blood count at baseline level. 3. Remain without other evidence of infection (e.g., cough productive of thick, tenacious sputum; cloudy appearing urine; pain, redness, and swelling at invasive monitoring and intravenous sites).	• Implement measures to reduce risk of infection. ◆ Maintain sterile technique for all procedures involved in ICPM. ◆ Maintain aseptic technique for all invasive procedures: – Endotracheal/tracheostomy tube care and management. – Foley catheter care. – All invasive lines: pulmonary artery catheter; triple lumen catheters (CVP or central lines); all peripheral intravenous lines. ◆ Prevent urinary retention. – Monitor the following parameters: temperature; all intravenous sites for signs of redness, swelling, warmth, pain, and tenderness. – Assess for wound drainage—quantity and quality. – Monitor cough and sputum production. – Monitor WBC profile. ◆ Assess for signs of meningeal irritation: increased restlessness; presence of Kernig or Brudzinski signs; status of protective reflexes; cough, gag, epiglottal closure. ◆ Obtain culture and sensitivity on body	• An increase in body temperature of 1°F can increase cerebral cellular metabolism by 10 per cent. ◆ ICPM is a highly invasive diagnostic approach placing the patient at serious risk of infection (e.g., meningitis, encephalitis). – Artificial airways compromise the normal physiologic functions of the respiratory tract including the warming, filtering, and humidifying of inhaled gases. ◆ The physiologically compromised patient is at risk of urinary infection. ◆ Status of protective reflexes needs to be monitored because aspiration is a common risk in the compromised patient. ◆ Cultures and sensitivity ensure

Contd...

Problem	R	Objective	Nursing Interventions	Rationales
	/		discharges, secretions, wounds, and puncture sites. – Initiate prescribed antibiotic therapy and monitor response to therapy. ◆ All staff caring for compromised patient should execute meticulous handwashing; visitors should be taught to do likewise.	that the appropriate antibiotic is prescribed.
			◆ Monitor nutrition status.	◆ Neurologically compromised patients are at risk of malnutrition; an appropriate dietary regimen should be initiated as early as possible.
			– Hyperalimentation should be initiated early in treatment.	– Hyperalimentation provides necessary protein for tissue repair and rebuilding; necessary carbohydrates and lipids for energy; and necessary minerals and vitamins for cellular metabolism.

Head Injury or Craniocerebral Trauma

Head injury includes any trauma to the scalp, skull, or brain tissues either singly or collectively. The term head trauma is used primarily to signify craniocerebral trauma, which includes alteration in consciousness, no matter how brief. Head trauma has a high potential for poor outcome. Death from head injury trauma occurs at three time points after, injury, immediately after injury, within 2 hours after injury, and approximately 3 weeks after injury. The majority of deaths after a head injury occur immediately after the injury, either from the direct head trauma or from massive haemmorrhage and shock. Death occurring within a few hours of the trauma caused by progressive worsening of the head injury or from internal bleeding. An imemdiate note of change in neurologic status and surgical intervention are critical in the prevention of deaths at this point. Death occurring 3 weeks or more after injury results from multisystem failure. Expert nursing care in the weeks following the injury are crucial in decreasing mortality. Factors that predict a poor outcome include the presence of an intracranial haematoma, increasing age of the patient, abnormal motor responses, impaired or absent eye movement or pupil light refluxes, early sustained hypertension hypoxaemia, or hypercapnia and ICP level higher than 20 mm Hg.

Aetiology

The variables that influence the extent of the injury to the head include the following.

- Status of the head at impact-moving or still.
- Location and direction of the impact.
- Rate of energy transfer.
- Surface area involved in the energy transfer.

Blunt head injuries will occur due to motor vehicle collision, pedestrian event, fall, assault and sports injury. Penetrating head injuries are due to - gunshot wound arrow and such types.

Pathophysiology

Mechanisms of trauma to the head are of general types, deformation, acceleration-deceleration and rotation.

- *Deformation* results from the transmission of energy to the skull of the energy is sufficient, the skill is deformed of fractured.
- *Acceleration-deceleration* injuries typically occur when the acceleration skull moving in a motor vehicle, suddenly decelerates when it hits an immobile object as the steering wheel or windshield.
- *Rotational* forces also distort the brain and can cause tension, stretching and diffuse shearing of brain tissues. Often the forces of acceleration, deceleration and rotation occur together, affecting both the brain and spinal cord.

Injuries vary from minor scalp wound to concussions and open skull fractures with severe brain injury.

- *Scalp lacerations* are the most minor of the head trauma, because the scalp contains many blood vessels with poor constructive abilities. Most scalp lacerations associated with profuse bleeding. The major complication associated with it is infection.
- *Skull fractures* are a common form of primary craniocerebral trauma. Fracture of the skull may be linear or depressed, simple or communuted, or combine and closed or open.
  i. Linear fractures caused by low-velocity injuries in which break is continuity of bone without alteration of relationship of parts.
  ii. Depressed fractures caused by powerful blow, in which inward dentation of skull is seen.
  iii. Simple fractures are caused by low to moderate impact in which linear or depressed fracture without fragmentation or communicating lacerations are present.

iv. Communuted fractures are caused by direct high momentory impact, in which multiple linear fractures with fragmentation of bone into many places are seen.

v. Compound facture is a severe head injury in which there will be a depressed skull fracture and scalp laceration with communicating pathway to intracranial cavity.

The location of the fracture alters the presentation of the clinical signs and symptoms. Clinical manifestation of the skull fractures by location are as follows:

Location		*Syndrome or Sequelae*
i. Frontal Fracture	:	• Exposure of brain to contaminatants through frontal air sinus. • Possible association with air in forehead tissue. • CSF rhinorrhoea or pneumocranium.
ii. Orbital fracture	:	• Periorbital ecchymosis (raccoon eyes).
iii. Temporal fracture	:	• Boggy temporal muscle because of extravasation of blood, benign oval-shaped bruise behind ear in mastoid region (Battles sign). • CSF otorrhoea.
iv. Parietal fracture	:	• Deafness. • CSF or brain otorrhoea. • Bulging of tympanic membrane caused by blood or CSF. • Facial paralysis. • Loss of taste. • Battle's sign.
v. Posterior fossa fracture	:	• Occipital bruising resulting in cortical blindness end visual field defects. • Rare appearance of ataxia or other cerebellar signs.
vi. Basillar skull fracture	:	• CSF or brain otorrhoea, bulging of tympanic membrane caused by blood or CSF. • Battle's sign. • Tinnitus or hearing difficulty. • Facial paralysis. • Conjugate deviation of gaze. • Vertigo.

The major potential complication of skull fractures are intracranial infections and haemotoma, as well as meningeal and brain tissue damage.

Brain injuries are categorized as being minor or major.

i. *Minor head injury*: Concussion is considered as minor head injury. Concussion refers to a sudden transient mechanical head injury with disruption of neural activity and a change in level of consciousness. Signs of concussion include:
   - Brief disruption in LOC.
   - Amnesia regarding the event (retrograde amnesia) and
   - Headache.

The manifestations are generally of short duration. A loss of consciousness may occur that is instant or delayed, and the person usually recovers rapidly. Any person who exhibits alteration in consciousness after a blow to the head should be closely observed, after the injury, because the extent of the damage is not always immediately apparent. The postconcussions syndrome is seen anywhere from 2 weeks to 2 months after concussion. The symptoms include:

- Persistent headache, dizziness and fatigue.
- Lethargy.
  Personality and behavioural changes.
- Shortened attention-span-impaired concentration.
- Decreased short-term memory and memory impairment.
- Changes in intellectual ability.

ii. *Major head injury*: Major head injury includes contusions and laceration. Both injuries represent severe trauma to the brain. Contusion and laceration associated with closed injuries.

A *contusion* is the bruising of the brain tissue within a focal area that maintains integrity of the pia mater and archnoid layers. It is structural alteration characterized by extravasation of blood into the brain. A contusion develops areas of necrosis, infarction, haemorrhage and oedema. A contusion frequently occurs at the site of the fracture. It may be at the site of impact or on the opposite side of a camp-contra camp injury. Contusions often damage cerebral cortex. Bleeding around the contusion site is generally minimal, and the blood is reabsorbed slowly. Neurologic assessment demonstrates focal findings and generalized disturbance in the LOC. Seizures are a common complication of brain contusion.

Lacerations involve actual bearing of the brain tissue and occur frequently in association with depressed and compound fractures and penetrating injuries. Tissue damage is severe, and surgical repair of the laceration is impossible., because of the texture of the brain tissue. If bleeding is deep into the brain parenchyma, focal and generalized signs are noted.

When major head injury occurs, many delayed responses are seen including haermorrhage, haematoma formation, seizures and cerebral oedema. Intracerebral haemorrhage is generally associated with cerebral laceration. This haemorrhage manifests as a space-occupying lesion accompanied by unconsciousness, hemeplegia on the contralateral side and dilated pupil on the ipsilateral side. As the haematoma expands, syptoms of increased ICP become more severe. Prognosis generally poor with a large intracerebral haemorrhage.

Diffuse Axonal Injury (DAI) caused by rapid movement of the brain during which delicate axons are stretched and damaged. This damage interferes with nervous transmission and can cause extensive diffuse deficits.

Complications

Secondary injury occurs as a result of the body response to the initial trauma, which include cerebral oedema, increased ICP and haematoma formation.

Cerebral oedema. In response to local injury, bleeding and systemic disturbances in circulation that result in hypoxia, the brain becomes oedematous. Cell damage and systemic hypoxia cause cell membranes to fail, leading to cytotoxicoedma, cell lining the blood vessels are damaged and capillaries become more permeable, allowing fluid to leak out into the interstitial space. This is called vasogenic oedema.

Increased ICP, Vasogenic oedema contributes to increased ICP.

Haematoma Formation

- An epidural haematoma results from bleeding between the dura and the inner surface of the skill.
- A subdural haematoma occurs from bleeding between the duramater and the arachnoid layer of the meningeal covering of the brain. It results from injury to brain substance and its parenchymal vessels (Venous brain).
- Intracerebral haematoma occurs from bleeding within the parenchyma.

This usually occurs within the forntal and temporal lobes possibly from the rupture of intracerebral vessels at the time of injury. A burst lobe in an intracerebral or intracerebellar haematoma that is in extension of subarchnoid haemorrhage. This type of intracerebral haematoma is thought to result from haemorrage of supracortical vessels.

Nursing Management During Emergency

Assessment may be done as with other naurological assessment procedures, and diagnostic studies. Accordingly, findings of the assessment during emergency management will include.

i. *Surface findings*:
   - Scalp laceration.
   - Fracture or depression in skull.
   - Bruises or contusions on face, Battle's sign (Bruising behind ears).
   - Reccon eyes (dependent bruising around eyes).

ii. *Respiratory findings*:
   - Central neurogenic hyperventilation.
   - Cheyne-stokes respirations.
   - Decreased oxygen saturation.
   - Pulmonary oedema.

iii. *Central nervous system*:
   - Unequal or dilated pupils.
   - A symmetric facid movements.
   - Garbled speech and abusive speech.
   - Confusion.
   - Decreased level of consciousness.
   - Combativeness.
   - Involuntary movements.
   - Seizures.
   - Bowel and bladder incontinence.
   - Flaccidity.
   - Depressed or hyperactive reflexes.
   - Decerebrate or decorticate posturing.
   - Glasgow coma scale 12.
   - CSF leaking from ears or nose.

The nursing intervention during initial stage and ongoing monitoring are as follows:

In an initial stage:

- Ensure patent airway.
- Stabilize cervical spine.
- Administer oxygen via nasal cannular or non-rebreather mask.
- Establish IV access with two large bore catheters to infuse normal saline or lactated Ringer's solution.
- Control external bleeding with sterile pressure dressing.
- Assess for rhinorrhoea, scalp wounds.
- Remove patient's clothing.

Ongoing monitoring includes:

- Maintain patient warmth using blankets, warmth IV fluids, overhead warming lights and warm humidifying oxygen.
- Monitor vital signs, level of consciousness, oxygen saturation, cardiac rhythem, Glasgow coma score, pupil size, and reactivity.
- Anticipate need for intubation if gag reflex is absent.
- Assume neck injury with head injury.
- Administer fluids cautiously to prevent fluid overload and increasing ICP.

Nursing Management

Assessment: The patient with head injury is always considered to have potential for development of increased ICP. The data collected generally include information gathered for unconscious patient, which include Glasgow Coma scales, monitory neurological status and determining the leakage of CSF, etc.

Nursing Diagnosis will be:

- Altered tissue perfusion, cerebral related to interruption and cerebral blood flow associated with cerebral haemorrhage, haemotomy and oedema.

- Hyperthermia related to increased metabolism, infection and loss of cerebral integrative function secondary to possible hypothalmic injury.
- Sensory/perceptual alteration related to cerebral injury and ICU environment.
- Pain related to headache, nausea and vomiting.
- Impaired physical mobility R/T decrease LOC and treatment imposed and bedrest.
- Risk for eye injury R/T loss of protective reflexes.
- Risk for infection R/T and environmental contamination.
- Anxiety R/T abrupt charges in health status, hospital environment.
- Self-esteem disturbance R/T altered appearance of head and face.

Planning: The voerall goals are that the patient with an acute head injury will:

- Maintain adequate cerebral perfusion.
- Remain normothermic.
- Be free from pain, discomfort and infection and
- Attain maximum cognitive, motor and sensory function.

Nursing Intervention

The following nursing intervention to be installed when taking care of person with closed head injury.

1. Promote rest.
   - Provide with quiet environment.
   - Observe frequently.
   - Administer anticonvulsants as ordered.
   - Medication for pain as necessary.
2. Maintain temperature.
   - Give tepid sponge bath if hyperthermic.
   - Administer antipyretic as ordered.
   - Use hypothermia blanket if ordered.
   - Reduce or increase temperature in patient's room as needed.
3. Promote adequate respiration
   - Suction only as necessary to provide adequate airway.
   - Elevate head of bed to 30 degrees.
   - Administer supplemental oxygen if ordered.
   - Place patient in side-lying position.
4. Observe for drainage from ears and/or nose.
   - Make no attempt to clean out orifice.
   - Do not suction nose if drainage is present.
   - Test drainage for presence of CSF and refer immediately if present.
5. Control of cerebral oedema:
   - Administer diuretics as ordered.
   - Elevate head of bed to 30 degrees.
   - Perform neurological checks as ordered.
6. Maintain electrolyte balance
   - Observe for inappropriate hydration or dehydration.
   - Monitor electrolytes.
7. Maintain elimination
   - Keep accurate intake and output record.
   - Restrict fluid if ordered.
   - Monitor output.
   - Remove catheter as soon as possible.
8. Provide emotional support
   - Give specific guidelines for appropriate behaviour.
   - Give positive feedback.
   - Allow patient adequate time to complete tasks.

Table 11.2: Care plan for the patient with acute head injury

Problem	*R*	*Objective*	*Nursing Interventions*	*Rationales*
Nursing Diagnosis #1 Alteration in cerebral perfusion pressure, related to: 1. Cerebral/oedema. 2. Potential intracranial bleeding and haematoma formation.		Patient will: 1. Maintain: • Cerebral perfusion pressure > 60 mmHg. • Intracranial pressure < 15 mmHg. • Mean arterial blood pressure ~80 mmHg. 2. Exhibit intact level of consciousness and mentation. • Oriented to person, place, time. • Memory intact. 3. Demonstrate intact sensorimotor function.	♦ Monitor for signs and symptoms of increasing intracranial pressure. ♦ Maintain the integrity of the intracranial pressure monitoring system.[3] ♦ Implement measures to prevent and/or reduce intracranial pressure: Maintain optimal positioning. – Prevent increase in cerebral blood flow. – Limit or decrease cerebral oedema. – Minimize cellular metabolism. – Plan nursing care activities to prevent cumulative increase in intracranial pressure.[4]	• Refer to Table 8-2 for presentation of the following nursing interventions/rationales.

Contd...

Problem	*R*	*Objective*	*Nursing Interventions*	*Rationales*
		• Distinguish pinprick from crude pressure. • Purposeful response to painful stimuli.		
Nursing Diagnosis #2 Breathing pattern ineffective, related to: 1. Brainstem compression associated with: a. Cerebral oedema. b. Rapidly expanding mass lesion (e.g., subdural hematoma).		Patient will demonstrate effective breathing pattern: 1. Respiratory rate <25/min. 2. Rhythm and depth of spontaneous breathing—eupneic. • Tidal volume >1-10 ml/kg. • Vital capacity >12-15 ml/kg. 3. Adequate alveolar ventilation: • $PaCO_2 < 30$-35 mmHg. • $PaO_2 > 80$ mmHg. • pH 7.35–7.45.	• Assess airway patency and spontaneous ventilatory effort. • Implement measures to maintain airway patency. • Implement measures to improve breathing pattern.	• Refer to Table 9-1, Nursing Diagnosis #2, for specific nursing interventions/rationales including:
Nursing Diagnosis #3 Airway clearance ineffective, related to: 1. Compromised cough. 2. Thick tenacious secretions.		Patient will: 1. Maintain patent airway with normal breath sounds. 2. Demonstrate secretion-clearing cough (unless contraindicated by increased intracranial pressure).		• Refer to Table 9-1, Nursing Diagnosis #3, for specific nursing interventions/rationales.
Nursing Diagnosis #4 Imapired gas exchange, related to: 1. Neurogenic pulmonary oedema (i.e., adult respiratory distress syndrome [ARDS] of neurogenic origin): • Right to left shunting. • Ventilation/perfusion mismatch. • Diffusion defect.		Patient will: 1. Be alert and oriented to person, place, time. 2. Demonstrate appropriate behaviour. 3. Maintain effective cardiovascular haemodynamics: • Mean arterial blood pressure within ~10 mmHg of baseline. • Cardiac output ~4-8 liters/min. • Haematocrit > 30-35 per cent. • Haemoglobin > 10 g/100 ml. 4. Maintain optimal arterial blood gases: • $PaCO_2$ ~ 30 mmHg. • $PaO_2 > 80$ mmHg. • pH 7.35–7.45.	• Establish baseline assessment parameters for neurologic, respiratory, and cardiovascular function. • Administer prescribed humidified oxygen therapy. • In addition: • Implement positive end-expiratory pressure (PEEP) as prescribed, carefully-monitoring effect on intracranial pressure. • Perform ongoing intracranial and arterial pressure monitoring. • Assess effectiveness of interaction of intracranial and haemodynamic phenomena in terms of maintaining adequate cerebral perfusion pressure (>60 mmHg; ideally 80-90 mmHg).	• Refer to Table 34-3, Nursing Diagnosis #1, for specific nursing care activities including: • Consequent increase in intrathoracic pressure impedes venous outflow from the cranial vault via the venous sinuses, internal jugular veins, and superior vena cava; the resulting increase in intracranial volume may cause a precipitous rise in intracranial pressure in patients with unstable intracranial pressure and reduced brain compliance.
Nursing Diagnosis #5 Alteration in fluid and electrolyte balance:		Patient will:		• See Chapters 23 and 30.

Contd...

Problem	*Objective*	*Nursing Interventions*	*Rationales*
1. Fluid volume excess with associated: • Cerebral oedema. 2. Fluid volume deficit, related to: • Diuretic therapy. • Diabetes insipidus. 3. Altered electrolytes, related to: • Diuretic therapy. • Corticosteroid therapy. • Acid-base imbalance.	1. Maintain effective haemodynamic function: • Mean arterial blood pressure ~80 mmHg. • Heart rate at baseline for patient. • Cardiac rhythm regular, without dysrhythmias. 2. Demonstrate intact level of consciousness and mentation: • Oriented to person, place, time. • Memory intact. • Appropriate responses to verbal commands. 3. Maintain balanced intake and output: • Daily weight stable at patient's baseline (unless contraindicated). • Urine output > 30 ml, <200 ml/hr. • Urine specific gravity 1.010-1.025. 4. Maintain laboratory parameters within acceptable range: • Haematocrit, haemoglobin. • Serum electrolytes, BUN, and creatinine. • Serum osmolality.	◆ Monitor for signs and symptoms of diabetes insipidus. ◆ Implement measures to maintain adequate fluid intake to prevent dehydration (in the scenario of diabetes insipidus). ◆ Administer prescribed medications (to treat diabetes inalpidus).	• Refer to Table 9-1, Nursing Diagnosis #5, for presentation of the following nursing interventions/rationales.
Nursing Diagnosis #6 Alteration in oral mucous membranes, related to: 1. Dehydration (diabetes insipidus). 2. Compromised nutritional intake.	Patient will maintain oral mucous membranes that are intact, moist, and free of infection.	• Assess for evidence of dehydration including the following parameters: ◆ Assess vital signs; intake and output; skin turgour over forehead or sternum; presence of sunken eyeballs. ◆ Assess mouth and oropharynx for dryness, cracking, fissures, bleeding, or other lesions. • Provide supportive care: ◆ Maintain hydration as prescribed. ◆ Provide oral hygiene at frequent intervals. ◆ Apply Vaseline or swabs with glycerin.	• Dry, cracking, or fissured mucous membranes reflect dehydrated state. ◆ Ongoing assessment assists in determining changes in the mucosa and response to fluid therapy. ◆ Ideally, the patient is maintained in a slightly dehydrated state to minimize risk of cerebral oedema. ◆ Provides comfort, is aesthetically appealing, reduces risk of oral infection in compromised patient (e.g., Candida albicans). ◆ Prevents cracking and fissure formation.
Nursing Diagnosis #7 Potential for injury: Seizures, related to:	Patient will:	◆ Assess characteristics of seizure activity.	• Refer to Table 9-1, Nursing Diagnosis #6, for presentation of the following nursing interventions/rationales.

Contd...

Problem	*R*	*Objective*	*Nursing Interventions*	*Rationales*
1. Cerebral hypoxia associated with: • Increased intracranial pressure. • Reduced cerebral perfusion pressure. 2. Cerebral irritation, associated with: • Craniocerebral trauma. • Surgical manipulation of fragile brain tissue. • Cerebral oedema. • Infection (e.g., meningitis).		1. Remain seizure-free. 2. Maintain effective serum levels of phenytoin (Dilantin). • Usual serum levels: 10-20 μg/ml.	♦ Implement safety measures during actual seizure activity. ♦ Implement safety measures to prevent seizure activity. – Avoid activities that increase intracranial pressure. – Monitor for signs of meningeal irritation. – Initiate and maintain seizure precautions. – Administer prescribed anticonvulsant therapy, and monitor response to therapy.	
Nursing Diagnosis #8 Potential for infection: Meningitis, related to: 1. Open, penetrating wound/trauma with leakage of cerebrospinal fluid. 2. Surgical disruption of integrity of meninges. 3. Iatrogenic causes via invasive procedures.[2] 4. Compromised immune response associated with corticosteroid therapy.		Patient will: 1. Maintain body temperature ~98.6°C (37°C). 2. Remain free of signs of meningeal irritation: negative Kernig's/ Brudzinski's signs. 3. Demonstrate normal cerebrospinal fluid analysis including WBC and protein levels. 4. Maintain serum WBC within normal range.	♦ Monitor for signs and symptoms of infection (meningeal irritation). ♦ Assess for rhinorrhoea and otorrhoea. ♦ Assist with lumbar puncture. ♦ Implement measures to prevent infection. ♦ Administer prescribed course of antibiotics, and monitor response to therapy.	• Refer to Table 9-1, Nursing Diagnosis #7, for presentation of nursing interventions/rationales including. ♦ See Table 49-7.
Nursing Diagnosis #9 Potential for alteration in body temperature, related to: 1. Cerebral oedema with altered hypothalamic function. 2. Infection.		Patient will maintain optimal body temperature ~98.6°F (37°C).	♦ Monitor body temperature. ♦ Assess for signs and symptoms of hyperpyrexia. ♦ Obtain specimens of body fluids and discharges for culture and sensitivity. ♦ Inspect all invasive sites and wounds for signs/symptoms of infection. ♦ Implement measures to reduce body temperature.	• Refer to Table 9-1, Nursing Diagnosis #8, for presentatioan of nursing interventions/rationales including.
Nursing Diagnosis#10 Alteration in nutrition: Less than body requirements,lated to: 1. Catabolic state. 2. Compromised nutritional intake associated with: • Altered state of consciousness.		Patient will: 1. Maintain body weight within 5 per cent of patient's baseline. 2. Maintain total serum proteins: 6-8.4 g/100 ml. 3. Maintain laboratory data within acceptable range: BUN, serum creatinine, electrolytes, fasting serum glucose, haematology profile, total protein (albumin).	• Arrange consultation with nutritionist and collaborate to perform nutrition assessment. ♦ Assess specific parameters: general state of health; baseline body weight. – Physiologic factors: age, height, weight, triceps skin fold; mild-upper arm circumference. (See Fig. 53-3). – Caloric requirements of the critically-ill patient. – Laboratory data: fasting serum glucose; BUN, creatinine, serum electrolytes, total protein (serum albumin); haematology profile.	• For details regarding the nutrition assessment, see Chapter 53. • Adequate nutritional intake is essential to meet the metabolic needs of the catabolic state. – Nutritional deficiencies (especially in the elderly) are often associated with underlying chronic disease.

Contd...

Problem	*Objective*	*Nursing Interventions*	*Rationales*
• Compromised protective reflexes (i.e., cough, gag, and epiglotial closure).		• Maintain optimal nutrition with prescribed enteral and/or parenteral feedings. ◆ Special considerations: – Methods of enteral and parenteral administration. – Mechanical complications associated with enteral feeding tubes or with parenteral lines.	◆ Patients receiving mechanical ventilation therapy are highly stressed and require additional nutritional supplements to meet hypermetabolic needs.
		• Place patient in optimal position for enteral feedings (semi-Fowler's position). ◆ Assess status of protective reflexes. ◆ Assess for bowel sounds.	• Proper patient positioning and intact protective reflexes reduce risk of aspiration. ◆ The presence of a paralytic ileus is a contraindication for enteral approach because of increased risk of aspiration; abdominal distention may compromise diaphragmatic excursion.
		◆ Confirm placement of nasogastric tube in stomach before initiating enteral feedings.	◆ Proper placement of nasogastric tube helps prevent aspiration.
		• Provide frequent mouth care and other comfort measures.	• May be aesthetically pleasing to patient and family; reduces risk of oral infection (e.g., candida albicans) in the compromised patient; keeps mucous membranes moist and intact.
		• Monitor daily weight (unless contraindicated because of intracranial hypertension) and fluid intake and output.	
		• Assess bowel function: ◆ Auscultate bowel sounds. ◆ Implement prescribed bowel regimen. – Gastrointestinal decompression. – Adequate fluid intake. – Use of stool softeners.	• Presence of a paralytic ileus may predispose to foecal impaction; measures need to be employed to minimize straining at stool because Valsalva's maneouver can increase intracranial pressure.
Nursing Diagnosis#11 Potential for physiologic injury: Acute upper gastrointestinal haemorrhage, related to: 1. Stress of catabolic state. 2. Corticosteroid therapy.	Patient will remain without gastrointestinal bleeding: 1. Haematology profile stable at patient's baseline. 2. Nasogastric drainage and stools negative for occult blood. 3. Nasogastric secretions: pH > 4.5. 4. Vital signs stable; arterial blood pressure and heart rate at patient's baseline.	• Assess the conditon. • Test blood, stools and napogastric secretions. • Check vital signs.	• Refer to Table.
Nursing Diagnosis#12 Alteration in comfort: Headache, related to: 1 Meningeal irritation. 2. Surgical scalp incision. 3. Anxiety.	Patient will: 1. Verbalize and/or indicate comfort. 2. Demonstrate relaxed facial expression and demeanour. 3. Maintain intracranial pressure < 15 mmHg.	• Assess patient for signs of pain and discomfort. • Implement measures to reduce discomfort. – Administer analgesics and sedatives as prescribed, monitor response to therapy. – Position patient to relieve muscle tension. – Monitor dressing for tightness and constriction. – Provide a quiet environment. – Provide periods of uninterrupted sleep. – Provide much therapy; speak softly in soothing voice. – Employ diversional and comfort measures.	• Refer to Table Nursing Diagnosis #4, for presentation of the following nursing interventions/rationales.

Contd...

Problem	*Objective*	*Nursing Interventions*	*Rationales*
Nursing Diagnosis#13			
Impaired physical mobility, related to: 1. Altered state of consciousness. 2. Restricted activity associated with intracranial hypertension. 3. Sedation. 4. Neuromuscular impairments (e.g., hemiparesis). 5. Pain.	Patient will: 1. Maintain full range of motion. 2. Remain without contractures. 3. Verbalize and/or indicate comfort.	• Assess neuromuscular function. ◆ Assess for limitations in range of motion, in coordination of movement, and presence of sensorimotor dysfunction. ◆ Assess for the presence of pain, fear, and anxiety. • Consult with physical therapist regarding patient's neurologic and musculoskeletal status. • Implement measures to improve mobility: ◆ Include passive range of motion exercises in planning care. ◆ Avoid cumulative effect of activities; too many activities within a short time span predispose to increase in intracranial pressure. ◆ Provide rest periods between patient care activities. ◆ Use hand/wrist splints as prescribed. ◆ Maintain optimal positioning; avoid crossing one leg over the other; avoid pillows under knees. ◆ Offer praise and encouragement.	• The degree of musculoskeletal activity should be guided by intracranial pressure measurements. ◆ Fear of precipitating pain or causing injury can significantly compromise musculo-skeletal function. • In the patient at risk of developing an increase in intracranial pressure, all activities should be guided by intracranial pressure monitoring measurements. ◆ Prevents pooling of blood in extremities. ◆ Exercise periods should be incorporated into daily care and planned around other patient care activities. ◆ Positioning is important in patients with reduced brain compliance to allow free flow of blood and cerebrospinal fluid from cranial vault. ◆ Minimizes risk of thrombophlebitis or thromboembolic episodes.
Nursing Diagnosis#14			
Potential for injury to eyes: Abrasions, related to: 1. Inability to close eyes, or keep eyes closed, associated with: • Altered state of consciousness. • Neurologic deficit (cranial nerves). • Periorbital oedema.	Patient's eyes will remain intact without inadvertent abrasions.	• Assess patient's ability to close eyelids and keep them closed. ◆ Assess for corneal reflex. • Implement measures to protect eyes. ◆ Administer lubricants for the eyes (e.g., Tearisol). ◆ Gently tape eyes in closed position if necessary. ◆ Cleanse around eyelids to prevent crusting of secretion.	• Disturbance in cranial nerve function can place eyeballs at risk of injury. ◆ Cranial nerve III dysfunction causes ptosis of upper eyelid on ipsilateral side. ◆ Cranial nerve VII dysfunction alters ability to close eyelid on ipsilateral side. ◆ Cranial nerve V dysfunction impairs corneal reflex. • Help to protect eyes and minimize risk of infection.
Nursing Diagnosis#15			
Impairment of skin integrity: Potential, related to: 1. Immobility associated with intracranial hypertension	Patient will: 1. Maintain intact skin with good turgour over forehead and sternum. • Absence of lesions, irritations, pruritus, or infection.	• Assess skin, especially reddened areas over bony prominences where skin is thin. ◆ Assess for dependent oedema associated with immobility. • Implement measures to prevent skin breakdown.	• In patients with reduced brain compliance, turning, positioning, and nursing care activities should be guided by intracranial pressure measurements. • Promote circulation and prevents venostasis. If reddened areas at

Contd...

Problem	*R*	*Objective*	*Nursing Interventions*	*Rationales*
and altered consciousness. 2. Altered nutritional state. 3. Increased skin fragility associated with compromised health status.		• Absence of pressure (dermal) ulcer.	◆ Pressure relief device: air mattress, sheepskin, Clinitron bed and others. ◆ Local skin care: Keri lotion, Granulex, Duoderm, Travase, Debrisan, others. ◆ Turning and positioning.	pressure points do not blanch within less than 30 minutes, avoid using the position except for short periods at less frequent intervals. ◆ Also assist to mobilize secretions and prevent pooling.
			• Assess nutritional status.	
Nursing Diagnosis#16 Alteration in thought processes, related to: 1. Cerebral ischaemia and hypoxia. 2. Sedation.		Patient will: 1. Demonstrate improvement in thought processes. • Oriented to person, place, time. • Improved memory. • Increased attentiveness. • Improved ability to problem-solve and make decisions.	• Assess for alterations in mentation and thought processes. ◆ Assess the following parameters: – State of awareness or cognition. – Behaviour: restlessness, irritability, reduced attentiveness. – Impaired memory, confusion. – Ability to problem solve.	• Disruption in thought processes suggests hemispheric lesion; alterations in arousal and cognition reflect disruption of reticular activating system.
			• Confirm recent behavioural or personality changes with family members/significant others.	• Helps to ascertain patient's base-line capabilities, and to plan care.
			• Implement measures to assist patient in thought processes: ◆ Reorient patient as follows: – Reorient to person, place, and time. – Call by name when talking with patient. – Orient to immediate environment, but minimize stimuli at any given moment. ◆ Repeat instructions and information, allowing adequate time for communication, explanations. – Encourage to ask questions; use clear simple sentences.	
			◆ Plan patient's activities and write out schedule for patient to refer to: – Involve in problem-solving.	◆ Writing out instructions or schedules reinforces verbal communication.
			◆ Allow to choose between simple options (e.g., bathing and bedding change before or after meals). – Monitor patient's readiness and ability to learn. – Ascertain patient's comprehension.	◆ Provides patient with a sense of control of his/her body.
			◆ Provide continuous encouragement and feedback, and praise positive gains made by patient. ◆ Assist with self-care as indicated. ◆ Encourage patient to be independent, but provide close supervision. ◆ Involve family members and/or significant others in care plan.	◆ Assists in motivating patient regarding selfcare. ◆ Assists patient in gaining self-confidence regarding his/her capabilities.
			◆ Offer reassurance regarding alterations in intellectual and emotional functions.	◆ Depending on magnitude of insult and secondary injury, the patient may have memory loss and personality changes, which may persist for several months or longer.
			◆ Be realistic when offering explanations and providing information.	
Nursing Diagnosis#17 Sensory-Perceptual alterations, related to: 1. Sensory deprivation:		Patient will: 1. Demonstrate appropriate interactions with	• Assess patient's ability to interact with environment.	• Depending on the extent and location of insult, a disruption in sensation might be anticipated.
			◆ Identify specific sensory deficits:	◆ Major sensory capabilities

Contd...

Problem	*R*	*Objective*	*Nursing Interventions*	*Rationales*
• Restricted environment. • Altered communication capabilities. 2. Sensory overload: • Complexity of intensive care environment. • Needs of Critically-ill Patients • Patient Stressors in the ICU).		people and environment using sensory perceptions. 2. Verbalize restfulness and relaxed feeling.	– Visual perception: need for glasses ro contact lenses. – Auditory perception: presence of language disorder (e.g., receptive dysphasia, expressive dysphasia), need of hearing aid.	include: visual, auditory, kinesthesia (spatial sense, perception of movement), tactile, gustatory, and olfactory.
			◆ Tactile perception: hyperesthesia, hypo-esthesia.	◆ *Hyperesthesia* is an overly acute sensitivity to touch, pain, temperature, or other stimuli. ◆ Hypoesthesia is a diminished sensitivity to sensory stimuli.
			◆ Identify previous coping abilities and influence on behaviour. • Provide usual necessary aids (e.g., glasses, hearing aid). • Arrange environment to compensate for deficits: ◆ Reorient to environment as needed. – Keep articles and equipment in the same place. – Remove unnecessary materials from bedside. – Use safety measures to prevent accidents.	• A comprehensive patient's clinical history helps to identify the patient's baseline capabilities and limitations.
			• Implement measures to reduce sensory deprivation: ◆ Encourage communication by the patient as tolerated. – Allow visits by family members as tolerated.	• Fatigue may compromise patient's capabilities, leading to frustration, withdrawal, and depression.
			◆ Provide frequent, undisturbed rest periods. ◆ Provide occasional changes in routine and sensory stimuli. – Provide soothing music/other radio programs. – Provide diversional activities depending on patient's status (e.g., reading, television). – Encourage conversations with the client; update patient on what's happening, and other covnersational topics of interest to the patient.	◆ Minimizes fatigue and conserves strength. ◆ Ask family members about the patient's preferences, likes and dislikes. Familiar stimuli may motivate increased participation.
			• Implement measures to reduce sensory overload: ◆ Set priorities in care. – Arrange patient care activities to allow for undisturbed rest periods. – Provide periods of uninterrupted sleep with lights off and minimal noise. – Alter environmental activities (e.g., avoid constant use of radio or television). – Encourage verbalization regarding concerns, annoyances. – Allow to decide on care activities and environmental stimuli.	• Minimizing distractions enables the patient to concentrate on more per-tinent stimuli. Ability to problem-solve and tolerate frustration decreases as the number of stimuli impacting on the individual increase.
			• Recognize and accept patient's perception of stimuli (e.g., delusions and hallucinations). – Reinforce reality. – Maintain continuity of care.	

INFECTIONS AND INFLAMATION OF BRAIN

The nervous system may be attacked by a variety of bacteria and virus. The infection may wall off and create an abscess or the meningitis. Meningitis and sometimes the brain itself may become involved. Organisms reach the nervous system in various routes. Chronic otitis media, sinusitis, and mastoiditis and fracture of any bone adjacent to the meninges can be the source of infection. Some organisms such as the tubercle bacillus, reach the nervous system by means of the blood or the lymph system. Infection can also occur as a complication of invasive procedures such as lumbar puncture. The exact route by which some infectious agents reach CNS infections. Meningitis, encephalitis and brain abscesses are the more common inflammatory conditions of brain and spinal cord. Inflammation can be caused by bacteria, viruses, fungi and chemical (e.g. contrast media used in diagnostic tests) or blood in the subarachnoid space. As stated earlier, CNS may occur via the blood stream by extension from a primary site, by extension along cranial and spinal nerves or in vitero. Bacterial infections are the most common, and the organism usually involved are streptococcus pneumoniae, haemophilus influenza, neisseria meningitides, staphylococcus aureus, and meningococcis.

Meningitis

Meningitis is an acute inflammation of the piamater and the arachnoid membrane surrounding the brain and spinal cord. Therefore, meningitis is always cerebrospinal infection.

Aetiology

Bacterial meningitis affects the leptomeninges, thepia and arachnoid layers and the CSF. The most common pathogens causing meningitis are hemophilus influenza, nisseria meningitides, and streptococcus pneumoniae. The causative organism is very significantly at different ages. *Haemophilus* is common in young children, and often follows an upper respiratory infection or ear infections.

Nisseria has its highest incidence in children and young adults and can cause an overwhelming septicaemia. *Streptococcus Pneumonia* causes pneumococcal form of meningitis which is common in adults. Viral meningitis also called septic meningitis caused by viral and nonviral sources.

Pathophysiology

Organisms and viruses reach the nervous system by many routes. The most common route is the blood stream and bacteria in the nasopharynx may enter the blood stream during an upper respiratory infection. Once the organism reaches the brain, the CSF in the subarachnoid space and the arachnoid membrane become infected. The infection then spreads rapidly throughout the meninges and eventually invades the ventricles. The inflamatory response to the infection tends to increase CSF production with a moderate increase in pressure. In bacterial meningitis, the purulent secretion produced quickly spreads to other areas of the brain through the CSF. If this process extends into the brain parenchyma or if concurrent encephalitis is present, cerebral oedema and increased ICP become more problem. Pathological alteration includes hyperaemia of the meningea vessels, oedema of brain tissue, increased ICP and generalized inflammator reactions with exudation of white blood cells into the subarachnoid. Hydrocephalus may be caused by exudate blocking the small passages between ventricles.

Clinical Manifestation

- Fever.
- Severe headache.
- Nausea and vomiting.
- Nuchal rigidity (Resistance to flexion of the neck).
- Positive Kerning's sign (inability of the patient to extend the legs when the knee is flexed at the hip).
- Positive Brudzinski's sign (the hip and knee flex when the neck of patient's neck is flexed).
- Photophobia.
- A decreased LOC.
- Signs of increased ICP.
- Coma is associated with poor prognosis.

Headache becomes progressively worse and may be accompanied by vomiting and irritability. If the organism is meningococcus, a skin rash is common and petechiae may be seen.

Complications

The most common complications of meningitis is residual neurologic dysfunction. Cranial nerve dysfunction (III, IV, VI, VII or VIII) and cranial nerve irritation (II, III, IV, VI, VII, VIII). Accordingly, sensory loss occurs. And hemiparesis dysphasia and hemianopia may also occur. These signs usually resolve. If resolution does not occur, a cerebral abscess, subdural empheyema, subdural effusion, or persistent meningitis is suggested. Acute cerebral oedema may occur with bacterial meningitis causing seizures, CN III palsy, bradycardia, hypertensive coma and death. And non-communicating hydrocephalus may occur if the exudate causes adhesions that prevent the normal flow of the CSF from the ventricles. A complication of the menigococcal meningitis is the Waterhouse-Friderichsen syndrome.

Diagnostic Studies

- History and Physical examination.
- Analysis of CSF.
- CBC, coagulation profile, electrolyte levels, glucose, platelet count.
- Routine urinalysis.
- Blood culture (twice).
- Urine specific gravity (4th hourly).
- CT scan, MRI, EEG, skull X-Ray studies, brain scan.

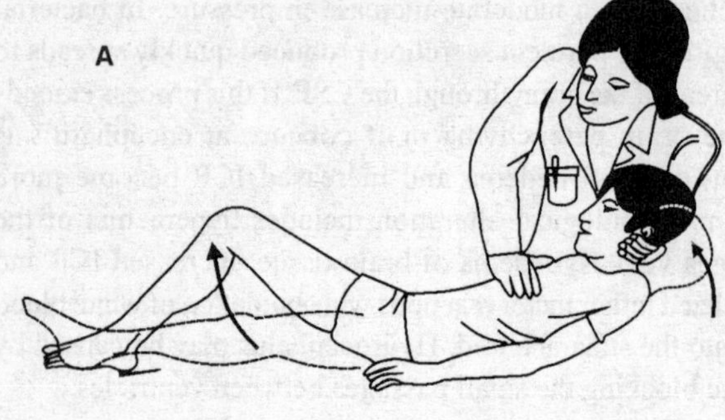

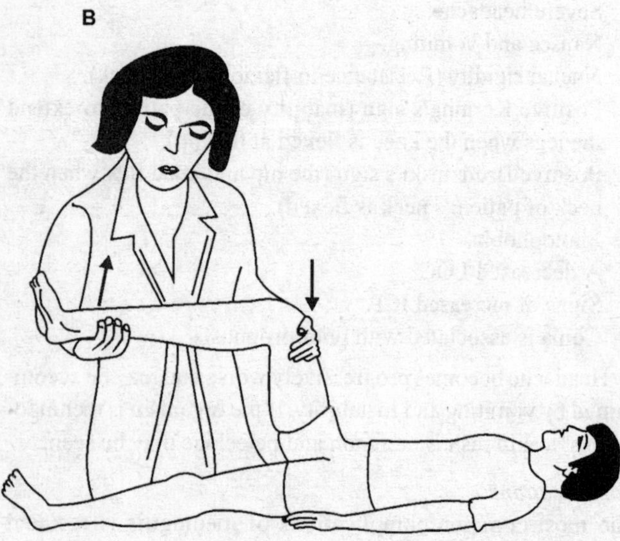

Fig.: 11.1: Signs of meningeal irritation include nuchal rigidity, a positive Brudzinski's and Kernig's signs. To elicit Brudzinski's sign; place the patient supine and flex the head upward. Resulting flexion of both hips, knees, and ankles with neck flexion indicate meningeal irritation. To test for the Kernig's sign, once again place the patient supine. Keeping one leg straight, flex the other hip and knee to a bent knee to form a 90 degree angle. Slowly extend the lower leg. This places a stretch on the meninges, resulting in pain and spasm of the hamstring muscle. Resistance to further extension can be felt.

Management

Meningitis can cause a medical emergency. When meningitis is suspected antibiotic therapy (Penicillin, ampicillin, ceftraxine, cefotaxamine) is instituted after the collection of specimens for culture, even before the diagnosis is confirmed. Diagnostic measures include lumbar puncture and analysis of CSF. The fundus of the eye should be examined via Opthalmoscope for Papilloedema before lumbar puncture for identification of possibly-increased ICP.

Treatment of bacterial infections consist of antibiotic therapy for the causative organism and determine by culture of CSF. Parenteral antibiotic at least 10 days. Antibiotic may be given direct i.e. intrathecally. Steroids may be given to reduce oedema.

General treatment measures include suggestive care to control and reduce fever, balance fluids and electrolytes and promote comfort.

The patient with meningitis is usually actualy ill. The fever is high and head pain is severe. Irritation of the cerebral cortex may result in seizures. The changes in mental status and LOC depend on the degree of increased ICP. Assessment of vital signs, neurologic evaluation, fluid intake and output and evaluation of the lung field and skin should be performed at regular intervals based on the patient's condition and recorded carefully.

Encephalitis

Encephalitis is an acute inflammation of the brain and is usually caused by virus, can also be caused by bacteria or fungi.

Aetiology

Viral infection is the most common, typically caused by the arbovirus or Herpes Simplex (HSV). Many different viruses have been implicated in encephalitis, some of them are associated with certain seasons of the year and endemic to certain geographic area. Epidemic encephalitis is transmitted by ticks and mosquitos. Nonepidemic encephalitis may occur as a complication of measles, chickenpox and mumps.

Pathophysiology and Clinical Manifestations

Encephalitis causes degenerative changes in the nerve cells of the brain and produces scattered areas of inflammation and necrosis. Some inflammation of the meninges is also typically present. The symptoms vary significantly from virus to virus. But often include fever, headache, seizures, stiff neck and a declining level of consciousness that can progress from lethargy and restlessness to coma. Manifestations resemble those of meningitis. A wide variety of local neurological signs can also be present. The mortality rate for encephalitis also varies subsequentally, but most of the patients experience some degree of residual deficit. Deficits include decreased cognitive functioning, personality changes, paralysis, and dementia. Patients can also be left deaf and blind.

Diagnosis and Treatment

Early diagnosis and treatment of viral encephalitis are essential for favourable outcomes. Brain imaging techniques such as MRI, and PET along with polymerase chain reaction tests for the HIV, DNA levels in CSF allow for earlier detection of viral encephalitis.

Collaborative and nursing management is symptomatic and supportive. Cerebral oedema is a major problem and diuretics (mannitol) and corticosteroids (dexamethasone) are used to control it. The decrease is characterised by diffuse damage to the nerve cells of the brain. Perivascular cellular infiltration, proliferation of glial cells and increasing cerebral oedema. The sequelae of encephalitis include mental deterioration, amnesia, personality changes and hemiparesis.

Acyclovir (20 Virax) and vidarabine (Vire-A) are used to treat encephalitis caused by HIV infection. Long-term symptoms, memory impairment, epilepsy, anosmia, personality changes, behavioural abnormalities and dysphasia. For maximal benefit, antiviral agents should be started before the onset of coma.

Brain Abscess

Brain abscess is an accumulation of pus within the brain tissue that can result from a local or a systemic infection.

Aetiology

Direct extension from ear, tooth, mastoid, or sinus infection is the primary cause. Other causes for brain abscess formation include spetic venous thrombosis from a pulmonary infection, bacterial endocardities, skull fracture, and nonsterile neurologic procedure. Streptococci and staphylococci are the primary infective organisms.

Clinical Manifestation

Manifestations are similar to those of meningitis and encephalitis and include headache and fever. Signs of increased ICP may include drowsiness, confusion, and seizures. Focal symptoms may be present and reflect the local area of the abscess. For example visual field defects or psychomotor seizures are common with-temporal lobe abscess, whereas an occipital abscess may be accompanied by visual impairment and hallucinations.

Management

Antimicrobial therapy is the primary treatment for brain abscess. Other manifestations are treated symptomatically. If drug therapy is used effective, the abscess needs to be drained, or removed if it is encapsulated. In untreated, treated cases, mortality rate is 100 per cent. Seizures occur in 30 per cent cases.

Nursing measures are similar to those for management of meningitis or increased ICP for surgical drainage or removal is the treatment of choice, nursing care is similar to that described under cranial surgery.

Other infections of the brain include subdural empheyema, oestiomyelitis of the cranial bones, epidural abscess and venous sinus thrombosis after periorbital cellulitis.

INTRACRANIAL TUMOURS

Tumours of the brain may be primary, arising from tissues within the brain or secondary, resulting from a metastasis from malignant neoplasm elsewhere in the body. Brain tumours are generally classified according to the tissue from which they arise. If malignant, the tumour is graded according to general cancer staging procedures.

Classification of Intracranial Tumours

Brain tumours may be classified as those arising inside the brain substance as follow:

1. *Gliomas*
   - *Astrocytoma* arises from supportive tissue, glial cells and astrocytes. Usual location is the white matter of frontal and temporal lobes in adults, lateral and cerebellar lobes in children. This is and moderately malignant grades I and II.
   - *Glioblastoma multiforomea* arises from primitive stem cell (glioblast) usual location is cerebral hemisphers. This is highly malignant and invasive and grades III and IV.
   - *Oligodendroglioma* arises from glial cells and dendrites. Usual location are cerebral hemispheres, most in frontal lobe, some in basal ganglia and cerebellum. Most are benign (encapsulation and calcification).
   - *Ependymoma* arise from ependymal epithelium usually occurs in lateral and fourth ventricles in children and young adults. They are benign to highly malignant, most benign and encapsulated.
   - *Medulloblastoma* arise from supportive tissue, usually at posterior fossa, fourth ventricle, brainstem in children. They are highly malignant and invasive, metastatic to spinal cord and remote areas of brain.
2. *Menigioma* arise from endothelial cells, fibrous tissues elements, transitional cells and angioblasts. Usual locations are arachnoid villi dura, half over convexity of hemisphere and half at base of hemisphere. They are usually benign, encapsulation outside brain substance.
3. *Acoustic neuroma* (neurofibroma) arise from Schwann cells inside auditory meatus on vestibular (sheath of vestibular portion of III CN) occurs at site between pons and cerebellum. They are usually benign or low grade malignancy encapsulation.
4. *Pituitary adenoma* arise from pituitary glandular tissue, located at pituitary gland, usually benign.
5. *Vascular tumours* (Hemangioblastoma, arteriovenous malformation) arises from overgrowth of arteries and veins enlarging from feeder vessels. Usual location is parietal cortex near middle cerebral vessels. They are benign.
6. *Metastatic tumours* due to cancer cells spread to the brain via circulatory system from lungs, breast, kidney, thyroid and prostate. Usual location is cerebral cortex and diencephalone. They are malignant.

Pathophysiology

The clinical manifestation of intracranial tumours are generally caused by the local destructive effects of the tumours, the resulting accumulation of metabolites, the displacement of structures, the obstruction of CSF or, and the effects of oedema and increased ICP on cerebral function. The rate of growth and the appearance of manifestations depend on the location, size and miotic rate of the cells of the tissue of origin.

Clinical Manifestations

A wide range of possible manifestations are associated with brain tumours with the classic feature being progressive manifestations of clinical symptoms. Symptoms can be generalized as well as specific to the tumour location and the structures of the brain that are compressed. The general symptoms are:

- "Pressure" headache (generalized or periorbital).
- Nausea and vomiting unrelated to food intake.
- Symptoms of increased ICP.
- Visual changes:
  - Blurred vision.
  - Diplopia (with III, IV and VI nerve compression).
  - Visual field alteration (with tumour compression of the optic chasam or optic pathways).
  - Enlarged blind spot related to papillaedema.
- Seizures.
- Speech difficulty (when the tumour affects the language area in the dominant hemisphere).
- Weakness or hemiparesis (when the tumour affects the motor cortex).
- Alteration in level of consciousness (with a midbrain tumour).
- Personality changes (with frontal tumours).

Tumour location and associated presenting symptoms are as given below:

- *Cerebral hemispheres*
  - Frontal lobe (unilateral): unilateral hemiphlagia, seizures, memory deficit, personality and judgment changes; visual disturbances.
  - Frontal lobe (bilateral): Symptoms associated with unilateral frontal lobe, and ataxic gait, aphasia (Motor dysfunction).
  - Parietal lobe: Speech disturbance, (if tumour is in the dominant hemisphere, inability to write, inability to replicate pictures, spatial disorders, unilateral neglect). Loss of right-left discrimination, seizures, paresthesic sensory-perceptual deficits.
  - Occipital lobe: Visual disturbances (blindness), headache and seizures.
  - Temporal lobe complex or partial seizures, with automatic behaviour.
  - Halluciations (Olfactory, visual or gustatory), Aphasia (receptive, sensory).
- *Subcortical*: Hemiplegia, other symptoms may depend on are of infiltration.
- *Meningeal tumours*: Symptoms associated with compression of the brain and depends on tumour location.
- *Metastatic tumours*: Headache, nausea or vomiting because of increased ICP other symptoms depend on location of tumour.
- *Thalamus and sellar tumours*. Headache, nausea, or and papillidaema, nystagamus occur from an increased ICP diabetes incipedus may occur.
- *Fourth Ventricle and cerebellar tumours*: Headache, nausea, and papilloedema mystagamus, occur from an increased ICP, ataxic gait and changes in coordination.
- *Cerebellopontine tumours*: Tinnitus and vertigo deafness.
- *Brainstem tumours*: Headache upon awakening, drowsiness, vomiting, ataxic gait, facial muscle weakness, hearing loss, dysphagia, dysarthria, "Crossed eyes" or other visual changes and memiparesis.

SPINAL CORD TUMOURS

Depending upon the nerves involved:

- Cervical: Pain, weakness or muscle wasting in arms, back, neck or legs.
- Thoracic: Pain accentuated with deep breathing and coughing, lack of bowel or bladder control may occur depending on tumour location.

Management of Intracranial and Spinal Cord Tumors

The nurse works collaboratively with other members of the health care team to implement the prescribed medical therapy. Because the nurse has a major role in discharging planning and patient teaching. Nurses also has the responsibilities to assist in diagnostic studies.

Diagnostic Studies

An extensive history and a comprehensive neurologic examination must be done in the work-up of a patient with a suspected brain tumour. A careful history and physical examination may provide data with respect to location. Diagnostic studies are similar to those used for a patient with increased ICP. The sensitivity of MRI allows detection of very small tumours. Other diagnostic studies include CT scan, skull X-rays, cerebral angiography EEG, brain scan, PET and lumbar Puncture myelogram.

An initial nursing assessment similar to that of unconscious patriot. In addition, assessment should be structured to provide baseline data of neurologic status and the information LOC. Areas to be assessed include the LOC and content consciousness, motor abilities, sensory perception, integrated function (include bowel and bladder functions, balance and proprioception and coping abilities of the patient and family. Watching a patient perform ADL and listening to the patient conversation are convenient ways are to perform part of neurological assessment. The possible *nursing diagnosis* are:

- Altered tissue perfusion: cerebral related to cerebral oedema.
- Pain (headache) R/T cerebral oedema and increased ICP.

- Self-care deficit R/O altered neuromuscular junction.
- Anxiety R/T diagnosis and treatment.
- Potential for seizures R/T abnormal electrical activity of brain.
- Potential for increased ICP R/T presence of tumour.

The overall goals are that the patient with brain tumour will:

1. Maintain normal ICP.
2. Maximize neurological functioning.
3. Be free from pain and discomfort and
4. Be aware of the long-term implication with respect to prognosis and cognitive and physical function. Determination of the presence of seizures, syncope, nausea and vomiting pain and headache or other pain is important in planning care for the patient.

Drug Therapy is used in the management of brain tumour, both to treat the tumour with chemotherapy and to manage symptoms. The common medication used and nursing intervention are as follows:

1. Phenytoin (Dilantin) used to prevent seizures. In this, the nurse has to assess for gingival hyperplasia, administer drug on schedule and assess for signs of toxicity and rash.
2. Dexamethasone (Decadran), used to reduce cerebral oedema. In this the nurse has to monitor for increased blood glucose, Taper dosage after long-term therapy.
3. Laxatives/stool softener are used to prevent constipation. The nurse should monitor fecal impaction and instruct patient not to strain.
4. Ranitidin or Famotidin are used to decrease gastric acid secretion. This is usually safe and without significant side effects.

Radiation therapy lengthens survival in patient with malignant gliomas especially when it is combined with partial surgical removal.

Diet therapy: No special diet is prescribed for the patient with brain tumour. Regular diet may be recommended with modification according to condition of the patient.

Surgical therapy i.e., surgical removal is the preferred treatment for brain tumour. Cranial surgery is as follows:

INTRACRANIAL SURGERY

A surgical opening through the skull is known as craniotomy. This procedure is used to treat any pathology requiring surgical intervention within the cranial cavity. Person with tumours, strokes, subarchnoid haemorrhage and trauma requiring surgical repair may also undergo craniotomies. The basic preparation of the patient before surgery and care in the immediate postoperative period are virtually the same, regardless to underlying conditions.

Indication for Cranial surgery are as follow:

1. Intracranial infections caused by bacteria. In these early findings, include stiffneck, headache, fever, weakness, seizures, and later finding include seizures, hemiplegia, speech disturbances, occular disturbances, changes in LOC. Surgical Procedure is excision of drainage of abscess.
2. *Hydrocephalus* due to overproduction of CSF, obstruction to flow, defective reabsorption. In these early findings are, mental changes, disturbance in gait later findings are memory impairment. Urinary incontinence, increased tendon reflexes and Surgery will be on placement of ventriculaterial or ventriculopenitoneal shunt.
3. *Intracranial tumours* due to benign or malignant cell growth. Manifestation included are change in LOC, pupillary changes, sensory or motor deficit, papilloedoma, seizures, personality changes. Surgical procedure will be excision or partial resection of tumour.
4. *Intercranial bleeding* due to repture of cerebral vessels because of trauma or cardiovascular accident. In epidural haemorrhage, there will be momentary unconsciousness, lucid period, then rapid deterioration. In subdural, there will be headache, seizures and pupillary changes, for which, is surgical evaluation through burr holes or cranotomy.
5. *Skull fractures* due to trauma to skull. Here we find headache, CSF leakage, cranial nerve deficit. Surgical procedure performed here are debridement of fragments and necrotic tissue, elevation and realighment of bone fragments.
6. *Arteriovenous malformation* may be due to congenital tangle of arteries and veins (frequently in middle cerebral artery). Symptoms are headache, intracranial haemorrhage, seizures, mental deterioration. Excision of malformation is the surgical procedure.
7. *Aneurysm repair*. Due to dilatation of weak area in arterial wall, (usually near anterior portion and circle of Willis). Manifestation before rupture are headache, lethargy, visual disturbance. After rupture, violent headache, decreased LOC, visual disturbances, motor disturbances. Here dissection and clipping of aneurysm is the surgical procedure.

The types of cranial surgery performed are:

1. *Burr hole:* It is the opening into cranium with a drill, used to remain localized fluid and blood beneath the dura.
2. *Craniotomy:* Opening into the cranium with removal of a bone flap and opening the dura to remove lesion, repair a damaged area, drainblood or relieve increased ICP.
3. *Craniectomy:* Excision into the cranium to cut away a bone flap.
4. *Cranioplasty:* Repair of a cranial defect resulting from trauma, malformation, or previous surgical procedure: artificial material used to replace damaged or lost one.
5. *Stereotaxis.* Precision localization of a specific area of the brain using a frame or a frameless system based on 3-dimensional coordination: procedure is used for biopsy, radiosurgery, or dissection.

6. *Shunt procedures*: Provide an alternative pathway to redirect CSF from one area to another using a tube or implanted device. Examples include ventriculoperitoneal shunt and CSF reservoir.

The following guidelines are used for preoperative care of the patient having intracranial surgery:

1. Baseline data of neurological and physiological status are recorded.
2. Patient and family are encouraged to verbalize fears.
3. Treatment and procedures are explained fully, even if unsure whether patient understands.
4. If head is shaved, it usually is done in the operating room.
5. An antiseptic shampoo may be ordered at the night before the surgery.
6. If hair is shaved, it is saved and given to patient or family.
7. Family is prepared for appearance of patient after surgery:
   – Head dressing.
   – Oedema and ecchymosis of face common.
   – Possible decrease in mental status.

And following guidelines of care should be used for postoperative care of patient after intracranial surgery.

1. Perform monitoring-
   • Assess neurological status, including ability to move, level for orientation and alertness and pupil checks.
   • Assess degree and character of drainage.
     – Amount of drainage and bleeding should be minimal.
     – Initial head dressing can be reinforced as necessary.
     – Often incision is left open to air after first several days.
2. Promote mobility
   • Turning to either side is permitted.
   • If supratentorial surgery was performed, the head of the bed is kept elevated at elast 30-degrees.
   • Early ambulation is encouraged to prevent complications of bedrest. Observe carefully for signs of postural hypotension; raise head of bed gradually; patient should always sit on edge of bed before standing.
3. Promote decreased intracranial pressure.
   • Space nursing activities to allow patient to rest between them.
   • Coughing and vomiting shall be avoided.
   • Suctioning should be performed only as necessary and then gently and cautiously.
4. Protect safety of patient.
   • Use soft hand restraints if restraints are necessary.
   • Use mittens as alternative to restraints. Change Mitt. fourth hourly provide range of motions to hand at this time.
   • Keep side rails up at all times.
5. Promote electrolyte balance.
   • Perform accurate intake and output with measurement of specific gravity. Do frequent testing for blood glucose.
   • Have patient resume oral diet as soon as possible, assess for difficulty in swallowing or absence of gag reflex.
   • Monitor electrolytes for evidence of abnormality.
6. Promote comfort.
   • Medicate for comfort with codiene sulphate or non-narcotic analgesic.
   • Ice cap for headache may be helpful.

CEREBROVASCULAR ACCIDENT/STROKE

Cerebrovascular accident refers to any pathological process involving the blood vessels of the brain. Cerebrovascular accident (CVA) also referes to as stroke or brain attack, is a broad term that includes a variety of disorders that influence blood flow to the brain and results in neurologic deficits. Proper functioning of the brain depends on an adequate blood supply to deliver oxygen and glucose for neuronal activity and to remove the end product of metabolism. CVA results when there is inadequate supply of blood to the brain (cerebral ischaemea) or cerebral haemorrhage within the brain. Regardless of the cause, the damaged brain no longer performs cognitive, sensory, motor or emotional functions. The effects of CVA may vary from minor to severe disability.

Aetiology

CVA can be defined as a neurological deficit that has a sudden onset and lasts over 24 hours. Ischaemic strokes account for an estimated 85% of the total and this percentage can be further broken down into strokes resulting from atherosclerolic (20 per cent), cardiogenic (20 per cent), idiopathic (30 per cent) and other causes (15 per cent). Brief descriptions of these ischaemic strokes are as follows:

- *Atherosclerotic*: Atherosclerosis affects both the large extracranial and intracranial arteries. The lumen of the vessel narrows and can be a target site for thrombus formation. Transient ischaemic attacks (TIA) occur in about half of patients before the stroke.
- *Small penetrating artery thrombosis/lacuna/lacunar*: Thrombosis of a small penetrating brain artery causes a small damaged area of tissues in the deep white matter structures of the brain, called a lacuna. Lacunae typically occur in the basal ganglia, internal capsule, pons or thalamua.
- *Cardiogenic/embolic*: Most of these strokes are the result of emboli, usually of cardiac origin, that break off and travel in the arterial circulation until they reach a vessel that is too narrow to allow further passage. Atrial fibrillation is the most common cause of the emboli.
- *Other*: Ischaemic strokes can also result from vasospasm,

in inflammation coagulation disorders, and the effects of drug abuse, particularly cocaine.

- *Idiopathic.* No identifiable cause is establisehd in upto 30 per cent of all ischaemic strokes.

The risk factors associated with strokes can be divided into nonmodifiable and potentially modifiable. The non-modifiable include gender, age, race, hereditary. Modifiable are lifestyles, habits including excessive alcohol consumption, cigarette smoking, obesity, diet high in fat content, and drug abuse, increase the risk for stroke. Many pathologic conditions also increase the risk for stroke includes cardiac disease, diabetes mellitus, hypertension, migraine, headache, hypercoagulability states (e.g. high serum fibrinogen levels, increased hematocrit), polycethaemia, and sickle cell anaemia.

Pathophysiology

The cerebrovascular system is highly adaptive. It maintains constant blood flow to the brain in spite of significant changes in the systemic circulation. Blood flow must be maintained at 750 ml/min. (55 ml/100g) brain tissue) or 20 per cent of the cardiac output to ensure optimal cerebral functioning of blood flow to the brain in totally interrupted (e.g. cardiac arrest), neurologic metabolism is altered in 30 seconds, metabolism stops in 2 minutes, and cellular death occurs in 5 minutes. The factors that affect cerebral blood flow can be divided into extracranial (Systemic blood pressure, cardiac output and viscosity of the blood) and intracranial (Metabolic alteration, conditions of blood vessels supplying the brain, and intracranial pressure). Both extracranial and intracranial factors may be involved in a stroke. The initial insult may be related to one or more of these factors. For example, when an intracranial haemorrhage occurs, the continuity of the vascular system is interrupted. The lost blood and cerebral oedema secondary to the inflammatory process contribute to an increase in intracranial pressure. This interferes with cerebral perfusion, and carbon dioxide and hydrogen ion concentration increase, leading to further dilation of cerebral vessels and increased ICP. Atherosclerosis is common pathophysiologic process in stroke is usually involved in the development of a thrombosis and is often implicated in strokes caused by emboli.

Clinical Manifestations

A CVA ultimately affects many body functions including neuromotor activity, elimination, intellectual function, spatial-perceptual alterations, personality and affect, sensation and communication. The specific neurological defects that are produced by stroke reflect the location and severity of the ischaemia and the adequacy of the collateral circulation in the region. Many of the features overlap with other forms of brain injury.

Clinical manifestations of specific cerebral artery involvements are as follows:

1. *Middle cerebral artery involvement*
   – *Blockage of main stem*
     - Contralateral paralysis (hemiplegia).
     - Contralateral anaesthesia loss of proprioreception, fine tough, localization (hemiperesis).
     - Dominant hemisphere: Aphasia.
     - Nondominant hemisphere: neglet of opposite side, dysmetria.
     - Homonymaos hemianopsia and conjugate gaze paralysis.

2. *Anterior cerebral artery involvement*
   – *Occlusion* of stem.
   – *Occlusion* distal to anterior to communicating artery.
     - Contralateral sensory and motor deficit of foot and leg.
     - Contralateral weakness of proximal upper extremity.
     - Urinary incontinence (Possibly unrecognized by patient).
     - Apraxia.
     - Personality change: flat affect, loss of spontaneity and distractability.
     - Possible cognitive impairment.

3. *Posterior cerebral artery involvement*
   – Thalamogeniculate branch occlusion.
   – Contralateral sensory loss.
   – Temporary hemiparesis.
   – Homonymous hemianopsia.
   – *Paramedian branch occlusion: Central midbrain and thalamus.*
     - Weber's syndrome: oculomotor nerve palsy.
     - Contralateral hemiplegia.
   – *Cortical occlusion*: temporal and occipital lobe.
     - Incomplete homonymous hemianopsia.
     - Dominant hemisphere: dysphasia and anaemia.
     - Nondominant hemisphere: disorientation.
   – Upper basical occlusion (bilateral)
     - Visual disturbances (blindness, homonymous, hemianopsia, visual hallucinations, apraxia of ocular movements)
     - Anaemia: objects and inability to count.
     - Possible memory loss.

4. *Vertebrabasilar artery involvement.*
   - Bilateral motor and sensory deficits of all extremities.
   - Ipsilateral Horner's syndrome: miosis, ptosis, decreased sweating.
   - Hoarseness.
   - Dysphagia.
   - Nystagmus, diplopia and blindness.
   - Nausea, vomiting.
   - Ataxia.

The term stroke commonly evokes a classic mental picture of specific disabilities, but a wide variety of presentations can occur commonly encountered symptoms are as follows:

1. *Motor*
   - Hemiparesis or hemiplegia of the side of the body opposite the site ischaemia, initially flaccid, progressing to spastic.
   - Dysphagia: swallowing reflex may also be impaired.
   - Dysarthria.
2. *Bowel and bladder*
   - Frequency, urgency and urinary incontinence. Potential for bladder retraining is good if cognitively intact.
   - Constipation- Related more to immobility than to the physical effects of stroke.
3. *Language*
   - Nonfluent aphasia (also known as motor/expressive aphasia)—difficulty or inability to comprehend speech.
   - Fluent aphasia (also known as sensory/receptive aphasia)—difficulty ro inability to comprehend speech.
   - Alexia—inability to understand the written word.
   - Agraphia—inability to express self in writing.
4. *Sensory-perceptual*
   - Diminished response to superficial sensation—touch, pain, pressure, heat and cold.
   - Diminished proprioception—knowledge of position of body parts in the environment.
   - Visual defects—decreased acuity, diplopia, homonymous hemoanopsia.
   - Perceptual deficits.
     i. Unilateral neglet syndrome: A distortion in body image in which the patient ignores the affected side of the body (Distorted body image).
     ii Apraxia inability to carry out learned voluntary acts, i.e., loss of ability to carry out a learned sequence of movement or use objects correctly when paralysis is not present.
     Constructional: may not be able to sequence a planned act necessary for activities of daily living (e.g. dressing, brushing teeth and combing hair).
     iii. Agnosia—Inability to recognize a familar object by use of the senses, through senses sight (visual A) sound (auditory-A), touch (tactile A).
     iv. Anosognosia—Inability to recognise or denial of a physical deficit i.e., apparent unawareness or denial of any loss or deficition physical functioning.
     v. Special relationships—loss of ability to judge distances or size or localized object of space, impaired right-left discrimination.
     vi. Loss of proprioceptive skills: Lack of awareness or where various body parts are in relationship to each other, and the environment e.g. telling time, judging distance, right and left discrimination, memory of locationary object.
5. *Cognitive-emotional*
   - Emotional liability and unpredictability-behaviours may be socially inappropriate (e.g. crying, jags and swearing).
   - Depression.
   - Memory loss.
   - Short attention of span, early distiatibility.
   - Loss of reasoning, judgement and abstract thinking ability.

The clinical manifestation of transient ichemiottos attacks (TIA) are as follows.

1. Symptoms related to carotid involvement:
   - Visual disturbances: Temporary blindness in one eye, Blurred vision.
   - Motor disturbances: Hemiparesis, localized motor deficits in face or extremities.
   - Sensory disturbances: Hemianaesthesia, sensory deficits in face extremities.
2. Symptoms related to vertebral involvements:
   - Motor disturbances: Ataxia, dysarthria, dysphagia, unilateral or bilateral weakness.
   - Visual disturbances: Diplopia and bilateral blindness.
3. Other – Brief lapses in level of consciousness.
   – Sensory disturbances.
   – Dizziness.
   – Vertigo and
   – Tinnitus.

Management

As usual, diagnostic studies are carried out in stroke are

- Computed tomography scan for size and location of lesion.
- MRI—to differentiate hemorrhagic or nonhemmorhagic.
- EEG—For knowledge suggestive ischaemic infarction.
- PET—shows the chemical activity of brain and extent of tissue damage.
- Radionuclide scan.
- DSA (digital subtraction angiography)—Visualization of blood vessel involved and
- CSF analysis.

To know the evaluation of aetiology of CVA, the following are necessary.

- Cerebral blood flow-by doppler ultrasonographs, transcranial doppler carohd duplex and carohd angiography.
- Cardiac assessment-by ECG, cardiac enzyme, echocardiography and Holter monitor (evaluation of arrythmias).

Before diagnostic studies, proper history and thorough physical examination are necessary. For locating signs and symptoms listed in clinical manifestations, the nurses and health care team should take primary prevention as a priority for reducing morbidity and mortality associated with CVA. The goals of stroke prevention include health management for the well individual, modifiable risk factors, prevention of stroke for those with history of TIA, and prevention of additional stroke for those who have had a CVA. Health management focuses on (1) healthy diet, (2) weight control, (3) regular exercise (4) no smoking, (5) limiting alcohol consumption and (6) routine health assessments. Patients with known risk factors such as diabetes mellitus, hypertension, obesity, high serum lipids, or cardiac dysfunction require close management of their illness. Postmenopasal women on oestrogen therapy are less likely to experience a CVA as compared with women not on oestrogen therapy. Measures designed to prevent the development of thrombus or embolus are also used in patient at risk. Low dose aspirin is used as prophylactic dose of platelet inhibitor. Anticoagulation therapy for patient with atrial fibrillation. Treatment of underlying cardiac problem and surgical intervention for patients with aneurysm risk of bleeding i.e., with TIAs from carotid disease carotid endarectus, transluminal angioplasty and extracranial and intracranial bypass may be done as precaution.

Emergency Management of stroke carried out for patients with aetiology of sudden vascular compromise causing disruption of blood flow to the brain (may be thrombosis, trauma, aneurysm, embolism and haemorrhage). Assessment finding will reveal that patients are:

- Altered level of consciousness.
- Weakness, numbness, or paralysis of portion of the body.
- Speech or visual disturbances.
- Severe headache.
- Increased or decreased heart rate.
- Respiratory distress.
- Unequal pupils.
- Hypertension.
- Facial drooping on affected side.
- Difficulty in swallowing.
- Seizures.
- Bladder or bowel incontinence.
- Nausea and vomiting.

The nursing interventions carried on during emergency initially are:

- Ensure patent airway.
- Remove dentures.
- Administer oxygen via nasal cannula or nonrebreather mask.
- Establish IV access with normal saline to maintain BP.
- Remove clothing.
- Obtain CT scan immediately.
- Elevate head of bed 30 degrees of no symptoms of shock or injury.
- Institute seizure precautions.
- Anticipate thrombolytic therapy for ischaemic stroke.

Ongoing monitoring includes.

- Monitor vital signs, LOC, oxygen saturation, cardiac rhythm, GC scale pupil size and reactivity.
- Maintain patient warmth.
- Reassure patient and family.

Nursing Management

Nursing Assessment includes obtaining subjective and objective data of the person who had a stroke and will include:

- Health history including hypertension, and its management, history of coronary artery disease, diabetes and history of TIA.
- Medication in use, both prescription and over-the-counter drugs (OTC).
- Smoking history.
- Circumstances surrounding the stroke.
- Onset, nature and severity of symptoms.
- Presence of headache-nature and locaton.
- Visual ability-acuity, diplopia, blurred vision.
- Ability to concentrate and follow commands and memory.
- Emotion/affective response.
- Level of consciousness and response to tackle stimuli.
- Family and social support network, financial and insurance status and following to be observed:
- Motor strength—presence of and severeity of paresis or paralysis.
- Coordination—gait and balance.
- Ability to communicate.
- Cranial nerve assessment.
- Bowel and bladder control or incontinency.

Nursing diagnosis are determined from analysis of patient's data. The possible nursing diagnosis may include:

- Altered cerebral tissue perfuse R/T interruption of arterial blood flow.
- Risk for disuse syndrome R/T hemiparesis or hemiplegia.
- Self-care deficit: Feeding, bathing, toileting R/T neuromuscular and sensory perceptual impairment.
- Impaired swallowing, R/T oral and neck muscle weakness.
- Impaired verbal communication R/T residual aphasia.
- Sensory—perceptual alternated R/T altered sensory reception, transmission, integrated.
- Urinary incontinence R/T altered neurological stimulation.
- Impaired adjustment R/T residual disability necessary changes in lifestyle and independence.

Planning: The patient, family and nurse establish the goals of nursing care in a cooperative manner. These goals typically include that the patient will:

1. Maintain a stable or improved level of consciousness.
2. Attain maximum physical functioning.
3. Attain maximum self-care abilities and skills.
4. Maintain stable body functions (e.g. bladder control).
5. Maximize communication skills and abilities.
6. Maintain adequate nutrition.
7. Avoid complications of stroke.
8. Maintain effective personal and family coping.

Nursing Implementation

Monitoring Cerebral Perfusion

The nurse has to do continuous monitoring of patient's neurological status. Accordingly, the nurse has to maintain patient's patent airway and it is essential to support oxygenation and cerebral perfusion. Nursing intervention includes frequent assessment of airway patency and function, suctioning, patient's mobility, positioning of the patient to prevent aspiration, and encouraging deep-breathing. The environment is kept in quick and restful as possible, and all activities that are known to increase ICP such as coughing, straining, lying prone, isometric muscle contraction, emotional upsets and abrupt head or neck flexion are avoided or minimized. Administer prescribed medication and prevent thrombus formation.

Prevention of the Complications of Immobility and Disuse

Appropriate positioning is a key concern. Positioning is fundamental to preventing complication such as contractures and skin breakdown. Maintain alignment with support of pillows and footboards according to procedures, teach and assist family and patient with positioning techniques to prevent contractures. Administer active or passive range-of-motion exercises to affected extremities.

Promoting Independence in Self-Care

Assess document level of self-care to determine extent of problem and plan appropriate intervation. Encourage independence, provide supervision or assistance as needed to avoid development of dependency.

Promoting Safe Swallowing and Adequate Nutrition

The protective swallowing and gag reflexes usually return within a few days after the stroke, but the patient may have ongoing problems managing the complex act of swallowing. The following guidelines can be used for the patient with impaired swallowing.

1. Place the patient upright in bed or preferably sitting in a chair for meals.
2. Offer mouth care before meals to stimulate saliva flow; Strong-tasting or salty liquids also stimulate saliva flow.
3. Position the patient's head and neck slightly forward with the chin tucked in to prevent premature movement of food to the back of the mouth before it is adequately chewed.
4. Experiment with food texture. Most patients tolerate a mechanically soft diet better than liquids. Avoid thin liquids. Consider adding thickness to liquid if they are poorly tolerated.
5. Encoruage the patient to take small bites and chew food thoroughly.
6. If haemiplegia is present, food should be placed in the unaffected side of the mouth. If 'pocketing' of food occurs on the affected side, instruct the patient to sweep the affected side with a finger after each bite. Teach the patient to clean the affected side of the mouth with gauze wipes and perform mouth care after meals. Retained food causes mouth odours, infection and tooth or gum disease.
7. Position foods within the patient's visual field if haemianopia is present.
8. Keep an accurate intake and output record until the patient is drinking sufficient liquid daily. IV supplementation may initially be needed.
9. Monitor the patients weight weekly. Add supplements to diet or liquids to increase calorie and nutrient intake.

Supporting Communication

Communication problem following stroke may include both aphasia and dysarthria. Specific strategies for assisting the patients with aphasia are as follows:

i. *Nonfluent expressive Aphasia*
   - Allow the patient adequate time to respond. Establish a nonhurried atmosphere.
   - Be supportive and encouraging of the patient's efforts to communicate.
   - Use open-ended questions at intervals to assess spontaneous communication ability.
   - Involve the family or significant others in exercise to name objects used for routine self-care.
   - Express understanding and support to behavioural responses to frustration such as tears or anger. Remind the patient that speech skills will improve.
   - If the aphasia is severe, a picture board or book may be necessary to communicate by whatever means are successful (e.g. pointing, pantomime). Anticipate the patient's needs when appropriate and verify your interpretation of the patient's meaning.

ii. *Fluent sensory aphasia*
   - Face the patient and speak slowly and distinctly. Do not increase your volume: hearing is not the problem.
   - Break instructions into component parts and give them one at a time. Repeat as needed.
   - Use gestures appropriately to support your verbal messages.
   - Involve the family in planning and implementing all strategies.
   - Provide support and encouragement when the patient becomes frustrated.

iii. *General*
- Provide practice at times when the patient is rested and not fatigued.
- Offer liberal praise and reinforcement for efforts. Remind patient and family that small gains can still be made months into the rehabilitation process.

Compensatory for Sensory-Perceptual Deficits

A wide variety of sensory-perceptual deficits may be present following stroke; particularly strokes involving the right hemisphere. Specific intervention designed to address the major sensory-perceptual deficits in the following guidelines.

i. *Hemianopia* (loss of vision in a portion of visual field)
- Approach the patient from the side of intact vision.
- Position the patient in the room so that his or her intact visual field faces the door if possible.
- Teach the patient to move the head from side-to-side (scan) to compensate for diminished visual fields. Scanning is also important with meals.
- Place objects needed for self-care within the patient's intact visual field.

ii. *Denial/neglect and body image distortion*
- Encourage the patient to look at and touch the affected side. Verbally remind the patient to check the position and safety of the affected side during activity.
- Lightly touch and stimulate the affected side during care.
- Providing gentle but consistent reminders to include the affected side in care (e.g. bathing, dressing).
- Monitor the affected side for injuries when the patient is out of bed. A sling may be used to protect the affected side during ambulation.
- Use a full length mirror to assist the patient to reintegrate an intact body image and to assist with posture and balance.
- Assist the family to understand the nature of the patient's behaviour.

iii. *Agnosia/Apraxia*
- Encourage the patient to use all senses to compensate for problems in object recognition.
- Practise the recognition and naming of commonly used objects, and encourage the family to participate in the relearning process.
- Encourage the patient to participate in self-care.
- Correct the misuse of any object or task, guiding the patient's hand if necessary.
- Continue to verbally cue the patient about correct use of any object or self-care tasks.
- Be aware that memory deficits may make frequent reteaching necessary.
- Explain the nature of all deficits to the family.

Restoring Continence

Problems with urinary incontinence are common after stroke; but the chances for restoring continence are good because half of the innervation and control pathways to the bladder remain intact. Assess and record patient's continent and incontinent voidings to determine pattern and plan appropriate intervention. Note colour and character of urine daily-needed to ensure early detection of urinary tract infection and to prevent highly concentrated urine. Provide fluid intake of 2000 ml/day less contraindicated to foster adequate elimination of dilute urine. If indwelling catheter is used, give perineal cleaning and catheter care every shift and as needed to avoid infection and ensure uninterrupted urinary flow. Offer urinal or commode every 2 hours and encourage to empty the bladder and as needed to aid in establishing regular voiding pattern. Assure patient of your willingness to assist with urinary problem to avoid embarrassment and to demonstrate a caring attitude.

Constipation is the most common bowel problem after stroke. Regaining bowel incontinence is reasonable expectation for most patients if a pattern of constipation, impaction, and diarrhoea is not permitted to develop. The nurse needs to carefully monitor the patient's bowel elimination pattern and ensure that the patient received adequate daily fluid. A bowel program of stool softner, fiber laxatives and suppositories should be implemented at admission and modify as needed to support bowel regularity.

Promoting Effective Coping

The effects of stroke are usually life-altering and can be devastating to the patient and family. Depressions and despair are normal responses to stroke. The patient may experience significant difficulty in responding appropriately to any situation. He may be emotional and cry easily. Here, families need to be helped to understand that these behaviours are outcomes of the stroke and are not viotational acts by the patient. Distraction and shifting the patient's attention can be successful strategies for assisting the patient to regain control.

To evaluate the effectiveness of nursing intervention, compare the patient behaviour with those stated in the expected outcome objectives. Successful achievement of patients outcome for the patient with stroke is indicated by:

- Maintain stable vital sign and that he has no signs of increased ICP.
- Is able to move and transfer easily.
- Performs ADL independently.
- Consumes balanced oral diet without any problem.
- Communicate needs effectively.
- Uses technique to compensate for perceptual defects and injury.
- Maintain bladder and bowel continence.
- Participate with family in social interaction.

Table 11.3: Nursing care plan for the patient with a cerebrovascular accident (stroke)

Problem	*R*	*Objective*	*Nursing Interventions*	*Rationales*
Nursing Diagnosis #1 Alteration in cerebral perfusion pressure, related to: 1. Cerebral ischaemia. 2. Cerebral oedema. 3. Intracranial haemorrhage. 4. Vasospasm.		Patient will: 1. Maintain: cerebral perfusion pressure >60 mmHg. • Intracranial pressure <15 mmHg. • Mean arterial blood pressure ~80 mmHg. • Heart rate ~72/min; no dysrhythmias. 2. Exhibit intact level fo consciousness and mentation: • Oriented to person, place, time. • Memory intact. 3. Demonstrate neurologic function: • Pupils equal and reactive. • Sensorimotor functions intact (e.g., can discriminate between fine and crude touch; exhibits purposeful movement).	◆ Monitor for signs and symptoms of increasing intracranial pressure. ◆ Maintain integrity of intracranial pressure monitoring system. ◆ Implement measures to prevent and/or reduce intracranial pressure. – Maintain optimal positioning. – Prevent increase in cerebral blood flow. – Limit or decrease cerebral oedema. – Minimize cerebral cellular metabolism. – Plan nursing care activities to prevent cumulative increase in intracranial pressure. • Additional nursing considerations: ◆ Therapeutic approaches used to minimize risk of increased intracranial pressure are likewise implemented to prevent rebleeding in patients who have sustained an Intracranial haemorrhage.	
Nursing Diagnosis #2 Breathing pattern ineffective, related to: 1. Brainstem compression associated with haemorrhage or cerebral oedema. 2. Impaired chest excursion associated with hemipareals.		Patient will demonstrate effective breathing pattern: 1. Respiratory rate <25/min 2. Rhythm and depth eupnele: • Tidal volume>7-10 ml/kg. • Vital capacity >12-15 ml/kg. 3. Alveolar ventilation and gas exchange adequate. • $PaCO_2$ <30-35 mmHg. • PaO_2 >80 mmHg. • pH 7.35-7.45.	◆ Assess respiratory function. ◆ Implement measures to maintain airway patency. ◆ Implement measures to improve breathing pattern. ◆ Plan patient care activities to minimize a cumulative increase in intracranial pressure or increase risk of rebleeding. • Additional nursing considerations: ◆ Hyperventilation therapy has not been found to be overly effective in the treatment of the stroke patient probably because there is loss of autoregulatory mechanisms.	
Nursing Diagnosis #3 Airway clearance ineffective, related to: 1. Compromised cough. 2. Inability to handle tracheobronchial secretions. 3. Ineffective chewing/swallowing.		Patient will: 1. Maintain patent airway with normal breath sounds. 2. Demonstrate secretion-clearing cough (unless contraindicated by risk of incresed intracranial pressure or rebleeding).	• Assessment of respiratory function, and implementation of measures to maintain airway patency. ◆ Pneumonia is a frequent complication of stroke and usually develops on the paralyzed side, probably because of decreased thoracic excursion and altered pulmonary haemodynamics. To prevent pooling of secretions, it is recommended that the patient be repositioned hourly (unless contraindicated because of the risk of intracranial hypertension or rebleeding).	

Contd...

Problem	*R*	*Objective*	*Nursing Interventions*	*Rationales*
			– Side-lying position allows drainage of secretions from mouth and prevents aspiration. – Alternate positioning facilitates drainage of secretions from lung segments. – Positioning of patient should allow for maximum chest excursion.	
Nursing Diagnosis #4 Alteration in comfort: Headache, related to: 1. Meningeal irritation. 2. Surgical scalp incision.		Patient will: 1. Verbalize and/or indicate comfort. 2. Demonstrate relaxed facial expression and demeanour. 3. Maintain intracranial pressure <15 mmHg.	♦ Assess patient for signs/symptoms of pain and discomfort. ♦ Implement measures to reduce discomfort. ♦ Monitor head dressing for tightness or constriction. ♦ Provide quiet environment. ♦ Provide periods of uninterrupted sleep. ♦ Provide touch therapy; speak in a soft, soothing voice. ♦ Employ diversional measures.	
Nursing Diagnosis #5 Anxiety related to: 1. Fear of dying. 2. Potential sequelae associated with ischaemic or haemorrhagic cerebrovascular disease. 3. Intensive care setting.		Patient will: 1. Verbalize feeling less anxious. 2. Demonstrate a relaxed demeanour. 3. Perform relaxation techniques. 4. Verbalize familiarity with ICU routines and protocols.	♦ Assess for signs/symptoms of anxiety. ♦ Examine circumstances underlying anxiety. ♦ Assess patient/family coping behaviours and their effectiveness. ♦ Initiate interventions to reduce anxiety.	
Nursing Diagnosis #6 Alteration in fluid and electrolyte balance: 1. Fluid volume excess with associated • Cerebral oedema. 2. Fluid volume deficit, related to: • Diuretic therapy. • Diabetes insipidus. 3. Altered electrolytes, related to: • Diuretic therapy. • Corticosteroid therapy. • Acid-base balance.		Patient will: 1. Maintain haemodynamic function: • Mean arterial blood pressure ~80 mmHg. • Heart rate at patient's baseline; rhythm regular; no dysrhythmias. 2. Demonstrate intact level of consciousness and mentation: • Oriented to person, place, time. • Appropriate response to verbal commands. 3. Maintain balanced intake and output: • Stable baseline daily weight. • Urine output >30 ml <200 ml/min. • Urine specific gravity 1.010 to 1.025. 4. Demonstrate good skin turgour and moist mucous membranes. 5. Maintain laboratory parameters within acceptable physiologic range.	• Additional nursing considerations. • Prevent and/or minimize cerebral oedema. ♦ Restrict fluids as prescribed. ♦ Monitor intake and output; body weight, urine-specific gravity, and other laboratory parameters (e.g., serum electrolytes, osmolality, total protein, BUN, and creatinine). ♦ Administer prescribed medication regimen and monitor response to therapy. – Hyperosmolar agents, diuretics. – Corticosteroids. • Assess for signs of fluid overload or deficits.	• Hydration therapy is coupled with pharmacologic therapy to maintain the patient in a slightly dehydrated state to minimize cerebral oedema formation.
Nursing Diagnosis #7 Potential for injury: physiologic, related to:		Patient will: 1. Maintain vital signs at baseline values.	• Assess for signs and symptoms of diabetes insipidus.	• Diabetes insipidus is a frequent secondary complication of craniocerebral insult.

Contd...

Problem	*R*	*Objective*	*Nursing Interventions*	*Rationales*
1. Diabetus insipidus associated with craniocerebral insult. • Hypothalamic/ pituitary dysfunction.		2. Maintain desired hydration status: • Urine output >30 ml <200 ml/hr. • Urine specific gravity 1.010-1.025. 3. Remain without clinical signs of dehydration. 4. Maintain acceptable laboratory profile: • Serum electrolytes, BUN, creatinine. • Serum osmolality, serum proteins. • Haematology profile.	♦ Primary findings include: – Polyuria, polydipsia, dehydration, weight loss. – Urine specific gravity <1.010. ♦ Neurologic status: level of consciousness, mentation, cranial nerve and sensorimotor function and deep tendon reflexes.	♦ Cerebral oedema and/or intracranial haemorrhage may temporarily impair synthesis and release of antidiuretic hormone by the hypothalamus during the initial 48 hours post-insult.
			♦ Hydration status: strict hourly fluid intake/ output, body weight, urine-specific gravity; signs/symptoms of fluid overload or dehydration; laboratory data: serum electrolytes, serum osmolality; haematology profile (i.e., haematocrit, haemoglobin). ♦ Cardiopulmonary status: blood pressure, pulse, cardiac rate and rhythm. – Presence of adventitious sounds. – Ability to handle respiratory secretions; characteristics of sputum (e.g., thick tenacious).	♦ Patient with diabetes insipidus can quickly become dehydra-ted.
			• Identify patients at risk.	• Clinical manifestations of diabetes insipidus postinsult may be delayed because of limited endogenous stores of antidiuretic hormone.
			• Implement measures to maintain desired fluid status.	• Patient is usually maintained in a slightly dehydrated state to minimize risk of cerebral oedema and reduce blood pressure.
			♦ Administer prescribed medication regimen: vasopressin replacement therapy (e.g., vasopressin; desmopressin ace-tate); chlorpropamide, clofibrate, carbama-zepine; and corticosteroid therapy.	♦ These drugs may be prescribed to heighten the efficacy of antidiuretic hormone.
			♦ Administer prescribed fluid regimen. • Monitor effectiveness of overall thereapeutic regimen.	♦ Anti-inflammatory effect of steroid therapy may help to minimize cerebral oedema.
Nursing Diagnosis #8 Potential for injury: seizures, related to: 1. Intracranial haemorrhage. 2. Cerebral ischaemia. 3. Cerebral oedema.		Patient will: 1. Remain without seizure activity.	♦ Assess characteristics of seizure activity. ♦ Implement measures to protect patient during seizure activity. ♦ Implement measures to prevent seizure activity.	
Nursing Diagnosis #9 Potential for alteration in body temperature, related to: 1. Intracranial haemorrhage subarachnoid haemorrhage). 2. Infection.		Patient will: 1. Maintain optimal body temperature ~98.6°F (37°C).	♦ Monitor body temperature. ♦ Assess for signs and symptoms of hyperpyrexia. ♦ Obtain specimens of body fluids for culture and sensitivity. ♦ Inspect all invasive sites. ♦ Implement measures to reduce body temperature ♦ Offer reassurance	♦ Blood is very irritating to fragile brain tissue and predisposes to hyperpyrexia.
Nursing Diagnosis#10 Potential for infection, related to:		Patient will: 1. Maintain body temperature ~98.6°F (37°C).		

Contd...

Problem	*R* *Objective*	*Nursing Interventions*	*Rationales*
1. Meningeal irritation; surgical manipulation. 2. Iatrogenic (e.g., invasive lines/ procedures). 3. Pneumonia and urinary complications associated with immobility, catabolic state. 4. Compromised immune response possibly associated with corticosteroid therapy.	2. Remain free of signs of meningeal irritation. 3. Demonstrate normal cerebrospinal fluid analysis. 4. Maintain serum WBC within acceptable range. 5. Have normal breath sounds. 6. Urine clear, free of microorganisms on culture.	◆ Monitor for signs and symptoms of infection. ◆ Implement measures to prevent infection. ◆ Administer prescribed course of antibiotics. ◆ Provide reassurance to patient and family. • Additional nursing considerations.	
		• Identify patients at high risk of developing an infection.	• Patients with strokes are especially at high risk; many are elderly with underlying chronic and degenerative diseases.
		• Obtain baseline cultures of body secretions and drainage.	• In patients who are intubated, a baseline sputum specimen should be obtained for culture and sensitivity. Use of artificial airway and tracheobronchial suctioning contaminate the tracheobronchial tree, which is considered to be sterile below the level of the larynx.
		• Monitor for the following parameters: ◆ Body temperature. ◆ Haematology profile—evidence of leukocytosis.	• Early diagnosis with institution of timely therapy (including antibiotics) may help to prevent or minimize impact of infectous process on total body function.
		◆ Sputum for changes in colour, quantity, consistency, odour, and ability of patient to handle tracheobronchial secretions. ◆ Chest x-rays for pulmonary infiltrates.	◆ Patients with stroke are at high risk of developing a pneumonia because of compromised protective reflexes, altered sensorium, and immobility.
		◆ Urinary retention/distention; urinary incontinence.	◆ Altered state of consciousness and sensorimotor impairment may predispose to urinary retention with consequent infection.
		• Institute chest physiotherapy and bronchial hygiene (unless contraindicated by risk of intracranial hypertension or rebleeding).	• Secretion removal improves ventilation and reduces pooling of secretions, which may act as foci of infection.
		◆ Implement turning and positioning schedule.	◆ Positioning and turning help to mobilize secretions; positions used should protect the compromised patient from aspiration.
		• Use aseptic technique for patient care: tracheobronchial suctioning, urinary catheterization and Foley catheter care. • Maintain nutrition (anabolic state).	
Nursing Diagnosis#11 Nutrition, alteration in: Less than body requirements related to: 1. Catabolic state. 2. Compromised nutritional intake associated with: • Altered state of consciousness. • Compromised protective reflexes.	Patient will: 1. Maintain body weight within 5 per cent of baseline. 2. Maintain total serum proteins 6.0-8.4 g/100 ml.	◆ Arrange consultation with nutritionist and collaborate to perform nutritional assessment. ◆ Maintain optimal nutrition with prescribed nutrition regimen (e.g., oral, enteral, parenteral). – Maintain patient in optimal position for specific mode of nutrition intake (e.g., semi-Fowler's position in patients receiving enteral feedings). – Confirm placement of nasogastric tube in stomach before initiating feedings. ◆ Provide frequent mouth care and other comfort measures. ◆ Monitor daily weight (unless contraindicated by risk of increased intracranial pressure and/or rebleeding). ◆ Assess bowel function; implement prescribed bowel regimen.	

Contd...

Problem	*R*	*Objective*	*Nursing Interventions*	*Rationales*
• Ineffective chewing/ swallowing. • Fatigue. • Depression.				
Nursing Diagnosis#12 Impaired physical mobility, related to: 1. Comatose state. 2. Restricted activity associated with risk of intracranial pressure or rebleeding. 3. Haemostasis and/ or dependent oedema associated with immobility; neuromuscular impairment (e.g., hemiparesis).		Patient will: 1. Maintain full range of motion. 2. Remain without contractures. 3. Remain without incidence of thrombophlebitis.	• Consult with physician and physical therapist to assess neurologic and musculoskeletal status.	• The risk of intracranial hypertension and rebleeding must guide the type and extent of an activity program. A major objective is to maintain optimal function as dictated by patient's overall condition.
			• Plan and implement activity regimen: ◆ Initiate schedule of range-of-motion exercises.	◆ Exercise maintains muscle tone and prevents atrophy; stimulates circulation and prevents haemostasis.
			◆ Passive/active exercises should be performed as patient's condition warrants.	◆ Immobility associated with hemiparesis predisposes to thrombophlebitis.
			◆ Allow rest periods prior to and after exercise routines.	◆ Helps to conserve patent's energy and prevent feelings of frustration associated with inability to perform daily self-care.
			◆ Maintain optimal body alignment: – Use hand/wrist splints as prescribed. – Support affected extremities in functional position.	◆ Proper alignment is essential to prevent development of contractures and dependent oedema (sacral area, buttocks, extremities).
			◆ Use trochanter roll on outer aspects of thigh.	◆ Prevents external rotation.
			◆ Initiate turning and positioning schedule. – Encourage patient to deep breathe and cough (unless contraindicated).	◆ Turning, positioning, and deep breathing facilitate chest and lung expansion; mobilize oral and pulmonary secretions; prevent atelectasis.
Nursing Diagnosis#13 Skin integrity, impairment of, related to: 1. Immobility. 2. Catabolic state. 3. Altered sensation. 4. Incontinence.		Patient's skin will remain intact: • All reddened areas will blanch within 20-30 minutes of a position change.	• Implement skin care regimen. ◆ Inspect skin and all pressure point areas for compromised perfusion. ◆ Provide special skin care to back and joints and all pressure points. ◆ Provide pressure relief device (e.g., air mattress, sheepskin). ◆ Initiate pressure ulcer protocol if indicated: treat local skin areas with prescribed treatment (e.g., Skin Prep, Granulex, Duoderm, wet-to-dry dressings, other therapies).	• Maintain circulation to all areas; it is essential to prevent skin breakdown because the compromised patient is at high risk of developing an infection.
Nursing Diagnosis#14 Potential for physiologic injury: thrombophlebitis, related to: 1. Hemostasis associated with immobility.		Patient will: 1. Verbalize absence of calf tenderness. 2. Exhibit adequate peripheral circulation: • Usual skin colour; no cyanosis. • Extremities warm to touch. • Palpable pulses: pedal, popliteal, radial.	• Assess for signs/symptoms of venous thrombosis. ◆ Tenderness, pain, warmth, and peripheral pitting oedema.	• Deep venous thrombosis places patient at risk/of pulmonary embolism. ◆ Oedema is a characteristic manifestation of altered venous circulation.
			◆ Measure circumference of thighs and calves at designated points.	◆ Evidence of oedema is best assessed and monitored by determining the circumference of calves and thighs at designated points (use tape measure).
			◆ Skin colour and temperature.	◆ With altered venous circulation

Contd...

Problem	*R*	*Objective*	*Nursing Interventions*	*Rationales*
			– Observe extremities in both dependent and elevated positions.	a bluishred colour of skin may be observed.
			• Implement measures to minimize risk of thrombophiebitis/deep venous thrombosis.	◆ Temperature of skin is assessed by touch; unusually warm temperature in the lower extremities is commonly associated with venous thrombosis.
			◆ Maintain desired hydration state.	◆ While the patient with a cerebrovascular insult is usually maintained in a slightly dehydrated state, dehydration is to be avoided because it increases blood viscosity.
			◆ Apply antiembolic hose to both extremities; remove hose once per shift. ◆ Assist patient to perform range-of-motion exercises as appropriate.	◆ Exercise enhances "skeletal-muscular" pump, which functions to prevent pooling of blood in lower extremities (venous stasis), and increases venous return to heart.
			◆ Instruct responsive patient to avoid positions that compromise blood flow in the extremities (e.g., crossing of legs, prolonged sitting in one position, pillow under knees, or use of knee gatch).	◆ Positions that compromise blood flow can cause circulatory stasis.
Nursing Diagnosis#15 Alteration in self-concept, related to: 1. Changes in body image associated with neurologic deficits. 2. Low self-esteem (i.e., dependence on others to achieve activities of daily living). 3. Alteration in role and personal identity.		Patient will: 1. Verbalize feelings about self. 2. Maintain interpersonal relationships with family members and significant others. 3. Participate in decision-making. 4. Initiate activities of self-care.	◆ Encourage verbalization regarding patient's perceptions of changes in appearance and body function. ◆ Assist patient/family to identify coping patterns/strengths and weaknesses. ◆ Assess patient/family's readiness to participate in decision-making regarding care. ◆ Involve patient in making choices and decisions regarding self-care. ◆ Assist patient/family in initial goal-setting.	
Nursing Diagnosis#16 Thought processes, alteration in, related to: 1. Cerebral ischaemia and hypoxia. 2. Comatose state. 3. Sedation.		Patient will: 1. Demonstrate improvement in thought processes: • Oriented to person, place and time. • Improved memory. • Increased attentiveness. • Improved ability to solve problems and make decisions.	◆ Assess for alteration in mentation and thought processes. ◆ Confirm recent behavioural or personality changes. ◆ Implement measures to assist patient in thought processes.	
Nursing Diagnosis#17 Sensory-perceptual alterations, related to: 1. Sensory deprivation. 2. Sensory overload.		Patient will: 1. Demonstrate appropriate interactions with people and environment using sensory perception (e.g., converses with visitors).	◆ Assess patient's ability to interact with environment. ◆ Provide usual necessary aids (e.g., eyeglasses). ◆ Arrange environment to compensate for neurologic deficits. ◆ Implament measures to reduce sensory deprivation.	

Contd...

Problem	*Objective*	*Nursing Interventions*	*Rationales*
	2. Verbalize restfulness and relaxed feelings. 3. Demonstrate relaxed facies and body demeanour.	◆ Implement measures to reduce sensory overload. ◆ Recognize and accept patient's perceptions of stimuli-(reinforce reality).	
Nursing Diagnosis#18 Communication impaired, related to: 1. Aphasia (dysphasia). 2. Dysarthria (i.e., disturbance in articulation) (left cerebral hemisphere involvement).	Patient will: 1. Use language to verbalize or communicate needs or answer questions.	• Assess for difficulty in using language to verbalize needs and answer questions. ◆ Consult speech pathologist, if possible, to assess patient's clinical status and design a care plan.	• Primary speech center (Broca's) is predominantly in frontal lobe of left cerebral hemisphere. Cerebrovascular insult to this area can result in languge deficits.
		• Implement measures that enhance communication: ◆ Speak slowly, using simple sentences. ◆ Repeat questions or directions. ◆ Use supplemental gestures or pictures; blackboard or slate board. ◆ Face the patient directly when speaking.	• Directives here suggest some of the ways communication can be facilitated. In the clinical setting, ideally, speech therapy is conducted in collaboration with a speech pathologist so that specific communication problems can be addressed appropriately.
		◆ Avoid speaking too loudly.	◆ A language problem doesn't mean the patient can't hear.
		◆ Encourage patient to express his/her thoughts; avoid rushing the patient. ◆ Minimize distractions.	◆ Assist the patient to concentrate on communicating.
		◆ Offer encouragement; praise the patient for his/her accomplishments.	◆ Assist the patient in gaining self-confidence.
		• Anticipate patient's needs.	• May help to allay concerns regarding dependency on others.
Nursing Diagnosis#19 Coping, alteration in: Patent and family, related to: 1. Situational crisis. 2. Temporary family disorganization. 3. Inability to problem-solve. 4. Altered thought processes. 5. Catastrophic illness with long-term effects.	Patient/family will: 1. Identify useful coping mechanisms. 2. Demonstrate ability to assess, problem-solve, and make decisions. 3. Express realistic expectations of each other.	• Establish a rapport and trusting relationship with patient and family. ◆ Observe family dynamics and interactions. – Assess family relationships and communication pattern: usual coping mechanisms, usual decision-making process, especially during stressful or crisis situations. – Assess response of patient/family to stressful situations: identify strengths/weaknesses.	• These observations may help to identify strengths and weaknesses, and effective coping capabilities. Assisting patient/family to acknowledge their own strengths may help them cope more effectively.
		• Implement measures to assist in coping: ◆ Provide opportunity for patient and family members to express feelings and emotions: – Encourage honest communication among family members.	◆ Recognizing feelings and emotions helps one to deal with them.
		◆ Assist patient to prioritize daily activities.	◆ Reduction in level of stress assists in coping.
		◆ Encourage patient/family to assist in decision-making process regarding care: – Assist in identifying options and their consequences.	◆ Assists patient/family to be responsible for self-care, and level of health desired.
		◆ Advise patient/family regarding community resources.	◆ Sequelae from cerebrovascular disease can be catastrophic; it is essential for the patient/family to identify family and community resources.
Nursing Diagnosis#20 Unilateral neglect, related to:	Patient will:	• Assess sensorimotor function related to:	• It is essential to determine what deficits exist so that an appropriate

Contd...

Problem	*R*	*Objective*	*Nursing Interventions*	*Rationales*
1. Altered sensorimotor function associated with cerebrovascular accident. 2. Alterations in thought processes: perceptual.		1. Demonstrate awareness as to position or placement of all four extremities. 2. Demonstrate awareness of looking towards affected side in terms of: • Self-care (personal hygiene, grooming, dressing). • Safety measures. • Eating habits.	◆ Special senses: visual field defects, dysphasia (aphasia). ◆ General senses: pain and temperature, tactile sensations.	approach to therapy can be individualized for the patient. ◆ Often sensory deficits are permanent, necessitating that the patient learn what his/her deficits are, and how to accommodate actions and behaviours accordingly.
Nursing Diagnosis#21 Self-care deficits, related to: 1. Neuromuscular impairments (e.g., paresis, apraxia, visual/sensory defects, anosognosia) (right cerebral hemisphere involvement). 2. Reduced attention span.		Patient will identify: 1. Activities of daily living for which the patient requires some assistance. Patient will verbalize: 1. Feelings regarding dependency. Patient will: 1. Determine priorities. 2. Plan activities of daily living, leaving ample time to accomplish tasks.	• Implement measures to assist patient to learn what types of sensorimotor deficits exist, and the extent of the deficits in terms of self-care. ◆ Visual field deficits: – Teach patient to scan immediate environment and note the placement of objects and equipment. – Approach patient from intact side.	• It is important to involve patient and family members in patient care. ◆ Frequent praise encourages and motivates patient and family.
Nursing Diagnosis#22 Potential for injury: (Safety), related to: 1. Altered sensory/perceptual function. 2. Altered musculoskeletal function.		Patient will remain free from falls or other injury.	– Position bed so that the intact side can fully visualize the doorway. – Keep bedside uncluttered. ◆ Dysphasia: – Attempt to evaluate type of dysphasia. – Enlist the assistance of speech pathologist, if available, to establish program for patient, family members, and healthcare professionals working with patient, designed to facilitate communication. – Helpful measures may include: – Speak slowly and face the patient. – Use short, simple sentences. – Repeat directions or explanations as necessary. – Use gestures to further clarify what is being said. ◆ General sensorimotor functions: – Dressing and grooming: – Teach patient to care for affected side first when bathing or dressing; and to undress the affected side last. – Use sensory stimuli to help patient become aware of affected part of body. – Use exercises that enable affected side to cross midline. ◆ Reassure patient and family regarding progress: – Praise positive responses and activities.	– Prevents possible injury. ◆ Dysphasia (aphasia) is particularly associated with dominant cerebral hemisphere lesion (usually the left hemisphere). • Apraxia, unilateral spatial and visual neglect, and anosognosia are neurologic deficits associated with nondominant cerebral hemisphere involvement (usually the right hemisphere involvement). ◆ The patient's rehabilitation should begin during the acute phase; activities initiated during this period lay the foundation for patient/family participation in self-care.

Table 11.4: Nursing care plan for postoperative patient wth craniocerebral surgery

Problem	*R*	*Objective*	*Nursing Interventions*	*Rationales*
Nursing Diagnosis #1 Alteration in cerebral perfusion pressure, related to: 1. Cerebral oedema. 2. Potential intracranial bleeding with haematoma formation. 3. Compromised cardiovascular function.		Patient will: 1. Maintain • Cerebral perfusion pressure > 60 mmHg. • Intracranial pressure <15 mmHg. • Mean arterial blood pressure ~80 mmHg. 2. Exhibit intact level of consciousness and mentation; open eyes when name is called; be oriented to person and place. 3. Follow commands; differentiate pinprick from crude pressure.	♦ Monitor for signs and symptoms of increasing intracranial pressure. ♦ Maintain intracranial pressure monitoring system. ♦ Implement measures to prevent and/or reduce intracranial pressure. – Maintain optimal positioning. – Prevent increase in cerebral blood flow. – Limit or decrease cerebral oedema. – Minimize cellular metabolism. – Plan nursing care activities to prevent cumulative increase in intracranial pressure.	
Nursing Diagnosis #2 Breathing pattern ineffective, related to: 1. Brainstem compression associated with cerebral oedema (especially following infratenorial craniotomy). 2. Respiratory depression associated with anaesthesia, analgesia, and muscle relaxants.		Patient will demonstrate effective breathing pattern: 1. Respiratory rate <25/ min. 2. Rhythm and depth eupneic. • Tidal volume >7-10 ml/kg. • Vital capacity >12-15 ml/kg. 3. Adequate alveolar ventilation and gas exchange: • $PaCO_2$ < 30-35 mmHg. • PaO_2 >80 mmHg. • pH 7.35-7.45.	• Assess respiratory function hourly. ♦ Assess spontaneous respiratory effort: rate, depth, rhythm; use of accessory muscles; dyspnoea, tachypnoea; hyper or hypoventilation. ♦ Monitor arterial blood gases. • Implement measures to improve breathing pattern. ♦ Maintain patient in semi-Fowler's position. ♦ Maintain nasogastric decompression as indicated. ♦ Maintain mechanical ventilation and oxygenation. – Assess tidal volume and vital capacity.	• Adequate ventilation and oxygenation are imperative because hypercapnia and hypoxia cause cerebral vasodilation. In the patient with reduced intracranial compliance, an increase in cerebral blood flow may precipitate a significant rise in intracranial pressure. ♦ Reflect adequacy of ventilation and oxygenation. ♦ Permits maximal chest excursion and facilitates drainage of blood and cerebrospinal fluid from cranial vault via gravity. ♦ Prevents abdominal distention, which can compromise diaphragmatic excursion; minimizes danger of aspiration.
Nursing Diagnosis #3 Airway clearance ineffective, related to: 1. Compromised cough. 2. Thick, tenacious secretions.		Patient will: 1. Maintain patent airway. • Normal breath sounds on auscultation. • Absence of adventitious sounds (crackles, rhonchi, wheezes). 2. Demonstrate secretion-clearing cough (unless contraindicated by intracranial hypertension).	• Assess respiratory function hourly. ♦ Assess airway patency: status of protective reflexes: cough, gag, epiglottal closure. ♦ Auscultate breath sounds bilaterally. ♦ Assess characteristics of sputum (e.g., colour, tenaciousness and amount).	• Hypercapnia and hypoxia increase cerebral blood flow. ♦ Compromised protective reflexes place patient at risk of aspirat-ing tracheobronchial secretions. ♦ Presence of rales (crackles), wheezes, or rhonchi suggests increased pulmonary secretions (e.g., pulmonay oedema, infection) or inability to mobilize or clear secretions. Patient is at increased risk of developing a pneumonia.

Contd...

Problem	*R*	*Objective*	*Nursing Interventions*	*Rationales*
			◆ Assess hydration status.	◆ Dehydration causes tracheobronchial secretions to become thick, tenacious, and difficult to clear.
			• Implement measures to maintain airway patency: ◆ Humidify inspired air. ◆ Initiate suctioning of tracheobronchial secretions only when indicated; assess effect of suctioning on patient's intracranial pressure.	◆ Suctioning stimulates cough reflex and Valsalva's manoeuver; these responses are associated with an increase in intracranial pressure.
			◆ Follow appropriate suctioning technique, minimize suctioning time; hyperventilate with 100% oxygen via resuscitator prior to and between each pass, and after suctioning. – Monitor hydration status.	◆ Reduces risk of developing hypercapnia and hypoxaemia; minimizes risk of increasing intracranial pressure.
			◆ Turning and positioning measures. Plan for nursing activities to avoid a cumulative increase in intracranial pressure).	◆ Movement of the patient is guided by the status of intracranial pressure; turning the patient should be avoided when intracranial pressure is unstable.
Nursing Diagnosis #4 Alteration in comfort: Headache, related to: 1. Meningeal irritation. 2. Surgical scalp incision. 3. Anxiety.		Patient will: 1. Verbalize and/or indicate comfort. 2. Demonstrate relaxed facial expression and demeanour. 3. Maintain intracranial pressure <15 mmHg.	• Assess patient for signs of pain and discomfort. ◆ Symptoms may include: restlessness, agitation; clenched fist, tense facial expression; photophobia. ◆ Signs of discomfort may be reflected by increase in intracranial pressure, heart rate, blood pressure, and respiratory rate.	• The patient must be as comfortable as possible to prevent any increase in intracranial pressure. Pain, fear, anxiety, and muscle tenseness or rigidity can precipitate a rise in intracranial pressure and must be avoided.
			Implement measures to reduce discomfort. ◆ Administer analgesic or sedative as prescribed. Evaluate patient's response to medication. ◆ Position patient to relieve muscle tension and pressure on bony prominences.	• Nursing activities that limit sensory overload, prevent sleep deprivation and provide reassurance help to minimize changes in the patient's intracranial pressure status; such care minimizes cellular metabolic activities. reducing demand for oxygen and glucose, and thus the need for increase in cerebral blood flow.
			Make sure dressing is not too tight and constricting. ◆ Provide quiet environment. Minimize environmental stimuli: dim lights, reduce noise level, restrict visitors if necessary. ◆ Provide periods for uninterrupted sleep. ◆ Provide touch therapy; speak softly in a soothing voice. – Reassure patient you are there to anticipate and fulfill his/her needs. – Provide appropriate explanations. ◆ Employ diversional and comfort measures (e.g., soft music, mouth care, back rub, passive movement of extremities).	◆ Brain tissue itself is without free pain endings; pain experienced by patients is usually related to meningeal irritation and/or injury to scalp where free nerve endings are numerous.
Nursing Diagnosis #5 Alteration in fluid and electrolyte balance. 1. Fluid volume excess related to:		Patient will: 1. Maintain haemodynamic function. • Mean systemic blood pressure ~80-	• Monitor for signs and symptoms of diabetes insipidus: polyuria, polydipsia, and urine specific gravity <1.005; monitor fluid intake and output, weight; serum electrolytes and osmolality.	• Diabetes insipidus may occur secondary to craniocerebral trauma, infecton (e.g., meningitis), or pituitary tumours.

Contd...

Problem	*R*	*Objective*	*Nursing Interventions*	*Rationales*
• Cerebral oedema. • SIADH. 2. Fluid volume deficit related to: • Diuretic therapy. • Diabetes insipidus. 3. Altered electrolytes related to: • Diuretic therapy. • Corticosteroid therapy. • Acid-base imbalance.		100 mmHg. • Heart rate at patient's baseline; rhythm regular, without dysrhythmias. 2. Maintain balanced intake and output. • Stable baseline daily weight (unless contraindicated). • Urine output > 30 ml and <200 ml/hr. • Urine specific gravity 1.010-1.025. 3. Demonstrate good skin turgour and moist mucous membranes. 4. Maintain laboratory parameters within acceptable range. • Serum electrolytes, BUN, and creatinine. • Haematocrit, haemoglobin. • Serum osmolality. • Arterial blood gas studies; acid-base balance intact.	◆ Monitor for signs and symptoms of dehydration. • Implemnt measures to: ◆ Maintain adequate fluid intake to prevent dehydration. ◆ Administer prescribed medications: vasopressin replacement therapy; agents that enhance ADH secretion (e.g., chlorpropamide, carbamazepine).	◆ Cerebral oedema related to trauma or surgery may impair synthesis and release of antidiuretic hormone temporarily resulting in polyuria within 24-48 hours. As cerebral oedema subsides, symptoms also regress and diminish. • For information related to the diagnosis, treatment, and nursing management of diabetes insipidus.
Nursing Diagnosis #6 Potential for injury: Seizures, related to: 1. Cerebral ischaemia and injury associated with surgical manipulation.		Patient will: 1. Not have any seizures.	• Assess characteristics of seizure activity. ◆ Specific signs: onset (what triggers the seizure, type, locality, presence of aura, duration of seizure); type of movement: tonic, clonic, flaccid; associated changes in level of consciousness; pupillary size and reactivity; extraocular movements; associated vomiting or incontinence (urinary, fecal). • During seizure activity: ◆ Maintain safe environment. Remain with patient but do not restrain; provide reassurance. ◆ Do not force airway or other objects between clenched teeth. ◆ Keep resuscitative equipment at bedside. • Implement measures to prevent seizure activity. ◆ Avoid problems that cause an increase in intracranial pressure (e.g., headache, anxiety, hypoxia, hyperventilation, urinary retention, fecal impaction, hyperpyrexia). ◆ Monitor for signs of meningeal irritation (see Nursing Diagnosis #7). Initiate and maintain seizure precautions: oral airway; padded side rails and headboard; keep bed in low position with side rails in up position. ◆ Administer prescribed anticonvulsant therapy.	• Seizure activity can precipitate a significant increase in intracranial pressure; it increases cellular metabolism and the demand for metabolic substrates—oxygen and glucose; it raises body temperature. ◆ Postoperative seizure activity may be precipitated by hypoxia, hyperventilation, hyperpyrexia, meningeal irritation, and bladder distention. • A rise in intracranial pressure may precipitate seizure activity associated with cerebral ischaemia.

Contd...

Problem	*R*	*Objective*	*Nursing Interventions*	*Rationales*
			◆ Evaluate patient's response to anticonvulsant therapy. – Obtain serum levels of phenytoin. – Be familiar with effect of phenytoin on cardiovascular haemodynamics and adverse drug reactions.	◆ Diazepam, phenytoin, and barbiturates are commonly used to prevent and/or treat seizures. For specific information related to dose, route of administration, adverse reactions, and nursing implications for each of these drugs.
Nursing Diagnosis #7 Potential for infection: Meaningitis related to: 1. Craniocerebral trauma. 2. Surgical disruption of integrity of the meninges. 3. Iatrogenic causes via invasive procedures.		Patient will: 1. Maintain body temperature ~98.6°F (37°C). 2. Remain free of signs of meningeal irritation (nuchal rigidity, headache, photophobia, positive Kernig and Brudzinski's signs). 3. Demonstrate normal cerebrospinal fluid analysis (WBC and protein levels); serum WBC within normal range.	• Monitor for signs and symptoms of infection. ◆ Assess for meningeal irritation: hyperphrexia, chills, nuchal rigidity, photophobia, persistent headache, positive Kernig's sign (i.e., inability to extend lower leg when hip is flexed), positive Brudzinski's sign (i.e., flexion of hips and knees when head is flexed on chest). ◆ Assess for otorrhoea and rhinorrhoea. – Use of dextrostix to test for presence of glucose. – Observe for clear halo around serosan-guineous drainage from ear, nose, or dressing. – Observe for excessive swallowing or complaints of postnasal drip. ◆ Assist with lumbar puncture. – Observe colour of cerebrospinal fluid. – Record cerebrospinal pressure.	◆ Meningeal tears often accompany basal skull fractures. – Presence of glucose in nonbloody drainage from nose or ear suggests cerebrospinal leak. Nasopharyngeal secretions do not contain glucose. ◆ Presence of elevated levels of WBCs and protein in cerebrospinal fluid strongly suggests meningitis.
			• Implement measures to prevent infection. ◆ Specific nursing actions include: strict handwashing, sterile technique in managing all invasive procedures (e.g., intracranial pressure monitoring, ventricular shunts), sterile technique employed for all dressing changes (as per unit protocols). ◆ If rhinorrhoea or otorrhoea are present: – Caution patient not to cough, sneeze, blow the nose, or perform a Valsalva's manoeuver (e.g., straining at stool). – Instruct patient not to put fingers into ears or nose, and to lie quietly. – Allow free flow of drainage directly onto sterile pad; change pad as soon as it becomes damp. ◆ Have patient assume a position that facilitates free drainage (e.g., semi-Fowler's position) in the presence of rhinorrhea. ◆ Provide quiet environment; minimize stimuli.	• Disciplined aseptic technique is essential to prevent meningitis. ◆ These activities increase intracranial pressure and can place further stress on the dural tear. ◆ Free flow of drainage prevents pooling, which might otherwise provide a medium for bacterial colonization. ◆ Reduces risk of aggravating underlying dural tear.
			• Administer prescribed course of antibiotics. ◆ Evaluate response to therapy: – Monitor temperature, WBC profile. – Monitor neurologic function and signs of meningeal irritation. – Monitor intracranial pressure. • Provide reassurance to patient and family.	◆ Administration of corticosteroids to reduce cerebral oedema may compromise the immune response, placing patient at greater risk of developing an infection. Ongoing assessment for signs of infection must be diligent; aseptic technique must be impeccable.

Contd...

Problem	*R Objective*	*Nursing Interventions*	*Rationales*
Nursing Diagnosis #8 Potential for alteration in body temperature, related to: 1. Cerebral oedema with altered hypothaiamic function. 2. Infection.	Patient will: 1. Maintain optimal body temperature ~98.6°F (37°C).	• Monitor body temperature every 1-2 hours if unstable. ◆ Assess for signs and symptoms of hyperpyrexia (e.g., hot, dry skin; parched tongue; cool extremities; delirium). • Obtain specimens of body fluid (e.g., blood, urine, sputum, wound drainage) for culture and sensitivity. • Inspect all invasive sites and wounds for signs of infection (e.g., redness, warmth, swelling, pain, amount and characteristics of wound drainage). • Implement measures to reduce body temperature. ◆ Administer prescribed antibiotic and antipyretic therapy. – Evaluate patient's response to therapy by monitoring body temperature and WBC profile. ◆ Provide comfort measures. – Remove excess clothing and blankets. – Maintain room temperature at ~20°C (68°F). – Apply ice bags to groin and axilla; tepid bath. ◆ Provide diligent wound care. – Wash hands thoroughly. – Monitor all invasive sites and wounds for signs/symptoms of infection. – Provide wound care and dressings using aseptic technique; damp dressings should be changed promptly, and dry dressings should be applied as per unit protocol. • Implement hypothermia therapy as prescribed. • Offer reassurance to patient and family.	• Hyperpyrexia increases cerebral metabolism and cerebral blood flow; an increase in intracranial pressure may result from the consequent increase in intracranial blood volume. • In the scenario of a spiking body temperature (~39°C-41°C [102.2°F – 105.8°F]), obtain culture of body fluids prior to initiating prescribed antibiotic therapy. • When inducing an increase or decrease in body temperature, the change in temperature should not exceed 1°F (0.56°C) per 15-20 minutes.
Nursing Diagnosis #9 Potential for physiologic injury: Gastrointestinal bleeding associated with stress and corticosteroid tehrapy.	Patient will remain without gastrointestinal bleeding: 1. Haematocrit stable. • Male 45-52%. • Female 37-48%. 2. Haemoglobin stable. • Male 13-18 g/100 ml. • Female 12-16 g/100 ml. 3. Nasogastric drainage. • Negative for occult blood. • pH > 4.5. 4. Stool negative for occult blood. 5. Vital signs stable. • Blood pressure and heart rate at patient's baseline level.	• Assess GI bleeding • Monitor vital signs • Monitor lab valus of Hct, Hb% and others.	

Contd...

Problem	R	Objective	Nursing Interventions	Rationales
Nursing Diagnosis#10 Alteration in nutrition: Less than body requirements, related to: 1. Stress (cranlocerebral insult). 2. Compromised or absent protective reflexes (e.g., cough, gag, epiglottal closure). 3. Altered state of consciousness.		Patient will receive adequate nutritional intake. • Stable baseline body weight. • Balanced intake and output. • Stable laboratory parameters: serum protein (albumin) 3.5-5.0 g/100 ml, BUN, creatinine. • Positive nitrogen balance.	• Consult nutritionist to assess metabolic needs if needed. ◆ Take components of a Dietary History ◆ Take Protein Measurements. ◆ Take Correction Factors for Predicting Energy Requirements in Hospitalized Patient. ◆ Assess Caloric Requirements of the Critically ill. ◆ Have Large Bore vs. Small Bore Feeding Tubes. ◆ Use Method of Enteral Administration. ◆ Assess Mechanical Complications Associated with Enteral Feeding Tubes. ◆ Have Special Considerations for Specific Disease States.	
Nursing Diagnosis#11 Alteration in self-concept, related to: 1. Changes in body image associated with physical appearance (e.g., shaved head) or neurologic deficits (e.g., loss of sensorimotor function). 2. Loss of self- esteem (i.e., dependence on others to achieve activities of daily living). 3. Alterations in role and personal identity. 4. Stigma of seizure disorder.		Patient will: 1. Verbalize positive feelings about self. 2. Maintain interpersonal relationships with family members and significant others. 3. Participate in decision-making process regarding care. 4. Initiate activities related to self-care.	• Encourage verbalization regarding patient's perceptions of changes in appearance and body function. ◆ Observe nonverbal behaviour reflective of underlying feelings and concerns. ◆ Listen to patient's concerns. ◆ Provide information and explanations regarding patient's status and prognosis. Clarify misconceptions. ◆ Ascertain patient/family expectations and understanding regarding impact of illness on family lifestyle. ◆ Facilitate communication between patient, family, and significant others. • Assist patient/family to identify coping patterns/ strengths and weaknesses. • Assess patient/family's readiness to participate in decision-making process regarding care. • Involve patient in making choices and decisions regarding self-care. ◆ Readily identify and praise patient's accomplishments. Identify improvements in bodily functions as they occur. • Assist patient/family in initial goal setting. ◆ Refer to social worker. – Identify community resources. – Encourage use of community support groups (e.g., head injury support groups).	• Assist patient to increase self-awareness and to recognize and vent feelings of fear, anger, or frustrations. ◆ Often what the patient doesn't say is reflected in the body language. • Assist patient in maintaining a sense of control over his/her life. ◆ Positive reinforcement nurtures self-motivation. • Depending on underlying problem, a craniocerebral insult or injury can be catastrophic in terms of health-care costs, productivity, and quality of life for all concerned. ◆ Early referral to social worker and community agencies sho-uld be initiated.

EPILEPSY/SEIZURE DISORDER

A seizure is a paroxysmal, uncontrolled electrical discharge of neurons in the brain that interrupts normal functions. Seizures are frequently symptoms of an underlying illness. They may accompany a variety of disorders, or they may occur spontaneously without any apparent cause.

Epilepsy is a condition in which a person has spontaneously recurring seizures caused by chronic underlying conditions.

Aetiology

The most common causes of epilepsy during the first 6 months of life are severe birth injury, congenital defects involving the CNS infection and inborn errors of metabolism.

In patients between 2 and 20 years of ages, the primary causative factors are birth injury, infection, trauma, and genetic factors. In individuals between 20-30 years of age, epilepsy is a result of structural lesions, such as trauma, brain tumours or vascular diseases. After 50 years of age, the primary cause will be cerebrovascular lesions and metastatic brain tumours. Heredity may lead to epilepsy in a few cases. The common risk factors for epilepsy are as follows:

- Anoxia.
- Cerebral palsy.
- Perinatal problems (toxaemia, difficult delivery, low birth weight and hypoxia).
- Congenital central nervous system defects.
- Mental retardation.
- Febrile conditions.
- Family history of epilepsy.
- Head trauma.
- Central nervous system infections.
- Central nervous system tumours.
- Cerebrovascular disease.
- Alcohol or drug abuse.
- Metabolic distubrances.
- Exposure to toxins.
- Degenerative diseases (Alzheimer's disease).

Pathophysiology

A seizure can be caused by any process that disrupts the cell membrane stability of a neuron. The point at which the cell membrane becomes destabilized and an uncontrolled electrical discharge begins is known as seizures threshold. Some people have lower seizures threshold than others and are, therefore, more prone to seizures. In recurring seizures (epilepsy) a group of abnormal neurons (seizures focus) seems to undergo spontaneous firing. This firing spreads by physiologic pathways to involve adjacent or distant areas of the brain. If this activity spreads to involve the whole brain, generalized seizures occurs. The factor that causes this abnormal firing is not clear. Any stimulus that causes the cell membrane of the neuron to depolarize induces a tendency to spontaneous firing. Often the area of the brain from which the epileptic activity arises is found to have scar tissues (gloses). The scarring is thought to interfere with the normal chemical and structural environment of the brain neurons, making them more likely to fire abnormally.

Clinical Manifestations

The specific clinical manifestations of a seizure are determined by the site of electrical disturbance. In 1981, the International League Against Epilepsy (ILAE) proposed a revised classificatioan for epileptic seizures. The major categories are partial (focal) generalized and unclassified. Further, subdivisions within the categories based on the person's clinical behaviour during the *ictal* and *interictal* times. Ictal refers to the time during the seizure. *Interictal* refers to the time between seizure activity. Postictal refers to the time immediately after a seizure as the patient recovers.

The types of seizure and their signs and symptoms are as follows:

1. *Partial seizures*

i Simple partial seizures (Formerly focal) characterized by no impairment of consciousness, with symptoms of motor, somato-sensory or special sensory, autonomic and psychic, which includes focal twitching of extremity, speech arrest, specival visual sensations (e.g. seeing lights), feeling of fear or doom. There is no postictal state.

ii. Complex partial (Formerly psychomotor or temporal lobe seizures) is a simple partial seizure with progression to impairment of consciousness with no other features except features of simple partial seizure and automatism. That is it may begin as simple partial and progress to complex by showing automatic behaviour (e.g. lipsmacking, chewing, or picking at clothes). Postictal state as follows.

iii. *Complex partial generalized to generalized tonic-clonic seizures* begins as complex partial as above, then progresses to tonic-clonic as in generalized seizures. Postictal state presents.

2. *Generalized seizures*

Generalized seizures impair consciousness from the start.

i. *Absence seizures*: atypical seizures (formerly petit mal) do not include motor signs and may last less than 1-minute. There will be brief loss of consciousness, staring, unresponsive and no postictal state.

ii. *Tonic-clonic seizures* (formerly Grand mal). Tonic phase involves rhythmic jerking of muscles, possibly tongue biting and urinary and fecal incontinence. May be combination of tonic and clonic movement.

iii. *Atonic seizures*: In this, there will be impairment consciousness for only few seconds and brief loss of muscle tone, which may cause patient to fall or drop something referred to as drop attacks.

iv. *Myoclonic seizures*: There will be impaired consciousness for only few seconds or not at all and brief jerking of a muscle group which may cause the patient to fall.

Postictal states represent periods of recovery from the seizures. In this patients may have some degree of confusion, lethargies or inability to follow commands or speak clearly during this period. In some rare cases the patient may experience a prolonged period of weakness involving one or more extremities called Todd Paralysis.

Status epileptical is an episode of seizures activity lasting at least for 30 minutes or repeated seizures without full recovery between seizures. Seizures cause a marked increase in cerebral metabolic activity and demands. These demands may outpace the delivery of oxygen and nutrient from the cerebral blood flow. Prolonged seizures can lead to cellular exhaustion and destruction and lead to death if not effectively treated.

Management

The diagnosis of epilepsy is made from a careful history including the risk factors involved and physical examination supplemented by diagnostic tests (EEG, CT, MRI, PET). Antiepileptic drugs are used to control seizures. The common medications used, their actions and nursing interventions are as given below.

1. *Hydantoin*: (Phenytoin-Dilantin)- These blocks synaptic potentiation and propagation of electrical discharges in the motor cortex and blocks sodium transport and stabilize membrane sensitivity. They are used alone or in combination to manage tonic-clonic, simple partial and complex seizures. Therapeutic range is 10-20 mg/L N. saline takes at least 7-14 days to establish. The nursing intervention during this treatment with hydantoin are:
   - Monitor common side effects including nystagmus, ataxia, fatigue, drowsiness and cognitive impairment.
   - Gastrointestinal systems (nausea, anorexia, vomiting) are common. Drug may be given with meal.
   - Gingival hyperplasia is common side effect. Patients are taught the importance of scrupulous oral hygiene.
   - Regular follow-up for monitoring is encouraged.
2. *Barbiturates* (phenobarbitol- Luminal). It Depresses post-synaptic excitatory discharge. Used to manage tonic-clonic, simple partial and complex partial seizures and status epilepticus. During these stages, the nurse has to monitor side effects which include sedation, drowsiness and depression.
3. *Succinimides* (Ethosuximide) It depresses motor cortex and raises threshold to stimuli used to manage absence seizures. In this, nurse has to monitor side effects (e.g. Anorexia, nausia, vomiting and drowsiness) and caution the patient to never abruptly discontinue the drug. as this can precipitate status epilepticus.
4. *Others*
   - *Carbamazepine* (Tegretol) Is believed to reduce polysynaptic responses and blocks synaptic potentiation. This is used to manage tonic clonic, simple partial and complex partial seizures. In this the nurse has to monitor side effects i.e., drowsiness, dizziness, headache, nausea, anorexia, vomiting. Side effects tend to decrease in severity over time. Regular follow-up encouraged because drug can cause rare but severe bone marrow toxicities.

     Valpord acid (Depakene) Increases levels of gamma-amino-butyric acid for membrane stabilization. This is used to manage absence seizures or in combination with other drugs. For tonic-clonic and complex partial seizures. The nursing interventions include—monitor side effects (anorexia, nausea and vomiting). Teach patient to take drug with meal and watch for CNS side effects such as drowsiness, tremor and ataxia. Regular follow-up is encouraged because drug may cause liver dysfunction and blood dyscrasias.

Emergency Management of Tonic-Clonic Seizures

Tonic-clonic seizures may be caused by the following needs emergency management.

- Head Trauma: Haematuria of epidural, subdural, intracranial, cerebral contusion and traumatic birth injury.
- Drug-related process: Overdose, withdrawal of alcohol, opiods antiseizure drugs, ingestion and inhalation.
- Infectious process: Meningitis, septicimia.
- Intercranial event: Brain tumour, subarachnoid haemorrage and stroke, hypertensive crisis and increased ICP secondary to clogged shunt.
- Metabolic imbalance: Fluid and electrolyte imbalance and hypoglycaemia.
- Medical disorders: Heart, liver or kidney disease- systematic diseases.
- Others: Cardiac arrest, ideopathic, psychiatric disorder and high fever.

Assessment finding will reveal the:

- Aura- Peculiar sensation that preceds seizures.
- Loss of consciousness.
- Bowel and bladder incontinence.
- Tachycardia.
- Diaphoresis.
- Warm skin.
- Pallor, flushing or cyanosis.
- Tonic phase-continuous muscle contractions.
- Hypertonic phase-extreme muscular rigidity lasting 5 to 15 seconds.
- Clonic phase—rigidity and relaxation alternate in rapid succession.
- Postictal phase—lethargy, altered level of consciousness.
- Confusion and headache.
- Repeated tonic clonic seizures for several minutes.

Initial nursing interventions will include:

- Ensure patient airway.
- Assist ventilation if patient does not breath spontaneously after seizures. Anticipate need for intubation if gag reflex is present.
- Suction as needed.
- Stay with patient until seizures have passed.
- Protect patient from injury during seizures. Do not restrain. Pad side rails.
- Anticipate administration of phenobarbitol, phenytoin or benzodiazephine to control seizures.

- Remove or loosen tight clothing.

And ongoing monitoring instituted as follows.

- Monitor vital signs, LOC, O_2 saturation, GCS, pupil size and reactivity.
- Reassure and orient the patient after seizures.
- Never force an airway between a patient's clenched teeth.
- Give dextrose for hypoglycemia.

The following guidelines will help the nurse while taking care of patient in status epilepticus.

1. Protect airway and provide oxygen. Position the patient on side to prevent aspiration. Place on oral airway if the teeth are not clenched. Administer oxygen by mask of respiratory depression occurs from seizures or medication used to control seizures, intubation may be necessary.
2. Establish IV access for medication delivery and fluids.
3. Draw blood for electrolytes, arterial blood gases and toxicology to rule out metabolic causes for seizures.
4. Administer benzoidiazepines usually lorazepam (Ativan) 4 to 8 mg over 2 to 4 minutes or diazepam (valium) 5 to 20 mg over 5 to 10 minutes to stop seizures. These drugs are fast acting and will control seizures until anticonvulsant drugs reach therapeutic levels.
5. Administer anticonvulsants usually phenytoin 15 to 20 mg/kg in normal saline at 50 mg/min. maximum rate at the same time as the benzoidiazepines to begin establishing therapeutic levels. Phenytoin can cause significant hypotension and cardiac dysfunction. Place the patient on a monitor during loading doses.
6. Continue the search for an underlying cause of seizures.

Patient and Family Education

The patient with seizures disorders should be taught the following:

1. Medications must be taken as prescribed. Any and all side effects of medications should be reported to the health care provider. When necessary, blood drawings are done to ensure that therapeutic levels are maintained.
2. Use of nondrug technique, such as relaxation therapy and biofeedback training to potentially reduce the number of seizures.
3. Availability of resources and the community.
4. Need to wear a medic-alert bracelet, necklace and identification card.
5. Avoidance of excessive alcohol intake, fatigue and loss of sleep.
6. Regular meals and snack in between if feeling is shaky, faint or hungry.

Family members should be taught the following:

1. First aid treatment of tonic-clonic seizures. It is not necessary to call ambulance or send the patient to the hospital after a single seizure unless the seizure is prolonged, another seizure immediately follows or extensive injury has occurred.
2. During an acute seizure, it is important to protect the patient from injury. This may involve supporting and protecting the head, turning the patient to the side, loosening constricting clothing, and easing the patient to the floor if seated.

HEADACHE

Headache is probably the most common type of pain experienced by humans. Headache is a common symptom of many neurologic conditions and is also a separate disease process.

Aetiology

Headaches are classified by the international society on primary and secondary. Primary headaches are not associated with any other known pathological cause. Examples are *migraine, tension,* and *cluster* headaches. Secondary headaches are caused by known pathology such as meningitis, tumours or subarachnoid haemorrhage.

1. *Tension-type headache*. Occurs at any age and is associated with stress. Onset often in adolescence, related to tension or anxiety. There will be no family history. It is episodic, vary with stress; duration is variable. There is no prodrome (early manifestation) of impending disease. The pain is usually bilateral, occurring most often in the back of the neck. It is usually bilateral, occurring most often in the back of the neck. It usually does not interfere with sleep. The pain is often described as a tight, squeezing, bandline pressure. It is sustained, chronic, dull and persistent. The headache occurs intermittently for weeks, months or even years. Many patients have a combination of migraine and tension-type headache with features of both occurring simultaneously.
2. *Migraine-headache*. Migraine occurs more often in women than men and most commonly begins between adolescence and at the 40 years. They demonistrate a strong hereditary pattern, but no specific genetic link has been identified. It is episodic, tends to occur with stress or life crisis it lasts. Lasts hours to days. It occurs slowly. Pain becomes severe with one side of head affected more than other. There is prodromal i.e., vision field defects, confusion, paresthesia, and associated symptoms like nausea, vomiting, chills, fatigue, irritability, sweating and oedema. There are two types of migraine headache: migraine without aura (formerly called common migraine) and migraining with aura (formerly called classic migraine, i.e. with prodrome).

Migraine headaches in many cases have no precipitatory events. However, for other patients, the headache may be precipitated or triggered by stress, excitement, bright light, menstruation, alcohol or certain foods such as chocolate or cheese.

3. *Cluster Headache* is one of the most severe forms of head pain. No epidemiological pattern has been identified occurs in early adulthood, precipitated by alcohol or nitrate use, more common in older men. Episodes clustered together in quick succession for few days or weaks with remissions that lasts for months. It lasts a minute to a few hours. Pattern of pain is intense, throbbing, often unilateral pain begins in intraorbital region and spread to head and neck. There is no prodrome but associated with flushing, tearing of eyes, nasal stuffiness, sweating, swelling of temporal vessels.

Pathophysiology

The pathophysiology of headache is not full understood. Some structures of the head are incapable of sensing pain. The structures that are capable of feeling pain are, skin, muscles, periosteum of the skull, eyes, ears, nasal cavities and sinuses, meninges, cerebral blood vessels, and cranial nerves with sensory function. Pain is caused by traction, stretching of movement of structures or by vasodilation of blood vessels. Serotonin is the primary neurotransmitter found in the pathways involved in headache, but its role is not fully understood.

Migraine is believed to be caused when cerebral blood vessels narrow and blood flow is reduced to some areas of the brain. The initial vasoconstriction is followed by significant vasodilation and inflammation of the blood vessels which triggers a release of serotinin and causes headache. Migraine vary in duration, frequency and intensity from patient to patient and from episode to episode in the same patients.

Cluster headaches are thought to be similar to migrains but episodes are brief, usually lasting 45 minutes or less. They occur in 'Cluster' periods of weeks or months. Tension headaches are the results of the stress-induced muscle tension over the neck, scalp and face of the patient. These headaches are associated with the stresses of daily life. Some headaches are preceded by prodromal signs and symptoms called 'aurae'- The aura occurs before the acute attack and may include visual field defects such as "flashing lights" Photophobia, confusion or paresthsis. Aurae typically last for an hour or more. Their symptoms are associated with the reduction and cerebral blast flow that precedes the vasodilation of the migraine.

Clinical manifestations are discussed in types (see aetiology) and secondary headache, manifests associate an underlying disease.

Management

The diagnosis of headache is made from the patient's history, complete history, clinical examination (often negative). Inspect for local infections, palpation of tenderness, hardened arteries and bony swellings. Auscultation for bruits over major arteries. Assessment parameters for headache are development by the International Headache Society are as follows:

- *Headache characteristics*: Time of onset, location, frequency, severity, duration, quality (deep, superficial, steady, throbbing, stabbing, burning), situations or activities that make the headache better or worse.
- *Presence of an aura*. Duration, relation to onset of pain.
- *Associated symptoms* occuring before, during or after a headache: Nausea, vomiting, photophobia, visual disturbance, dizziness, incoordination, redness of the eye, facial symptoms (sweating, paleness, flushing), fatigue, or sleepiness, moodswings, weakness and paresthesia.
- Potential precipitating factors: Change in eating pattern, dietary substances (e.g. tyramines, nitrates), relationship to menstrual cycle, sexual intercourse, pregnancy, menopause, phychosocial stressors, change in sleep pattern, weather changes, hot or cold wind, attitude, lights and smog.
- *Activities of daily living patterns*: Eating, sleeping, exercise and relaxation.
- *Drug history*: Over-the-counter and prescribed headache medication, other medications (nitroglycerine, hormone replacement) alcohol and drug use and smoking history.
- *Medical history*: Asthma, peptic ulcer, motion sickness, head injury, seizure disorder, sleep walking. Raynaud's disease, irritable bowel syndrome, infertility, skin problems. Pain in neck, head or throat, abdominal distress: anxiety, depressions and insomnia.
- *Family history*: Hsitory of headache and other medical problems.

While nursing assessment, nurse should keep in mind the above stated parameters and she/he can suggest the patient keep a diary of headache episodes with specific details including complete description of each headache, precipitating events, associated symptoms, and in women, the relationship with menstrual cycles. This type of record can be of great help in determining the type of headache.

Nursing diagnosis for the patient with headache may include.

- Pain related to headache as manifested by complaint of steady throbbing or severe crushing pain.
- Anxiety related to lack of knowledge about headache details.
- Hopelessness related to chronic pain, alteration of lifestyles and ineffective treatment.
- Sleep pattern disturbance related to pain.

Planning. The overall goals are that the patient with headache will:

- Have reduced or no pain.
- Experience increased comfort and decreased anxiety.

- Demonstarte understanding of triggering events and treatment strategies.
- Use positive coping strategies to deal with chronic pain.

Nursing Intervention

Headaches may result from an inability to cope with daily stresses. The most effective therapy may be to help patients examine their lifestyle, recognize stressful situations and learn to cope with them appropriately. Precipitating factors can be identified and ways of avoiding them can be developed. Daily exercise, relaxation periods, and socializing can be encouraged, since each can help decreased the recurrene of headache. The nurse can surggest alternative ways of handling the pain of headache through technique such as relaxation, meditation, yoga, and self-hypnosis.

Medications for the treatment of headache fall into two broad categories: symptom relife and prevention.

i. *Symptomatic treatment.* Following drugs are used.
   a. Non-narcotic analgesics (aspirin, acetaminophen, and ibuprofen).
   b. Analgesic combinations (butalbital).
   c. Muscle relaxants.
   d. Serotonin receptor agonists (Sumatriptan, naratriptan, rizatriptan).
   e. Alpha-adrenergic blockers (ergatramine tartrate i.e., (afergot).
   f. Vasoconstrictors (isometheptone•-i.e. midrin).
   g. Corticosteroids (dexamethosone).
   (Note:- a, e, f, g are used in migraine and e.f. and oxygen used in cluster headache).
   h. Metodopramide (Reglan).
ii. *Prophylactic* treatment incldues the following:
   a. Tricyclic antidepressants (dexepin, amitriptyline).
   b. Beta-adrenergic blockers (Propranol-Inderal).
   c. Biofeedback.
   d. Muscle relaxation training.
   e. Psychotherapy (e.d.e. are not drugs).
   f. Calcium channel blockers (isoptin).
   g. Divalp..... (b, c, d, e, f, g, h are used in migraine).
   h. Yoga, meditation, electric counter stimulation).
   i. Corticosterroids (Prednosone).
   j. Lithium.
   k. Alpha-adrenaline blockers) (i,j,k,l are used in cluster headache).
   l. Serotinin antogonists.

Nursing intervention during medication are: advise the patients to take prescribed dose and the nurse has to observe the side effects as follows:

- *Ergot* alkoloids may be taken as soon as migraine symptoms begin. In this, nausea is common side effect. Patient may also need to use antiemetics. Ergot has a cumulative effect. Use sparingly and monitor for signs and symptoms of ergotism-numbness, and tingling, weakness, and muscle pain.
- *Metaclopnamide* increases gastrointestinal mobility to decrease the evidence of nausea and vomiting. During this medication, patients should avoid driving or other hazardous activity after taking drug.
- *Serotinin* receptor agonist, causes vasoconstriction. This drug contraindicates in pregnancy and coronary artery disease. Teach the patient to take drug at first sign of a headache.
- *Beta blockers* inhibit vasodilation and serotinin uptake. Prepranol is the first drug of choice for prophylaxis of migraine. This may cause cardiac dysfunction; monitor for bracycardia, orthostatic hypertension lethargy and depression.
- *Tricyclic antidepressants.* Block uptake of serotinin and catecholamies. They are most effective for migraine associated in tension headach. It is alternative if betablockers are not tolerated. These may cause dry mouth, drowsiness and urinary retention.

For the patient whose headaches are triggered by food, dietary counseling may be provided. The patient is encouraged to avoid foods that provoke headaches such as vinegar, chocolate, onions, alcohol (red wine) excessive cafeine, cheese, fermented or marinated food, monosodium glucamate and aspartane. Patients should avoid smoking and exposure to triggers such as strong perfumes, volatile solvents, and gasolene fumes. Cluster headaches' attacks may occur at high altitudes with low oxygen levels during air travel. Ergotamine, before the plane takes off, these may be decreased likelihood of these attacks. The following is the teaching guide for the patient with headache, used by the nurse while giving the patient and family education.

1. Avoid factors that can trigger a headache.
   - Food containing amines (cheese, chocolate), nitrates (meat), vinegar, onion, fermented or marionated food.
   - Monosodium glutamate.
   - Caffeine.
   - Nicotine.
   - Ice cream.
   - Alcohol (particularly red wine).
   - Emotional stress.
   - Fatigue.
   - Medications such as ergot-containing and monoamineoxidase inhibitors.
2. Able to describe the purpose, action, dosage and side effects of medication taken.
3. Able to self-administer sumatriptan subcutaneously if prescribed.
4. Use stress-reduction technique such as relaxation.
5. Participate in regular exercise.

6. Keep diary or calender of headaches and possible precipitatory event.
7. Contact health care provider if the following occur.
   - Symptoms become more severe, last longer than usual or are resistant to medication.
   - Nausea, vomiting, change in vision or fever occur with head ache.
   - Problem with medication.

MULTIPLE SCLEROSIS

Multiple sclerosis (MS) is a chronic, progressive, degenerative disorder of the central nervous system (CNS) characterized by inflammation of the white matter of the CNS.

Aetiology

The cause of MS is unknown, although an underlying viral infection has been suggested as a cause. It is also related to immunologic and genetic factors and is perpetuated as a result of intrinsic factors (e.g. faulty immunoregulation). The susceptibility to MS appear to be inherited, multiple unlinked genes confer susceptibility to MS.

The role of precipitating factors such as exposure to pathogenic agents in the aetiology of MS is controversial. The possible precipitating factors include infections, physical injury, emotional distress, excessive fatigue, pregnancy and a poorer state of health.

Pathophysiology

Multiple sclerosis causes scattered demyelination of the white matter of the CNS. It is characterized by chronic inflammation, demyelination and ghiosis (scarring) in the CNS. The primary neurophthologic condition is an immune-mediated inflammatory demyelinating process that some believe, may be triggered by a virus in genetically-susceptible individuals. The acute inflammation reduces the thickness of the myelin sheath that surround the axons and nerve fibers and impulse conduction is slowed and/or blocked. Astrocytes or scavenger cells that remove the damaged myelin and scar tissues form over the damaged areas. Natural healing may restore some of the functions of the myelin or the lesions may continue to interfere with nerve conduction. This partial healing accounts for the transitory nature of early disease symptoms. Eventually nerve fibers may generate so that permanent damage occurs and overt disabilities increase. The blood-brain barrier usually protects the brain from immune cell activity. In MS, however, the barrier is breached and activated T-Cells, antibodies and macrophages attack the fatty myelin sheath and the oligodendrocytes that produce it. The CNS damage is thought to be caused by a delayed type of hypersensitivity response, a cell-mediated immune response. The course of MS is highly variable and unpredictable. Site of inflammatory demyelination can occur usually anywhere in the brain and spinal cord and MS produces a greater range of signs and symptoms that any other neurological diseases.

Clinical Manifestation

The onset of MS is often insidious and gradual, with vague symptoms that occur intermittently over months or years. The clinical manifestations vary according to the areas of the CNS invoked. Some patients have severe long-lasting symptoms easily in the course of the disease. Other may experience only occasional and mild symptoms for several years after onset. A classification scheme that identifies the variety causing MS has been developed.

- *Relapsing/remitting* MS Disease: exacerbations occur over 1 to 2 weeks and then gradually resolve over 4 to 8 weeks, usually returning the patient to baseline or near-baseline functioning. It is characterized by clearly defined relapses with full recovery or with sequelae and residual deficit on recovery.
- *Relapsing/Progress* MS disease exacerbations occur, but the patient does not return to baseline and is left with increasing amounts of residual disability. It is characterized by the disease progression from onsets with occasional plateous and temporary minor improvement.
- *Secondary/chronic progressive MS* disease is characterized primarily by spinal cord and cerebellar symptoms which are progresive and rarely remit. It is characterized by replapsing-remittant followed by progression with or without occasional relapses, minor remissions and plateus.
- *Progressive relapsing/stable MS* is characterized by progressive disease from onset, with clear acute relapses, with or without full recovery; Periods between relapses are characterized by continuing progressing.

The following are the symptoms of multiple sclerosis.

1. *Sensory Symptoms*
   - Numbness and tingling on the face or extremities.
   - Decreased proprioception.
   - Paresthesis (burning, prickling).
   - Decreased sense of temperature, vibration and depth.
2. *Motor Symptoms*
   - Weakness or a feeling of heaviness in the lower extremities.
   - Paralysis.
   - Spasticity and hyper reflexes.
   - Diplopia.
   - Bowel and bladder dysfunction (retention, or urge, incontinence).
3. *Cerebellar Symptoms*
   - Spasticity and hyper reflexes.
   - Incoordination, ataxia, in lower extremities.
   - Slurred speech dysarthria.
   - Scanning speech (slow with pauses between syllables).

- Nystagmus.
- Dysphagia.

4. *Neurobehavioral symptoms*
   - Emotional liability, euphoria, depression.
   - Irritability.
   - Apathy.
   - Poor judgement, inability to solve problems effectively.
   - Loss of short-term memory.
5. *Others*
   - Opticneuritis (visual clouding and visual field deficits).
   - Impotence, sexual dysfunction.
   - Fatigue (extremely common, ranges from mild to disabling).

Management

Diagnosis is based primarily on history and clinical manifestation. Certain tests currently used are:

CSF analysis, evoked response test (AEP- auditory evoked potential VEP-visual evoked potential, SSEP- Somato-sensory evoked potential), CT scan and MRI (ask to see the sclerotic plaques).

Nursing assessment may be made by collecting subjective and objective data based on clinical manifestation. The possible nursing diagnosis will be:

- Impaired physical mobility: R/T muscle weakness.
- Self-care deficits R/T muscle spasticity and neuromuscular deficit.
- Risk of impaired skin integrity R/T immobility.
- Sensory-perceptual alteration R/T visual disturbance.
- Altered urinary eliminate (Retention or incontinence).
- Constipation R/T immobility.
- Sexual dysfunction R/T neuromuscular deficit.
- Self-esteem disturbance R/T prolonged debilitating conditions.
- Altered family processes R/T changing family roles, etc.

Drugs used for managing symptoms of MS are as follows:

1. *Spasticity*:
   - Baclofen (Licresal)
   - Dantrolene (Dantrium)
   - Diazepam (Valium).
2. *Tremors*
   - Hydraxyzine (Vistaril)
   - Isonaizid (INH)
   - Trihexyphenidyl (Artane)
   - Primidone (Mysoline).
3. *Spastic pladder and urge, incontinence:*
   - Oxybutynin
   - Imipramine (Tofranil)
   - Pro-pantheline (Probanthine)
4. *Urinary Retention*: Bethenicoal chloride (urecholine).
5. Antidepressants:
   - Amitriptyline (Elavil)
   - Imipramin (Tofranal)
   - Trazodone (Desuyrel)
   - Fluoxetin (Proleu)
   - Paroxetetin (Paxil)
   - Sertraline (Zoloft).
6. Fatigue:
   - Amantidine hydrochloride (Symmetrel)
   - Pemoline (Cylert).
7. Other
   - Stool softner
   - Laxatives.

The drugs used for reducing the frequency of severity of relapses of multiple sclerosis are as follows:

1. *Acute exacerbations*. Short course of high-dose corticosteroids are used, which include:
   - Methy, predoisoline (Medrol) IV daily for 3 to 7 days with or without the following taper of oral prednisoline.
   - Oral prednisoline tapered over 2 to 4 weeks.
   - Carticotrophine (ACTH) by IV infusion or IM gradually tapered over 2 to 4 weeks.
2. For decreasing relapses: usually used are:
   - Interferon beta-16 (Betaseron) SC.
   - Interferon beta-1a (Vvinex) 1g SC.
   - Copolymer 1 and injectable polyner (effecting if started early).
   - Azathioprene (Imuron)-an inti-inflamatory and immunosuppressive.
3. *For halting disease progression* drug used are:
   - Cyclophosphamide (Cytoxan)
   - Cyclosporine (Sandimmune)
   - Clad sporine (Leustatin), etc.

In addition, various nutritional measures that have been advocated in the management of MS include vitamin B_{12}, vitamin C and diet consisting of low-fat and gluten-free food and raw vegetables. A nutritious well-balanced diet is essential. Surgical measures are followed nursing management of neurosurgical nursing is carried out.

Patient education should be focussed on building general resistance to illness including, avoid fatigue, extremes of heat or cold, and expose to infection. The last measures involve avoiding exposure to cold climate and to people who are sick, as well as vigorous and early treatment of infection when it does occur. It is important to teach the patient to:

1. Achieve a good balance of exercise and rest,
2. Eat nutritious and well-balanced meals and,
3. Avoid the hazards of immobility (contractures and pressure ulcers).

Patient should know that treatment regimens, the side effects of medication and how to watch them, and drug interactions and new over the counter medications. The patient should consult a health care provider before taking any non-prescriptive drugs.

PARKINSON'S DISEASE

Parkinson's disease, a form of Parkinsonism is named after James Parkinson who in 1817 wrote a classic "shaking palsy" a disease for which the reason is still unknown. It is a chronic degenerative disorder that primarily affects the neurons of the basal ganglia. It is a syndrome that consists of slowing down in the initiation and execution of movement (Brady Kinesia), increased muscle tone (rigidity), tremor and impaired postural reflexes. The famous internationally known boxer Mr. Mohmed Ali suffered from this disease.

Aetiology

Parkinson's disease affects men and women about equally and usually occurs after the age of 50 with a median age of onset of about years. Actual aetiology of the disease remains unknown. The possible causes of Parkinson's disease may be:

- A genetic component has recently been proposed. (Heredity). The disease usually begins insidiously and then progresses.
- Primary Parkinson's disease is idiopathic, but variety of other categories exist.
- Symptoms of Parkinson's may develop in response to the use of antipsychotic drugs (or neuroleptic agents); following an encephalitis infection in response to brain trauma, tumours, hydrocephalis or ischaemia; in association with rare metabolic disorders; and in response to arteriosclerosis.
- Neurotoxin such as cyanide, manganese and carbon monoxide have also been proposed as possible causes of disease.

Drug-induced Parkinson's can follow reserpine (Hydropres)-methyldopa (Aldomet), haloperidol (Haldol) and phenothiazine (Thorazine) therapy.

Pathophysiology

The Pathology of Parkinson's disease is associated with the degeneration of the dopamine-producing neurons in the substantial nigra of neurun an area within the basal ganglia. Destructions of dopaminergic neurons in the substantia nigra significantly reduces the amount of available straital dopamine. Dopamine (DA) and acetylcholine (ACh) are primarily neurotransmitters that are responsible for controlling and refining motor movements and have opposing effects. Dopamine has inhibitory effect and acetylcholine has excitatory effects. When the excitatory activity of ACh is inadequately balanced by DA, and individual has difficulty in controlling and initiating voluntary movements. Cellular degeneration in Parkinson's disease also leads to impairment of the extrapyramidal tracts that control semiautomatic and coordinated movements.

Clinical Manifestations

The onset of Parkinson's disease is gradual and insidious, with a gradual progression and prolonged course. In the beginning stages, a mild tremor, a slight limp or a decreased arm swing may be evident. Later on the disease, the patient may have shuffling, propulsive gait with arms flexed and loss of postural reflexes. In some patients, there may be a slight change in speech pattern. The following are the 'classic' clinical manifestations of Parkinson's disease.

1. *Tremor*: (often the first-sign affects handwriting).
   - Non-intentional, present at rest but usually not during sleep.
   - Characterized by rhythmic movements of 4 to 5 cycles per second.
     - Movement of the thumb across the palm gives a "Pill rolling" character.
     - Tremor also seen in limbs, jaw, lips, lower facial muscles and head.
2. *Rigidity* (often the second sign)
   - Increased resistance to passive motion when the limbs are moved through their range of motion.
   - Muscles feel stiff and required increased effort to move.
   - Discomfort or pain may be perceived in muscle when rigidity is severe.
   - "Cogwheel" rigidity refer to ratchet-like rhythmic contractions of the muscle that occur when the limbs are passively stretched.
3. *Bradykinesia (Akinesia)*
   - Slowness of active movement.
   - Difficulty in initiating movement.
   - Often the most disabling symptom: interferes with ADK and predisposes patient to complication related to constipation, circulatory stasis, skin breakdown and other related complications of immobility.
4. *Postural instability*
   1. Changes in gait
      - Tendency to walk forward on the toes with small shuffling steps.
      - Once initiated, movement may accelerate almost to a trot.
      - Festination may occur, which propels the patient either forward or backward propulsively until falling is almost inevitable.
   2. Changes in balance:
      - Stooped-over posture when erect.
      - Arms are semiflexed and do not swing with walking.
      - Difficulty in maintaining balance and sitting erect.
      - Cannot 'right' or brace self to prevent falling, when balance is lost.

Complications

Many complications of Parkinson's disease are caused by the deterioration and loss of spontaneity of movements.

- Dysphagia leading to malnutrition or aspiration.
- Venereal debilitation leads to pneumonia, urinary track infection and skin breakdown.
- Decreased mobility affects gait.
- Lack of mobility leads to constipation, ankle oedema, and contractures.
- Orthostatic hypotension with loss of postural reflexes lead to fall on injury.
- Bothersome complications include seborrhoea, dandruff, excessive sweating, conjunctivitis, difficulty in reading, insomnia, incontinence and depressions.
- Side effects of drugs—dyskinacsia, weakness and akincsia.

The complication may be secondary manifestations of Parkinson's disease are as follows:

i. Facial appearance.
   - Expressionless.
   - Eyes store straight ahead.
   - Blinking is much less frequent than normal.
ii. Speech problems.
   - Low volume.
   - Slurred, muffled.
   - Monotone.
   - Difficulty with starting speech and word finding.
iii. Visual problems
   - Blurred vision.
   - Impaired upward gaze.
   - Blepharospasm - involuntary prolonged closing of the eyelids.
iv. Fine motor function
   - Microphagia-handwriting progressively decreases in size.
   - Decreased manual dexterity.
   - Clumsiness and decreased coordination.
   - Decreased capacity to complete ADL.
   - Freezing—sudden involuntary inability to initiate movement can occur during movement or inactivity.
v. Autonomic disturbance.
   - Constipation—hypomotility and prolonged gastric emptying.
   - Urinary frequency or hesitancy.
   - Orthostatic hypertention (dizziness, fainting and syncope).
   - Dysphagia (neuromuscular incoordination).
   - Drooling (results from decreased swallowing).
   - Oily skin.
   - Excessive perspiration.
vi. Cognitive/behavioural.
   - Depression.
   - Slowed responsiveness.
   - Memory deficits.
   - Visual-spacial deficits.
   - Dementia.

Management

The diagnosis of Parkinson's disease is made directly from the patient's history and symptoms. No definite diagnostic test exists, and the diagnosis may be confirmed primarily from the patient response to medication.

The common medications used for Parkinson's disease and their action and nursing intervention are as follows:

1. *Anticholinergics* are used to relieve tremors. They antagonize the transmission of acetylcholine in the CNS; most effective in decreasing rigidity, selective action but still have systematic anticholinergic effects. Example: Trihexyphenidyl, cycrimine, procyclidine, benztropine, biperiden. The side effects of these drugs, usually dry mouth, blurred vision, constipation, delirium, changes in memory, confusion, anxiety, agitation, hallucination. During this treatment, nurse has to monitor the incidence and severity of the side effects; avoidance of drugs with similar actions, (ex. antihistamine e.g. Sominex, antispasmodics like donnadral, bellergal, tricyclic antidepressants like tofoamil, elavil, etc.
2. *Antiviral* amantadine (Symmetril)-block the uptake and storage of catecholamines, allowing for the accumulation of dopamine. Positive effects may not be least beyond 3 months. Here, the nurses have to monitor for effectiveness and severity of side effects E.g. Mental confusion, visual disturbances, nervousness, insomnia, dry mouth, nausea, oedema orthostatic hypotension.
3. *Antihistamine* reduces the tremor and rigidity. The drugs used are: Diphenhydramine (Benedryl), orphenadrine, chlorphenaxamine, Phenindamine. Sedation is the side effect and the nurse has to take same precautions as for anticholenergic drugs.
4. *Dopamine agonists* include drugs such as bromocriptine merylate, pergolide (Permax), pramipexole (Mirapex), used to reduce bradykinaesia, and tremor and rigidity. They directly stimulate dopamine receptors and increase the effect of levadopa, minimize the fluctuations in drug responses. Possible side effects are: orthostatic hypotension, nausea, vomiting, toxic psychosis, limb oedema, phlebitis, dizziness, headache, insomnia. The nurse has to monitor the side effects and take precautions accordingly.
5. Dopaminergic (Ex. Levadopa, Carbidopa-Levadopa) used to relieve bradykinaesia, tremor and rigidity. They resotore deficient dopamine to the brain. Carbidopa blocks peripheral conversion of levadopa. Possible side effects are: Nausea, dyskinesia, hypotension. Palpitation, arrythmias, agitation, hallucination, confusion (older patient), drymouth, sleep disturbances. The nurse has to monitor side effects, take measures accordingly by using guidelines for safe use of levellopa-listed as given below (after MAO).
6. *Monoamine Oxidase inhibitors (MAO)* (E.g. Selegiline-(eldepryl)-MAO-blocks the metabolism of dopamine, may

slow the underlying disease process. This is also used for relieving symptoms like bradykinesia; rigidity, tremors. Side effects and precautions are taken similar todopaminergic drugs. Particularly, monitor for incidence of orthostatic hypotension. Do not exceed prescribed dose. The some may be given in combination with levadopa as the disease progresses.

The below given guidelines should be followed for the safe use of levodopa.

1. Levodopa is best absorbed in an empty stomach. If nausea occurs, it can be taken with food.
2. Dry mouth is common side effect. Chewing gum and hard candy can counter this effect.
3. Depression and moodswings may occur. Report the incidence of these or other cognitive-behavioural changes such as insomnia, agitation or confusion to health care provider.
4. Avoid the use of alcohol or minimize alcohol intake. It is believed to antagonize the effects of levodopa.
5. Avoid protein ingestion near the time for medication administration. Some protein aminoacids are believed to inhibit the absorption of levodopa. A pattern of low-protein breakfast and lunch with a high-protein dinner has improved symptoms in selected patients.
6. Be alert to the possibility of orthostatic hypotension. Change positions slowly. Avoid steam baths sauna, and hot tubs. Experiment with the use of support stockings to support venus return.
7. Avoid vitamin supplementation with products that contain Vitamin B6 (Pyridoxine). Pyridoxine increases the conversion of levodopa in the liver, which decreases the amount of available for conversion to dopamine in the brain.
8. Consult the primary care provider and pharmacists about the use of all other drugs. Levodopa has multiple adverse drug interactions.

The possible nursing diagnosis are as follow and perform nursing intervention and evaluation accordingly.

- Impaired physical mobility (R/T) rigidity, bradykinesia and akinesia.
- Self-care deficits R/T Parkinson symptoms.
- Impaired verbal communication R/T dysarthias and tremor or bradykinesia.
- Constipation R/T weakness of abdominal and perineal muscle, lack of exercise and side effects.
- Altered nutrition and body requirement R/T dysphagias.
- Diversional activity deficit R/T inability to perform usual recreational activity.
- Sleep pattern disturbance. R/T Medication's side effects.

In addition, the following health education is provided to the patient and family member, regarding activity, exercises, safety, nutrition, elimination, etc.

1. *Activity and exercise*

- Perform range of motion exercises to all joints for three times daily.
- Massage and stretch muscles to reduce stiffness.
- Use a broad base of support when ambulating, cautiously and consciously lift and down the feet when ambulating.
- Pay attention to posture. Try walking with the hands clasped behind.
- Explore the use of assistive devices.
- Avoid staying in one position for prolonged time and keep altering position regularly.

2. *Safety*

- Examine the home environment for risk of injury.
- Modify the environment to improve and remove hazards.
- Consider installing devices such as raised toilet seat, and grab bar.
- Change positions slowly if orthostatic hypotension develops.
- Be alert to the side effects of heat, stress and excitement on severity of symptoms.

3. *Nutrition*

- Monitor weight once a week.
- Evaluate dysphagia and modify diet to increase ease of chewing and swallowing if appropriate.
- Practice swallowing and take small bites.
- Provide an unhurried atmosphere and allow additional time for meal.
- Follow a plan of small, frequent meals, if fatigue is a problem during meals.
- Avoid eating high-protein meals at times of medication administration.
- Do not use supplements containing pyridoxine (Vit. B_6).
- Ensure adequate fiber and fluid intake to prevent constipation.
- Manage drooling problems with soft clothes.

4. *Elimination*

- Monitor bowel elimination pattern.
- Use diet, exercises and fluids to ensure regularity if possible.
- Use stool softeners if needed.
- Keep a urinal or commode at the bedside.
- Respond promptly to urge to urinate, and be sure to empty the bladder, at least every 2 to 4 hours. Bradykinesia may result in episodes of incontinence.

5. *Cognitive/behaviours*

- Monitor for depression. Report its presence to health care provides.

- Monitor change in sleep pattern, thought disorders, development of any other manifestations, convusion, hallucination—Report to health care provider.

6. *Communication*
- Exercise the voice regularly by singing or reading aloud.
- Attempt to project the voice and alter volume and pitch.
- Consult a speech therapist if vocal problems are severe.

MYASTHENIA GRAVIS

Myasthenia Gravis (MG) is a disease of the neuromuscular function characterized by the fluctuating weakness of certain skeletal muscle groups. It is a rare chronic disease that affects the myoneural junctions. The prevalence is estimated to be from 43 to 84 persons per million. (For example, unfortunately our Mega Star of the Millennium Mr. Amitab Bachchan is one among those who suffered from MG during 1980s).

Aetiology

Myasthenia Gravis is caused by an autoimmune process that results in production of antibodies directed against the Acetylecholone (ACh). Receptors and a reduction in the number of Ach receptor (AChR) sites at the neuromuscular junctions i.e., myoneural junctions. This results in the classic disease features of weakness and fatigue of selected voluntary muscles. The exact cause is not known but thymus tumour and viral infection are suspected as precipitating an attack.

Pathophysiology

Effective muscle contraction is contingent on adequate amounts of acetylecholin (ACh), a neuromuscular transmitter, being available at the postsynaptic membrane to generate an action potential that can spread along the length of the muscle and culminate in muscle contraction. Mitochondria in the motor nerve axons synthesize ACh, which is released when the nerve is stimulated. The ACh crosses the myoneural junction and binds with an ACh receptor (AChR) on the postsynaptic membrane to initiate the action potential. Acetylcholinesterase (ACh E) is also released into the synaptic cleft. The AChE breaks down the ACh, which limits the duration of the muscle contraction. The number of AChR sides are significantly reduced in persons with MG as a result of the destructive effects of an antibody mediated autoimmune attack that specifically target the AChR sites. As a result, the stimuli may lack sufficient amplitude to trigger an effective action potential in some muscle fibers. The strength of muscle responses is weakened and with the repeated stimuli to amount of ACh readily decreases resulting in muscle fatigue.

Clinical Manifestation

The classic symptoms of MG are muscle weakness and generalized fatigue. The primary feature of MG is easy fatigability of skeletal muscle during activity. Strength is usually restored after a period of rest. The muscle motor often involved are those used for moving the *eyes and eyelids*, *chewing, swallowing, speaking, and breathing*. Ptosis and diplopia are common early findings and the disease is occasionally limited to the eye muscles. Muscles innervated by the cranial nerves are often affected and it may be impossible for the patient to keep the mouth closed to chew and swallow for prolonged period. The mobility of the facial muscles also is affected and face may take on an *expressionless appearance*. Attempts to smile, may result in the classic myasthenic 'snarl'. The patient's voice is often weak, and as fatigue sets in, it may become difficult for the patient even to swallow saliva effectively. Weakness of the neck tends to cause the head to bend forward.

Weakness of the arm and hand muscles may first become apparent during self-care activities such as shaving or combing the hair. Symptoms develop rapidly but early in the course of the disease, they also are relieved easily with rest. As the disease progresses, fatigue becomes evident with less and less exertion. The muscles of the trunk and lower limbs may also become involved, creating difficulties with walking and even sitting. The distal muscles are rarely affected as severely as proximal muscles.

During a disease, exacerbation of muscle weakness of the intercostal and diaphragm may become so severe that intubation and mechanical ventilation are necessary. Exacerbations of disease can be triggered by upper respiratory infection, emotional stress, secondary illness, trauma, surgery, pregnancy and even menstruation. There is no accompanying sensory loss in the affected area.

The major complication of MG results from weakness in areas that affect swallowing, and breathing. Aspiration, respiratory insufficiency, and respiratory infection are the major complication. An acute exacerbation of this type is termed as "myasthenic crisis".

Management

The simplest diagnostic test for MG is to have the patient to look upward for 2 to 3 minutes. If the problem is MG, there will be an increased drop of the eyelids, so that the person can barely keep the eye open. After a brief rest, the eyes can open again. Complete history and physical examination (following fatigability and weakness). In addition, electromyogram (EMG) Tensilon test (reveals improved muscle contractability after giving AhE intravenously) are used to dignose MG.

Drugs used in MG are usually anticholenergic agents, corticosteroids and immunosuppressive agents. Surgical measure used in MG is thymectomy. Plasma pheresis is also used in the treatment of MG. The common drug used for MG is pyridostigmine (Mestinon).

The nurse can assess the severity of MG by asking the patient about fatigability, which body parts are affected, and how severely they are affected. The patient's coping abilities and understanding of the disorder should also be assessed. The objective rate should include respiratory rate and depth and oxygen saturation. ABG analysis, PFT and evidence of respiratory distress in patient with acute myasthenia crisis. Muscle strength of all face and limb muscles should be assessed on the basis of swallowing, speech (volume and clarity) and cough and gag reflexes.

The possible nursing diagnosis will be as follows:-

- Ineffective breathing pattern R/T intercostal muscle weakness (IMW).
- Ineffective airway clearance R/T intercostal muscle weakness and impaired cough and gag reflex.
- Impaired verbal communication R/T weakness of larynx, lips, mouth pharynx-jaw.
- Altered nutrition of body requirement R/T impaired swallowing and weakness.
- Sensory perceptional alteration R/T ptosis and gaze.
- Activity intolerance R/T muscle weakness and fatiguability.
- Body image disturbance R/T inability to maintain usual life style and role responsibility.
- The possible goals of nursing care will be to have return of normal muscle endurance.
- Avoid complication and
- Maintain quality of life appropriate to disease cause.

Nursing Intervention

The patients with MG who is admitted to the hospital usually has a respiratory tract infection or in an acute myasthenic crisis. Nursing care is aimed at maintaining adequate ventilation, continuing drug therapy and watching side effects of therapy.

As with chronic illnesses, care focuses on the neurologic deficits and their impact on daily-living. A balanced diet with food that can be chewed and swallowed easily should be prescribed. Semi-solid foods may be easier to eat than solid or liquid foods. Scheduling doses of medication, so that peak action is reached at meal time may make eating less difficult. Diversional activities that require little physical effort and interests of patients should be arranged.

Education should focus on the importance of following: medical regimen, potential adverse reactions to specific drugs. Planning activities of daily living to avoid fatigue, the availability of community resources and complication of disease and therapy and what to do about them. Following guidelines may be helpful in taking care of the patient with myasthenia Gravis.

1. Use of Mestinon (choice of dugs) safely and appropriately.
   - Take the drug with food or fluid.
   - Take the drug before meals to permit maximum effect for chewing and swallowing.
   - Adjust drug dosage and time of administration within set parameters in resposne to individual pattern of weakness.
   - Do not take any other medications, including over-the-counter products without proper approval of health care provider. Many drugs can compromise neuromuscular transmission and will worsen MG. (e.g. Local anaesthetics, aminoglucocides, beta blockers, calcium chanel blockers).
2. Modify diet as needed in response to swallowing problems.
   - A soft diet is usually well tolerated.
   - Eat slowly and take small bites.
3. Balance rest and activity throughout the day in response to weakness.
   - Plan for additional rest periods.
   - Seek out energy conservation strategies for routine activities.
4. Keep medical alert identification with you at all times.
5. Know the symptoms of cholenergic and myasthenic crisis and contact physically.
6. Be alert to disease response to periods of stress-infection, temperature extremes, and hormonal swings (e.g. menstruation or pregnancy).

ALZHEIMER'S DISEASE

Alzheimer's disease is a type of dimentia that is characterized by progressive deterioration in memory and other aspects of cognition.

Aetiology

The aetiology of Alzheimer's disease is still unclear. There is possibility of genetic aetiologies. At least four chromosomes (1,14,19,21) are involved in some forms of familial Alzheimer's disease. Inheritance of the apo E4 genotype is a major risk factor for developing this disease. Oestrogen protects against the development of disease and leads to slow progression of disease has been suggested and role of NSAIDs in reducing the risk of this disease. However, long-term NSAID leads to gastrointestinal and kidney problems.

Pathophysiology

Pathologic changes associated with Alzheimer's disease, include neurofibrillary tangles and beta-amyloid plaques in the cerebral cortex and hippocampus. The neuritic plaque is cluster of degenerating axonal and dendritic nerve terminals that contain an abnormal protein. (B-amyloid) Neurofibrillary tangles are seen in the cytoplasm of abnormal neurons. These bundles of protein are in the form of paired helical filaments. There is also excessive loss of cholinergic neurons, particularly in regions essential for memory and cognition.

Clinical Manifestation

An initial sign of Alzheimer's disease is a subtle deterioration in memory. Inevitably this progresses to more profound memory loss that interferes with the patients' ability to function. Recent events and new information cannot be recalled. Some patients develop psychotic symptoms. Personal hygiene deteriorates as does the ability to maintain attention. Later in the disease, long-term memories cannot be recalled, and patient loses the ability to recognize family members. Eventually, ability to communicate and to perform activities of daily living is lost. The progression of the deterioration which eventually leads to death, varies but can last as long as 20 years.

Management

The diagnosis of Alzheimer's disease is a diagnosis exclusive when all other possible conditions that can cause mental impairment have been ruled out and the manifestation of dementia persists the diagnosis of this disease can be made. CT scan and MRI scan may show brain atrophy and enlarged ventricles. Neuropsychologic testing can help document the degree of cognitive dysfunction in early stages.

Nursing assessment will include the following.

- Past health history : Repeated head trauma, exposure to metals (Alluminium Previous CNS infection).
- Medications : Use of any drug to mitigate symptoms, tranquilizers hypnotics, antidepressants and antipsychotics.
- Positive family history and emotional stability.
- Nutritional metabolic- Anorexia, malnutrition and weight loss.
- Elimination- incontinence.
- Activity exercise : Poor personal hygiene, gait instability, weakness, inability to perform ADL.
- Sleep-rest. : Frequent night-time awakening, day-time napping.
- Cognitive-perceptual : Forgetfulness, inability to cope with complex situation, difficulty in problem solving, depression, and suicidal ideation.
- General : Disheveled appearance and agitation.
- Neurologic : Loss of recent memory, disorientation to date and time, flat affect, lack of spontaneity, impaired abstraction, cognition, and memory, loss of remote memory, restlessness and agitation. Inability to recognise family members and friends, nocturnal wanderings, repetitive behaviour, loss of social graces, stubborness, paronea, belligerency, later on- Aphasia, agnosia, alexia, apraxia, seizures, limb rigidity and flexor posturing.

The possible nursing diagnosis are:

- Altered thought processes R/T effects of dementia.
- Self-care deficits R/T memory deficit.
- Sleep pattern disturbance R/T memory deficit.
- Risk for injury R/T impaired judgement—Possible gait instability.
- Rest for violence: Self or other-directed R/T sensory overload, misinterpretation.
- Ineffective individual coping R/T depression.
- Risk for ineffective management of therapeutic management.

AMYOTROPHIC LATERAL SCLEROSIS (ALS)

Amyotrophic Lateral Sclerosis (ALS) is a rare progressive neurologic disorder characterized by loss of motor neurons. It is also referred to as Loubehrig's disease after the, New York Yankee baseball player who died from this disease.

Aetiology

ALS occurs in 2 or 3 persons per 100,000 annually. Men have a higher incidence of ALS than women. The onset is between 40 and 70 years of age. The cause is unknown, but theories of causation includes exposure to heavy metals, vital infections, lympoma, gammopathy and hexosaminidase, and HIV infection.

Pathophysiology

The term amyotrophic refers to the weakness and atrophy that occur from the degeneration of alpha or lower motor neurons. For unknown reasons motor neurons in the brainstem and spinal cord gradually degenerate in ALS. The dead motroneuron cannot produce or transport vital signals to muscle. Consequently, electrical and chemical messages originating in the brain do not reach the muscles to activate them. ALS causes progressive degeneration of both the upper and lower motor neurons from demyelination and scar tissue formation. The disease gradually destroys motor pathways but leaves sensations and mental status intact. Lower mentors usually affect first resulting weakness and atrophy. The muscels of the upper body are affected much earlier than legs.

Clinical Manifestation

The primary symptoms are weakness of the upper extremities, dysarthria, and dysphagia. Muscle wasting and fasciculations result from the denervation of the muscles and lack of stimulation and use. The disease is relentlessly progressive and eventually involves the upper motor neurons, which causes increased weakness and spasticity in affected muscles. Hyperactive reflexes, jaw clonus, tongue fasciculations and a positive Babinski's reflex may be present. As the muscle of the neck, pharynx, and larynx becomes increasingly involved, slurring of the voice occurs, which gradually worsens to dysarthria and dysphagia. Paralysis is inevitable, and death usually results from pneumonia and respiratory failure within 5 years of diagnosis.

Management

ALS is diagnosed by a process of elimination because no definitive diagnostic tests exist. Muscle biopsies may be performed to determine the source of muscle weakness and an EMG will show muscle denervation fibrillation and fascioulation. Blood studies typically show elevation in the levels of creatinine phosphokinase.

There is no cure for ALS and treatment is primarily directed towards symptom relief. Rilusole (Rilutek) has recently been approved for use in ALS treatment. It is believed to extend the life of ALS patients. The specific interventions are directed at management of complications.

The focus of nursing care is on supporting self-care abilities of the patient and the coping resources of the entire family. General interventions are targeted at maintaining good general health, supporting nutrition, promoting adequated sleep, appropriately-balancing activity and rest, and introducing use of self-help devices as they become appropriate. And take measures according to symptom arising appropriately, and patient and family education also include taking of symptomatic measures accordingly.

GUILLAIN-BARRÉ SYNDROME

Guillain-Barré syndrome (GBS) is an acute inflammatory polyneuropathy characterized by varying degrees of motor weakness of paralysis. It primarily affects the motor components of the cranial and spinal nerves and is known by variety of other names, which include, *Landry-Guillain-Barré-Strohl syndrome, Postinfectious polyneuropathy, ascending polyneuropathic paralysis*. It affects the peripheral nervous systems and results in loss of myelin (a segmental demyelination) and oedema and inflammation of the affected nerves-causing a loss of neurotrans mission to the periphery.

Aetiology

GBS is a rare disorder with an incidence of 1.5 to 1.9 per one lakh population. The aetiology of this disorder is unknown, but it is believed to be cell-mediated immunologic reaction directed at the peripheral nerves. The syndrome is frequently preceded by immune system stimulation from a viral infection, trauma, surgery, viral immunization, human immunodeficiency virus (HIV) or lympoproliferative neoplasms. These stimuli are thought to cause an alteratiaon in the immune system resulting in sensitization of T-lymphocytes to the patient's myelin causing myelin damage.

Pathophysiology

In GBS an immune-mediated response triggers destruction of the myelin sheath surrounding the peripheral nerves, nerve roots, root ganglia, and spinal cord. Collections of lymphocytes and macrophages are believed to be responsible for the myelin stripping. Demyelination occurs between the nodes of Ranvier, which impair or blocks the transmission of impulse from node to node. The nerve axons are generally spared and recovery takes place, although process of re-mylination occurs slowly. In severe forms of the disease, Wallerian degeneration occurs that involves the axons, making recovery slower and more difficult. In a small percentage of patients the disease does not resolve and become chronic and recurrent. In this, lymphocytes are basically normal and return to complete functioning after an illness.

Clinical Manifestation

There are four major forms of GBS. Each reflects a different degree of peripheral nerve involvement.

i. *Ascending GBS* is the most common form. Weakness and numbness begin in the legs and progress upward. Fifty per cent of patients experience respiratory insufficiency. Sensory involvement is also usually present.
ii. Pure or motor GBS similar to the ascending form, but no sensory involvement is present. It is usually milder form of disease.
iii. Descending GBS begins with weakness in the muscles controlled by the cranial nerves and then progresses downward. The respiratory system is quickly impaired. Sensory involvement is present.
iv. *Miller-Fisher syndrome*; a variant of GBS is rare and primarily involves the eyes, loss of reflexes and severe ataxia.

Symptoms of GBS usually develop 1 to 3 weeks after an upper respiratory or gastrointestinal infection. The patients with GBS have symmetrical muscle weakness and flaccid motor paralysis. The paralysis usually starts in the lower extremities and ascends upwards to include the thorax, upper extremities and face. Progression of GBS to include the lower brainstem involves facial, abducens, oculomotor, hypoglossal, trigeminal and vagus nerves. This involvement manifests itself through facial weakness, extraocculomotor, eye movement difficulties, dysphagia and paresthesia of the face and patient may have difficulty in swallowing, speaking and breathing.

Pain and paresthesia are present when sensory nerves are involved. The pain can be categorised as paresthesias, muscular aches, and cramps, and hyperesthesias. Pain appears to be worse at night. Tingling or a pin and needle sensation is common. Pain may lead to a decrease in appetite and may interfere with sleep. Pain requires narcotics or analgesics.

Now autonomic dysfunction is recognized as a common problem with GBS and may include dysrythmias, blood pressure instability, tachycardia or bradycardia, flushing, sweating, urinary retention, and paralytic ileus. GBS does not affect the patient level of consciousness, alertness and cognitive functioning. GBS generally progresses through three stages. The initial period lasts from 1 to 3 weeks and ends when no further physical deterioration occurs. A plateau period follows, which lasts from a few days to few weeks. The recovery period can last from 6 months to well over 1 year. The remyelination of damaged nerves occurs during the recovery phase. Permanent dificits may remain.

Complications

The most serious complication of GBS is respiratory failure, which occurs on the paralysis progresses to other nerves that innervate thoracic area. Respiratory or urinary tract infections may occur. Fever is generally first sign of infection. Immobility from the paralysis may cause problem such as paralytic ileum, muscle atrophy, deep vein thrombosis, pulmonary emboli, skin breakdown, orthostatic hypotension and nutritional deficiency.

Management

The diagnosis of GBS is made from the clinical presentation supported by a history of recent viral infection, elevation in the levels of protein in the CSF and results of EMG studies.

The management of GBS is largely supportive and aimed at preventing complication until recovery process can begin.

- Respiratory support is always the priority intervention.
- Corticosteroid therapy is often used to attempt to reduce the autoimmune inflammation, but sterroid has not been proven to be beneficial.
- Plasmapheresis is used in first 2 weeks of GBS. With plasmapheresis, blood is removed and filtered of antibodies, immunoglobuline fibrinogens and other proteins.
- IV administration of high-dose immunoglobuline has also shown to be as effective as plasmopherons and has the advantages of immediate availability and greater safety.
- Recovery is accelerated by early institution of plasmapheresis and IV therapy.
- Carticosteroids and ACTH are used to suppress the immune response but appear have little effect on the prognosis and duration of disease.

Assessment of the patient is the most important aspect of nursing care during the acute phase. The nurse must monitor the ascending paralysis, assess respiratory function, monitor ABGs, and assess the gag, cornea and swallowing reflexes during the routine assessment. Monitoring blood pressure, cardiac rate and rhythm is also important in acute phase, and report and any autonomic disfunction also be assessed and reported to the concerned.

Nursing diagnosis of patient with GBS may be: Inability to sustain spontaneous ventilation R/T progression of disease process:

- Inability to sustain spontaneous ventilation R/T progression of disease process.
- Risk for aspiration R/T dysphagia.
- Pain R/T paresthesias.
- Impaired verbal communication R/o intubation or paralysis of muscles of speech.
- Fear R/T uncertain outcome.
- Self-care deficit R/T inability to use muscles to accomplish ADL.

Here nurse has to follow the measure to treat respiratory failure which may include endotracheal intubation, meticulous suctioning technique may be used to prevent infection. Through bronchial hygiene and chest physiotherapy, help clear secretions and prevent respiratory deterioration. If fever develops, sputum culture should be obtained and sent to laboratory. Good communication should be maintained with the patients. If urinary retention occurs, intermittent catheterization is preferred. Nutritional needs must be met in spite of possible problems associated with delayed gastric emptying, paralytic ileus and potential for aspirations if the gag reflex is lost. Throughout the course of illness, the nurse needs to provide support and encouragement to the family and patient because residual problem and relapses are common.

TRIGEMINAL NEURALGIA (TIC DOULOUREUX)

Trigeminal neuralgia affects the fifth cranial nerve and causes intense paroxysmal pain in one or more of the branches of trigeminal nerves. Then CN has both motor and sensory branches. The sensory branches are involved in trigeminal neuralgia. Primarily, the maxillary and mandibular branches.

Aetiology

No aetiology has been found for the disorder although variety of risk factors have been identified. Major initiating pathologic events may include nerve compression by tortuous arteries of the posterior fossa blood vessels, demyelinating plaques, herpes virus infection, infection of teeth and jaw, transmission infarction. The effectiveness of antiseizures drug therapy may be related to the ability of these drugs to stabilize neuron membrane and decrease paroxysmal afferent impulses of the nerve.

Pathophysiology

The trigminal nerve exists the pons and merges into the gassenar ganglion before it separates into its three major branches. It is the largest of the cranial nerve (CN) and has both motor and

Table 11.5: Nursing care plan: patient with guillain-barre syndrome

Problem	*R*	*Objective*	*Nursing Interventions*	*Rationales*
Nursing Diagnosis #1 Breathing pattern, ineffective, related to: 1. Compromised function of respiratory musculature. 2. Reduced diaphragmatic excusion. 3. Anxiety.		Patient will maintain adequate respiratory function: • Respiratory rate ~14-18/ min. • Respiratory rhythm: Eupneic. • Arterial blood gas values: pH 7.35-7.45 $PaCO_2$ ~35-45 mmHg. PaO_2 ~80 mmHg	• Assess respiratory function hourly. ◆ Specific parameters: – Rate, rhythm, depth, breath sounds, dyspsnoea; use of accessory muscles; status of pulmonary secretions: cough with sputum production.	• Progression of the underlying pathophysiologic process of Guillain-Barre syndrome is acutely reflected by increasing respiratory insufficiency. ◆ Guillain-Barre syndrome is an ascending disease of motor function; it enables the patient to be intubated prophylactically, rather than to have an emergency and potentially traumatic intubation.
			◆ Vital capacity and negative inspiratory force generated.	◆ Vital capacity and negative inspiratory force generated by the patient are especially crucial in identifying disease progression or improvement.
			• Prepare patient/family for possibility of intubation and mechanical ventilation therapy. ◆ Answer questions, take the time to explain what is happening. ◆ Establish alternative means of communication: blinking eyes-wiggle of finger, use of slate board or picture cards.	• Family and patient will accept initiation of mechanical ventilation therapy as part of the overall supportive therapy for patients with this syndrome.
			• Place patient on Roto-Kinetic bed.	• Use of the Roto-Kinetic bed helps to prevent pooling of tracheobronchial secretions.
			• Maintain optimal body alignment: ◆ Position patient so that chest is not restricted (e.g., if on his side, place arm slightly in front or back of patient).	◆ The weight of the patient's flaccid arms should be kept off his chest to allow for maximal chest wall excursion and lung expansion.
			• Notify physician of any changes in above assessment and document trends.	• By documenting data, trends can be followed and the stage of the disease progression can be pinpointed, facilitating quality of care.
Nursing Diagnosis #2 Airway clearance, ineffective, related to: 1. Compromised protective reflexes. 2. Weakness/paralysis of intercostal and abdominal muscles.		Patient will: 1. Maintain patent airway: • Normal breath sounds. • Absence of adventitious sounds (e.g., crackles, wheezes). 2. Demonstrate secretion-clearing cough.	• Assess airway patency hourly: ◆ Status of protective reflexes (cough, gag, epiglottal closure). ◆ Ability to handle tracheobronchial secretions.	• Cranial nerve dysfunction is commonly involved in the pathophysiology underlying Guillain-Barre syndrome. Involvement of cranial nerves VII, IX, X, and XII predisposes to compromised chewing, swallowing and speaking.
			• Maintain hydration state as prescribed. ◆ Humidity oxygen administered.	• Dehydration may enuse tracheobronchial secretions to become infected.
Nursing Diagnosis #3 Alteration in comfort: Pain, related to: 1. Sensorimotor dysfunction.		Patient will be able to verbalize relief from pain, and demonstrate a relaxed demeanour.	• Assess pain, including severity, location/radiation, and type or quality of pain.	• Pain is one of the most significant complaints made by patients with Gullain-Barre syndrome. It occurs in the most profoundly weakened muscles and is more intensified at night.
			• Provide comfort measures: ◆ Assist patient into positions of comfort and correct body alignment.	• Maintaining body in appropriate alignment may help to ease some of the ache.

Contd...

Problem	*R*	*Objective*	*Nursing Interventions*	*Rationales*
			◆ Remain with patient to reassure. ◆ Work with family members to help them understand what is happening and how they may best help their loved one. ◆ Enlist hospital volunteers/chaplain or others to spend some time with the patient.	◆ Families often feel helpless in this circumstance; allowing them to participate in the patient's care may be reassuring to both patient and family.
			• Administer analgesics as prescribed; monitor effectiveness in relieving pain.	• Pain may become severe enough to require narcotics for relief.
Nursing Diagnosis #4 Communication impaired, verbal/nonverbal, related to: 1. Intubatin. 2. Weakened muscles of speech. 3. Generalized muscle weakness/ paralysis.		1. Patient will be able to demonstrate alternative means of communication. 2. Patient will verbalize feeling comfortable with alternative means of communication. 3. Patient will verbalize why alternative means of communication may be necessary.	• Assess for difficulty in speaking.	• Cranial nerve involvement may compromise muscles of speech; eventually, the patient may not even be able to blink his eyes; yet, throughout this ordeal, the patient remain conscious and aware.
			• Keep patient/family appraised of expectations.	• Keeping patient/family abreast of what is happening may help them to adjust to dysfunctional changes more easily.
			• Constantly reassure patient that his needs will be met. • Initiate alternative means of communication before dysfunction occurs.	• Mr. L.'s constant bell ringing reflected his frustration with his dependency and his fear of not having his needs met.
Nursing Diagnosis #5 Self-care deficit, related to: 1. Dependent status necessitated by compromised sensorimotor dysfunction.		1. Patient will be able to verbalize feelings about being dependent on others. 2. Patient will identify activities requiring assistance. 3. Patient will set priorities as to which dependent activities will be accomplished first.	• Identify with patient/family those activities over which the patient can have control (e.g., when to bathe, when to turn, when to have visitors).	• Allowing patient to make decisions over care will help the patient to maintain some control over his body.
			• Work with family to assist the patient in some of his activities of daily living; assist the family to understand why they should respect the patient's need to maintain control of some of his care activities.	• If the patient refuses to see family members or states he doesn't want them to do anything for him, the patient's family should be reassured that it's okay for the patient to do these things and they should not feel rejected.
			◆ Encourage family members to verbalize thoughts and concerns. • Allow patient to ventilate frustrations about dependency.	◆ The patient's illness places a tremendous strain on family relationships, interactions, and lifestyle.

sensory fibres. Trigeminal neuralgia primarily affects the maxillary and mandibular brancehs of the nerve. The pain occurs abruptly lasts from few seconds to a few minutes and can recur at any time. Pain typically described as intense, piercing, burning or like a lightening bolt; the pain affects only one side of the face and there are no accompanying motor or sensory deficits in the region served by the nerve.

Clinical Manifestation

The classic feature of trigeminal neuralgia is an abrupt onset of paroxysms of excruciating pain described as a burning knife like or lightening, like shock in the lips, upper or lower gums, cheek, forehead or side of the nose. Intense pain, twitching, grimacing, and frequent blinking and tearing of the eye occur during the acute attack (giving rise to the term "tic"). The attacks are usually brief, lasting only from seconds to 2 or 3 minutes and are generally unilateral. Recurrences are unpredictable, they may occur several times a day or weeks or months apart. After the refractory (Pain free) period, a phenomenon known as clustering can occur. Clustering is characterized by a cycle of pain and refractoriness that continues for hours.

The painful expisodes are usually initiated by a triggering mechanism of light cutaneous stimulation at a specific point along the distribution of the nerve branches. Precipitating stimuli include chewing, teeth-brushing, a hot or cold blast of air on the face, washing the face, yawning or even talking. Touch and tickle seem to predominate as causative triggers rather than pain or changes in temperature. As a result, the patient may eat improperly, neglect hygienic practices, wear a cloth over the face, and withdraw from interaction with other individuals. The patient may sleep excessively as a means of coping with the pain. This pain disrupts the lifestyle, patients may even commit suicide.

Management

History and physical examination help to make diagnosis and

brain or CT scan, audiologic evaluation. EMG, CSF analgesics, arteriography, posterior myography and MRI are used as diagnostic measures.

There is no definitive treatment for trigeminal neuralgia. Treatment attempts to prevent or block the pain episodes in the most minimal invasive way. The majority of patients obtain adequate relief through antiseizure drugs such as carbamezepine (Tegretol), phenytoin (Bilantin) and valproate (Depekene). Clonazepam, Baclofen.

Nerve block is another possible treatment of trigeminal neuroliagia.

If a conservative approach is not effective, fitting surgical measures are available.

- Glycerol injection into one or more branches of trigeminal nerve.
- Retrogasserian rhizotomy for permanent anaesthesia.
- Suboccipital craniotomy.
- Percutaneous radiofrequency rhizotomy for total pain relief.
- Microvascular decompressing for pain relief without loss of sensation.
- Gamma knife radiosurgery.

The nursing intervention include assessment of attacks of pain and its characteristics, management of pain, maintenance of nutritional status of patient, and taking suitable hygienic measure and education. Patient and family regarding disorder and management.

BELL'S PALSY

Bell's palsy refers to a peripheral facial paralysis, acute benign cranial polyneuritis. It is a disorder characterized by a disruption of the motor branches of the facial nerve (CNVII) or one side of the face in the absence of any other diseases such as stroke.

Aetiology

The aetiology of disease is unknown; but it is generally believed to be a type of localized inflammatory reaction. There is evidence that reactivated herpes simplex virus (HSV) may be involved in majority of cases. The reactivation of HSV causes inflammation of oedema, ischaemia and eventually demyelination of the nerve, creating pain and alteration in motor and sensory function.

Pathophysiology

The facial nerve is primarily composed of motor nerve that innervates the muscles of expression on the face. Sensory branches supply the anterior two-thirds of the tongue. Bell's palsy is characterised by a rapid weakening or paralysis of the facial muscles on one side of the face, which creates a mask-like appearance. The eye on the affected side tears constantly, and the person has difficulty in swelling secretions. The paralysis may develop over a period of 24 to 36 hours or be fully present when a patient wakes from sleep.

Clinical Manifestation

The onsets of Bell's palsy is often accompanied by an outbreak of herpes vesicles in or around the ear. Patient may complain of pain around or behind the ear. In addition, manifestation may include fever, tinnitus, or hearing difficult. The paralysis of the motor branches of the facial nerve typically results in flaccidity of the affected side of the face, with dropping of the mouth accompanied by drooling. An inability to close the eyelid with an upward movement of eyeball when closure is attempted is also evident. A widened palpebral fissure (the opening between the eyelids), flattening of the nasolabial gold, and inability to smile, frown or whistle are also common. Unilateral loss of taste is common. Decreased muscle movement may alter chewing ability and although some patients may experience loss of tearing or excessive tearing, pain may be present behind the ear on affected side especially before the onset of paralysis.

Complication can include psychologic widhdrawal because of changes in appearance, malnutrition and dehydration, mucus membrane trauma, corneal abrasions, muscle stretching and facial spasms and contractures.

Management

There is no definitive test for diagnosing Bell's palsy. The diagnosis and prognosis are indicated by observatioan of the typical pattern of onset and signs and testing of percutaneous nerve exitability of EMG.

There is no definitive treatment for Bell's palsy, treatment for Bell's palsy includes moist heat, gentle massage and electrical stimulation of the nerve. Stimulation may maintain muscle tone and prevent atrophy. Care is primarily focussed on relief of symptoms and prevention of complication. Corticosteroid, especially predisone are started immediately and the best results are obtained if corticosteroids initiated before paralysis completes. When patient improves, they can be tapered off over 2-week period. Analgesics may be administered for pain management. Anti-HSV infection drug acyclovir, valacyclovir and Famiciclon are used if it is present.

The patient with Bell's palsy does not usually require inpatient hospitalization. The following nursing interventions are used throughout the course of disease.

- Mild analgesic can relieve pain.
- Hot wet packs can reduce the discomfort of herpic lesions aid circulation and relieve pain.
- The face should be protected from cold and drafts.
- Maintenance of good nutrition—Patient may be taught to chew food on unaffected side.
- Thorough oral hygiene.

- Teach patient to safely use of heat, massage and TENS at home.
- Instruct about safe use of corticosteroids.
- Teach importance of protecting eyes from infection and other supportive measures.

SPINAL CORD INJURY

The spinal column is a circular bony ring that provides excellent protection for the spinal cord from most low-intensity injury. The vertebrae are dense bony structures with multiple articulations that provide for a wide range of head and neck movements, but these articulations also create points of weakness that are vulnerable to a variety of types of injury. The close anatomical proximity of the spinal cord to the vertebrae, muscles and ligaments increases the chance of injury to any of the supporting structures will also result in injury to the cord itself.

Aetiology

Spinal injuries occur most commonly when excessive force is exerted on the spinal column, resulting in excessive flexion, hyperextension, compression or rotation.

The population at risk for spinal cord injury is primarily young adult men between ages of 15 and 30 years and those who are impulsive or risk taken in daily living. Individuals at risk for spinal cord injury include motor cyclists, skydivers, football players, police personnel, divers and military personnel. Coordination exists between alcohol and drug abuse and spinal injuries that substantial abuse is present in the majority of motor vehicle accidents that result in spinal cord injury (SCI) as well as many other accidents' diving incidents, and episodes of violent trauma.

Events that cause abrupt forceful acceleration and deceleration are common initiating factors for SCI. Injuries to the spinal cord can be classified in a variety of ways that take into account damage to both the vertebrae and the underlying spinal cord. Most injuries are the results of sudden and often violent external trauma, but the persons who have chronic conditions affecting the vertebrae such as stenosis, arthritis, or osteoporosis are also at a high risk for injury.

Mechanisms of Injury

- *Hyperflexion injuries* are frequently the result of sudden deceleration as might be experienced in a head on collision or from a severe blow to the back of the head. The head and neck are forcibly hyperflexed and then may be snapped backward into forced hyperextension. These injuries are typically seen in C-5-6 area of the cervical spine. They may result in fracture of the vertebrae, dislocation and or tearing of the posterior ligaments.
- *Hyperextension injuries* are frequently acceleration injuries as are seen in rear-end collisions or as the result of falls in which the chin is forcibly struck. These injuries tend to cause significant damage because the downward and backward area of the head's movement is so great. C-4-5 is the area of the spine most commonly affected.
- *Compression injuries* cause the vertebrae to squash or burst. They usually involve high velocity and affect both the cervical and thoracolumbar regions of the spine. Blows to the top of the head and forceful landing on the feet or buttocks can result in compression injury.
- *Rotational injuries* are caused by extreme lateral flexion or twisting of the head and neck. The tearing of ligaments can easily result in dislocation as well as fracture, and soft tissue damage frequently complicates the primary injury. The result can be a highly unstable spinal injury. Many SCI involve more than one type of directional force.

Types of Spinal Cord Damage

The injuries that can affect the spinal cord are concussion, contusion, laceration and transection.

- *Cord concussion*. The cord is severely jarred or squeezed as is frequently seen with sports-related injuries e.g. football. No identifiable pathological changes are detectable in the cord but a temporary loss of motor or sensory function, or both can occur. The dysfunction resolves spontaneously within 24-48 hours.
- *Cord contusion*. This injury is frequently caused by compression. Bleeding into the cord results in bruising and oedema. The extent of damage reflects the adequacy of the overall perfusion to the cord and then severity of the inflammatory response.
- *Cord transection*. A complete or incomplete severing of the spinal cord with loss of neurological function is below the level of the injury. The cord segment in which neurological function is preserved.

Spinal Cord Syndrome

There are many unique and specific syndrome can occur in SCI. They represent types of localized spinal damage although it is unusual to see any of these syndromes in their pure form.

- *Central cord syndrome* reflects damage primarily to the central gray or white matter of the spinal cord. It is believed to be resulting from oedema formation that occurs in response to the primary injury and puts pressure on the anterior horn cells. It usually occurs in older adults who experience a hype extensive injury, typically in the cervical region. The resulting motor deficit is more severe in the upper extremities than in the lower, particularly in the hand. The amount of sensory impairment is highly variable. Bowel and bladder function may or may not be affected. Improvement over the time is expected.

- *Anterior cord syndrome* typically results from injury or infarction involving the anterior spinal artery, which perfuses the anterior two-thirds of the spinal cord. It can also result from tumours and acute discherniation. The resultant damage includes motor paralysis with loss of pain and temperature sensation. Position, vibration, and touch sensation remain intact.
- *Posterior cord syndrome* is an extremely rare syndrome in which proprioceptive sensation is the position and vibration are lost due to damage to the posterior column of the spinal cord.
- *Brown sequare syndrome* results from unilateral injury usually of the penetrating type, that involves just half of the spinal cord. There is a resulting loss of motor ability plus touch, pressure, and vibration sensation on same side as the injury but loss of pain and temperature sensations on the opposite side.
- *Conus medullaris syndrome* results from damage to the sacral region of the spinal column and the lumbar nerve roots that comprise the cauda equina. It creates a lower motor neuron injury with flaccid paralysis of the bowel and bladder and loss of sexual function. Motor function in the sensory involvement is rarely present.

Pathophysiology

Trauma to the spinal cord produces both primary and secondary injury processes. The primary damage results from the initial mechanical insult and is usually irreversible. Bruising and compression are the most common types of injury. The cord is rarely transected at the time of primary injury, but the initial insult initiates a self-destructive process that frequently results in a worsening of the injury. This is primarily the result of a progressive slowing of blood flow to the cord.

The primary compression, stretching, jarring or tearing of the spinal cord causes small haemorrhages in the gray matter of the cord. Oedema causes the blood blow to the cord to slow in a matter of minute. Hypoxia develops rapidly which often leads to tissue necrosis.

Secondary cord injury results from the body's natural responses to injury and inflammation, which can have dramatic negative consequences for the spinal cord. Capillary permeability increases in response to traum which allows fluid to move into interstitial spaces. Oedema impairs the microcirculation and worsens the ischaemia. The developing hypoxia stimulates the release of vasoactive substances such as catecholamines, histamin and endorphins from the injured tissue, which further decreases blood flow in the microcirculation and may induce vasospasm. Proteolytic and lypolytic enzymes are also released from the injured cells. Which can clog the microcirculation and worsen the oedema, ischaemia and necrosis. The enzymes actively work to clear cellular debris, which can include removal of neural tissue that is then incapable of regeneration.

This secondary injury process can destroy the full thickness of the spinal cord at the level of injury and further extends its effects severe and cord segments above and below the original level of injury. The process of secondary injury is initiated immediately after the original insult and progresses rapidly. Blood flow to the injured spinal cord is further compromised by the upset of spinal shock.

Spinal Shock

Spinal shock represents a temporary but profound disruption of spinal cord functions, which occur immediately after injury, typically within 30 to 60 minutes. It is a state of a reflexion characterized by the loss of all neurological function below the level of the injury. Spinal shock causes a complete loss of the motor, sensory, reflexes, and autonomic functioning. The severity of shock varies depending on the extent and level of the primary injury, but injuries at T6 or above usually result in more severe forms. Spinal shock is the direct result of the neuronal injury and is not preventable. The clinical manifestation of spinal shock are as follows:

- Flaccid paralysis: Affects all skeletal muscles below the level of injury.
- Loss of spiral reflex activity: Paralytic ileus, loss of bowel and bladder tone.
- Sensory loss below the level of injury: Pain, temperature, touch, pressure and proprioceptive senses, somatic and visceral sensations. Bradycardia (results from unopposed parasympathetic vagal (slowing of the heart).
- Bradycardia (results from venous pooling in lower extremities and splanchnic circulation, related to loss of vasomotor tone).
- Loss of temperature control.
  - warm, dry skin
  - inability to shiver or perspire.
  - Poikilothermia: the body assumes the temperature of the external environment.

Clinical Manifestations

The clinical manifestations of the spinal cord injury are dependent on the level of the injury and whether the injury is complete or incomplete. The terms paraplegia' tetraplegia (previously quadriplegia) are used to describe the functional consequence of spinal cord injury (SCI).

Generally there will be poikilothermia and warm, dry-flushed extremities below the level of injury (Spinal shock). Other manifestations related to level and degree of injury are as follows: RS Lesions at C_1 to C_3 give rise to apnoea, inability to cough.

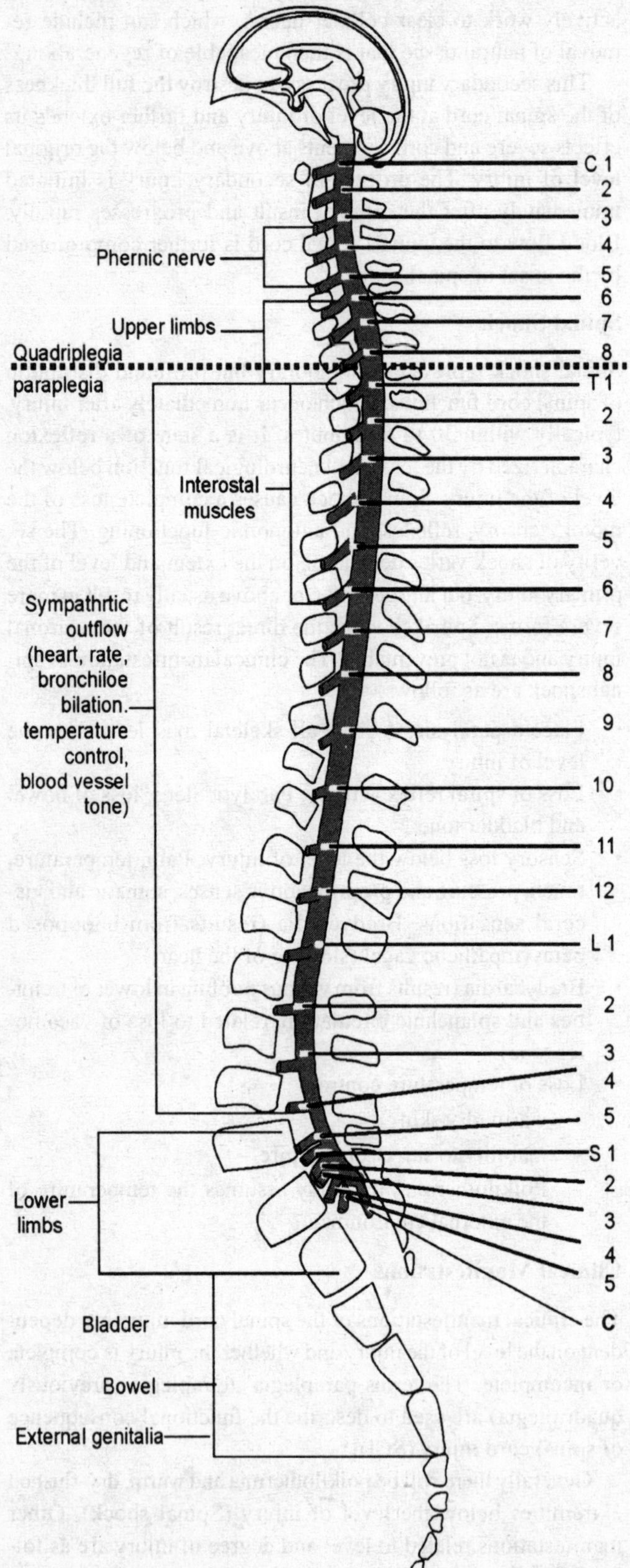

Fig.11.2: Spinal Cord Innervation

- Lesion at C_4 gives rise to poor cough, diaphragmatic breathing.
- Lesion at C_5 to T_6 give rise to hypoventilation, decreased respiratory reserve.
- Lesions above T_5 leads to bradycardia, hypotension, postural hypotension, and absence of vasomotor tone.
- Lesion above T_5 also leads to decreased or absent bowel sounds (paralytic ileum) abdominal distension, constipation, fecal incontinence and fecal impaction.
- Lesions between T_1, L_2 leads to flaccid bladder (acute stages) spasticity with reflex bladder emptying (later stages).
- Lesion above C_8: resulting in flaccid paralysis and anaesthesia. Below the level of injury resulting in tetraplegia.
- Lesion below C_8 leads to hyperactive deep tendon reflexes, bilaterally positive Babinkis test.

Mixed loss of voluntary motor activity and sensations and muscle atomy (in flaccid state), contractures (in spastic state) will be present. In addition, priapism, loss of sound functions also occur.

Management

The initial goals for the patient with a spinal cord injury are to sustain life and prevent further cord damage. Spinal cord injury is initially diagnosed on the basis of the presenting symptoms. Systemic, neurogenic and spinal cord shock must be treated. For injury at the cervical level, all body systems must be maintained until the full extent of the damage can be evaluated. Treatment of spinal cord injury may be medical or surgical.

Emergency Management

Patient may come to hospital with blunt injury or penetrating injuries. Blunt injuries include, compression, flexion, extension, or rotational injuries to spinal column, due to motor vehicle accidents pedestrian accidents, falls and diving.

Penetrating injuries may be stretched, torn, crushed or lacerated spinal cord due to gunshot wounds and stab wounds.

During this, the nurse has to make the following assessment of findings.

- Pain, tenderness, deformities or muscle spasms adjacent to vertebral column.
- Numbness, paresthesias.
- Alterations in sensation; temperature, light, touch, deep pressure and proprioception.
- Weakness or heaviness in limbs.
- Weakness, paralysis or flaccidity of muscles.
- Spinal shock.
- Cuts, bruises, open wounds overhead, face, neck or back.
- Neurogenic shock, hypotention, bradycardia, dry flushed skin.
- Bowel and bladder incontinence.

- Urinary retention.
- Difficulty in breathing.
- Priapism.
- Diminished rectal sphincter tone.

Nursing Intervention

- Ensure patent airway.
- Stabilize cervical spine.
- Administer oxygen via nasal cannula or nonbreather mask.
- Establish IV with two large-bone catheters and infuse normal saline or lactated Ringer's solution as appropriate.
- Assess for other injuries.
- Control external bleeding.
- Obtain cervical spine radiographs or CT scan.
- Prepare for stabilization with cranial tong and traction.
- Administer high-dose methyl prednisolone, and ongoing monitoring includes
  - Monitor vital signs, level of consciousness, oxygen saturation, cardiac rhythm, urine output.
  - Keep warm.
  - Monitor for urinary retention and hypertention.
  - Anticipate need for intubation if gag reflex is absent.

Following emergency management, patient should be prepared and assisted to perform the following diagnostic measure:

- Complete neurologic examination.
- ABG analysis.
- Electrolytes, glucose, haemoglobin, and haematocrit levels.
- Urinalysis.
- Anteroposterior, lateral and odontoid spinal X-ray studies.
- CT Scan.
- Myelography.
- MRI.
- EMG to measure evoked potentials.

Following measures should be taken if confronted with cervical cord injury.

- Immobilisation of vertebral column by skeletal traction.
- Maintenance of heart rate (Example atropine) and blood pressure (e.g. dopamine).
- Methylprednisolone therapy to reduced oedema.
- Insertion of nasogastric tube and attachment to suction.
- Intubation (if indicated by ABGs).
- Administration of oxygen by high humidity mask.
- Introduction of indwelling catheter.
- Administration of IV fluids.

In addition, following ambulatory care should be followed.

- Stress ulcer prophylaxes.
- Physical therapy (range of motion exercises).
- Occupational therapy (splints and ADL training).

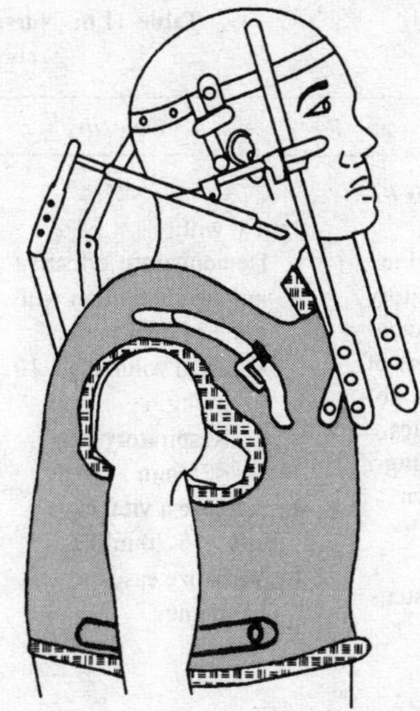

Halo vest traction

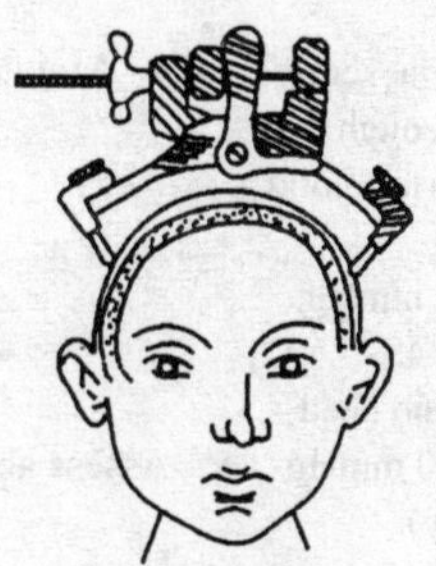

Crutchfield traction tongs

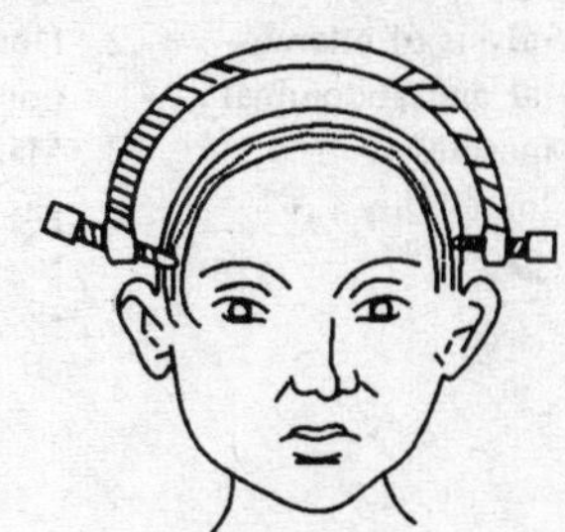

Gardner-Wells traction tongs

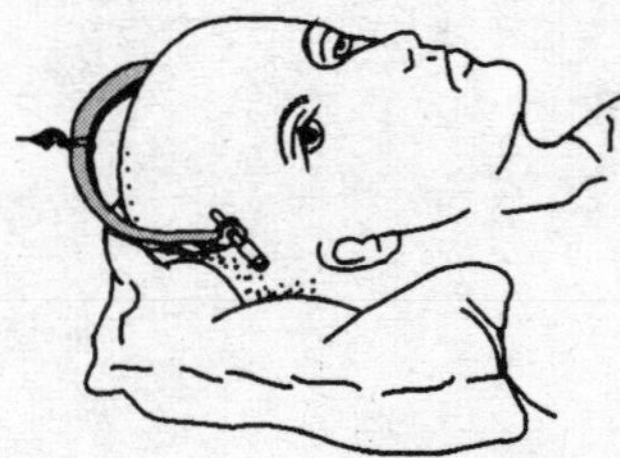

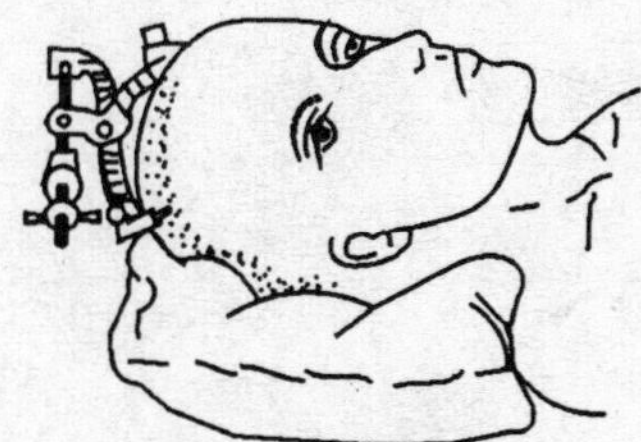

Fig.11.3: Cervical traction

Table 11.6: Nursing care plan for the initial management of the spinal cord-injured patient (cervical cord injury)

Problem	*R*	*Objective*	*Nursing Interventions*	*Rationales*
Nursing Diagnosis #1 Breathing pattern, ineffective, related to: 1. Altered ventilatory mechanics associated with paralysis of intercostal and abdominal muscles. 2. Limited diaphragmatic excursion associated with paralytic ileus (abdominal distention). 3. Immobility.		Patient will: 1. Demonstrate effective minute ventilation with trend of improving: • Tidal volume > 7-10 ml/kg. • Respiratory rate <25/min. 2. Achieve a vital capacity >15-20 ml/kg. 3. Verbalize ease of breathing.	• Perform a comprehensive respiratory assessment.	• Major goal of airway management is to establish and/or maintain adequate alveolar ventilation.
			◆ Airway patency.	◆ Baseline data are essential to evaluate effectiveness of therapeutic interventions and to follow trends.
			◆ Rate, rhythm, depth of breathing.	◆ Increased rapid, shallow respirations may signal deterioration of respiratory function.
			◆ Chest and diaphragmatic excursion.	◆ C_{3-5} cervical cord injury may disrupt innervation of diaphragm; paralysis results in respiratory arrest.
			◆ Use of accessory muscles.	
Nursing Diagnosis #2 Airway clearance, ineffective, related to: 1. Ineffective cough associated with paralysis of intercostal and abdominal muscles. 2. Immobility.		Patient will: 1. Demonstrate clear breath sound on auscultation. 2. Demonstrate a secretion-clearing cough. 3. Maintain arterial blood gas values: • PaO_2 > 80 mmHg. • $PaCO_2$ 35-45 mmHg, if no head injury (<30 mmHg with injury). • pH 7.35-7.45.	◆ Auscultation of breath sounds.	◆ May detect evidence of secretion of secretion accumulation; airway obstruction.
			◆ Monitor arterial blood gases (ABGs).	◆ Determine baseline respiratory function and monitor adequacy of ventilation/oxygenation. ◆ Hypoxaemia in the spinal cord-injured patient is most commonly caused by retained secretions.
			• Assess ability to cough and clear secretions.	• Loss of intercostal and abdominal muscles compromise the patient's ability to cough effectively.
			◆ Status of protective reflexes: cough, gag, and epiglottal closure.	◆ Loss of protective reflexes places patient at risk of developing aspiration pneumonia; a moist-sounding, unproductive cough signals retention and pooling of pulmonary secretions.
			◆ Monitor quality, quantity, colour and consistency of sputum. – Obtain sputum for culture and sensitivity.	◆ Baseline data enable changes in sputum production and characteristics to be identified. Infection or other pulmonary insult may increase quality and quantity of sputum; a pulmonary embolism may cause hemoptysis.
			◆ Assess secretions-for state of hydration or need for mucolytic therapy.	◆ Thinning of secretion's facilities, mobilization and clearance of secretions.
			• Monitor serial pulmonary function tests: ◆ Tidal volume. ◆ Vital capacity.	• Serial monitoring enables trends to be identified; progressive decline in pulmonary function may signal need for elective intubation and mechanical ventilation.
			• Assess neurologic status:	• Hypoxia may be reflected by changes in patient's mental status or

Contd...

Problem	*R*	*Objective*	*Nursing Interventions*	*Rationales*
			◆ Level of consciousness; mentation.	behaviour (e.g., restlessness, irritability).
			• Implement measures to ensure adequate respiratory function:	
			◆ Establish and maintain airway patency.	◆ Airway obstruction frequently occurs with spinal cord injury or injuries involving head and neck.
			◆ Maintain head and neck in straight alignment without hyperflexion or hyperextension.	◆ Reduces risk of further neurologic damage; allows for unimpeded flow of blood and cerebrospinal fluid from cranial vault; head injury often accompanies traumatic cord injuries.
			◆ Implement intubation and mechanical ventilation as per unit protocol.	◆ Elective intubation and mechanical ventilation are often performed with cervical injury $C_{5\text{-}6}$ and above.
			◆ Initiate oxygen therapy to maintain arterial blood gases within physiologically acceptable range.	
			◆ Initiate measures to clear secretions. – Provide humidified oxygen. – Maintain hydration.	
			◆ Implement nasotracheal suctioning as necessary to maintain airway patency.	◆ Vagal stimulation may cause severe bradycardia in the spinal cord-injured patient who is already bradycardic.
			◆ Initiate chest physiotherapy techniques as tolerated. – Postural drainage. – Percussion and vibration.	◆ Loosens and dislodges secretions and enhances movement toward trachea from where they are accessible to removal by coughing and/or suctioning. ◆ Quad-assist coughing method may be helpful in patients with weakened cough (see text for details).
			◆ Encourage deep breathing and coughing.	
			◆ Instruct patient in use of incentive spirometry (see Table 32-2).	◆ Increases vital capacity; helps to more evenly match ventilation with perfusion. ◆ Use of incentive spirometry encourages deep breathing, reducing risk of atelectasis.
			◆ Ensure hydration status. – Monitor intake and output, daily weight.	◆ Adequate hydration moistens, loosens, and liquefies secretions.
			◆ Insert nasogastric tube.	◆ To decompress stomach: Helps to prevent aspiration and allows for full diaphragmatic excursion.
			◆ Use a calm, reassuring approach. – Anticipate needs. – Be accessible; offer explanations.	◆ Anxiety is a major problem in the spinal cord-injured patient who may be fearful of drying.
Nursing Diagnosis #3 Cardiac output, alteration in: Decreased, related to: 1. Decreased venous return associated with spinal shock (pooling of blood in dilated vasculature)		Patient will: 1. Maintain stable haemodynamics: • Blood pressure within 10 mmHg of baseline. • Heart rate > 60 < 100/min.	• Assess for presence of neurogenic or spinal shock: Blood pressure, pulse, body temperature, skin; orthostatic hypotension.	• Complete transection of spinal cord at T4-6 and above precipitates spinal shock with loss of sympathetic autonomic reflex activity. ◆ Hypotension occurs due to loss of sympathetic vasomotor tone with resultant vasodilation of systemic vasculature.

Contd...

Problem	*R*	*Objective*	*Nursing Interventions*	*Rationales*
2. Orthostatic hypotension 3. Bradycardia.		• Cardiac output ~ 4 - 8 litres/min. • Central venous pressure 0-8 mmHg. • Pulmonary capillary wedge pressure 8-12 mmHg.		◆ Bradycardia occurs due to unopposed parasympathetic (vagal) tone to the heart.
			• Rule out conco haemorrhagic, hypovolaemic shock: ◆ Neurogenic shock: Hypotension, bradycardia, warm dry skin. ◆ Haemorrhagic shock: Hypotension, tachycardia, thready pulse, cool clammy skin.	• Infrequently, spinal cord trauma may be accompanied by internal injuries with possible bleeding.
			– Assess for signs of bleeding in spinal cord-injured patient who is tachycardic.	◆ Presence of internal bleeding may be difficult to detect in the insensate patient: a high degree of suspicion and meticulous assessment are essential.
			• Perform ongoing cardiovascular assessment: ◆ Continuous cardiac monitoring.	◆ Cardiac and cerebral tissue hypoxia can occur with hypoxemia precipitating dysrhythmias.
			◆ Continuous haemodynamic monitoring.	◆ Offers significant data regarding cardiopulmonary function: access for serial blood gas measurements.
			– Arterial, central venous pressure (CVP) and pulmonary capillary wedge pressure (PCWP).	– PCWP assists in determining hydration status: the patient in neurogenic or spinal shock is not hypovolaemic and should not receive large amounts of fluids; overhydration may increase. Oedema formation at site of injury.
			– Cardiac output.	– Positive pressure mechanical ventilation increases intrathoracic pressures, which impedes venous return and reduces cardiac output.
			• Implement measures to stabilize cardiopulmonary function: ◆ Initiate prescribed intravenous fluid therapy ~ 75 ~ 100 ml/hr to maintain systolic blood pressure ~ 100 mmHg.	• CVP and PCWP should be monitored to determine trends and to evaluate patient's response to hydration therapy.
			– Monitor fluid intake and output.	◆ Intact mental status, and acceptable urine outputs ensure adequate tissue perfusion.
			◆ Initiate activities to minimize orthostatic hypotension: – Apply antiembolic stock – Abdominal binder.	◆ Orthostatic hypotension results from venous stasis associated with impaired vasomotor tone and skeletal muscle paralysis.
			– Gradual increase to vertical position (sitting up at 90°) as tolerated.	◆ Observe patient carefully when sitting up; syncopal episodes secondary to hypotension may occur.
Nursing Diagnosis # 4 Injury, potential for, related to: 1. Vertebral instability. 2. Spinal cordoedema.		Patient will: 1. Maintain immobilization of head, neck, and back. 2. Maintain and/or improve neurologic function.	• Determine extent of injury and baseline assessment data. • Patient history: ◆ Obtain information regarding circumstances of injury/accident: Mechanism of injury? Neurologic status post-injury?	◆ Knowledge of mechanism/location of spinal cord injury assists

Contd...

Problem	*R*	*Objective*	*Nursing Interventions*	*Rationales*
3. Stress.	3.	Demonstrate effective ventilatory effort.		in determining type and extent of spinal injury and the presence of other injuries.
			◆ Did the patient lose consciousness? If so, for how long? Was there seizure activity? Was the patient incontinent—bowel? bladder?	◆ Concomitant head injury is always a possibility especially with cervical cord injury.
			◆ Type of treatment administered at scene of injury: Medications? Fluids? – Mode of transportation to the hospital? How long a delay between occurrence of injury and admission to emergency department? – Patient's status on arrival to the hospital?	◆ Interview EMTs, and family member if present, about the circumstances of the injury.
			◆ Obtain pertinent information regarding the patient's past history: Pre-existing disease: Pulmonary, cardiac, renal, endocrine, neurologic, mental/emotional/psychologic; known allergies?	◆ A thorough assessment and database assist in developing a treatment plan and individualizing care.
			◆ Use of medications?	
			• Physical examination:	
			◆ Estimate extent of cord involvement. Level and areas of neurologic deficits can be delineated by checking sensation, muscular strength, and reflexes.	◆ Knowledge regarding level of cord injury assists in determining level of function and in anticipating problems. Example: Impending danger of phrenic nerve dysfunction with cord injury at C_{3-5} or above. Documentation of this information is critical to the continuity of patient care.
			◆ Grade muscle strength with scale of 0-5. 0 = no movement. 5 = movement against reflexes.	◆ Organized approach ensures thoroughness of testing all major muscle groups.
			◆ Test for sensory function using touch and pinprick as stimuli.	◆ To assist in demarcating areas of function from areas of altered sensation progress from area of neurologic deficit to area where sensation is intact.
			◆ Assess patient's neurologic status every 1 to 2 hours during initial 48-72 hours postinjury.	◆ Neurologic deterioration with additional loss of function may be caused by spinal cord oedema, haemorrhage, compromised blood supply, and tissue ischaemia.
			◆ Examine patient thoroughly to determine if any other injury has been sustained.	◆ The neurologically compromised patient may not be able to tell you that other problems exist.
			◆ Look for signs of internal and/or external bleeding if tachycardia is present.	◆ Thoracolumbar injury is frequently associated with internal abdominal complications caused by sheer violent force of such injuries.
			• Establish baseline laboratory and other diagnostic studies: serum glucose, electrolytes, BUN, creatine; CBC with differential, haemoglobin, haematocrit; type and crossmatch, coagulation studies; baseline urinalysis, Haematuria.	• To be used for comparison in evaluating patient's status and response to therapy.
			• Obtain pertinent x-rays.	• Patient should not be moved until cervical spine X-rays have been

Contd...

Problem	*R*	*Objective*	*Nursing Interventions*	*Rationales*
				carefully evaluated and the patient's status has been determined. Cervical vertebrae: All seven must be definitively viewed.
			Note: Once the patient's condition is stabilized, a more extensive history in terms of the patient's functional health patterns should be obtained.	
			• Implement measures to stabilize cervical spine. ◆ Use principles-underlying traction: – Weights are never removed, but must be allowed to hang freely at all times. – When turning, positioning, or moving patient, obtain adequate assistance; patient should be lifted using a sheet. ◆ Implement nursing measures in caring for the patient with a halo immobilization brace.	• To prevent further neurologic damage. – Skeletal traction must be in effect at all times. ◆ For details regarding the care of the patient with a halo brace.
			• Monitoring for neurologic changes associated with spinal cord oedema. ◆ Assess respiratory function: rate, rhythm, depth, and pattern of breathing; arterial blood gas studies. ◆ Monitor response of patient to corticosteroids. ◆ Perform serial neurologic assessments comparing sensory and motor function with the baseline data.	• In cervical spinal cord injury, ascending oedema may compromise phrenic nerve innervation to diaphragm, precipitating respiratory arrest. It may be necessary to intubate patient and initiate mechanical ventilation. ◆ Steroids have been found to be efficacious in incomplete cord transections. May reduce inflammation and oedema.
			• Monitoring gastrointestinal function. ◆ Monitor pH of gastric solutions. ◆ Monitor response to antacids. ◆ Monitor haematest gastric secretions. ◆ Monitor stool for guaiac.	◆ Steroids predispose to stress ulcer development. Exogenous steroids may potentiate effect of endogenous steroids in this regard. (Actual role played by steroids in this regard remains controversial.)
Nursing Diagnosis # 5 Anxiety, related to: 1. Loss of sensorimotor function below level of lesion. 2. Immobilization. 3. Impact of lifestyle.		Patient will: 1. Verbalize feeling less anxious. 2. Demonstrate a relaxed demeanour. 3. Verbalize familiarity with ICU routines and protocols. 4. Initiate attempts to discuss magnitude of this catastrophe and what it means to the patient.	◆ Assess for signs and symptoms of anxiety. ◆ Examine the circumstances underlying anxiety. ◆ Assess patient/family coping. ◆ Initiate interventions to reduce anxiety.	
Nursing Diagnosis # 6 Ineffective thermoregulation associated with autonomic dysfunction. *Nursing Diagnosis # 7* Potential alteration to body temperature.		Patient will: 1. Maintain body temperature ~98.6°F (37.0°C). 2. Verbalize comfort and absence of chilling or diaphoresis above the level of lesion.	• Monitor body temperature and complaints of chilliness or sweating. • Maintain a constant room temperature. ◆ Use of extra blankets should be guided by patient's temperature. – Avoid drafts. – Avoid use of excessive beeding.	• Impaired homeothermia causes the patient's body to assume environmental temperature. • This is the most effective way of controlling patient's temperature. ◆ Drafts can precipitate an episode of autonomic dysreflexia in patients with spinal cord injury above C_7-T_1.

Contd...

Problem	*R*	*Objective*	*Nursing Interventions*	*Rationales*
Nursing Diagnosis #8 Urinary retention, related to atonic bladder associated with spinal shock. *Nursing Diagnosis # 9* Urinary elimination, alteration in.		Patient will: 1. Have a urine volume of < 400-450 ml on intermittent catheterization program. 2. Demonstrate absence of suprapubic distention. 3. Balance intake with output.	• Monitor urinary function. ◆ Assess for bladder distention hourly. ◆ Insert Foley catheter if prescribed. – Avoid overdistended bladder. – Provide meticulous aseptic catheter care. – Minimize duration of use of indwelling catheter.	• Urinary retention predisposes to complications of infection and autonomic dysreflexia. ◆ During spinal shock, atonic bladder predisposes to urinary retention and urinary tract infection. – Indwelling Foley catheters place patient at high risk of infection. ◆ Prolonged use of indwelling catheter may contribute to bladder atony, compromising efforts to train bladder for reflex emptying.
			• Initiate intermittent catheterization program as early as possible. ◆ Establish necessary criteria: fluid intake < 2000 ml/24 hr; absence of urinary infection on culture and sensitivity.	• Minimizes renal/urinary complications associated with infection. ◆ Intermittent catheterization program should be initiated as early as possible, even during acute state if feasible. This simulates normal bladder filling and emptying and facilitates bladder training.
			◆ Monitor fluid intake. – Limit fluid intake after the evening meal. Avoid beverages that have a diuretic effect (e.g., caffeinated colas, tea, coffee).	◆ Efforts to establish effective urinary management require a collaborative approach involving patient, family and/or significant others, and health-care providers.
Nursing Diagnosis#10 Alteration in fluid and electrolytes: Fluid volume deficit, related to nothing-by-mouth (NPO) status associated with weakened protective reflexes and paralytic ileus.		Patient will: 1. Maintain baseline body weight. 2. Balance fluid intake with output. 3. Have stable vital signs, clear breath sounds, absence of peripheral or dependent oedema. 4. Maintain laboratory studies (e.g., electrolytes, BUN, creatinine, total protein, haematology profile) within acceptable physiologic range.	• Maintain fluid and electrolyte balance. ◆ Monitor intravascular fluid volume to maintain systemic blood pressure (systolic). ◆ Assess for fluid volume deficit. Signs and symptoms include: – Weakness, listlessness: diminished urinary output; decreased central venous pressure. – Hypotension, rapid thready pulse, increased heart rate respiratory rate. – Poor skin turgor over sternum and forehead; sunken eyeballs. – Weight loss.	◆ Adequate renal perfusion maintains glomerular filtration and renal function. ◆ Haemoconcentration may predispose to electrolyte imbalance, increased viscosity of blood, thromboembolic complications.
			◆ Assess for fluid volume overload: Signs and symptoms include: – Confusion, dillutional hyponatraemia, elevated central venous pressure. – Neck vein distention in upright position (45°). – Shortness of breath, rales, hypertension, bounding pulse, dependent oedema, weight gain.	◆ Fluid volume overload increases risk of pulmonary congestive heart failure. ◆ Haemodilution may predispose to electrolyte imbalance. ◆ Can potentiate cord oedema.
			• Prevent fluid and electrolyte imbalance. ◆ Administer fluids based on fluid losses (include Insensible losses) and state of hydration.	• *Note:* Disruption of sympathetic vasomotor tone precipitates a hypotensive state, which triggers an

Contd...

Problem	*R*	*Objective*	*Nursing Interventions*	*Rationales*
				increased secretion of aldosterone, with sodium retention.
			• Administer electrolytes as indicated by clinical and laboratory status.	• Nasogastric decompression results in loss of hydrogen and chloride ions: hypokalaemia may occur because the kidneys retain hydrogen ions while excreting potassium ions.
			• Signs/symptoms of hypokalaemia: Weakness, paralysis, respiratory arrest, mental status disturbances, paralytic ileus, coma; arrhythmias; ECG changes.	• May be difficult to differentiate some symptomatology in the spinal cord injured patient. • An inability to perspire due to disruption of sympathetic innervation contributes to fluid and electrolyte imbalance.
Nursing Diagnosis#11 Bowel elimination, alteration in: Constipation, related to atomic bowel (paralytic ileus) associated with spinal shock.		Patient will: 1. Remain without constipation and fecal impaction. 2. Establish regular bowel elimination management regimen.	• Prevent complications of gastrointestinal function.	• Level of cord injury determines the extent of gastrointestinal and bowel dysfunction. • Entire gastrointestinal tract becomes atonic with onset of spinal shock 24 to 48 hours post injury.
			• Insert nasogastric tube to decompress gastrointestinal tract. – Relieve distention associated with paralytic ileus. – Prevent vomiting/aspiration.	• Prevents aspiration of gastric contents. Abdominal distention may limit diaphragmatic excursion.
			• Assess patient with high degree of suspicion. – Measure abdominal girth. – Be alert for signs/complaints of "referred" pain. – Auscultate in all quadrants.	• With loss of sensation, patient may be unaware of signs of bleeding, ileus, impaction.
			• Assess for signs of constipation: Dull sound over descending colon on percussion; palpation of hard, rigid stool over areas of bowel.	
			• Be suspicious of diarrhoea. – Haematest gastric secretions, stool for guaiac.	• It may signal presence of fecal impaction.
			• Initiate bowel continence program post-spinal shock and resolution of paralytic ileus: • Establish regular routine: Dulcolax suppository inserted, digital examination.	• Critical care nurse can be instrumental in initiating and maintaining bowel and bladder program.
			– Same hour of day, usually after breakfast. – Maintain appropriate diet.	• Takes advantage of peristalsis initiated by eating.
Nursing Diagnosis#12 Skin integrity, impairment of: Potential, related to: 1. Immobility. 2. Urinary and bowel incontinence. 3. Catabolic state.		Patient's skin will remain intact.	• Assess for alteration in skin integrity.	• Loss of mobility and sensation, impaired circulation, and inadequate nutrition predispose to skin breakdown.
			• Identify areas at risk (weight-bearing bony prominences depending on position assumed) (i.e., supine, prone, and so forth)	• Pressure develops when there is lack of continuous movement and distribution of weight. • Pressure most concentrated between bone and skin surfaces that support body weight.
			• Inspect skin after each position change.	• Reddened areas should blanch within 20-30 minutes after a position change.

Contd...

Problem	*R*	*Objective*	*Nursing Interventions*	*Rationales*
			♦ Inspect for open or ulcerated areas and localized oedema (dependent/orthostatic edema).	♦ Dependent oedema is incriminated in the pathophysiology of skin breakdown; it interferes with cellular nutrition and increases susceptibility of tissues to the effects of pressure. Susceptibility increased during period of spinal shock.
			• Implement measures to promote tissue perfusion.	• Meticulous systematic surveillance of all pressure points from body position, bed, or traction equipment, is the key to maintaining intact skin integrity.
			♦ Provide therapeutics: – Turning and positioning at least every 2 hours. – Document rotation of positions. – Maintain proper alignment. – Passive range-of-motion exercises with dorsiflexion of feet. – Use footboard—splints. – Provide pressure relief device: Air mattress, sheepskin, and so forth. – Administer lotion to bony and reddened areas.	♦ Prevents stasis and tissue ischaemia. – Prevents further neurologic damage, contractures, frozen joints. – Prevents foot drop. – Helps to displace weight more evenly and soften surfaces in contact with pressure points. – Stimulates circulation.
			• Monitor and evaluate response to therapy; monitor nutritional intake.	• Anticipate and prevent problems; intervene early on.
Nursing Diagnosis#13 Potential for physiologic injury: Deep venous thrombosis; related to: 1. Haemostasis associated with immobility; 2. Loss of skeletal muscle pump; 3. Pooling of blood in dilated capacitance vessels (e.g., absence of vasomotor tone during spinal shock).		Patient will: 1. Exhibit adequate peripheral circulation: • Usual skin colour; no cyanosis. • Extremities warm to touch. 2. Maintain consistent calf and thigh circumference measurements. 3. Maintain effective respiratory function. 4. Maintain stable vital signs.	• Monitor for signs and symptoms of deep venous thrombosis. ♦ Assess skin colour and temperature. ♦ Assess calf and thigh circumference.	• Venous stasis, skeletal muscle paralysis, and immobilization place patient at risk of developing deep venous thrombosis and pulmonary embolism. ♦ Assessment for deep venous thrombosis is difficult because of sensorimotor deficits in spinal cord-injured patient. ♦ A slowly increasing circumference suggests a possible underlying thrombosis.
			• Monitor for signs and symptoms of pulmonary embolism ♦ Assess sudden onset of respiratory difficulties (e.g., tachypnoea, dyspnoea, cough with hemoptysis); altered pulmonary function tests: tidal volume, vital capacity; neurologic findings: restlessness and lethargy.	
			• Implement measures to minimize risk of deep venous thrombosis and pulmonary embolism. ♦ Maintain desired hydration. – Monitor intake and output. – Monitor daily weight. – Hematology profile. ♦ Apply antiembolic stocking to both lower extremities. ♦ Institute exercise program. – Passive range-of-motion exercises with dorsiflexion of feet. – Maintenance of proper body alignment.	♦ Prevents increase in blood viscosity, which predisposes to a hypercoagulable state.

Contd...

Problem	*Objective*	*Nursing Interventions*	*Rationales*
		– Use splints as directed. – Avoid crossing legs, using knee gatch, or pillow under knees. – Avoid prolonged sitting or lying in one position. ◆ Administer prophylactic heparin therapy as prescribed.	
Nursing Diagnosis#14 Alteration in nutrition: Less than body requirements, related to: 1. Nothing-by-mouth (NPO) status during spinal shock associated with paralytic ileus. 2. Weakened or absent protective reflexes (e.g., cough, gag, epiglottal closure). 3. Anorexia associated with depression, or inability to self-feed.	Patient will: 1. Maintain baseline body weight within 5 per cent of baseline. 2. Maintain triceps skinfold measurements within baseline range. 3. Maintain laborarory parameters within acceptable physiologic range: • BUN, creatinine. • Total protein, albumin. • Haematology profile. 4. Verbalize increase in appetite. 5. Remain free of infection.	• Obtain a complete nutritional assessment within 24-48 hours of admission. ◆ Baseline nutrition status. ◆ Nutritional requirements of the compromised state. ◆ Blood chemistry and haematology. ◆ Height and weight. ◆ Pre-injury nutritional status: dietary habits, likes, and dislikes.	• Baseline nutritional needs must be identified to ensure adequate nutritional intake; individualized care. ◆ Stress increases energy needs by 50 per cent. ◆ Baseline data assist in planning a nutrition program specific to the needs and desires of patient.
		• Consult with nutritionist. Determine anthropometric data.	
		• Establish and maintain a balanced nutritional state—positive nitrogen balance.	• Balanced nutritional intake promotes wound healing and prevents complications.
		◆ Administer nutritional supplements: (as per unit protocol); parenteral nutrition (TPN and PPN) during period of spinal shock and paralytic ileus. ◆ Initiate nasogastric tube feedings when paralytic ileus subsides but protective reflexes are still compromised. – Assess location/patency of naxogastric tube prior to each feeding. ◆ Evaluate patient's response to therapy: emphasis placed on prevention of complications. ◆ Document daily caloric intake, fluid intake and output, daily weight, vital signs including temperature. ◆ Assess blood chemistry and haematology. ◆ Assess would healing, skin integrity. ◆ Assess patient's overall physical, mental, emotional state.	◆ Depression can cause anorexia.
Nursing Diagnosis#15 Potential for physiologic injury: Episode of autonomic dysreflexia, related to noxious stimuli (e.g., distended bladder or rectum, others.	Patient will not experience an episode of autonomic dysreflexia. • Stable vital signs; without pounding headache and profuse diaphoresis.	• Assess for presence of signs and symptoms of autonomic dysreflexia: Classic manifestations include: paroxysmal elevation in systolic blood pressure (> 240 - 300 mmHg); pounding headache with blurred vision; anxiety, fright, nausea; profuse diaphoresis.	• Vasomotor tone to areas above cord lesion can receive signals from higher brain centers. When blood pressure rises, the sympathetic tone is reduced and vasodilation of these vessels occurs. This accounts for the profuse diaphoresis, headache, and flushing above lesion. ◆ *Below* the lesion, an intense sympathetic response remains as inhibition from higher brain centers is blocked. Blood vessels, therefore, remain severly constricted, resulting in skin palor and coolness, pilomotor erection (i.e., goose bumps), and paralytic Ileus.
		• Implement emergent measures to treat autonomic dysreflexia.	

Contd...

Problem	R	Objective	Nursing Interventions	Rationales
			◆ Follow protocols. – Place patient in upright position. – Monitor blood pressure and heart rate. – Notify physician.	◆ Helps to lower blood pressure. – Physician should be notified if blood pressure is severely elevated (>240 mmHg) and/ or unresponsive to therapy. – This is best treatment for a autonomic dysreflexia.
			– Identify underlying cause and remove if possible. – Administer prescribed antihypertensive drug therapy. – Stay with patient, provide reassurance and emotional support. – Monitor blood pressure every 4 hrs post crisis and for 24 hours thereafter.	◆ Anxiety and fright increase catecholamine secretion, potentiating massive sympathetic response.
			• Implement preventive nursing interventions.	
Nursing Diagnosis#16 Sensory perceptual alteration: Visual, tactile, related to : 1. Immobilization. 2. Sensory deficits associated with disruption of ascennding nerve pathways at level of cord lesion.		Patient will: 1. Verbalize comfort in visualizing people and objects within immediate visual field. 2. Verbalize areas where tactile sensation is perceived.	• Assess underlying reason for alteration in sensory perception. • Assess patient's view of immediate environment. ◆ Consider type of spinal stabilization and use of specialized bed (e.g., Roto-Rest, Clinitron bed). – Skeletal traction. – Halo immobilization brace.	• Viewing immediate environment from patient's perspective assists in arranging environment so desired materials are accessible to patient. ◆ Nurses caring for the patient with a halo should receive continuing education regarding how to maximize effectiveness of brace and prevent complications.
			• Implement measures to make immediate environment accessible to patient's field of vision. ◆ Arrange desired objects as patient requests. ◆ Position mirrors to enhance patient's view.	◆ Helps to provide increased visualization and stimulation.
			◆ Place self within patient's field of vision when speaking to patient. Direct others to do same.	◆ Reduces sensory deprivation.
			• Assess patient's tactile and pain sensation. ◆ Use touch and pinprick stimuli: – Test for sensory perception progressing from area of deficit to area of intact function. – Frequently touch patient in areas demarcated as having sensory perception intact. – Touch patient with different textured objects.	• Touching patient in areas of intact sensation helps to provide stimulation.
			• Implement measures to reduce sensory overload. ◆ Set priorities in care.	• Minimizing distraction helps patient to concentrate on more pertinent stimuli, and on how best to perceive environment from a new vantage point.
			◆ Allow patient choices and options.	◆ Helps to give patient a feeling of some self-control.
			◆ Encourage verbalization: carefully observe facial expression; provide a listening ear.	◆ What is not verbalized may be reflected in patient's facial expression.

Contd...

Problem	*R*	*Objective*	*Nursing Interventions*	*Rationales*
Nursing Diagnosis#17 Coping, alteration in: Patient and family, related to: 1. Situational crisis. 2. Temporary family disorganization.		Patient/family will: 1. Identify useful coping mechanisms. 2. Demonstrate ability to assess, problem-solve, and make decisions. 3. Express realistic expectations of each other.	• Establish a rapport and trusting relationship with patient and family. • Observe patient/family dynamics and interactions. ◆ Assess family resources: usual coping mechanisms. • Implement measures to assist in coping: ◆ Provide opportunity for patient and family members to express feelings and emotions. – Encourage honest communication. – Provide emotional support and relieve anxieties by making appropriate explanations. ◆ Keep patient and family informed: – Be honest and realistic. – Be accessible to patient/family. – Allow time for questions to be asked and feelings vented. ◆ Increasingly include patient/family in decision-making process as they demonstrate a readiness to do so (e.g., the ability to verbalize and discuss feelings).	• These observations may help to identify strengths, weaknesses, and effective coping capabilities. ◆ Long-term rehabilitation places tremendous burden on family resources. ◆ Recognizing feelings and emotions is the first step in dealing with them. – Support and reassurance assist patient/family to cope with catastrophic event. ◆ Enables patient to feel useful, to have some control. ◆ Promotes involvement in the rehabilitation process.
Nursing Diagnosis#18 Social isolation, related to: 1. Immobility. 2. Prolonged hospitalization. 3. Depression.		Patient will: 1. Demonstrate desire to interact and maintain relationships. 2. Verbalize feelings of isolation. 3. Participate in diversional activities.	• Assess patient's usual degree of social interaction. • Assess for signs/symptoms suggestive of social isolation. ◆ Specific signs/symptoms might include: Expression of loneliness or feelings of rejection; flat affect; depression; uncommunicative; withdrawn, preoccupied. • Encourage verbalization regarding patient's sense of isolation. ◆ Assess patient's feelings about self: Sense of being "out of control": hopelessness. • Develop a plan of action to decrease feelings of social isolation. ◆ Provide effective alternative method of communication. ◆ Encourage interactions with significant others. ◆ Assist patient to set up visiting schedule with family/friends. ◆ Encourage participation in diversional activities. ◆ Initiate referrals to appropriate resources (e.g., occupational, recreational therapist when feasible).	• It is important to establish a therapeutic nurse/patient relationship, one in which the patient is able to comfortably air thoughts and concerns. ◆ Helps to reassure that his/her needs are being met, and they have not been forgotten. ◆ Knowing when to expect a visit or call can be reassuring.

Health Education-Patient and parents regularly, autonomic dysreflection Halo-vest-care, skin care, and Bowel managers after signal card injury are very impressive. The following guidelines are helpful for health events.

1. *Autonomic dysreflexin*

Patient and family must know in signs and sympton of autonomic dysreflection, so that provides intervention can occur. These induce the following:

- Sudden onset of acute headache.
- Elevation in blood pressure and/or reduction to pulse rate.
- Flushed race and upper chest above the level of the lesion and pale extremies (below the level of the lesion).
- Sweating above the level of the lesion.
- Nasal congestion.
- Feeling of apprehension.

Immediate intervention include the following:

- Raise the person to a sitting position.
- Remove the stimulus (local imagiction, kinked urinary catheter).
- Call the primary care provides of above action do not relieve signs and mystery.

Efforts to decrease the likelihood of autonomic dysreflection includes the following

- Maintain regular bowel function.
- If manual rectal stimulation is used, local anaesthetic may reduce stimulation of autonomic dysreflectic.
- Monitor urine output.
- Wear a medic-alert bracelet indicating a history of autonomic dysreflection.

2. *Halo vest care*

The following reacting guidelines for a rational with a halo vest:

- Inspect the pins on the halo traction ring. Report to health care provider that your pins are loose or of there are signs of infection inducing redness, tenderness, swelling or damage at the insertion sites
- Clean around pin sites carefully with hydrogen peroxide on a catton swab. Repeat the procedure using water.
- Use alcohol swabs to cleanse pin sites of any dranage.
- Apply antibiotic ointment as prescribed.
- To provide skin care, have the patient lie down on a bed with his or her head resting on a pillow to reduce pressure on the brace.

Loosen one side of the vest, gently wash the skin under the with soap and water, resent, and then dry not thoroughly. At the same time, check the skin for pressure points, redness, swelling bruising, or chafing close the open side and repeat the proceed on his opposite side.

- If the vest becomes wet or damage not can be carefully dried with a blow dryer.
- An assistive device (of cane or walker) may be used to provide greater balance. Flat shoes should be worn.
- Turn the entire body, not just the head and neck. When trying to view sideways.
- In case of emergency, keep a set of wrenches close to the halo vest at all times.
- Marie the vest swap such than consistent budding and fit can be maintained.

3. *Skincare for patient with SCI*

Skin breakdown is a potential problem following SCI. The following measurers are used to decrease this possibility.

i. Change positions frequently
   - If in a wheelchair, lift self up and shift weight every 15 to 30 minutes
   - If in bed, a regular turning schedule (at least every 2 hours) than includes sides, back and abdomen in enraged to charge position.
   - Use special mattresses and wheelchair cushions.
   - Use pillows to protect bony-prominences when in bed.

ii. Monitor skin condition
   - Inspect the skin frequently for areas of redness, swelling, and breakdown.
   - Keep finger nails trimmed to avoid scratches and abrasions.
   - If a wound develops follow wound care management, which includes keeping wound, open to air and applying treatments as prescribed.

4. *Bowel managements*

The following are some guidelines for a patient with a signal card injury:

- Optimal nutritional intake includes:
  3 well-balanced meals each day.
  2 servings from the milk groups.
  2 or more savings from the major group, including beef, poultry, eggs and dish.
  4 or more serving from the vegetable and fruit groups.
  4 or more serving from the broad and cereal group.
- Fibre intake should be approximately 20 to 30 g per day gradually increase amaine and fiber eaten over 1 to 2 weeks.
- Three quasts of fluid per day should be consumed unless contaminated water or fruit juice, should be used and caffenated beverages such as coffee, tea and cola should be avoided. Fluid softens hard stools caffeine stimulates fluid loss through urination.
- Food thus produce gas (beans) or upper GI upset (spicy foods) should be avoided.
- Timing: A regular schedule for bowel evacuation should be established. A good time is 30 minutes after the first meal of the day.
- Position: If possible, an upright position with feet flat on the floor or a steps stool enhances bowel evacuation. Staying on the toilet, commode, or bedpan the longer than 20 to 30 minutes causes skin breakdown. Based on stability someone may need to struck with the patient.
- Activity: Exercise is important for bowel function. In addition to improving muscle tone, not also increases GI transit time and increases appetite. Muscles should be exercised. This

includes stretching, range-of-motion and position changing.

- Drug Treatment: Laxatives, including suppositories may be necessary to stimulate a bowel movement. However, these drugs can be habit forming and thus should only be taken when necessary. Manual stimulation of the rectum may also be helpful in initiating defections.

Management and Neurogenic Bladder

Diagnosis
- Neurological examination
- Cysto metropram
- IV pyelogram
- Urine culture

Drug Therapy
- Bethanechol (urecholine) for increasing detrusor muscle strength
- Asoribic acid (vit. C) for acidification of urine
- Methenamine mandelete (Mandelamine)—and urinary antisystetic
- Relaxation of urethral syswinter

Nutrition
- Low calcium diet (< 1g/day).
- Fluid intake a 1800-2000 ml/day.

Urine drainage
- Reflex reasoning
- Intermittant catherization
- Indwelling catheter
- Urinous diversion surgery

Table 11.7: Nursiwng care plan for the patient with spinal cord compression

Problem	*R Objective*	*Nursing Interventions*	*Rationales*
Nursing Diagnosis # 1 Potential for injury, related to: 1. Sensory deficits.	Patient will: 1. Remain free from injury while hospitalised.	• Keep siderails up at all times. • Have call light and personal items within patient's reach. Instruct patient to call for assistance if desiring to get out of bed. • Assess level of consciousness as indicated. • Assess sensory level q shift.	• Patients receiving narcotics for pain relief may have an altered sensorium. • Loss of sensation places patient at increased risk of injury
Nursing Diagnosis # 2 Alteration in comfort: Acute pain, related to: 1. Damaged spinal cord.	Patient will: 1. Utilize measures effective in managing pain. 2. Verbalize relief from pain. 3. Present relaxed facies and overall demeanour.	• Assess patient for intensity, radiation, and character of pain. • Inform patient and/or significant others of available methods of pain relief. • Administer pain medication as requested and prescribed. Assess for effect in 10-20 minutes. • Explain importance of pain medication in patient's progress. • Collaborate with physician and patient in altering pain medication as needed. • Suggest alternate positions. • Log roll when needed. • Position on eggerate mattress or other pressure relief device.	• Pain associated with spinal cord compression may be especially severe. • Patient should be encouraged to request pain medication early on instead of waiting until the pain becomes unbearable.
Nursing Diagnosis # 3 Alteration in bowel and urinary elimination: incontinence and/or constipation, related to: 1. Nerve disruption. 2. Immobility. 3. Narcotic administration.	Patient will: 1. Maintain regular bowel elimination without constipation or fecal impaction.	• Explain need for scheduled bowel elimination program. • Monitor intake and output q shift. • Instruct patient on need for good hydration. • Force fluids as necessary unless contraindicated.	• It is essential for the patient to establish and maintain regular bowel elimination. The patient's usual bowel habits should be assessed and incorporated into daily schedule. • Patient/family should be able to explain the importance of hydration and diet high in fiber, in terms of overall bowel function. • Patient/family should be aware of signs and symptoms suggestive of

Contd...

Problem	*R*	*Objective*	*Nursing Interventions*	*Rationales*
				constipation: Abdominal fullness or distention, loss of appetite, nausea, headache, feeling of fullness in rectum. • Appearance of diarrheal stool may suggest the presence of fecal impaction.
			• Administer stool softeners/laxatives as needed and prescribed. • Consult dietician to increase fiber in foods.	
		2. Adhere to a bladder control program.	• Offer fluids to patient q 2 hr. • Offer bedpan or assist patient to bathroom q 2 hr. • Palpate bladder for distention.	• Urinary retention can predispose to infection.
			• Explain importance of bladder program.	• Patient/significant others should be able to check for urinary retention of which the patient may not be aware.
Nursing Diagnosis # 4 Potential impairment of skin integrity, related to: 1. Decreased mobility.		Patient will: 1. Be free from skin breakdown.	• Inspect patient's skin integrity q shift.	• Loss of mobility and sensation, immunosuppressed state, and altered nutrition place patient at greater risk of skin breakdown. • Meticulous surveillance of pressure areas is essential to maintain skin integrity.
			• Encoruage/assist patient to turn q 2 hr while in bed. • Apply lotion to dry skin q shift. • Apply eggerate mattress or sheepskin to bed. • Force fluids as necessary unless contraindicated.	
Nursing Diagnosis # 5 Impaired physical mobility, related to: 1. Motor neuron damage.		Patient will: 1. Maintain muscle tone and coordination. • Demonstrate active range of motion of all extremities. • Verbalize importance of exercise and avoidance of fatigue.	• Inspect muscles of arms and legs for atrophy and involuntary movements. • Assess for muscle coordination. • Perform active and/or passive ROM exercises to all extremities qid. • Encourage activity as prescribed/tolerated. • Collaborate with Rehabilitation Department regarding mobility and an individualized exercise plan.	• A baseline assessment should be performed to establish the patient's physical capabilities. • Actions should be performed to maintain muscle strength, and mobility. • Family participation in exercise regimen should be encouraged.
Nursing Diagnosis # 6 Alteration in self-concept, related to: 1. Incontinence and immobility.		Patient and/or significant other will: 1. Begin accepting the change in usual function. • Verbalize feelings • Initiates discussion of disease and impact on lifestyle.	• Explain to patient and/or significant others reasons for changes in muscle control. • Assess patient's/significant other's usual coping mechanisms, encouraging positive ones. • Encourage patient and/or significant other to discuss their feelings regarding these changes.	• Recognizing one's feeling and emotions is the first step in dealing with them. • Observing patient/family/significant other interactions may assist in determining strengths and effective coping capability.
Nursing Diagnosis # 7 Alteration nutrition: less than bone requirements, related to: 1. Presence of a neoplasm in the		Patient will: 1. Meet the estimated nutrients: • Calories per day • Grams of protein per day as established by	*Parenteral nutrition* • Monitor daily intake and output, calorie count, and weights. Notify physician for weight gain greater than 2 lb in 24 hr. • Monitor blood glucose levels and ketone levels in urine q 6 hr.	• Monitors effectiveness of therapy. • The increased glucose load may overtax the pancreas and its ability

Contd...

Problem	*R*	*Objective*	*Nursing Interventions*	*Rationales*
GI tract preoperatively and NPO status postoperatively.		the nutritional support service. 2. Maintain body weight within 5 per cent of baseline. 3. Maintain laboratory data within acceptable range: BUN, creatinine, electrolytes, glucose, albumin, and transferrin levels.		to produce insulin. Patient may require regular insulin coverage.
			• Monitor lab values (while on TPN): ◆ Hematology profile. ◆ Serum glucose and electrolytes, calcium, phosphorus. ◆ BUN and creatinine. ◆ Liver profile. ◆ Serum cholesterol, triglycerides. ◆ Total protein and serum albumin, transferrin. ◆ Coagulation profile.	• Obtain full compliment of blood work prior to initiation of TPN for baseline values. Repeat weekly. ◆ Monitors adequacy of replacement therapy.
			• Maintain a constant IV infusion via infusion pump. Should therapy be interrupted, run dextrose 10W at the TPN rate.	• Allows pancreas to adjust to a high glucose level.
			• Administer vitamin K 20 mg IM once per week as prescribed.	• Provides nutritional supplement.
			• Infuse lipids (10 or 20%) and amino acids daily as prescribed.	
			Enteral tube feedings	
			• Monitor daily intake and output, calorie counts. ◆ Weigh patient 3 times per week. ◆ Monitor serum glucose and ketone levels in urine q 6 hrs.	• Monitors effectiveness of therapy.
			• Monitor laboratory values: CBC with differential, albumin, and TIBC, electrolytes, BUN, and glucose.	• Obtain full complement weekly.
			• Place continuous tube feeding on infusion pump, keep load of bud elevated 30•, check residual volume of feeding q 4 hours. If > 150 cc, discontinue feeding for 1 hour. If feeding held for more than 2 hours notify physician	
			◆ Irrigate feeding tube with at least 20 cc water q 4 hours.	◆ Patients receiving enteral nutrition in high osmolar concentrations require free water to prevent dehydration.
			• Notify physician if patient develops diarrhoea.	• Indicates patient's intolerance to glucose and/or osmolar concentration. May require either a decrease in rate or concentration. Patient may require antidiarrhoeal medication to prevent fluid and electrolyte imbalance.
			• Administer formula at room temperature. Discard unusued feeding q 4 hr.	
			• Provide frequent mouth care.	• Aesthetically pleasing to patient. Keeps mucous membranes moist and intact.
Nursing Diagnosis #8 Potential for infection, related to: 1. Central line and TPN infusion.		Patient will: 1. Be free from catheter and infusion-related infections.	• Monitor for symptoms of infection, i.e. fever, tachycardia, increased WBC count.	• Patients receiving TPN are susceptible to infection due to high glucose concentration.
			• Perform central venous line site care as per unit protocol. The area is cleansed with accetone and betadine and redressed with a transparent and occlusive dressing.	• TPN solution is a media for bacterial growth. The central line allows for systemic access into the patient.
			• Assess dressing integrity and catheter site q shift for redness, swelling, pain, or drainage. Obtain cultures as needed. Tubing changes are done daily. TPN bottles are discontinued after 24 hours.	

Contd...

Problem	*R*	*Objective*	*Nursing Interventions*	*Rationales*
			• Note: Once a central line is dedicated for TPN use, it should not be used for additional medication, infusions, CVP readings, or blood aspiration.	• Allows for additional entry of bacteria into system.
Nursing Diagnosis #9 Social isolation related to prolonged hospital stay.		Patient will: 1. Maintain social contacts developed prior to surgery.	• Encourage verbalization regarding social contacts. • Consult social service when indicated. • Promote privacy for patients and visitors.	• Identifies contacts that the nursing staff may make on behalf of the patient while in ICU.

*PROCEDURE 11.1 *ASSISTING THE PATIENT UNDERGOING A LUMBAR PUNCTURE.*

Equipment: Sterile lumbar puncture set, Xylocaine 1-2 per cent., Sterile gloves, Band aid

STEPS OF PROCEDURE

Nursing action	*Rationale*
Preparatory Phase	
1. Before procedure, the patient should empty bladder and bowel.	1. To enhance comfort.
2. Give a step-by-step summary of the procedure. For lying position : See accompanying figure.	2. Reassures the patient and gains cooperation.
Technique of Lumbar	
3. Position the patient on side with a small pillow between legs. Patient should be lying on a firm surface.	3. The spine is maintained in a horizontal position. The pillow between the legs prevents the upper leg from rolling forward.
4. Instruct the patient to arch the lumbar segment of back and draw knees upto abdomen, chin to chest, clasping knees with hands.	4. This posture offers maximal widening of the interspinous spaces and affords easier entry into the subarachnoid space.
5. Assist the patient in maintaining this position by supporting behind the knees and neck. Assist the patient to maintain the posture throughout the examination.	5. Supporting the patient helps prevent sudden movements, which can produce a traumatic (bloody) tap and thus impede correct diagnosis.
For Sitting Position	
6. Have the patient straddle a straight-back chair (facing the back) and rest head against arms, which are folded on the back of the chair.	6. In obese patients and those who have difficulty in assuming an arched side-lying position, this posture may allow more accurate identification of the spinous processes and interspaces.
Performance Phase (By the physician)	
1. The skin is prepared with antiseptic solution, and the skin and subcutaneous spaces are infiltrated with local anaesthetic agent.	1. To reduce risk of contamination and decrease pain.

Contd...

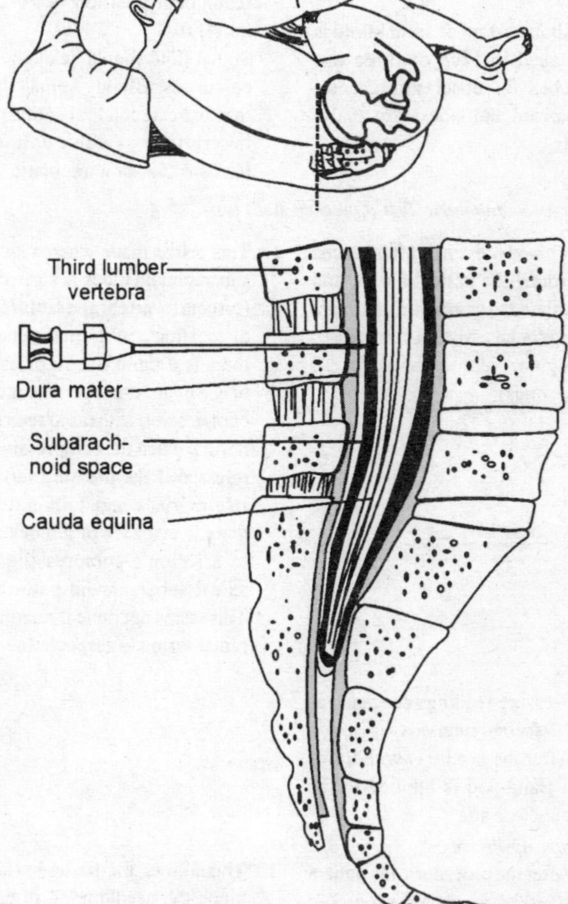

Fig.11.4: Technique of lumbar puncture.

2. A spinal puncture needle is introduced at the L3-L4 interspace. The needle is advanced until the "give" of the ligamentum flavum is felt and the needle enters the subarachnoid space. The manometer is attached to the spinal puncture needle.	2. L_3-L_4 interspace is below the level of the spinal cord.
3. After the needle enters the sub-	3. This manoeuvre prevents a false

Contd...

Nursing action	*Rationale*
arachnoid space, help the patient to slowly straighten legs.	increase in intraspinal pressure. Muscle tension and compression of the abdomen give falsely high pressure.
4. Instruct the patient to breathe quietly (not to hold breath or strain) and not to talk.	4. Hyperventilation may lower a truly elevated pressure. Talking can elevate CSF pressure.
5. The initial pressure reading is obtained by measuring the level of the fluid column after it comes to rest.	5. With respiration there is normally some fluctuation of spinal fluid in the manometer. Normal range of spinal fluid pressure with the patient in the lateral recumbent position is 70-200 mm H_20.
6. About 2-3 ml of spinal fluid is placed in each of three test tubes for observation, comparison and laboratory analysis.	6. Spinal fluid should be clear and colourless. Bloody spinal fluid may indicate cerebral confusion, laceration, subarachnoid haemorrhage or a traumatic tap.
Lumbar Manometric Test (Quecken stedt test).	
1. A blood pressure cuff is placed around the patient's neck and inflated to a pressure of 20 mm Hg (or an assistant compresses jugular vein or veins for 10 seconds).	1. This test is made when a spinal subarachnoid block is suspected (tumour, vertebral fracture or dislocation), in normal persons there is a rapid rise in pressure of CSF in response to jugular compression with rapid return to normal when the compression is released if the pressure fails to rise or rises and falls slowly, there is evidence of a block due to a lesion's compressing the spinal subarachnoid pathways. This test is not done if an intracranial lesion is suspected.
2. Pressure readings are made at 10-second intervals.	
3. After the needle is withdrawn a Band-Aid is applied to the puncture site.	
Follow-up Phase	
1. After the procedure, the patient is asked to remain prone (on abdomen) for about 3 hours.	1. This allows the tissue surfaces along the needle track to come together to prevent cerebrospinal fluid leakage.

PROCEDURE 11.2. INTRACRANIAL PRESSURE MONITORING (ICP)

Equipment: Sterile gloves
Airway
Ambu Bag
ICP Monitoring system (intraventricular, subarachnoid and epidural)
IV pole or standard on which to mount the system
IV solution as ordered
IV high pressure tubing
Burr hole tray for insertion or as needed.
Topical anaesthetic.

STEPS OF PROCEDURE

Nursing action	*Rationale*
Preparatory Phase	
1. Explain the need for extensive, continuous assessment and appropriate nursing intervention to the family and patient.	1. Explanations will decrease anxiety, allow patient and family a sense of control, and encourage compliance with procedure.
2. Gather and assemble equipment. Flush lines with ordered solution according to manufacturer's directions.	2. Availability of equipment will enhance success of procedure.
3. Calibrate equipment according to directions.	3. Accurate interpretation of ICP values and wave patterns will depend on appropriate baseline function.
4. Perform neurologic assessment.	4. Patient baseline must be established to determine changes and guide therapy.
5. Administer light sedation/ analgesia if patient is agitated.	5. Procedure is invasive and injury may result with excessive patient movement.
Performance Phase	
1. Establish head of bed at 30 degrees.	1. Facilitates venous drainage decreasing intracranial volume and prevents collapse of the ventricles if ventricular placement.
2. Shave and cleanse the operative site.	2. Removes bacteria from the site, reducing the risk of infection.
3. Establish the sterile field.	3. A sterile field reduces the risk of infection.
4. Assist with burr hole and placement of intracranial monitoring system.	4. Direct monitoring of intracranial pressure allows for early detecion of decompensation and management of complications.
5. Connect monitoring catheter to transducer/monitoring equipment according to directions.	5. Allows for conduction of intracranial and cerebral perfusion pressures to the interpretive component of the system.
6. Observe numerical readings and wave patterns. Adjust characteristics to obtain optimal visual reading.	6. Changes in baseline readings indicate alterations in intracranial pressure or problems with the mechanics of the monitering system.
7. Cover the catheter insertion site with a sterile dressing. Observe for possible CSF drainage depending on the placement of the cathether.	7. The skull and meninges have been penetrated leaving the patient at risk for infection.
8. Adjust alarm system according to ordered parameters.	8. Alarms should be on at all times to alert the nurse away from the bedside of ongoing adverse changes.
Follow-up Phase	
1. Frequently assess the patient and the system to ascertain neurologic status and patency of the system.	1. Manipulation of the system may inadvertently close the system, leaving the patient without the benefit of monitoring.
2. Irrigate the system using sterile technique according	2. Irrigation helps maintain the patency of the system.

Contd...

Nursing action	*Rationale*
to policy or p.r.n. as indicated to maintain patency.	
3. Report dampened wave forms, and have 1 cc of normal saline available for irrigation if indicated.	3. The tip of the catheter may have migrated against the ventricular wall or cerebral tissue depending on location, or ventricular collapse may be imminent, irrigation is done by the healthcare provider in this case.

Nursing action	*Rationale*
4. Assess head dressing for CSF drainage, change dressing according to policy.	4. Because of its high glucose content, CSF is an excellent media for bacterial growth.
5. Adjust the height of the transducer of the system to the level of the patient's ventricles (inner canthus of eye and tip of ear) with every position change for accurate readings.	5. Position of the transducer in relation to the ventricles will influence the accuracy of the readings because of fluid gradient pressures.

Haematological Nursing

HAEMATOLOGICAL NURSING

Haematology is the study of blood and blood forming tissues. This includes the blood cells, the bone marrow, the spleen and the lympth system. A basic knowledge of haematology is useful in clinical settings to evaluate the patient's ability to transport oxygen and carbon dioxide coagulate blood, and combat infection. Another important homeostatic function of the blood cells is removing old and dead cells. This functions is accompanied by the mononuclear phagocyte system (MPS). This is formerly known as the reticuloendothelial system (RES) is composed of monocytes and macrophages. Diseases associated with MPS are diverse in their underlying pathological manifestations disease course, and response to treatment. Most often the accompanying symptoms result from interference with normal development and function of the blood components; erythrocytes (RBCs) thrombocytes (platelets) leukocytes (WBCs) and altered haematopoiesis (blood cell production).

Normally, homeostasis is maintained through a balance between the rate of production of normal blood cells and the rate of destruction. Disorders of blood occurs when the balance is lost. Disturbances of the coagulation mechanism also result in blood disorder. Nurse has to play an important role in management of these conditions associated with haemotological disorders.

ASSESSMENT OF THE HAEMATOLOGICAL SYSTEM

Most of the evaluation of the haematologic system is based on a thorough health history. In addition other key points to include are family history, drug history, exposure to chemicals and general nonspecific complaints offered by the patient.

Health History

A thorough history inccludes detailed information about the person's symptoms and through review system. The vagueness symptomatology of disorders of the haemotological system makes a thorough assessment is essential, common symptoms include, shortness of breath, fatigue, bruising, tarry stools, constipation, lymphadenopathy, flue-like illness, and musculoskeletal pain. Unfortunately these symptoms occur in a vast number of other common disorders. The cause of any haematological abnormality must be assiduously pursued. The importance of accurate diagnosis, combined with the diverse and usually nonspecific signs and symptoms, makes it likely that the person will become involved in arduous diagnostic process. It is also important to learn whether the patient has had prior haematological problem (mononuclosis, malabsorption, liver disorders, thrombosis and spleen disorders and leukaemia, etc.).

Family History

The existence of inherited haematological disorders such as sickle cell disease, and malignant tumours, requires detailed family history. Questions regarding disease or presence of symptoms among relatives should include reference to parents and siblings. Most specific disorders such as haemophilia may involve questions to grand fathers, uncles and nephews. For other disorders, female relatives need to be considered. Information regarding instances of severe or prolonged bleeding after trauma, dental extractions or surgery and occurrence of jaundice or anaemia in relatives also should be obtained.

Drugs and Chemical

Drugs may induce or potentiate haematological disease. Most notable are the haematological effect of the cytotoxic drugs used in cancer therapy and the neutropoenia associated with chloromphenical. Do not negate the importance of over-the-counter medication. Certain chemicals may exist a potentially harmful effect on haemopoietic system. To obtain a history of exposure to chemicals, an occupational history is useful. Some drugs affecting the haematologic function and laboratory values are as follows:

- Antituberculin (e.g. PAS) leads to leukocytes secondary to hypersensitivity and INH leads to neutropoenia.
- Antifungal (e.g. amphotaracin B) leads to anaemia.
- Antiseizure (e.g. carbomazephin) leads to anaemia, leukopnoea, thrombocytopoenia.
- Antibiotic (e.g. chloromphenical)–Anaemia, neutrepoenia, thrombocytoponea.
- Antihypertensin (e.g. Aldos terone) haemolytic anaemia.
- Anti-inflammatory (e.g. phenylbutazone)–anaemia, leukopoenia, neutropoenia, thrombocytopoenia.
- Diuretics (chlorothiazic)–Thrombocytopoenia (occasional).
- Antiarrhythmic (e.g. procainamad HCL)–Agranulocytosis.

- Antibacterial (e.g. bacterim, septran)–Anaemia, leukopoenia, neutropoenia thrombocytopoenia).
- Antineoplastics (immunosuppression)–Anaemia leukopoenia, neutropoenia and thrombocytopoenia).
- NSAIDs—Inhibition of platelet aggregation
- Analgesia, antipyretics—Reduced platelet aggregation, prolonged bleeding time

History of Fever, Fatigue and Malaise

Fever is common manifestation of many haematological disorders and information about history of fever should be obtained. In addition, information about fatigue and malaise are also obtained.

Physical Examination

A complete physical examination is necessary to accurately examine all systems that affect or are affected by the haematologic system. It is useful to recognize target organs and alteration that may reflect haematological disease. The nurse must be aware of signs and symptoms can be caused by haematological problems, even though these are not the obvious causes. The common assessment of abnormalities of haematologic systems and their causes include:

Skin

- Pallor of skin or nailbeds–Decrease in quantity of haemoglobin (anaemia).
- Flushing–Increase in haemoglobin (polycythaemia).
- Jaundice–Accumulation of bile pigments caused by rapid or excess haemolysis.
- Purpura, petachiae, ecchymois, haematoma–Haemostatic deficiency of platelets or clotting factors resulting haemorrhage into skin.
- Excoriation and pruritus–Scratching from intense pruritus secondary to disorders such as Hodgkin diseases; increased bilirubin.
- Leg ulcers–Common in sickle cell disease, especially prominent on the malleoli on the ankles.
- Brownish discolouration–Haemosiderin and melanin from the breakdown of erythrocytes, iron deposits, secondary to transfusional iron overload.
- Cyanosis–Reduced haemoglobin.
- Telengiectasis–Hyperemic spots caused by capillary or small artery dilation, small angioma with a tendency to haemorrhage.
- Angioma–Benign tumour consisting primarily of blood or lymph vessels.
- Spider nevus–Breached growth of dilated capillaries resembling a spider associated with liver disease and elevated oestrogen levels as in pregnancy.

Nails

- Rigid longitudinally, flattened concave–Chronic severe iron-deficiency anaemia.

Eyes

- Jaundiced sclera–Accumulation of bile pigments because of rapid or excessive haemolysis.
- Conjunctival pallor–Reduction in quantity of haemoglobin (anaemia)
- Retinal haemorrhage–More frequent in concurrent states of thrombocytopoenia and anaemia than with thrombocytopoenia alone.
- Dilation of veins–Polycythaemia.

Mouth

- Pallor–Reduction in quantity of haemoglobin (anaemia)
- Gingival and mucosole ulceration–Neutropoenia, severe anaemia.
- Gingival infiltration (swelling, reddening bleeding)–Leukaemia caused by impeded movement of granulocytes and monocytes through gingivia tooth attachment into mucous membrane or by inability of impaired leucocytes to combat oral infections.
- Gingival or mucosal bleeding–Haemorrhagic disease, thrombocytopoenia.
- Smooth tongue texture–Pernicious and iron deficiency anaemia.

Lymph Nodes

- Lymphadenopathy, tenderness–Normal response to infection in infants and children, cancerous invasion is causative factor in adult's enlargement caused by infection, foreign infiltrates, or metabolic disturbances especially with lipids.

Chest

- Widened mediastinum–Enlarged lymphnodes.
- Generalized sternal tenderness–Leukaemia resulting from increased bone marrow cellularity causing increase in pressure and bone erosion.
- Localized sternal tenderness–Multiple myeloma as result of stretching periosteum
- Tachycardia–Compensatory mechanism in anaemia to increase cardiac output.
- Murmurs–Usually systolic murmur in anaemia caused by increased quantity and speed of low viscosity blood going through pulmonic valves.
- (Carotid bruits)–Anaemia caused by increased flow of ion viscosity blood swirling through blood vessels.
- Angina pectoris–anaemia.

Abdomen

- Hepatomegaly–leukaemia, cirrhosis or fibrosis secondary to iron overload from sickle cell or thalassaemia.
- Splenic bruits and rubs–splenic infarction.
- Increasing abdominal girth–Hepatomegaly, splenomegaly, abdominal bleeding.

Nervous System

- Pain and touch. Position and vibratory sensation, tendon reflexes.
  - Impaired nervous system functions because of cobalamin deficiency or compression of nerve by masses.
- Decreasing level of consciousness–intracranial haemorrhage needs thorough neurological examination.

Back and Extremities

- Backpain—Acute haemolytic reaction from flank pain because of renal involvement with haemolysis; multiple myeloma from enlarged tumours that stretch periosteum or weaken suppressive tissue causing ligament strain, muscle spasm, and sickle cell diseases.
- Arthralgia–Leukaemia as a result of aching in bones that contain marrow, sickle cell disease from haemarthosis.
- Bone pain–Bone invasion by leukaemia cells, bone demineralisation resulting from various haematoptotic and solid malignancies enhancing possibility of pathological fracture; sickle cell disease.

Diagnostic Studies of the Haemotological System

The nurse should recognise the need to thoroughly explain any diagnostic procedures to the patient. It is common for patient to be anxious when faced with illness. Therefore, instructions must be simple, clear and repeated when necessary to decrease anxiety and ensure the patient's compliance with preparatory protocol. Whether studies are performed on an outpatient or an inpatient basis. Written instruction regarding the procedure facilitates compliance. If a diverse ethnic population is served, it is helpful to have instructions translated into the patient's dominant language.

The repeated acquisition of blood specimen may be distressing for the patient. Some patients and staff members become concerned that amount of blood withdrawn for tests could lead adverse effects. Although multiple blood studies may be uncomfortable, it anoys in rate situation that diagnostic blood withdrawal predisposes the patient to significant volume loss. The nurse must capitalize on all appropriate opportunities to use independent nursing assessment and clinical judgement. For example, when there is suspicion of bleedings, it is important to perform guaiac test of the stool, nasogastric secretions or emesis and hematest of the urine.

The complete blood count studies and their purposes and normal values are as follows:

A. *RBC Count*

1. *Haemoglobin* (Hb) is a measurement of gas-carrying capacity of the red blood cells. Normal values male 13-18 g/100 ml, female 12-16 g/100 ml.
2. *Haematocrit* (Hct) is a measure of packed cell volume of RBCs expressed as a percentage of the total blood volume (Normal values male: 45-52 per cent Female 37-48 per cent).
3. Total RBC counts: Count of number of circulating RBCs (Male 4.6-6.1 million/mm, Female 4.0-5.4 million/mm).
4. *Red cell indices:* Mean corpuscular volume (MCV).

$$= \frac{\text{Hct} \times 10}{\text{RBC} \times 10^6}$$

- MCV is the determination of relative size of RBCs, low MCV reflection of microcytosis, high MCV reflection of macrocytosis (Normal 80-95).
- Mean corpuscular Hgb (MCH) is a measurement of average weight of Hb/RBC; low MCH indication of microcytosis or hypochromia, high MCH indication of macrocytosis (Normal 27-33 Pg).

$$\text{MCH} = \frac{\text{HB} \times 10}{\text{RBC} \times 10^6}$$

- Mean corpuscular high concentrate (MCHC) is an evaluation of RBC saturation with Hb; Low MCHC indication of hypochromia high-MCHC evident in spherocytosis (Normal 32-36 per cent).

$$\text{MCHC} = \frac{\text{Hb}}{\text{HCt}} \times 100.$$

B. *WBC counts*

1. *WBC total count* (TC) is the measurement of total number of leukocytes (normal 5000 to 10,000/mm).
2. *WBC differential count* (DC) is the determination of whether each kind of WBC is present in proper proposition, determination of absolute value by multiplying percentage of cell type to a total WBC count and dividing by 100 (Neutrophile 55-70 per cent, eosinophils 1-4 per cent, basophils 0-1 per cent, monocyte 2-6 per cent and lymphocyte 25-40 per cent) DC count totals 100 per cent.

C. *Platelet counts* is the measurement of number of platelets available to maintain platelet clotting functions (not measurements of quality of platelet function). Normal value of platelets is 150,000-400,000/mm.

D. *Erythrocytic sedimentation* rate (ESR)

ESR measures the sedimentation or setting of RBCs and used as a nonspecific measure of many diseases, especially inflammatory condition. Increased ESR are common during acute and chronic inflammatory reactions when cell destruction is increased. The normal ESR in males–1-15 mm in 1 hour; females–1-20 mm in 1 hour.

E. *Blood typing and Rh Factors*

ABO blood groups are named for the antigen found on the RBCs compatibility is based on the antibodies present in the serum.

Blood group	*RBCs Aggluti-nogen(s)*	*Serum Aggluti-nogen(s)*	*Compatible Donor blood groups*	*Incompatible Donor blood groups*
A	A	Anti-B	A & O	B & AB
B	B	Anti-A	B & O	A & AB
AB	A and B (universal reciepient)	Neither	A, B, AB & O	None
O	Neither (universal donor)	Anti A & anti B	O	A, B & AB

Other Haematological Studies

1. *Urine studies*

Bence Jones protein studies is an electrophoretic measurement used to detect the presence of Bence Jones protein, which is found in most cases of multiple myeloma. Negative findings indicate patient is normal. Nurses should acquire random urine specimen for urine study.

2. *Radioisotope studies*
   - *Liver/spleen scan*—Radioisotope is injected intravenously. Images from the radioactive emissions are used to evaluate the structure of the spleen and liver. Patient is not a source of radioactivity.
   - *Bone scan* Same procedure as spleen scan except used for the purpose of evaluating the structures of bone.
   - *Isotopic lymphangiography* Radionuclide study is used to assess lympth nodes and lymph system. Tectinetium 99 m is used. Technique is less invasive than radiographic lymphangiograph.

     No specific nursing responsibilities for radioisotopic study.

3. *Radiologic studies*

- *Lymphangiosgraphy* The purpose is to evaluate deep lympth nodes. Radiopaque oil-based dye is infused slowly into the lymph vessels via small needles in the dorsum of each foot. Radiographs are taken immediately and on the next day.

  The nursing responsibilities include:

  - Inform the patient about what to anticipate.
  - Obtain consent form.
  - Assess for iodine sensitivity.
  - Give preparatory sedation, if indicated.
  - Instruct that patient's urine will be blue from the dye exretion for 1-2 days.
  - Inform patient that transient fever–general malaise may be experienced for 12-24 hours.
  - Watch for signs of oil embolus to lung (hacking cough, dyspnoea, pleuritic pain and haemoptysis.
  - Computed tomography (CT) A noninvasive radiologic examination using computer-assisted X-ray evaluates the spleen, liver, or lymph nodes. No specific nursing responsibility required.
- *MRI* is the noninvasive procedure for sensitive images of soft tissue without using contrast dyes. No ionizing radiation is required. Technique used to evaluate spleen, liver and lymph nodes. Here nurse instructs patient to remove all metal objects and asks about any history of surgical insertion of staples, plates, or other metal appliances. Inform patient of need to lie still in small chamber.

4. *Biopsies*
   - *Bone marrow*—Technique involves removal of bone marrow through a locally anaesthesized site to evaluate the status of the blood-forming tissue. It is used to diagnose multiple myeloma, all types of leukaemia, and some lymphomas and to stage of some tumours (e.g. breast cancer). It is also done to assess the efficacy of leukaemic therapy.

In these procedures, nurses have to explain the procedure to patient, obtain signed consent form, consider pre-procedure, analgesic administration to enhance patient's comfort and cooperation. Apply pressure while dressing after procedure. Assess biopsy site for bleeding.

- Lymph node biopsy—The purpose is to obtain lympth tissue for histologic examination to determine diagnosis and therapy. *Open test* is performed in operative room with direct visualization of the area and closed (needle) test is performed at bedside or in office. In this, the nurse must explain procedure to the patient. Obtain signed consent form. Use sterile technique in dressing changes after procedure. Carefully evaluate for wound for healing. Assess patient for complications, especially bleeding and oedema.

5. *Coagulation studies*
   - Platlet count—Count of number of circulatory platelet (normal value) 1,50,000 to 4,00,000.
   - Prothrombin test—Assessment of extrinsic coagulation by measurement of factors I, II, V, VII, X (PT: 12-25 seconds).
   - *International normalized ratio (INR)*: Standardised system or reporting PT based on reference calibration model and calculated by comparing the patient with PT with a central value. (The desired level of anticoagulation regimen 2.0-3.0).
   - *Activated partial thromboplastin time* (APTT): Assessment of intrinsic coagulation by measuring factors I, II, V, VIII, IX, X, XI, XII, longer with use of heparin (30-45 seconds).
   - *Automated coagulation time* (ACT): Evaluation of intrinsic coagulation status; more accurate than APTT, used during dialysis, coronary artery bypass procedure artenogram (Normal 150-180).

- *Thromboplastin generation test* (TGT)—Reflection of generation of thromboplastin; if abnormal, second stage done to identify missing coagulation factor (Normal less than 12 seconds (100 per cent).
- *Bleeding time* (BT) Is measurement of time small skin incision bleeds; reflection of ability of small blood vessels to constrict (Normal: 1-6 minutes).
- *Thrombin time* (TT)—Reflection of adequacy of thrombin; prolonged thrombin time indication that coagulation is inadequate secondary to decreased thrombin activity (Normal 8-12-seconds).
- *Fibrinogen:* Reflection of level of fibronogen; increase in fibrinogen possible indication of enhancement of fibrin formation, making patient hypercoagulable; decrease in fibrinogen indicates that patient possibly predisposed to bleeding (Normal 200-400 mg/dl).
- *Fibrin split products*: Reflection of degree of fibrinolysis; reflection of excessive fibrinolysis and predisposition to bleeding (if present); possible indication of disseminated intravascular coagulation (Normal: less than 10 mg/L).
- *Clot retraction*: Reflection of clot shrinkage or retraction from sides of test tube after 24 hours; used to confirm platelet problem (Normal 50-100% in 24 hours).
- *Capillary fragility test* (Tourniquet test, Leeds test): Reflection of capillary integrity when positive or negative pressure is applied to various areas of the body. Positive test indicates thrombocytopnoea, toxic vascular reaction (Normal: No petechia or negative).
- *Protamine sulphate test*: Reflection of presence of fibrin monumer (Portion of fibrin remaining after elements that polymerize and stabilize detach); Positive indication of predisposition to bleed and possible presence of dissemination intravascular coagulation (Normally it is negative).

HAEMATOLOGICAL DISORDERS

Management of persons with problems of the haematological system present challenges to the nurse because of the diversity and vagueness of the presenting symptomatology. Disease processes are as diverse as the components that make up the haematological system. For this reason, the nurse performs a complete and thorough ongoing assessment of the patient to determine the aetiology of the patient's health concerns. Interventions should be focussed on supporting the patient's return to optimal function and resolution of haematological alterations. The nurse is responsible for assisting the patient to a better understanding of the haematological system and the complexities therein to obtain an optimal level of health.

DISORDERS OF ERYTHROCYTES

Common disorders of erythrocytes include underproduction (anaemia) overproduction (erythrocytosis) and impaired haemoglobin synthesis (haemoglobinopathies).

Anaemia

The term anaemia refers to a deficiency in the number of circulating red blood cells available for oxygen transport. Anaemia is a reduction below the normal in the number of erythrocytes, the quantity of haemoglobin, and the volume of packed red cells (Hct) caused by rapid blood loss, impaired production of RBCs, or increased destruction of erythrocytes. Because RBCs transport oxygen, crythrocytic disorder can lead to hypoxia. This hypoxia accounts for clinical manifestations of anaemia. Anaemia is not a specific disease, it is a manifestation of pathologic process.

Aetiology

Anaemia can result from primary haemotologic problems or can develop on a secondary consequence of defects in other body systems. The many kinds of anaemia can be grouped according to either as a morphologic or an aetiological" classification. *Morphologic* classification is based on descriptive objective laboratory information about erythrocyte size and colour. *Aetiologic* classification is related to the clinical condition causing the anaemia such as decreased erythrocytic production, blood loss or increased erythrocytic production. The aetiologic classification of anaemia are as follows:

i. *Decreased erythrocyte production*
   - Decreased haemoglobin synthesis
     - Iron deficiency (chronic blood loss and inadequate intake)
     - Thalassaemias (decreased haemoglobin synthesis)
     - Sideroblastic anaemia (decreased prophyrin)
   - Defective DNA synthesis
     - Cobalamin (vitamin B_{12}) deficiency of megaloblastic anaemias.
     - Folic acid deficiency.
   - Decreased number of erythrocyte precursors (secondary to impaired production).
   - Aplastic anaemia (drugs, chemicals, radiation, chemotherapy, virus congenital autoimmune mechanisms).
   - Anaemia of leukaemia and myelodysplasia.
     - Chronic disorders or diseases.

ii. *Secondary to blood loss*
   - Acute
     - Trauma
     - Blood vessels rupture (haemorrhage).
   - Chronic
     - Gastritis, gastrointestinal bleeding, or other malignancy.
     - Bleeding ulcers, bleeding haemorrhoids.
     - Menorrhagia (menstrual flow).

iii. *Increased erythrocytes destruction (Haemolysis)*
- Intrinsic
  - Abnormal haemoglobin (Hbs-sickle cell disease (anaemia) genetic haemoglobinopathy).
  - Enzyme deficiency (G6PD) deficiencies or glucose-6 phosphate dehydrogenase.
  - Membrane abnormality (paraxysmal nocturnal haemoglobinuria).
  - Hereditary spherocytoses (inherited as autosomal dominant trait).
- Extrinsic
  - Physical trauma (prosthetic heart valves and extra-corporeal circulation).
  - Antibodies (isoimmune and autoimmune-drug induced autoimmune response).
  - Infectious agent and toxins (malaria).

Although the morphologic system is more accurate means of classifying anaemias, it is easier to discuss patientcare by focussing on the aetiologic problem. The relationship of morphological classification and aetiologies of anaemia are as given below.

1. *Normocytic, normochromic* anaemias may be due to acute blood loss, haemolysis, chronic renal disease, cancers, sideroblastive anaemias, refractory anaemia, diseases of the endocrine dysfunction, aplastic anaemia pregnancy.
2. *Macrocytic, normochromic anaemias* may be due to cobalamin (Vit B_{12}) deficiency, folic acid deficiency, liver disease (including effects of alcohol abuse) postsplenectomy.
3. *Microcytic, hypochromic* anaemia may be due to iron-deficiency anaemia, thalassaemia lead poisoning.

Clinical Manifestations

The clinical manifestations of anaemia are primarily caused by the body response to tissue hypoxia. The intensity of the manifestations varies depending on the severity of the anaemia and presence of coexisting diseases. The severity of anaemia can be determined by the Hb level:

i. *Mild states* of anaemia (Hb 10 to 14 g/dl) may exist without causing symptoms. If symptoms develop, they are usually caused by an underlying disease or a compensatory response to heavy exercise. These symptoms include palpitations, dyspnoea and diaphoresis.

ii. *Moderate* states of anaemia (Hb 6 to 10 g/dl) the cardiac pulmonary symptoms may be increased and may be associated with rest as well as activity.

iii. Severe anaemia (Hb less than 6/dl) displays many clinical manifestation involving multiple body systems, which include:
- Skin, pallor, jaundice, pruritus, (Jaundice and pruritus due to haemolysis).
- Eyes–Retinal haemorrhage, blurred vision, icteric conjunctiva and sclera (dueo haemolysis).
- Mouth–Glossitis and smooth tongue
- Cardiovascular–Palpitations (mild and moderate), tachycardia, increased pulse pressure, systolic murmurs, intermittent claudication, angina, CHF and MI.
- Pulmonary–Exertional dyspnoea (mild), dyspnoea (moderate), tachypnoea, orthopnoea and dyspnoea at rest.
- Neurologic–Headache, vertigo, irritability, depression, impaired thought process.
- Gastrointestinal–Anorexia, hepatomegaly, splenomegaly, difficulty in swallowing and sore mouth.
- Muscutoskeletal–Bone pain.
- General–Sensitivity to cold, weight loss and lethargy.

Management

The numerous causes of anaemia necessitate different nursing interventions specific to the needs of the patient. Nevertheless there are certain general components of care for all patients with anaemia. The main problems are activity intolerance, alteration in nutrition, ineffective management of the respective regimen and hypoxaemia. The plan of exercising care designed according to problems. However, dietary and lifestyle changes can reverse some anaemias. Acute intervention for severe anaemia include blood transfusion, drug therapy (e.g. erythropoetin, vitamin supplements) and oxygen therapy and patient education regarding awareness care with therapy.

Iron Deficiency Anaemia

Iron is present in all RBCs a heme in haemoglobin and is stored form. The heme in haemoglobin accounts for two-thirds of the body's iron. The other one-third of iron is stored as ferritin and haemosiderin in macrophages in the bone marrow, spleen and liver. Normally 1.5 mg of iron is lost daily through GI tract, sweat and urine. When the stored iron is not replaced, haemoglobin production is reduced, leads to iron-deficiency anaemia.

Aetiology

Iron deficiency may develop from inadequate dietary intake, malabsorptions, blood loss of haemolysis. The body loses approximately 1.5 mg iron daily; this loss is usually compensated for with daily dietary intake. This tenuous balance may be compromised by chronic blood loss, either physiological such as menstruation; or pathological form gastrointestinal or other bleeding. This compromise results in an iron deficiency anaemia.

Common cause of gastrointestinal blood loss in adult are peptic ulcer, gastritis, oesophagitis, diverticuli, haemorrhoids and neoplasia, genitouterine blood loss occurs primarily from menstrual bleeding. The average monthly menstrual blood loss is about 45 ml and causes the loss of about 22 mg of iron. Pregnancy contributes to iron deficiency because of the diversion of iron to the foetus for erythropoiesis, blood loss at delivery and lactation. In addition chronic renal failure, dialysis may induce anaemia.

Clinical Manifestation

In the early course of iron deficiency, the patient may be free of symptoms. As the disease becomes chronic any of the general manifestations of anaemia may develop. In some persons, in addition to pallor, specific symptoms may occur. Mild cases may develop fatigue and exertion dyspnoea. Severe anaemia causes the nails to become brittle and shaped (concave) and develop longitudinal ridges. Glossitis (Inflammation of tongue–The papillae of the tongue atrophy, and tongue has a smooth shiny, bright-red appearance and cheilosis (inflammation of lips–The corners of mouth may be cracked, reddened and painful). In addition, the patient may complain about headache, paresthesia, and burning sensation of the tongue, all of which are caused by the lack of iron in the tissues.

Management

The cells are characteristically phypochromic and microcytic and may be detected by observation of the peripheral blood smears or by blood cell indices (Het, Hb.KBC). Diagnosis may be confirmed by a low serum iron levels and elevated serum iron-binding capacity or by a low serum ferritin level or absent iron stores in the bone marrow endoscopy, colonscopy may be used to detect GI bleeding.

The main goal of management is to treat the underlying disease that is causing reduced intake (malnutrition, alcoholism) or absorption of iron. In addition, efforts are directed towards replacing iron. This may be done through increasing the intake of iron. The patient should be taught which foods are good sources of iron. The role of nutrients is erythroporesis and their sources are as follows:

1. *Cobalamin* (Vit B_{12}) has role in RBC maturation, found in red meats, especially liver.
2. *Folic acid* also has role in RBC maturation found in green leaves, vegetables, liver, meat, fish, legumes and whole grains.
3. *Vitamin* B_6 has role in haemoglobin synthesis, found in liver and muscle meat, eggs dried fruits, legumes, dark green leafy vegetable, whole grain and bread enriched with cereals, potatoes.
4. *Amino acids* have role in synthesis of nucleoproteins, found in eggs, meat, milk and milk products (Cheese, ice creams, poultry, fish, legumes and nuts).
5. *Vitamin C* has role in conversion of folic acid to its active forms aids in absorption found in citrus fruits, leafy green vegetables, strawberries and cantaloupe.

The first step in medical therapy is to determine and correct the cause of anaemia. Repletion of iron stores in the body may then be accomplished by the administration of iron. Oral iron supplements usually is given in the form of ferrous sulphate. Patient teaching is very essential for newly diagnosed patient, because ferrous sulphate may be irritating to GI tract. It should be taken after meals and with orange juice or vitamin C to increase the absorption. The person is told that the stools will be black or tarry and that symptoms of diarrhoea or nausea should be reported to health care provider. Constipation is the major side effect of iron supplementation and a stool softener may be needed. When the patient cannot tolerate oral iron preparation or is unable to absorb iron properly, parenteral iron is administered by IM or IV administration of iron. Nutritional education is essential. Transfusion of packed RBCs in selected cases.

Megaloblastic or Macrocytic Anaemia

Megaloblastic anaemias refer to anaemia with characteristics morphological changes caused by defective DNA synthesis and abnormal RBC maturated. The RBCs are large (macrocyte) and abnormal and are referred to as *megaloblasts*. Macrocytic RBCs are early destroyed because of their fragile membranes. Although the overwhelming majority of megaloblastic anaemias result from cobalamin and folate deficiencies; their type of RBCs deformity can also occur from suppression of DNA synthesis by drugs from inborn errors of cobalamin and folic acid meta-bolism and from erythroleukaemia (malignant disorder charac-terised by proliferation of erythropoiesitic cell in bone marrow). The common forms of megaloblastic anaemia and their causes are as follows:

1. Cobalamin (vitamin B_{12}) deficiency can result from dietary deficiency, deficiency of gastric intrinsic factor (due to gastrectomy, and pernicious anaemia), intestinal malabsorption and increased requirement.

The deficiency results in impaired synthesis of DNA, resulting morphological changes in blood and bone marrow. General symptoms of anaemia related to cobalamin deficiency develop because of tissue hypoxia (as stated earlier). Gastrointestinal manifestation includes a sore tongue, anorexia, nausea, vomiting and abdominal pain. Typical neuromuscular manifestation includes weakness, paresthesias of the feet and hands, reduced vibratory and position senses, ataxia, muscle weakness, and impaired thought process ranging from confusion to dementia. Because cobalamin deficiency-related anaemia has an insidious onset, it may take several months for these manifestations to develop.

Diagnosis of pernicious anaemia is confirmed by an abnormal Schilling test result which demonstrates, the inability to absorb vitamin B_{12} unless intrinsic factor is also administered. Treatment consists of parenteral administration of vitamin B_{12}, usually once in a month by nurse in outpatient setting. The most common cause of relapse in person with pernicious anaemia is that reluctance to continue therapy for life. Patient teaching is a focus of nursing care and discharge planning. In addition to general measures for anaemia, the nurse should ensure that injuries are not sustained because of the diminished sensation to heat and pain resulting from the neurologic impairment. The patient must be protected from burns and trauma. If heat therapy is required, the patient's skin must be evaluated at frequent intervals to detect redness. Irritation from nasogastric tubes and restrictive clothing may not be procurred by the patient because of reduced pain sensations. A careful follow-up is required.

2. *Folic acid deficiency* also causes megaloblastic anaemia. Folic acid required for DNA synthesis leading to RBC formation and maturation. Common causes of folic acid deficiency include the following.
   - Poor nutrition, especially a lack of green leafy vegetables, liver, citrous fruits, yeast, dried leaves, nuts and grains.
   - Malabsorption syndrome, particularly small-based disorders.
   - Drugs that impede the absorption and use of folic acid (e.g. methotrexate, oral contraceptives), as well as antiseizure agents (e.g. phenobarbital, dephenylhydantine).
   - Alcohol abuse and anorexia (chronic alcoholism).
   - Haemodialysis patients, because folic acid is dialyzable.
   - Malnutrition.
   - Pregnancy causes increase in need for and use of folic acid. Deficiency during pregnancy may result in neural tube defects.
   - Increased requirement.

The clinical manifestation of folic acid deficiency is similar to those of cobalamin deficiency. This disease develops insidiously and the patient's symptoms may be attributed to other coexisting problems such as cirrhosis or oesophageal varices. GI disturbances include dyspepsia and a smooth beefy red tongue. The absence of neurologic problem is an important diagnostic finding. This lack of neurologic involvement differentiate folic acid deficiency from vitamin B_{12} deficiency.

Laboratory findings include macrocytic anaemia, megaloblastic changes in the bone marrow and a low serum folate level. Most persons respond promptly to oral folic acid and well-balanced diet. Daily requirements for folic acid and 100 to 200 mg. The body is able to store approximately a 4-month supply of folic acid. Persons with anaemia caused by a dietary deficiency can be treated with 1 mg of folic acid for 3-month period. Locate the cause and avoid or by corrective measures. Patients should be instructed in food rich in folic acid including organ meat, eggs, cabbage, broccoli, citrus fruits and brussels, sprouts. Boiling, steaming and canning forlolic acid-rich foods reduces the amount of available vitamin persons who consume large amounts of are susceptible to folic acid deficiency. Advise patients to reduce or avoid alcohol.

Further, there are other forms of megaloblastic anaemia which include:

- Drug-induced suppressions of DNA synthesis-resulting from folate antagonists. Metabolic inhibitions, alkylating agents, nitrous xoide.
- Inborn errors–heredity defective folate metabolisms Lesch-Nyham syndrome, defective of cobalamins.
- Erythroleukaemia.

Thalassaemia

Thalassaemia is one of the common inherited single gene disorders in the world. As in iron-deficiency, it is a disease of inadequate production of normal haemoglobin. Haemolysis occurs in thalassaemis, but insufficient production of haemoglobin is the predominant problem. In contrast to iron deficiency anaemia, in which haemesynthesis is the problem, thalassaemia involves problem with the globin protein.

Aetiology

Thalassaemias are a group of autosomal recessive genetic disorder commonly found in certain ethnic groups. An individual with thalassaemia may have a heterozygous or homozygous form of the disease. A person who is heterozygous has one thalassaemic gene and one normal gene and is said to have thalassaemia minor or thalassaemic trait, which is mild form of disease. A homozygous person has two thalassaemia genes, causing severe condition known as thalassaemia major.

Pathophysiology

Thalassaemia is characterized by a decreased synthesis of one of the globin chains of haemoglobin. The beta chain is most often affected. As a result, there is decreased synthesis of haemoglobin and an accumulation of the alpha globin chain in the erythrocyte. These alterations result in decreased RBC production and a chronic haemolytic anaemia.

Clinical Manifestation

The patient with thalassaemia minor is frequently asymptomatic because the patient adjusts to the gradually acquired chronic state of anaemia. Occasionally splenomegaly may develop in this patient, and mild jaundice may occur if malfored erythrocytes are rapidly haemolysed. The person who has thalassaemia major is pale and displays general symptoms of anaemia. In addition, the person has pronounced splenomegaly. Jaundice from RBC haemolysis is prominent. Chronic bone marrow hyperplasia leads to expansion of the marrow space. This may cause thickening of the cranium and maxillary cavity leading to an appearance resembling Down's syndrome. Thalassaemia major is a life-threatening disease in which growth of both physical and mental are often retarded.

Management

Thalassaemia minor requires no treatment because the body adapts to the reduction of normal haemoglobin. At present only treatment of thalassaemia major is transfusion therapy and chelation therapy (therapy to reduce the iron overloading that sometime occurs with chronic transfusion therapy). No specific drug or diet therapies are effective in treating thalassaemia. The nurse must be familiar with transfusion therapy and sensitive to the emotional needs of the patient who receive frequency transfusions. Avoid hopelessness and depression among population. Couple should be referred to genetic counselling.

Aplastic Anaemia

One of the most severe forms of anaemias related to reduced or impaired erythrocyte production is a group of disorders termed "aplastic" hypoplastic or pancytopoenic "anaemias". These anaemias are life-threatening stem cell disorders, characterized by hypoplastic, fatty bone marrow and that result in pancytopoenia.

Aetiology

Aplastic anaemia is to an extent is a misnomer because in most cases, all marrow elements–erythrocyte, leukocytes and platelets are quantitatively decreased, although they are qualitatively normal.

Aetiology

Aplastic anaemia affects all age groups and both genders. The incidence is low, affecting approximately 4 persons per one million. There are various aetiological types of aplastic anaemia, but they can be divided into the major groups i.e. congenital (idiopathic) or acquired.

1. *Congenital* origin caused by chromosomal alterations. (approximately 30 per cent of the aplastic anaemia that appear in childhood). Fancohis syndrome, Dyskertosis congnita, Schwactimen-diamond syndrome.
2. *Acquired* as a result of exposure to:
   - Ionizing radiation, chemical agents (e.g. benzene, insecticide-DDT, arsenic, alcohol).
   - Viral and bacterial infections (e.g. hepatitis, parvovirus, miliary TB).
   - Prescribed medication (e.g. alkalating agents, antiseizure agents, antimetabolite, antimicrobial and gold).
   - Pregnancy.
   - Idiopathic.

Pathophysiology

Aplastic anaemia usually is characterised by depression or cessation of activity of all blood-producing elements. There is a decrease in white blood cells (leukopoenia) a decrease in platelets (thrombocytopoenia) and decrease in the formation of RBC, which leads to an anaemia. The process may be chronic or acute depending on the causative factor of the anaemia.

Clinical Manifestation

Aplastic anaemia usually develops insidiously. Clinically, the patient may have symptoms caused by suppression of any or all bone marrow elements general manifestations of anaemia such as pallor, fatigue, and dyspnoea as well as cardiovascular and cerebral responses may be seen. Pallor of skin and mucous membranes is characteristic in addition to fatigue, palpitation and exertional dyspnoea. Infection of the skin and mucous membrane occur with severe granulocytopoenia; haemorrhagic symptoms (bleeding into the skin and mucous membranes and spontaneous bleeding from the nose, gums, vagina and rectum) occur with severe thrombocytopoenia.

Management

The diagnosis is confirmed by laboratory studies. Results of physical examination often are normal. The CBC characteristically reveals a pancytopoenia (a marked decrease in the numbering of cell types). The reticulocyte count is low. Definitive diagnosis made by bone marrow examination and biopsy.

Management of aplastic anaemia is based on identifying and removing the causative agent (when possible) and providing appropriate care until the pancytopoenia reverses. In the past, treatment of aplastic anaemia was aimed at mainly at stimulating haematopoiesis through and administration of steroids and androgens therapy. It has shown limited value and can produce toxic effects.

In recent years, bone marrow transplantation from a donor with identical human leukocyte antigen has emerged as the treatment of choice for the person younger than 40 years with severe aplastic anaemia. The remainder of persons are treated with immunosuppressive therapy. The prognosis of persons depending on severity and method of treatment. Patients who are not successfully treated often die of complications associated with haemorrhage and infection.

Nursing care is based on careful assessment and management of complications of pancytopoenia, primarily focused on preventing infection and monitoring signs of bleeding. To prevent infection in the hospitalised patient who is immunosuppressed, the following intervention should be included in the plan of care.

- Private room
- Protective isolation
- Provide and instruct the patient on meticulous hygiene
- Assessment and maintenance of oral care regimen
- Monitor invasive lines for signs of infection
- Avoid bladder catheterization.
- Instruct family and visitors on careful handwashing.

Nursing intervention aimed at the prevention of bleeding episodes include the following:

- Monitoring invasive line sites
- Testing urine and stools for blood
- Minimizing venipuncture and injections
- Avoiding rectal temperatures, medication and enaema
- Instructing the patient on use of soft sponges for oral care.

Decreasing oxygen-carrying capacity of the blood diseases, oxygen supply to the tissues, will lead to fatigue with activity. Measures to prevent fatigue include provide frequent rest periods, avoiding fatigue-producing activities, and monitoring the patient for signs of excessive fatigue or shortness of breath with activities. Patients are often hospitalised for several weeks depending on the type of treatment received. The nurse needs to assist the patient's developing coping strategies to deal with the anxiety and isolation of prolonged hospitalisation. Music and art therapies are helpful strategies to assist the patient in coping positively with the disease and treatment.

Education of the patient and family members is the cornerstone in the prevention of infection and avoidance of bleeding episodes. Teaching the person with aplastic anaemia includes the following:

a. *Prevents infection*
   - Use good handwashing technique
   - Avoid sharing eating utensils and bath linens.
   - Take bath everyday (for every other day if skin is dry). Keep perineal area clean.
   - Use good oral hygiene
   - Eliminate intake of raw meat, fruits or vegetables
   - Report signs of infection immediately to health care provider.

b. *Prevent haemorrhage*
   - Observe for signs such as bloody urine, stool and patechae and report
   - Use a soft toothbrush or swab for mouth care and avoid the use of dental floss.
   - Keep mouth clean and free of debris
   - Avoid enemas or other rectal insertions
   - Avoid pricking or blosing the note forcefully
   - Avoid trauma, falls, bumps, and cuts, avoid contact with sports
   - Avoid use of aspirin preparations (anticoagulant effect)
   - Use an electric razor
   - Use lubrication and be gentle during sexual intercourse.

c. *Prevent fatigue*
   - Take frequent rest periods between ADL and activity
   - Avoid excessive work load or heavy lifting, and ask for assistance with sternum activity.
   - Increase time necessary for routine care.
   - Decrease activity if shortness of breath, dizziness or sensations of heaviness in extremities occurs.
   - Report signs of increased fatigue with activity to health care provider.

Haemolytic Anaemias

Haemolytic anaemia is defined as the premature destruction of erythrocyte occurring at such a rate that the bone marrow is unable to compensate for the loss of cells. Haemolysis can occur either extravascularly or intravascularly.

In cases of extravascular haemolysis, the spleen removes erythrocytes from circulation at a much more rapid rate, usually because of some perceived problems with the erythrocyte. Examples are autoimmune anaemias and hereditary spherocytosis. Extravascular haemolysis takes place in the macrophages of the spleen, liver and bone marrow.

Intravascular haemolysis is secondary to the erythrocyte lysing and spilling the cell contents into the plasma. This occurs as a result of an enzyme deficiency in the erythrocyte membranes or mechanical factors such as dialysis or prosthetic heart valves, which can prematurely weaken the erythrocyte. Haemolytic anaemias can also develop as a result of abnormal haemoglobin synthesis as in the thalassaemia and sickle cell disease. Intravascular haemolysis occurs within the circulation.

Aetiology

The causes of haemolytic anaemias may be acquired form or hereditary forms as briefed below.

A. *Acquired forms*
   - Immune system–mediated haemolysis is caused or associated with transfusion reactions, haemolytic disease of the newborn, and autoimmune haemolytic anaemia. The mechanism of RBC destruction will be antibody mediated erythrocytes by enzymes of the complement system.
   - *Traumatic haemolysis* is caused by presence of prosthetic heart valves; structural abnormalities of the heart; haemolytic uremic syndrome; disseminated intravascular coagulation and haemodialysis.. Here physical destruction of erythrocytis by "mechanical" means (trauma).
   - *Infectious haemolysis* are due to bacterial infection (clostridia, cholera, typhoid). Destruction occurs as a result of infection of erythrocytes.
   - *Toxic (chemical) haemolysis* occurs as a result of exposure to toxic chemical agents; haemodialysis or uremia; and venoms. Destruction due to chemical injury of erythrocytes. The chemical such as oxidative drugs, arsenic, lead, copper and snake venom.
   - *Physical haemolysis* are due to burns and radiation, destruction of erythrocyte by heat or radiation injury.
   - *Hypophosphatemic haemolysis* are due to hypophosphatemia (phosphate deficiency in plasma). Destruction, RBCs by diminished cellular production of substances required for erythrocyte life and function.

B. *Hereditary form*
- *Structural defects* i.e., plasma membrane defects, destruction due to fragility of the erythrocyte.
- *Enzyme deficiency* i.e. deficiency of glycolytic enzymes and deficiency of metabolic enzymes (i.e., glucose-6-phosphate dehydrogenase). Destruction by diminished cellular function.
- *Defects of globin synthesis or structure* associated with:
  - Sickle cell anaemias–There is increased membrane fragility and deformation during sickle cell crisis.
  - Thalassaemia–There is defective haemoglobin structure and function.
  - Miscellaneous Hb defects–Defective Hb structure and function.

Pathophysiology and Clinical Manifestation

In warm-reacting anaemias, antibodies (IgG) develop against an individual's own erythrocytes. These antibodies combine more readily at body temperature. Antibody-coated RBCs are destroyed by the reticuloendothelial system, particularly the spleen symptoms depend on the onset. In episodes of severe haemolysis dyspnoea, palpitations and congestive heart failure occurs. Jaundice, pallor and splenomegaly are common.

In cold-reacting disease, IgM antibodies react, with antigens on the erythrocyte, optimally in cold temperature (less than 31°C) ischaemia occurs when red cells clump in the capillary beds, causing cyanosis, pain and paresthesias. Haemoglobinuria also occurs.

Autoimmune reaction results when individuals develop antibodies against their own erythrocytes. Autoimmune haemolytic reactions may be idiopathic developing with no prior haemolytic history as a result of the immunoglobulin IgG covering of RBCs or secondary to other autoimmune disease (e.g. SLE), leukaemia, lymphoma, or drugs (penicillin, indomethacin, phenylbutazone, phenacetin, quinidine, quninine and methyldopa).

Management

Diagnosis is confirmed by demonstrating the presence of the antibody or complement on the RBCs (direct Coomb's test) or in the serum 'indirect Coomb's test). Additional laboratory test findings will show a decreased Hct, increased reticulocytes, and an increased bilirubin.

Treatment depends on the cause of haemolysis. Mild cases require no treatment. Treatment and management of acquired haemolytic anaemias involve general supportive care until the causative agent can be eliminated or at least rendered loss injurious to the erythrocytes. Supportive care includes administering corticosteroids and blood products or removing the spleen.

Nursing management consists of teaching the patient about the drug therapy, preparing the patient for surgery if indicated and helping the patient and family to cope with the illness. The patient and family need to be instructed regarding precipitating factors associated with autoimmune haemolytic anaemias. Teaching should include preventive measures such as avoiding exposure to cold for persons with cold-reacting anaemias.

Hereditary Spherocytosis

Hereditary spherocytosis (HS) is the most common problem of alteration in erythrocyte shape. It is inherited in an autosomal dominant trait it is characterised by a membrane abnormality that leads to osmotic swelling of the RBC and susceptibility to destruction by the spleen.

This anomaly occurs in 1 of every 5000 persons irrespective of their sex or race. It is usually detected in childhood; but, may appear initially in adulthood.

In this disease, there is deficit in the proteins that form the structure of the erythrocyte. This malformation of protein gives the cells a thick spherical appearance. This abnormal cell then becomes increasingly permeable to sodium, leading to increased energy demands by the cell. The circulating spherocytes become trapped in the spleen, where increased energy demands cannot be met and the cell dies.....

Symptoms include those typically associated with anaemia (Pallor, fatigue, exceptional dyspnoea), jaundice from the increased serum bilirubin level, and enlarged spleen from the increased RBCs destruction.

Diagnosis depends on observations of spherocytes in the peripheral blood smear and by laboratory demonstration of increased osmotic fragility of the RBCs. The reticulocytes count usually elevated, as is the serum bilirubin level.

The treatment for hereditary spherocytosis is splenectomy, which will correct the haemolytis, for the underlying sperocytosis will persist. The gallbladder is often also removed because of the increased incidence of gallstones in patients with HS.

Routine postoperative care is indicated for person who has undergone splenectomy or cholecystectomy. Nursing interventions include careful monitoring for infection and continuing monitoring for signs of anaemia. Patient education should include wound management of surgery. Genetic counselling is indicated for couples considering childbirth. Energy conservation technique should be included in the teaching plan.

Enzyme Deficiency Anaemia

Deficiency of enzymes in the pathways that metabolise glucose and generate adenosine triphosphate (ATP) commonly leads to premature RBC destruction, known as enzyme deficiency anaemia. A most common clinically significant enzyme abnormality is that of "Glucose-6-phosphate dehydragenase" (G6 PD)

Aetiology

Haemolytic episodes in G6PD deficiency can be caused by viral and bacterial infection or oxidant drugs (antimalarial, antipyretics, sulfonamides, quinidine, vitamin K derivatives and phenacetin, choromphenical.

Pathophysiology

The enzyme G6PD is responsible for the antioxidant reactions in the RBCs. The lack of this enzyme causes the cell to be susceptible to oxidizing agents. This exposure results in damage to the haemoglobin in RBC membrane and the subsequent release of haemoglobin into the circulation G6PD deficiency is a sex-linked disorder and directly affects the erythrocyte ability to resist oxidative damage consequently when G6PD is reduced there is a decrease in glucose used by the RBCs. If erythrocytes are exposed to oxidative foods and drugs the metabolic needs of RBC increases. However, G6PD deficiency interferes with glucose metabolism and leads to damage of older RBCs, which are then destroyed by haemolysis.

Clinical Manifestation

Haemolytic episodes persists for 7 to 10 days after exposure to oxidating agents. The patient may experience back pain, jaundice, and haemoglobinurin as evidence of haemolytic process.

Management

Diagnosis is established by assay for the enzyme. Managing the haemolysis seen in G6PD deficiency is realtively easy. Because, only older RBCs are destroyed by the oxidative agents, the younger cells survive. The cause of the haemolytic reaction must be removed. During the period of acute haemolyis, the patient will require rest, adequate hydration and assessing kidney function. Attention should be focussed on preventing haemolytic disorders by treating infections promptly and screening high risk individuals of G6PD deficiency before giving an oxidative drug.

Treatment is in the recognition of the disorder and cessation of the offending drugs. During a haemolytic episodes, hydration and blood transfusion may be necessary. Prompt treatment of infection is also important in managing patients. Nursing care includes management of episodes and educating patient and family on the precipitating factor of disorder, and its prevention. Teaching also focuses on the bacterial and viral illnesses and avoiding precipitating drugs.

Sickle Cell Disease (SCD)

Normal haemoglobin is composed of heme (red) and globin (protein component). The globin portion comprises of two pairs of polypeptide chains–alpha and beta. Each of the polypeptide chains has a specific amino acid sequence and number. Any deviation in the normal number of sequence of essential amino acids results in abnormal haemoglobin (Hgb) synthesis. Disorders of haemoglobin synthesis are categorised as "haemoglobinopathies". They result from abnormalities in one or both of the polypeptide chain or in any one of the more than 500 amino acids. One of the most common haemoglobinopathies is sickle cell disease (Hbs) or sickle cell anaemia.

Aetiology

Sickle cell disease (SCD) is a family of genetic disorder caused by abnormal properties conveyed to sickle cell RBC by mutant sickle cell haemoglobin (Hbs). It is an incurable disease that is often fatal by middle age.

Sickle cell anaemia, one type of SCD is an autosomal recessive genetic disorder in which the person is homozygous for Hbs, Characterized by a chronic haemolytic anaemia, sickle cell anaemia occurs predominantly in the black population e.g. Afro-American.

Some persons may have sickle trait, a mild condition that may be asymptomatic. A person with sickle cell trait is heterozygous, with approximately 1/4 of the haemoglobin in the abnormal S from and 3/4 in the normal A form. If two parents have sickle cell trait, there is 25 per cent chance with each pregnancy that the child will have sickle cell anaemia.

Different terms are used with discussion of sickle cell anaemia. Only the homozygous condition of *HbS* describes the classic form of the disease called *Sickle Cell Anaemia*. The heterozygous state HbSA refers to the often asymptomatic condition called sickle cell trait. In addition, a category of sickling disorders called sickling syndrome is associated with presence of HbS. The phenotypes of sickle cell are:

Genetic relationship	Hb	SCD
• Homozygous dominating	HbA, HbA	sickle cell Disease
• Heterozygous	HbA, HbS	Sickle cell tract
• Homozygous recessive	HbS HbS	Sickle cell anaemia

Pathophysiology

The mutation that causes sickle cell haemoglobin (HbS) to develop, involves one amino acid. The basic abnormality lies within the haemoglobin fraction of the haemoglobin (Hgb), where a single amino acid (valine) is substituted for another (glutamic acid) in the sixth position of the beta chain. This single amino acid substitution profoundly alters the properties of the Hgb molecule. This substitute leads to an abnormal linking reaction that causes development of deformed crescent-shaped (sickle shape) cells when oxygen tension is lowered.

However, when the oxygen tention of RBCs decreases, HbS polymerizes causing the Hgb of distort and realign the RBC into sickle shape. The sickle cell in circulation leads to increased blood viscosity, which prolongs circulation time. This decrease in circulation time causes an increase in the hypoxic time of the cell, promoting further sickling. The development of sickle cells leads to plugging, the small circulation further decreasing the cellular pH and oxygen tension. Anaerobic metabolism occurs with resulting tissue ischaemia in any organ.

When hypoxia occurs in a patient with sickle cell anaemia, the RBCs containing HBs changes from a biconcave disk to an elongated, crescent or sickle cell. These sickling cell may clog the small capillaries. The resulting homeostasis promote a self-perpetuating cycle of local hypoxia, deoxygenation of more erythrocytes and more sickling. As blood vessels are occluded, thrombosis occurs. This can ultimately lead to ischaemia and necrosis of the infarcted tissue from lack of oxygen. With repeated infarction there is gradual involvement of all body systems, especially the spleen, lungs, kidney and brain. The abnormal shape of the haemoglobin is recognised by the body and the cell is haemolysed. Sickle cells are also destroyed randomly. Initially sickling is reversible on reoxygenation but eventually becomes irreversible with cells being haemolysed and haemolytic anaemia develops.

Clinical Manifestation

Infant with sickle cell anaemia do not manifest symptoms until 10 to 12 weeks of age at which time most of the foetal haemoglobin (HbF) has been replaced by HbS. RBCs with high levels of HbF are resistant to sickling. Children with sickle cell disease manifest a general impairment of growth and development and a failure to thrive.

The effect of sickle cell disease varies greatly from person to person. Many of them with SCD possess reasonably good health. The typical patient is anaemic but asymptomatic except painful episodes. Anaemia usually is severe, chronic and haemolytic.

Patients manifest the clinical manifestations of chronic anaemia with *pallor* of mucous membranes, fatigue and decreased exercise tolerance. Because of the haemolyser jaundice is common patients are prone to gallstones (cholelithiasis). The painful vaso-occlusive episodes are the most common events in SCD. The *pain* is the manifestation of localised bone marrow necrosis affecting juxta-articular areas of the long bones, spine, pelvis, ribs and sternum. The painful episodes occur once a year or twice a year; the duration of episode lasts from 1 to 10 days. Physical and probably emotional (stress) factors precipitate a painful episode. Physical factors include events that cause dehydration or change the oxygen tension in the body such as infection, overexertion, weather changes (cold), high Hgb levels, ingestion of alcohol and smoking.

Persons with SCD are particularly susceptible, primarily because most experience as anaemia meningitis, sepsis, pneumonia and urinary tract infections. The sudden exacerbation of sickling can bring about a condition known as sickle cell crisis. Sickle cell crisis may be thrombotic, aplastic, megaloblastic or splenic sequestration. Shock is a possible development for sickle cell crisis.

To sum up, clinical manifestation of SCD are:

Acute Episodes

- *Pain* Usually in back, chest or extremities, may be localised migratory or generalised.
- *Fever* Low grade, 1-2-days after onset of pain.
- *Vaso-occlusive crisis* Occlusion of blood vessels by the sick cells may occur in area such as the brain (CVA), chest, liver or penis, leads to:
  - Acute chest syndrome: fever, chest pain, cough, dyspnoea, pus infiltrate pulmonary infarction leads to pulmonary hypertension heart failure.
  - Priapism (condition of prolonged or constant erection of penis)
  - Jaundice caused by increased RBC destruction and release if bili rubin vaso-occlusive crisis are triggered by stress, cold water exposure, dehydration, hypoxia, and infection.

Chronic Problem

- Leg ulcers, usually of the medial malleolus.
- Renal problems is renal insufficiency from repeated infarction.
- Occular problem of microinfarctions of the peripheral retina, leading to retinal detachment and blindness.
- Musculoskeletal: The painful bone infarction of the hand-foot syndrome (painful swelling and hands over foot), necrosis of femoral heads.

The major causes of mortality are renal and pulmonary failure.

Management

The diagnosis of sickle cell anaemia should be considered with any black patient who has haemolytic anaemia. In addition, routine CRC, Hct, Hb levels and others, the common screening test for sickle cell is peripheral blood smear, sickle cell preparation, sickle cell, haemoglobin electrophores have been useful in diagnosis.

There is no specific treatment for the disease. Patients with sickle cell disease should be advised to avoid high altitudes, adequate fluid intake, and treat infections promptly. Pneumovax and H-influenza vaccine should be administered. Therapy is usually directed towards alleviating the symptoms from complication of the disease. For example, chronic leg ulcers may be treated with bedrest, antibiotics, warm saline soaks, mechanical or enzyme debridements and grafting if necessary.

Patient should be assessed for infarction; and thrombosis resulting from anoxia may occur in brain, kidneys, bone marrow and spleen. He/she should be watched for complication such as:

- Increased intracranial pressure (Brain-CVA)
- Infections–lungs, urinary tract and bones
- Leg ulcers
- Bony complications–avascular necrosis in shoulder and hips
- Pulmonary complications
- Cardiovascular complication–arrythmia and murmurs.

- Priapism (prolonged and painful erection)
- Haemorrhage and shock.

Take measures to correct them accordingly–which includes taking nursing measures to promoting comfort and oxygenation; promoting hydration preventing infection; promoting tissue perfusion; promoting activity tolerance; facilitating family planning and genetic counselling; facilitate coping. In addition, teaching the person with sickle cell anaemia includes:

- Knowledge of the disease
- Avoidance of situation that causes crisis (infection, high altitude, overexertion, emotional stress, alcohol, cigarette smoking and avoidance of trauma.
- Importance of adequate fluid intake.
- Availability of psychological support services and social resources.
- Need for medical checking.

ERYTHROCYTOSIS

Erythrocytosis refers to an abnormal increase in erythrocytes. The increase may be secondary to hypoxia (from high altitude or from pulmonary and cardiac disease) or certain erythroproteins producing tumours or *primary disorder* (polycythaemia vera). With hypoxia, RBCs increase as a compensatory mechanism to carry additional oxygen.

Polycythaemia Vera

Polycythaemia vera is a myeloproliferative disorder of the pluripotent stem cell. Polycythaemia is the production and presence of increased number of RBCs. The increase in erythrocytes can be so great that blood circulation is impaired as a result of the increased blood viscosity (hyperviscocity and volume (hypervolumea).

Aetiology

There are two types of polycythaemia and includes primary polycythaemia and secondary polycythaemia. Although this aetiology and pathogenism differ, clinical manifestation and complication are similar.

Polycythaemia vera is considered a myeloproliferative disorder arising from a chromosomal mutation in a single pluripotent stem. Due to this there will be thrombocytosis and leukocytosis.

Secondary polycythaemia is caused by hypoxia rather than increase in the development of the RBC. Hypoxia stimulates erythrocyte production. The need for oxygen may be due to high altitude, pulmonary disease, cardiac vascular disease, alveolar hypoventilation, defective oxygen transport, or tissue hypoxia.

Pathophysiology

Polycythaemia vera is a bone marrow disorder characterised by erythrocytosis, usually with a simultaneous leukolytosis and thrombocytosis, hypervolaemia, increased blood viscosity from the increased RBC mass and platelet dysfunction occur.

Clinical Manifestation

Symptoms usually are absent in early stage, circulatory manifestation of polycythaemia vera occur because of the hypertension caused by hypervolaemia and hyperviscosity. They are often the first symptoms and include subjective complaint of headache, vertigo, dizziness, tinnitus, and visual disturbances. In addition, patients may experience angina, CHF, intermittent claudication and thrombophlebitis, which may be complicated by embolisation. These manifestations are caused by blood vessel distension, impaired blood flow, circulatory studies, thrombosis and tissue hypoxia caused by the hypervolaemia and hyperviscosity. The most serious complications is CVA secondary to thrombosis. Generalised pruritus may be striking symptoms and is related to histamine release from an increased number of vasophils and mast cells.

Haemorrhagic phenomena caused by either vessel rupture from overdistention or inadequate platelet function may result in petechae, ecchymosis, epistaxis or GI bleeding. Haemorrhage may be acute or catastrophic.

Hepatomegaly and splenomegaly from organ engorgements may contribute to patient complaints of satiety and fullness. The patient also experiences pain from peptic ulcer. Plethora (ruddy complexion) may also be present. Hyperuricaemia is caused by the increase in RBC destruction that accompanies excessive RBC products. Uric acid is one of the products of cell destruction. This may cause secondary form of gout (a form of arthritis).

Management

Polycythaemia confirmed by lab test of blood where there is increase in Hgb, Hct, WBC (basophilia), platelets and platelet dysfunction, leucocyte alkaline phosphate, uric acid, cobalamin levels and histamine levels. Bone marrow examination in polycythaemia vera shows hyper cellularity of RBCs, WBCs and platelets, splenomegaly also are found.

Once the diagnosis of polycythaemia vera is made, treatment is directed towards reducing blood volume and viscosity and bone marrow activities. The goal of therapy is to decrease the red cell mass. Treatment options are phlebotomy (for diminished blood values) alkalating agents (busulfan, hydroxyurea, melphalan), radioactive phosphorous or interferon to inhibit bone marrow activity. Usual treatment is periodic phlebotomy aimed at maintaining the Hct and Hgb at normal level.

When acute exacerbations of polycythaemia vera develop, the nurse has several responsibilities. Depending on the institutional policies, the nurse may either assist with or perform phlebotomy, fluid intake and output must be evaluated during hydration therapy to avoid overload (which further complicate the circulatory congestion) and underdehydration (which can cause the blood to become even more viscus). If myelosuppressive agents are used, the nurse must administer the drug as ordered, observe the patient and teach the patient above medication and side effects. Teach about importance of combined medical care, blood tests and phlebotomy. Repetitive phlobotomy may lead to iron deficiency and take measures accordingly. The complications are treated accordingly.

ANAEMIA CAUSED BY BLOOD LOSS

Anaemia resulting from blood loss may be caused by either acute or chronic.

Aetiology/Pathophysiology

Acute blood loss occurs as a result of sudden haemorrhage causes of acute blood loss include trauma, complications of surgery and diseases that disrupt vascular integrity. There are two clinical concerns in such situation. First, there is sudden reduction in the total blood volume that can lead to hypovolaemic shock. Second, if the acute loss is more gradual, the body maintains its blood volume by slowly increasing the plasma volume. Consequently, the circulating fluid volume is preserved. But the number of RBCs available to carry oxygen is significantly diminished.

The sources of chronic blood loss are similar to those of iron deficiency (e.g. bleeding ulcer, haemorrhoids, menstrual and postmenopausel blood loss).

Clinical Manifestation

The clinical manifestation of acute blood loss are caused by the body's attempt to maintain adequate blood volume and meet O_2 requirements. Clinical manifestation of acute blood loss according to varying degrees of blood volume loss as follows:

Volume loss	*Clinical manifestation*
10%	None
20%	No detectable signs or symptoms at rest, tachycardia with exercise and slight postural hypertension.
30%	Normal supine blood pressure and pulse at rest, postural hypertension and tachycardia with exercise.
40%	Blood pressure, central venous pressure, and cardiac output below normal at rest, rapid, threading pulse and cold and clammy skin.
50%	Shock and potential death.

Management

When blood volume loss is sudden, the body reacts by vasoconstriction. In this stage, erythrocyte, Hb, and Hct levels are usually low and reflect the blood loss. Care of these patients induce replacing blood volume to prevent shock and identify the sources of haemorrhage and stopping blood loss. IV fluid used in emergency includes dextran, hetastarch, albumin, or crystalloid electrolyte solution such as lactated ringers. Blood transfusion (Packed RBCs) may be needed of the blood loss is significant. The patient also needs supplemental iron because, the availability of iron affects the marrow production of erythrocytes. When anaemia exists after acute blood loss, dietary sources of iron will probably not be adequate to maintain iron pools. For every 2 ml of blood lost, 1 mg iron is also lost. Therefore, oral or parenteral iron prepared are administered. Nursing intervention includes treating shock in acute blood loss and locating the cause and take measures everyday in both acute and chronic blood loss.

DISORDERS OF HAEMOSTASIS

The haemostatic process involves the vascular endothelium, platelets, and coagulation factors, which normally function in concert to arrest haemorrhage and repair vascular injury. Disruption of any of these may result in bleeding or thrombolic disorders. The common disorders associated with platelet and coagulation are:

1. *Platelets*
   - Thrombocytopoenia – Decreased numbers of platelets.
   - Thrombocytosis – Increased number of platelets.
   - Bleeding syndrome – Disorders of platelet functions.
2. *Coagulation*
   a. *Congenital*
   - Haemophilia A – Decrease of factor VIII
   - Haemophilia B – Decrease of factor IX
   - Von Willebrands disease – Decrease of factor VIII defective platelet aggregation.

   b. *Acquired*
   - Vitamin K deficiency – Decrease of factors II, VII, IX and X.
   - Disseminated intravascular coagulation – Stimulates first the clot--ting process then fibro-analytic process.

THROMBOCYTOPENIA

Thrombocytopenia is defined as a lower than normal number of circulating platelets (Ranges of 150,000 to 400,000).

Aetiology

Platelet disorders can be inherited (e.g. Wiskott-Aldrich syndrome) but vast majority are acquired. Acquired disorders occur because of decreased platelet production, or increased platelet production and many abnormalities occur following ingestions of some foods and drugs.

1. Decreased Platelet production.
   a. *Inherited*

- Fanconi's syndrome (Pancytopoenia).
- Hereditary thrombocytopoenia.

b. *Acquired*
- Aplastic anaemia.
- Haematologic malignant disorder.
- Myelosuppressive drugs.
- Chronic alcoholism.
- Exposure to ionizing radiation.
- Viral infections.
- Deficiencies of cobalamin and folic acid.

2. Increased Platelet Distruction

a. *Nonimmune*
- Thrombotic thrombocytopoenia purpura.
- Pregnancy.
- Infection.
- Drug induced.
- Severe burns.

b. *Immune*
- Immune thrombocytopoenic purpura.
- Human immunodeficiency virus infection.
- Drug induced.

c. *Splenomegaly.*

3. *Drugs, spices and vitamin causing abnormalities in platelet function*

a. Suppression of platelet production.
- Thiazide diuretics, alcohol, oestrogen and chemotherapeutic drugs.

b. Abnormal platelet aggregation.
- NSAIDS: Ibuprofen, indomethacin naproxen.
- Antibiotics: Penicillin and cephalosperins.
- Analgesics: Aspirin and aspirin containing drugs.
- Spices: Ginger, cumin, turmeric, cloves and garlic.
- Vitamins: Vitamin C and vitamin E.
- Heparin.
- Other drugs, chroquine, digitoxin, methyldopa, oral hypoglycaemic agents, phenobarbital, quinidone, quinine, refampin and sulphana.

Pathophysiology

The major signs of thrombocytopoenia observable by physical examination are petechiae, ecchymosis, and purpura. Petechae occur only in platelet disorders. The person may give a history of menorrhagia, epistaxis and gingival bleeding. The patient is questioned about recent viral infections which may produce a transient thrombocytopoenia; drugs in current use; and extent of alcohol ingestion.

Clinical Manifestations

In spite of different aetiologies, clinical manifestation of thrombocytopoenia, are similar. Thrombocytopoenia most commonly manifested by the appearance of small, flat, pin-point red or reddish brown microphages termed "Petechiae". When the platelet count is low, RBC may leak out of the blood vessels and into the skin to cause Petechiae, when petechiae are numerous, the resulting reddish skin bruise is termed "purpura". Larger purplish lesions caused by haemorrhage are termed ecchymoses. Ecchymoses may be flat or raised, pain and tenderness are sometimes present.

Prolonged bleeding often routine procedures such as venipuncture or IM injection may also indicate thrombocytopoenia. Because this bleeding may be internal the nurse must also be aware of manifestations that reflect the type of blood loss including weakness, fainting, dizziness tachycardia, abdominal pain and hypertension.

The major complication of thrombocytopoenia is haemorrhage. The haemorrhage may be insidious or acute and internal or external. It may occur in any areas of the body, including the joints, retina, and brain. Cerebral haemorrhage may be fatal.

Management

Diagnostic studies include complete laboratory studies to ascertain the status of all blood components. The most commonly used test for assessment of platelets are platelet count, peripheral blood smear and bleeding bone. In addition, bone marrow examination is performed to determine the presence of megakaryocyte (Precursor of platelets in the bone marrow), and other abnormalities such as neoplastic invasion, aplastic anaemia or fibrosis.

The primary treatment modalities for immunothrombocytopoenia purpura (ITP) are cortosteroid therapy and splenectomy. Steroids appear to decrease both antibody production and phagocytosis of the antibody-coated platelets. Splenectomy removes the principal organs involved in destruction of the antibody-coated platelets. To sum up, the treatment modalities according to different aetiologies are:

1. Immune thrombocytopenic purpura (ITP).
   - Corticosteroids.
   - Platelet transfusions.
   - Intravenous immunoglobulin.
   - Danazol (an androgen).
   - Immunosuppressives (cyclophosphomide and azathioprine).
   - Splenectomy.
2. Thrombotic, thrombocytopenic purpura (TTP).
   - Plasma infusion.
   - Plasmapheresis and plasma exchange.
   - High dose prenisone
   - Splenectomy.
3. Decreased production problems.
   - Identification and treatment of cause.
   - Corticosteroids.
   - Platelet transfusion.
   - Thrombopoietin (investigational).

The goal during acute episodes of thrombocytopenia is to prevent or control haermorrhage. The nurse has to assess the bleeding sites and take measures accordingly as practised institutional policies and follow standard guidelines to prevent and control bleeding. In a woman with thrombocytopoenia, menstrual blood may exceed the usual amount and duration. Counting sanitary napkins used during menses is another important intervention to detect blood loss. Fifty milli litres of blood will completely soak a sanitary napkin. Suppression of menses with hormonal agents may be indicated during predictable period of thrombocytopoenia.

The proper administrations of platelet transfusion is an important nursing responsibility. Platelet concentrates, derived from fresh whole blood, can increase in the platelet level effectively. One unit of platelets, a yellow liquid that is usually 30 to 50 ml in volume can be derived by centrifuging 500 ml. of whole blood. Platelet concentrates from multiple units of blood (usually from 6 to 8 different donors) can be pooled together for a single administration. Platelet transfusion can also be prepared by pheresing *single* donors This may be indicated when HLA matched platelets are needed, especially for patients requiring multiple platelet transfusions. Transfusion often must be administered twice weekly.

A primary concern in the nursing care of persons with a decreased number of platelets is the concomitant bleeding tendency. Bleeding associated with trauma is likely with a platelet count less than 60,000/mm. Spontaneous haemorrhage may be a life-threatening possibility when the platelet count is less than 20,000/mm. Ongoing nursing assessment of the patient is essential and includes alertness of increased ecchymoses, petehiae, bleeding from other sites and any change in mental status. The need for avoiding trauma is obvious. Person with platelets counts below 20,000/mm should have bleeding precautions instituted. These include the following:

- Test all urine and stools for blood (guaiac).
- Do not take temperature rectally.
- Do not administer intramuscular infections.
- Apply pressure to all venipunctures sites for 5 minutes and to all arterial puncture sites for 10 minutes.

In addition, the nurse has the responsibility of teaching the person with thrombocytopenia which includes the following.

a. Nature fo the disorder.
b. Signs of decreased platelets (Petechaie, ecchymosis, gingival bleeding, haematuria, menorrhagia).
c. Name, dosage, frequency and side effects of prescribed medications (corticosteroids) and importance of not stopping corticosteroids abruptly.
d. Measures to prevent injury:
   - Use a soft toothbrush or swab for mouth care.
   - Do not use dental floss.
   - Keep mouth clean and free of debris.
   - Avoid intrusion into rectum (e.g. rectal medication and enemas).
   - Use electric shaver.
   - Apply direct pressure for 5 to 10 minutes if any bleeding occurs.'
   - Avoid contact sports, electrice surgery and tooth extraction.
   - Avoid blood thinning drugs such as Aspirin, that decreases sticking ability of platelet.
   - Increase knowledge of contents of over-the-counter (OTC) medications and effects on platelets functioning. Read labels on OTC drugs.
e. Need for follow-up medical care..

THROMBOCYTOSIS

Thrombocytosis is defined as the presence of an abnormally high number of circulating platelets.

Aetiology Pathophysiology

Mild bleeding syndrome may be caused by quantitatively normal but functionally defective platelets. The most common cause of platelet abnormality in drugs, particularly aspirin. Aspirin inhibits, the release of intrinsic platelet adenosine diphosphate (ADP) and produces a defect in platelet aggregation. The defect remains for the lifespan of the platelet.

Thrombocytosis can be categorised as reactive (hyperactive bone marrow) or essential (myeloproliferative syndrome). The associated conditions include polycythemic vera, myelofibrosis, splenectomy, iron deficiency anaemia, chronic inflammatory diseases, haemorrhagic thrombocythermea, and advanced carcinoma.

Clinical manifestation includes thrombosis, increased bleeding tendencies, platelet counts more than 1000,000/ml.

Management

The abnormality may be detected by a test of bleeding time or more sensitively, by platelet aggregation tests. Patients with disorders of platelet function have clinical manifestation and patient care needs similar to these of persons with thrombocytopoenia. Treatment of thrombocytosis include the control of underlying cause, myelosuppressive drug therapy, plasmapheresis to reduce circulating number of platelets; and antiplatelet agents (e.g. Aspirin, dipyridamole).

DISORDERS OF COAGULATION

Haemophilia

Aetiology/Pathophysiology

Haemophilia is a hereditary bleeding disorder caused by defective or deficient coagulation factors. The two major forms of haemophilia which can occur is mild to severe forms are haemophilia A (Classic haemophilia, factor VIII deficiency) and haemophilia B (Christmas disease, factor IX deficiency). The disorder termed "von Willebrand's disease" is a related disorder involving a congenitally acquired deficiency of von Willebrand compilation proteins. Factor VIII is synthesized in the liver and circulates complexed to von Willebrand's protein (VWP). And one more haemophilia C (Factor XI deficiency).

Haemophilias are inherited as sex-lined recessive disorders and are therefore almost exclusively limited to males. The incidence of haemophilia A (1:10,000) haemophilia B (1:100,000) of the male population. Haemophilia C is rare with incidence 2 per cent to 3 per cent.

The inherent pattern of these haemophilion are as follows:

- Haemophilia A: Recessive sex-linked (transmitted by female carriers, displayed almost exclusively in men).
- Haemophilia B: Recessive sex-linked (transmitted by female carriers, displayed almost exclusively in men).
- von Willebrand disease: (VWP dysfunction) Autosomal dominant, seen in both sexes, recessive (in severe form of the disease).

Clinical Manifestation

Clinical manifestation and complications related to haemophilia include:

- Slow, persistent, prolonged bleeding from minor trauma and small cuts;
- Delayed bleeding after minor injuries (the delay may be for several hours or days);
- Uncontrollable haemorrhage after dental extractions or irritation of gingiva with a hard-bristle tooth brush;
- Epistaxis, especially after blow to the face;
- GI bleeding from ulcers and gastritis;
- Haematuria from GU trauma and splenic rupture resulting from fall or abdominal trauma.
- Ecchymoses and subcutaneous haematomas (common);
- Neurologic signs, such as pain, anaesthesia and paralysis which may develop from nerve compression caused by haematoma formation and
- Haemarthrosis (bleeding from joints) which may lead to joint deformity severe enough to cause unresolvable crippling (most commonly in knees, elbows, shoulders, hips and ankles).

Life-threatening bleeding involves retroperitoneal, intracranial soft tissue haemorrhages.

Management

A diagnosis of haemophila is made by specific assays for factors VIII, IX and XI. The partial thromboplastotime (PTT) which reflects the intrinsic pathway of coagulation, is prolonged in haemophilia A, haemophilia B and haemophilia C. The platelet count and prothrombic time is normal.

Treatment is replacement of the deficient coagulation factor. When bleeding episodes do not respond to local treatment, i.e., ice bags, manual pressure or dressings, immobilization, elevation, or topical coagulate such as fibrin foam and thrombin.

Fresh frozen plasma once commonly used for replacement therapy is rarely used now. Cryoprecipitate which primarily contains factor VIII and fibrinogen is prepared for plasma, frozen rapidly and kept frozen until used. Before administration, the cryoprecipitate is thawed slowly.

The standard therapeutic products i.e. concentrate factor used in treating haemophilia today are:

1. Factor VIII
   - Plasma derived products: Monoclate, Hemofil, Profilate, Huma
   - Recombination products: Recombinates, Kogenate,
2. Factor IX
   - Plasma-derived products: Alpha-Nine, Mononine, Ronyne, Profilinine.
   - Recombination products: Bebulin, autoplex, FEIBA and Hyate.

Nursing interventions are related primarily to controlling bleeding and include the following.

- Stop the topical bleeding as quickly as possible by applying direct pressure or ice packing the area with Gelfoam or fibrin foam, and applying topical haemostatic agents such as thrombin.
- Administer the specific coagulation factor concentrate ordered to raise the patient's level of the deficient coagulation factor.
- When joint bleeding occurs it is important to totally rest the involved joint, in addition to administering antihemophilitic factors to help prevent crippling deformities from haemarthrosis. The joint may be packed in ice, analgesics are given to reduce joint pain. However, aspirin and aspirin containing compounds should never be used.
  As soon as bleeding ceases, it is important to ROM exercises and physical therapy. Actual weight bearing is avoided until all swellings has resolved and muscle strength has returned.
- Manage any life-threatening complication that may develop as a result of haemorrhage. Example includes nursing intervention to prevent or treat airway obstruction from haemorrhage into the neck and pharynic, as well as early assessment and treatment of intracranial bleeding.

In addition, the nurse must provide ongoing assessment of the patient's adaptation to the illness. Psychosocial support and assistance should be readily available as needed. Most of the long-terms are related to patient education. The patients with haemophilia must be taught to recognize disease-related problems and to learn which problem can be resolved or borne and which require hospitalization. Immediate medical attention is required for severe pain or swelling of a muscle or joint that restricts movement or inhibits sleep and for a head injury, a swelling in the neck or mouth, abdominal pain, haematuria, melena and skin wound needed for suturing.

Daily oral hygiene must be performed without causing trauma. There are many potential sources of trauma. The patient can learn to prevent trauma by using gloves whenever needed to prevent cuts or abrasion from knives, hammer and other tools. The patient should wear a medic-alert tag to ensure that health care providers know about the haemophilia in case of an accident. Since the haemophilia is hereditary, genetic counselling is necessary as preventive measures if needed.

Vitamin K Deficiency

Vitamin K, a fat soluble vitamin, is a cofactor in the synthesis of clotting factors II, VII, IX and X. Approximately 50 per cent of required vitamin K is obtained from a normal diet and 50 per cent is produced by intestinal bacteria.

Vitamin K deficiency can be anticipated in persons who have a decrease intake and who are given broad-spectrum antibiotics, (such as neomycin sulphate that decreases the growth of intestinal bacteria. Interference with vitamin K, absorption occurs with primarily intestinal disease (Ulcerative colitis, Crohn's disease) biliary disease and malabsorption syndrome drugs such as large doses of salicylates, quinine and barbiturates interfere with vitamin K function.

Symptoms are those of anaemia superimposed on the underlying disorders that is bleeding of the mucus membrane and into the tissue. Postoperative haemorrhages may be observed. In severe cases, GI bleeding may be massive.

Management

Diagnostic features of vitamin K deficiency are prolonged PT and PTT. There is also a decrease in the levels of vitamin K dependent clotting factors.

Treatment consists of therepy for the underlying disorder and cessation of causative drugs. For mild disorders, a water soluble vitamin K preparation (menadione) is given orally or parenterally. In severe disorders, fat-soluble vitamin K preparation (Phytonadione) may be given. Fresh frozen plasma will partially correct the disorder immediately whereas, vitamin K therepy takes 6 to 24 hours to be effective and does not have the complication of fresh frozen plasma.

Nursing management includes monitoring of vital signs and teaching regarding safety precautions to prevent bruising, eipsodes. The patient should be instructed to avoid tramatising brush, avoid intramuscular injections and apply direction immediately on any bleeding site.

DISSEMINATED INTRAVASCULAR COAGULATION (DIC)

Disseminated intravascular coagulation (DIC) is a serious bleeding disorder resulting from abnormally initiated and accelerated clotting.

Aetiology

DIC is not a disease, it is an abnormal response of the normal clotting cascade stimulated by another disease process or disorders. The diseases and disorders are known to predispose in patient with DIC are as follows:

1. *Acute DIC*
   - Shock-Haemorrhagic; Cardiogenic; Anaphyloctic.
   - Septicaemia.
   - Haemolytic process – Transfusion of mismatched blood.
     – Acute haemolysis from infection or immunologic disorders.
   - Obstetric conditions:
     - Abruption placenta.
     - Amniotic fluid embolus.
     - Toxaemia.
     - Septic abortion.
   - Tissue damage.
     - Extensive burns and trauma.
     - Heat stroke.
     - Severe head injury.
     - Transplant rejections.
     - Postoperative damage, especially after extracorporeal membrane oxygenation.
     - Fat and pulmonary emboli.
     - Snake bites.
     - Glomerulonephritis.
     - Acute anoxia (e.g. after cardiac arrest).
     - Prosthetic devices.
2. *Subacute DIC*
   - Neoplastic disease – Adenocarcinoma, acute leukaemias, metastatic cancer and pheochromocytoma
   - Obstetric – Retained dead foetus.
3. *Chronic DIC*
   - Liver disease.
   - SLE.
   - Localized malignancy.

   Others include vascular disease like aortic aneurysm and fat embolus, vasculitis and crush injuries, brain injury; burns ischaemia.

Pathophysiology

The primary disease initiates the clotting process. The response is generalized and occurs throughout the vascular system, creating state of hypercoagulability. The fibrinolytic processes which normally operate to limit clot extension and dissolve clots are then stimulated. As clotting factors are depleted and fibrinolysis continue a state of hypocoagulability develops.

The most common sequela of DIC is haemorrhage. This paradox is caused by (1) decreased platelets (2) depletion of clotting factors, II, V, VIII and fibrinogen in the process and (3) the production of fibrin degradation products (FDP) through fibrinolysis. The FDP act as anticoagulants and increase the haemorrhagic tendency. As the disorder progresses, clinical manifestation may include bleeding of the mucus membranes and tissues (petechiae, ecchymosis); oral, gastrointestinal genitourinary and rectal bleeding and bleeding after injections and venipuncture may occur. Hypoxia, tachypnoea, haemoptysis, hypotension, acidosis and fever may also be presented. The generalized clinical manipulation of DIC includes the following.

a. *Neurological*
   - Confusion
   - Irritability
   - Headache
   - Dizziness
   - Seizures
   - Fevers
   - IICP
   - Vertigo
   - LOC.
b. *Sensory*
   - Blurred vision
   - Intraoccular haemorrhage
   - Inner ear-bleeding
   - Conjunctival haemorrhage
   - Epistaxis
c. Cardiovascular
   - Tachycardia
   - Chest pain
   - Hypotension
   - Abscess and peripheral pulses
   - Abnormal or increased bleeding from venipuncture or IV insertion sites.
d. Genitourinary
   - Progressive oliguria
   - Haematuria
   - Renal failure
   - Bleeding around-indwelling poley catheter
   - Severe bleeding during menstruation
   - Vaginal bleeding
   - Proteinuria.
e. Gastrointestinal
   - Melena
   - High-pitched bowel sounds
   - Nausea
   - Vomiting
   - Abdominal distension
   - Haematemesis.
f. Integumentary
   - Cool, moist skin
   - Cyanosis
   - Petechiae
   - Mottling
   - Ecchymosis
   - Purpura.
g. General
   - Acidosis
   - Acral cyanosis.

Management

Diagnosis of DIC is confirmed by laboratory findings. Abnormal RBCs may be found on peripheral smear, fibrinolysis reflected in increased fibrin split products D-dimers and prolonged prothrombin time. Fibrinogen level plabectomy is decreased. PT, PTT and TT are prolonged. Assay shows decreased levels of factors V, VIII and LX.

The management of DIC always begins with treatment of primary disease. Once this has been inhaled, the goal is to control the bleeding and restore normal levels of clotting factors. Blood products such as fresh frozen plasma, platelet packs, cryoprecipitate, and fresh whole blood may be administered, to replace the depleted factors. Heparin has been used to inhibit the underlying thrombotic process; however, it too often promotes rather than decreases bleeding and its use is controversial.

Nursing managment of the patient with DIC is extremely challenging. The person who develops DIC is critically ill and commonly has numerous sites of bleeding. The amount and nature of drainage from chest and nasogarstric tubes, oozing from surgical incisions and progressive discoloration for the skin should be noted and recorded. Continual observation for new bleeding site and for an increase or decrease in bleeding is an integral part of the nursing care plan, especially heparin therapy is being used. The susceptibility of these persons to bleeding present special problems. Medication should be given or ally or intravenously if at all possible; and small guage needles should be used when other injections are necessary. All precautions to be taken to prevent haemorrhage as described earlier (Thrombocyopoenia). Maintaining fluid balance is very essential. Person with DIC usually lose large quantities of blood and receive frequent transfusions and other fluid replacement. In addition to monitoring blood infusion rates carefully, the nurse must be alert to signs of fluid overload such a slow-bounding pulse, and increasing central venous pressure. Intake and output are to be maintained accurately.

Generally the patient is comotose and the presence of purpura, numerous intravenous lines, and drainage tube makes patient appear may upset the family members. Emotional support should be given by the nurse to family. And family to be educated accordingly regarding disease process and other treatment modality and precautionary guidelines.

DISORDERS OF WBCS

The white blood cells (WBC-Leukocyte) system is composed of neurophils, lymphocytes, monocytes, basophils and eosinophils. All but lymphocytes are derived from a common stem cell. The primary function of WBC is to provide humoral and cellular response to infections. Neutrophils are primarily responsible for phagocytosis and the destruction of bacteria and the infectious organism. Lymphocytes are the principal cells involved in immunity, which is responsible for the development of delayed hypersensitivity and the production of antibodies. Any compromise in the integrity of the WBC system renders a person susceptible to infection.

Leukopoenia refers to a decrease in the total WBC counts (granulocytes, monocytes and lymphocytes). Granulocytopoenia is a deficiency of granulocytes which incldue nutrophils, eosinophils and basophils.

Neutropenia

The neutrophilic granulocytes, which play a major role in phagocytizing pathogenic microbes are closely monitored in clinical practice as an indicator of patient's risk for infection. A reduction in neutrophils is termed "neutropenia" or granulocytopoenia. Neutropenia is defined as a neutrophil count of less than 2000/mm.

Aetiology

Neutropenia is not a disease, it is a syndrome that occurs with variety of conditions and can also be an expected effect, side effect, or unintentional effect of taking certain medication includes the following:

a. *Haematological disorders*
   - Idiopathic neutropoenia.
   - Cyclic neutropoenia.
   - Aplastic anaemia.
   - Leukaemia.

b. *Autoimmune disorders*
   - Systemic lupus erythematous.
   - Fettyis syndrome.
   - Rheumatoid arthritis.

c. *Infections*
   - Viral (e.g. hepatitis, influenza; HIV, measles).
   - Fulminant bacterial infections (e.g. typhoid fever, military tuberculosis).

d. *Drug-induced causes*
   - Antitumour antibiotics (daunorubicin, doxorubicin).
   - Alkylating agents (nitrogen mustard, busubfan and Chlorombucil).
   - Antimetabolites (methotreate, 60-mercaptepurine).
   - Anti-inflammatory drugs (phenylbutazone).
   - Antibacterial drug (chloromphenicol, trimethoprime sulfamethoxazole Penicillin).
   - Anticonvulsant drugs (Phenytoin).
   - Antithyroids.
   - Hypoglycaemia (tolbutamide).
   - Phenothiozines (chloropromazine).
   - Psychotropics (and antidepressants (Clozapine, imipramine).
   - Miscellaneous (gold, penicillamine, mepacrine and amodiaquine).
   - Zidovudine (AZT).

e. *Miscellaneous*
   - Severe sepsis.
   - Bone marrow infiltration (e.g. carcinoma, tuberculosis, lymphoma).
   - Hypersplenism (e.g. Portal hypertension, Fetty's syndrome, Storage diseases (Gaucher's disease).
   - Nutritional deficiency (Cobalamin and Folic Acid).

Pathophysiology

The patient with neutropoenia is predisposed to infection with non-pathogenic organism that normally constitute normal body flora, as well as opportunistic pathogens. When the WBC count is depressed or immature WBCs are present, normal phagocytic mechanisms are impaired. Because of the diminished phagocytic response, the classic signs of inflammation—redness, heat, swelling—may not occur. WBCs are the major components of pus; therefore, in the patient with neutropoenia pus formation is also absent. Therefore, the presence of fever is of great significance in recognizing the presence of infection in a neutropoenic patient.

Clinical Manifestation

When fever occurs in the neutropoenic patient, it is generally assumed to be caused by infection and requires immediate attention because the immunocompromised, neutropoenic condition can lead to a rapid, sometimes fatal progression of minor infections to sepsis. The mucus membranes of the throat and mouth, the skin, perineal area and pulmonary systems are common entry points for pathogenic organisms susceptible to hosts. Clinical manifestation related to these sites includes complaints of sore throat and dysphagia, appearance of the ulcerative lesions of the pharyngeal and buccal mucosa, diarrhoea, rectal tenderness, vaginal itchings, or discharge, shortness of breath, and non-productive cough. These seemingly minor complaints can progress to fever, chills, sepsis, and systic shock if not recognized and treated in early stages.

Management

The primary diagnostic test for assessing neutropoenia are the periheral WBC count and bone marrow aspiration and biopsy. A peripheral smear is used to assess for immature form of WBCs. The Hct level, reticulocyte count, and platelet count are done to evaluate general bone marrow function. Bone marrow aspiration or biopsy includes cultures of nose, throat sputum, urine, stool, blood as indicated and chest X-ray also is necessary to confirm concerned infection.

The factors involved in the nursing care and collaborative care of patients with neutropoenia include:

- Determining the cause of the neutropoenia.
- Identifying the offending organisms if an infection has developed.
- Instituting prophylactic, empiric or therapeutic antibiotic therapy and
- Administering haematopoietic growth factors (e.g. granulocyte colonystimulating factor (G-CSF); and
- Instituting protection isolation practices such as strict handwashing, visitors' restrictions, private room, high-efficiency particulate air (HEPA) infiltration, or laminar air flow (LAF) environment.
- Occasionally the cause of the neutropoenia can be easily removed. (e.g. by termination of the medications by drug-induced condition).
- Patient teaching about precaution to prevent neutropoenia.

Neutrophilia

Neutrophilia is defined as a neutrophilia greater than 10,000/m. Such an increase is normal response to infections primarily bacterial infections. Prolonged elevation of neutrophil count, especially in the absence of an apparent cause, demands a diligent search for the underlying cause. Persistent elevated neutrophil counts are associated with polycythemia vera, myeloid metaplasia and various systemic and inflammatory disorders.

LEUKAEMIAS

Leukaemia is the general term used to describe a group of malignant disorder, affecting the blood and blood-forming tissues of the bone marrow lymph system and spleen. Leukaemia occurs in all age groups. It results in an accumulation of dysfunctional cells because of a loss of regulation in cell division. It follows a progressive course that is eventually fatal if untreated.

Aetiology

The aetiology of leukamia is unknown. Regardless of the specific type of leukaemia, there is generally no single causative agent in the development of leukaemia. Most results from combination of predisposing factors including genetic and environmental influences. Persons with specific chromosomal aberrations such as occurs with Down syndrome, Von Recklinghausens neurofibromatosis and Fanconi's anaemia, have an increased incidence of acute leukaemia. Chromic exposure to chemicals such as benzene, drugs that cause aplastic anaemia, and radiation exposure have been associated with an increased incidence of disease. An increased risk for development of acute leukaemia has been noted after cytotoxic therapy for Hodgkin's disease, non-Hodgkin's lymphoma, multiple myeloma, polycythmia vera and breast, lung and testicular cancers.

Classification of Leukaemia

The leukaemias are classified as acute or chronic and are further divided according to cell type or maturity.

- *Acute leukaemia* is characterized by the clonal proliferation of immature haematopoitia cells. The leukaemia arises following malignant transformation of a single haematopoiestic progenitore followed by cellular replication and expansion of the transformed clone. The most prominent characteristic of the neoplastic cell in acute lekaemia is a defect if maturation beyond the myoloblast or promyelocyte level in AML and the lymphoblast level as ALL. Acute leukamias are subclassified as acute lymphoitic leukaemia (ALL) or acute nonlymphoitic leukaemia (ANLL) according to the specific morphology of the leukaemia cell. ANLL further classified as acute myelogenous leukaemia (AML) Promelocytic leukaemia, monocytic leukaemia and other varieties according to cell type.
- Chronic leukaemia may be lymphocytic as in chronic lymphocytic leukaemia (CLL) or granulocytic as in chronic granulocytic or myelogenous leukaemia (CMD).

1. Acute Lymphocytic Leukaemia (ALL)

Acute lymphocytic leukaemia, usually occurs before 14 years of age, peak incidence is between 2-9 years of age and is older adults.

Pathophysiology

Acute lymphocytic leukaemia is malignant disorder arising from a single lymphoid stem cell, with impaired maturation and accumulation of the malignant cells in the bone marrow. Diagnosis is confirmed by bone marrow aspirations or biopsy, which typically shows different stages of lymphoid development, from very immature to almost normal cells. The degree of immaturity is a guide to the prognosis, the greater the number of immature cells, the poorer will be the prognosis.

Clinical Manifestation

Signs and symptoms of ALL include anaemia, bleeding, lymphadenopathy and a predisposition infection. Clinical manifestation include fever, pallor, bleeding, anorexia, fatigue and weakness; bone, joint and abdominal pain; generalized lymphadenopathy; infections of respiratory tract, anaemia bleeding of mucus membrane, ecchymoses; weight loss; hepatomegaly; headache, mouth sores; neurologic manifestation including CNS involvement increased intracranial pressure, secondary to meningeal infiltration.

Management

Diagnostic findings reveals low RBC count, Hb, Hct, low platelet count low normal or high WBC count, transverse line of refraction at end of metaphysis of long bones on X-ray; hypercellular bone marrow with lymphoblasts. Lymphoblasts are also possible in CSF. A blood smear show immature lympth blasts.

Treatment of ALL include use of chemotherapeutic agents. Untreated patients have a median survival from MST) of 4 to 6 months with current chemotherapeutic regimen MST is close to 5 years. Chemotherapic protocol for ALL involve three phases:

1. *Induction*: Often using vincristine and prednisone.
2. *Consolidation*: Using modified course of intensive therapy to eradicate any remaining disease, and
3. *Maintenance*: Usually combination of drugs including the antimetabolites 6-mercaptopurine and methotrexate.

The use of prophylactic treatment of the CNS (intrathecal administration of methotrexate with or without craniospinal radiation). Intrathecal administration and/or craniospinal radiation with eradicate leukaemic cells.

The patients are advised to eat diet that contains high in protein, fiber and fluids; avoid infection (by handwashing, and avoiding crowds) and injury; take measure to decrease nausea and to promote appetite; maintain oral hygiene. Smoking and spicy and hot foods may alter taste or irritate buccal mucus membrane. These foods should be avoided and teach the patient about medication.

2. Acute Myelogenous Leukaemia (AML)

Acute myelogenous leukaemia (AML) is a disease of the pluripotent myeloid stem cell. The cause of AML is unknown. AML occurs at any age but occurs most often at adolescence and after the age of 55. There is increase in incidence with advancing age—peak incidence and is bet-ween 60-70 years of age.

Pathophysiology

AML arises from a single myeloid stem cell and is characterized by the development of immature myeloblasts in the bone marrow.

Clinical Manifestation

Clinical manifestations are similar to ALL, which includes fatigue, and weakness; headache, mouth sores, minimal hepatomegaly and lymphadenopathy anaemia, bleeding, fever, infection and sternal tenderness.

Management

Diagnostic findings reveal low RC count, Hb, Hct low platelet count, low to high WBC count with myeloblasts greatly hypercellular bone marrow with myeloblasts.

Treatment includes the use of cytarabine, 6-thioquanine, and doxorubicin or daunomycin. Treated patients MST is in 2 to 3 years. In the untreated or patient unresponsive to therapy the MST is 2 to 3 months. Some studies show bone marrow transplantation may benefit the clients.

The patient and family should be instructed to avoid sources of potential infection. Signs of potential infection should be recognized and reported to health care provider. Precaution to minimize bleeding should be emphasized (soft bristled tooth brush and electric razor). The patient should be instructed to avoid possible injury or trauma (e.g. blow nose gently, avoid constipation). Dietary instruction should include the basics of nutritionally adequate diet, particularly high protein and high fiber foods. Adequate amounts of fluids (2000 to 3000 per day). Patients should be instructed about medication, effects, side effects and nursing measures.

3. Chronic Lymphocytic Leukaemia (CLL)

The incidence of CLL increases with ages and is rare under the age of 35. It is common in men than women.

Pathophysiology

Chronic lymphocyte leukaemia (CLL) is neoplasm of activated by lymphocytes. The CLL cells which morphologically resemble mature, small lymphocytes of the peripheral blood, accumulates in the bone marrow, blood lymph nodes and spleen in large number. CLL is characterized by proliferation of small, abnormal, mature B lymphocytes, often leading to decreased synthesis of immunoglobulin and depressed antibody response. The accumulation of abnormal lymphocytes begins in the lymphnodes then spreads to other lymphatic tissues and the spleen. The number of mature lymphocytes in peripheral blood smear and bone marrow are greatly increased.

Clinical Manifestation

Usually there is no symptom. Detection of disease is often during examination for unrelated conditions, chronic fatigue, anorexia, splenomegaly, lymphadenopathy and hepatomegaly. The onset is insidious with weakness, fatigue and lymphadenopathy. Symptoms include pruritic vesicular skin lesions, anaemia, thrombocytopoenia, and enlarged spleen. The WBC count is elevated to a level between 20,000 to 100,000. This increases blood viscosity, and a clotting episode may be the first manifestation of disease. Bone marrow briefly shows infiltration of lymphocyte.

Management

The MST of person with CLL is 4.5 to 5.5 years. As a general rule, persons are treated only when symptoms, particularly anaemia, thrombocytopoenia, or enlarged lymph nodes and spleen appear. Chemotherapeutic agents used in the treatment of CLL are most often one of the alkylating agents, such as chlorambucil and the glucocorticoids. Although no treatment is curative, remission may be induced by chemotherapeutics or rataliation of the thymus, spleen or entire body. Patient and family education is that described for AML.

4. Chronic Myelogenous Leukaemia (CML)

Chronic myelogenous leukaemia (CML) occur between 25-60 years of age. Peak incidence is around at 45 years of age. Although the aetiology of CML is unknown, benzene exposure and high doses of radiation have been associated with CML. Philadelphia Chromosome (translocation of chromosome 22 and 9) is identified in person diagnosed with CML.

Pathophysiology

The primary defect in CML is in abnormal cell leading to uncontrolled proliferation of the granulocytic cells. As a result, proliferation, the number of circulating granulocytes increases sharply.

Clinical Manifestation

There is no symptoms in disease. The classic symptoms of chronic types of leukaemia also exist in CML. These include fatigue, weakness, fever, sternal tenderness, weight loss, joint pain, bone pain, massive splenomegaly and increase in sweating. CML commonly changes from a chronic indolent phase into a fulminant neoplastic process some time indistinguishable from acute leukaemia. The accelerated phase of the disease (blostic phase) is characterized by increasing number of granulocytes in the peripheral blood. There is a corresponding anaemia and thrombocytopoenia. Fever and adenopathy also may develop.

Management

Diagnostic findings reveal low RBC count, Hb, Hct, high platelet count early, lower count later; increase in polymorphonuclear neutrophilis, normal number of lymphocytes, and normal or low number of monocytes in WBC differential; low leukocyte alkaline phosphate, presence of philadelphia-chromosomes.

The overall survival rate is poor. Only 30 per cent patients will survive 5 years after diagnosis. After the onset of blast crisis the life expectancy decreased to 2 to 4 months and prognosis is grave.

The goal of therapy of CML is to control proliferation of WBC. The commonly used drugs are hydroxyurea and busulfan (monitor of WBC count needed with therapy). Once CML is converted into blastphase of disease, anthracyclines and cytosine arabinocyde have been used. The only potential curative therapy of CML is the bone marrow transplant.

Nursing intervention of leukaemia patients include taking measures to prevent infection, promoting safety, providing oral hygiene, preventing fatigue, promoting effective coping; and patient and family education regarding disease process, oral care, medications and follow-up care.

5. Lymphedema

Lymphedema is an abnormal accumulation of lymph within the tissue caused by destruction in flow.

Lymphedema can be classified as primary or secondary.

- Primary lymphedema results from hypoplastic, aplastic or hyperplastic development of the lymphatic vessels. Symptoms may manifest at birth, during puberty or in middle age.
- Secondary or acquired lymphedema most often develops from trauma to the lymph nodes. Common cause sinclude surgical removal of lymph node, radiation-induced fibrosis, inflammation, lymphomas and parasitic infection (filarial infection).

Pathophysiology

The lymphatic vessels carry lymph from the tissue back into venous circulation. This system is made up of small, thin, vessels that are found throughout the body in close proximity to the veins. The lymphatics begin as capillaries that drain the tissue of lymph (fluid similar to plasma) and tissue fluid that contains cells, cellular debris and proteins. The lymph flows through oval bodies called lymph nodes, which remove nucleus agents such as bacteria and toxin. The flow that drain into the thoracic duct and right lymphatic duct, which empty into the junction of the internal jugular vein and subclavian vein.

Pathophysiological changes may include (1) roughening of the surface of the symptomatic vessel, (2) dilation of some lymph channels with thickening and oedema of the lymphatic tissue and (3) fibrosis and separation of elastic fibers that may present in inflammatory state. Recurrent episodes of lymphoedema may cause fibrosis and hyperplatia of lymph vessels, leading to severe enlargement of the extremity called elephant basis.

Clinical Manifestation

Lymphedema of the lower extremities begin with mild swelling at the ankle, which gradually extend to the entire limb. Initially, the oedema is soft and pitting, but it then progresses to firm, rubbery, non-pitting oedema. Left leg swelling is more common than right leg swelling. This condition is aggravated by prolonged standing, pregnancy, obesity, warm weather and menstruation.

Management

Diagnostic test includes the use of lymphangiography. Radioisotope lymphography involves injections into the foot with subsequent scanning A CT Scan may show a honey comb pattern in the subcutaneous compartment.

Treatment consists of elevating the foot of the best on blocks at a height of 8 inches, wearing compression support stockings, and using an intermittent pneumatic compression device. Monitoring the circumferences of the extremities can help in determining the effectiveness of treatment.

Diuretics can be prescribed to temporaily decrease the size of the limp. Long-term antibiotic therapy may be indicated to control recurrent cellulitis and infection. Surgery is restricted to severe cases of lymphedoma that are unsuccessfully treated by medical management. Surgery also may be used to decrease the incidences of recurrent infection. Microsurgery involving vein grafting to small lymph vessels has been successful.

There is no special diet to treat lymphedema. However, the patient's receiving diuretic therapy required adequate potassium. Salty and spicy foods that predispose to fluid retention and oedema should be avoided. Avoid standing still for long periods of times. If infection is present, advise bedrest with legs are elevated.

LYMPHOMAS

Lymphomas are malignant neoplasm originating in the bone marrow and lymphatic structures resulting in proliferation of lymphocytes. The cause for the currently rising incidence is not entirely understood. Two major types of lymphoma are—Hodgkin's disease and non-Hodgkin's disease.

1. Hodgkin's Disease

Hodgkin's disease is a malignant disorder of lymph nodes first described by Thomas Hodgkin in 1832. It is characterized by proliferation of abnormal gaint, multinucleate cells called Reed-sternberg cells which are located in lymph nodes.

Aetiology

The aetiology of the Hodgkin's disease is unknown, but there may be several factors that are thought to play a role in its development. The main interactive factors include infection with Epstein Barr virus (EBV), genetic predisposition and exposure to occupational toxins. The first peak incidence in 30-40 years and second peak incidence occur at 55 to 77 years.

Pathophysiology

The presence of the Reed-Sternberg (RS) cell is the pathological hall mark of the disorder, but four histological substances of Hodgkin's disease have been recognized: Lymphocyte, predominant, nodular sclerosis, mixed cellularity and lymphocyte depletion.

Clinical Manifestation

The onset of symptoms in Hodgkin disease is usually insidious. The initial development is most often enlargement of cervical, axillary or inguinal lymph nodes. This lymphadenopathy affects discrete nodes that remain movable and nontender. The enlarged nodes are not painful unless pressure is exerted on adjacent nerves.

The patient may notice weight loss, fatigue, weakness, fever, chills tachycardia or night sweats. A group of initial findings include fever, night sweats and weight loss (termed B symptoms) correlate with a worse prognosis. After the ingestion of even small amounts of alcohol, individuals with Hodgkin disease may complain of a rapid onset of pain at the site of disease. The cause for the alcohol-induced pain is not known. Cough, dyspnoea, strider, and dysphagea may all reflect mediastinal node involvement.

In more advanced disease, there is hepatomegaly, and splenomegaly. Anaemia results from increased destruction and decreased production of erythrocytes. Other physical signs vary depending on where the disease has spread. For example, intrathoracic involvement leads to superior venacava syndrome; enlarged retroperitoneal nodes may cause palpable abdominal masses or interfere with renal function; jaundice may occur from liver involvement and spinal cord compresses lead to paraplegia may occur with extradural involvement. Bone pain occurs as result of bone involvement.

Management

Peripheral blood analysis, lymph node biopsy, bone marrow examination and radiological evaluation are important means of evaluating Hodgkin's disease using all the information from the various diagnostic studies, a stage of disease is determined as given below:

Stage I: Involvement of a single lymph node or a single extranodal site.

Stage II: Involvement of two or more lymph node regions on the same site of the diaphragm or localized involvement of an extranodal site and one or more lymph node regions of the same side of the diaphragm.

Stage III: Involvement of lymph node regions on both sides of the diaphragm may include a single extranodal site, the spleen, or other, now subdivided into lymphatic involvement of the upper abdomen in the spleen (ophiceliac and portal nodes). Stage III (1) and the lower abdomen nodes in the periaortic, mesenteric and iliac region (Stage III 2).

Stage IV: Diffuse or disseminated disease of one or more extralymphatic organs or tissues with or without associated lymph node involvement; the extranodal side is identified as H-hepatic, L. lung, P-Pleura, M-Marrow, D-Dermal and O-Osseous.

Treatment decisions made on the basis of stages of diseases as follows:

Stage	Recommended Therapy
• I, II (A or B)	: Radiation
• I, II (A or B with mediastinal mass 7-1/3 diameter of Chest)	: Combination chemotherapy followed by radiation to involved field.

• III A (Minimal abdominal disease)	:	Combination of chemotherapy with radiation to involved sites.
• III B	:	Combination chemotherapy
IV (A or B)	:	Combination chemotherapy.

The two chemotherapeutic regimens for Hodgkin's disease includes

Drugs	*Schedule*
MOPP	
• Nitrogen mustard	Days 1 and 8
• Vincristine (Oncorin)	Days 1 and 8
• Procarbazine	Days 1 and 14
• Predisone (Circle 1 and 4 only)	Days 1 and 14
ABVD	
• Dexorubiun (Adriamycin)	Days 1 and 15
• Bleomycin	Days 1 and 15
• Vinblastin	Days 1 and 15
• Dacarbazine	Days 1 and 15.

The nursing care of the Hodgkin's disease is largely based on managing pancytopoenia and other side effects of the therapy. The patient undergoing radiotherapy will need special nursing intervention. Psycholosocial considerations are just as important as they are with leukoemia. The regimen of drug administration is a 2-week course each month or as ordered by the physician.

Non-Hodgkin's Lymphoma (NHL)

Non-Hodgkin's lymphoma (NHL) is a heterogenous group of malignant neoplasms of immune system affecting all ages.

Aetiology

The cause of NHL is unknown, although viruses have been implicated. An association between the development of NHL and immunosuppressed status particularly with AIDS and organ transplant recipient has been reported. An increased incident has also been reported in persons with certain autoimmune disorders such as Sjögren's syndrome. Men once more are coming affected usually after 60 years. Burkitt's lymphoma, high grade tumour, is more common in children and persons with AIDS.

Pathophysiology

NHL's classified according to different cellular and lymphnode characteristics. As more information about the cell types is discovered, evolving schemes have been used to describe different subtypes. A variety of clinical presentation and courses are recognized from indolent (slowly developing) to rapidly progressive disease. Common names for different types of NHLs include BURKITT's lymphoma, reticulum cell sarcoma, and lymphosarcoma.

Once classification separates the NHLs into lymphocytic, histocytic and mixed cell types each of which may appear as nodular or diffuse on microscopic examination. These have been subdivided into "favourable" and "unfavourable" histology as follows:

i. *'Favourable' Histology*
- Nodular poorly differentiated lymphocytic lymphoma (NLPD).
- Nodular mixed lymphocyte and histiocytic lymphoma (NML).
- Well-differentiated lymphocytic lymphoma of the nodular (NLWD) or diffused type (DLWD).

ii. *'Unfavourable' Histology*
- Nodular histiolytic (NHL).
- Diffuse poorly differentiated lymphocytic (DPDL).
- Diffused histiocytic lymphoma (DHL).
- Diffused mixed lymphoma (DML).
- Diffuse undifferentiated lymphoma (DUL).

In general, a nodular pattern of cell structure conveys more favourable prognosis than a diffuse pattern. All NHL involve lymphocytes arrested in various stages of development, but there is no hall mark feature in NHL that parallels the Reed-Sternberg cell of Hodgkin's disease.

Clinical Manifestation

NHL originate outside the lymphoid, the method of spread can be unpredictable, and the majority of patients have widely disseminated disease at the time of diagnosis. Primary manifestation is painless lymphoid enlargement. Patients most often have nonreader peripheral lymphadinopathy that may appear bulky. The liver and spleen may be moderately enlarged the symptoms that may occur include unexplained fever, night sweats, and weight loss plus symptoms of affected organs.

Management

The diagnosis of NHL is made by examination of pathological lymphoid tissue. Lymphoid biopsy establishes the cell type and pattern. Once the diagnosis is made, the extent of the disease (staging) must be determined. As with Hodgkin's disease, accu-rate staging is a staging work-up similar to Hodgkin's disease.

Treatment of NHL involves radiotherapy and chemotherapy. Ironically, more aggressive lymphomas are more responsive to treatment and more likely to be cured. In contrast, indolent lymphomas have naturally long course. But, are difficult to effectively treat. Radiotherapy alone may be effective treatment of stage I disease, but combination of radiation therapy and chemotherapy is used for other stages.

Initial chemotherapy uses allocating agents such as cyclophos phonormid and chlorambutil. However, numerous combinations have been used to try to overcome the resistance nature of the disease. The most common chemotherapeutic regimen is CDVP (Cyclophosphemide, doxoribicin, vincristine, prednisone). Other combination therapies include cyclophosphomide, (CVP) and cyclophoshamide vincristine (oncovin) procarbozine and prednison (CVPP). Furthermore, high dose therapy with peripheral blood stem cell or bone marrow transplantation is also commonly employed.

Biologic therapy such as interferon, interlukin-2 and tumour necrosis factor is also being investigated for treating NHL.

The nurse has a crucial role in assisting patients to develop a realistic approach to the illness and to meet successfully the demands and limitations imposed by illness and its treatment. The nurse has to provide some of the needed support and guidance as the person learns to incorporate the illness into daily life. For which patient teaching needs as points covered in Hodgkin's disease.

Infectious Mononucleosis

Infectious mononucleosis is an acute disease caused by a herpes-like virus, the Epstein-Barr virus (EBV). It occurs more often in young persons with the highest incidence occurring between 15 to 30 years of age.

It is a benign disease with favourable prognosis. The onset may be subtle, appearing almost as flu-like symptoms. Malaise is a common early complaint, and it is often accompanied by fever, lymphadenopathy, sore throat, headache, generalized aches, and pains resembling those of influenza and moderate enlargement of the liver and spleen. Pruritus, palatal petechias, jaundice and rash may be present. The mode of transmission is via intimate contact with the spread of virus through the saliva. Rupture of the spleen and encephalis are rare complications.

Management

Diagnosis of infection mononucleosis is established by the heterophil agglutination or monospot blood test. Other lab tests show there is an increase in atypical lymphocytes. At the height of the disease the WBC count may range between 10,000 to 20,000 cells/mm.

Infectious mononucleosis is self-limiting and with rest. Affected persons usually recover spontaneously within 2 to 3 weeks'. Effectiveness of antiviral therapy has not been established. The use of corticosteroid may be indicated in severe cases with tonsillar enlargement and potential airway obstruction. Acetaminophen is effective in relieving fever, sore throat, and myalgias. Most persons can return to activities that do not require heavy exertion in 1 to 2 weeks and to normal activities in 4 to 6 weeks. Some persons have persistant fatigue for several months. Nursing management is supportive and focusses on the relief of symptoms and promotion rest.

The patient is instructed to avoid heavylifting or contact sports at least one month until splenomegaly resolves. An enlarged spleen is susceptible to rupture. Additional teaching includes the need for increasing fluids and to use appropriate handwashing to prevent the spread of disease. Person with this disease is to be cautioned against donating blood and avoid events that oral secretions of the infective person should not spread to others. Take precautions accordingly.

Multiple Myeloma

Multiple myeloma or plasma cell myeloma is a condition in which neoplastic plasma cells infiltrate the bone marrow and destroy bone.

Aetiology

There are many predictions regarding the aetiology of this condition, including chronic inflammation, chronic hypersensitivity reactions, and viral influences, but no actual cause has been found.

Pathophysiology

The disease process involves excessive production of plasma cells. Plasma cells are activated B Cells, which produce immunoglobulins (antibodies) that normally serve to protect the body. However, in multiple myeloma malignance plasm cells infiltrate the bone marrow and produce abnormal and excessive amount of immunoglobulin.

(Usually IgG, IgA, IgD, IgE). This abnormal immunoglobulin formed as *myeloma protein*. Furthermore, plasma cell production of excessive and abnormal amounts of cytokins (IL-4, IL-5, IL-6) also plays an important role in pathological process of bone destruction. As myeloma protein increases normal plasma cells are reduced which further compromises the body's normal immune response. Ultimately the plasma cell destroys bone and invades the lymph nodes, spleen and kidneys.

Clinical Manifestations

The condition develops slowly and insidiously. The patient often does not manifest symptom until the disease advanced at which time, skeletal pain is the major manifestation. Pain in the pelvis, spine and ribs is particularly common. Diffuse oestroporesis develops as the myeloma protein destroys more bone. Osteolytic lesions are seen in the skull, vertebrae and ribs. Vertebral destruction can lead to collapse of vertebrae with ensuing compression of the spinal cord, requiring emergency measures to prevent paraplegia (radiation, surgery, chemotherapy). Loss of bone integrity can lead to pathological fractures. Bony degeneration also causes calcium to be lost from bones, eventually causes hypercalcemia.

Hypercalemia may cause, renal, GI, or neurologic changes such as polyuria, anorexia and confusion. Later hyperuricemia and renal failure may occur. There may be symptom of anaemia, thrombocytopoenia, and granulocytopoenia, all of which are related to the replacement of normal bone marrow elements with plasma cells.

Management

Diagnosis conformed by required laboratory, radiologic and bone marrow examination.

Treatment includes administering pamidronate (for skeletal pain) and maintaining an adequate hydration are primary nursing considerations to minimize hypercalaemia. In addition, weight bearing helps bones reabsorb some of the circulation. Calcium and corticosteroids may augment the excretion of calcium. Once chemotherapy is initiated, the uric acid levels rise because of the increased cell destruction. Hyperuricemia must be resolved by ensuring adequate hydration and using allapurinol.

Suitable analgesics may be used to reduce pain. There may be potential for pathological fracture, the nurse must be careful when moving and ambulating the patient. Braces, especially for spine may also help to control pain. The patient's psychosocial needs require skilled management sometime.

Disorders of Spleen

The spleen performs many functions and is affected by many illnesses. The term "hypersplenism" refers to the occurrence of splenomegaly and peripheral cytopoenia (Anaemia, leukopoenia, thrombocytopoenia).

There are many different causes of splenomegaly which includes:

- Hereditary haemolytic anaemias: Sickle cell disease, Thalasaemia.
- Autoimmune cytopoenia: Acquire hymolytic anaemia, Immune thrombocytopoenia.
- Infections and inflammation: Bacterial endocarditis. Infectious mononucleosis, SLE, sarcoidosis, HIV infection and viral hepatitis.
- Infiltrative diseases: Acute and chronic leukaemia, lymphemias, polycythaemia cera.
- Congestion: Cirrhosis of liver, congestive heart failure.

When the spleen enlarges, its normal filtering and sequestering capacity increases. Consequently, there is often a reduction in the number of circulating blood cells. A slight to moderate enlargement of the spleen usually asymptomatic and found during a routine examination of the abdomen. Even massive splenomegaly can be well tolerated, but the patient may complain of abdominal discomfort and early satiety. Other techniques to assess the size of the spleen includes TC colloid liver-spleen scan, CT scan and ultrasound scan.

Occasionally laperotomy and splenectomy are indicated in the disorder or treatment of splenomegaly. Splenectomy can have a dramatic effect in increasing peripheral RBCs, WBC and platelet count. Another major indication of splenectomy is splenic rupture. The spleen may rupture from trauma, inadvertent tearing during other surgical procedure and diseases such as mononucleosis.

Nursing responsibilities for the patient with spleen disorders vary depending on the nature of the problems.

BLOOD COMPONENTS THERAPY (BLOOD TRANSFUSION)

Traditionally the term Blood Transfusion meant the administration of whole blood. Blood transfusion now has broader meaning because of the ability to administer specific components of blood, such as platelets, RBCs, or plasma. *Blood component therapy* is frequently used in managing haemotologic diseases. Many therapeutic and surgical procedures depend on blood product support. However, blood component therapy only temporarily supports the patient until the underlying problem is resolved. Because transfusions are not free from hazards, they should be used only if necessary. Nurses must be careful to avoid developing a complacent attitude abouit this common but potential dangerous therapy.

Type of Blood Components

The type of blood components and their indications for use are as given below.

1. *Red Blood Cells*
   i. *Packed RBCs* (PRBCs): RBCs separated from plasma and platelets. Packed RBCs are prepared from whole blood by sedimentation or centrifugation. One unit contains 250-350 ml. PRBCs indicated for severe or symptomatic anaemia, and acute or moderate blood loss. Use of RBCs for treatment allows remaining components of blood (e.g. platelets, albumin and plasma) to be used for other purposes. There is less danger of fluid overload as compared with whole blood. PRBCs are preferred RBC source because they are more components or specific.
   ii. *Autologous PRBCs* are used in elective surgery for which blood replacement is expected. These units may be stored for upto 35 days.
   iii. *Washed RBCs*: RBCs are washed with sterile isotonic saline before transfusion. These are used when previous allergic reactions to transfusion. These are used when previous allergic reactions to transfuson. There is increased removal of immunoglobulins and proteins.
   iv. *Frozen RBCs*: Frozen RBCs prepared from RBCs using glycerol for protection and frozen. They can be stored for 3 years at –188.6°F (–87°C). Frozen RBCs are indicated when autotransfusion is needed, or patient with previous febrile reactions to transfusion. There are infrequently because filters remove WBCs i.e. they relatively free from leukocytes and microemboli, but they are expensive.

Since RBCs are frozen in a glycerol solution, cells are washed after thawing to remove glycerol. They must be used within 24 hours of thawing. Successive washing with saline removes majority of WBCs and plasma proteins.

v. *Leukocyte-poor RBCs*: RBCs from which most leukocytes have been removed. It is used when client has previous sensitivity to leukocyte antigens from prior transfusions or from pregnancy. In this, fewer RBCs than packed RBCs washed leukocyte poor RBCs units have more RBCs than nonwashed.

vi. *Neocytes*: RBC units with high number or reticulocytes (young RBCs. They are used in transfusion-dependent anaemias. There will be fewer problems with iron overload, but expensive.

2. *Other Cellular Component*

i. *Platelets*

- *Random donor packs*: Platelets are prepared from fresh whole blood within 4 hours after collections. One unit contains 30-60 ml of platelet concentrate. In this, platelets are separated from RBCs by centrifuges: given in 50 ml of plasma. Platelets are used when bleeding caused by thrombocytopoenia, Thrombocytopoenia, and disseminated intravascular coagulation (DIC). In this, plasma base is rich in coagulation factors. Platelets preparation can also be packed, washed or made leukocyte poor.
- *Pheresis Packs*: Multiple units of platelets can be obtained from one donor by platelet pheresis. Platelets from an HLA-matched donor are separated by apheresis. They can be kept at room temperature for 1-5 days depending on type of collection and *storage bag used*. It is used for allosensitized persons with thrombocytopoenia. The bag should be agitated periodically. Expected increase is 10,000/mkl/u. Failures to have rise may be due to fever, sepsis, splenomegally or DIC.

ii. *Granulocytes*: Granular leukocytes separated by apheresis. It is used for granulocytopoenia from malignancy or chemotherapy. Allergen sensitization may occur with chills and fever.

3. *Plasma Components*

i. *Fresh Frozen Plasma (FFP)*: Freezing of plasma within 4 hours of collection. Here, liquid portion of whole blood separates from cells and frozen. One unit contains 200-250 ml. Plasma is rich in clotting factors but contains no platelets. It may be stored for one year. It must be used within 2 hours after thawing. It may be indicated when bleeding is caused by deficiency in clotting factors (e.g. DIC clotting deficiencies, haemorrhage, massive transfusion, liver disease, haemophilia, defibrination. It should be administered through a filter. Use of plasma in treating hypovelemic shock is being replaced by pure preparations such as albumin plasma expanders.

ii. *Factor Concentrate VIII and IX*: Prepared from large donor pools. Heated to inactivate HIV. It is used in VIII; haemophilia A and IX haemophilia B. There is increased risk of hepatitis (VIII, IX) and thromboembolism (IX). It can be given in small volumes.

iii. *Cryoprecipitate*: Precipitated material obtained from FFP when thawed. It is used for haemophilia A. Infection of burns, hypofibrinogenaemia, uremic bleeding. It contains factor VIII, XIII and fibrinogen.

iv. *Serum Albumen*: (Normal serum albumin, plasma proteinfraction).

In this albumin is chemically processed from pooled plasma. Albumin is prepared from plasma. It can be stored for 5 years. It is available in 5 per cent or 25 per cent solution. Albumin 25g/100 ml is osmotically equal to 500 ml of plasma. Hyperosmolar solution acts by moving water from extravascular to intravascular space. Serum albumin is used in hypovolemic shock, hypoalbuminaemia, burns and haemorrhagic shock. Its use has no risk of the hepatitis, does not require ABO compatibility, but lack of clotting factors, hypotension may occur if PFF is given faster than 10 ml/min.

v. *Immunoserum Globulin*: Obtained from plasma of preselected donors with specific antibodies. It is used in hypogammaglobinaemia and used as prophylaxis for hepatitis A and tetanus. It is given intramuscularly.

Administrative Procedure of Blood Components

Blood components can be administered safely through a 19-gauge or larger needle into a free-flowing IV line. Larger size needles (e.g. 19 gauge) may be preferred if rapid transfusions are given. Smaller size needles can be used for platelets, albumin and cryoprecipitates. Peripherally inserted central catheters (PICCs) are not recommended because of increased incidence of clogged lines due to slow blood flow. The blood administration tubing with a filter should have a stop cock or other means to develop a closed system, with blood open to one part and isotonic saline solution infusing through the other. Dextrose solutions or lacted ringers should not be used because they induce RBCs haemolysis. No other additives (including medications) should be given via the same tubing unless the tubing is cleaned with saline solution.

When the blood or blood components have been obtained from the blood bank, positive identification of the donor blood and recipient must be made. Improper product to patient identification causes transfusion reactions, thus placing a great responsibility on nursing personnel to carry out the identification procedure appropriately. The nurse should follow the policy and procedure at the place of employment (Hospital or institution or nursing home). The blood bank is responsible for typing and crossmatching the donors' blood with the recipients blood.

The blood should be administered (Procedure-Page No......) as soon as it is brought to the patient. It should not be refrigerated on the nursing unit. If the blood is not used in right way, it should be returned to the blood bank.

During the first 15 minutes or 50 ml of blood infusion, the nurse should stay with the patient. If there are any untoward reactions, they are most likely to occur at this time. The rate of infusion during this period should be not more than 2 ml/minute. Blood should not be infused quickly unless an emergency exists. Rapid infusion of cold blood may cause the patient to become chilled. If rapid replacement of large amounts of blood is necessary, a blood warming device may be used.

After the first 15 minutes, the rate of infusion is governed by the clinical conditions of the patient and the product being infused. Most patients not in danger of fluid overload can tolerate the infusion of 1 unit of packed RBCs over 2 hours. The transfusion should not take more than 4 hours to administer. Blood remaining after 4 hours should not be infused because of the length of time it has been removed from refrigeration.

If a blood transfusion reactions occur, the following steps should be taken:

- Stop the blood transfusion.
- Maintain a patent IV line with saline solution.
- Notify the blood bank and the physician immediately.
- Recheck identifying tags and numbers.
- Monitor vital signs and urine output.
- Treat symptoms as per physician's order.
- Use the blood bag and tubing and send them to blood bank for examination.
- Complete transfusion reaction reports.
- Collect required blood and urine specimens at intervals stipulated by hospital policy to evaluate for haemolysis.
- Document on transfusion reaction form and patient chart.

The blood bank and laboratory are responsible for identifying the types of reaction.

The major non-immunological transfusion reaction include the following:

1. *Circulatory overload*: Can occur when blood is given too rapidly or in large quantities. The elderly are particularly vulnerable. Patient develops signs of fluid overload and pulmonary congestion. The transfusion is stopped and oxygen and diuretic may be administered. The signs and symptoms of circulatory overload includes:
   - Dyspnoea
   - Chest tightness
   - Headache
   - Hypertension
   - Cough
   - Cyanosis
   - Peripheral oedema
   - Jugular vein distention
   - Rales
   - Abnormal heart sounds.
   - Hypertension
2. *Sepsis*: Bacterial contamination may occur at any time during the collection or handling of blood. Signs of sepsis begin almost immediately. The transfusion is stopped and the patient receives antibiotics and treatment for shock if it occurs. The signs of sepsis include:
   - Fever greater than 40°C.
   - Abdominal Cramps.
   - Nausea.
   - Vomiting.
   - Diarrhoea.
   - Septic shock.
3. *Disease transmission*: Hepatitis, CMV, and HIV are the most common diseases transmitted by blood transfusion. Hepatitis A and B are effectively identified with current screening capabilities but hepatitis C is still readily transmissible.

The following points are to be kept in mind when patient is receiving a blood transfusion.

- Carefully check all of the following:
  - Identity of patient to receive transfusion.
  - The label of the unit of blood for the name of the person for whom it is intended; make certain that if matches the patient's wrist band before administering the blood.
  - Expiration date of the blood.
  - Colour and consistency of blood (if bag appears to have clots, gas or a dark purple colour, it could be contaminated and should not be infused).
- Obtain base line vital signs and check again at frequent intervals throughout the procedure.
- Administer all blood products through micron mesh filters.
- Assess patient for any unusual sensation felt throughout the transfusion (This information helps with early identification of any reaction that occurs).
- Infuse blood within 4 hours after it is taken from the blood bank (to prevent bacterial growth).
- If blood cannot be infused within 4 hours, return it to the blood bank for proper refrigeration.
- Follow facility guidelines for proper disposal of empty blood bag and tubing.
- Record patient's response to the infusion.
- Report any adverse effect to the primary care provider immediately.
- Return the blood bag and tubing to the laboratory for testing if a reaction occurs.

Complication of Blood Transfusion

The complications of transfusion therapy may be significant and necessitate judicious evaluation of the patient. The common immunological reaction to blood transfusion and identification, management are as follows:

1. *Acute haemolytic reactions* caused by transfusion of

ABO-incompatible blood. This is an example of a type II Cytotoxic hypersensitivity reaction. When infusion of ABO-incompatible whole blood, RBCs or components containing 10 ml or more RBCs antibodies in the recipient's plasma attach to antigens on transfused RBCs causing RBC destruction. The chemical manifestations include chills, fever, low-backpain, tachycardia, tachypnoea, hypotension, vascular collapse, haemoglobinuria, haemoglobinaemia, bleeding, acute renal failure, shock, cardiac arrest and death.

When it occurs following measures to be taken immediately.

- Treat shock if present.
- Draw blood samples for serological testing slowly. To avoid haemolysis from the procedure, use a new venipuncture (not an existing central line and avoid small gauge needles. Send urine specimen to the laboratory.
- Maintain BP with IV colloid solution. Give diuretics as prescribed to maintain urine flow.
- Insert indwelling catheter or measures voided amounts to monitor hourly urine output. Dialysis may be required if renal failure occurs.
- Do not transfuse additional RBC containing components until the transfusion service/blood bank has provided newly cross-matched unit.

Acute haemolytic reactions can be prevented by meticulously verify and document patient identification from sample collections to component infusion and transfuse blood slowly for first 15-20 minutes with nurse is at patient's side.

2. *Febrile, nonhaemolytic reaction:* reactions are most common. It may be due to sensitization to donor WBCs, platelets or plasma proteins. There will be sudden chills and fever (Rise in temperature of greater than 1°C), headache, flushing, anxiety, muscle pain. When it occurs measures to be taken immediately include:
   - Give antipyretics as prescribed—Do not give aspirin to thrombocytopoenia patients.
   - Do not restart transfusion unless physician orders.
   - This reaction can be prevented by considering and administering leutocyte-poor blood products (filtered, washed, or frozen) for patients with a history of two or more such reactions.
3. *Mild allergic* reactions may be due to sensitivity to foreign plasma proteins. There will be flush in, itching, urticaria (hives). The nursing intervention included here are:
   - Administering antihistamine as directed.
   - If symptoms are mild and transient, transfusion may be restarted slowly.
   - Do not restart transfusion if fever or pulmonary symptoms develop.

This reaction can be prevented by prohylactic treatment with glucocorticosteroids or antihistamines. (Decadron, Benydryl) given 30-60 minutes before blood transfusion.

4. *Anaphylactic and severe allergic reaction* are due to sensitivity to donor plasma proteins and/or infusion of IgA proteins to IgA-deficient recipient who has developed IgA antibody. In this, there is anxiety, urticaria, wheezing, tightness and pain in chest, difficulty in swallowing, progressing to cyanosis, shock and possible cardiac arrest. This can be managed with following measures.
   - Initiate CPR if indicated.
   - Have epinephrine ready for injection (0.4 ml of a 1: 1000 solution S.C. or 0.1 mk of 1:1000 solution diluted to 10 ml with saline for I.V. use).
   - Do not restart transfusions.

This reaction can be prevented by transfusing extensively-washed RBC products from which all plasma has been removed. Alternatively use blood from Ig A deficient donor. Use antologous components.

5. *Delayed haemolytic reactions*: In this there is fever, chills, backpain, jaundice, anaemia, haemoglobinurea. Nursing intervention includes: monitor adequately urinary output and degree of anaemia, treat fever with tybenol (PML). May need further blood transfusions. This will be prevented by doing more specific type and crossmatch when giving patient blood.
6. *Post-transfusion graft-versus-host disease.* There will be anorexia, nausea, diarrhoea, high fever, rash, stomatitis, liver dysfunction. For which there is no effective treatment. Administer steroids. This can be prevented by giving irradiated blood products.
7. *Noncardiac Pulmonary Oedema*: There will be fever, chills, hypotension cough, orthopnoea, cyanosis, shock. Here, stop transfusion; continue IV saline; administer steroids as directed; give furosemide (Lasix) and epinephrine as ordered.
8. *Cardiac Overload*: Occurs when fluid administered faster than the circulation can accommodate. Due to this, cough, dyspnoea, pulmonary congestion, headache, hypertension, tachycardia and distended neck vein occurs. When it occurs, nursing measures inclucde:
   - Place patient upright with feet in dependent position.
   - Administer prescribed diuretics, oxygen and morphine.
   - Phlebotomy may be indicated.

   Cardiac overload can be prevented by
   - Adjusting transfusion volume and flow rate based on patient size and clinical status.
   - Have blood bank divide unit into smaller aliquots for better spacing of fluid input.
9. *Sepsis*: Occurs when transfusion of bacterially-infected blood components. There will be a rapid onset of chills, high fever, vomiting, diarrhoea, marked hypotension or shock. Nursing interventions here include:
   - Obtain culture of patient's blood and send bag with remaining blood and tubing to blood bank for further study.

- Treat septicaemia as directed-antibiotics, IV fluids and vasopressors.

Sepsis can be prevented by collection, process storing and transfusion of blood products according to blood banking standards and infusion within 4 hours of starting time.

Prevention is the key to management of transfusion. Accurate prescreening of potential donors, meticulour laboratory testing, and close patient monitoring are all essential components of care. The common screening guidelines for *blood donors* includes that persons with any of following are not permitted to donate blood.

- History of infectious diseases such as hepatitis HIV infection and AIDS tuberculosis, syphilis or malaria.
- Malignant diseases.
- Allergies or asthma.
- Polycythaemia Vera.
- Abnormal bleeding tendencies.
- Hypotension (current).
- Anaemia (current).
- Recent pregnancy or major surgery.
- Men with at least one homosexual or bisexual contact since 1975 (Concern for AIDS).
- International travel to malarial areas or high risk countries (concern for AIDS).
- Blood transfusion during last 6 months.
- History of jaundice.
- Diseases of the heart, lung or liver.
- Immunizations or vaccinations with attenuated viral vaccine rubella or rabies vaccine.
- Haemoglobin level below 13.5 g/dl for men, or 12.4 g/dl for women.
- Abnormalities in vital signs particularly fever.

Endocrinological Nursing

The endocrine system is an integrated chemical communication and coordination system that enables reproduction, growth and developement with the nervous and immune systems, the endocrine system maintains the internal homeostasis of the body and coordinates response to external and internal environment changes. The endocrine system is composed of glands and glanduler tissues that synthesize, store and secret chemical messengers (hormones) that travel through the blood to specific target cells throughout the body. The specificity of the system is determined by the affinity of reception on the target organs and tissues for a particular hormone, the 'lock and key' mechanism.

The endocrine system consists of the hypothalamus, anterior and posterior pituitary, thyroid, parathyroid,adrenal cortex, adrenal medulla pancreas, gonads, peneal body and thymus glands. Specialized endocrine cells are also located along the gastrointestinal tract. The hormones from these glands are vital to this important life transactions of the organism, including differentiation, reproduction, growth and development, metabolism adaptatation and sexual function.

ASSESSMENT OF THE ENDOCRINE SYSTEM

Normal function of all the hormones influence four broad domains which include maintenance of a normal internal environment, energy production, storage and utilization; growth and development; and reproductive and sexual functions. Hormones affect every body tissue and system causing great diversity in the signs and symptoms of endocrine dysfunction. Therefore, assessment of the endocrine system is often difficult and requires keen clinical skills to detect mainfestations because of disruption in maintenance of normal internal enviornment, inadequate energy production, storage and utilization, abnormal growth and development and abnormal reproductive and sexual function.

Systemic assessment of multiparameters is necessary to define the healthiness of a person's endocrine system or needs. The anatomical location of endocrine glands preludes their direct assessment. Endocrine dysfuntion may result rom deficient or excessive hormone secretion, transport abnormalities, and inability of the target tissue to respond to a hormone, or inappropriate stimulation of the target tissue to respond to a hormone, or inappropriate stimulation of the target tissue receptor. A thorough history from the patient or significant others is absolutely necessary. Special attention should be paid to the patient history, regarding fluid and nutritional intake, elemination pattern, energy level, perceptions of changes in body characteristics, reproductive and sexual function and tolerance to stressors.

Fluid/Nutritious intake: May be increased or decreased intake may not be associated with weight loss or weight gain, and also cover quantity and quality of food and fluids including alcohol and tolerance of foods

Elimination patterns: Includes frequency, approximate amount, and colour of urinary elminations the pressence of nocturia or dysuria the frequency of the colour of bowel movements, eonstipation, diarrhoea, etc.

Energy level: Performing proper activity of daily living, etc. Perception of changes in body-includes changes in hair distribution, body proportions, voice, skin pigmentation, etc.

Reproduction and sexual related problems: Fragility, menstruation and pregnancy in females and impotence in males.

Tolerance to stressors: Physical and psychological stressors such as intolerance to heat and cold infection, irritation, euphoria, depression,crying and anger.

The collection of objective data about endocrin system requires a complete physical examination which includes inspection, palpation and other assessment skills.

The nurse should observe the patient's general appearance and appropriateness of dress for ambient temperature. Assessment should include the following.

1. *Body size:* Height and weight compared to the table of standards or estimation of normality, size of the hand and extremities, proportionality and posture and facial features.
2. *Skin:* Skin colour, pigmentation, texture, coarseness, leathery texture excessive thinness, size of the sweat glands, diaphoresis, acne, strial, echymoses and vitiligo,
3. *Hair:* Texture, distribution, brittleness and lopecia.
4. *Face:* Colour, erythema, especially on cheeks (Plethora), pained, anxious expression.

5. *Eyes:* Eyebrows, hair distribution,visusl scuity, lens opacity, shape, position, movement of eyelids, lid lag, visual fields, extraocular movements, oedema.
6. *Nose:* Mucosa, noisy breathing.
7. *Mouth:* Buccal mucosa, condition of teeth, malocclusion and mottling, tongue size and fasciculations (localized, uncoordinated uncontrollable twitching of single muscle groups) shape and size of jaw.
8. *Voice:* Huskiness or hoarseness,volume, pitch and slurring.
9. *Neck:* Symmetry; alignment; forceful carotid pulsation, unusual bulging of thyroid lobes behind the sternoleidomatoid muscles; trachia in midline, dullness, thickening, flabbiness of vocal cords, polyps, gray-brain hyperpigmentation on posterior neck and axilae (acanthosis nigricans); when inspecting the thyroid gland observations should be made first in the normal position, preferably with side lighting,then slight extentions and then as the patient swallows some water.
10. *Extremities:* Size, shape, symmetry, proportionately (distance from symphysis pubis to foot; approximately half of total height) odema.
    a. *Hands:* Tremors (a piece of paper is placed on outstretched fingers, palmdown, to assess fine tremor), muscle strength grip, thenar (ball of the thumb, westing, dupuytrens, constracture, clubbing muscle wasting.
    b. *Legs:* Muscle weakness (assessed by having the seated patient extend one leg to a horizontal position; ability to hold this position for 2 miniutes usually indicates normal muscle strength) bowing, colour and amount of hairs, size of feet, corns, celluses and pedal pulses.
    c. *Toes:* Masceration, fissures, deformities, toe nails with fungal infection
    d. *Reflexes:*Particularly deep tenden reflexes, relaxation time
    e. *Pulses:* Rate and rhythm.
    f. *Thorax:* Gynecomastia in men.
    g. *Abdomen:* Increased pigmentation of scars, purplish pain on light palpation.
    h. *Genitalia:* Decreased hair distribution (diamond pattern in women may indicate virillizing adrenal tumour) size of the testes, clitoral enlargement.

Inspection and palpation are used to check skin turgor, mucous membrane moisture, and jugular vein distention and to check for the presence of edema. These data will give information about the fuid and electrolyte status of the person which can be charged with almost any endocrine problem routine palpation required for thyroid, parathyroid gland and routine palpation required for thyroid, parathyroid gland and panreas to determine the size, shape and symmetry. In addition, assessment of vital signs (TPR,BP heart sound) routine done.

Diagnostic Studies of the Endocrine System

Accurately performed laboratory tests aid and confirm diagnosis of problems of the endocrine system. The commonly used tests are as follows:

Pituitary Studies

- *Serum studies:* include test of growth hormone, somatomelin (insulin-like growth factor (1); GH release after exercise; insulin-induced hypoglycemea, prolactin level; FSH an LH; water deprivation tests.
- *Radiological studies:* Still X-Ray, CT scan, MRI.

Thyroid Studies

- *Serum studies:* Include test for T4,T3,T3 resin uptake, Free T4 Free T3, radioactive iodine uptake TSH and calcitonin.
- Radiological studies- Thyroid scan.

Parathyroid

- Serum studies: parathyroid hormones (PTH), Total serum calcium phosphorous, 125-Dihydroxy vitamin D3 tests
- T Radiological: Skeletal X-ray. CT scan

Adrenal Studies

- Serum studies: Cortisol, aldosterone, ACTH stimulation, dexamthosone suppression (overnight), metyrapone suppression tests.
- Urine studies: 17-Ketosteroid, aldosteron, free cortisol vanillymandelic acid.

Pancreatc Studies

- Serum studies- FBS, oral glucose tolerance, capillary glucose monitoring and glylosylates Hb.
- Urine studies- Glucose (Sugar), ketone, glucose and acetone tests.

DISORDERS OF PITUITARY GLAND

Hyperfunction of the Pituitary Gland (Hyperpituitarism)

The hypothalamus and pituitary gland form a unit that controls the function of several endocrine glands- thyroid, adrenals, and gonad as well as a wide range of physiological activities.

Aetiology

Hyperfunction of the anterior portion of the pituitary gland may involve one or more hormones. A cause from the pituitary gland itself is deemed primary. If the cause is from interference with the pituitary pathway (i.e.if cause of stems from the hypothalamus) the problem is considered *secondary*.

Tumours of the pituitary gland are common cause of hyperfunction. pituitry hyperfunction also can result from pituitary hyperplasia.

The cause of hyperplasia is not always known, but may be due to altered feedback signals cause the hypersecretions.

Diminished feedback from target organ secretions can result in hyperplasia and hypersecretion.

The cause of pituitary tumours or adenomas are unknown pituitary adenomas and functioning or nonfunctioning, depending on whether or not they secrete a homone. Most adenomas are benign, but can be come quite aggressive and grown to large sizes. They are classified according to the hormone being secreted. For examples, prolactinomas and growth hormons secreting tumour adenomas also are classified according to tumour size as given below.

- Enclosed- No invasion into the floor of the Sella turcica.
- Invasive- Destruction of part or all of the Sella turcica.
- Microadenoma- Enclosed tumour less than 10mm in diameter.
- Macroadenoma- Enclosed tumours greater than 10mm diameter; these tumour may show suprasellar extension.

Pathophysiology

Pituitary adenomas may depend on intrasellar adenomas, less than 1 cm in diameter that present with manifestations of hormonal excess without sellar enlargement or extraseller extension. Panhypopituitarism does not occur. Macroadenomas are the tumours larger than 11 cm in diameter and caused generalized sellar enlargement. Tumour 1 to 2 cm in diameter and confined to the sell turcica. These tumour can usually be sucessfully treated. Larger tumours esecially those with suprasellar, sphenoid sinus or lateral extension are much difficult to manage and treat. panhypopituitarism (insufficiency of pituitary hormone caused by damage or deficiency of pituitarygland), and visual loss increase in frequency with tumour size and suprasellar segment. Alteration is physiological functioning that occurs with pituitary tumours result from the presence of space occupying mass in the cranium and from the effects of the excessive secretions of hormones by functional neoplasm. In contrast, another alteration may result from the compression of glandular tissues by the tumour mass, that can cause a decrease in the secretion of one or more anterior pituitary hormones and is caused by a nonfunctional adenoma. Alteration may be neurological and endocrine alteration.

Neurological alteration occurs because the growing tumour presses on the dura, diapharagm sellae, or adjascent structure, including optichiaasm, caranial nerve II, III, IV and VI may be involved causing visual defects. Tumour may involve the neighbouring bony structure and lobes further may compress or infilltrate hypothalamus. Sudden increase in size with rapid onset of neurological signs may lead to pituitary apoplexy haemorrhage into the tumour.

Endocrine alterations are depending on which hormone the adenoma is secreting a variety of effects may be seen.

Clinical Manifestation

The clinical mainifestation of pituitary hormone secreting tumours include the following:

Neurological Manifestation

- Visual defects often is first seen as losses in superior temporal quadrants with progression to a hemianpia or scotomas and finally to total blindness.
- Headache
- Somnolence
- Rarely signs of increased intracranial pressure (hydrocephalus and Papilledema)
- With very large tumours, disturbance in appetite, sleep, temperature regulation, and emotional balance becuse of hypothalamic involvement.
- Behvioural changes and seizures with expansion causing compression of the temporal or frontal lobe (very rare).

Endocrinal Manifestations

a. Prolactin Hyper secretion

In females

- Menstrual disturbances, such as irregular menses, anovulatory periods, oligomenorrhea or amenorrhea.
- Infertility.
- Galactorrhoea.
- Manifestations of ovarian steroid deficit; such as dyspareunia, vaginal mucusal atrophy, decreased vaginal lubrication and decreased libido.

In males

- Decreased libido and possible erectile dysfuntion.
- Reduced sperm count and infertility.
- Gynecomastia
- Galactorrhoea.

And both males and females have depressed levels of gonadal steroids.

b. Growth hormone hypersecretion (acromegaly)

- Macroadenoma with resultant headache and visual changes.
- Changes in facial features (coarsening of features; increased size of nose, lips and skin folds; prominence of supraorbital ridges; growth of mandible resulting in prognathism and widely-spaced teeth;soft tissue growth resulting in facial puffiness.
- Increased size of the hands and feet and weight gain.
- Deepening of voice from thickening of vocal cords.
- Increased vertebral bodies resulting in thoracic kyphosis.
- Enlarged tongue, salivary glands, spleen, liver, heart, kidney and other organs; cardiomegaly results in increased blood pressure and signs and symptoms of congestive cardiac failure.
- Elevated blood pressure even without cardiac failure.
- Snoring, sleep apnoea and respiratory failure.
- Dermatological changes; Acne, increased sweating, oilness, development of skin tags.
- Hypertrophy progressing to atrophy of skeletal muscles.
- Backache, arthralgia, or arthritis from point damage and bony overgrowth.

- Peripheral nerve damage, such as corpal tunnel syndrome or neuropathies, from bony overgrowth and change in nerve size.
- Imapired glucose tolerance progressing to diabetes mellitus.
- Changes in fat metabolism resulting in hyperlipidaemia.
- General changes in mobility; presence of lethargy and fatigue
- Oesteoporosis.
- Radiographic findings indicative of bony proliferation in hands, feet,skull, ribs and vertebrae.
- Electolyte change, increased urinary excretions of calcium; elevated blood phosphate level.

Gonadotrophic hypersecretion: The incidence of gonadotrophic hypersecretion occurs more in male than female, highest incidence is in middle age, in which follicle-stimulating hormone (FSH) is more common and also luteinizing hormone (LH) secretion. The clinical mainfestation, the ptient will have history of normal pubertal development and fertility, but there will be hypersecretions of only FSH result in secondary to hypogonadism.

Management

In addition to history and physical examination, diagnosis is confirmed by routine pituitary studies.

Pituitary adenomas are treated with surgery, radiation or drugs to suppress hypersecretion by adenoma. Pituitary surgery is initial therapy of choice by many surgeons, and the transphenoidal microsurgical approach to the sell turcica in the procedure of choice. Transfrontal craniotomy is required only in the occasional patient with massive suprasellar extension of the adenoma.

Pituitary radiation is usually reserved for patients with larger tumours who have had an incomplete resectin of large pituitary adenomas. Both surgery and radiation have its own advantages and complications. The common complication in hypopituitarism, damage to optic nerve mechanism, seizures, radionecroses of brain tissue.

Medical management of pituitary adenoma became feasiblity with the availability of bromocriptive, a dopamine agonist, bromocriptine a dopamine agonist. The drug is most sucessful in the treatrment of hyperprolactinemia and is also useful in selected patients with acromgaly or Cushing's disease. Octreotide acetate, a analogy is used in the therapy of acromegaly and TSH secreting adenomas.

The patient with pituitary adenoma will need teaching and support to deal with a variety of issues including body image, changes, anxiety, sexual functioning, active tolerance and homegoing medications.

The patients who have undergone surgery with transphenoidal resection are advised to avoid activities causing incrased intracranial pressure. Bending over at the waist, blowing to the nose forcefully, coughing and straining with defecation can increased intracranial pressure. Teaching should be inclusive of strategies to prevent constipation and its avoidance of such activity. Assistance may be needed with activities of daily living.

PROLACTIN HYPERSECRETION

Prolactin (PRL) hypersecretion is the most common endocrine abnormality caused by hypothalamic-pituitary disorders and PRL is the hormone most commonly secreted in excess by pituitary adenoma.

Aetiology

The causes of prolactinaemia are physiological, pathological and pharmacological and include the following;

i. *Physiological:* prolactinoma, primary hyperthyroidism chronic renal failure, polycystic ovarian syndrome; Cushing's disease; hypothyroidism, acromegly, chest wall trauma; spinal cord injury and idiopathic.
ii. *Pharmacological*
   - Psychotrophic agent: Neuroleptics (phenothiazone, chloropromozon and haloperidol.
   - Antidepressants: Trycyclics, impiramine, monoamino oxidase inhibitors.
   - Anxiolytics; Benodiazephnes.
   - Antiemetics: Metoclopramide, sulpiride.
   - Opiates: Methodone, morphine.
   - Gastrointestinal agents: Metodopramide, cisapride, dompiridone
   - Bet Blockers-Ranitidine, cemetidine, femotidine
   - Antihypersensive: Resrpin, methyldopa.
   - Calcium Channel Blocker: Verapamil
   - Hormones: Estrogens, Thyrotrophin-releasing hormone (TRH).

Pathophysiology and Clinical Manifestation

Normal serum prolactin levels are usually less than 20 mg/m1. Prolactin is a natural contraceptive (inhibits gonadotropin releasing hormone (GRH) and is necessary for lactation.

The clinical manifestations of PRL excess are the same regardless of cause. The classic features are galactorrhoea and aminorrhe a in women and galactorrhoea, decreased libido or erectile dysfuntion in men.

Pathophysiological mechnism of prolactin hypersecretion include dopamine disorder, hypersecretion includes dopamine disorders, hypersectretion of pituitary tumours, hypothalamic thropin, releasing hormones stimulation, neugenic secretions triggered by chest irritation (rib fracture) anoracotomy, or herpes zosteur) and decreased clearance of prolactin as seen in chronic renal failure.

Management

The assessment of patient with galactorrhoea or unexplained gonodal dysfunction with normal or low plasma gonadeotrophin levels should include a history regarding menstrual status, pregnancy, fertility, sexual function and symptoms of hypothyroidism or hypopituitarism. Current and previous use of medication shall be documented.

All patients with PRL- secretioning macroadenomas should be treated, because of the risks of further tumour expansion. hypopituitarism and visual imairment. Treatment for patient with microadema is also recommended to prevent early osteoprosis.

Surgical treatment of choice is resection of the aenoma with the trans-sphenoidal approach. Medical treatment consists mainly of brococriptine, a potent domaine against the stimulate, dopamine and affects hypothalaemia and pituitary levels. The dosage2,5 to mg/dl orally in divided doses. Side effects such as dizziness postural hypertension, nausea, that can be minimised by gradually increasing the dose. Another drug used is pergolide Mesylatexd (dose 25 to 300 mg/dl).

The teaching needs of the hypeprolactimea are similar to those of person with hyperpituitarism.

GROWTH HORMONE HYPERSECRETION

Growth hormone (GH), an anabolic hormone promotes protein synthesis and moblilizes glucose and free fatty acids. Overproduction of GH which is usually caused by a benign pituitary adenomea (tumour) causes gigantism or acromegaly chracterized by soft tissue and bony overgrowth.

Pathophysiology

In acromegaly, chronic GH hypersecretion is usually related to a pituitary adenoma. The secretion remains episodic, although the number, amplitude, and duration of secretory episodes increased and occur randomly. The chracteristic nocturnal surge is absent, and there are abnormal responses to suppression and stimulation. Therefore, glucose suppressibility is lost and GH stimulation by hypoglycaemia, is usually absent. Most of the deterious effects of chromic GH hyperscecretion are caused by its stimulation of excessive amount of insulin-like growth factor1(IGF-1 a protein secreted by the liver) and palsma levels of this are increased in acromegaly. The growth promoting effects of IGF -1 lead to the chracteristic proliferation of bone, carilage and soft tissues and increase in size of other organs to produce the classic clnical manifestation of acromegaly. The insulin resistance and carbohydrate intolerance seen in acromegaly appear to be direct effect of GH and not due to IGF-1 excess.

Clinical Manifestation

Symptoms of acromegaly begin insidiously in the third and fourth decades of life and both genders are affected equally. When the problem develops after epiphysal closure bones increase in thickness and width. Physical features include enlargement of the hands, feet and paranasal and frontal sinuses include enlargement of the hands , feet and paranasal and frontal sinuses and deformities of the mandible and spine. In addtion, enlargement of the soft tissue (e.g.tongue,skin, abdominal organs causes mainfestation such as speech difficulties and hoarseness, coarsening of facial features, abdominal distention and sleep apnoea. The sleep a pnoea may be related to upper airway narrowing or may be central in origin. Persons with acromegaly may have hypertension, cardiomegaly, left ventricular hypertrophy, diaphoresis, oily skin, peripheral neuropathy, proximal muscle weakness, and joint pain, women exhibit menstrual disturbances.

The enlarged pituitary gland can exert pressure on surrounding structures, leading to visual disturbances and headaches. HG mobilizes stored fat for energies; it increases free fatty acids levels in the blood and predisposes patients to atherosclerosis. Prolonged secretion of GH is diabetogenic which leads to hyperglycemia.

Management

Diagnostic measures include evalution of plasma GH and IGF 1 levels, IGF binding protein 3 (IGF BP-3), oral glucose tolerance tests. MRI, CT scan for lacating tumour and opthalmologic examination.

The therapeutic goal in accromegaly and giagantism is to return GH levels to normal . This is accomplished by surgery, radiation, drug therapy, or combination of the three.

Surgery is most commonly accomplished with trans sphenoidal approach, in which an incision is made in the inner aspects of the upper lip and gingiva. The Sella turcica is entered through the floor of the nose and sphenoid sinuses. The goal of transphenoidal microsurgery removes only the GH - Secreting adenoma. Sometimes pituitary gland may be destroyed and removed, which result in deficiency of hormone of anterior pituatany which requires parental administration of the essential hormones produced by target organs (glucocorticoids, thyroid hormone and certain sex homones

Conventional radiotherapy is also sucessful, although a much longer period is required to reduce GH levels to normal streotactic radiosurgery (gamma surgery) may be applied to small, surgically inaccessible pituitary tumours.

Drug therapy may include the use of bromocriptine (parlodel), a dopamine agonist or octreotide (Sandostatin), a somastatin analog that reduce GH levels to within the normal range in many patients. The GH-lowering effects of these drugs are seldom complete or permanent and they are often used adjuvant to other therapies or to reduce tumour size before surgery.

Nursing interventions include assessment of signs and symptoms of abnormal tissue growth and evaluates physical size of each patient from time to time, and physical application, symptom of diabetes mellitus and cardic vascular disease.

The individual treated surgically needs skilled neurosurgical nursing care and must be prepared before surgery for postoperative care. Nursing intervention includes preoperative instillation of bacteracin nose drops, discussion of mouth breathing, mouth care, ambulation, pain control, activity and hormone replacement. The patient should be instructed to avoid vigorous coughing, sneezing and straining at stool (valsalva meneouver) to prevent CSF leakage from the point at which sella turcica was entered, and skilled postoperative neurosurgical care should be procide. The complication of surgical intervention includes transient diabetes insipidus, menigitis, infection, CSF rhinorrhea and hypopituitarism. Dieting and activities recommended according to problem rised. e.g. DM. CHF, etc.

HYPOPITUITARISM

Hypopituitarism is a rare disorder that involves a decrease in one or more of the anterior pituitary hormones. (i.e, Growth Hormones (GH) Adrenocorticotrophic hormone (ACTH), Gonadotropic hormone (GTH), Protactin (PRL), Thyroid stimulation hormone (TSH) and non-functioning pituitary adenomas). Any combination of deficit of the six major harmones may occur in hypopituitarism.

Aetiology

Hypopituitarinism may be classified in number of ways, isolated, partial or panhypopituitary transient or permanent Idiopathic or organic, and primary (Pituitary) or secondary (affecting hypothalemic releasing factors). Several disorders can interfere with the function of interior pituitary gland and cause hyposecretion of one or more hormones or hypoptuitarism which includes the following.

- *Tumours:* Craniopharyngioma; primary CNS tumours; nonsecreting pituitary tumour.
- *Ischemic changes:* Sheehan's syndrome 'Ischemic changes following postpartum hemorrhage or infections resulting shock
- *Developmental abnormalities:*
- *Infections:* Viral encephalities, bacteremia and tuberculosis.
- *Autoimmune disorders*
- *Radiation:* Damage, particularly after treatment of secreting adenomas of pituitary gland.
- *Trauma:* Including surgery.

Pathophysiology

In hypopituitarism, the symptoms vary widely depending on the cause and the endocrine dysfunction present. If tumour is the cause, symptoms resulting from growth of a space-occupying lesion in the cranium, effects resulting from pressure on the optic chiasm and potential disturbances of the cranial nerves III, IV,and VI. If the tumour arises from regions surrounding the pituitary such as Rathke's pouch (craniopharyngiomas), the hypothalamus, or the third ventricle, the neurological signs and symptoms will be more severe and include manifestation of increased intracranial pressure.

The endocrine dysfunction may be the result of hypothalamic damage of primary pituitary disease. The most frequent pathophysiological alteration results from lack of synthesis and secretion of ganodotropin. The patients with hypopituitarism exhibit all or only selected aspects of these hormonal deficiency. Usually the pathological altration progresses slowly.

Clinical Manifestations

Clinical findings associated with pituitary hypofunction vary with the degree and speed of onset of pituitary dysfunction and are related to hyposecretion of the target glands. The symptoms are often and commonly included weakness, fatigue, headache, sexual dysfunction fasting hypoglycaemia, dry and skin, diminished tolerance stress, and poor resistance to infection. In the adults, premature wrinkling around the eyes and mouth is common. Psychiatric symptoms include apathy, mental slowness, delusions, orthostatic hypertension. The common clinical manifestation of hypopitutarism include the following:

i. Manifestation based on causes, such as bacteremia, viral hepatis, autoimmune disorders and trauma.
ii. Manifestation such as vision changes, papillaedema or hydrocephalus if cause is tumour
iii. Manifestation of gonadotropin deficiencies.
   - Decreased Serum levels of FSH, LH and gonadal steroids.
   - Children- delayed puberty.
   - Adults.
     a. Women-oligomenorrhoea, or amenorrhoea, uterine and vaginal atrophy, potential atrophy of breast tissue, loss of libido, decrease in body hair and decreased breast size.
     b. Man- loss of libido, decreased sperm count, possible erectile dysfunction, decreased testicular size, decreased total body hair, impotence.
iv. *Manifestations of Growth hormone deficiency.*
   a. Children.
      - Stunted growth (below third percentile) with normal body proportions, excessive subcutaneous fat, poor muscle development.
      - Immature facial features and immature voice.
      - Slow growth of nails and thin hair.
      - Delayed puberty but eventual normal sexual development.
      - Decreased level of GH.
   b. Adults
      - Severe, short stature.

- Immature faces
- Moderate obesity
- Decreased muscle mass and weakness
- Lassitude
- Emotional liability.
- Decreased basal levels of GH or decreased response to provocative testing.
- Some person my have norml GH level with low level somatomeding (IGF-1)

v. Manifestations of prolectin deficiency.
- Failure to lactate in the postpartum women (Sheehan's syndrome).
- decreased serum levels of prolactin.

vi. Manifestations of Thyroid stimulating hormone (TSH) deficiency. signs and symptoms of secondary hypothyridism-anorexia, bulimia.
- Decreased serum levels of TSH and thyroid hormone.

vii. Manifestation of ACTH deficincy
- Signs and symptoms of secondary ACTH insufficiency; no hyperpigmenation
- Decreased levels of ACTH, glucocorticoids and adrenal and ogens (aldosterone levels may be normal).

Management

The decision to treat a patient is based on symptoms of a mass lesion including headache, impaired vision, and cranial nerve palsy and other factors include concerened hormonal deficiency. Treatment of hypopituitarism consists of surgery, or radiation for tumour removal, permanent target gland hormone replacement and nutrition dietory plan. Replacement therapy is carried out with corticosteroids, thyroid hormone, and sex hormones. Gonadotropin can some time restore fertility.

A primary nursing role in anterior pituitary insufficiency is assessment and recognition of subtle signs and symptoms. Nursing care focusses on assisting the patient to effectively cope with change in the body image and teaching about treatment protocol. Some symptoms are reversible once the treatment is initiated. Treatment with sex steroids helps to initiate the development of sexsual chracteristics and adolescent entering puberty. Treatment with sex steroids restores secondary sexual chracteristics in adults, and treatment with gonadotropins restores fertility in the women with normal menstrual cycles. Helping patients identify their strength, coping strategies may help them to deal with body image disturbances and decreased self esteem that may result from their illness.

Patient education is another focus of nursing care. The patient must be prepared for various diagnostic tests including blood tests and roentgenograms, CT scans, or MRI of the head. If a tumour is a cause of the deficiency, the tumour is removed. Hormonal replacement of therapy with gonadal steroids and gonadotropin in adolecents and in adults are individualized. The patient needs to be taught about precribed dedication GHs are given subcutaneously. Gonadal steroids are given orally to restore sexual chracteristics and gonadotropin or clomiphene is used in women to induce ovulation if pregnancy is desired. Patients should be taught that steroids are effective in preventing premature bone demineralization. Patient who declines hormone therapy, particularly women, need to be monitored periodically for accebrated bone loss and must take adequate calcium.

HYPERFUNCTION OF POSTERIOR PITUITARY

The hormone secreted by the posterior pituitary are antidiuretic (ADH) hormones, is also called arginine vasopressin (AVP) and oxytocin. These hormones are formed in the hypothalmus and stored in the posterior pituitary. ADH contributes to fluid balance by contolling renal reabsorption of free water, It also has potent vasoconstriction properties. *Oxytocin* controls lactation and uterine contraction. Oxytocin excess is not recognized as a clinical problem. This hormone is administered pharmacologically in the management of labour.

SYNDROME OF INAPPROPRIATE ANTI-DIURETIC HORMONE (SIADH)

Syndrome of inappropriate anti-diuretic hormone is (SIADH) also called Schwartz-Bartter syndrome occurs as a result of the excessive release of ADH (vasopressin), resulting in fluid and electrolyte imbalance of those indicated by the plasma osmotic pressure.

SIADH is characterized by fluid retention, serum hypoosmality, dilutional hyponatraemia, hypochloremia, concentrated urine in the presence of normal or increased intravascular volume and normal renal function.

Aetiology

SIADH has various causes which include the following.

- *Pulmonary disorders*: Malignant neoplasms (e.g. Oat cell adenocarcinoma of lung), tuberculosis, ventilator patients receiving positive pressure and lung abscesses pneumonia, COPD.
- *Other malignancies*: Duodenum, pancreas, prostatic lymphoma, sarcoma, leukaemia, Hodgkin's lymphoma, non Hodgkin lymphoma and Thymonia.
- *CNS disorders*: Tumours infection (meningitis), trauma (subarachnoid haemorrhage), cerebrovascular accident, surgery GBS, SLE, encephalitis and skull fracture.
- *Endocrine disorders:* That result in hypovolaemia and impair free water excretion, particularly if associated with fluid replacement (adrenal insufficiency and anterior pituitary insufficiency).
- *Drugs:* Such as clofibrate, chlorpropamide, thiazides, vineristine, cyclophosphomide, morphine, general anaesthetic agents, opiods, trycyclic antidepressants and carbamazopine, oxytocin and narcotics.

- *Stressors*: Fear, a cute infections, pain, anxiety, trauma and surgery.

Pathophysiology

In patients with SIADH total body water increases because of water retention and hypo-osmolar state results from hyponatraemia. ADH release follows one of four patterns.

- ADH release is erratic and unrelated to plasma osmolality.
- ADH release varies with plasma osmolality, but osmostat has been reset, and ADH release occurs at lower plasma osmolality.
- ADH release is normal, but the patient is more sensitive to the released ADH or some unmeasured factor, that increases water retention is released. ADH or some unmeasured factor, that increases water retention is released.
- The abnormally-released ADH or the increased sensitivity of cells to ADH increases the permeability of the distal renal tubules and collecting ducts to water, and water reabsorption by the kidney increases. Intravascular volume increases but oedema does not occur due to natriuresis (urinary sodium excretion). Natriuresis is a result of enhanced glomerular filtration and decreased proximal tubular sodium reabsorption, even with hyponatraemia. Hyponatraemia results in hypoosmolality and creates an osmolar gradient across the blood brain barrier and other cellular membrane. This osmolar gradient results in water movement into the brain and other cells and cellular hydration.

Clinical Manifestation of SIADH

- *Early symptoms*: Anorexia, nausea, vomiting, weight gain, muscle weakness, irritability, mild disorientation, malaise, hostility, anxiety unco-operativeness.
- *Late symptoms*: Lethargy, headache, decreased deep tendon reflexes coma and seizures.
- *Fluid and electrolyte changes*:
  - Decreased plasma sodium and plasma osmolality.
  - Increased urinary sodium and urinary osmolality.
  - Decreased urinary volume.
  - Absence of oedema.

Management

The treatment goal is to restore normal fluid volume and osmolality medical management of acute SIADH focuses on treating the aetiologic factor (e.g. carcinoma or Infection) and correcting or at least restoring toward normal, the plasma sodium level and plasma osmolality. Water restriction is the first priority. Water may be restricted to as little as 500 ml/day oral salt intake is increased if the patient is able to take oral nutrients.

In chronic SIADH, water restriction of 800 to 1000 ml/day is recommended. Regardless of aetiology, demeclocyclin (Occlimycin) a tetracyclin that causes nephrogenic diabetes insipidius is useful. This drug blocks the action of ADH source, Severe hyponatraemia is treated with hypertonic saline and loop diuretic such as lasix.

Nursing care of the person with SIADH includes the following:

Perform Careful Nursing Assessment

- Identify patietns at high risk.
- For high-risk patient, monitor daily weights, daily intake and output accurately, daily serum and urinary sodium levels and osmolality, vital signs and neurological states every 4 hours. Report any decrease below normal and serum sodium (1-1.25 m Eq/L) any signs of fluid retention (increased weight and decreased output) and any neurological changes (Headache, or nausea or decreased responsiveness or LOC.
- For patients with diagnosed SIADH being treated aggressively with hypertonic sodium or loop diuretics, the frequency of monitoring is increased to every 1 to 2 hours. Any deterioration in neurological status is reported immediately.
- For patients with Chronic SIADH, monitor weight daily to weekly and report any increase not attributed to dietary changes or any complaint of nausea, headache or lethargy. Monitoring by the nurse in OPD is the same as for the hight risk person.

Provide Supportive Care

- Restrict fluids as prescribed until normalization of serum sodium (if appropriate).
- Control discomfort from thirst:
  - Space fluid intake throughout the 24 hours period.
  - Use inches, which allow more frequent relief of thirst with less fluid intake.
  - Provides frequent mouth care.
- Administer drugs and fluids as ordered.
- Positioning head of bed. Flat or with no more than 10 degrees of elevation to enhance venous return to heart and increase left atria filling pressure and reducing antidiuretic hormone release.
- Positioning side rails up because of potential alteration in mental status.
- Turning of patient every 2 hours, proper positioning, range of motion exercise, massage (if patient is bedridden.)
- Use of seizure precautions such as padded side rails and dimlighting.
- Assistance with ambulating.
- Provision from frequent oral hygiene.

Patient and family teaching should include the information about the following:

- Review the purpose and management of fluid restriction.

- Review self-monitoring required on a long-term basis (intake and output measurement, weight change).
- Discuss drug therapy as appropriate.

DIABETES INSPIDIOUS (DI)

Pituitary Diabetes Inspidious (DI) results from lack of sufficient ADH either from inadequate levels of circulating ADH, insufficient pituitary release of ADH or accelerated degradation of circulating ADH. Central DI occurs where any organic lesion of the hypothermia. In fundibular, stem or posterior pituitary interferes with ADH synthesis, transport, or release.

Aetiology

The cause of pituitary DI may be central brain or pituitary tumours, head trauma, encephalitis, meningitis, hypophysectomy or cranial surgery. The cause is often idiopathic. Nephrogenic DI is a second form of the disorder and results from failure of the renal tubules to respond to ADH. The cause of nephrogenic DI may be chronic renal failure, sickle cell anaemia, and Sjogrens syndrome. Diabetes inspidious may be transient or permanent. Postsurgical DI is permanent, transient DI associated with pregnancy is caused by an excessive amount placental secreted vasopressinase that neutralises ADH activity.

Pathophysiology

The lack of adequate ADH or an ineffective kidney response to ADH results in insufficient water reabsorption by the kidney. The loss of excessive water from the body (Polyuria) stimulates the perception of thirst (polydipsia). If the problem stimulates the perception of thirst (polydipsia). If the problem is long standing, diabetes inspidious can result in an increased bladder capacity and hydronephrosis. When inadequate water replacement occurs, CNS and vascular changes from hyperosmolality and volume depletion can occur.

Clinical Manifestation of DI

Polyuria: Increased urination, as much as 20. frequencies of urine per day may be excreted; Urine is dilute with specific gravity of 1.005 or less osmolality of 200 or less.

Polydipsia: Increased thirst, patient favours cold or ice drinks.

- Only slightly elevated serum osmolality because of water intake usually is maintained. (Most patients compensate for fluid loss by drinking large amount of water).
- Abnormal results of tests for urine concentration
  - Water deprivation test; No increase in urine concentration with either pituitary or nephrogenic DI.
  - ADH replacement; Increase in urine osmolality with pituitary
  - DI, but no response with nephrogenic DI.
- Sleep disturbance from polyuria.
- Inadequate water replacement results in:
  - Hyperosmolality; irritability, mental dullness, coma, hyperthermia
  - Hypovolemia: hypertension, tachycardia, dry mucus membrane, poor skin turger. Weight loss, shock and constipation

Management

The therapeutic goal is maintained of fluid and electrolyte balance. This goal may be accomplished by IV administration of fluid (saline and glucose) and by hormone replacement with ADH (vasopressi) administer either SC, IM or IV. In acute DI, fluids should be administered at rate that decreases the serum sodium by about 1 mEq/2 every 2.hours. Clofibrate Atrmoid), Carbamazepine (Tegretol) and thiazide may also be prescribed for symptomatic DI. For long term therapy, desopress in acetates. An analoge of ADH that is administered as a nasal preparation and does not have the vasconstrictive effects, is the preferred therapy.

Nursing care of the patient with DI is based n the clinical symptoms. Fluid volume deficit manifested by hypertension, techycardia and rapid, shallow respiration can be detached early by frequent assessment. Polyuri and nocturi can cause disturbances in rest and sleep pattern. Nursing intervention for the person with Diabetes Inspidious focus on the following.

a. Maintain fluid and electrolyte balance.
   - Monitor intake and output, daily weight, urine specific gravity, vital signs (orthostic), skin turgor, and neurological status every 1 to 2 hours during the acute phase, then every 4 to 8 hours untill discharge and again return to physician or OPD clinics.
b. Provide fluids be sure patient can reach them.
c. Administer drugs as ordered, which includes
   - Arginine vasopressin 0.25-0.5 mg SC or IM
   - Lysin vasopressin (Dypressin) 3-8 dose/24hr.-nasal spray.
   - Pitressin tannate in oil, 10-40 mg /1-3 doses/week IM.
   - Desmopressin (DDAVP) s-10 mg/dose/1-2-doses/24 hr. Nasal inhalation.

Except desmopressin, other preparations mentioned here interact with V1 and V2 receptors. This pressor side effects can occur including abdominal cramping, hypertension and angina.

In addition, patient and family teaching should include inform about diagnostic test, drug therapy and side effects and instruction regarding self-management.

Table 13.1: Nursing care plan for the patient with syndrome inappropriate secretion of antidiuretic hormone (SIADH)

Problem	*R*	*Objective*	*Nursing Interventions*	*Rationales*
Nursing Diagnosis # 1 Fluid volume, alteration in: Excess related to: 1. Increased secretion of ADH in presence of low serum osmolality.		Patient will maintain stable: 1. Neurologic status: • Mental status alert, oriented to person , place, and date. • Appropriate behaviour • Without seizure activity, tremors, weakness. • Deep tendon reflexes brisk.	(For a detailed presentation of pertinent nursing interventions and their rationales related to fluid volume excess, See earlier NCPs in other chapters. In addition, consider the following: • Assess for signs and symptoms of SIADH: ◆ Specific symptomatology reflects alterations in cerebral function: ◆ Assess for confusion, disorientation, irritability, restlessness, lethargy; tremors, seizure activity, hyper-reflexia.	• Excess water of SIADH is distributed almost entirely to intracellular compartment; clinically, the patient presents with CNS manifestations reflective of cerebral swelling. • Hyperosmolality of intracellular compartment creates osmotic grandient for free water to flow from ECF to ICF space.
Nursing Diagnosis # 2 Electrolyte imbalance, related to: 1. Hyponatraemia (dilutional). 2. Water intoxication.		2. Haemodynamic status; • Weight within 2-5% of baseline. • BP within 10 mmHg of base line. • Pulse strong >60<100 beats/min. • Haemodynamic parameteres: CVP—mean 0-8 mm Hg. PCWP—mean 8-12 mm Hg. CO—4-8liters/min. 3. Renal status: • Hourly urine output >30 ml/hr. • Laboratory studies; • BUN and creatinine at baseline • Serum osmolality—285–295 mOsm/kg. • Serum sodium—135-148 mEq/liter.	◆ Haemodynamic status: Vital signs—arterial blood pressure, peripheral pulses, heart rate and rhythm; respiratory rate and patter; body temperature. – Body weight. – Signs of fluid overload. ◆ Laboratory parameters: – Serum osmolality: <280 mOsm/kg. – Serum sodium: <130Eq/liter. ◆ Urine osmolality:–to serum osmolality. ◆ Urine sodium:>180mEq/liter. – Urine specific gravity: 1.030. – Other serum electrolytes: Potassium and chloride.	◆ Water intoxication of SIADH is largely distributed to cells (intracellular); in extracelular compartments (i.e. interstitium, intravascular space), fluid volume is diminished. Therefore, classic signs/symptoms of fluids overload may not be observed (e.g., pulmonary congestion, congestive heart failure, neck vein distention, pitting oedema, hypertension, bounding pulse, and 50 forth) at least intially. ◆ Early signs and symptoms of SIADH are highly nonspecific; therefore, a high index of suspicion is necessary in assessing patient's overall status. A gradual onset may progress rapidly to muscle cramps, twitches and seizures. ◆ Hallmarks of SIADH: production of concentrated urine in the presence of low serum osmolality; dilutional hyponatraemia. ◆ Urine osmolality equal to or greater than serum osmolality is classic finding highly suggestive of SIADH. ◆ Continued elevation in urinary sodium. If present, assists in differential diagnosis.
Nursing Diagnosis # 3 Thought processes, alteration in, related to 1. Hyponatraemia (dilutional) and. water intoxication.		Patient will: 1. Demonstrate improved neurologic status: • Alert, oriented to person, place, date. • Longer attention span, • Improved memory; speech intact. • Relaxed demeanour.	• Assess thought/behavioural process. ◆ Specific neuralgic parameters: – General cerebral functions: Consciousness and mentation. – Immediate memory-Ask patient to repeat another series of numbers backwards; ability to calculate; abstractm reasoning. – Thought content: Spontaneous, logical; flight of ideas, inappropriate recurrent thoughts, or excessive repetition of thoughts. ◆ Inquire of family/significant others us to recent change in behaviour or personality. Have such changes occurred suddenly or gradually? Are	• Ascertaining usual behaviour of patient as sists in establishing baseline data with which to evaluate subsequent reponses.

Contd...

Contd...

Problem	*R*	*Objective*	*Nursing Interventions*	*Rationales*
			the changes in behaviour response associated with some event? • Implement measure to foster optimal thinking and expression of thoughts: ◆ Specific considerations: – Provide quiet environment with minimal distractions. – Allow adequate time for communication; be accessible to patient/family – Provide explanations in clear, concise terms; repeat questions or directions to the patients understanding ◆ Involve patient and family/significant others in decision making regarding care and activities.	• Involvement in decisionmaking regarding care raises awareness and consciousness in self care; participation in self-care increases interest in what is happening and stimulates thinking processes.
Nursing Diagnosis # 4 Coping, ineffective, individual/family, related to: 1. Strict fluid restrictions.		Patient/family will be able to: 1. Explain need for fluid restriction. 2. Develop schedule for fluid intake. 3. Decide on nutritional fluids for intake.	• Collaborate with patient and family/significant others to develop/implement prescribed therapeutic regimen: ◆ Fluid restrictions: – Discuss reasons for strict fluid intake, balanced with output. – Encourage patient/family to ask questions and express concerns. – Assist patient/family to develop plan as to when and how much fluid will be gested per 24–hour schedule. – Teach patient/family how to record intake and output accurately.	◆ The significance of fluid restriction therapy in SIADH cannot be overestimated. If patient's neurologic status is unstable, the family can be involved in assisting with implementation of fluid restriction.
		• Serum potassium—3.5-5.5 mEq/liter. • Serum chlorides—100-106 mEq/ liter. • Urine specific gravity-1.010-1.025. • Urine sodium—80-180 mEq/liter. • Serum glucose—70-110mg/100 ml. • Haematology profile: Haeamatrocrit, Haemoglobin	• Implement therapeutic regimen: ◆ Fluid intake: – Initial intake limited to urine output/24 hr. – As serum sodium level moralize and CNS symptoms additional fluid is given equal to that estimated insensible losses (i.e.fluid lost via skin, lungs). ◆ Aggressive fluid therapy: ◆ Administration (IV) of 3% hypertonic saline. ◆ Administer/monitor diuretic therapy: ◆ Furosemide therapy in conjunction with prescribed fluid replacement therapy.	• Approach to therapy is guided by CNS symptomatology and hyponatraemia status: initial goal is to relieve CNS dysfunction. ◆ Aggressive fluid therapy may be necessary in the face of severe CNS symptomatology: seizures, coma, and serious cardiac dysrhythmias. ◆ Hypertonic saline will reverse hyponatraemia quickly as fluid is drawn into intravascular space; overly rapid correction can precipitate congestive heart failure; continuous cardiac monitoring is essential. ◆ Furosemide therapy is accompanied by rapid losses of sodium and potassium and requires close monitoring of serum electrolytes. ◆ Correction of serum sodium to levels that relieve CNS symptomatology

Contd...

Contd...

Problem	*R*	*Objective*	*Nursing Interventions*	*Rationales*
			• Hypertonic peritoneal dialysis may be considered to relieve fluid excess. • Close ongoing monlitoring of the following is necessary to evaluate effectiveness of therapy – CNS function – Intake/output and body weight – Cardiac status, cardiopulmonary function: Syspnoea, tachpnoea, productive cough with pink-tinged sputum, presence of adventitious breath sounds-crakles, wheezes. – Laboratory parameters (as above)	is primary goal of therapy; serum sodium need not be totally corrected • Use of hyperosmolar glucose dialysate solutions functions osmotically to pull fluid into the peritoneal cavity. From these it can be drained from the body.
Nursing Diagnosis # 5 Nutrition, alteration in: Less than body requirements, related to: 1. Reduced oral and nutritional intake.		Patient will: 1. Maintain body weight between 2% and 5% of patient's baseline. 2. Maintain serum electrolytes within acceptable range: • Sodium >135 mEq/litre. • Potassium 3.5-5.5 mEq /litre 3. Verbalize why it is necessary to restrict fluid intake. 4. Develop schedule of fluid intake for each 24-hour period including amount and types of foods taken:	• Emphasize importance of daily weight – Identify fluids especially enjoyed by patient. • Offer praise for accomplishments in implementing fluid restricion. – Remain accessible to patient/family. – Lend a listening and concerned ear. • Consult nutritionist to perform comprehensive nutritional assessment • Implement fluid restriction on nutritional regimen as prescribed. • Explain therapeutic regimen to patient/family. • Encourage fluids/foods with high sodium content	• Body weight, taken daily, is best indicator of fluid status. • It is very difficult for family/significant others to cope when their loved one is limited to an intake of 500 ml of fluid / 24 hour. Reassurance and encouragement may be helpful. Family members can often be a positive influence on the patient's compliance with therapeutic regimen. • Fluid restricion prevents further fluid intake retention • Hyponatraemia underlies CNS symptomatology; when hyponatraemia is corrected, CNS dysfunction will abate.
Nursing Diagnosis # 6 Injury, potential for, related to: 1. Seizures/convulsions.		Patients will remain injury-free.	• Perform assessment of patient's immediate environment for potentially injurious equipment or materials. • Minimize neurologic/neuromuscular stimulation. • Institute seizure precautions: Bed in low position, side rails padded; pharyngeal airway and suction equipment at beside.	• Assessment of patient's immediate beside evironment helps to reduce risk of injury by removal of potentially hazardous objects. • CNS dysfunction associated with hyponatraemia may include seizures and altered stapes of consciousness.

Table 13.2: Nursing care plan for the patient with diabetes insipidus

Nursing diagnosis	*R*	*Desired patient outcome*	*Nursing intervention*	*Rationales*
Nursing Diagnosis # 1 Fluid volume deficit: Actual, related to: 1. Decreased ADH synthesis and/or secretion. 2. Defective osmoreceptors 3. Altered immunologic function (Presence of ADH antibodies) 4. Unresponsiveness of cells in the late distal tubules and collecting ducts to action of ADH (nephrogenic DI).		Patient will maintain stable. 1. Hydration status: • Body weight within 5% of baseline, • Balanced intake and output *Laboratory studies.* • Serum osmolality: ~285-295 mOsm/kg. • Urine specific gravity: ~1.010-1.025 2. Neurologic status: • *Alert, oriented* to person, place, and date. • Visual fields at baseline for patients • Motor function muscle tone and strength intact; absence of twitching or seizure activity. • Deep tendon reflexes brisk	(For a detailed presentation of the nursing interventions and their rationales related to fluid volume deficit, see earlier NCPs in other chapter). In addition, consider the following: • Assess for signs and symptoms of DI: ◆ Specific symptomatology includes: – Polyuria (urine output: 4-6 litres/24 hr or more). – Polydipsia (fluid intake: 4-6 liters/24 hr or more). – Weight loss. – Signs of dehydrations: Sunken eyeballs, poor skin turgor, dry mucous membranes, hypotension, rapid pulse ◆ Laboratory findings: – Serum osmolality: >295 mOsm/kg. – Serum sodium:>148 mEq/liter. – Urinary sodium:<20 mEq/liter. – Urine specific gravity:~1.005. • Collaborate with other health care providers to implement and monitor therapeutic regimen. ◆ Monitor neurologic function: Mental status; level of conciousness sensory motor function; deep tendon reflexes ◆ Implement measures to protect patient from injury caused by altered sensorium, seizure activity. – Pharyngeal airway and suction intact at bedside; padded side rails; bedside free of potential hazards (unnecessary equipment/ furniture, electrical appliances, and so forth).	• DI is a state of reduced ADH synthesis and/or secretion, or diminished response of cells of the distal tubules and collecting ducts of kidneys to the actions of ADH. Osmoreceptors may be impaired. • Loss or absence of ADH compromises water reabsorption, resulting in excretion of large volumes of water despite a high serum osmolality (e.g., >295 mOsm/kg). • Excretion of water without concomitant excretion of sodium and other solute predisposes to hypernatraemia and high serum osmolality. Urine excreted is therefore, very dilute (e.g., low-specific gravity) and urinary sodium is reduced as it is reasorbed in renal tubules. • DI may result in total body water deficit. Alterations in cerebral function may reflect cerebral intracellular dehydration with cell shrinkage (crenation).
Nursing Diagnosis # 2 Cardiac output, alteration in: decreased, related to: 1. Severely contracted intravascular volume.		3. Haemodynamic status: • Blood pressure within 10 mmHg of baseline. • Pulse strong; rate >60, <100neats/min, • Haemodynamic parameters: CVP- mean 0-8 mmHg. PCWP-mean 8-12 mmHg. Co-4-8 liter/min.	• Monitor haemodynamic status: ◆ Vital signs: Heart rate, peripheral pulses arterial blood pressur. ◆ Haemodynamic parameters: CVP, PCWP and CO. ◆ Hydration status: Hourly fluid intake and output; daily weight; urine-specific gravity.	• Severe dehydration reduces circulating in travascular blood volume, diminishing venous return to the heart and compromising cardiac output. ◆ Progressive of hypovolemic state to hypotensive shock and circulatory collapse can occur rapidly in the setting of DI.
Nursing Diagnosis # 3 Electrolyte imbalance, related to: 1. Excess water loss with hypernatraemia.		4. Renal status: • Hourly urine outputs: >30, <200 ml/hr. *Laboratory studies:* • BUN and creatinine at baseline for patient. • Serum sodium: 135-148 mEq/liter. • Urinary sodium: *80-180 mEq/liter.*	• Implement fluid replacement regimen. ◆ Administer hypotonic fluids initially. • Monitor all vital parameters during fluid replacement therapy. • Monitor serial laboratory studies: serum electrolytes, osmolality,	• Major goal of therpy in treating DI is to prevent hypovolaemia and dehydration. • Fluid therapy is precribed to correct hypovolaemia and dehydration ◆ Hypotonic fluids intialy allow for more vigorous treatment of hyperosmolar state; provide aptient with access to cpopious amouts of fluid because of intense thirst.

Contd...

Contd...

Nursing diagnosis	*R*	*Desired patient outcome*	*Nursing intervention*	*Rationales*
		• Other electrolytes within acceptable range for patient • Serum glucose: 70-110 mg/100ml. • Haematology profile within acceptable range (haematocrit, haemoglobin).	BUN and creatinine, haematology profile; urinary sodium and osmolality. ◆ Monitor cardiac status: cardiac output, peripheral pulses (quality, amplitude, contour); neck vein distention. – Overhydration: Full, bounding pulse; neck vein distention. – Dehydration: Weak, thready pulse; flat neck veins	◆ Aggessive fluid replacement therapy can predispose to fluid overload; elderly patients (>65 years) are more suceptible to fluid overload because their total body water (TBW) is lower than in young persons. ◆ Overhydration can precipitate congestive heart failure and pulmonary oedema
			• Administer ADH replacement therapy as prescribed; monitor response to therapy. ◆ Pharmacologic, preparations include vasopressin (Pitressin), vasopressin tannate, lupressin (Diapid), and desmopressin acetate (DDAVP). ◆ Monitor for side effects: – Vasopressin may cause diaphoresis, tremor, pounding headache; nausea, abdominal/uterrine cramps, diarrhoea; hypertension, angina, angina, water intoxication.	◆ Vasopressin drug therapy should be accompanied by water ingestion to minimize side effects of nausea and abdominal cramps. ◆ Vasopressin preparations in oil base require warning the ampule and shaking vigorously to disperse medication evenly in the oil medium ◆ Subcutaneous and intramuscular injections may be painful a large needle is recommended.
			– Rhiorrhoea, nasal congestion, headache, increased blood pressure, flushing of skin, and abdominal cramps may accompany use of lypressin and desmopressin.	– Lypressin and desmopressin acetate are administered intranasally. These drugs should not be inhaled; keep refrigerated.
		5. Respiratory status: • Respiratory rate <25-30 breaths/min. • Rhythm: Euppeic • Breath sounds: Clear to ausculation. • Absence of adventitious sounds.	• Administer prescribed thiazide diuretic therapy.	• Antidiuretic response may be poteintiated by concomitant administration of chlorpropamide, clofibrate, or carbamazepine. ◆ Thiazides promote sodium excretion, which may help to prevent hypermatroemia in the face of excessive water loss. ◆ Thiazides may be prescribed in nephrogenic DI to promote water reabsorption via mechanisms independent of ADH effect.
			• Monitor respiratory function: presence of tachypnoea, dyspnoea. ◆ Presence of adventitious breath sounds—crackles (rales), wheezes. ◆ Presence of cough, productive or non-productive?	◆ Presence of crackles /rales may suggest pulmonary congestion associated with overly aggressive fluid replacement. ◆ Overhydration: Thin, copious secretions.Dehydration: Thick, tenacious secretions.
			• Establish regimen for positioning, turning, deep breathing, and coughing; chest physiotherapy and bronchial hygiene.	• These activities as tolerated by the patient assist in mobilizing and removing secretions by coughing and/or suctioning.

Contd...

Contd...

Nursing diagnosis	*R*	*Desired patient outcome*	*Nursing intervention*	*Rationales*
Nursing Diagnosis #4 Oral mucous membranes, alteration in related to: 1. Dehydration state.		Mucous membranes will remain clean, moist, and without cracking or fissures.	• Monitor integumentary status: ◆ Assess skin/mucous membranes. ◆ Initiate oral hygiene regimen.	◆ Patients with DI are at great risk of becoming dehydrated when they are no longer able to maintain fluid intake to match fluid loss. ◆ Severely dehydrated patient is at increased risk of infection; wound healing may be compromised.
Nursing Diagnosis #5 Skin intergrity, impairment; potential related to: 1. Dehydration diarrhoea.		Skin warm and dry; turgor over sternum or forehead, elastic; skin intact.	◆ Initiate skin care regimen: – Frequent turning and positioning . – Active/passive ROM exercises. – Initiate pressure relief device (air mattress, sheepskin, other). ◆ Monitor nutritional intake.	◆ Maximizes tissue perfusion, prevents stasis of blood and decubitus ulcer formation.
Nursing Diagnosis # 6 Bowel elimination, alteration in, related to: 1. Diarrhoea (possible side effect of vasopressin therapy).		Patient will establish and maintain effective bowel function. 1. Bowel pattern to return to patient's baseline. • Stool formed and soft. • Absence of diarrhoea and abdominal cramping. 2. Bowel sounds approprite throughout all quadrants.	• Assess gastrointestinal function: ◆ Specific symptomatology includes: – Anorexia, nausea, vomiting, abdominal cramping and distention; and diarrhoea. – Increased bowel sounds associated with increased peristalsis. • Implement measures to maintain optimal gastrointestinal function with least discomfort. ◆ Provide coplous amounts of fluid at patient's disposal. – Monitor strict intake and output. – Monitor electrolytes.	◆ Abdominal cramping, increased gestrointestinal mobility, and diarrhoea are associated with large doses of vasopressin. ◆ Gastrointestinal symptomatology may be associated with hypernatreamic state. ◆ Severe thirst requires large fluid intake to prevent dehydration. ◆ Water taken in conjunction with ADH replacement therapy may help to minimize side effects of abdominal cramping.
Nursing Diagnosis # 7 Sensory perceptual alteration: visual, related to: 1. Pressure on optic chasm associated with pituitary tumour oedema as occurs with head injury or hypophysectomy.		Patient will: 1. Demonstrate awareness of visual field defect if present. 2. Demonstrate maneuvers in activities of daily living to compensate for defect. 3. Verbalize improvement in vision.	• Assess visual function: ◆ Specific parameters include: – Visual acuity. – Extraocular movement. ◆ Visual fields. – Direct consensual light reflex. – Pupil shape, size, reactivity, and accommodation. • Implement measures to minimize risk of injury due to visual field defect. ◆ Teach patient to become aware as to where "blind spots" are in the overall field of vision, and how to compensate for defect by turning the head. ◆ Keep patient's immediate environment uncluttered, free of necessary equipment, furniture, and so forth. ◆ Teach patient to place personal articles within reach. ◆ Assist patient with activities of daily living.	• It is important to establish baseline function to measure patient's response to therapy. ◆ Bitemporal hemianopsia: Blindness temporal half of the visual field in each eye. This is a most frequently occuring disturbance in patients with pituitary pathology because of structurl contiguity between optic chiasm and sella tursica and its contents (i.e., pituitary gland).

Contd...

Contd...

Nursing diagnosis	*R*	*Desired patient outcome*	*Nursing intervention*	*Rationales*
Nursing Diagnosis # 8 Nutrition alteration in: Less than body requirements, related to: 1. Anorexia, nausea associated with hypernatraemic state. 2. Abdominal cramping associated with ADH replacement therapy. 3. Fatigue associated with excessive thirst fluid intake.		Patient will: 1. Maintain body weight between 2% and 5% of patients's baseline. 2. Maintain serum electrolytes within acceptable range: • Sodium: 135-148 mEq/liter. 3. Maintain serum proteins within acceptable range: • Total protein: 6-8.4 g/100 ml. 4. Verbalize dietary restrictions: • Low sodium diet.	• Collaborate with nutritionist to perform comprehensive nutritional assessment. • Implement nutrional regimen as prescribed: • Monitor parameters reflective of nutritional status. – Weigh daily under same conditions. – Monitor intake and output. – Monitor serum electrolytes, plasma proteins, and serum osmolality.	• Provides baseline for planinng nutrition • Major objectives of nutritional therapy: 1. Provide sufficient calories to prevent protein catabolism. 2. Provide sufficient protein to ensure tissue healing and to prevent breakdown. 3. Limit salt intake untill fluid and sodium balance stbilizes
			• Provide comfort measures: ◆ Assist with frequent oral hygiene. ◆ Encourage family to bring patient's favorite foods, if possible. ◆ Offer a variety of fluids. ◆ Provide frequent rest periods.	• May assist in improving appetite ◆ Home-cooked food, coupled with company at mealtime, may improve nutritional intake ◆ Fluid intake of 4-6 or more liters/24hr may be fatiguing.
			• Initiate patient/family education regarding nutritional requirements and dietary limitations. ◆ Limits salt intake.	◆ Hypernatraemia associated with excess water loss can be significant. Efforts need to be directed toward limiting sodium in take until fluid and electrolyte balance is re-estblished.
Nursing Diagnosis # 9 Injury, potential for physiological: Thrombophlebitis, deep venous thrombosis pulmonary embolism, related to: 1. Immobility. 2. Haemoconcentration associted with severe water deficit and dehydration.		Patient will remain without thromnoembolic complications 1. Absence of calf pain, tenderness,swelling 2. Peripheral pulses palpable. 3. Usual skin colour and temparature in exeremities.	• Assess for signs/symptoms of venous thrombosis: ◆ Symptomatology may include: ◆ Tenderness, warmth pain – Changes in skin colour and temperature. – Increase in mid-thigh or mid-calf circumference	◆ Positive Homan's sign reflects pain in calf when the knee is placed in a flexed positions and the examiner abruptly dorsiflexes the ankle. This maneuver will elicit pain in some patients with deep venous thrombosis (DVT). However absence of calf pain does not rule out DVT; the presence of pain may also occur with herminated lower intervertebral disks or lumbosacral problems.
			• Implement measures to reduce risk of thromboembolic disease: ◆ Encourage position changes at frequent intervals. ◆ Avoid positions that compromise blood flow (e.g.crossing legs, use of knee gatch or pillow under knees). ◆ Assist with ROM exercise for 5-10 min every 1-2 hr. ◆ Apply antiembolic stockings if appropriate.	◆ Venous stasis coupled with haemoconcentration increase the risk of thromboembolic disease. Exercise increases venous return and reduces risk of pooling of blood in the extremities.
			◆ Monitor haematology profile.	◆ Serial haematocrit/haemoglobin studies help to evaluate fluid status.

Contd...

Contd...

Nursing diagnosis	*R*	*Desired patient outcome*	*Nursing intervention*	*Rationales*
Nursing Diagnosis # 10 Coping, ineffective, Individual,related to: 1. Excessive thirst and the need to drink large volumes of fluid.		Patient will. 1. Verbalize feelings regarding thirst and fluid status. 2. Idenify approach to fluid intake: When, how much, how often and what kinds of fluids.	• Collaborate with patient and family/ significant others to define the magnitude of the water imbalance and to explore how the problem can best be addressed. ◆ Specific measures: – Discuss the importance of balancing intake with output. – Teach patient/family how to record intake and output accurately. – Emphasize importance of daily weight. – Identify fluids and other sources of water (e.g., watermelon) that appeal to patient. ◆ Encourage participation in decisions regarding care (e.g., what to drink or eat, how much, how often).	• Hypovolemic and dehydration can progress rapidly to hypovolmic shock and circulatory collapse. ◆ Involving patient and family/significant others in decision-making process regarding care enables the patient to assume responsibility for self-care and may increase compliance with prescribed therapeutic regimen.
Nursing Diagnosis # 11 Anxiety, related to: 1. Excessive thirst and its underlying cause.			(For pertinent nursing interventions and theri rationales in the care of the patient exhibiting anxiety, the reader is referred to earlier NCPs in other chapters)	

Table 13.3: Nursing care plan for the patient with hyperthyroid crisis

Problem	*R*	*Objective*	*Nursing Interventions*	*Rationales*
Nursing Diagnosis # 1 Cardiac output, alteration in: Decreased, related to: 1. High output cardiac failure associated with increased demand and exaggerated adrenergic effect. 2. Cardiac dysrhythmias 3. Reduced circulating blood volume associated with excessive diaphoresis vomiting, diarrhoea.		Patient will maintain: 1. Usual mental status: Alert, oriented to person, place, date; deep tendon reflexes brisk. 2. Adequate cardiovascular function: • Cardiac rate and rhythmheart rate >60, <100 beats/min, rhythm-regular sinus without symptomatic dysrhythmias. Haemodynamic status: • CVP: 0-8 mmHg mean. • PCWP: 8-12 mmHg mean. • CO: 4-8 liters/min. • Arterial blood pressure within 10 mmHg of baseline supine and upright. 3. Renal status: • Urine output >30 ml/hr.	• Maintain adequate cardiovascular function. ◆ Assess the effect of hypermetabolic state on cardiovascular function: cardiac rate and rhythm; occurrence of chest pain and/or palpitations. ◆ Assess changes in heart sounds, extra heart sounds S3 and S4) murmurs. ◆ Breath sounds: abnormal, or adventitious breath sounds (e.g., crackles, wheezes). ◆ Assess haemodynamic parameters: Arterial blood pressure (supine/ upright);widened pulse pressure; CVP, PCWP,CO, systemic vascular resistance(SVR).	• Hypermetabolic state increases myocardial oxygen consumption predisposing to ischaemia; cardiac ischaema may precipitate cardiac dysrhythmias and /or anginal pain. ◆ Reflect increased force of myocardial contraction; may be associated with cardiac dysrhythmias ◆ Increased risk of developing hypovolaemic shock due to dehydrated state. ◆ Widening pulse pressure reflects increase in stroke volume and decrease in systemic vascular resistance. ◆ Haemodynamic parameters reflect cardiac status; assist in evaluating fluid state and response to overall therapy.

Contd...

Contd...

Problem	*R*	*Objective*	*Nursing Interventions*	*Rationales*
		4. Respiratory status: • Respiratory rate and breathing pattern: < 25-30 breaths min; eupnoea.	• Assess predisposition to congestive heart failure, pulmonary oedema. • Monitor for symptomatic cardiac dysrhythmias. Which can predispose to cardiogenic shock: – Supraventicular tachyarrhythimias: paroxysmal atrial tachycardia; atrial tachycardia with rapid ventricular response.	• Related to cardiac oxygen demand in excess of adequate supply, with tissue ischaemia and injury; high output cardiac failure related to hypermetabolic demands.
			– Symptomatic bradycardia, heart block, and conduction disturbances. – Ventricular dyrhythmias: Premature ventricular contractions, ventricular tachycardia, ventricular fibrillation.	• Conduction disturbances and bradycardia may be associated with propranolo therapy.
			• Anticipate the occurrence of potential lethal dysrhythmias. The following equipment should be available at bedsides – Antiarrhythmia drugs. – Pacemaker and insertion equipment – Equipment for cardioversion/ defibrillation. • Monitor cardiac rate and rhythm continuously.	• Patients in hyperthyroid crisis are at increased risk of catastrophic events related to potential lethal dysrhythmias.
			• Implement prescribed drug regimen to reduce thyroid hormone synthesis and release and to inhibit adrenergic hyperactivity.	
			• Administer therapy to block thyroid hormone synthesis: – Propylthiouracil (PTU).	• PTU functions to reduce circulating levels of thyroid hormone over days to weeks by blocking a strategic step in the synthesis of thyroid hormones.
			• Administer via nasogastric tube if patient is unable to swallow or to cooperate.	– PTU is not available in parenteral form.
			• Assess the patient for adverse drug reactions.	– Patients can develop minor side effects such as urticaria, epigastric distress, granulocytopoenia, and over the long term, lupus like syndrome. Hepatitis has been known to occur.
			• Administer antithyroid drug of choice, which acts to block thyroid secretion:	– Abrupt withdrawal can precipitate thyroid crisis.
			• Sodium iodide.	• Iodides have an immediate effect in reducing serum. Levels of thyroid hormone; full therapeutic effect takes 10-14 days.
			• Establish any prior incidence of allergy to iodine preparations; contrast dye.	• Presence of allergy to iodine may require an alternative approach to therapy.

Contd...

Contd...

Problem	*R*	*Objective*	*Nursing Interventions*	*Rationales*
			• Assess the patient for adverse drug reactions. • Administer beta adrenergic blocker to inhibit adrenergic overactivity. – Propranolol is the drug choice.	• Patient can develop minor side effects urticaria or other skin lesions. • Propranolo markedly reduces the effects of excessive thyroid hormone on cardiovascular function by competing with epinephrine and norepinephine for beta-adrenergic receptors. • Propranolol is available in oral and parenteral preparations; this drug may be life saving because its therapeutic effects, via intravenous use, are achieved rapidly. • Intravenous propranolol warrants thorough and continuous monitoring of vital signs and cardiac rhythm. • Propranolol acts to reduce heart rate, cardiac contractility and oxygen consumption; it reduces mycocardia irritability and associated supraventicular tachyarrhythmias; it ameliorates clinical manifestations of adrenergic overactivity including palpitations associated with forceful heart contractions, nervousness, tremors, profuse diaphoresis, and heart intolerance • Untoward reactions to beta adrenergic blockage may include a symptomatic bradycardia; heart block, heart failure, and respiratory insufficiency.
			• Establish baseline vital sign parameters; closely monitor heart rate, rhythm, blood pressure, apical and peripheral pulses, respiratory rate and pattern. Observe for desired and adverse effects. • Be cognizant of contraindications to the use of propranolol.	• Contraindications to the use of propranolol include: Asthma, chronic obstructive pulmonary disease; nonhyperthyroidal heart failure; symptomatic sinus bradycardia; atriventricular heart block. • Beta-adrenergic blockade causes bronchiole constriction. • Tachyarrhythmias may remain refractory to therapy until the underlying hyperthyroidism is under control. • Intravenous propranolol can have sudden adverse effects: Sudden bradycardia; hypotension (orthostatic); syncope; evidence of congestive heart failure, dyspnoea, respiratory compromise, and cardiac arrest.

Contd...

Contd...

Problem	*Objective*	*Nursing Interventions*	*Rationales*
		• Maintain the following drugs within easy access: – Atropine for symptomatic bradycardia – Vasopressors (e.g.,dopamine) for hypertension – Isoproterenol (positive inotropic effect). – Aminophylline for bronchospasm. – Digoxin for heart failure – Furosemide (diuretic).	
		• Monitor serum glucose (serially)	• Propranolol may mask signs of insulin overdosage in patients receiving insulin therapy and may prolong hypoglycemic effects.
		• Administer other prescribed medications if use of propranolol is contraindicated: – Reserpine	• Reserpine reduces synthesis of norepinephrine, and competitively inhibits its reuptake in storage granules.
		• Guanethidine	• Guanethidine acts to displace stored norepinephrine from storage granuies; acts as a"false neurotransmitter" that effectively blocks adrenergic actions of norepinephrine.
		• Administer prescribed glucocorticosteroid therapy.	• Potential accelerated turnoverand degradation of glucocorticosteroids in hyperthyroid crisis warrants the administration of "stress-dose" replacement therapy.
		– Dexamethasone – Hydrocortisone sodium succinate (Solu Cortef).	• Dexamethasone also inhibits peripheral conversion of T_4 to T_3.
		• Evaluate effectiveness of antithyroid hormone therapy: – Improvement in clinical signs: Temperature reduction; clearing of mental status; reduced heart rate; stable blood pressure, pulse, respiratory rate and rhythm; reduction in palpitations, tremors, nervousness, profuse diaphoresis.	• The effects of antithyroid therapy and diminished adrenergic response should be come clinically obvious within 6-12 hours after initiation of therapy.
		• Improvement in laboratory studies: – Serum T4, T3RIA, RT3U,	• Serum levels of thyroid hormone do not significantly drop for several days after initiation of therapy; initial improvement in clinical status is probably due to the diminished adrenergic response.
		– Improvement in liver function and other studies.	• Overall treatment plan may need to be modified continuously to meet the changing needs of the patient.
		– Absence of adverse reactions to therapy.	• In evaluating laboratory data, it must be remembered that serum tests are measurements of thyroid hormone levels at only one point in time. It is possible for an isolated thyroid hormone value to reflect intake of exogenous iodine whether in diet or medications. It is important to

Contd...

Contd...

Problem	*R*	*Objective*	*Nursing Interventions*	*Rationales*
				question the patient regarding the intake of exogenous iodine because this may be reflected in the laboratory results.
		Patient will maintain effective fluid and electrolyte balance:	• Note if the patient has any allergies to iodine containing substances. • Assess if established protocols for specific tests are followed.	• It is important to follow established protocols for testing to ensure that test results are valid.
Nursing Diagnosis # 2 Fluid volume deficit Actual related to: 1. Hypermetabolic state with hyperpyrexia associated with profuse diaphoresis. Nursing Diagnosis # 3 Electrolyte imbalance, related to: 1. Severe dehydration. 2. Haemoconcentration with hypernatraemia.		1. Neurologic status: Alert, oriented to person, place, date; deep tendon reflexes brisk. 2. Haemodynamic status: (As in Nursing diagnosis #1 above) 3. Body weights will stabilize within 5% of patient's baseline. 4. Renal status: urine output>30 ml/hr. 5. Gastrointestinal status: absence of anorexia, nausea, vomiting, and diarrhoea. 6. Laboratory data: • Serum osmolality:~285-295 mOsm/kg. • Serum sodium:>3.5<5.5 mEq/liter. • Serum glucose, BUN, creatinine, and hamatology profile at optimal levels for patient.	For patient nursing interventions and their rationales in the care of the patient in hyperthyroid crisis who is experiencing hyperpyrexia accompained by fluid and electrolyte imbalance, see the related nursing diagnosis in earlier chapters. In addition, consider the following nursing interventions/rationales: • Maintain fluid and electrolyte balance ◆ Assess the effect of hypermetabolic state on body fluid balance: ◆ Assess for sign/symptoms of fluid volume deficit: Nonproductive cough; flat neck veins, dry, parched mucous membranes. ◆ Assess for signs/symptoms of fluid volume excess: – Auscultate breath sounds (crackle). – Productive cough, frothy, pink-tinged sputum; neck vein distention. ◆ Monitor intake and output, urine specific gravity; serial weights. ◆ Prevent fluid imbalance. – Administer fluids based on fluid losses (include insensible losses) overall state of hydration and serum electrolyte values. – Continue to monitor closely intake and output, daily weight, vital signs, serum electrolytes, urine output and other parameters reflective of fluid state.	• The hypermetabolic state may predispose to widely fluctuating imbalance in total body fluids ◆ Depleted fluid state, dehydration may be due to profuse diaphoresis associated with hyperpyrexia and to disturbances in gastrointestinal function vomiting, and/or diarrhoea. ◆ Fluid volume overload increases the risk of congestive heart failure and pulmonary oedema. ◆ Overly aggressive fluid replacement therapy can predispose to fluid volume excess. ◆ Body weight is a good indicator of insensible fluid loss. ◆ Haemocoentration or haemodilution can predispose to electrolyte imbalance.
			• Consider the effects of hypermetabolic state on serum electrolytes. ◆ Monitor for hypokalaemia: – Assess signs/symptoms: General malaise, fatigue, anorexia, nausea and vomiting, diarrhea, abdominal cramps, muscle weakness, hyporeflexia; hypotension, dysrhythimas' presence of U wave on 12-lead electrocardiogram; apathy, restlessness, irritabillity. – Monitor serial serum potassium levels. – Administer potassium supplements and assess clinical response.	◆ Gastrointestinal symptoms of vomiting and diarrhoea and excessive administration of diuretics to the patient with fluid overload are largely responsible for the occurrence of hypokelaemia. – Intravenous potassium must be administered slowly to avoid lethal cardiac dysrhythmias or standstill; oral potassium supplements can cause gastrointestinal irritation.

Contd...

Contd...

Problem	*R*	*Objective*	*Nursing Interventions*	*Rationales*
			• Monitor for hyponatraemenia: – Assess for sign/ symptoms of dilutional state such as: Headache, faintness, muscle cramps; mental confusion; seizures, convulsions, coma. – Monitor intake and output; serial electrolyte and osmolality levels. – Restrict fluids as per medical therapeutic plan and monitor response.	• Hyponatraemia is usually delusional in origin, occurring due to excess in body fluid volume or hypo-osmolar state (water intoxication). Delusional hyponatraemia: Due to water excess. • Depletional hyponatraemia may occur in hyperthyroid crisis because of profuse diaphoresis associated with hyperpyrexia. Depletional hyponatremia: Due to sodium loss.
			• Monitor for hypercalcaemia – Assess signs/symptoms including: Drowsiness, fatigue, anorexia, thirst, nausea, vomiting, constipation, neuromuscular changes are reflected in hypotonicity of muscles, with weakness; deep bone pain; central nervous system depression may be reflected by depression, lethargy, psychosis, and coma.	• Hypercalceamia is related to increased activity of osteoclasts causing bone resorption and demineralization. • Constipation is related to depressed one of smooth muscles within the bowel; reduced peristalsis may progress to paralytic ileus.
			• Monitor serial serum levels; observe for ECG changes reflected by a shortened OT interval, and dyshythmias; maintain strict intake and output.	• Large amounts of calcium may be lost in urine and stool; long-term effect often involves pathologic fractures due to demineralization of bone; and renal calculi.
			• Implement prescribed therapeutic plan and monitor patient's response to therapy: • Intravenous saline and diuretics.	• Sodium diruresis promotes renal excretion of calcium.
			• Administration of therapeutic plan an monitor patient's response to therapy: • Administration of intravenous or oral phosphates. • Administration of glucocorticoids.	• Phosphates induce calcium excretion, and together with glucocorticoids, inhibit calcium absorption.
Nurisng Diagnosis # 4 Hyperthermia, related to: 1. Hypermetabolic rate, 2. Enlarged adrenergic activity.		Patient's body temperature will stabilize at~ 37°c (98.6F).	• Administration of sodium bicarbonate.	• Increases fraction of calcium that is protein bound.
			• Dialysis. • Initiate range of motion exercise as condition stabilizes.	• Inactivity contributes to bone resorption.
			• Evaluate status of body temperture. • Assess the effect of hypermetabolic state on body functions: signs/symptoms may in clude the following: • Fever as high as 106° F (41°c). – Resting tachycardia; supraventricular tachyarrhythmia; congestive heart failure; hypovolemic shock.	• Hyperpyrexia develops when the compensatory mechanisms of peripheral vasodilatation, diaphoresis, and polyuria are no longer able to dissipate excessive heat production of the hypermetabolic state.
			– Nausea/vomiting, diarrhoea; liver failure abnormal liver function tests. – State of physical, mental, emotional exhaustion. – Coma.	• Excessive heat production (thermal energy) largely results from exceedingly enhanced lipolysis and oxidation of fatty acids stimulated by increased circulating thyroid hormone.

Contd...

Contd...

Problem R	Objective	Nursing Interventions	Rationales
			• Body temperature may fluctuate rapidly; sudden increase or fall in body temperature stresses irritability and serious ventricular dysrhythmias. • Untreated hyperthyroid crisis can cause death from excessive fever, cardiac and/ or liver failure; exhaustion-cellular "burn out".
		– Monitor rectal temperature hourly or continuously if rectal probe available.	• Assists in evaluating trends in body temperature and response to therapy.
		– Assess the state of hydration: Body weight, urine specific gravity; hourly intake and output; extent of diaphoresis.	
		• Institute fever-reducing therapy. • Administer antipyretic agents (acetaminophen is drug of choice).	• Aspirin (acetylsalicylic acid) worsens hyperthyroid crisis by displacing thyroid hormones from serum protein thyroid hormone binding receptors, resulting in an increase in free circulating thyroid hormone.
		• Implement body surface-cooling measures (for temperature 38 °C, 102° F). • Hypothermia blanket. • Ice packs to axilla and groin area.	• When body temperature exceeds 38°C in a patient with pre existing hyperthyroidism, it may signal that a state of physiologic decompensation and disequilibrium is in the process of evolving
		• Cool environment with minimal bed covers. • Use fans, if available, to circulate air.	• Lowered body temperature decreases metabolic needs.
		• Administer oxygen therapy if necessary	• Hypermetabolic state causes increased oxygen demand and consumption.
		• Provide supportive nursing measures: • Scrupulous skin care with frequent tepid sponge baths and adequate skin drying.	• Potential for impairment of skin integrity is increased by the catabolic state; skin is thin, friable, and easily injured.
		• Frequent turning and changes in position.	• Increases circulation to prominent bony areas and pressure points.
		• Assess for shivering; muscle relaxants and /or sedation may be necessary.	• Shivering increases metabolic needs.
Nursing Diagnosis # 5 Oral mucous membranes, alteration in.	Patient's mucous membranes will remain: 1. Clean, moist and without cracking or fissuring.	• Assess status of oral mucous membranes and skin integrity.	• The high metabolic state can deplete body fluid rapidly leading to an alteration in mucous membranes with fissuring and cracking; skin becomes fragile especially over pressure points.
Nursing Diagnosis # 6 Skin intergity impairment: Potential for.	Patient's skin will remain warm and dry; good turgor over forehead or sternum.	• Implement measures to maintain the intactness of mucous membranes and skin: • Provide frequent mouth care; prevent encrustation; keep lips moist.	• Scrupulous skin care should be provided with frequent tepid sponging and drying.
		• Initiate pressure relief device (e.g., airmatress, sheepskin, egg crate mattress). • Execute plan for turning/positioning every 2 hours. • Monitor nutritional status.	• Helps to maximize perfusion, catabolic state predisposes to thin, friable, and easily injured skin and mucous membranes.

Contd...

Contd...

Problem	*R*	*Objective*	*Nursing Interventions*	*Rationales*
Nursing Diagnosis # 7 Breathing pattern, alteration in related to: 1. Weakness of pulmonary musculature, and fatigue.		1. Patient will maintain arterial blood gas parameters as follows: • pH: 7.35-7.45(room air) • PaCo 2:35-45 mmHg • HCO_3: 22-26 mEq/liter • $PaCo_2$:>60 mmHg 2. Patient will verbalize ease of breathing.	• Maintain effective respiratory function. ◆ Assess the effects of hypermetabolic state on respiratory function: ◆ Respiratory rate and rhythm. – Tachypnoea, dyspnoea – Use of accessory muscles of respiration.	• Ineffective-breathing pattern may be associated with muscle weakness and exhaustion due to hypermetabolic state.
			◆ Pulmonary function parameters: – Tidal volume, vital capacity ◆ Auscultation of breath sounds. ◆ Evidence of cyanosis.	• Pulmonary congestion oedema is associated with high cardiac output congestive heart failure. • Extreme vasodilatation in response to hypermetabolic state causes skin to be flushed and warm; presence of cyanosis in lips, mucous membranes, earlobes, and nailbeds suggests decreased oxygenation related to hyperventilation and/or impaired gas exchange.
			◆ Arterial blood gas–trend.	• A change in the patient's breathing pattern from hyperventilatory to hypoventilatory coupled with a rising P_aCO_2 (From <35 mmHg to >45 mmHg) strongly suggests that the patient is decompensating.
			◆ Obtain specimen of sputum for culture and sensitivity.	• Pulmonary infection is a frequent precipitating factor in the occurrence of hyperthyroid crisis.
			• Provide supportive therapy ◆ Administer oxygen therapy.	◆ Oxygen therapy will assist in meeting the increased demand for oxygen caused by the hypermetabolic state; it may help to relieve dyspnoea.
			◆ Assist patient to assume a position that facilitates breathing ◆ Provide a quiet environment with frequent rest periods ◆ Provide explanation and feedback regarding progress of course.	◆ All efforts are directed towards assisting the patient to conserve strength and prevent a state of exhaustion.
			• Initiate antibiotic therapy to treat suspected and/or diagnosed infection.	• Infection may be an underlying cause of hyperthyroid crisis.
Nursing Diagnosis # 8 Nutrition,alteration in: Less than body requirements,related to: 1. Hypermetabolic state		1. Patient's body weight will stabilize within 5% of baseline 2. Serum proteins will be maintained within acceptable physiologic range: ~6.0 to 8.4 g/100ml 3. Serum glucose: 70-110 mg/100ml. 4. Urine negative for glucose and acetone.	• Maintain adequate nutrition to meet tissue requirements of the hypermetabolic state. ◆ Consult with nutritionist regarding alterations in nutrition caused by hypermetabolic state. ◆ Assess overall nutritional status and potential alterations associated with hypermetabolic state. – Assess for hyperglycemia:	◆ Elevated circulating levels of thyroid hormone greatly enhance glycogenolysis and reduce serum insulin levels; increased adrenergic activity can impair insulin secretion and/or diminish tissue response to the effects of insulin.

Contd...

Contd...

Problem R	Objective	Nursing Interventions	Rationales
		• Signs symptoms include: Polydipsia, glycosuria, polyuria, nocturia, weakness, muscle cramping; irritability; lethargy, depression.	• Polydispsia, glycosuria, and polyuria are related to the osmotic diuretic effect of elevated serum glucose.
		• Monitor serum glucose levels; urine for sugar and acetone.	• Glycosuria may be the only symptom of altered glucose metabolism.
		• Administer prescribed insulin/glucose: – Glucose with insulin in small amounts to control hyperglycemia.	• This therapy provides an essential nutrient and ensures its use by cells–insulin is necessary for absorption and utilization of glucose by liver, muscle, and adipose tissues; the availability of glucose diminishes the occurrence of a catabolic state due to glucoeogenesis.
		• Maintain prescribed caloric intake.	
		• Provide necessary electrolytes and soluble vitamin B complex and vitamin C supplements.	• Hypermetabolic rates rapidly deplete stores of vitamins and trace metals, which are vital coenzymes in many biochemical interactions.
		• Maintain prescribed lipid intake.	• Excessive lipolysis and oxidation of free fatty acids largely accounts for hyperpyrexia due to inability of body to dissipate excessive heat generation.
		• Maintain positive nitrogen balance: – Monitor BUN creatinine.	• Protein catabolism occurs at greater rate than protein synthesis. Goal of therapy is to prevent negative nitrogen balance. • Enhanced gluconeogenesis contributes largely to negative nitrogen balance.
		• Assess signs/symptoms including: Weakness, fatigue, weight loss, muscle wasting and hypoalbuminaemia.	• Continued weight loss may indicate inadequacy of treatment in meeting energy needs of hypermetabolic state.
		• Monitor body weight and serial serum protein levels.	• Reduced levels of serum proteins exacerbate effect of excessive thyroid hormones due to additional free, unbound quantities of thyroid hormone.
		• Provide adequate nutritive intake to meet needs of hypermetabolic state. – Essential amino acids and trace metals in addition to caloric intake.	• Complete nutritional and supportive therapy must be provided simulataneously with therapeutic modalities to decrease serum levels of thyroid hormone.
		Minimize energy expenditure by coordinating overall patient care activities and allowing for uninterrupted rest periods.	• Protein catabolism produces weakness in all muscle groups. Fatigue increases stress.
		• Assess effects of hypermetabolic state on gastrointestinal function: • Assess for signs/symptoms such as nausea, vomiting, diarrhoea, abdominal pain, hepatomegaly.	
		• Monitor mental status and presence of protective reflexes (cough andgag).	• Intravenous therapy may be indicated if there is risk of aspiration.
		• Provide frequent, small feedings.	• Frequent small feedings may help to diminish epigastric distress.
Nurisng Diagnosis # 9 Injury potential for, related to: 1. Altered neurologic function associated with hypermetabolic state. 2. Exopthalmopathy	Patient will: 1. Demonstrate usual mental status: • Alert, oriented to person, place. • Increased attentiveness.	• Maintain integrity of neurologic, physical, and psychologic processes. • Assess effect of hypermetabolic state on neurologic function.	• Symptomatology related to central nervous system function is attributed largely to the hypermetabolic activity within neurons.

Contd...

Contd...

Problem	*R*	*Objective*	*Nursing Interventions*	*Rationales*
		2. Remain injury free • Without seizure activity. • Corneas intact, without erosions or ulcerations.	◆ Perform neurologic assessent every 1-2 hr during acute phase of illness. Signs/symptoms may include: – Mental status: Blunted level of consciousness; disorientation, confusion agitation, restlessness, irritability, coma. – Cranial nerves: Sluggish pupillary response; impaired protective reflexes (cough, gag). – Motor function: Hypokinesis, easy fatigability, muscle weakness; seizures activity. – Hyper reflexia.	• Rapid fluctuations in neuralgic status can occur; changes in neuralgic status may reflect patients response to therapy.
			• Employ safety measures to prevent injury: ◆ Seizures precautions: Padded bed rails; oral airway and suction at beside; bed in low position; soft protective restraints.	– Seizure activity may reflect deterioration in the patient's condition.
			• Orient to person, date ,and place; provide clock and calendar in patient's room; confirm reality. • Maintain cool, quiet environment with occasional soft, soothing music.	
			• Allow for frequent undisturbed rest periods.	• Goal of therapy is to maximize the resting state to minimize cellular metabolic needs.
			• Avoid sensory overload.	• A reduction in stimuli diminishes state of hyperactivity and cellular metabolism.
			• Administer prescribed sedation, and monitor patient's response to therapy.	• Hyperactivity needs to be reduced because it exacerbates the hypermetabolic • Use of sedatives is avoided if possible because they can mask changes in the patient's neurologic status.
			• Assess status of exophthalmopathy. ◆ Protect exposed corneas: – Administer prescribed methylcellulose eyedrops. – Tape eyes shut if necessary while patient sleeps.	• Exophthalmopathy associated with long-standing hyperthyroidism may prevent patient from closing eyelids completely.
			◆ Encourage verbalization of fears and concerns regarding injury to eyes and overall appearance.	◆ Verbalization of feelings and concerns may assist the patient in coping with what might be a chronic problem.
Nurisng Diagnosis # 10 and # 11 Rest activity pattern infective sleep-pattern disturbance,related to: 1. Hyperactive state associated with increased metabolic rate.		Patient will: 1. Demonstrate performance of activities of daily living without fatigue. 2. Verbalize ability to sleep and feelings of rest and relaxation.	• Examine nursing care considerations concerned with fostering rest relaxation: ◆ Identify factors that contribute to fatigue and assist patient to cope within his/her limitations. – Help patient /family to identify signs of fatigue, and those activities that are especially tiring to the patient. – Help to plan rest periods between patient activities to minimize ftigue.	

Contd...

Contd...

Problem	*R*	*Objective*	*Nursing Interventions*	*Rationales*
			◆ Provide diversional activities.	◆ Such activities help to channel some of the otherwise unusable energy associated with overwhelming adrenergic response and the direct effect thyroid hormonal action on overall metabolic rate.
			◆ Initiate relaxation exercise when patient's condition stabilizes.	◆ Hyperthyroidism is often a long-term chronic illness; relaxation techniques may assist in coping.
			◆ Ascertain patient's usual sleep habits: – Identifies disruptions in usual sleep pattern caused by illness and hospitalization.	◆ Enhance adrenergic response predisposes to restlessness, agitation, irritability.
			– Encourage patient to verbalize feelings about sleeping capability, and ways to improve sleeping.	◆ It may also be helpful to verbalize the patient's feelings of frustration; the patient may be reassured that he/she is not all alone; that others understand and care.
			– plan for quite, restful period prior to sleeping. – Promote a quite, cool, and soothing atmosphere at sleep time. – Allow for flexibility in the patient's daily routine.	◆ Involving the patient in planning for sleep enables the patient to exert some control over his/her status. Patient's control over his/her status. Patients sometime describe that they can't sit still; that their mind/body seems to be racing.
			◆ Administer prescribed sedative if necessary; monitor effectiveness of therapy in relaxing patient and facilitating sleepfulness.	
Nurisng Diagnosis # 12 Thought processes, alteration in, related 1. Enhanced adrenergic activity.		Patient will: 1. Maintain baseline mental status: • Alert, oriented • Mentation: Memory intact; able to concentrate. • Behaviour appropriate. • Usual personality (as per family or significant others).	• Assess effect of hypermetabolic state on psychologic status: ◆ Assess for signs/symptoms including: Insomnia, fear, anxiety, emotional liability: apathy, depression, personality changes; psychosis.	• Severe hypermetabolic state coupled with excessive adrenergic activity may predispose to psychosis and coma.
			◆ Elicit information from family members regarding patient's usual personality and behaviour.	◆ Eliciting history from family members or significant others assists in determining patient's baseline status including behavioural and personality characteristics.
			◆ Monitor neurologic and psychologic status hourly	◆ Monitoring of patient's status at regular intervals assists in determining the effectiveness of therapy; enables the patient to be appraised of progress.
			• Implement therapeutic measures: ◆ Explain all ongoing procedures and reasons underlying therapy (e.g., use of hypothermia blanket). Explanations should be brief and repeated as necessary	◆ Appropriate explanations may help to alleviate heightened anxiety.
			• Encourage verbalization of fears, questions, concerns; take the time to listen.	
Nurisng Diagnosis # 13 Knowledge deficit, regarding underlying disease process, and factors that may trigger an exacerbation of the illness		Patient /family will: 1. Demonstrate a readiness to learn: • Interest and willingness to examine optimal level of health desired.	• Provide patient/family education to assist in developing and implementing prophylactic health-care practices. • Assess patient/family knowledge regarding disease process and therapy • Assess readiness to learn	• Understanding of underlying disease processes assists the patient/family to cope with and adjust to the limitations imposed by the diseases.

Contd...

Contd...

Problem	*R*	*Objective*	*Nursing Interventions*	*Rationales*
		2. Verbalize details of plan of care including need for diligent follow-up care.	• Implement teaching program to include the following topics: – Pertinent anatomy and physiology of thyroid gland. – Underlying pathophysiology of thyroid disease as it pertains to the patient's status. – Identification of stressors that precipitate or predispose to hyperthyroid crisis in the patient with hyperthyroidism. – Identification of stressors that precipitate or predispose to hyperthyroid crisis in the patient with hyperthyroidism.	• Hyperthyroidism has an impact on all members of the family; interested and supportive family members should be included in the educational processes.
			• Recognition of signs and symptoms of hyperthyroid crisis. • Understanding of medication regimen: – Indications for antithyroid and antiadrenergic medications – Dosage and administration. – Adverse side effects.	• Patient/family must appreciate the importance of seeking timely medical assistance when a stressful event occurs, of hyperthyroid crisis.
			• Understanding of importance of continuous medical follow-up with appropriate periodic blood testing. Initiation of self-care practices to prevent recurring – Usefulness of behavioural modifications and/or relaxation techniques.	• The importance of maintaining therapeutic blood levels must be stressed; noncompliance with drug regimen can predispose to hyperthyroid crisis.
Nursing Diagosis # 14 Self concept, disturbance in: Body image, related to: 1. Exophthalmopathy 2. Other changes in physical appearance: • Hyperpigmentation • Pretibial odema. • Muscle weakness wasting. • Menstrual irregularities, decreased libido in women. • Impotence in men. • Emotional lability.		Patient will: 1. Be able to verbalize feelings regarding body changes. 2. Be able to explore feelings associated with self-perception. 3. Identify own strrengths/weaknesses. 4. Identify coping options.	• Assist patient/family to examine their values and expectations; and the desired level of health.	• Hyperthyroidism is an especially compromising condition because often it becomes chronic, and patients often become noncompliant with prescribed therapeutic regimen.
			• Encourage patient to identify and verbalize feelings regarding self (capabilities). • Assist patient/family to identify coping strengths and weaknesses.	• Helps patient to begin to examine self, and to begin self acceptance.
			• Assess support system within family and friends/neighbours/significant other. • Be accessible to patient/family: – Provide a listening ear. – Praise accomplishments. – Assist in realistic goal-setting.	– Patient's family and significant others can be helpful accepting the patient as he/she is; positive support reinforces the patient's self esteem.
			• Encourage expression of honest feelings about self. – Be nonjudgmental; accept patient as he/she is.	• Being honest with oneself helps to promote relationships with others. • Verbalizing feelings of self increases self-awareness.
			• Involve in divisional activities as condition permits.	• Helps the patient to avoid dwelling on self limitations and indequacies.

DISORDERS OF THE THYROID GLAND

Thyroid hormone, thyroxine (T_4) and triode thyroxine (T_3) which is the more active form, regulate energy metabolism and growth and development. Alterations in the thyroid gland may be associated with hypersecretion, hyposecretion of normal secretion of thyroid hormone. Thyroid disorders are manifested as hyperfunction (thyrotoxicosis), hypofunction, inflammation or enlargement (goiter may interfere with surrounding structures and can be associated with increased, normal or decreased hormone production.

HYPERTHYROIDISM

Hyperthyroidism is defined as sustained, increased synthesis and release of thyroid hormone by the thyroid gland. Thyrotoxicosis is hypermetabolism that results from excess circulating levels of T_4 T_3 or both. Hyperthyroidism and thyrotoxicosis usually are together as in Grave's disease. However, in some forms of thyroiditis, thyrotoxicosis may occur without hyperthyroidism.

Aetiology

The incidence of hyperthyroidism is 4 to 10 times greater in women and the highest frequency is in the 30—50 years age group. The cause and definitions of different hyperthyroidism includes the following.

1. *Toxic diffuse goiter* (Grave's disease) is an autoimmune disorder characterized one or more of the following diffuse goiter, hyperthyroidism, infiltrate opthalmopathy and infiltration dexmopathy. The aetiology is unknown. The patient who is genetically susceptible becomes sensitized to and develops antibodies (TSABs) against various antigens within the thyroid gland and often other tissue as well. TSABs (thyroid stimulating antibodies) stimulate the TSH receptor on the thyroid hormone. Precipitating factors such as insufficient iodine supply, infection and stressful life events may interact with genetic factors that control immunology and metabolic abnormalities to cause Grave's disease.
2. *Toxic multinodular goiter* (Plummer's disease) is a disorder characterized by the presence of many thyroid nodules and a milder form of hyperthyroidism is seen with Grave's disease. Plummer's disease frequency is highest in women and it is more common in iodine deficient areas.
3. *Toxic adenoma* Single or occasionally multiple adenomas of follicular cells that secrets and function independent of TSH.
4. *Thyroiditis* is an inflammatory process in the thyroid and can have several causes such as subacute granulomatus (de Querrains) thyroiditis which is due to bacterial or fungal infection. There is increased amount of T_4 and T_3 released during acute inflammatory process; transient hyperthyroid states followed by return to state, and eventually to hyperthyroid state chronic immune thyroid. (Mashimotos thyroiditis) as a gland is destroyed by the recurring inflammatory exacerbations; hyperthyroid state usually requires no treatment.
5. *T_3 thyrotoxicism* T_3 level elvated but cause is unknown. T_4 but have signs and symptoms of thyrotoxicosis.
6. *Hyperthyroidism caused by metastatic thyroid cancer* Rare because thyroid cancer cells do not concentrate iodine efficiently may occur and may large follicular carcinoma.
7. *Pituitary hyperthyroidism* Rare pituitary adenomas may secrete excesses TSH; treatment involves removal of pituitary tumour.
8. *Chronic hyperthyroidism* Chronic gonadotropin has weak thyrotropin activity; tumours such as choriacarcinoma, embrayonal cell carcinoma and hydatixform mole have high concentrations of chotionic gonadotropins that can stimute T_4 and T_3 secretions; hyper thyroidism disappear with treatment of tumour.
9. *Struma ovaril* Ovarion dermoid tumour made up of thyroid tissue that secretes thyroid hormone.
10. *Factitious hyperthyroidism* Results from ingestion of exogenous thyroid extraction.
11. *Iodine induced hyperthyroid* Over production of thyroid hormone resulting from administration of supplemental iodine to a person with endemic goiter.

Pathophysiology

In hyperthyroidism from any cause, the normal regulating control of thyroid function is lost, resulting in an increased concentration of thyroid hormone and increased peripheral manifestations of thyroid hormone excess. Thyroid hormone increases metabolic rate and calorigenises alters protein, fat and carbohydrate metabolism, directly stimulate some body systems such as bone and bone narrow and increase sympathetic (adrenergic) activity. The underlying pathophisiology of all manifestations is not known. However, the effects of hyperthyroidism on body system are well known and occur in large part because of the interaction of the hypermetabolic static, increased circulation and adrenergic stimulation.

In Grave's disease, opthalmopathy, may precede, coincide with are following hyperthyroidism. The changes may be infiltrative or noninfiltrative or both. In infiltrative, the eye balls protrude from the orbits (exaphthalmos proptosis). This is due to impaired venous drainage from the orbits which causes increased fat deposits and fluid (odema) in retro-orbital tissues. Because, if increased pressure, the eyeballs are forced to outward and *protrude*. In noninfiltrative, the upper lids are usually retracted and elevated with sclera above the iris visible. When the eyelids do not close completely, the exposed corneal surfaces become dry and irritated. Serious consequences such as corneal ulcer and eventual loss of vision occur.

Clinical Manifestation

The manifestation of thyroid hyper functions are systemwise and include the following.

Cardiovascular Systolic hypertesion; increased rate and force of cardiac contractions; bound and rapid pulse; increased cardiac output; cardiac hypertrophy; systic murmurs; arrhythmias; Palpitations; atrial fibrillation (in order adult); angina.

Respiratory Increased respiratory rate; dyspnoea on mild exertion.

Gastrointestinal Increased appetite, thirst; weight loss; increased peristalsis; diarrhoea, frequent defecation; increased bowel sound; splenomegaly and hepatomegaly.

Integumentary Warm, smooth, moist skin; thin, brittle nails detached from nail bed (nydrolysis); hair loss (may be patchy); acropachy (clubbing), Palmer erythema; fine silky hair premature graving (in mendioaphoresis; vitiligo).

Muscutloskeletal Fatigue, muscle weakness especially proximal, Proximal muscle wasting; pretibial nyxedema; dependant oedemas osteoporosis.

Nervous system Difficulty in focussing eyes. Nervousness; fine tremor (of fingers and tongue); insomnia; liability of mood, delirium; restlessness; personality changes of irritability, agitation; exhaustion; hyper reflexion of tendon reflexes; depression, fatigue, apathy (in older adult); Lack of ability to concentrate; stupor; and coma.

Reproductive Menstrual irregularities; amenorrhoea; decreased libido;

Others Intolerance to heat; increased sensitivity to stimulant drugs; elevated basal temperature, lidlag, stare, eyelid retraction, exopthalmos, goiter, raid speech.

Ophthalmopathy in Grave's Disease

Signs

Bright -eyes stare: results from retraction of the upper eyelid.

- Lidlag-on downward gaze, upper lidlag, behind the globe movement and scelera seen between lid and limbus.
- Globelag: globelag behind lid with upward gaze.
- Lid movement; Jerky and spasmodic.
- Eyes partly open when sleeping.
- Periorbital oedema.

Symptoms

- Sense of irritation and excessive tearing.
- Feeling of pressure behind eyes.
- Complaints of blurred or double vision, easy tiring of eyes.

Complication

- Corneal ulceration.
- Optic nerve involvement (optic neuropathy).
- Myopathy of extraocular muscles.

Management

When hyperthyroidism is suspected, various diagnostic tests are necessary to confirm diagnosis in addition to history and physical examination and ophthalmologic examination, which includes ECG and laboratory tests such as serum T_3 Ru, T_4, free T_3, TSH levels, and TRH stimulation test, and thyroid scan also is useful.

Three classes of medications are used in the treatment of hyperthyroidism, which include the following:

i. *Antithyroids* of thiomide, which inhibit the synthesis of thyroid hormone and prophylthiouracil (PTU) and methimazole (Tapezole)
ii. *Iodides* Which primarily inhibits the release of thyroid hormone Eg-Radioactive iodine (RAI) RAI therapy are being increasingly used because:
   - It can be given on outpatient basis.
   - It is safer for wider range of patients including elderly persons who are poorer surgical runs.
   - It can result in faster improvement in thyroid function than antithyroid drug therapy and
   - Although still controversial, can be used in women of childbearing age.

   It is administered orally in one dose, average dose 80 to 90 per/g. of thyroid tissue. Treatment can be repeated after six months.
iii. Beta-adrenergic blockers such as propranolol (Inderal) calcium antagonists the effect; thyroid hormone on body cells.

Surgery is no longer the treatment of choice with Grave's diseases, if indicated, surgical techniques include the removal of one lobe (subtotal thyroidectomy) or removal of the gland (Total thyroidecromy).

Nursing Management

A restful, calm, quick room should be provided because of increased metabolism causes sleep disturbances. Provision of adequate rest may be a challenge because of the patient's irritability and restlessness. Nursing intervention may include:

- Placing the patient in a cool room, away from very ill patients and noisy high traffic areas;
- Using light bed coverings and changing the linen frequently if the patient is diaphoretic;
- Encouraging and assisting with exercise involving large muscle groups (tumours can interfere with small muscle coordination) to allow the release of nervous tension and restlessness.

- Restricting visitors who upset the patient and
- Establishing a supportive, trusting relationship to help the patient to cope with aggravating events and lessen anxiety.

If exophthalmos is present, there is potential for corneal injury related to irritation and dryness. The patient may have orbital pain. Nursing intervention to relieve eye discomfort and prevent corneal ulceration include applying artificial tears to soothe and moisten conjunctival membrane, salt restriction may help to reduce pre-orbital oedema. Elevation of the patient's head promotes fluid drainage from the preorbital area; the patient should sit upright as much as possible. Dark glass reduces glare and prevent irritation from smoke, air currents, dust and dirt. If the eyes cannot be closed, they should be lightly taped for sleep. To maintain flexibility, the patient should be taught to exercise the intraocular muscles several times a day, by turning eyes in the complete range of motion. Good grooming can be helpful in reducing the loss of self-esteem that can result from an altered body image. If the exophthalmos is severe, treatment may include suturing the eyelids together, administering corticosteroids, radiation of retro-orbital tissues, orbital decompression, or corrective lid or muscle surgery.

If surgery is scheduled, the patient must be adequately prepared to avoid postoperative complications, Routine nursing intervention followed according to surgical procedure.

The person receiving radiation therapy of the thyroid gland should be taught the following:

- Flush the toilet two or three times after each use.
- Increase intake of fluids to aid in RAI's excretion.
- Use separate eating utensiles and separate towels and wash clothes. Wash these and underclothes and bedlinen separately.
- Rinse bathroom sinks and tube thoroughly after use, and wash hands carefully after using the bathroom.
- Sleep alone for few days and avoid kissing and intercourse (although amount of radiation in the patient's body is minimal).
- Avoid prolonged physical contact with anyone.
- Do not breastfeed.
- Delay pregnancy for 6 months after therapy.
- RAI should not be used in pregnant women because of the teratogenic effects on foetus, and the placenta transports iodine early

The following measures to be taken when the person with thyroid crisis or storm by the nurses include:

- Monitor the patients temperature, intake output, neurological status and cardiovascular status every hour.
- Initiate an IVLine for medication and fluids.
- Administer increasing doses of oral prophilthiouracil as ordered (200 to 300 mg every 6 hours may be given) after a loading dose of 800 to 1200 mg orally.
- Administer iodine preparation as ordered. Sodium iodine given IVtwice daily or an oral preparation may be ordered.
- Administer propranolol 1to 20 to 80 mg per oral or 2 to 10 mg IV as ordered. Propranolol can worsen asthma or CHF because it constricts bronchial smooth muscles and causes a decrease in cardiac output.
- Initiate measures to lower body temperature, including external cooling devices, cold baths and acetaminophen. Salicylates are contraindicate because they inhibit thyroid hormone binding to protein carries and thus increase free thyroid hormone levels.
- Initiate other supportive therapy as ordered, including oxygen, cardiac glycosides, and treatment measures for the precipitating event.
- Maintain quiet, calm, cool, private environment until crisis is over.
- Maintain continuity of care.
- Decrease stressers by use of patient education, comfort measures or family support.

As recovery ensures, the nurse must continue to provide intervention that addresses the outcomes related to hyperthyroidism. These include but or not limited to:

- Initiate other supportive therapy as ordered, including oxygen, cardiac glycosides, and treatment measures for the precipitating event.
- Maintain quiet, calm, cool, private environment until crisis is over.
- Maintain continuity of care.
- Decrease stressers by use of patient education, comfort measures of family support.

As recovery ensures, the nurse must continue to provide intervention that addresses the outcome related to hyperthyroidism. These include but or not limited to:-

a. Promote adequate rest.
    - Provide a quite, comfortable enviornment.
    - Provide back rubs.
    - Use home remedies such as hot milk to assist in promoting sleep.
    - Encourage quiet periods even if the patient does not sleep
b. Maintain increase activity tolerance.
    - Encourage short walks if cardiac output is stable.
    - Space activity between rest periods.
c. Maintain adequate nutrition intake.
    - Monitor intake and output every 8 hours
    - Weight daily
    - Monitor nutritional intake
    - Provide frequent high-protein and high caloric meals.
d. Promote good eye care.
    - Perform visual assessment every shift.
    - Initiate appropriate measures such as using dark glasses, or elevating head of bed; using artificial tears and tapping the eyelids closed at various intervls.
    - Report any new complaints immediately.

e. Facilitate improved coping. Offer patient's intervention to help them relax, such as music, backrubs, and distraction.
f. Enhance patient knowledge – regarding diseases-signs and symptoms, explain medication use, purpose, dosage, schedule and side effects; precaution during RAIT, self monitoring.

HYPOTHYROIDISM

Hypothyroidism is a metabolic state resulting from a deficiency of thyroid hormone that my occur at any age. Congenital hypothyroidism results in a condition called *Cretinism.*

Aetiology

Hypothyroidism may result from the following.

- *Loss or atrophy of thyroid tissue* Autoimmune thyroiditis, ablative therapy for hyperthyroidism, thyrotoxic drugs, congenital agenesis, maldevelopment, or radiation for head and neck malignancy.
- *Loss of trophic stimulation* Pituitary dysfunction (pituitary or secondary hypothyroidism) or hypothalamus dysfunction.
- *Miscellaneous alterations* Deficit in hormone biosynthesis; peripheral resistance to thyroid hormone, idiopathic factors or environment factor (iodine deficiencies).

The most frequent causes and their brief description are as follows:

1. *Hoiter* Any enlargement of the thyroid gland is not associated with hyperthyroidism hypothyroidism, cancer or inflammation is referred to as *Simple* goiter; *Endemic* goiter due to iodine deficiency. Sporadic goiter occurs sporadically in regions that are not the locus of the endemic goiter. Mostly seen in females and family history of goiter.
2. *Thyroiditis*
   - *Acute thyroiditis (*acute pyogenic thyroiditis) results from infection of thyroid by pyogenic organisms: symptoms include pain, and tenderness in thyroid, dysphasia, fever, malaise, treatment, symptomatic.
   - *Subacute nonsuppurative thyroiditis* (Dequavain thyroiditis and Granulomatous thyroditis) results from vital infections of thyroid gland, may follow an upper respiratory infection, most often seen in 4th and 5th decades of life, symptoms include pain in the thyroid, fever, hoarseness, dysphasia, pallitations, nervousness; lassitude, thyroid moderately enlarged, subsides in few months, treatment usually symptomatic, aspirin for mild cases, glucocorticoids when disease is unresponsible to other measures.
   - *Subacute lymphocytic thyroiditis* (Painless thyroiditis, lymphocytic thyroiditis). It is a form of thyroiditis increasing in frequency; aetiological factor unknown but possible autoimmune symptoms include self-limiting form of hyperthyroidism and nontender enlarged thyroid gland, which may be followed by hypothyroidism treatment symptomatic during hyperthyroidism phase may include betadrenergic blockers but not propylthiouracid (not effective) monitor annually for hypothyroidism.
   - *Chronic thyroiditis* (Hashimoto's thyroditis, Riedel's thyroiditis) is a rare form of thyroiditis, cause is unknown. Extensive fibrosis gland occurs; symptoms include insidious onset, symptoms form compression of traches, oesophagus, and recurrent laryngeal nerve, gland enlarged hard; hypothyroidism can occur, treatment is symptomatic with surgery for symptoms of compression, and thyroid replacement for hypothyroidism.
3. *Ablative therapy* Total thyroidectomy, hypophysectomy, and radiation therapy of pituitary or thyroid gland cause is iatrogenic hypothyroidism. Patients undergoing these treatments must take thyroid hormone replacement for life.

Pathophysiology

The patients with hypothyroidism may or may not have a goiter. An enlarged thyroid gland is seen when the disease results from thyroiditis. Defective hormone biosynthesis, peripheral resistance to thyroid hormone, and environment factors. All these conditions reduce thyroid hormone production and as a result, TSH secretions is increased because of lack of negative feedback. Increased thyroid mass then results from the increased stimulation. In contrast, hypothyroidism results from lack of TSH, (secondary hypothyodism) growth of the thyroid gland are not stimulated. The three types of thyroiditis are acute. subacute, chronic occur (already briefed in aetiology). And regardless of the cause, lack of thyroid hormone results in a general depression of basal metabolic rate and slows the development of functioning of the every system of the body. Alteration in the integumentary cardiovascular, nervous, musculoskeletal, alimentary and reproductive system are seen one of the major changes in accumulation of hyaluronic acids and alterations of the ground substances producing mucinous–oedema Myocoedema and third space fluid effusions. Myocodedema coma represents the most severe form of hypothyroidism and ultimately can occur in any patient with untreated prolonged hypothyroidism. Precipitating factors include, sedatives narcotics, exposure to cold, surgery, infection and trauma.

Clinical Manifestations

The major manifestations of cretinism are defective physical development and mental retardardation in infants/children. Affected infants may exhibit a large posterior fontanels, squinting, excessive sleeping, thickened skin and lips, enlarged tongue, abdominal distention, vomiting and a hoarse cry. Dull facial expression, feeding and respiratory difficulty, peripheral cyanoses, and supraclavicular and periorbital oedemas umbilical herneas and hypothermia. Hypothyroids in childhood is due to autoimmune thyroiditis (Symptom explained in earlier pages).

Hypothyroidism in the adult is characterized by an insidious and non-specific slowing of body process. The system-wise clinical manifestation of hypothyroidism are as follows:

- *Cardiocasular;* Increased capillary fragility, decreased pulse rate, varied changes in blood pressure; cardiac hypertrophy, weak contractility, distant heart sounds, anaemia, tending to develop CHF, angina and MI.
- *Resparatory;* Dyspnoea; decreased breathing capacity.
- *Gastrointestinal:* Decreased appetite, nausea and vomiting; weight gain, constipation, distended abdomen and enlarged scaly tongue.
- *Integumentary:* Dry, thick inelastic, cold skin; brittle nails; dry, spares, coarse hair, poor turgor of mucosa; generalized interstitial oedema; puffy face and decreased sweating; pallor.
- *Musculoskeletal:* Fatigue; weakness; muscular aches and pains; slow movement; arthralgia.
- *Nervous: Apathy;* lethargy; forgetfulness; slowed mental processes; hoarseness; slow, slurred speech; prolonged relaxation of deep tendon muscles; stupor, coma, parenthesis; anxiety, depression; polyneuropathy
- *Reproductive:* Prolonged menstrual periods or amenorhoea; decreased libido and infertility
- *Others:* Increased susceptibility to infection; increased sensitivity to narcotics, barbiturates, and asthenia, intolerance to cold, decreased hearing; sleepiness and goiter.

Management

Studies of thyroid function useful for diagnosing hypothyroidism include serum T_3 RU, $T_{3,}$ T_4 serum cholesterol, ECG. Serum cholesterol, ECG, Serum TSH, and TSH stimulation tests. Other tests may be needed to determine the true hormonal status.

The therapeutic objective in hypothyroidism is restoration of a euthyroid state as safely and rapidly as possible with hormone replacement in the adult, a low-calòric diet is indicated to promote weight loss. Synthetic oral thyroxine synthroid, levothyroid is the drug of (sodium-levo-thyroxine) choice to treatment of hypothyroidism. In the young, otherwise, healthy patient, maintenance of replacement dose can be started at once. In the older adults, patients, and person with compromised cardiac status, a small initial dose (12.5 to 25 mg.L) is recommended because the usual dose may increase myocardial angine and cardiac arrhythmia's. Any chest pain experienced by a patient starting thyroid replacement should be reported immediately and ECG and cardiac enzyme tests are performed.

Treatment consists of pharmacological therapy described. Surgery may be performed for large goiter, particularly those compressing adjacent tissues and organs.

Nursing Management

Assessment of the patient who is suspected of having hypothyroiditis based on clinical manifestations that usually occur. If the patient has any oedema, coma, mechanical respiratory support will be necessary as well as cardiac monitoring. The nurse will be administering all medications IV since the paralytic ileus associated with myxoedema causes unreliable absorption of oral medications. If the patient is hyponatcremic, hypersonic saline may be infused. The nurse should monitor hypothermia. For the assessment of the patient progress vital signs, body weight, fluid intake and output visible oedemas should be monitored. Cardiovascular assessments also follow, and take measures accordingly as in acute interventions.

The nursing interventions required by the patients with hypothyroidism vary greatly depending on the severity of disease. Because the hypothyrodic state is reversed slowly, the patient will not return to the premorbid health state for 2 to 3 months. Potential nursing intervention include the following:

a. Promote activity to the level of patient tolerance. At first the patient will have a very limited tolerance and only be able to move around in the room. Activities should be increased gradually.
   - Monitor the cardiovascular response to new activities. If the patient complains of chest pain or develops an unacceptable heart rate, stop the activity and then resume at a slower rate.
   - Monitor blood pressure, pulse and respirations before, during and after each activity.
b. Promote positive body image.
   - Provide information that helps the patient and significant others understand the relationship of body changes to hypothyroidism.
   - Educate about reversible body changes.
   - Stress the positive changes that have occurred.
c. Promote normal bowel elimination.
   - Monitor bowel elimination.
   - Maintain adequate fluid intake
   - Increase bulk in the diet.
d. Treat hypothermia
   - Monitor temperature every 2 to 4 hours.
   - Maintain environment temperature that is comfortable for the patient
   - Use blankets to increase body temperature if necessary.
e. *Facililitates* Intake of a nutritional diet that is low in calories and includes food from all food groups.
f. *Promote comfort*
   - Use nonmedicinal comfort measures such as massage, cool or warm heart and distraction to pain control.
   - If medications are used, monitor carefully. Patient will have a lower tolerance for sedatives and depressant medications.

g. *Provide* for self-care needs. At first the patient may require complete care for hygiene, toileting and dietary needs.
h. *Facilitate* patients understandings of the relationship between the sexual problems and the hypothyroidism.
i. *Maintan skin intergrity:*
   - Monitor skin condition each shift.
   - Institute preventive care measures such as sheepskin pads and soft sheets.
   - If patient is unable to or does not turn be on his/her own, assist in turning in every hour.
j *Facilitate* safe environment and orientation to environment.
   - Monitor neurological status every shift.
   - Reorient that patient frequently uses resources such as current events, clocks and newspapers.
   - Maintain a safe environment; remove any clutter, keep bed low, and keep bed rails up.
   - Check on patient frequently, especially at night, and use night-lights to prevent confusion.
   - Inform significant others of relationship between mental status and hypothyroidism.
   - Involve patient as much possible as in decision about care.

In addition, the nurse helps the patient and family caregivers learn how to continue the plan of care after discharge. The importance of compliance with medications and follow-up care should be stressed.

CANCER OF THE THYROID GLAND

Cancer of the thyroid gland less prevalent than other forms of cancer and only very small percentage of thyroid neoplasm are malignant. Two general types of malignant neoplasm are found which include:

1. Those arising from follicular epithelium (Papillary, follicular, medullar and anaphasic.
2. Those arising from parafollicular tissue. Thyroid-lymphoma. The characteristics of the five forms of primary malignant neoplasms of the thyroid include the following:
   i. *Papillary* The incidence of this cancer is 65% usually occurs in young persons, more in females than males. The prognosis is good. Rarely causes death in young person if occult or intrathyroidal. Metastasis is intra-glandular lymphathics, slows growing tumour.
   It is asymptotic. Occult (Less than 1.5 cm in diameter) Intrathyroidal (greater than 1.5 diameter, but does not extend through surface and extrathyroidal extends through thyroid surface. It is well differentiated psammoma body found in 40% of tumours and virtually diagnostic of malignant nature. Tumours appear as a cold sport on thyroid scan. Growth partially depends on TSH.
   ii. *Follicular* The incidence of this cancer is 20%. Usually occurs after 40 years; more in female. Metastasis occurs early by blood vessels in sites bones, lung, liver. Prognosis is good if minimally invasive lesion; symptom of goiter may have been present for years; Tumour is well differentiated to poorly differentiated, cyst formation and calcification; tremors may appears as "hot" areas on thyroid scan. Suppressive thyroid therapy can cause regression of metastatic lesion.
3. *Aaplastic:* The incidence of this cancer is 5% usually occurs after 60 years more in females than males; Metastasis by direct invasion to adjacent structures; highly malignant prognosis varies with cell type (giant cell-6 months, and small cells-5 years symptoms include hoarseness, inspiratory strider, pain dysphasia signs of invasion adjacent areas. Two cell forms of tumour, giant cell and small cell.
4. *Thyroid lymphoma:* The incidence of this cancer is 5%. Occurs usually after 40 years, more in women than men. Metastasis by lymphatic system; gland fixed to other structures. Prognosis is good. Patient may have long history of previous goiter, rapid enlargement of goiter, hoarseness, dysphasia, pressure sensation dyspnoea and some pain: Tumour usually is in nodular histocytic form. It is strongly associated with hashimotos thyroiditis.
5. *Medullary:* The incidence of this type of cancer is 5% usually occurs after 50 years, both in male and female equally. Metastasis is by interglanular lymphatic and blood vessels. Prognosis is moderate (10 years survival estimated). Because of tumour produces hormone, possible survival is estimated). Because of tumour produces hormone, possible, paraendocrine manifestation such as carcinoid syndrome, watery diarrhoea, Cushing's syndrome, tumour of C-cells of thyroid, not accelerated, some appear as 'cold' spots on the thyroid scan; may produce ACTH, prostaglandin for carcinoembryonic antigen. It occurs as a familial form as apart of multiple endocrine neoplasia (MEN).

Management

Diagnosis of the thyroid cancer has been simplified by the acceptance of the fine-needle biopsy and obtaining tissue samples from solid tumours or fluid cysts. Radionuclide imagery, ultrasound tests and thyroid suppression tests are helpful in thyroid cancer.

Medical management of person with thyroid cancer includes use of all modalities of cancer treatment: surgery, radiation, hormoneal suppression, and chemotherapy (see topic oncological nursing chapter).

Care of the patient with thyroid nodule first focuses on helping patient through the diagnostic process. Thyroid nodule occurs frequently, and most are not to be concerned. No one diagnostic test is completely reliable. Depending on the patient characteristics, various tests may be performed. The nurse prepares the patient for each test, focusing particularly on education.

When surgery is indicated, nurse has to prepare the patient for surgery by performing required routine measures preoperatively and postoperatively, which includes patient teaching regarding general preoperative and postoperative care. Particularly in thyroid surgery, patient needs to,learn how to cough, and move the head and neck postoperatively without placing strain on the suture line. Thus, the patient is taught preoperatively to support the neck by placing both hands behind the neck when moving the head or when coughing.

The nursing intervention during postoperative care of the person after thyroid surgery includes the following:

A. Monitor for and report signs of complications.
  a. Laryngeal nerve damage; hoarseness and weak voice.
  b. Haemorrhage of tissue swelling
    - Bleeding on dressing; check back of dressing by slipping hand gently under the neck and shoulders.
    - Choking sensation.
    - Difficulty in coughing or swallowing.
    - Sensation of dressing being too tight even after it loosened.
  c. Calcium deficiency (tenany)
    - Early signs: tingling around mouth or of toes and fingers. decreasing serum calcium levels.
    - Later signs: positive Chrostek's and Tousseau's signs and grand malseizures.
  d. Respiratory distress associated with any signs just listed.
B. Provide emergency care.
  a. Keep emergency supplies readily available.
    - Tracheotomy set for Laryngeal nerve damage. Oxygen and suction equipment suture removal set for respiratory obstruction haemorrhage.
    - IV calcium gluconate or calcium chloride (for tetany)
  b. For acute respiratory diseases:
    - Call for immediate medical help.
    - Raise head of bed.
    - Loosen dressing over incision.
    - Give calcium as ordered, if signs and symptoms of tetany present.
    - If loosening dress does not relieve symptoms of respiratory distress and if medical help is not readily available, remove clips or sutures as instructed.
  c. Provide comfort
    - Avoid tension on suture lines: encourage patient to support head when turning by placing both hands behind neck.
    - Give prescribed analgesics as necessary.
  d. Maintain nutritional status
    - Start soft foods as soon as tolerated only fluids may be tolerated initially.
    - Encourage a high carbohydrate and high-protein diets.
  e. Teach patient
    - ROM exercises to neck when suture line healed to prevent permanent limitations.
    - Need for life-long thyroid hormone replacement therapy after a total thyroidectomy.
    - Any special care measures related to the underlying disease.
    - Need for follow-up care.

DISORDERS OF PARATHYROID GLAND

Hyper Parathyroidism

Hyper parathyroidism is a condition involving increased secretion of parathyroid hormone (PTH) PTH has following functions.

- Maintenance of normal serum calcium.
- Regulate bone resorption of calcium.
- Regulates reabsorption of calcium from glomerular filtrate.
- Regulates phosphate and bicarbonate excretion in kidney tubule.
- Regulates calcium absorption in intestine; influenced by oestrogen, drestrogen in women and activated vitamin D (1,25-dehyaroxy-choledlciferol calcitrol.)
- Calcium regulates pores of cell membranes, movement of sodium, and thus depolarization and resultant action potential in nerves and muscles.

In short, PTH helps regulates calcium, and phosphate levels by stimulating bone resorption, renal tubular reabsorption of calcium and activation of vitamin D.

Aetiology

Hyperparathyroidism is classified as primary, secondary, or tertiary.

- Primary parathyroidism is due to an increased secretion of PTH leading to disorders of calcium, phosphate, and bone metabolism. The excessive concentration of circulating PTH usually leads to hypocalcaemia and hypophoshataemia. The most common cause is a benign neoplasm or a single adenoma in the parathyroid gland. It is most common in women and usually occurs between 30 to 70 years.
- Secondary hyperparathyroidism appears to be compensatory response to states that induce or cause hypocalcaemia, the main stimulus of PTH secretion. Disease condition associated with secondary hyperparathyroidism include vitamin D deficiencies, malabsorption, chronic renal failure and hyperphosphataemia.
- Tertiary hyperparathyroidism occurs when there is hyperplasia of parathyroid glands and the loss of feedback from circulating calcium levels. Thus, there is autonomous secretion of PTH, even with normal calcium levels. It is observed in the patient who has had a kidney transplant after a long period of dialysis treatment of chronic renal failure.

Pathophysiology

Primary hyperparathyroidism is result of one or two major problems. The exageration of the normal effects of PTH on skeletal, renal and gastrointestinal system and the associated hypercalcemia. Hypersecretion of PTH results in continued stimulation of target organs and elevates serum calcium. The normal negative feedback of serum calcium on PTH and secretion is lost or ineffective. Increased PTH, increased bone resorption enhances the reabsorption of calcium from the glomerular filtrate, and increases calcium absorption through the gastrointestinal tract.

In the *skeletal system* There are increased PTH, increased bone resorption resulting in oesteopoenia and in very severe cases, cysts and fractures. From osteitis fibrose cystica. Joint changes also occur. In the renal system, increased PTH enhances the reabsorption of calcium from the glomerular filtrate, reabsorption of phosphate and alteration in the excretion of bicarbonate. Production of activated vitamin D increases elevated PTH effects the GI tract are indirect and occur through the action of vitamin D. The activated vitamin D results in increased agent of vitamin D. The activated vitamin D. The activated vitamin D results in increased calcium absorption through GI tract. These processes result in elevated serum calcium which in itself leads to neurological, musculoskeletal, cardia, GI and renal alteration.

In both secondary and tertiary hyperparathyroids, the calcium level is chronically low. In chronic renal failure the low calcium results from hyperphosphataemia, a decreased production of activated vitamin D and a decrease in calcium absorption. There also may be a decreased sensitivity of bone to the action of PTH. This process results in hyperplasia and excessive production of PTH are usually able to keep the calcium level close to normal, but at the expense of bone destruction The bone lesions are characterized by osteomalacia, osteosclerosis and osteitis fibrosa cystica.

Clinical Manifestation

Hyper parathyroidism has varying symptoms. The sytem-wise clinical manifestations are as follows.

- *Cardiovascular:* Arrhythmia's, shortened QT interval on ECG, and hypertension.
- *Gastrointestinal*: Vague abdominal pain, anorexia, nausea and vomiting, constipation, pancreatitis, peptic ulcer disease, cholelmthiasis, weight loss and appetite.
- *Integuentary:* Skin necrosis and moist skin.
- *Musculoskeletal:* Skeletal pain, backache, weakness, fatigue, pain on weight bearing; osteoporosis, pathologic fracture of long bones; compressed fractures spine and decreased muscle tone
- *Neurologic:* Personality disturbances, emotional irritability, memory impairment, psychosis, delirium confusion, coma; incoordinations; hyperactive deep tendon reflexes; abnormalities of gait; psychomotor retardation and headache.
- *Renal:* Hypercalciuria, kidney stones (nephrolithiasis), urinary tract infection and polyuria.
- *Others:* Corneal calcification on slit-lamp examination, serious complications are renal failure, pancreatitis, collapse of vertebral bodies, cardiac changes and long bone and rib fractures.

Management

An increased serum PTH levels and persistent hypercalcaemia are criteria for establishing diagnosis of PHPT and other causes of hypercalcaemia and increased serum ruled out. PTH measured by radio immuno assay. Serum calcium level will exceed 10 mg/dl Elevation in other lab test include urine calcium, serum chloride, uric acid, creatinin amylase bone changes are detected by radiological studies-Ray, MRI, CT scan ultrasound for location and adenoma.

The treatment objectives are to relieve symptoms and prevent complication caused by excess PTH. The choice of therapy complications causes excess PTH. The choice of therapy depends on the urgency of clinical situation, the degree of hypercalcaemia, the underlying disorder, the status of renal, renal and hepatic function, the clinical presentation of patient.

Plicamycine mithracin and antihypercalcemic agent, lowers the serum calcium in 48 hours, used for metastatic parathyroid carcinoma and svere bone diseases . It has many side effects. Biophosphonate such as pamidronate (Aredia) used to inhibit oestoclastic bone resorption. Destrogon progesteron can reduce calcium levels in postmenopausal woman. Oral phosphate can be used to inhibit calcium absorption effects of vitamin D in intestine. Diuretic may be given to increase the urinary excretion of calcium. In several cases to correct fluid volume deficit and promote calcium excretion by administration of saline, lasix and drugs as ordered.

Parathyroid tumours should be removed surgically. The goal is to restore normal parathyroid function and hypercalcaemia or hypocalcaemia. The amount of parathyroid tissue removed depends upon the appearance of each gland.

Nursing care of the patient depends upon the treatment. During the acute preoperative period, patients are treated medically which consists continuing hydration, administration of loop diuretics, replacement of electrocytes and administration of sodium chloride and other prescribed medication.

Postoperatively, the care requirements are very similar to these required after thyroidectomy. Potential physiological complication includes haemorrhage, hypocalcaemia and airway obstruction. The patients respiratory, cardiovascular, neurological and fluid volume state are monitored routinely.

The nursing intervention includes.

- Have a tracheotomy set and IV Calcium preparation readily available.
- Report any signs of haemorrhage, hypocalcaemia, or airway obstruction.

- Assess mental status and motor strength.
- Perform complete respiratory assessments. Keep head of bed elevated 30 degrees to facilitate respiration. Encourage deep breathing, coughing and tuning 2-4th hourly.
- Increased ambulations at patient's tolerance take into account mental status and weakness.
- Maintain fluid intake at prescribed levels or enough to achieve 1000 ml or more if serum calcium levels are normal or 2000 mls or more if they are higher.
- Teach patient and significant others about:
  - Prescribed drug.
  - Prescribed diet if any
  - Electrolyte replacement if any.
  - Fluid intake requirements.
  - Wound care.
  - Symptoms to report: those indicating infection, hypercalcemia, or hypercalcemia.
  - Follow-up care requirements.

HYPOPARATHYROIDISM

Hypoparthyroidism or inadequate circulatory PTH, is characterized by hypocalcemia resulting from lack of PTH to maintain serum calcium levels. It may be pseudohyparothyroidism (idiopathic) or true hypoparathyroidism (iatrogenic)

Aetiology

The causative factors of true hypoparathyroidism may be classified into three major categories surgically induced, idiopathic and functional:

- The most common cause of hypoparathyroidism is iatrogenic that is accidental removal of parathyroids or damage to the vascular supply of the glands during neck-surgery (e.g thyroidectomy, radical neck surgery).
- Idiopathic hypoparathyroidism resulting from the absence, fatty replacement or atrophy of the glands as a rate disease that usually occurs early in life and may be associated with other endocrine disorders because many of these persons have abnormal antibodies directed against parathyroid gland. The cause is unknown.
- Functional hypoparathyroidism is the result of chronic hypomagenesemia, which may be seen in malabsorption or alcoholism, and appear to impair PTH release.
- In pseudohypoparathyroidism, the excretion and release of PTH are normal. But there is target tissue resistance to PTH. The cause is unknown may cause by genetic defect resulting in hypocalcemia in spite of normal or high PTH levels is often associated with hypothyroidism and hypogonadism.

Pathophysiology

A deficiency of tissue resistance to PTH results in decreased bone resorption, decreased activation of vitamin D and thus decreased intestinal absorption of calcium, increased renal excretion of calcium and decreased renal phosphorus. The result is hypocalcemia and hyperphosphataemia, The major physiological alterations result from the effect of low calcium levels on neuromuscular irritability, nerves show decreased threshold of excitation, repeated responses to a single stimuli and in severe cases continuous activity of muscular spasms (tetany). Cardiac activity is altered. Calcification of basal ganglia and lens of the eye may occur. The severity of the hypocalcemia and chronicity of the problem indicate the sign and symptoms seen with true hypoparathyroidism. In mild cases which results in any slightly decreased serum calcium levels, the patient may be asymptomatic.

The patient with pseudohypoparathyroidism may have the same signs and symptoms as seen with true hypoparathyroidism. In addition, such patients may have skeletal and developmental abnormalities including short stature, round face , short neck, stocky body, and discrete bone lesions. The most common bone lesion is unilateral or bilateral shortenings of the fourth of fifth metacorpal or metatarsal bone. Mental retardation may also be present. The patient has low serum calcium and high serum phosphorus levels with normal to PTH level on radioimmunoassay.

Clinical Manifestation

The clinical features of acute hypoparathyroids are due to slow serum calcium levels. Sudden decrease in calcium concentration gives rise to syndrome called *tetany.* This is characterized by tingling of the lips, fingertips, and occasionally feet and increased muscle tension leading to paresthenias and stiffness. Painful tone spasms of smooth and skeletal muscles particularly of the extremities and face dysphagia, a constricted feeling of throat and laryngospasm. Chrostek's sign (facial muscle spasm when the face is tapped below the temple) and trousseau's sign (carpopeda spasm when arterial circulation is interrupted by applying BP Cuff.

To sum up, the true hypoparathyroidism and clinical manifestation includes the following.

1. *Neuromuscular manifestation:* Changes in nerve activity affect peripheral motor and sensory nerves.
   - Numbness and tingling parasthesia around mouth, tips of fingers and some times in the feet.
   - Tetany with positive Chrostek's and Trousseau's sign, spasms of wrists, fingers, forearm feet and toes.
   - Fatigue, weakness, painful cramps, osteosclerosis, soft tissue calcification and difficulty in walking
   - Convulsions that may consist of tonic spasms of the total body or the more typical tonic clonic activity.
   - Laryngeal stridor and dyspnoea.
   - Other neurological signs: headache, painful oedema, elevated CSF pressure, local signs and symptoms, including gait changes, tremors, rigidity, and spasms; possible signs of Parkinsonism, hyperactivity, deep-tendon reflexes paresthesia of perioral area, hands and feet.

2. *Emotional:* mental manifestation-Irritability, depression, anxiety, emotional liability, memory impairment, confusion, frank psychoses, personality changes, disorientation, etc.
3. *Cardiovascular manifestation*
   - Decreased contractility of heart muscle.
   - Decreased cardiac output from congestive heart failure.
   - Prolonged QT and ST intervals and occasional dysrhythmias (ECG
   - Resistance to effect of digitalis preparations.
4. *Eye manifestation:* Eye changes including lenticular opacities, cataracts, papill oedema. Eventualy there will be loss of total sight.
5. *Dental manifestation*:
   - Enamel defects seen on the tooth crown.
   - Delayed or absent tooth eruption.
   - Defective dental root formation.
6. *Integumentary:* Dry, scaly skin, hair loss on scalp and body, thin patchy hair, brittle nails, fragile nails, vitiligo, skin infection (Candidiasia).
7. *GI and Renal Manifestation* Abdominal cramps and urinary and fecal incontinence, urinary frequency, malabsorption, and steatorrhoea.

Management

The main objectives of treatment are to treat tetany when present and prevent long-term complication by maintaining normal serum calcium level (eucalcaemea). The first priority of trachea in correcting calcium levels to prevent tetany. This is achieved by giving IV calcium gluconate or calcium chloride. Airway pathway must be maintained.

Tetany is treated with IV infusion or slow push of calcium salts (calcium salts can cause hypotension and cardiac arrest-thin slow push) long-term therapy consists of the administration of vitamin D and possibly supplemental calcium and oral phosphate binders.

The cause of hypoparathyroid is the identified and long-term therapy is started as soon as possible. Normal serum calcium levels are maintained by supplemental dietary and elemental calcium by dietary phosphate restriction and phosphate-binding agents such as aluminium hydroxide and by vitamin D therapy to increase GI absorption of calcium. Vitamin D preparation includes ergocalciferol, or calcitrol, or calderol.

Nursing care of the patient with hypoparathyroidism requires close assessment for signs of tetany. The patient may experience anxiety and in effective breathing pattern as a result of the signs and symptoms of the disease. The nurse should be readily available to answer the patient questions. The patient should be kept in a room from where the nurses' station can be visible. The patient's call light should be answered promptly. The nurse needs to keep attending on any patient complaint. Hyperventilation which can accompany anxiety worsens the hypocalcaemia because hyperventilation causes respiratory alkalosis, which in turn causes more of the ionized calcium to bind to serum protein. The decrease in ionized calcium exacerbates symptoms of hypocalcemia. Thus, a patient should be supported to prevent hyperventilation. Keeping patient informed of their serum calcium levels will also help them feel in control and lesser anxiety. The patients are assessed for following by the nurse:

- Chrostek's and Trousseau's signs.
- Airway patency.
- Mental status orientation.
- Emotional status; anxiety and irritability
- Vital sign: Pulse rate and rhythms.

Any abnormal changes should be reported immediately so that treatment can be instituted and prevent seizure. Safety precaution to prevent nature of disease; need for long-term therapy, medication, administration, monitoring signs of:

- Infective treatment: recurrence of tetany.
- Signs of hypercalcaemia: thirst, poluria, lethargy, muscle tone, constipation.
- Complication: Renal stones (flank pain i.e.pain radiating down into groin) and need for continual follow-up care and dietary changes.

DISORDERS OF ADRENAL GLAND

The adrenal gland is essential to life. Without the hormone cortisol and aldesterone produced in the adrenal cortex, the body's metabolic processes responds inadequately to even minimal physical and emotional stressors such as changes in the temperature, exercises or excitement. More severe is stressors such as serious infections, surgery, or extreme anxiety would possibly result in shock and death. The adrenal medulla secretes hormones are also produced by sympathetic nervous system although more slowly.

There are three main classifications of adrenal steroid hormones.

- *Glucocorticosteroids* Regulate metabolism, increased blood glucose level and are critical in the physiologic stress response. In humans, the primary glucocorticoids is *Cortisol.*
- *Mineralo Corticosteroid* Regulate sodium and potassium balance. The primary in mineralcorticoid is *aldosterone*.
- *Androgens* Contribute to growth and development of both genders and to sexual activity in adult women.

The term corticosteroids refers to any one of these three types of hormones produced by the adrenal cortex. Dysfunction of the adrenal gland can be manifested as increased or decreased function of the cortex or increased function of the medulla.

CUSHING'S SYNDROME

Hyperfunction of the adrenal cortex, cortisol excess leads to Cushing's syndrome. Cushing's syndrome is spectrum of clinical abnormalities caused by excess corticosteroids particularly glucocorticoids.

Aetiology

The causes of Cushing's syndrome may be divided into three major groups.

1. Primary Cushing's syndrome: Excessive cortisol production resulting from adrenal adenoma or carcinoma also called adrenal Cushing's syndrome.
2. Secondary Cushing's syndrome: Excessive cortisol production resulting from adrenal hyperplasia, because of excessive ACTH production. These excessive ACTH production results from either.
   Increased release of ACTH from the pituitary gland because of pituitary of hypothalamic problem also called Cushing's disease or pituitary Cushing's syndrome.
3. Iatrogenic Cushing's syndrome: Excessive cortisol levels resulting from chronic glucocorticoid therapy.

Pathophysiology

The major result of Cushing's syndrome is excessive production of cortisol early in the nonlatrogenic disorders, the most prominent alteration is loss of the normal diurenal secretory pattern. With loss of diurenal pattern, the morning level of cortisol production may not be abnormally elevated, but levels during the day do not show the normal decrease below the morning peak, at later stages cortisol elevated at all times.

The pathophysiological factors associated with cortisol excess primary result from exaggeration of all the known actions of glucocorticoids and includes alteration in the :

- Protein, fat and carbohydrates metabolism.
- Inflammatory and immune responses.
- Water and mineral metabolism.
- Emotional stability.
- RBCs and platelets levels.

Excessive cortisol may disturb secretion of other anterior pituitary hormones (Prolactin, thyrotropin, LH and GH) and cause alteration in sleep patterns. Some of these alterations may contribute to the clinical picture. In many instances, cortisol excess is also associated with excessive production of androgen, this results in virilization in females. Adrenal tumours may secrete cortisol, androgens and aldosterone in various proportion depending on the hormone-produced excess clinical manifestation occurs.

Clinical Manifestation

The clinical manifestation of Cushing's syndrome can be body systems and are related to excess levels of corticosteroids. Although manifestation of glucocorticoids excesses usually predominated symptom of minor corticoids and regan excess may also be seen. They are as follows:

1. Glucocorticoids (Cortisol)
   - *General appearance:* Truncal centripedal obesity, thin extremities, rounding of face (moon face) fat deposits, on back neck and shoulder (Buffalo hump).
   - *Integumentary* Thin fragile skin, purplish-red striae, Potential haemorrhages; bruises; cheeks plethora, acne, poor wound healing.
   - *Cardiovascular:* Hypervolaemia, hypertension, oedema of lower extremities.
   - *Gastrointestinal* Increase in secretion of pepsin and hydrochloric acid and anorexia.
   - *Urinary:* Glycosuria, hypecalciuria and kidney stones
   - *Musculoskeletal:* Muscle waisting in extremities, and proximal muscle weakness; fatigue, osteoporesis, awkward gait, back and first pain weakness and growth retardation in children.
   - *Immune:* Inhibition of immune response
   - *Haematologic* leukocytosis, lymphopoenia, polycythaemi and increased coagubility.
   - *Fluid Electrolyte:* Sodium and water retention, oedema, hypokalaemia
   - *Metabolic* Hyperglycemia, negative nitrogen balance, dyslipidemia.
   - *Emotional* Psychic stimulation, euphoria, irritability, hypomania, to depression, emotional liability, mood-swings.
2. *Mineral corticoid* (Aldosterone)
   - Fluid Electrolyte: Marked sodium and water retention, tendency toward oedema marked hypokalaemia.
   - Cardiovascular: Hypertension, hypervolaemia, dysrhythmia and CHF.
3. Androgens
   - Integumentary: Hirustism acne, loss of scalp hair and coat hair on face and total body.
   - *Reproductive:* menstrual irregularities oligomenorhoea enlargement of clitoris in females, gynacomastia and testicular atrophy in males and changes in libido.
   - *Musculoskeletal:* Increase in muscle development.

Management

Medical management is focussed on identifying the cause of the problem and removing the cause of cortisol excess if possible. Various diagnostic procedures are preformed to confirm the diagnosis and differentiation among the various causes of cortisol excess. Abnormal signs include granulocytosis, lymphocytopoenia, eosinopaenia, hyperglycaemia signs include granulocytosis, lymphocytopaenia, eosinopaenia, hyper glycaemia glycosuria, hypercalsuria, and osteoporosis, hypokalaemia, alkalosis, etc.

The treatment of choice for Cushing's disease is transphenoidal surgical removal of the pituaitary ademosis hyperphysectomy. Adrenolectomy is indicated for adrenal tumour or hyperplasia. Currently transperitonial or retroperitoneal laparoscopic surgery) is performed to remove adrenal tumour less than 5 cm in size.

Those who do not cope with surgery, are treated with mitotine (Lysoeren). This drug suppresses cortisol production, alters peripheral metabolism of cortisol and decreases plasma and urine corticosteroid level. This action results as "medical adrenality" Metyrpone, ketoconazole and cytadren may be used to inhibit cortisol synthesis. And long-cortico steroid therapy lead in the cause of the problem. Gradually it should reduce to complete the side effects of anticortisol should be monitered, which includes anorexia, nausea, vommiting, GI bleeding, depression, vertigo, skin rashes and diplopia.

If surgery is anticipated the patient should be brought to optimal physical condition. Hypoglycaemia and hypertension must be controlled and hypokalaemia is corrected with diet and potassium supplements. A higher protein diet meal plan helps correct the protein depletion. Vitamin A supplementation may be given to counteract the problem of delayed healings.

Nursing Management

The patient with excessive cortisol secretion needs skilled nursing care. The patient can be crtically ill. During the acute period, the primary focus of care is on high-priority needs of supporting coping, restoring fluid balance, and preventing infections and injuries. While providing physical care of the patients, the nurse has to take following measures.

a. *Decrease controllable stressors*
   - Provide continuity care.
   - Explain all procedures slowly and carefully.
   - Spend time with patient and listen carefully.
   - Avoid sudden noises, temperature changes, drafts and unnecessary invasion of privacy.

b. *Monitor physiological coping*
   - Ensure blood pressure and pulse remain stable.
   - Take vital signs at least every 2 to 4 hours.

c. *Control fluid volume excess.*
   - Restrict fluids as prescribed; distribute fluid throughout the 24 hours; use ice chips to prevent thirst.
   - Provide a diet low in sodium as necessary.
   - Provide potassium replacement as ordered oral-intake foods high in potassium.
   - Monitor daily weight, intake and output for every 4 to 8 hours and laboratory values of sodium, potassium, chloride, bicarbonate and pH.

d. *Prevent infection and falls*
   - Monitor temperature every 4 hours.
   - Assess mouth, lungs and skin every shift for early signs of infection and report signs immediately.
   - Limit staff and visitors with signs and symptoms of upper respiratory infection.
   - Institute preventive care; sterile technique for invasive procedures routine turning, coughing and deep breathing every 2 hours; oral hygiene. Before breakfast, after meals, and at bed time.

If person undergoing adrenal surgery following intervention to be followed during preoperative and postoperative period.

a. *Preoperative*
   - Provide supportive care.
   - Assist patient with usual preoperative care.
   - Maintain nutritional status with a high protein, prescribed calorie diet with adequate minerals and vitamins.
   - Assist with correction of fluid and electrolyte imbalance.
   - Assist with hormonal therapy as prescribed.
   - Assist with measures used to prevent or treat crisis of adrenal hormonal excess of deficit.
   - Administer prescribed IV fluids and glucocorticoids before surgery

b. *Postoperative*
   1. Establish monitoring schedule, detect complications of surgery and adrenal crisis, blood pressure alterations, blood glucose alterations fluid and electrolyte imbalances.
   2. Because the patient may have unusual activity intolerance, pace postoperative activities with alternate periods of rest and a gradual increase in self care.
   3. Provide measures to minimize effects of postural hypertension:
      - Supply ace bandages or elastic stockings.
      - Assess effects of posture on blood pressure.
      - Assist or accompany the patient during ambulation while blood pressure remains labile.
   4. Provide measures to decrease risk of infection in the immunosuppressed patient (e.g.strict surgical asepsis, deep breathing and avoiding contact with person with infections).
   5. Administer cortisol replacement as typically prescribed:
      - IV route for first 24 to 48 hours .
      - Oral route when patient is able to tolerate food by mouth.
   6. Administer mineralocorticosteroid (fludocortisone) replacement, if prescribed, this is typically prescribed when cortisol replacement is less than 40 to 50 mg/24 hours in the patient with bilateral adrenalectomy.
   7. Assist patient and family in learning about required hormonal replacement:
      - Bilateral adrenalectomy- Maintenance dose of cortisol and mineralocorteoids.
      - Untilateral adrenalectomy doses of cortisol dependent on degree of suppression of HPA axis.

IATROGENIC CUSHING'S SYNDROME

Iatrogenic Cushing's syndrome occurs when a patient takes large doses of exogenous glucocorticoids for their therapeutic anti- inflammatory effects. The clinical situation in which glucocorticoids might be used for their anti-inflammatory and immunosuppressive effects include the following:

- Eyes surgery or trauma: usually given as drops, ointment, or intraorbital systemic effects minimal.
- Dermatologic disorders: used as ointmetns; can have systematic effects if used over large parts of the body or used daily.
- Autoimmune diseases: Rheumatoid arthritis, systemic lupus erythematosus and scleroderma.
- Rheumatoid arthritis, systemic lupus erythematosus scleroderma.
- *Haematological disorders:* Haemolytic anaemias, thromhocytopoenia, lymphomas leukaemias.
- *Allergic reaction:* Anaphylaxis, contact dermatitis, transfusion reaction.
- *GI disorders:* Ulcerative colitis, Crohn;s diseases, hepatitis
- *Nephrological disorders: Nephrotic syndrome.*
- *Neurological diseases*: head trauma and surgery to prevent cerebral oedema and increased intracranial pressure.
- *Cardiopulmonary diseases:* Asthma, COPDs myocarditis.
- *Transplantation:* Renal, liver, heart, beta-cell transplantation.
- *Others:* part of many protocols for various malignancies.

Pathophysiology: Long-term therapeutic doses of glucocortioids can result in the full clinical picture of Cushing's syndrome. Bone changes are great in Iatrogenic Cushing's syndrome. Syndrome often develops vascular nacrosis. There are mild fluid and electrolyte imbalance. Severe myopathy may occur. Peptic ulcer occurs more often. Patients who receive glucocorticoids are very susceptible to cataract formation and are susceptibe to all types of infections.

Management

A different type of problem, cortisol deficit can occur when glucocorticoids are given for a prolonged period. They must be withdrawn slowly to remove adrenal insufficiency. Blood glucose levels may be monitored frequently if there is a history of diabetes mellitus. For hyperglycemia the experience of most of the people can increase in appetite. If the weight gain is a problem, a calories restricted diet may be necessary. To prevent GI problem steroids should be taken with food or antacids. Stools should be guiac-tested regularly to monitor early signs of GI irritation. If fluid retention problem, sodium restriction diet is prescribed. Take measures to prevent fluid and electrolyte problem accordingly. In addition, monitor signs of infection and assessment of psychological and emotional status, anxiety, depression and mood swings.

Patient receiving prolonged therapeutic glucocorticoid therapy need considerable teaching to be able to manage therapy and to identify signs and symptoms of complication which include the following.

a. Take drug as prescribed.
   - Do not miss a dose or stop medication suddenly.
   - Drug must be withdrawn slowly under physician's supervision.
   - If nausea and vomiting occur and drug cannot be taken, notify physician immediately.
   - Keep sufficient tablets always to avoid missing a dose.
   - Take drug with food or antacids
   - With every other day, therapy, take twice the normal dose every other day at 8 hours.
   - If travelling, carry medication with one does'nt keep (do not ship them).
b. Monitor self and report side effects of weightgain, oedema, behaviour changes, GI bleeding, increased urination, or thirst or signs of infections.
c. Check blood glucose levels if directed.
d. Prevent infection:
   - Avoid persons, especially children, with infections.
   - Avoid crowded, poorly ventilated places.
   - Care of wounds carefully.
   - Report any signs which may include feelings of increased weakness, feeling poorly and having less energy.
e. Maintain a nutritious diet, including foods from all groups, follow direction for any prescreibed diet (low calorie, high potassium, low sodium).
f. Carry out a regular exercise program: walking helps to strengthen muscles and decrease bone problem.
g. Have yearly eye examination.
h. Consult physician regularly as instructed.

ALDOSTERONISM

Aldosteronism or aldosterone excess can be either primary (Conn's syndrome) or secondary. *Primry aldosteronism* results from bilateral nodular hyperplasia or from a single aldosterone, producing adenoma. *Secondary aldosteronism* occurs frequently and results from the presence of exogenous conditions, that stimulate the renin angiostenism-aldosterone system which includes:

- Cardiac failure
- Liver disease
- Nephrosis
- Renal artery stenosis
- Bartter's syndrome
- Idiopathic cyclic oedema
- Pregnancy.
- Hypovolaemic states.
- Oestrogen therapy.

Pathophysiology

In primary aldosteronism, excessive aldosterone is secreted and stimulate the reabsorption of sodium in kidney in exchange for potassium and hydrogen, which results water retention, further volume expansion and hypertension. Further and hydrogen, which results water retention, further volume expansion and hypertension. Further, retinopathy develops headache in clinical findings. The loss of intracellular and extracellular potassium changes the excitability of muscle membrane, resulting in muscular weakness, intermittent parenthesis and sometimes diminished deep tendon reflexes. Paralysis may occur. Severely low levels of potassium leads to loss of concentrating ability of the kidney tubules leading to increased water loss, polyurea, nocturia, and polydipsia. Further, it leads to hypernatraemia excessive loss of hydrogen results in hypokalaemia alkalosis, producing signs and symptoms of tetany.

Secondary aldosteronism results when increased renin secretion is stimulated by the various pathological factors, which leads to hypokalaemia and alkalosis and hypertension depending on the severity of the exogenous cause.

Management

Blood test and urine tests reveal alteration in serum electrolytes. Hypertension and hyperkalaemia are key factors; these should be treated accordingly as described concerned chapters.

- If primary aldosteronism results froma an aldosterone secreting adenoma treatment of choice in surgical resection i.e. untilateral adrenalectomy.
- In blatant hyperplasia medical treatment with sodium-restriction potassium replacement therapy and spironolactone the choice of treatment.
- In secondary aldosteronism, medical treatment for the abnormal secretion and water retention is sodium restriction. K_2 replacement and diuretics provide nursing care accordingly.

ADDRENOCORTICAL INSUFFICIENCY ADDISON'S DISEASE

Adrenocortical insufficiency (hypofunction of the adrenal cortex) may be primary (Addison's disease) or secondary from a lack of pituitary ACTH.

Aetiology

Inadequate secretion of cortisol may occur as a result of

1. Insufficient secretion of ACTH resulting from hypothalamic pituitary disease (secondary).
2. Insufficient secreation of ACTH and adrenal atrophy resulting from suppression of hypothalamic- pituitary function by long-term exogenous glycocorticoids given in therapeutic doses (iatrogenic) or
3. Destruction of the adrenal cortex itself (primary)

Primary insufficiency also called Addison's diseases can result from several causes which include:

- Idiopathic atrophy, probably caused by autoimmune abnormality.
- Infiltration of adrenal glands with cancer.
- Impairment of blood flow from vasculitis or thrombosis.
- Haemorrhage and infarction secondary to septicemia (waterhouse-Fridrichse syndrome).
- Destruction of adrenal glands by chemical such as mitotane.
- Congenital hypoplasia.
- Surgical removal of adrenal glands.
- Metastases to adrenal glands.

Pathophysiology

Primary adrenocortical insufficiency deprives the body of both minerlocorticosteroids and glucococorticoids. These hormonal losses decreases body's ability to retain sodium and secrets potassium. The loss of sodium decreases extracelluler electrolytes and fluid volume. The decreased volume along with decreased vascular tone, diminished cardiac output, and decreased renal perfusion. Excretion of waste products is inhibited. The loss of glucocorticoids in Addison's disease decrease hepatic gluconeogeneses and increases tissue glucose uptake. Muscle strength is lost. Various GI disorders may occur and mental and emotional functioning and stability are impaired. The loss of negative feedback of glucocorticoids with pituitary secretion of ACTH results uncontrolled ACTH release along with lipoprotein. Various changes in sexual characteristics may result from a decrease in adrenal androgen or from the general debility associated with insufficiency.

Secondary adrenal insufficiency results in similar pathophysiological disturbance except that the fluid and electrolytic imbalance because of aldostereone in response to the renin – angiotensin system. Adrenal crisis (Addisonian crisis) is a severe exacerbation of adrenal insufficiency, occurring in any person with chronic insufficiency regardless of the cause.

Clinical manifestations of acute or chronic adrenal insufficiency can include the following.

Mental and emotional changes are some of the symptoms and may include lethargies, loss of vigour, depression, irritability and loss of ability to concentrate. Patient can become increasingly apathetic and be unable to participate in and ADL.

The clinical manifestations of adrenal insufficiency also can be seen in most body systems and related to deficit levels of corticosteroids, which also include symptoms of aldosterone and androgen.

1. *Glucocorticoids*
   - *General appearance*- Weight loss.
   - *Integumentary*- Bronzed or smoky hyperpigmentation of face, neck, hands, especially creases, buccal

membranes, nipples, genitalia and scars (if pituitary function normal), vitiligo, alopecia.
- *Cardiovascular:* Hypotension, tendency to develop refractory shock; vasodilators.
- *Gastrointestinal:* Anorexia, nausea, vomiting, cramping, abdominal pain diarrhoea or constipation.
- *Urinary:* No glycosuria
- *Musculoskeletal:* Fatigability.
- *Immune:* Propensity toward autoimmune diseases.
- *Haematologic:* Anaemia, lymphocytosis.
- *Fluid and Electrolyte:* Hyponatraemia, hypovolaemia, and dehydration, hyperkalaemia.
- *Metabolic:* Hypoglycaemia, insulin sensitivity and fever.
- *Emotional:* Neurasthenia, depression, exhaustion or irritability confusion, and delusions.

2. Aldosterone:
   - *Fluid and Electrolyte:* Sodium loss, decreased volume of extracellular fluid, hyperkalaemia and salt craving.
   - *Cardiovascular:* Hypovolaemia, tendency toward shock, decreased cardiac output and decreased heart size.
3. Androgens
   - *Integumentary:* Decreased axillary and pubic hair (women).
   - *Reproductive*: No effect in men. Decreased libido in women.
   - *Musculosketal:* Decrease in muscle size and tone.

Management

In addition to clinical feature, a diagnosis of Addison's Disease can be made when cortisol levels are subnormal and fail to raise over basal levels with ACTH stimulation tests. Tests under plasma cortisol serum electrolyte, Tuberculin test, CT scan are MRI also used.

Pharmacological treatments of adrenal crisis include the following.

- Administration of glucocorticoids and mineral corticoids, e.g. Decadran, hydrocortisone, fluid cortisone.
- Initiation of volume replacement, e.g. IV normal saline.
- Administration of glucose, e.g. IV dextrose.
- Administration of vasopressors.

Treatment includes identification of precipitating factors and initiate treatment accordingly. Nursing care that is related to nursing diagnosis includes promoting activity, facilitates coping, promoting comfort, balance, preventing injury, promoting good nutrition, promoting comfort, improving self exteem, and patient teaching regarding disease and treatment and follow-up.

DISORDERS OF ADRENAL MEDULA

Pheochromocytoma is catecholamine producing tumour of the sympathetico-adrenal medullary system that causes hypertension. If a person with an undiagnosed pheochromocytoma has surgery or an accident, he or she mat die from a hypertension crisis.

Pathophysiology

Pheochromocytomas of the adrenal medula release excessive amounts of catecholominas both epinephrines and non-epinephrines. A tumour of the sympathetic nervous system's in turn releases excessive amounts of nonepinephrine. The hormone release may be constant or episodic producing constant or episodic clinical manifestation. A proxysm or crisis may be precipated by any lifting, straining, bending or exercise that increases intra-abdominal pressure or moves abdominal contents. Palpation of the abdomen may also precipitate paroxysm. Anxiety or stress doest not usually precipitate an attack. In some patients has no specific precipitating factor is identified.

Clinical Manifestation

Hypertension is the key feature of phenochromocytoma. The manifestation frequently presents include.

- Signs of cardiac stimulation tachycardia, palpitation, chest pain, ECG changes and angina.
- Headaches that are throbbing and severe.
- Increased metabolic manifested by heat tolerance. Sweating, fever, wasting of fat stores, and weight loss.
- Elevated blood glucose level
- Nausea, vomiting, epigastric pain
- Flushing
- Pallor
- Tachypnoea
- Nervousness or anxiety.

Nephrosclerosis and retinopathy may result from uncontrolled sustained hypertension. Untreated pheochromocytomas may lead to diabetic mellitus, cardiomyopathy and manifestation uncontrolled hypertension and death.

Management

The diagnosis is confined by assays of catecholamines and other metabolites of the urine. Treatment consists of surgical removal of the tumour. Surgery may be done via laparoscopic adrenalectomy or by open abdominal incision. Preoperatively sympathetic blocking agents (e.g. Phenoxybenzamine, prazisin, terozosin or doxazosin are administered to reduce the blood pressure and alleviate other symptoms of catecholamine excess).

Preperatively nursing case is focussed on instituting measures to help stabilize the patient's haemodynamic status, monitor the clinical state, prepare the patients for tests and surgery, and prevent edpisodes of hypertension. Patient experiencing hypertentive crisis should be in an intensive care unit because frequent cardiac, blood pressure, and neurological monitoring are required.

If phentolamine infusion is necessary, the blood pressure is checked every 15 miniutes and the drug is given by controlled infusion at a rate to keep the blood pressure at a prescribed level. During this time, the patient must be informed about planned diagnostic and planned treatment and is prepared for surgery. Activities that precipitate paroxysm such as bending, valsalva manoevre, palpating the abdomen and lifting should be limited.

The patient continues to need close monitoring of blood pressure, pulse, cardiac rhythm, neurological status and the effectiveness of the treatment postoperatively, after the hypertensive period, hypotension may occur. This nursing care is focussed on continual monitoring and administration of fluids or plasma as prescribed.

For patient treated medically or surgically, patient without remission of symptoms, nursing care is focussed on helping the patient attain the skill necessary for self care. It is achieved by proper prompt patient teaching by the nurse.

DISORDERS OF PANCREAS

The pancreas is along, tapered, labular, soft gland that between 60 to 90g. It lies behind the stomach and anterior to the first and second vertebrae, The pancreas perform exocrine and endocrine function.The islets of Langerhans are the areas of endocrine activity and they release their secretions into the portal circulation. However, the secretions are also pancrine. Pancrine diffuse to neighbouring cells to exert their action, rather than travelling to their target tissues through the blood like endocrine secretions. The islets account for less than 2% of the gland and alphs, beta and delta cells. Glucon is synthesized by the alpha cells, insulin, by the beta cells gastrin and somaltostatin by the delta cells. Any deficiency in the endocrine function of the pancreas insulin leads diabetes mellitus.

DIABETES MELLITUS (DM)

Diabetes mellitus is a group of metabolic diseases characterized by hyperglycaemia resulting from defect in insulin secretion, insulin action or both. The basis of the abnormalities in carbohydrate, protein and fat matabolism in diabetes is the deficient action of insulin on the target tissue of skeletal muscle, adipose tissue, and liver. Uncontrollable DM may result in long term damage, dysfunction, and failure of various organs. especially the heart, kidneys and eyes.

Aetiology and Classification of DM

The diagnosis label of diabetes mellitus (DM) carries many physiologic and socio-economic ramification and therapeutic requirement. Therefore, accurate classification of the degree of glucose tolerance and type of diabetes are important, In July 1997, a new diagnostic and classification system for diabetes was published by an expert committee on the diagnosis and classification of diabetes mellitus of the American Diabetes Association. The new system reflects the aetiology and pathophysiology of diabetes with two major categories being type 1 diabetes mellitus, (previously termed insulin-dependent DM or Juvenile onset DM) and type 2 diabetes mellitus (previously termed "noninsulin dependent DM or maturity-onset DM).

The classification of diabetes and other disorders of glucose tolerance with the defining characteristics are as follows:

Type 1 Diabetes Mellitus

Type one diabetes mellitus is characterized by autoimmune beta-cell destruction, which is attributed to a genetic predisposition coupled with one or more viral agents and possible chemical agents. It is immune mediate. The characteristics include:

- Insulinopence (insulin deficit) and dependent on exoginous insulin sustain life.
- Onset generally before age 30, but may occur at any age, including old age.
- Person's body built is generally lean, rarely obese.
- Variable rate of beta-cell destructions.
- Clinical presentation is usually rapid (polyuria, polydipsia, polyphagia weight loss).
- Majority of persons (85-90%) have one or more of the following auto antibodies present at the time when fasting hyperglycaemia is initially detected.
- Islet cells autoantibodies (ICA)
  - Insulin autoantibodies. (IAA)
  - Glutamic acid decarboxylase autoantibodies (GAD).
  - Tyrosine phosphatase IA-2 or IA 2B autoantibodies,
  - Strong human leukocyte antigen (HLA) associations
    - Linkage of DQA and B genes.
    - Influenced by DRB genes.

Idiopathic diabetes has some defined characteristics; which include the following:

- No immunological evidence for beta cell destruction
- No HLA association
- Strongly inherited
- Most individuals effected are of African or Asian origin.
- Episodic ketoacidosis with varying degrees of insulin deficiency below episodes.

Type 2 Diabetes Mellitus

Majority of 90% of people with diabetes mellitus have Type 2 has strong genetic influences but has no correlation with HLA type has been found. The defining characteristics will include:

- The absolute requirement of exogenous insulin is episodic.
- No requirement for exogenous insulin to sustain life at least initially.
- Ranges form a picture of predominantly insulin resistance with mild relative insulin deficiency to a picture of more severe insulin secretory defects with insulin resistance.

Table 13.3: Nursing care plan for the patient in adrenal crisis (addisonian crisis)

Problem	*R*	*Objective*	*Nursing Interventions*	*Rationales*
Nursing Diagnosis # 1 Cardiac output, alteration in: Decreased, related to: 1. Reduced circulating blood volume and decreased venous return. 2. Dysrhythmias associated with hyperkalaemia.		Patient will maintain: 1. Usual mental status: • Alert, oriented to person, place, date. • Behaviour appropriate. • Usual personality (as per family/significant others).	• Establish and maintain effective cardiovascular function. ◆ Establish assessment data of overall body function	• A brief but highly scrutinized assessment of the patient and family faciliates early diagnosis with institution of timely and effective therapy; once the patient's condition is stabilized, a comprehensive investigation of the patient and patient / family-environment interaction should be performed. A thorough database facilitates treatment and rehabilitation.
		2. Effective cardiovascular function: • Heart rate>60 <100 beats/min. • Cardiac rhythm: regular sinus, without symptomatic dysrhythmias haemodynamic parameters:	• Examine for presence of Medic-Alert identification tag or bracelet. • Thoroughly document all findings	• Such identification facilitates immediate diagnosis and treatment. • Provides basis for compositions; assists in evaluating response to therapy; steroids therapy may precipitate dysrthymias because of sudden shifts in electrolytes.
		• CVP: 0-8 mmHg. • PCWP: 8-12mmHg • CO:4-8 liter/min. • Arterial BP within 10 mm Hg of base line. 3. Renal status: • Urine output:>30ml/hr. 4. Respiratory status: • Respiratory rate: <25-30 breaths/min. • Breathing pattern: Eupnoea.	• Maintain continuous assessment of vital parameters: ◆ Cardiac rate and rhythm. Apical/radial pulse deficit. ◆ Haemodynamic parameters: central venous pressure: pulmonary artery pressure; pulmonary capillary wedge pressure; arterial pressure; cardiac output; orthostatic hypotension. • Arterial blood gases. ◆ Serum electrolytes.	• Sudden shifts in fluid and electrolytes may precipitate serious dysrhythmias. ◆ Hyperkalaemia may precipitate serious dysrhythmias. ◆ Assist in determining fluid status; prevents overhydration from too aggressive fluid replacement therapy; hypertension congestive heart failure with pulmonary oedema are potential complications of hypervolaemia. ◆ Assist in evaluating adequacy of alveolar ventilation and gas exchange. ◆ Diminished aldosterone secretion predisposes of hyponatraemia hyperemia, and extracellular fluid volume deficit.
			• Institute prescribed fluid replacement: Dextrose 5% in saline; plasma expanders. • Administer vasopressors (dopamine) maintain resuscitation equipment at beside. • Institute immediate corticosteroid therapy.	• Prevents hypovolemic shock; the amount of fluid administered is guided by haemodynamic parameters. • Administered to relieve severe hypotension and hypovolaemic shock. • Immediate administration of corticosteroids may prevent cardiovascular collapse.
			◆ Administer drug regimen in highly individualized manner. ◆ Consider underlying pathophisiology; – Pulmonary disease; heart disease; diabetes mellitus.	◆ Goal of corticosteroid replacement therapy is maximize efficacy while minimizing adverse effects. – Minimize mineralocorticoid activity; major concern is fluid overload with concomitant risk of congestive heart failure and pulmonary oedema.
			◆ Hepatic disease or hepatic dysfunction with an associated endocrine disorder (e.g., diabetes mellitus; hypothyroidism).	– Liver may be unable to completely activate enterally administered exogenous steroids – Liver disease may impair ability to clear or metabolize exogenous steroids. • The presence of other endocrine disorders may exaggerate response to steroids by alteration in steroid metabolism.

Contd...

Contd...

Problem	*R*	*Objective*	*Nursing Interventions*	*Rationales*
			• Review mode of corticosteriod administration.	• All corticosteroids can be given parenterally except prednisone, which is available only in oral form.
			◆ Intravenous cortisol should be given very slowly (e.g.100mg IV over 10-20 minutes).	• Rarely, rapid infusion can result in shock and anaphylaxis in-patients with acute bronchospasms.
			◆ Continuous monitoring of cardiac and haemodynamic parameters is essential with intravenous administration of large dosage of steroids. ◆ Continuous monitoring of serum electrolytes and serum glucose is absolutely essential.	• Dysrhythimas may be precipitated by sudden electrolyte shifts induced by steroids; fluid overload may be precipitated by increased by steroids; fluid overload may be precipitated by increased levels of mineralocorticoid activity.
			◆ Ongoing monitoring of serum proteins	• Steroids are >90% protein bound serum proteins should be closely monitored.
			• Assess prescribed drug regimen and risk of adverse drug interactions.	• To prevent undesired complications, it is esential to determine the presence of incompatibility of therapeutic measures or potential alterations in physiologic processes.
			• Monitor potassium level carefully inpatient receiving furosemide or other diuretics.	• The enhanced secretion of potassium caused by these drugs, coupled with the potassium wasting effects of steroids, may predispose to hypokalaemia; major concern with digoxins use.
			• Monitor for masked infections when administering broad spectrum antibiotics (e.g.,tetracycline).	• Antibiotic administration can predispose to opportunistic infections, the signs of which can be masked by steroids.
			• Carefully monitor the therapeutic effects of steroids in patients receiving medications such as barbiturates, phonation, isoniazid, rifampin.	• Such drugs diminish the efficacy of steroids by stimulating increased hepatic microsomal enzymatic activity, which metabolizes steroids to inactive compounds.
			• Monitor ongoing administration of steroids for associated complications. These may include. ◆ Metabolic: Metabolic alkalosis, potassium depletion, sodium retention, glucose intolerance, adrenal suppression, ◆ Cardiovascular oedema, hypertension ◆ Neurologic: Insomnia, euphoria, muscle weakness, irritability, depression, personality changes. ◆ Gastrointestinal; Peptic ulcer disease, gastritis, haemorrhage. ◆ Other: impaired wound healing increased vulnerability to infection, depressed WBC, osteoporosis muscle wasting, glaucoma/cataracts, moon face, abdominal fat pad.	• Despite careful administration, steroids always have the potential of causing complications.
Nursing Diagnosis # 2 Fluid volume deficit: Actual, related to: 1. Hyponateaemia associated with hyposecretion of aldosterone.		Patient will maintain effective fluid and electrolyte balance: 1. Neurologic status: • Alert, oriented to person, place, date. • Behaviour appropriate.	For pertinent nursing interventions and their rationales related to fluid and electrolyte balance, see related NCPs.	

Contd...

Contd...

Problem	*R*	*Objective*	*Nursing Interventions*	*Rationales*
Nurisng Diagnosis # 3 Electrolyte imbalance, related to: 1. Hyponatraemia and hyperkalaemia associated with hyposecretion of mineralocorticoids (e.g., aldosterone) and glucocorticoids (e.g., cortisol).		• Usual personality (as per Family) • Deep tendon reflexes brisk. 2. Haemodynamic status: • See Nursing diagnosis # 1, above. 3. Renal status • Urine output (hourly) 30ml/hr. 4. Respiratory status: • Respiratory rate: <25-30 breaths/min. • Breathing pattern: Eupnoea • Breath sounds clear; absence of adventitious sounds (e.g.,) crackles, wheezes). 5. Gastrintestinal status: • Absence of anorexia, nausea, vomiting, diarrhoea, bleeding 6. Laboratory data: • Serum osmolality 285-295 mOsm/kg. Sodium: >135 <148 mEq/liter. Potassium 3.5-5.5 mEq /liter Glucose: 70-110 mg/100 ml. Haematology profile. Urine-specific gravity: 1.010-1.025.	In addition, consider the following: • Maintain fluid and electrolyte balance. ◆ Assess for signs and symptoms of hyperkalaemia >6.0 mEq/liter. – Signs and symptoms related to neuromuscular function: Muscle weakness, paralysis, paresthesias, twitching hyperreflexia, bradycardia proceeding to cardiac arrest, ventricular fibrillation, oliguria.	• Hyperkalaemia may precipitate serious dysrhythmias; a decreased serum mineralocoticoid level predisposes to hyperkalaemia due to increased reabsorption of potassium via the kidney tubules in the presence of hyponatraemia.
			• Monitor serial electrolytes	• Patients taking digitalis are at high risk of lethal dysrhythmias in the presence of hyperkalaemia.
			• Monitor for hypoglycaemia	• Fluid volume deficit can decrease cerebral perfusion, which together with hypoglycaemia can predispose to coma.
			• Assess for fluid volume deficit: ◆ Cardiovascular: Decreased haemodynamic pressure, hypotesion, tachycardia, tachypnoea, and haemoconcentration. ◆ Neuromuscular parethesias weakness listlessness. ◆ Renal: Decreased urine output. ◆ General; Poor skin turgor over sternum or forehead, sunken eyeballs, weight loss.	• Patients with underlying cardiac or renal disease are especially at high risk to develop complications associated with fluid deficit or excess.
			• Assess for fluid volume excess. ◆ Cardiovascular Elevated haemodynamic values neck vein distention in upright position (45°), hypertension, bounding pulse, dependent oedema. ◆ Neurologic: Confusion associated with dilutional hyponatraemia. ◆ Pulmonary: Dyspneoea, rales. ◆ General: weight gain.	• May occur with overly aggressive fluid replacement; haemodynamic parameters should be monitored very closely.
			• Monitor intake and output (hourly); daily weight. • Include all gastrointestinal fluid losses. • Insensible losses, especially in presence of fever.	• Assist in evaluating fluid status; body weight is an excellent guide to fluid state.
Nursing Diagnosis # 4 Tissue perfusion alteration in : Cerebral, related to: 1. Fluid volume deficit 2. Electrolyte disturbance • Hyponatraemia • Hyperkalaemia.		Patient will: 1. Exhibit intact level of consiousness and mentation. • Alert, oriented to person , place, date • Memory intact. 2. Demonstrates intact sensorimotor function. 3. Deep tendon reflexes brisk. 4. Respiratory rate: <25-30 breaths/min. • Breathing pattern: Eupnoea.	• Maintain integrity of neurologic and psychologic processes. ◆ Establish baseline neurologic function: – Mental status: Changes in level of consciousness, disorientation, confusion, agitation, irritability, coma	◆ Symptomatology is related to hypoglycaemia and decreased cerebral perfusion is due to cardiovascular instability
			◆ Sensory function: presence of paresthesias. ◆ Motor function: muscle weakness, paralysis, hyper-reflexia.	◆ May be difficult to differentiate signs and symptoms of alterations in neurologic function associated with hypoglycaemia and decreased cerebral perfusion from those associated with hyperkalaemia.
			• Establish baseline psychological function of both patient and family. ◆ Assess level of anxiety. ◆ Assess level of knowledge regarding disease.	◆ Provides a base to build on because anxiety can be used constructively in certain situations.

Contd...

Contd...

Problem	*R*	*Objective*	*Nursing Interventions*	*Rationales*
			• Estimate development level.	• Age and developmental level may not necessarily be the same.
			• Record emotional/personality changes; speak with family regarding such changes in the patient: • Specific changes; when did they begin to appear? Were they associated with specific stressor or stressful event?	
			• Assess coping capabilities: Role of patient in family nucleus: independent? Dependent? Active, decision-maker? Passive personality?	• Role of patient in family nucleus with influence rehabilitative process for all members.
			• Identify family resources and significant others.	• Observation of interactions between patient and family/significant others may provide valuable cluses as to how they are coping, which may impact on the rehabilitative process.
			• Assess readiness to learn.	• Teaching can be geared to level at a which patient and family can best learn.
			• Therapeutic consideration: • Minimize stressors. – Quiet, comfortable environment – Anticipate needs – Relaxed atmosphere.	• A minimum of stimuli reduces risk of aggravating underlying pathophysiology.
			• Conserve energy – Maintain bedrest; avoid activities that may precipitate orthostatic hypotension. – Frequent rest periods.	• Conservation of energy helps to lessen demands of an already high catabolic state with diminished stores of muscle and liver glycogen.
			• Encourage verbalization of fears and concerns.	• It may help to identify underlying problems or areas of particular concerns.
			• Observe for nonverbal communication: Eye contact, posture, movements and touch.	• Nonverbal communication is especially helpful in assessing patient/family interactions.
			• Provide informations in manageable amounts provide opportunity for discussion and feedback.	• Patient may feel overwhelmed with too much information raising anxiety levels.
			• Remain accessible to family members or significant others should they request to speak alone with the health care provider.	• Feedback is important to enable clarification and verification of what has been said.
			• Enlist assistance of social worker or psychiatric liasion should in such services be indicated or requested by patient, family, or significant others.	• Consensual validation assist in minimizing inaccurate assumptions.
			• Explain all ongoing procedures and reasons underlying therapy.	• Appropriate explanations may help to alleviate heightened anxiety.
			• Applaud patient/family efforts to cope.	
Nursing Diagnosis # 5 Nutrition alteration in: Less than body requirements related to: 1. Catabolic state.		1. Patient's body weight will stablize within 5% of baseline. 2. Serum protein will be maintained within acceptable physiologic range: 6.0-8.4 g/100 ml. • Serum albumin: 3.5 -5.0 mg/100ml 3. Serum glucose: 70-110 mg/ 100ml.	• Maintain adequate nutrtion to meet the demands of the catabolic state. • Consult nutritionist and physician to determine nutritional needs of catabolic state. – Baseline nutritional status. – Nutritional requirements of compromised state. – High carbohydrate. – High protein. • Liberal salt intake. • Serum electrolytes, glucose, and total body proteins must be monitored	• Baseline nutrtional needs must be identified to ensure adequate nutritional intake prevent hypoglycaemic episodes, and reduce risk of infection. – Patient is prone to hypoglycaemia; It is a important to establish positive nitrogen balance and decrease muscle wasting. – Liberal salt intake offsets loss of sodium via kidneys. – These data assist in monitoring response to therapy

Contd...

Contd...

Problem	*R*	*Objective*	*Nursing Interventions*	*Rationales*
		4. Urine negative for glucose and acetone.	on a regular basis; haematology studies are necessary. ◆ Intake and output; daily weight • Note therapeutic considerations when the patient can tolerate dietary intake. ◆ Establish which foods are best tolerated; offer nourishment between meals and at bedtime	– Valuable parameters for determining fluid status. • Foods appealing to patient may help to increase intake; smaller, more frequent meals may be better tolerated; hypoglycemic reactions may be avoided.
			◆ Create environment conducive to eating.	• Activities that promote nutritional intake should be encouraged food brought from home may help to ensure necessary nutritional intake.
			◆ Avoid fasting or meal delays.	• A severe hypoglycaemia reaction may be triggered by extending the fasting state or delaying meals; an increased sensitivity to insulin coupled with a low serum glucose may precipitate a hypoglycemic reaction.
Nursing Diagnosis # 6 Potential for infection, related to: 1. Catabolic state. 2. Compromised immune response.		Patient will. 1. Maintain body temperature within acceptable range ~ 98.6° (37°). 2. Maintain white blood count: ~ 5000-10000/ mm³ 3. Remain without signs/symptoms of infection: Pain redness, swelling, suppuration. 4. Lungs clear to auscultation; chest x-ray without infiltrates. 5. Cultures negative: Blood, urine, sputum, wound, intravenous access sites.	• Provide supportive measures to reduce risk of infection ◆ Assess for signs of infection. ◆ Vigilant assessment of all invasive lines is critical. – Observe for redness, pain, swelling at all invasive sites; dressing changes of invasive lines should occur every 48 hr or according to unit protocol. – Culture catheter tips.	◆ Infection presents a serious pressure capable of inducing circulatory collapse if untreated – Steroids suppress the immuneresponse and place patient at greater risk of developing infection the anti-inflammatory effects of steroids may mask signs of infection by decreasing pain, swelling, redness, and other signs of infection. – Temperature may be low grade or normal and may not reflect an underlying infectious process. Antipyretic agents may be prescribed.
Nursing Diagnosis # 7 Oral mucous membranes, alteration, related to: 1. Dehydrated state.		Mucous membranes will remain moist and intact.	• Provide comfort measures ◆ Assist in personal hygiene. ◆ Assess intergity of skin for pressure areas, swelling, ecchymosis. – Apply lotion.	• Measures need to be implemented to maximize circulatory and pulmonary functions while conserving energy; such measures may help to reduce risk of infection. ◆ Increase in capillary fragility is associated with protein wasting.
Nursing Diagnosis # 8 Skin intergity, impairment, Potential.		Skin will remain intact with good turgor. Patient will verbalize concerns/ feelings regarding body changes.	◆ Assist with turning and positioning; apply antiembolic stockings. ◆ Encourage deep breathing ◆ Passive range of motion exercise ◆ Provide frequent rest periods.	◆ Frequent turning and breathing assist in mobilizing pulmonary secretions and preventing atelectasis; these activities are helpful in preventing pulmonary complications including pneumonia or pulmonary embolism. ◆ Limited musculoskeletal activities maintain muscle tone and decrease resorption of bone calcium; such activities improve circulation and increase venous return.
Nursing Diagnosis # 9 Self-concept, alteration in: body image related to: 1. Increased pigmentation. 2. Hirustism. 3. Fat distribution: "Moon face" "buffalo hump" masculinizing (women), gynecomastia (men).			• Encourage verbalization of fears and concerns regarding body changes. • Exhibit acceptance of patient as individual. • Offer reassurance; be accessible.	• It may help identify problems or area of concern • Encourages patient to talk about self.

- Persons usually are obese; those who are not obese by traditional criteria, usually have abdominal adiposity.
- Onset usually after 40, but may occur at any age.
- No autoimmune HLA association.

Other Disorders of Glucose Tolerance

a. *Genetic defects of beta cell function:* Previously termed maturity onset diabetes of youth (MODY) imapired insulin secretion without defects in insulin action. Autosomal dominant inheritance is present. Abnormalities in the three genetic loci have been determined to date.
b. *Genetical defects in insulin action:* Not available.
c. *Diseases of the exocrine pancreas*: Pancreatitis, trauma and infection, pancreatectomy, pancreatic carcinoma, cystic fibrosis and haemochromatosis.
d. *Endocrinopathis:* Acromegaly, Cushing's syndrome, glucagonoma, pheochromocytoma.
e *Drug induced*
   - Permanent destruction of beta cells (vacorcrat poison) IV Pentamidine.
   - Impairment of insulin action (nicotinic acid, glucocorticoids) thiazidediuretics.
   - Impairment of insulin secretion, thready precipitating DM in an individual with insulin resistance (e.g. drug-induced hypokalaemia)
f. *Infections:* Congenital rubella and cytomegalarirus.
g. *Uncommon forms:* immune mediatal: stiffman syndrome, anti-insulin receptor antibodies.
h. *Genetic syndromes associated with DM:* Turner's syndrome, Down syndrome and Klinefelter's syndrome.
i. *Gestation DM:* Pregnancy related.
j. *Impaired Glucose tolerance (IGT):* Glucose levels are higher than normal but do not meet diagnostic criteria for DM. Generally obese person will have insulin resistant and are at increased cardiovascular risk.
k. *Impaired fasting glucose:* Fasting glucose levels are higher than normal but lower than those in IGT or DM.

Pathophysiology

The hallmark of diabetes is insulin deficiency, either absolute or relative. In *absolute* insulin deficiency, the pancreas produces either no insulin or very little insulin, as seen in type 1 DM. In *relative* insulin deficiency the pancreas produces either normal or excessive amounts of insulin, but the body is unable to use it effectively, such that glucose levels remain elevated. This latter deficit is called "Insulin that glucose levels remain elevated. Resistance and is seen in type 2 DM. Basically it is failure of the pancrease to produce enough insulin to overcome this insulin resistance that participates clinical type 2 DM. Basically it is failure of the pancrease to produce enough insulin to overcome this insulin resistance that participates clinical type 2 DM in predisposed individuals.

This absolute or relative insulin deficiency results in significant abnormalities in the metabolism of the body fuels. The body needs fuel for all its functions. For building new tissue, and for repairing tissue. The fuel comes from the food that is ingested which is composed of carbohydrates, protein and fats. It is important to understand and emphasize to patient that diabetes is not a disease of glucose alone although the patient that diabetes is not a disease of glucose alone, although the diagnostic criteria that have been devised use the serum glucost level as the marker of diagnosis and control of the diseases. It is important that nurse helps patients understand that diabetes is a disease that effects how the body utilizes all foods carbohydrates, fats and protein.

The insulin-requiring organs are the liver-skeletal muscles and adipose tissue. The consequences of either absolute or relative insulin deficiency at the levels of these organs are as follows:

i. *Liver:* Hyperglycaemia, hypertriglyceridaemia, and ketone production
ii. *Skeletal Muscle:* Failure of glycost uptake and amino acid uptake;and
iii. *Adipose tissue:* Lipolysis resulting in elevated free fatty acids level in the circulation.

This situation is worsened by the consumption if dietary carbohydrates which are metabolized into glucose and fail to be utilized by the liver and skeletal muscles, with resultant progressive hyperglycaemia and glycost when the blood glucose level reaches the renal threshold (approximately 180 mg/dl) in normal kidney, the kidneys cannot keep up with reabsorbing the glucose from the glomerular filtrate and glycosuria results. Glucose attracts water and an osmotic diuresis occurs, resulting in polyuria (increased urination). This polyuria rsults in the loss of water and electrolysis, particularly sodium a chloride, potassium and phosphate. The loss of water and sodium results in thirst and increases fluid intake (Polydispsia) are triggered as the cell becomes starved of their fuel. This glycosuria leads to rapid weight loss in Type 1 DM and pathological metosia in Type 2.1 in both types, dehydration and electrolyte disturbances lead to fatigue and listlessness. Serum lipid abnormalities (TGs) very-low density lipoprotein (VLDLS) and some time cholesterol may be elevated. This leads to depletion in all electrolytes K, Na, CI.) if is not treated, complications will develop. Actually, the patient can develop nausea, and vomiting, and conditions can advance to hyperglycaemic coma or diabetic ketoacidosis (DKA). Chronically, the patient can develop milovascular and macrovascular complication or neuropathy.

Clinical Manifestation

Early symptoms include polyuria, polydipsia, polyphagia, visual blurring, fatigue, weight loss and late signs and symptoms include coma and chronic complications. Normally insulin and its counter regulatory hormones maintain blood glucose within range of 70 to 110 mg/dl. Elevated blood glucose level produce symptoms related to the degree of actual or relative insulin deficiency. When absolute insulin deficiency of decreased insulin activity occurs, glucose is not used properly. Glucose remains in the blood stream and produces an osmotic effect on intracellular and interstitial fluid. This shift in fluid balance results in clinical manifestation of frequent urination (polyuria) and thirst (polydipsia). Without sufficient insulin, the patient may experience hunger (polyphagia) as the body turns to other energy resources besides glucose; First fat and then protein. Acute and chronic complications from hyperglycaemia are closely associated with the type of diabetes mellitus and circumstances in which it occurs.

Management

Management of diabetes mellitus is primarily aimed at achieving a balanced diet, activity, and medication together with appropriate monitoring, patient, and family education. These components are equally necessary for effective control of diabetes.

Diagnosis of diabetes mellitus can be made on the basis of the following:

m0p3

- Complete history and physical examination.
- Blood tests, including fasting blood glucose, postprandial blood glucose, glycocylated, haemoglobin, cholesterol and triglyceride levels, blood urea nitrogen and serum creatinine, electrolysis.
- Urine for complete urinalysis, microalbuminuria, culture and sensitivity glucose and acetone.
- Funduscopic examination—delayed eye examination.
- Neurologic examination.
- Blood pressure.
- Monitoring of weight
- Doppler scan.

Treatment of Type 1 DM

Treatment of Type 1 DM involves a insulin, diet and exercise. The discovery of insulin by *Banting and Best* in 1921 occupies as major place in medical history. Today common insulin used for DM are as follows.

- Quick-acting insulin lipro, regular (bufferal).
- Intermediate acting insulin: NPH, Lente.
- Combination insulin 70% NPH and 30% regular.

Insulin differes in speed of effect onset time of greater action (peak) and how they act duration. Insulins are classified as quick, intermediate, and long acting. Dietary carbohydrate and activity must be coordinated with insulin action so that:

1. Insulin is available for optimal metabolism when the food that was eaten is absorbed and
2. Food is available while insulin is acting to prevent hypoglycaemic reactions.

Two principles are useful in coordinating food and insulin.

1. The carbohydrate intake must be coordinated with insulin actions.
2. Regular or quick-acting insulin requires that a supplemantal snack of 15 gram of carbohydrate be given to match the peak action of the insulin. For example, (1) 10 AM injection of regular insulin in plan.

The nurse must clarify the insulin prescription in terms of the type strength and species. Any change in any one of the properties may lead to difference in action. When the insulin prescription is changed, careful patient monitoring is necessary to identify clinical effect. The *steps of administration of insulin* are as given below.

- Wash hands thoroughly.
- Roll intermediate or long-acting insulin between palms of hands to mix insulin. Note: Always, insulin bottle before using for first time. Make sure that it is proper type and concentration, expration date not over and top of the bottle is in perfect condition.
- Prepare insulin injection is same manner as for any injection.
- Select proper injection sites and inject following procedure for any subcutaneous (SC) injection. In site where SC tissue is adequate, inject commercial insulin needles at 90-degree angle. For sites with minimal SC tissues pinches up skin and insert needle at 45-degree angle.
- If blood appears in syringe after needle insertion, select new site for injection. Aspiration is not necessary.
- After injecting insulin, apply some pressure, with dry cotton ball (or 2X2) at site when withdrawing needle.
- Hold cotton ball in place for a few seconds but do not massage.
- Destroy and disposeor single –use syringe safely. Note: When instructing patient to self-inject insulin, use the following guidelines (if appropriate).
- Aspiration does not need to be done before injection.
- Disposable syringe can be used for several injections.

Problems with insulin therapy are hypoglycaemia, allergic reactions, lipodystrophy and the somogyi effect.

Treatment of Type 2 DM

Currently four classes of medication are available to improve diabetes control for patient with type 2 DM. The common oral medication type 2 DM. Includes the following.

- *First generation sulfonylureas:* Which stimulate release of insulin from pancreatic islets; decrease glycogenolysis and gluconeogenesis and enhance cellular sensitivity to insulin. They are tolbutamide (Orinse) acetohexamide (Dymelar), tolazamide (Tolinase), chloropropammide (Diabenase).
- *Second –generation sulfonylurea:* which stimulate release of insulin from pancreatic islets, decreased glycogenolysis

and gluconeogenic, enhance cellularsensitivity to insulin. They are glipizide (Glucotrol)glybunde.

- *Megiitinides* stimulate a rapid and short-lived release of insulin from pancreas. E.g. Repoglunide (Prandin).
- *Biguanide* Decrease the rate of hepatic glucose production and augments glucose uptake by tissues. E.g.Metformin (Gulucophage).
- *Alpha-Glucosidase Intubitory* works on the brush border of the small intestine to slow the breakdown of disacarides and polysaccharides into monosaccarides; delays subsequent ansorption of glucose. Examples acarbone (Precose), miglitol (Glyset).
- *Thiozolidinidiones* decreases peripheral insulin resistance in skeletal muscle without stimulating insulin secretion. E.g.Troglitazone (Rezulin).

Oral agents are not oral insulin or substitute for insulin. The patient must have some functionary endogenous insulin or for oral agents to be effective. They may be combination of oral agencies or with insulin to achieve goal-ranged control. Dietary control should be provided before starting oral agents. The hypoglycaemic action of oral medications can be enhanced are prolonged by means of the concurrent administration of drug such as anticoagulants, salicylates, alcohol and propranalol. Drugs that can suppose oral agent action include thyroid preparation, corticosteroids, and thiazide diuretics.

Therapy is the cornerstone of care of person with diabetes mellitus. The recommended diet can only be defined as a dietary prescription bases on nutritional assessment and goal. Nutritional assessment is used to determine what the individual with diabetes is able and willing to do. Sensitivity to cultural, ethnic and financial consideration is important when developing meal-planning approaches. The overall goal is to assist persons with diabetes in making changes in nutrition and exercise habits leading to improved metabolic control. The specific goals of nutritional therapy include:

- Maintenance of normal blood glucose level as possible by balancing food intake and insulin or glucose-lowering medication and activity and
- Achievement of optimum serum lipid level.
- Provision of adequate calories for maintaining or attaining reasonable weight for adults, normal growth and development rate in children, and adolescents, increased metabolic needs during pregnancy, and lactation, or recovery from catabolic illness.
- Prevention and treatment of acute complications, such as hypoglycaemia, and long-term complication such as renal disease, neuropathy, hypertension and cardiovascular disease.
- Improvement of overal health though optimal nutrition.

Principles that the nurse should teach the patient and reinforce, including the following:

1. Eat according to the prescribed meal plan: A dietary need related to the specific patient's body weight, occupational age activities and type of diabetes individual response to a dietary prescription should be monitored and appropriate adjustment should be made when necessary.
2. *Never skip meals* This is particularly important for patient taking insulin or oral agents. The body requires food at regularly-spaced intervals throughout the day. Insulin and oral agents prescribed to fit the schedule. Omissions or delay of meals can result hypoglycaemia.
3. Learn to recognize, appropriate, food portions; can result in accurate portion allotments.

Exercise

Regular, consistent exercise is considered an essential part of diabetic management. Exercise contributes to weight loss, reduces tryglycerides and cholesterol, increases muscle tone, and improves circulation. Exercise plans for persons with diabetes should keep in minerals both benefit and risks of exercise as follows:

1. *Benefits* of exercise for the person with diabetes include:
   - Improves insulin sensitivity.
   - Lowers blood glucose during and after exercise.
   - Improves lipid profile.
   - May improve some hypertension.
   - Increased energy expenditure; Assists with weight loss, preserve lean body mass.
   - Promotes cardiovascular fitness.
   - Increases strength and flexibility.
   - Improves sense of well-being.
2. Risks of exercises for the person with diabetes.
   - Precipitation or exacerbation of cardiovascular disease, angina, dysrhythmias and sudden death.
   - Hypoglycaemia if taking insulin or oral-agents.
     - Exercise-related hypoglycaemia.
     - Late onset postexercises hypoglycaemia.
   - Hyperglycaemia after every strenuous exercise. Strenuous exercise.
   - Worsening of long-term complication
     - Proliferative retinopathy.
     - Peripheral neuropathy.
     - Autonomous neuropathy.

Before entering titany type of exercise program, all patient should have a complete history in physical examination, with particular attention to the cardiovascular system and any existing long-term complications. An exercise stress ECG is recommended for all persons over 30 years of age. The general guideline for exercise program for the person with diabetes includes the following:

i. *Exercise type:* Aerobic (Low impact for type 2 DM) start with light level.
ii. *Exercise session*: Each session should eventually include:
    - 5 to 10 minutes of warm-up stretching and limbering exercises.

- 20-30 minutes of aerobic exercises and heart rate in target zone (as defined by the physician) or perceived exercise rating.
- 15-20 minutes of light exercise and stretching to cool down.

iii. *Exercise frequency:* 3 to 5 times per week.

iv. Special precautions:
- Consider the insulin/oral agent regimen (may need to decrease insulin).
- Consider the plan for food intake—Discuss with health care provider. May need to take extracarbohydrates before exercise.
- Check blood glucose before, during, afterward (for baseline).
- If glucose is over 250 mg/dl, check urine ketones; if negative, okay to exercise; if positive, take insulin; dont not exercise until ketones are negative.
- Exercise should not cause shortness of breath and should be stopped with any onset of chest pain or dyspnoea.
- Carry diabetic ID card and bracelet.
- Carry source easily absorbed carbohydrates (three glucose tablets or hard candies).
- Do not exercise in extreme heat or cold.
- Inspect feet daily and after exercise.

v. Precautions for selected persons:
- Person with insensitive feet should choose good shoes for walking and avoid running and jogging. Swimming and cycling may also be included.
- Persons with proliferate retinopathy should avoid exercises associated with valsalva manoeuvers or that cause jarring and jointing of head or exercises with head in low position.
- Persons with hypertension should avoid exercises associated with valsalva maneuvers and exercise involving intense exercises of tarso and arms (Exercises involving the lower extremities preferred).

Exercise does not have to be vigorous to be effective. The blood glucose-reducing effects of exercise can be attained with mild exercise such as brisk walking. The exercise selected should be enjoyable to foster regularity. Exercise is best done after meals, when the blood glucose level is rising.

COMPLICATIONS OF DIABETES MELLITUS

The complications of DM are classified as acute and chronic. Acute complications include hypoglycaemia, diabetes ketoacidism (DKA), and hyperglycaemic hyperosmalor nonketonic coma (HHNC).

Diabetic Ketoacidosis (DKA)

Diabetic ketoacidosis are referred to as diabetic acidosis and diabetic coma may develop quickly or over several days or weeks. It can be caused by too little insulin accompained by increased calorie intake, physical or emotional stress or undiagnosed diabetes, may be due to indequate treatment of existing DM; insulin is not taken as precribed; infection; change in diet; insulin or exercise regimen. DKA mostly likely to occur in Type 1 DM and also seen in Type 2 DM.

In DKA, an assessment finding includes the following needs immediate intervention.

- Dry mouth
- Thirst
- Abdominal pain
- Nausea and vomiting
- Gradually increasing restlessness, confusion, Lethargy
- Flushed dry skin
- Serum glucose greater than 300mg/dl.
- Eyes appear sunken
- Breath orders of ketones
- Rapid, weak pulse.
- Laboured breathing (kussmauls respiration)
- Fever
- Urinary frequencies
- Glycosuria and knenouria.

Diagnostic measures include blood work (immediate blood glucose, CBC, Keton pH, electrolytes. BUN, ABG, urinalysis including Sp. Gr. PH sugar assessment.

The preferred treatment for DKA is the low dose insulin. IV infusion method. In this method 5 to 10 units of insulin per hour is normal salin solution is administered until ketodosis is reversed. This insulin therapy is continued until a blood glucose level of 250 mg/dl is reached. When the glucose level is reached in level, a solution contains 5% dextrose in saline is given to prevent hypoglycaemia along with IV or SC insulin as needed to maintain in blood glucose level fluid and electrolyte therapy aimed at replacing extracellular and intracellular water and deficits of sodium, chloride, bicarbonate, potassium, phosphate magnesium and nitrogen. Ongoing monitoring includes monitoring vital signs, level of consciousness cardiac rhythm, oxygen saturation, and urine output. And assess breath sound for fluid overload, monitor serum glucose and serum potassium, and anticipated posssible administration of sodium bicarbonate with severe acidosis (pH lesser than 7-0).

HYPERGLYCAEMIC HYPEROSMOLAR NON-KETONIC COMA (HHNC)

HHNC in the acute complication of Type 2 DM. It occurs in the patient with diabetes, who is able to produce enough insulin to prevent DKA but not enough to prevent severe hyperglycaemeia, Osmotic diuresis and extracellular fluid depletion. Increasing hyperglycaemeia causes intracellular dehydration because of a shift of the fluid from the intracellular to the extracellular space. This causes neurologic abnormalities such as somnolence, coma, seizures, hemiparesis, and aphasia. There is usually a history if indequate fluid intake, increasing mental depression and polyuria.

Table 13.4: Nursing care plan for the patient with diabetic ketoacidosis (DKA)

Problem	*R*	*Objective*	*Nursing Interventions*	*Rationales*
Nursing diagnosis # 1 Fluid volume deficit: Actual (total body dehydration), related to: 1. Osmotic diuresis caused by extreme glycosuria associated with hyperglycaemic state. 2. Ketosis and ketonaemia associated with enhanced lipolysis caused by insulin insufficiency. Nursing Diagnosis # 2 Electrolyte imbalance, related to: 1. Profound osmotic diuresis caused by extreme glycopsuria 2. Acidemia and ketnoaemia associated with enhanced lipolysis; and lactic acidosis associated with tissue hypoxia. 3. Profound dehydration and hypovolaemia. 4. Nasogastric suctioning. 5. Profuse diaphoresis.		Patient will maintain stable: 1. Neurologic status: • Alert, oriented to person place, and date. • Appropriate behaviour • Usual personality (per family). • Sensorimotor function intact. • Deep tendon reflexes brisk. 2 Haemodynamic status: • BP within 10mmHg of baseline. • Heart rate> 60, <100 beats/min. • Cardiac rhythm: Regular sinus haemodynamic parameters: • CVP mean 0-8 mmHg. • PCWP mean 8-12 mmHg. • Cardiac output: 4-8 liters/min. 3 Renal status: • Body weight within 5% of baseline • Urine output >30 ml/hr. 4. Laboratory status: Serum: • Osmolality: 285-295 mOsm/kg. • Sodium: 135-148 mEq/liter. • Potassium: 3.5 –5.5 mEq/liter.	For pertinent nursing interventions and their rationales related to fluid volume deficit and electrolyte imbalance, sec earlier NCPs in this text. In addition, consider the following: • Assess impact of osmotic diuresis on total body fluid and electrolyte status. • Assess neurologic status: – Mental status, level of consciousness – Behaviour and personality. – Sensorimotor function. – Deep tendon reflexes.	• Extreme glycosuria related to hyperglycemic state precipitates profound fluid loss via a glucose osmotic diuresis. • As an osmotically active molecule, the presence of glucose in the glomerular filtrate after the renal tubules have reabsorbed the maximum amount possible requires an obligte loss of water. • Severe hyperosmolality related to hyperglycaemia can predispose to alterations in neurologic function.
			• Assess fluid status: – Body weight, vital signs. – Intake and output – Skin turgor, signs of dehydration: Dry, parched skin and mucous membranes; sunken eyeballs. – Gastrointestinal fluid losses; nasogastric suctioning; diarrhoea. – Insensible fluid losses via lungs and skin (excessive ventilatory effort of Kussmaul respiration can lead to considerable fluid loss). – Stress, fever, excessive diaphoresis.	• Hypovolaemic state is reflected by decreased arterial and venous blood pressures; pulse may be rapid and therapy; potential risk of hypovolaemic shock must be anticipated and carefully assessed for. • Severe dehydration further exacerbates creations of stress hormones (e.g., glaucagon, cortisol, and epinephrine) which function to increase tissue resistance to the action of insulin.
			• Laboratory tests; serum osmolality; electrolytes; serum glucose, phosphorus and calcium.	• Laboratory values may appear elevated due to haemoconcentration (i.e.severe volume construction related to total body dehydration).
		• Chloride:100-106 mEq/liter • Calcium: 8.5-10.5 mg/100 ml. • Phosphorous: 3.0-4.5 mg/100 ml. • Glucose: 70-110 mg/100ml. • haematology profile • Total protein. *Urine:* • Sodium: 80-180 mEq/liter. • Specific gravity: 1.010-1.025. • Negative for glucose and acetone.	• BUN and creatinine. – Haematology profile: Haematocrit, haemoglobin. – Total protein (blood) – Urine specific gravity. – Urine glucose and acetone. • Assess sources of electrolyte loss: – Profound osmotic diuresis with sodium loss.	• Decreased renal perfusion diminishes the glomerular filtration rate, predisposing to oliguria and placing the severely dehydrated patient at risked developing acute renal failure. • Loss of sodium contributes to hyperkalaemia because there is a decrease in potassiùm secretion in the distal

Contd...

Contd...

Problem	*R*	*Objective*	*Nursing Interventions*	*Rationales*
				renal tubules in the absence of sodium reabsorption. • In the presence of acidemia, there is shift of potassium ions from the intra-to extracellular space in exchange for hydrogen ions. • Shift of potassium ions from the intra-to extracellular compartment in exchange for hydrogen ions contributes significantly to hyperkalaemia. • It is estimated that for every 0.1 decrease in Ph, the serum potassium concentration increases by 0.6 mEq/ liter. • While hyperkalaemia might be anticipated in the initial clinical presentation of ketoacidaemia, normokalaemia is equally as common and hypokalaemia is not uncommon.
			• Losses of sodium and chloride occur with vomiting and nasogastric suctioning	• Serum electrolytes must be evaluated in terms of total body water status because such values, if assessed seperately, may not reflect the true electrolyte status. For example, while hypernatraemia might be anticipated in the face of significant osmotic diuresis, the osmotic effect of the glucose load within the extracellular fluid compartment causes water to be extracted from the intracellular compartment, expanding the extrcellular fluid volume. Thus actually, a dilutional hyponatraemia may occur. – A formula developed to compensate for this dilutional hyponatraemia secondary to the osmotic effect of glucose in the ECF compartment may be a helpful assessment tool. A 1.6.3.0 mEq/liter reduction in serum sodium occurs per every 100 mg elevation of serum glucose.
			– In the presence of severe ketoacidaemia, a concomitant increase in the urinary excretion of phosphates may predispose to hypophosphataemia.	– Phosphorus is a major constituent of ATP. Excessive deficit of phosphorous reduces ATP energy stores and predisposes to alterations in cellular metabolism. At serum phosphorous levels less than 1.0mg/100ml, muscle weakness may become sufficiently profound to depress myocardial contractility or produce respiratory arrest. – Reduction in stores of 2,3-diphosphglycerate (DPG) within red blood cells compromises oxygen delievery to tissues. In the absence of 2,3-DPG, haemoglobin unloads very little oxygen

Contd...

Contd...

Problem	R	Objective	Nursing Interventions	Rationales
				at the tissue level contributing to tissue hypoxia. A decrease in 2,3-DPG stores causes the oxyhaemoglobin-dissociation curve to shift to the left.
			• Implement prescribed fluid replacement regimen:	• Rapid rehydration with isotonic saline (0.9 N saline) is the treatment of choice; use of hypotonic saline (0.45 N saline) may produce a precipitious fall in extracellular fluid shifts and cerebral oedema.
			◆ Administer aggressive fluid therapy. – Overall goal of fluid restoration is the rapid and effective correction of the fluid volume deficit.	◆ Because patients with DKA manifest varying degrees of fluid and electrolyte imbalance, fluid and electrolyte replacement therapy must be individualized and guided by continuous monitoring and assessment.
			◆ Monitor for signs/symptoms of fluid excess: Cardiac rate and rhythm; haemodynamic parameters-CVP, PCWP, CO, – Physical signs: Extraheart sounds (gallop rhythm); full bounding pulse; neck vein distention at 45° (upright position); dependent oedema.	◆ Rapid fluid replacement necessitates close monitoring of vital signs and haemodynamic function to avert overhydration with its attendant danger of CHF and pulmonary oedema. Patients with compromised cardiac and /or renal function are especially at high risk.
			◆ Closely monitor for hypoglycaemia, hypokalaemia, and cerebral oedema. – Serial serum glucose studies.	◆ When serum glucose levels approach 250 mg/100ml, dextrose 5% in 0.45 N saline is substituted for normal saline to avoid precipitating a hypoglycaemic reaction.
			◆ Insert Foley catheters during the acute phase to more closely monitor urine output.	◆ Accurate assessment of urinary output is essential to assess renal function and to dectrimine fluid and electrolyte therapy. ◆ Precise documentation of fluid intake and output is necessary to determine fluid replacement therapy and the patient's response to such therapy.
			• Restore and maintain electrolyte balance. ◆ Implement electrolyte replacement therapy.	• Serum sodium and potassium concentrations are variable, but total body concentrations are severely depleted.
			◆ Administer prescribed saline therapy.	◆ Provides necessary sodium and water replacement.
			◆ Assess for signs and symptoms of hyperkalaemia. – Monitor ECG for peaked T-wave and S-T segment changes. – Monitor serum electrolytes and pH.	◆ Hyperkalaemia is associated with profound osmotic diuresis with haemoconcentration; shifting of potassium ions from intra-to extrcellular space due to ketoacidaemia;and retension of potassium ions in intravascular compartment in the absence of insulin.
			◆ Assess for signs and symptoms of hypokalaemia. – Monitor ECG for inverted or flattened T-wave; appearance of U-wave; prolonged Q.T intervals.	◆ Hypokalaemia becomes manifest within 2-4 hours of initiation of insulin, fluid, and electrolyte replacement therapies. Physiology underlying the total body potassium deficit; Dilutional factor with rehydration;

Contd...

Contd...

Problem	*R*	*Objective*	*Nursing Interventions*	*Rationales*
			– Monitor serum electrolytes and pH.	reduction in ketoacidaemia related to insulin therapy—shift from fatty acid to glucose metabolism; movement of potassium ions into cells with glucose in the presence of insulin. Increase. in the presence of insulin; increases. In renal perfusion with consequent fluid and electrolyte loss.
Nursing Diagnosis #2 (cont.)			• Administer potassium replacement therapy as prescribed. One approach is the following: – *Hyperkalaemia:* withhold initial potassium therapy until serum potassium level returns to within normal physiologic range. – *Normokalaemia:* Potassium chloride 10-20 mEq/hr is added to intravenous replacement fluids. – *Hypokalaemia:* Initial potassium replacement therapy is more aggressive; 20-40 mEq/hr administered with intravenous approach. – In the absence of cardiac dysrhythmias and with good renal perfusion, potassium replacement therapy may be safely initiated even before the serum potassium is known. Recommended dose: 10-15 mEq/hr.	• Goal is to restore and maintain normal extracellular potassium concentrations during the acute period. – Severely dehydrated patients who present with oliguria upon admission should be observed for underlying renal disease. – In patients who remain oliguric despite sodium repletion, a trial with furosemide should be attempted. If oliguria persisits, intrinsic renal diseases becomes highly suspect and further fluid and electrolyte replacement therapy must be administered cautiously.
			– Continuous monitoring of ECG and serial serum potassium levels is critical	– Close monitoring of serum potassium and ECG changes is essential because alterations in serum potassium can precipitate serious/lethal dysrhythmias.
			• Administer phosphate replacement therapy usually in conjunction with potassium therapy.	• Total body phosphate depletion is usually associated with severe DKA. – Initial hyperphosphataemia followed by precipitous fall with hypophosphataemia postimplementation of fluid and insulin therapy. – Overly aggressive phosphate replacement therapy unnecessay. – Phosphates given in conjuction with potassium replacements therapy; potassium chloride is alternated with potassium phosphate during the intial phase of therapy. – There are no definitive consequences of hypophosphataemia. – Caution must be taken to prevent hyperphophataemia (overshoot) because this in turn may predispose to hypocalcaemia and hypomagnesaemia.

Contd...

Problem	*R*	*Objective*	*Nursing Interventions*	*Rationales*
			• Implement prescribed insulin replacement therapy. ♦ Low-dose regular insulin regimens are usually prescribed.	• Goal is to ensure a sustained, progressive reduction in serum glucose levels. ♦ Insulin therapy requires that serum glucose be monitored at frequent intervals. In DKA, prolonged insulin therapy is required after serum glucose levels reach 250 mg/100ml, because correction of ketoacidaemia takes longer to resolve.
Nursing Diagnosis # 3 Acid–base balance, alteration in related to: 1. Ketoacidosis associated with insulin insufficiency. 2. Enhanced lipolysis 3. Lactic acidaemia associated with reduced tissue perfusion and tissue hypoxia.		1. patient's arterial blood gases will normalize as follows • pH:7.35-7.45 • PaCO2: 35-45 mmHg, or optimal for patient. 2. Anions will stabilize as follows: • HCO3: 22-26 mEq/liter. • Chloride: 100-106 mEq/liter. • Anion gap: <12-15 Eq/liter.	• Implement measures to restore and maintain acid-base balance. ♦ Monitor acid-base balance: – Serial arterial blood gases. – Serial electrolytes. – Calculation of anion gap: The major two anions are chloride (Cl^-)and bicarbonate (HCO_3^-). They account for all but 10-15 mmol/liter of the total anion charge in the body. To calculate; Anion gap=$Na^{+}-(CL^{-}+HCO_3^{-})$. – Normal anion gap: <15 mmol / liter. ♦ If pH is < 7.0 bicarbonate therapy may be prescribed. Approach to therapy: – Administer 1 ampule of sodium bicarbonate (44.6 mEq/liter) at a time; follow blood study results carefully. When pH is >7.0, discontinue bicarbonate therapy. ♦ Monitor ketoacidotic state: – Presence of prominent gastrintestinal symptomatology: Epigastric distress, nausea, vomiting; abdominal pain, distention, ileus. – Heavy, labored breathing (kussmaul) – Flushed skin; fruity odour to breath.	• Ketoacidaemia is a major distinctive finding in DKA with marked depression of the arterial pH(<7.20) due largely to ketosis. ♦ Serum and urine are highly positive for acetoacetic acid, beta-hydroxybutyric acid, and acetone. Note: ketostix test for acetoacetic acid and acetone does not test for beta hydroxybutyric acid. Thus, in the patient with predominantly elevated levels of this latter ketone, a severe ketoacidemia may exist without a positive serum acetone. – An anion gap greater than 15 mmol / liter indicates existence of another anions(s). In DKA, the source of these additional anions are the ketones, acetoacetic and beta-hydroxybutyric acids and acetone. ♦ If bicarbonate therapy is initiated (for pH <7), caustion must be taken to avoid too rapid restoration of pH; this may predispose to alterations in cerebral functions due to paradoxical cerebrospinal fluid (CSF) acidosis. Remember: Carbon dioxide penetrates the blood-brain barrier much more easily than the bicarbonate ion (HCO_3) does.
Nursing Diagnosis # 4 Cardiac output, alteration in: Decreased, related to: 1. Severe volume depletion with reduced venous return. 2. Cardiac dysrhythmias.		Patient will maintain stable 1. Neurologic status. 2. Haemodynamic status. 3. Renal status. 4. Laboratory parameters.	• Restore and maintain effective cardiovascular, neurologic, and renal function. ♦ Establish baseline data reflective of cardiovascular/renal function: cardiac rate and rhythm: haemodynamic parameters-arterial BP, CVP, PCWP, cardiac output, peripheral pulses.	• Of immediate concern in the clinical setting of severe DKA with intra- and extracellular fluid volume depletion is the imapct on cardiovascular and renal function. ♦ Baseline assessment data provide a basis for comparison and assist in evaluating the patient's response to therapy.
Nursing Diagnosis # 5 Tissue perfusion, alteration in cerebral, peripheral, related to: 1. Hypovolaemic state severe dehydration.			♦ Urine output: Hourly measurement of urine output; specific gravity; fluid intake; bodyweight (daily). ♦ Establish baseline data reflective of neurologic function: Mental status,	

Contd...

Contd...

Problem	*R*	*Objective*	*Nursing Interventions*	*Rationales*
2. Extreme hyperosmolality with haemoconcentration.			state of consciousness; behavior/ personality; sensorimotor function; deep tendon reflexes.	
			◆ Assess cardiovascular function for signs/ symptoms of fluid overload.	◆ Sudden shifts in fluid and electrolytes may precipitate fluid excess; careful ongoing assessment (following trends) helps to obviate overhydration from too aggressive fluid replacement therapy; hypertension, congestive heart failure with pulmonary oedema are potential complications of hypervolaemia.
			◆ Assess for evidence of hypovolaemic shock: – haemodynamic: hypotension; tachycardia (weak, thready peripheral pulses), decreased hemodynamic pressures. – Neurologic: Altered state of consciousness, weakness, paresthesias. – Renal: hourly urine output. – Skin: cool, clammy, motted	◆ Plasma expanders and vasopressors (dopamine) in addition to isotonic saline therapy may be necessary to maintain perfusion to vital tissue during hypovolemic shock state.
			◆ Administer fluids, volume expanders (e.g. dextrose, blood plasma, albumin), vasopressors (as prescribed).	◆ Very careful, ongoing assessment of vital parameters forms the basis for fluid and pharmacologic resuscitation.
Nursing Diagnosis # 6 Skin integrity, impairment of, related to: 1. Compromised peripheral perfusion associated with volume depletion and reduced cardiac output. 2. Immobility. 3. Catabolic state. 4. Peripheral neuropathy.		Patient's skin will maintain 1. Dry and warm to touch 2. Without cyanosis or mottling. 3. With peripheral pulses palpable and full. 4. Intact, without evidence of pressure areas or skin break down. 5. With capillary refill spontaneous. 6. With minimal or absent pain of diabetic neuropathy. 7. Without oedema.	• Maintain intergrity of skin and mucous membranes ◆ Inspect skin and mucous membranes. – Establish state of turgor, moisture oedma (pitting, dependent), pressure areas, cracking, fissuring, lesions. – Monitor circulation to extremities. – Peripheral pulses, capillary refill.	• Vascular insufficiency associated with diabetes increases risk of injury to skin especially in lower extremities. ◆ Sensory /motor deficits due to peripheral vascular disease increase risk of injury.
			◆ Apply therapeutic measures: – Lubricate skin – Keen skin clean and dry. – Use egg-crate mattress, air mattress, or sheepskin. – Avoid very hot water when bathing.	◆ Lubricating skin helps to improve circulation and protects from infection. ◆ Pressure relief devices. ◆ Scalding can easily occur in presence of sensory deficits often experienced by patients with diabetes.
Nursing Diagnosis # 7 Oral mucous membranes, alterations in, related to: 1. Severe dehydrates state 2. Catabolic state.		Patient's mucous membranes will remain clean, moist, and without cracking or fissuring.	◆ Provide supportive care and comfort measures: Assist in personal hygiene; in turning and positioning; encourage deep breathing. – Apply antiembolic stockings. – Active /passive range-of-motion exercises as tolerated; early ambulating. – provide for frequent rest periods in a quiet milieu. – Encourage gradual increase in self-care.	◆ Supportive and comfort measures need to be implemented to maximize circulatory and pulmonary function and reduce risk of infection. ◆ Venous thrombosis and disseminated intravascular coagulation (DIC) are serious complications associated with DKA. Major contributing factors. – Dehydrates state with hemoconcentration, and elevated serum protein with consequent increase in blood viscosity. – Altered haemodynamics associated with peripheral vascular disease and venous stasis.

Contd...

Contd...

Problem R	*Objective*	*Nursing Interventions*	*Rationales*
			– Altered platelet adhensiveness and aggregation – Alteration in level of clotting factors
		• Minimize pain associated with diabetic neuropathy: Aching and burning sensation in extremities especially at night. – Encourage walking (if possible) to relieve pain; use of foot cradle. – Maintenance of serum glucose within therapeutic range.	• Prevents contact of extremities with bed clothes. • Neuropathic pain is most often associated with increased serum glucose levels.
Nursing Diagnosis # 8 Breathing pattern, ineffective: Hyperventilation (Kussmaul breathing) related to: 1. Severe ketonaemia and acidaemia associated with excessive lipolysis in the absense of insulin (pH <7.20). 2. Tissue hypoxia associated with impaired perfusion.	Patient will: 1. Maintain ventilatory efforts as follows: • Respiratory rate: <25-30 breaths/min. • Tidal volume (TV): >5-7ml/kg. • Vital capacity (VC): >15 ml/kg. 2. Demonstrate eupneoea without use of accessory muscles of breathing 3. Avoid fatigue with reduced work of breathing.	• Establish baseline assessment database: • Assess pertinent parameters of respiratory function: – Respiratory rate, rhythm, and pattern of breathing. – Hyperventilation (kussmaul) – tachypnoea, dyspnoea. • Use of necessary muscles of respiration. • Pleuritic pain. • Pleuritic function parameters: • Pulmonary function parameters: – Tidal volume. – Vital capacity. • Auscultation of breath sounds.	• Goal of therapy is to maintain effective respirartory function as guided by arterial blood gas, tidal volume, vital capacity, and neurologic function. • Infective breathing pattern often associated with muscle weakness caused by hypokalaemia; patient is at great risk of developing respiratory arrest. • Kussmaul breathing associated with severe ketoacidaemia; it is compensatory response of the body to blow off excess CO_2 and thereby increase arterial pH. • Use of accessory muscles may cause undue fatigue. • Severely dehydrated state may predispose to pleuritic friction rub.
Nursing diagnosis # 9 Gas exchange impaired related to: 1. Tissue hypoxia associated with decreased tissue perfusion. 2. Increase in ventilation/perfusion mismatch 3. Diffusion defect.	The patient's parameters will stabilize as follows: 1. Arterial blood gases: • pH>7.35 • PaO2> 80mmHg • PaCO2 return to baseline (normally 35-45 mmHg). Haemoglobin oxygen saturation: >95%. 2 Neurologic status: Oriented to person, place date: protective reflexes (cough, swallowing) intact. 3 Skin and mucous membranes—No cyanosis.	• Arterial blood gases: Trends • Cyanosis of lips, mucous membranes, and nailbeds • Acetone odour to breath • Neurolgic status.	• Adventitious sounds (rales, rhonchi; wheezes) may signal pulmonary congestion progressing to pulmonary oedema wheezing reflects congested airways due in part to inability of patient to handle secretions. • A rising $PaCO_2$ suggest decresing ventilatory capability. – A $PaCO_2$ <60 mmHg predisposes to tissue hypoxia. • Cyanosis reflects decreased tissue oxygenation related to altered ventilation. • Reflects ketogenesis. • Ongoing neurologic assessment is essential to detect cerebral function due to paradoxic CSF acidosis.
		• Provide supportive therapy. • Administer humidified oxygen. • Assist patient to assume a position that facilitates breathing. • Encourage deep breathing.	• May assist in relieving tissue hypoxia; prevents thick tenacious secretions of dehydrated state. • Efforts must be directed towards assisting patient to conserve strength. • Insertion of nasogastric tube may be necessary to prevent gastric dilation, which limits diaphramatic excursion and increases the risk of aspiration pneumonia. • Deep breathing minimizes atelectasis.

Contd...

Contd...

Problem	*R*	*Objective*	*Nursing Interventions*	*Rationales*
			◆ Initiate ventilatory assistance if indicated (respiratory arrest).	◆ Position changes minimize pooling of secretions. ◆ Ventilatory support may be needed in presence of altered state of consciousness, ineffective breathing pattern, inability to handle secretions.
Nursing Diagnosis #10 Anxiety related to: 1. Fear of dying 2. ICU setting 3. Seriousness of compromised health state. 4. Personal and social responsibilities (e.g., effect of illness on job.)		1. Patient and family will be able to verbalize fears and concerns regarding current illness, diabetes mellitus, and its complications. 2. Patient and family's behaviour will demonstrate less apprehension or withdrawal; increased interest in learning about illness state.	• Maintain integrity of neurologic and psychological process. ◆ Establish baseline neurologic function: – Mental status: Changes in level of consciousness, disorientation, confusion, agitation, irritability, coma. – Cranial nerve function. – Sensory function: Parenthesis. – Motor function: muscle weakness, paralysis, hyper-reflexia – Seizure activity. ◆ Establish baseline psychologic function including patient and family: – Assess level of anxiety, apprehension. Does behavior reflect withdrwal, disinterest, apathy?	◆ Alterations in neurologic function realted to hyperglycaemia with extreme hypersomolaity, and severe acidaemia. ◆ It is essential to appreciate that the patient with DKA can shift from a coma state hypoglycaemia shock without regaining consciousness. Neurologic status must be carefully evaluated in conjunction with cardiovascular function and serum glucose levels.
Nursing Diagnosis # 11 Communication impaired: Verbal, related to: 1. Altered state of consciousness associated with severe dehydration and acidotic state.		1. Patient will remain alert and oriented to person, place, date. 2. Patient will verbalize needs and whether they have been met.	◆ Estimate developmental level. ◆ Assess coping capabilities: Role of patient family nucleus: Dependent, independent? Decision-maker? – Identify family resources and significant others.	◆ Age and developmental level may not necessarily be the same. ◆ Role of patient in family nucleus will influence rehabilitative process for all members.
Nursing Diagnosis # 12 Thought processes, alteration in, related to: 1. Altered state of consciousness related to severe hypersmolality (hyperglycaemia): severe volume depletion.		1. Patient will exhibit appropriate behaviour and thought processes intact. 2. Patient will demonstrate the ability to think and make decision regarding care, likes and dislikes.	◆ Assess readiness to learn. ◆ Consider the following when providing care: – Be an attentive interested caring listener.	◆ Teaching can be geared to level at which patient and family can best learn. Observation of interactions between patient and family may provide valuable cluses as to how they are coping, which could be an important consideration in the rehabilitative process.
Nursing Diagnosis # 13 Self-concept, disturbance in body image, self-esteem, related to: 1. Chronic illness.		Patient will feel comfortable talking about what diabetes means and how it will effect lifestyle and optimal level of health desired.	◆ Encourage verbalization of fears and concerns. ◆ Involve patient/ family in decision-making process. – Support patient/family efforts in coping – Remain accessible to patient and family. – Provide emotional support to patient and family.	◆ It may help to identify problems or areas of concern. ◆ Appropriate explanations may help alleviate heightened anxiety. ◆ Management of diabetes a chronic disease syndrome requires self-care health practices by patient and family; their active involvement is essential if they are to evolve a meaningful life within the constraints of the disease.
Nursing Diagnosis # 14 Nutrition alteration in: Less than body requirements, related to: 1. Catabolic state 2. Insulin lack.		Patient's condition will stabilize as follows: 1. Body weight will stabilize within appropriate range. 2. Positive nitrogen balance will be maintained. 3. Combination of insulin, diet, and exercise, therapies will maintain serum glucose levels within optimal range.	• Implement prescribed nutritional regimen. ◆ Perform an abdominal assessment: – Subjective: Anorexia, nausea, voimiting, epigastric discomfort and abdominal pain. – Objectives: tender, distended abdomen, absence of bowel sounds, paralytic ileus; limitation of diaphagmatic excursion. ◆ Insert nasogastric tube.	◆ Alterations in serum potassium and severe acidaemia predispose to impaired gastric motility and abdominal discomforts and symptomatology. ◆ Limitations of diaphragmatic excursion may compromise ventilatory effort, increasing risk of atelectasis. ◆ Gastric decompensation reduces abdominal discomfort and risk of aspiration.

Contd...

Problem	*R*	*Objective*	*Nursing Interventions*	*Rationales*
		4. Abdominal discomfort will be minimized; gastric aspiration will be averted.	♦ Monitor serum glucose, ketones, electrolyte levels, and arterial blood gases. ♦ Monitor intake, output; daily weight. ♦ Initiate dextrose 5% in 0.45 N saline infusion when serum glucose drops to 250 mg/dl in the presence of insulin therapy. ♦ Consult with nutritionist, physician, patient, and family to determine specific nutritional nees.	♦ With initiation of insulin therapy metabolism shifts from fatty acids to glucose with a resultant drop in serum glucose and ketones. ♦ Overall goals of nutritional therapy: 1. Meet the basic nutritional requirements. 2. Attain and/or maintain ideal body weight 3. Prevent complications (e.g. hypoglycaemia).
Nursing Diagnosis # 15 Knowledge deficit: Nutritional /insulin therapy regimen		Patient and family will: 1. Discuss underlying principles of diabetic diet therapy 2. Specific dietary restrictions and their significance. 3. Relate how diet therapy coincides with insulin and exercise regimens. 4. Demonstrate proficiency in performing and intepreting test for serum glucose. 5. Identify action to be taken in the event of gastrointestinal disorder or significant stressor. 6. Verbalize concerns regarding the diseases syndrome and overall anti-diabetes therapy regimen.	– Baseline nutritional needs. • Initiate teaching program regarding dietary therapy for the diabetic patient. ♦ Involve patient/family in diet planning and decision-making. ♦ Provide booklets and pamphlets to reinforce teaching. ♦ Stress importance of regularity of diet and exercise; rest, sleep, and relaxation. ♦ Encourage verbalization of feelings regarding impact of diabetes on family lifestyle and the integrity of each individual.	♦ Therapeutic anti-diabetes treatment regimen requires that diet therapy coincide with insulin and exercise regimen. ♦ Ideal body weight should be established and maintained. ♦ Diet therapy is an essential aspect of antidiabetes therapy. ♦ Self–care is an absolute requirement for successful management of diabetes. Participation in decision making and planing increases motivation and compliance.
Nursing diagnosis # 16 Injury, physiologic, potential for: Hypoglycaemia, related to: 1. Ineffective dietary/ insulin regimen 2. Non-compliance with therapeutic regimen. 3. Stressful event.		1. Patient will maintain optimal serum glucose levels: • Fasting serum flucose: 70-110 mg/100 ml • 1-2 hr postprandial: <160-180 mg/100 ml 2. Patient will be able to verbalize signs and symptoms of hypoglycaemic and hyperglycaemic state.	• Teach the importance of, and how to document, significant data, including: ♦ Insulin dosage, time. ♦ Site of injection. ♦ Serum glucose (glucometer or dextrostix). ♦ Urinary sugar and acetone. ♦ Diet. ♦ Exercise. ♦ Stressors.	♦ Data assist in evaluating response to therapy so that appropriate adjustment can be made as necessary.
Nursing Diagnosis # 17 Potential for infection, related to: 1. Catabolic state associated with insulin insufficiency.		Patient will: 1. Remain nonfebrile. 2. Keep white blood count within acceptable physiologic range. 3. Verbalize a general feeling of well-being. 4. Remain without signs/symptoms of infection: Pain, redness, swelling suppuration. 5. Have lungs clear on auscultation. 6. Have negative cultures: blood, urine, sputum, wound, intravenous access sites.	• Implement activities to reduce the risk of infection. ♦ Assess for signs of infection. ♦ Vigilant assessment of all invasive lines is critical. – Observe for redness, pain, swelling at all invasive sites; dressing changes should occur every 48 hrs. or according to unit protocol. – Culture catheter tip. ♦ Assess lungs for adventitious sounds of pulmonary congestion or increased secretions. ♦ Examine urine for cloudiness or unusual odour. – Assess body temperature. – Monitor white blood count. ♦ Culture all body fluids/secretions in presence of increased body temperature. – Blood, septum, urine, wounds. ♦ Administer antibiotic therapy as prescribed assess for response to therapy.	♦ Infection is a serious stressor, which can disrupt diabetic control and precipitate DKA.

HHNC constitutes a medical energy. The management of both DKA and HHNC is similar except that HHNC requires greater fluid replacement. Diagnostic measures followed as in DKA. The primary management of HHNC involve intravenous Rehydration with hypertonic solution (OUS Normal saline). Hypertonic solutions are indicated, because patient is hyperosmolar. As the patient is rehydrated, the hyperglycaemia resolves. Intravenous insulin is generally not needed. Once the patient is stabilized, attempts to detect and correct the underlying precipitating cause should be initiated.

When hospitalized, the patient (DKA or HHNC) is closely monitored with appropriate blood and urine tests. The nurse is responsible for monitoring blood glucose and urine output and ketones as well as using laboratory data to direct care. Areas that need monitoring are administration of IV fluids to correct dehydration, administration of insulin therapy to reduce blood glucost and serum acetone, administration of electrolytes to correct electrolyte imbalance, assessment of renal status, assessment of cardiopulmonary status related to hydration and electrolyte levels, and monitoring the level of consciousness. And vital signs should be assessed often to determine the presence of fever, hypovolaemic shock, tachycardia and Kussamaul's breathing.

According to assessment, proper reporting and recording are maintained to take measures of any deviation accordingly. *Hyperglycaemia* may be caused by intake of too much food; too little or no diabetic medication; inactive and emotional physical stress; and poor absorption of insulin.

The clinical manifestation of hyperglycaemia, include the following:

- Elevated blood glucose
- Increase in urination
- Increase in appetite followed by lack of appetite
- Weakness, fatigue.
- Blurred vision.
- Headache
- Glucosuria
- Nausea and vomiting
- Abdominal cramps
- Progression of DKA or HHNC.

Treatment of hyperglycaemia includes;

- Physician attention.
- Continuation of diabetic medication as ordered.
- Frequent checking of blood and urine specimen and recording results.
- Hourly drinking of fluids.

Preventive measures for hyperglycaemia include:

- Taking of prescribed dose of medications at proper time.
- Accurate administration of insulin or oral agents
- Maintenance of diet.
- Maintenance of personal hygiene
- Adherence to sick-day rules when ill.
- Checking of blood for glucose as ordered.
- Contacting physician regarding ketonuria
- Wearing diabetic identification.

CHRONIC COMPLICATIONS OF DM

The chronic complication of diabetes mellitus are classified microvascular (small blood vessels) and macrovascular (large blood vessels).

These are consequences of the duration and degree of hyperglycaemia. These changes of:

i. Microvascular-Diabetic retinopathy, diabetic nephropathy, neuropathy systemetrical sensory peripheral polyneuropathy, painful peripheralneuropathy, mononeuropathy, radioculopathy and amyotrophy.

ii. *Macroovascular:* Dyslipidaemia, hypertension, (coronary artery diseases). The signs and symptom of different diabetic neuropathy as follows:

i. Peripheral sensory polyneuropathy
   - Classic symmetrical glove-and stocking distributions.
   - Paresthesia, hyperesthesias.
   - Pain (characteristics vary; may be sharp, stabbing lancinating, aching, etc.)
   - Loss of sensation to pinprick, vibration and temperature.
   - Loss of deep tendon reflexes.
   - Muscle wasting and weakness.

ii. *Autonomic*
   - Orthostatic hypertension.
   - Cardiac denervation.
   - Anhidrosis.
   - Gustatory sweating.
   - Gastroparesis, with delyed gastric emptying , nausea, emesis.
   - Diarrhoea.
   - Bladder atony/annoyance.
   - Erectile dysfunction.

iii. *Mononeuropathy*
   - Cranial nerve palsy (III, IV, VI and VII).
   - Ulnar nerve palsy.
   - Corpal tunnel syndrome.

iv. Amyotrophy
   - Acute anterior thigh pain or numbness.
   - Weakness to hip flexion on examination.
   - Quardriceps wasting.

v. *Radioculopathy*
   - Follows dermatomal distribution on trunk
   - Paresthesis.
   - Hyperesthesia.
   - Pain.
   - Numbness.

Treatment of diabetic neuropathy by medication, particular as painful diabetic neuropathy, includes

	Min.	*Max*
• Prepoxyphene with Darvon (Darvocet N-100)-Min	1tabQID	2 tab4th Hrly
• Amitryptyline HCL (Elavil)		
• Carbemazepine (Tegreso)	25 mg tid	100 mg tid

• Phenotoin (Dilantin)	100mg hrs	100mg gid.
• Gabapentin (neurontin)	300mg h	600mg QID.
• Capsaican (zostrex)	Apply topically.	

HYPOGLYCAEMIA IN DM

Hypoglycaemia or low blood glucose occurs when proportionately too much insulin is in the blood for the available glucos. This causes the blood glucose to drop to less than 50 mg/ dl.

The cause of hypoglycaemia include the following.

- Alcohol intake with food.
- Too little food –delayed-omitted, -inadequate intake.
- Too much exercise without compensation.
- Diabetes medication or food taken at wrong time.
- Loss of weight with change in medication.
- Use of beta blockers interfering with recognition of symptoms.
- A decrease in available blood glucose can result sypathetic nervous system activation and the release of epinephrine. This results in manifestations of cold sweats, weakness, trembling, nervousness, irritability pallor. And increased heart rate. The clinical manifestation of hypoglycaemia varies with each patient. The brain depends on a constant supply of glucose because it is unable to stone glucose or glycogen. If that supply is indequated, the patient will experience confusion, fatigue, and abnormal behaviour that can resemble alcohol intoxication.

The clinical manifestation of hypoglycaemia includes the following:

- Blood glucose less than 50 mg/dl.
- Cold, clammy skin
- Numbness of fingers, toes, mouth
- Rapid heart beat
- Emotional changes
- Headache
- Nervousness
- Faittness, dizziness
- Unsteady gait, slurred speech
- Hunger
- Changes in vision
- Seizures, coma.

Treatment of hypoglycaemia needs:

- Immediate ingestion of 5-20 gm of simple carbohydrates.
- Ingestion of another 5-20 gm of simple carbohydrates in 15 minutes if no response or relief.
- Contacting of physician if no relief is obtained.
- Discussion with physician with medication dosage.

Preventive measure of hypoglycaemia includes:

- Taking of prescribed medications at proper time.
- Accurate administration of insulin or oral agents.
- Ingestion of all ordered diet foods at proper time.
- Provision of compensation for exercise.
- Ability to recognise and know symptoms and treat them immediately.
- Carrying of simple carbohydrate (Sugar).
- Education of friends, family employees about symptoms and treatment.
- Checking blood glucose as ordered.

HYPOGLYCAEMIA IN NON-DM

Hypoglycaemia in the nondiabetic person is characterised by subnormal plasma glucose, generally less than 50 mg/dl. It may be asymptotic, may cause adrenergic symptoms (anxiety, irritability, palpitation, diaphoresis, and pallor) or may cause neurologlycopoenic symptoms with more severe hypoglycaemia. Neurologlycopenic symptoms include mental confusion, seizures, and coma may be associated with severe trauma (e.g. motor vehicle accidents). A firm diagnosis rests with the documents of Whipple's traid.

1. Appropriate signs and symptoms.
2. Appropriate abnormal blood glucose and
3. Responses to normalised blood glucose with carbohydrate ingestion.

Classification

Hypoglycaemia in nondiabetics may be broadly classified as either fasting or nonfasting (reaction) hypoglycaemia. Fasting hypoglycaemia generally results in neuroglycopoenic symptoms whereas ready hypoglycaemia generally results in neuroglycopoenic symptoms whereas ready hypoglycaemia is usually associated with mere adrenergic symptoms.

The cause *fasting hypoglycaemia* includes the following:

1. *Insulin Excess*
   - Exogenous insulin surreptitiously.
   - Sulfomylurea ingestion (accidental in individual without DM, surreptitious use and pharmacy dispensation error).
   - Insulin producing islets cell tumour insulinomo-benign or malignant).
   - Islets hyperplasia.
   - Neridioblastosis.
2. *Increased hepatic glucose production*
   - Advanced renal disease.
   - Advanced liver disease.
   - Ethnol use, especially in the setting of poor nutrition.
   - Severe sepsis.
   - Secure malnutrition.
3. Counter regulatory hormone deficiency.
   - Hypopituitarism
   - ACHT deficiency.
   - GH deficiency.

Table 13.5: Nursing plan for the patient with hypoglycaemia (hypoglycaemic shock)

Problem	*R*	*Objective*	*Nursing Interventions*	*Rationales*
Nursing Diagnosis # 1 Cerebral function, alteration in related to: 1. Hypoglycaemia		Patient's condition will stabilize: 1. Neurologic status: • Mental status: Oriented to person, place, date. • Level of consciousness: Arousal and awareness intact. • Cranial nerve function intact • Cerebellar function intact • Sensorimotor function intact. • Deep tendon reflexes brisk. 2. Vital signs: • Arterial blood pressure within 10 mmHg of patient's baseline • Heart rat: >60, <100 beats/min. • Cardiac rhythm; Regular sinus. • Respirations: <25-30 breaths/min. • Breathing pattern: Eupnoea. 3. Serum glucose: Stable at 70-110 mg/100ml.	• Implement patient care to stabilize glucose metabolism ◆ Establish baseline neurologic function: neuroglycopoenia. – Mental status: changes in level of consciousness, disorientation, confusion; headache, lightheadeness visual disturbances, irritability, leyhargy; inappropriate behaviour, convulsions, paralysis, coma. ◆ Cranial nerve function. ◆ Cerebellar function – Sensory/motor function: parehemiparesis, paralysis, seizure convulsions. Deep tendon reflexes. ◆ Establish baseline adrenergic function: Vital signs-Blood pressure, heart rate pulses, respiration, temperature. ◆ Administer 50 ml of 50% dextrose in water intravenously as prescribed – If venous access is not available, administer glucagon 1 mg. intramuscularly. – Infusion of 10% dextrose should be initiated to maintain serum glucose levels between 100 and 200 mg/100 ml; and until the patient can safely ingest oral intake. – Keep emergency dose of glucose at bedside. ◆ Monitor all vital signs and ECG throughout acute phase. ◆ Carefully monitor serum glucose levels.	• Primary energy substrate for the brain is glucose. Serum glucose levels < 55 mg/100 ml can produce alterations in cerebral functions; appropriate and timely treatment is necessary to avert permanent neurologic damage. ◆ Appropriate cranial nerve and cerebellar functions reflect an intact brainstem. • Adrenergic stimulation is a compensatory reaction by the body in response to hypoglycaemia; it is largely responsible for symptomatology that occurs early in the course of hypoglycaemia. • Draw blood sample prior to administration of glucose for retrospective diagnosis. • A rapid and dramatic response should be expected upon glucose administration; if coma persist in spite of therapy, suspect cerebral oedema.' • Establish that protective reflexes-gag, swallowing, cough are intact before offering food/drink for oral consumption, to prevent aspiration. ◆ Wide fluctuations in serum glucose can occur rapidly. • Assist in evaluating response to therapy.
Nursing Diagnosis # 2 Injury, potential for: seizures, related to: 1. Altered neuronal cellular metabolism associated with hypoglycaemia.		Patient will remain seizures free and without injury.	• Implement measures to protect patient from potential injury associated with seizure activity and neuroglucopoenia. ◆ Identify patient at risk of developing seizures. ◆ Assess for seizure activity: – Patient's activity at time of seizure – Precipitating event. – Description on onset and progression note any changes in pupil size and reactivity; urinary or bowel incontinence. – Duration of apneic periods if generalized seizure.	• Precautions can be taken to avert seizure activity and to protect the patient from injury. • An alteration in the level of consciousness may occur due to a variety of circum-stances. Careful assessment and description of seizure activity may be helpful in diagnosing and treating the underlying problem.

Contd...

Contd...

Problem	*R*	*Objective*	*Nursing Interventions*	*Rationales*
			– Duration of seizure activity. – Patient's post-seizure behaviour. ◆ Institute seizure precautions: – Side rails padded and kept in up position. – Bed placed in low position if possible – Oral airway conspicuously placed at head of bed. – Suction equipment available for emergency care. – Available oxygen source. – Removal of potentially harmful objects from bedside.	
Nursing Diagnosis # 3 Nutrition, alteration in less than body requirements, related to: 1. Altered glucose metabolism.		Patient's condition will stabilize: 1. Serum glucose levels maintained within normal physiologic range: 70-110 mg/100 ml. 2. Body weight will stabilize within appropriate range positive nitrogen balanced will be maintained. 3. Patient will verbalize an increase in strength and improved appetite. 4. Patient will verbalize the effect of alcohol on glucose metabolism.	• Implement patient care activities to assist patient/family to understand execute prescribed nutritional regimen. ◆ Assess patient for the following: – Anorexia, nausea, vomiting, diarrhoea hunger, weakness, diaphoresis, tremors. – Inquire of patient and /or family if this adrenergic symptomatology occurred at home and under what circumstances.	• Hypoglycaemia stimulates sympathetic nervous system activity; such symptomatolgy suggest at low serum glucose. ◆ It is essential to identify the precipitating cause of hypoglycaemic episodes in order to determine how they can be prevented.
			◆ Consult with nutritionist, physician, patient, and family to determine nutritional needs. – Baseline nutritional status. – Must include patient/family past eating habits, food preferences, and preparation.	◆ Baseline nutritional needs must be identified to ensure adequate nutritional intake: (1) maintenance of glucose homeostasis; (2) prevention of recurring hypoglycaemic episodes; (3) and reduction of risk of infection or other stressor.
			◆ Involve patient and family in planning immediate and long-term treatment regimen.	• In the presence of diabetes, nutritional regimen must coincide with insulin or oral hypoglycaemic therapy and exercise regimen. • Involving patient and family in decision-making process fosters compliance
			◆ Consider 6 small meals per day plan.	• Helps to maintain serum glucose within acceptable range; prevents wide fluctuations with periods of hypoglycaemia alliterating with hyperglycaemia.
			◆ Use of anticholinergic therapy.	Used in conjunction with small meals, anticholinergic therapy can reduce rapid gastric emptying. • Rapid gastric emptying and accelerated intestinal glucose absorption can provoke hypoglycaemia in some patients. While the underlying mechanism is unclear, gastrointestinal hormones may contribute to an exaggerated

Contd...

Contd...

Problem	*R*	*Objective*	*Nursing Interventions*	*Rationales*
			◆ Encourage patient and family to verbalize feelings regarding alcohol consumption. – Discuss use of alcohol and imapact on patient's overall status.	glucose-initiated insulin release. The triad of gastrointestinal disease, early onset of hypoglycaemia after eating (within 1-3 hours) and the excessive discharge of insulin characterize the syndrome of alimentary of "intestinal-hurry" hypoglycaemia. • Alcohol interferes with hepatic gluconeogenesis, decreasing availability of glucose during the postabsorptive state.
Nursing Diagnosis # 4 Knowledge deficit regarding underlying diseases, and overall therapeutic regimen: Nutritional/insulin or hypoglycaemic therapy/exercise. Nursing Diagnosis # 5 Health management alteration in.		Patient will be able to: 1. Related hypoglycaemia with level of health desired. 2. Specific major underlying principles regarding therapeutic regimen; Diet, insulin or oral hypoglycaemia and exercise. 3. Explain why it is necessary to carry a rapid-acting sugar source, and usefulness of wearing a Medic-Alert tag. 4. State the early signs in symptoms of hypoglycaemia and actions to be taken. 5. Demonstrate self-care activities: Monitoring blood/urine; self-medication.	• Determine the presence of knowledge deficit regarding overall treatment regimen, and diet particular. • Initiate teaching program regarding diet therapy with emphasis on self-care. ◆ Patient/family should become familiar with signs of hypoglycaemia and institute treatment immediately on their appearance. • Assess patient/family knowledge regarding disease syndrome and its essential long-term therapy. ◆ Assess readiness to learn. • Implement teaching program on self-care health–care practices.	• Knowledge of overall therapeutic regimen will facilitate self-care and health management; complications will be minimized. ◆ Patient should verbalize the need to carry a rapid acting sugar source on his or her person at all times a Medic-Alert braciet or wallet card is important to have at all times. • Understanding of underlying disease processes assist patient and family to cope with and to adjust to the limitation imposed by the illness.
Nursing Diagnosis # 6 Noncompliance: Denial.		Patient will be able to: 1. Admit he/she has hypoglycaemic disorder. 2. Ask pertinent questions regarding care. 3. Actively plan necessary changes in lifestyle to include underlying illness. 4. Verbalize need for continued and regular follow-up care. 5. Report on available resources within the family and community setting.	• Assess patient's attitude regarding chronic illness. • Allow patient and family to verbalize fears and concerns regarding underlying disease. • Encourage patient to make decisions regarding care. ◆ Have patient/family explain the significance of continued follow-up care.	• Fostering a positive attitude helps to ensure compliance. • Verbalization assists in identifying misconceptions and unwarranted fears; patient and family attitudes regarding the health state desired can be ascertained. • When patient feels in control, he/she may readily assume responsibility for self-care.

4. Hypothyroidism C.
5. Nonislets cell tumors; Mesenchymal tumour.
6. Autoimmune disease, Antibodies that stimulate the insulin receptor (rare).

Reactive hypoglycaemia generally occurs 3 to 5 hours after meals, related to either primary delay in insulin secretion (idiopathic) or rapidly rising postprandial glucose related to rapid gastric emptying postgastric surgery. Failure of the pancreas to keep pace with this rapidly rising postprandial glucose results in later insulin hypersecretion and hypoglycaemia. Reactive hypoglycaemia person have an increased of type 2 DM.

Management of these hypoglycaemia detects the cause and correct the hypoglycaemia. Fasting hypoglycaemia person using insulin or sulfonylureas surreptitiously should be educated regarding deleterious effects and referred for counseling. Reactive hypoglycaemic persons need focus on a prevention or hypoglycaemia episodes by:

1. Delaying the postprandial glucose rise through increased dietary fiber and the use of complex carbohydrates and
2. Enhancing insulin sensitivity through exercise and weight reduction towards desirable body weight.

THE DIABETIC FOOT

One of the complications of DM is diabetic foot. Three major factors play a role in the diabetic foot: neuropathy, ischaemia, and sepsis. Amputation commonly results.

Sensory impairment leads to painless trauma and potention for ulceration. Motor impairment contributes to wasting of intrinsic muscles in the feet, resulting in foot deformity. Foot deformities alter the normal gait and pressure distribution. Friction and resultant callosities may develop and result in fractures in the ankle or forefoot and ultimately there is a significant deformity called a Charcot foot. Anhidrosis as manifestation of autonomic neuropathy can result in excessive dryness and cracking of the skin, which also contributes to infection. A macrovascular and microvascular alteration produces tissue ischarmia and may lead to sepsis. The traid of neuropathy, ischaemia, and sepsis result in gangrene and ultimately leads to amputation.

Gangrene may be classified as dry or wet. *Dry gangrene* occurs when tissue death is not associated with inflammatory changes. Aggressive glycaemic control and hospitalization for IV antibodies to limit spread of infection are necessary. Amputation of effected toes is often necessary.The area must be kept dry to prevent wet gangrene. *Wet gangrene* is gangrene coupled with inflammation, septicaemia, and shock may occur. Paediatric care is critical to attain and maintain a health proper toe nail trimming and use of orthotic extra depth. Extra-width of custom-moulded shoes can prevent ongoing trauma and ultimately the amputation associated with the diabetic foot.

Prevention of microvascular disease, neuropathy, and macrovascular disease should be major focus of the diabetic care. Thorough interim histories, interim physical examination, and measurements of laboratory parts meters will allow for early diagnosis. Therefore, allowing for early intervention and risk factor modifications and prevention of end-stage diseases.

Proper care of the feet is crucial for the patient with peripheral vascular disease. The guidelines for patient teaching regarding foot care includes the following:

- Wash feet daily with a mild soap and warm water. Test water temperature with hand first.
- Pat feet dry gently especially between toes.
- Examine feet daily for cuts, blister, swelling and red, tender areas. Do not depend on feeling sores. If eye sight is poor have lanolin
- Use on feet to prevent skin from drying and craking. Do not apply between toes.
- Use mild foot powder on sweaty foot. Powder feet only, not shoes.
- Do not use commercial remedies to remove calluses or corns.
- Cleanse cuts with warm water and mild soap, covering with clean dressing. Do not use iodine, rubbing alcohol, or strong adhesives.
- Report skin infections or non-healing sores to health care provider immediately.
- Cut toenails even with rounded contour of toes. Do not cut down corners. Soak nails before cutting.
- Separate overlapping toes with cotton or lamp's wool.
- Break in new shoes slowly. Avoid open toe, open-heal, and high-healed shoes. Leather shoes are preferred to plastic ones. Wear slippers with soles. Do not go barefoot. Shake out shoes before use.
- Wear clean, absorbent (cotton or wool) socks or stockings that have not been mended. Coloured socks must be colorfast.
- Do not wear clothing that leaves impressions, hindering circulation.
- Do not use hot water bottles or heating pads to warm feet. Wear socks for warmth.
- Guard against frostbite.
- Exercise feet daily either by walking or by flexing and extending feet in suspended position. Avoid prolonged sitting, standing, or crossing of legs.

Urological and Renal Nursing (Renourological Nursing)

Urology is the study of urinary tract and renal is related to kidneys. Urological and renal nursing (Reno-urological nursing) in the study of the urinary tract and kidneys and nursing management of disorders of urinary tract as well as kidneys. Nursing professional have played an vital role in this area and needs to have an understanding of terminology assessment, pathophysiology and treatment concessesfor disorders of urinary system to enhance the delivery of adequate and appropriate care to respective patient.

ASSESSMENT OF URINARY SYSTEM

Subjective renal assessment begins with an assurance begins with an assessment of the patient's overall state of health and perceptions of what constitutes good health, rather than merely listening of documented health problems and concerns. The interview that explores any patient concerns or health problems especially any urinary tract symptoms which includes.

- Dysuria : Pain/burning with voiding.
- Frequency : Voids multiple times during the day either in large or small amounts.
- Nocturia : Awakens to void; abnormal when it occurs multiple times during the sleep cycle.
- Haematuria : Red blood cells in the urine may be gross (visible to eye) or microscopic (detectable with urine screen and microscope)
- Hesitancy : Difficulty initiating voiding.
- Polyuria : Urine output greater than 3000 ml/24 hours.
- Oliguria : Urine output less than 400 ml/24 hours.
- Anuria : Urine output less than 100 ml/24 hours.
- Urgency : The need to void immediately.
- Urine odour : Foul smell associated with urine.
- Frothing : Excessive foaming of urine.
- Myoglobinuria : Red-brown at times black, pigment in the urine.

When a kidney problem is suspected, the nurse asks the patient directly about the symptoms, moderate or severe renal disease can cause significant observable pathological changes.

The clinical significance of urinary tract symptoms are as follows.

- Dysuria : Found in urinary tract infection (UTI).
- Frequency : Urinary tract infection, retention, hyperglycaemia with increased fluid intake, prostatic hypertrophy.
- Urgency : UTI, bladder irritation, trauma, and tumour.
- Nocturia : Diuretics, prostatic hypertrophy, renal failure/insufficiency, increase fluid intake and congestive heart failure.
- Hesitancy : Partial urethral obstruction, posturinary catheter removal, CNS or spinal cord disease, postprostatectomy and laxity of perineal muscles in older women.
- Frothing : Presence of protein in the urine.
- Foul odour : Urinary tractinfections.
- Polyuria : Diabetes mellitus, hormonal abnormality, diabetes inspiduous high output renal failure.
- Oliguria : Renal failure, urinary retention/obstruction.
- Anuria : Renal failure, total obstructions (trauma, mass).
- Myoglobinuria : Muscle tissue breakdown following extreme physical exertion or massive trauma (myoglobin in muscle Hb) can result in renal failure.
- Haematuria : Renal calculi, urinary tract infection, inflammation of the kidney or bladder, trauma to the kidney or urinary tract. Posturinary catheter removal and menses.

The patient should be questioned about the presence or history of disease that are known to be related to the renal or other urologic problems, which includes hypertension, diabetes mellitus, gout or other metabolic disorders, connective tissue disorders, skin or upper respiratory tract infections of streptococcal origin, tuberculosis, viral hepatitis, congenital disorders, neurologic condition and specific urinary problems such as cancer, infections, BPH, calculosis, etc.

Diagnostic Studies

Diagnostic studies are important in locating and understanding the problems of the urinary system. The nursing responsibilities related to diagnostic studies include providing the patient with an adequate information of the procedure. The period during a diagnostic work-up is typically a time of anxiety for most patients for which patient should be explained regarding the diagnostic procedure and also should be instructed on personal responsibility during particular study according to procedures. Diagnostic studies of the urinary system often cause embarrassment and emotional stress. Examination of the urinary system may be perceived as intrusion on a personal body area. The nurse should alleviate anxiety by providing privacy and protecting the patient's modesty.

Here are the usual diagnostic studies and the routine responsibilities of nurses.

URINE STUDIES

i. Urinalysis

This is a general examination of urine to establish baseline information or provide data to establish tentative diagnosis and determine whether further studies are to order. Here, the nursing responsibilities are:

- Try to obtain first urinated morning specimen.
- Ensure that specimen is examined within 1 hour of urinating.
- Wash perineal area if soiled with menses or foecal material.

ii. Creatinine Clearance

Creatinine is a waste product of protein-breakdown (Primary body muscle mass). Clearance of creatinine by the kidneys approximates the GFR. Normal finding is 85-135 ml/min.

Nursing responsibilities in this test are to:

- Collect 24-hours urine specimen.
- Discard first urination when test is started.
- Save urine from all subsequent urination for 24 hours and add specimen to collections container.
- Ensure urine collection container used.

iii. Urine Culture (Clean Catch "Midstream")

This study is done to compress suspected urinary tract infection and identify causative organisms. Normally bladder is sterile, but urethra contains bacteria, and a few WBCs. If properly collected, stored and handled: < 10,000 organisms/ml usually indicate no infections. But > 100,000/ml indicates infection.

When collecting a *mid-stream* urine specimen, the nurse has to collect needed equipments which include:

- Sterile container for the urine.
- Three sponges (cotton or gauze) saturated with cleansing solution and follow general direction.
- Touch only the outside of the collecting container.
- Collect the urine in container well after urinary stream is started and follow special directions as given below.

For Female

- Keep labia separated throughout the procedure.
- Cleanse the meatus with one front-to-back motion with each of the three cleansing sponges.

For Males

- Retract the foreskin of man in uncircumcised.
- Cleanse the glans with each of the three cleansing sponges.

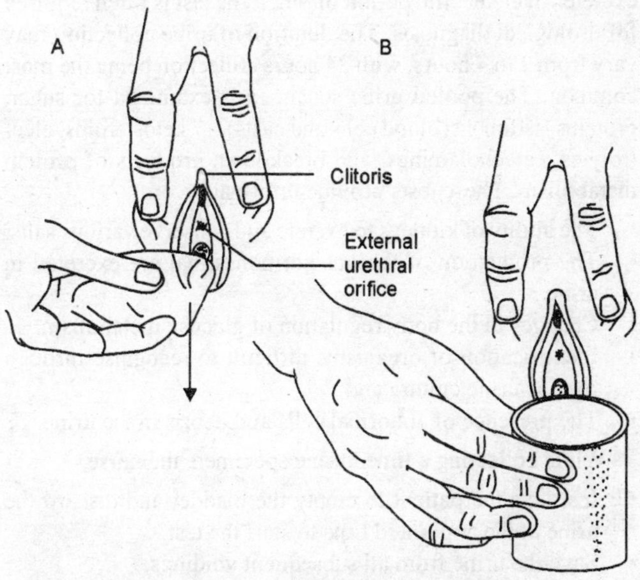

Fig. 14.1: Obtaining a clean-catch midstream urine specimen in the female patient. (A) Instruct the patient to hold the labia apart and wash from high up front toward the back with gauze soaked in soap. (B) The collection cup is held so that it does not touch the body, and the sample is obtained only while the patient is voiding with the labia held apart.

The collected specimen are ideally transported to the laboratory within 30 minutes or promptly refrigerated.

iv. Concentration Test (Fishberg)

This study evaluates renal concentration ability. The test is used to determine ability of kidney to conserve fluid and to establish differential diagnosis for diabetes insipidus and psychogenic polydypsia. The normal readings are:

- Urine volume 300 ml/12 hours.
- Specific gravity 1.020 to 1.035.
- Urine osmolity of 850 m. om or greater.

In this test, instruct patient to fast after given time in evening (in usual procedure). No fluid can be taken during test period. For period 8-12-hours usually during night. First morning void ensures maximal concentration. Three-hourly urine specimen are collected for volume, specific gravity, and osmolality after test period. Patient should be observed for signs of vascular collapse.

v. Urine Cytology

This study is to identify charges in cellular structure indicative of malignancy, especially bladder cancer. Here obtain urine and send immediately to laboratory. The first morning specimen should not be used.

vi. Timed Urine Collection

A timed urine collection involves pooling of all the urine patient excretes over specific period of time. The test is often required for urological diagnosis. The duration of urine collection may vary from 2 to 4 hours, with 24 hours collection being the most common. The pooled urine specimen is examined for sugar, proteins, sediment (blood cells and casts). 17 ketosteroids, electrolytes, catecholamines, and breakdown products of protein metabolism. These tests provide information on:

- The ability of kidneys to excrete and conserve various salts.
- The production of various hormones that are excreted in urine.
- Changes in the body regulation of glucose metabolism.
- Identification of organisms difficult to recognise through routine urine culture and
- The presence of abnormal cells and debris in the urine.

While collecting a timed urine specimen, the nurse

- Instructs the patient to empty the bladder and discard the urine at the appointed time to start the test.
- Save the urine from all subsequent voidings.
- Provide specific directions for storing the urine. Some specimen need to be kept cold during the collection period, and some need preservatives and some need no special care.
- Instruct the patient to void into a separate receptacle before defecating to avoid contaminating the specimen.
- Instruct the patient to empty the bladder and add the urine to the collection at the appointed time to end the test.
- Send the designated amount (properly labeled) to the laboratory.

Timed urine test also may involve collecting urine from more than one source (ex. through the nephrostomy tube) follow instructions accordingly.

Blood Chemistries

i. *Blood Urea Nitrogen* (BUN). This study is most commonly used to identify presence of renal problems. Concentration of urea, in blood is regulated by rate at which kidney excretes urea. The normal finding is 5.20 mg/100 ml. Test indicates ability of kidneys to excrete nitrogenous wastes. BUN can be affected by high protein diet, blood in GI tract and catabolic state (injury, infection, fever and poor nutrition). Be aware that when interpreting BUN, nonrenal factors may cause increase (e.g. rapid cell destructions from infection, GI bleeding, trauma, athletic activity with excessive muscle breakdown and corticosteroid therapy).

ii. *Serum Creatinine*. This is more reliable than BUN as a determinant of renal function. Creatinine is end product of muscle and protein metabolism and is liberated at a constant rate. Normal finding in men: 0.85-1.5 mg/100 ml and in women 0.7-1.25 mg/100 ml. Test indicates ability of kidneys to excrete creatinine. Serum creatinine gives a rough estimate of GFR. No specific preparation needed for test. Diet and metabolic rate have little effect on creatinine values.

iii. *Uric acid*. This study is used as a screening test primarily for disorders of purine metabolism but can indicate kidney disease as well. Values depend on renal function and rate of purine metabolism and dietary intake of food rich in purines. Normal values is 2.5-5.5 ml/dl in women and 4.5-6.5 ml/dl in men.

iv. *Sodium* (Na^+). It is main extracellular electrolyte determining blood volume. Usually values stay within normal range until late stages of renal failure. Normal findings are 135-145 mEq/litre.

v. *Potassium* (K^+) Kidneys are responsible for excreting majority of body's potassium. Potassium determinations are critical because potassium is one of the first electrolytes to become abnormal. Elevated K^+ levels of > m Eq/L can lead to muscle weakness and cardiac arrythmias. Normal findings is 3.5 - 5.5 m Eq/L.

vi. *Calcium* (Ca^+) Calcium is main mineral in bone and helps in muscle contraction, neuro transmission, and clotting. In renal disease, decreased absorption of calcium leads to renal osteodystrophy. Normal findings is 9-11 mg/dL (4.5-5.5 mEq/L).

vii. *Phosphorous*. Phosphorous balance is inversely related to a calcium balance. In renal disease, phosphorous levels are elevated because the kidney is the primary excretary organ. Soft tissue calcification may occur in both phosphorous in C^{a-1} are elevated. Normal findings is 2.8-4.5 mg/dl.

viii. *Bicarbonate* (HCO^{-3}): Most patients in renal failure have metabolic acidosis and low serum HCO^3 levels. Normal finding is 20-30 mEq/L.

Radiological Studies

i. KUB (Kidney Ureter, Bladder) X-ray films. This study involves flat-plate X-ray examination of abdomen, and pelvis and delineates size, shape and position of kidneys. In this gross visualization of KUB location of calcifications and stones are possible. For this test bowel cleansing sometimes is ordered.

ii. *IVP* (Intravenous Pyelography): X-ray examination visualizes urinary tract after IV injection of contrast material (dye).

The purposes of IVP are:

- Determination of size and location of kidneys.
- Demonstrations of presence of cysts or tumours.
- Outline of filling of renal pelvis.
- Outline of ureters and bladder.

In this procedure:

- X-ray film of abdomen (KUB) taken to identify size and position of kidneys.
- Radiopaque dye given intravenously.
- X-ray films of kidneys taken at 3-, 5-, 10 and 20-minutes interval.

For this procedure, preparation includes:

- Evening before procedure, give cathartic or enema to empty colon of feces and gas.
- Keep patient on NPO status 8 hours prior to the procedure.
- Before the procedure, assess the patient for any history of allergy to iodine, shelfish, or dyes to avoid anaphylactic reactions.
- Inform patient that a feeling of warmth, flustering of the face, and salty taste in the mouth may occur as the dye is injected.
- Inform the procedure involved, lying on table and heavy serial X-rays taken.
- Inform patient that numerous X-ray and films are taken during the procedure. This does not indicate a problem.
- During the procedure, patient should be carefully monitored for signs and symptoms of a reaction to dye, including respiratory distress, diaphoresis, urticaria, instability of viral signs or unusual sensations. Emergency equipment should be available.
- After the procedure, fluids are forced to help excrete or flush out the contrast material and prevent renal failure.

iii. *Nephrotomogram.* X-ray is taken with rotating tubes. Multiple exposures are taken to visualize specific sections of the kidney after IV injection of contrast material (dye). Explain procedure and prepare patient as for IVP.

iv. *Retrograde Pyelography.* This is performed for visualization of urinary tract. X-ray of urinary tract is taken after the injection of contrast material into kidneys, cystoscope is inserted and urethral catheters are inserted through it into renal pelvis. Contrast material (Radiopaque matter is injected through the catheters. X-ray films are taken of renal collecting structure. Here also prepare patient as for IVP and

- Inform patient that pain may be experienced from distension of pelvis and discomfort from cystoscope.
- Inform patient that general anaesthesia may be given for procedure.

v. *Cystogram:* In this, contrast material is instilled into bladder via cystoscope or catheter. Its purpose is to visualize bladder and evaluate vesicoureteral reflux. Nursing responsibility is as in cystoscope.

vi. *Renal Angiography*. The purpose of this test is to visualization of renal circulation. Particularly, useful in evaluating renal contrast material (dye) often injected directly into femoral artery by passing a catheter through artery to level of renal arteries.

Nursing implications are the same as for IVP.

- Patient must be observed for dye-induced acute renal failure and bleeding at arterial puncture site especially in the first 4 hours.
- The pressure dressing should be checked for fresh bleeding.
- The puncture site should be checked for tenderness or swelling.
- Vital signs and distal pulses must be assessed frequently for every 15 minutes and 4 hours.
- Bed rest should be maintained for 8 hours after the procedure.

vii. *Ultrasound.* In this,small external ultrasound probe is placed on patient's skin. Conductive gel is applied to the skin. Non-invasive procedure involves passing sound waves into body structure and recording images as they are reflected back. Computer interprets tissue density based on sound waves and displays it in picture form. Study is most valuable in detection of renal or perirenal masses. Differential diagnosis of renal cysts, solid masses and identification of obstruction It can be used safely in patients with renal failure. Since this procedure is painless and noninvasive. A full bladder is required to delineate the abdominal structure.

viii. *CT Scan*. This study provides excellent visualization of kidneys and renal circulation using an X-ray beam rotated around body. A kidney size can be evaluated, tumours, abscesses, suprarenal masses (e.g. adrenal tumours, pheochromocytomas) and obstruction can be detected.

Advantage of CT over ultrasound is its ability to distinguish subtle difference in density. Use of IV administered contrast material during CT accentuates density of renal tissue and helps differentiate masses. Whole body CT scanner segments kidneys. If dye is used, the same nursing implications apply as listed in IVP.

ix. *MRI*. Computer-generated films rely on radio waves and alteration in magnetic field. It is useful for visualization of kidneys. It has not been not proven useful for detecting urinary calculi or calcified tumours. In this, there is need to explain procedure to the patient. Have patient removed all metal objects. Patient with a history of claustraphobia needs to be sedated.

x. *Renal Radionuclide Imaging (RRI).* In renal scan, radioactive isotopes are injected. IV radiation detector probes are placed over kidney and scintillation counter monitors radioactive material in kidneys. Purpose is to show blood flow, glomerular filtration, tubular function and excretion. Radioisotope distribution in kidney is scanned and mapped. Test is usual in showing location, size and shape of kidney and in general assessing blood perfusion and its ability to secrete urine. Abscesses, cysts and tumours may appear or coast spots because of presence of non-functioning tissue.

This procedure requires no dietary or activity restriction. Inform patient that no pain or discomfort should be felt during test.

Endoscopy

Endoscopy: i.e.,Cystoscopy study involves use of tubular-lighted scope to inspect bladder. Lithotomy position is used. It may be done using local or general anaesthesia. The nursing responsibilies include:

- Before the procedure, force fluids or give IV fluids if general anaesthesia is to be used.
- Ensure that consent form is signed.
- Explain procedure to the patient.
- Give preoperative medication.
- After procedure, explain that burning on urination, pink-tinged urine and urination frequency are expected effects after cystoscopy.
- Do not let patient walk alone immediately after the procedure because orthostatic hypotension may occur.
- Offer warm site bath, heat and mild analgesics to relieve discomfort.

Urodynamics

Urodynamics: i.e. Cystometrogram. This study involves insertion of catheter and instillation of water or saline solution into bladder. Measurement of pressure exerted against bladder wall is recorded. Purpose is to evaluate bladder tone, sensations of filling, and bladder (detrusor) stability. This test needs explain procedure to the patient and observe patient for manifestation of urinary tract infections after the procedure.

Invasive Procedure

Invasive procedure: i.e., Renal biopsy is the technique usually done as a skin (percutaneous) biopsy through needle insertion into lower lobe of kidney. Prupose is to obtain renal tissue examination to determine type of renal disease or to follow progress of renal disease. Before the procedure, ascertain coagulation status through patient history, medications, history, CBC, haematocrit, prothrombin time and bleeding and clotting time, type and crossmatch for patient's blood. Ensure that consent form is signed. Be aware that IVP or ultrasound study is done before biopsy. After procedure, apply pressure dressing to biopsy site and check frequently for bleeding. And

- Bedrest must be maintained with the patient flat, in a supine position and motionless for 4 hours after renal biopsy.
- Coughing is avoided for first 4 hours after biopsy.
- Blood pressure and pulse should be taken on the following schedule.
  - Every 15 minutes for 1 hour, every 30 minutes for 1 hour, every hour for 2 hours until it becomes stable.
- Bedrest should be maintained for 24 hours.
- Urine is observed for haematuria for first 24 hours and biopsy.
- Patient should avoid heavy lifting for 10 days after biopsy.
- Assess patient for flank pain. Monitor haematocrit levels.

INFLAMMATORY DISORDERS OF URINARY SYSTEM

Urinary Tract Infections (UTI)

Infections of the urinary tract may appear as a variety of disorders. Infections may be broadly classified as upper and lower UTI, based on the patient's symptoms. Terminology may specifically delineate the site of inflammations or infection. Examples of terms are 'pyeloenephritis' (involvement of kidneys and kidney pelvis) and cystitis (involvement of bladder). Lower UTIs involve the urinary bladder (cystitis), urethra (Urethritis) and prostatitis. Upper UTS may involve kidney and renal pelvis (Pyelonephritis).

Aetiology

The urinary tract above the urethra is normally sterile. Several physiologic and mechanical defense mechanisms assist in maintaining sterility and preventing UTIs. These defenses include normal voiding with complete emptying of the bladder. Normal antibacterial ability of bladder mucosa and urine, ureterovesicle junction competence, and peristaltic activity that propels urine towards bladder. An alteration in any of these defence mechanisms increases the risk of contracting a UTI.

Common micro-organisms causing urinary tract infections are:

- Escheria coli
- Enterococci
- Klebsiella
- Enterobacter
- Serratia
- Proteus
- Pseudomonas
- Staphylococci
- Candida

The risk factors associated with development of urinary tract infections are:

i. Female due to : Short urethra, close proximity to vagina and anus.
: Postmenopausal decrease in oestrogen and loss of vaginal lactobacilli, which prevent infection.
: Diminished ureteral peristalsis (e.g. pregnancy).
: Use of diaphragm.

ii. Structural abnormality
   - Stricture urethra.
   - Incompetent ureterovesical function anomalies.

iii. Obstruction
   - Compression of growing uterus against ureter, compression of growing uterus against ureters. (e.g. tumour, fibroids).
   - Presence of tumours, calculi, prostatic hypertrophy.
   - Iatrogenic causes.

iv. Impaired bladder innervation
   - Congenital spinal cord malformation.
   - Spinal cord injury.
   - Multiple sclerosis.
   - Urinary stasis.
   - Neurogenic bladder.

v. Chronic diseases
   - Gout, diabetes mellitus, hypertension, sickle cell disease.
   - Polycystic kidney disease, multiple myeloma.
   - Glomerulonephritis.
   - Immunosuppression.

vi. Instrumentation
   - Catheterization.
   - Diagnostic procedures.
   - Incomplete-bladder emptying.

vii. Age
   - Decreased acidity of urine.
   - Anaemia and malnutrition.

viii. Renal scarring from previous UTIs.

The mode of entry of bacteria into the genitorurinary tract can always be traced with certainty. There are four major pathways exist:

i. *Ascending infection* From the urethra it is the most common cause of genitourinary tract infection in men and women. As the female urethra is short and rectal bacteria tend to colonize the perineum and vaginal vestibule, females are especially susceptible to ascending urinary tract infections. A common factor contributes ascending infection is urologic instrumentation (catheterization-cystoscopy). Sexual intercourse has been shown to be a major precipitating factor of UTI in women. Sexual intercourse promotes milking of bacteria from vagina and preineum and may cause minor urethral trauma that predisposes women to UTIs. UTIs associated with sexual intercourse can develop as quickly as 12 hours after intercourse.

ii. *Haematogenous spread* Occurs infrequently. With the exception of tuberculosis, renal abscesses are perinephric abscesses. Bacteraemia is more likely to complicate UT when structural and functional abnormalities exist and when the urinary tract is normal.

iii. *Lymphogenous spread is rare* Bacterial pathogens travel through the rectal and colonic lymphatics to the prostate and bladder through the preuterine lymphatic in the female genitourinary tract.

iv. Direct extension from another organ occurs with extraperitoneal abscesses, especially those associated with inflammation, bowel disease, fulminant, pelvic inflammatory disease in women, paravesical abscesses and genitourinary tract fisutla and pyelonephritis.

Pathophysiology

Normally urine produced in kidneys flows unobstructed through urinary tract. Urine is sterile unit which reaches urethra. Most UTIs result from gram-negative organisms, such as E-coli-klebsiella, proteus or pseudomonas, that originate in the persons own intestinal tract and ascend through the urethra to the bladder. During micturition urine may flow back the ureters (vesicoureteral reflux) and carry bacteria from the bladder up through the ureters to the kidney pelvis. Whenever urinary stasis occurs, such as with incomplete emptying of the bladder, renal calculi, or genitourinary obstructions, the bacteria have a greater opportunity to grow. Urinary stasis also promotes a more alkaline urine which facilitates bacterial growth. UTI occurs primarily when host resistance is impaired due to above stated causes.

Clinical Manifestation

The symptoms that bring the person with UTI seek medical attention typically include frequency, urgency, dysuria, (burning on urination) cloudy or foul-smelling urine, suprapubic discomfort, and haematuria, becteriuria, upper UTIs and pyelonephritis are associated with fever, flank pain, costovertebral angle tenderness, nausea, and vomiting. Most persons, however, are asymptomatic or minimally symptomatic. In these persons, UTI is identified only on routine examination of the urine. Bacteriuria and positive urine cultures serve as basis for diagnosing lower UTIs.

Management

Diagnostic test includes urinanalysis, culture and sensitivity test before starting medication. If necessitated, advance test like IVP cystogram.

Medication typically used is the treatment of urinary tract infections include anti-infectives, analgesics and anticholenergies.

i. Trimethoprimsulf a methoxazole (Bactrim, Septran) is folate antoganist, enzymatic inhibition of bacterial synthesis, when patient is on the medication:
   - Increase fluid intake to 1500 ml/day.
   - Monitor intake and output.
   - Observe for adverse reactions (rash, hives, etc.).

ii. *Nitrofurantoin* interferes with bacterial enzyme systems. When patient is on this medication.
   - Administer with food or milk.
   - Avoid exposure of the drug to light.
   - Space dose equally around the clock.

iii. *Ciprofloxacin* inhibits DNA-gyrase, preventing bacterial DNA replication. During this treatment, nurse:
  - Instructs the patient to avoid antacids.
  - Encouirage intake of at least 1500 ml/day.
  - Monitor intake and output.
  - Assess nausea, vomiting and diarrhoea.

iv. *Amoxicillin* inhibits mucoprotein synthesis in the cell wall of rapidly dividing bacteria. During this treatment, the nurse, should:
  - Observe for urticaria or rash.
  - Assess renal, hepatic, and haematological function.
  - Administer round the clock without skipping doses.

Analgesics such as penozopyridine (Pyridin, urogenic), local anaesthetic action on urinary mucosa. Administer after meals. Instruct patient that urine may turn orange and will stain fabrics. Avoid use more than 5 days.

Anticholenergic such as propantheline bromide (Probanthin). Potent antimuscarinic activity, decreases bladder spasm. Administer one hour before meals do not crush medications, assess bowel sounds, and postural hypertension.

Additional treatment includes increasing fluid intake to 3 to 4 liters per day unless it is contraindicated. Increased fluid intake helps to dilute the urine, lessens irritation and burning, and provides a continued flow of urine to minimize stasis and multiplication of bacteria in the urinary tract. Sitz bath may provide comfort for individual with urethritis. And regular intake of vitamin C in sufficient dose to be excreted in the urine can reduce bacterial growth due to ascorbic acid. Lemon juice may be provided to increase ascorbic acidity to prevent growth of bacteria.

Health education to be given to the public to reduce urinary tract infections in the community are regarding:

- Symptoms of urinary tract infections.
- Need for prompt medical attention when symptoms of UTI occurs.
- Need to continue drug therapy even though symptoms abate.
- Importance of following care and repeat urine culture.
- Maintenance of fluid intake of 3 to 4 L/day if patient's health permits as increased fluid intake helps flush bacteria out of the urinary system.
- Avoidance of bubble bath, powders, and harsh soaps in the perineal area.
- Wearing of cotton underpants as nylon and synthetic fabrics do not allow ventilation and may facilitate bacterial growth.
- Avoidance of tight-fitting pants that may irritate the urethra.
- For women, importance of wiping perineal area from front to back to prevent introducing bacteria into the urethra.
- Need to shower instead of tubbath for persons with recurrent urinary tract infections.
- Need to increase fluid intake before and after sexual intercourse and empty the bladder immediately after intercourse.
- Avoidance of urinary stasis by voiding approximately every 2 to 4 hours.
- Need for regular intake of vitamin C or cranberry juice or lemon juice to help prevent urinary tract infections.

Cystitis

Cystitis is the inflammation of the urinary bladder.

Aetiology

The incidence of cystitis is very high in women followed by older men and young children especially in girls. These age and sex variation in the frequency of cystitis are related to anatomic differences or pathologic changes in the groups at risk. The adult female urethra is short and the proximity to rectum and vagina predisposes women to the risk of bladder contamination. Bacterial contamination of the bladder can be the result of poor personal hygienic practices and sexual intercourse.

In children, vesicoureteral reflux is usually the pre-existing abnormality. In men, the longer urethra (of which the proximal two-thirds is normally sterile) and the antibacterial property of prostatic secretions provide protection from bacterial infections, unless there are predisposing causes such as BPH.

Pathophysiology

Once cystitis has occurred, it may remain localized in the urinary bladder for years without ascension to the kidneys or may be completely resolved after initial treatment. Although the bacterial infection may be self-limiting, the urinary tract should be evaluated if there is recurrence, even in the patients who have no symptoms. The risk of recurrent symptomatic infection is increased when there are urinary tract abnormalities. Asymptomatic bacteriuria can occur and is no synonymous with UTI. It indicates that bacteria can be present in the urine. Tissue invasion must occur for an infection to exist. Pyuria (the presence of WBCs in the urine) usually signals this occurrence and is the characteristic laboratory findings in symptomatic UTI.

Clinical Manifestation

The manifestation of cystitis are frequency and urgency of urination, suprapubic pain, dysuria, foul-smelling urine and pyuria. Haematuria may or may not occur in symptomatic UTI. The presence of fever, nausea, vomiting, and flank tenderness usually indicates pyelonephritis. About half of all persons with significant bacteruria have no symptoms or may reflect nonspecific signs such as increased fatigue, anorexia, or changes in cognitive ability. The incidence of asymptomatic bacteriuria increases greatly with age. Asymptomatic bacteriuria is more likely to occur in women over 65 years of age.

Diagnostic studies

- Urinalysis for presence of WBC.
- Urine for gram stain.
- Urine for culture and sensitivity with clean-catch urine.
- IVP, cystoscopy if indicated.

The nurse should be aware that noninfectious agents also cause irritative bladder symptoms similar to UTI and intravesical chemotherapy or pelvic radiation.

Management

Uncomplicated cystitis are treated with antimicrobial therapy which includes, bactrim, septra, nitrofurantoin and cephalexin, of which single time therapy or 1 to 3 days or therapy. Prophylactic antibiotic therapy is given to prevent recurrence of after treatment of UTI. Acute intervention for a patient with cystitis includes an adequate fluid intake if this is not contraindicated which helps increase feelings or urgency and frequency and also dilute the urine to reduce irritation in the bladder. Potential bladder irritants like coffee, alcohol, citrus juices, chocolate and highly-spiced food or beverages should be avoided. The patient should be instructed to take complete course of treatment as prescribed and periodical urine examination should be done, i.e. gross or microscopic haematuria. Presence of WBCs, malodor and sediment and follow health education as in UTI. Acute intervention for a patient with cystitis includes an adequate fluid intake if this is not contraindicated which helps increased feeling of urgency and frequency and also dilutes the urine to reduce irritation and the bladder.

Pyelonephritis

Pyelonephritis usually is an infectious inflammatory disease that involves both the parenchyma and the kidney pelvis. In other words, it is an acute or chronic inflammatory process of the renal pelvis and parenchyma of the kidneys.

Aetiology

Generally the inflammatory process is caused by bacterial invasion. Most infections are caused by the normal inhabitation of the intestinal tract (e.g. E. coli, proteus, klebsiella and enterobacter). Pyelonepohritis is most frequently associated with cystitis, pregnancy or obstruction, instrumentation or trauma of the urinary tract. Pregnant women with bacteriuria are at significant risk for developing pyelonephritis. Other risk factors include septicaemia or chronic health problem, including diabetes analgesic abuse, polycystic kidney disease and hypertensive kidney disease.

Pathophysiology

Pyelonephritis usually ascends from the lower urinary tract. A pre-existing factor is often present in children, associated with vesicoureteral reflux or other urinary tract abnormalities. In adults, common pre-existing factors are bladder tumours, prostate hyperplasia, strictures, urinary stones and pregnancy. Infection of the kidney occurs in both acute and chronic forms. Acute pyelonephritis may temporarily affect renal function, but rarely progresses to renal failure. Repeated attacks of acute pyelonephritis especially in the presence of abnormalities can result in chronic pyelonophritis. The infection commonly starts in the renal medulla and spreads to the adjacent cortex. The infected portion of kidney heals resulting in fibrosis and scarring. The process of developing chronic renal failure from repeated kidney infections occurs over a number of years or after several extensive and fulminant infections.

Clinical Manifestations

The normal functions of the kidney is the regulation of fluids, electrolytes, and blood pressure and also excretion of metabolic wastes. The clinical manifestations of acute pyelonephritis vary from mild lassitude to the sudden onset of chills, fever, vomiting, malaise, flank pain, dysuria and frequent urination. Symptoms of cystitis may or may not be present. Costovertebral tenderness will be present on the affected side. The clinical manifestation usually subsides within a few days or even without specific therapy. However, bacteriuria or pyuria may persist. The results of CBC shows leukocytosis and a shift to the left with an increase in banded neutrophills. Urinalysis shows pyuria, bacteriuria and varying degrees of haematuria. White cell casts may be found in the urine.

In chronic pyelonephritis, the only symptom may be persistent bacteriuria until extensive scarring and atrophy result in renal insufficiency, as manifested by hypertension, increased blood urea nitrogen (BUN) and decreased creatine clearance. Bacteraemia can occur secondary to a UTI ascending to the kidney and can reuslt in sepsis. Some patient may develop septic shock as a result of endotosin produced by gram-negative bacteria that are released in the blood.

Management

Optimal treatment of pyelonephritis includes early detection of the bacterial infection through urine culture, antibacterial therapy based on identified sensitivities and detection and treatment of any underlying systemic disease or urinary abnormalities.

The routine diagnostic test includes urinalysis, urine culture and sensitivity (Gram stains), IVP, ultrasound or CT scan and WBC count. Blood cultures (if bacteria suspected) and palpation of flank pain are needed.

For mild symptoms, outpatient management of short hospitalization for IV antibiotics, administration of oral antibiotics for 14-21 days (e.g. Bactrim, septra, cephalxin, ciprofloxacin, nitrofurantoin, norflaxacin, ofloxacin—and any one of them) i.e. the course of antibiotic therapy may extend over weeks. The urine is recultured 2 weeks after drug therapy has been discontinued and monthly for several months thereafter. If infection becomes chronic, maintenance of drug therapy may continue indefinitely; the goal is to reduce and control the bacterial population of the urinary tract to prevent renal damage. If bacteraemia is a possibility, close observation and vital sign monitoring are essential. Prompt recognition and treatment of septic shock may prevent irreversible damage.

For severe symptoms, hospitalization is very essential for administrational parenteral antibiotics. It is important to maintain sufficient urinary flow to remove by-products of the inflammation and to prevent urinary stasis with further bacterial growth. Fluid intake of 3 L/day is encouraged in persons with normal excretory function. During the acute phase, the patient is encouraged to rest. Prescribed analgesics may be given for flank pain. Back massage often gives short-term relief. Pain ceases as the inflammation resolves.

Nursing interventions vary depending on the severity of symptoms. These interventions include teaching the patient about the disease process with emphasis on:

- The need for continuing medication as prescribed.
- The need for follow-up urine culture to ensure proper management and
- Identification recurrence of infection or relapse.

Persons with pyelonephritis may be treated at home, therefore teaching is very important. Instructions to patient include:

- Continue antibiotic therapy even after symptoms resolve.
- Drink 3 L/per day (at least 8 glasses of fluids) of fluids unless otherwise instructed.
- Monitor urinary output: report to the physician if output is considerably less than fluid intake.
- Weigh self daily: report if a sudden weight gain to physician.
- Take measures to prevent infection: report signs of urinary infection (increased flank pain, fever, chills, frequency, urgency) to physician.
- Continue with medical follow-up and have follow-up urine culture as instructed.

Urethritis

Urethritis is an inflammation of the urethra is often difficult to diagnose, but the clinical manifestations are the same as those for cystitis. The female urethra may be extremely tender or there may be a discharge especially in men. Inflammatory changes may make recovery of bacteria difficult because they become entrapped in urithral tissues and do not appear in the urine.

Aetiology

The causes of urethritis include a bacterial or viral infection, Trichomonas and monilial infection (especially in women), chlamydia and chlamydia and gonorrhoea (especially in men). Urethritis may coexist with cystitis.

Management

Any urethral discharge may confirm a diagnosis of urethritis. Cultures on split urine collections taken at beginning of urine flow and then midstream are helpful. Detection of chlamydial organisms requires tissue culture or immunological testing for Chlamydial antigen in urethral or cervical specimens. Chlamydial infection is less likely to cause haematuria and suprapubic pain than bacterial infection.

Treatment is based on identifying and treating the cause and providing symptomatic relief.

- Bactrim septran, nitrofurants for bacterial infection.
- Flagal for treating trichomonas infection.
- Nystatin of flucanizol of moniliasis infection.
- Doxycyclein for chlamydial infection.

Women with negative urine culture and the pyuria do not respond to antibiotics. Hot sitz bath without perfumed bath oil or bath salts may relieve the symptoms. The patient should be instructed to avoid the use of vaginal deodorants sprays, to properly cleanse the perineal area after bowel movements and urination and to avoid intercourse until symptoms subside.

Renal Tuberculosis

Renal tuberculosis is a secondary infection caused by pulmonary tuberculosis.

Aetiology

Mycobacterium tuberculosis is the causative agent of renal tuberculosis.

Pathophysiology

Renal tuberculosis occurs after the M. tuberculosis invades the kidney. Early in the disease, renal cortex or medulla is affected. Tissue damage is progressive and eventually the renal cortex can rupture into the renal pelvis and infection can spread via the mucosa to the remainder of the urinary tract. If infection involves ureters, strictures can develop complicating the infection by causing an obstruction. In addition, blood supply will also be affected due to the destruction of kidney tissues by masses of the tubercles. Initially, collateral circulation will become insufficient and the kidney will become ischaemic.

Clinical Manifestation

Clinical manifestations of renal tuberculosis are mild and usually include loss of appetite, unexplained weight loss and intermittent fever. Haematuria may also be present. Diagnostic tests usually include screening for pulmonary tuberculosis. The patient will have psoitive Mantoux skin test. Urine samples also are obtained and screened for the presence of M. tuberculosis.

Management

Treatment usually involves antituberculosis medication. Medications typically used include isonaizid, rifampin and ethambutol. Drug therapy is usually given for 9 to 24 months. If the spread of infection has caused structural damages, a nephrectomy or urinary diversion may be necessary. Nursing care is focussed on managing pain and discomfort and education regarding the medication regimen. Patient must be instructed to continue entire causes of medication even after symptoms subside. Educating the patient and family and community regarding the risk factors and prevention of tuberculosis.

Chemical-Induced Nephritis

Chemical-induced nephritis is an idiosyncratic reaction that results in damage to the kidney tubules and interstitium.

Aetiology

This disease process was first noted in patient's sensitiveness to the sulfonamides. The many other substances are now associated with chemical-induced nephritis which are as follows:

i. Solvents
- Carbon tetrachloride
- Methanol
- Ethyline glycol.

ii. Heavy metals
- Lead
- Arsenic
- Mercury

iii. Antibiotics
- Kanamycin
- Gentamycin
- Amphoteracin B
- Calistin
- Neomycin
- Phenazopyridine.

iv. Pesticides and poisonous mushrooms.

Pathophysiology

Chemical-induced nephritis usually begins within 15 days exposure to the chemical. The inflammatory process disrupts the ability of the glomeruli to filter. Furthermore, the capillary membrane becomes permeable to plasma proteins and RBCs which result in proteinuria and haematuria.

Clinical Manifestation

The signs and symptoms of the nephritis include fever, eosinophilia, haematuria, mild proteinuria and rash. Oliguria or urine output of 400 ml or less in a 24 hours period occurs. Urinalysis used to demonstrate protein or RBCs in the urine. Serum toxicology screening may identify the source of the nephritis.

Management

Medical management includes immediate withdrawal of the suspected chemical. Haemodialysis may be required to remove the nephrotoxin from the blood. Steroids are often administered because of their anti-inflammatory effect. If renal function is severely compromised, dietary sodium and protoein restriction may be instituted. The patient is assessed for fluid and electrolyte imbalance, including presence of oedema, blood pressure changes, and adventious breath sounds. The person needs to know the rationale for maintenance of fluid balance and any sodium restriction.

Education of the patient focuses on prevention. Patients should be instructed to keep solvents in well-ventilated areas. All household chemicals should be clearly labelled. The health care professional including nurses must be aware of the causative agents and signs and symptoms associated with chemical-induced nephritis. With early detection and removal of causative agent as soon as possible, the prognosis improves. A major risk factor is industrial exposure to chemicals. Occupational health professional should be aware of potential risks and should educate employees regarding appropriate preventive measures.

Glomerulonephritis

Glomerulonephritis is a disease, that affects the glomeruli of both kidneys i.e. inflammation of the glomeruli. Although the glomerulus is the primary site of inflammation, tubular, interstitial, and vascular changes also occur.

Aetiological factors are many and varied; they include:

- Immunological reactions (systematic lupus erythematosus and streptococcal infection).
- Vascular injury (hypertension).
- Metabolic disease (diabetes mellitus) and
- Disseminated intravascular coagulation.

Glomerulonephritis is divided into a number of classifications which may describe:

- The extent of damage (diffuse or focal).
- The initial cause of the disorder (systematic lupus erythematosa, streptococcal infection, scleroderma, and/or
- The extent of change (minimal or widespread).

Glomerulonephritis exists in acute, latent and chronic form.

Acute Glomerulonephritis

Acute poststreptococcal glomerulonephritis (APSGN) is most common in children and young adults, but all age groups can be affected.

Aetiology

APSGN develops 5 to 21 days after an infection of the pharynx or skin (e.g. Streptococcal sore throat, impetigo) by certain nephrotoxic strains of group A beta-haemolytic streptococci. The person produces antibodies to the strepotcoccal antigen. The antigen-antibody complexes are deposited in the glomeruli and activated compliment. Compliment activated causes an inflammatory reaction to the injury. This response to the injury is also a decrease in the filtration of metabolic waste products from the blood and an increased permeability of the glomerulus to larger protein molecules.

Pathophysiology

APSGN is a result of an antigen-antibody reaction with glomerular tissue that produces swelling and death of capillary cells. The antigen-antibody reaction activates the complement pathway, resulting in chemotaxis of polymorph nuclear leukocytes with release of lysosomal enzymes that attack the glomerular basement membrane. The responses in the membrane is an increase in all three types of gloemrular cells (i.e. endothelial, mesangial, and epithelial) causing an increase in membrane porosity with resultant proteinuria and haematuria. Renal function is depressed by scarring and obstruction of the circulation through the glomerulus. Signs and symptoms reflect damage to the glomeruli with leaking of proteins and RBCs into the urine and varying degrees of decreased glomeruli filtrations, with retention of metabolic wastes products, sodium and water.

Clinical Manifestations

Typical patient complaints include shortness of breath, mild headache, weakness, anorexia, flank pain. The early clinical manifestation of APSGN includes haematuria, proteinuria, azotemia, increased urine-specific gravity, elevated ESR, oliguria, elevated antistreptolysine *'O titer*. Later chemical manifestations include circulatory congestion, hypertension, oedema and end-stage renal failure. Signs and symptoms which may include generalized body oedema, hypertension, oliguria, haematuria with a smoky or rusty appearance, and proteinuria. Fluid retention occurs as a result of decreased glomerular filtration. The oedema appears initially in low pressure tissue such as around the eyes (Periorbital oedema), but later, progresses to involve total body as ascitis or peripheral oedema in the legs. Smoky urine is indicative of bleeding in the upper urinary tract. The degree of proteinuria varies with severity of glomerulonephropathy. Hypertension primarily results from increased ECF.

Management

The diagnosis of APSGN is based on a complete history and physical examination and laboratory studies to determine the presence or history of a group. A extrahaemolytic streptococci in a throat or skin lesion. Urinalysis provides important data such as presence of proteinuria, haematuria and cell debris. Serum BUN and urine creatinine clearance test indicates renal function status. Test to determine infection includes ESR and anistreptolysis 'O'titter, and *rena l* biopsy is indicated.

The management of APSGN focuses on lymptomatic relief. Rest is recommended until the signs of glomerular inflammation (Proteinuria, haematuria) and hypertension subside. Oedema is treated by restricting sodium and fluid intake and by administering diuretics. Severe hypertension is treated with antihypertensive drugs. Dietary protein intake may be restricted if there is evidence of an increase in nitrogenous wastes (e.g. elevated BUN value). The restriction varies with proteinuria.

Persistent infection is treated promptly to help prevent an increase in antigen-antibody complex formation. Patients with poststreptococcal glomerulonephritis are given a course of prophylactic antibiotics, the drug of choice is penicillin. Prophylactic therapy may be continued for months after the acute phase of illness. Diuretic therapy is implemented when severe overload develops. Elevated blood pressure is controlled by antihypertensive drugs only after fluid control has proved to be unsuccessful.

There is no specific treatment for APSGN. General management focussed on prevention, i.e. early defection and prompt treatment of URTI. Fluid retention is often managed by dietary sodium restrictions and nurse should be constantly alert for signs and symptoms of fluid overload and bedrest is prescribed during the acute phase of illness.

The recovery period for acute glomerulonephritis may be as long as 2 years; therefore, patient teaching is important. Proteinuria, haematuria and cellular debris may exist microscopically even when other symptoms subside. Although fatigue may be present, these persons usually feel well. They often need to be convinced of the importance of follow-up care.

Teaching includes:

- Nature of illness and effect of diet and fluids on fluid balance and sodium retention.
- Diet teaching regarding prescribed sodium and fluid restrictions.
- Medication regimen: dose, frequency, side effects, need to continue regimen as prescribed.
- Need to balance activities with rest of fatigue present.
- Avoidance of infection which may exacerbate illness.
- Signs and symptoms indicating need for medical attention (haematuria, headache, oedema, or hypertension).
- Importance of follow-up care.

Chronic Glomerulonephritis (CGN)

Chronic glomerulonephritis is a syndrome that reflects the end stage of glomerular inflammatory disease.

Aetiology

Most types of glomerulonephritis and nephrotic syndrom can eventually lead to chronic glomerulonephritis (CGN). Although CGN may follow the acute disease, most of the persons have no history of the disease or source of predisposing infection. Some persons with minimal impairment in renal function continue to feel well and show little progression of disease. The progression of renal deterioration may be insidious or rapid, resulting in end stage of renal disease.

Pathopysiology

Chronic glomerulonephritis is characterized by progressive destruction (sclerosis) of glomeruli and gradual loss of renal function. The glomeruli having varying degrees of hypercellularity and become sclerosed (hardened). The kidney decreases in size. Eventually there is tubular atrophy, chronic interstitial inflammation, and arteriosclerosis.

Clinical Manifestation

Various symptoms of renal dysfunction may lead the person to seek health care, including headache, especially in the morning; dyspnoea on exertion, blurred vision, lassitude, weakness or fatigue. Other signs of CGN include oedema, nocturia, and weight loss. Early in the disease process, urinalysis may reveal albumin, casts and blood despite normal renal function tests. The ability of kidneys to regulate internal environment will begin to decrease as more glomeruli become scarred resulting in fewer functional nephrons. The syndrome is characterized by proteinuria, haematuria and the slow development of uremic syndrome as a result of decreasing renal function.

Management

CGN is often found coincidentally when an abnormality on urinalysis or elevated blood pressure is detected. It is common to find that the patient has no recollection or history of acute nephritis or any renal problems. A renal biopsy is performed to determine the exact cause and nature of the glomerulonephritis. However, now some of them use ultrasound and CT scan as diagnostic measure.

No specific therapy exists to arrest or reverse this disease process. Treatment is supportive and symptomatic. Hypertension and urinary tract infections should be treated vigorously. With any exacerbation of haematuria, hypertension and oedema, the patient is returned to bedrest, and treatment is similar to that of acute glomerulonephritis is instituted. Signs of pulmonary oedema and congestive cardiac failure are closely monitored. Women with CGN who become pregnant appear to be susceptible to toxaemia and to spontaneous abortion, needs close observation by obstetrician. Protein and phosphate restrictions may slow the rate of progression of renal failure.

For prevention or to reduce risk, known infection should be treated promptly. Care involves teaching the patient to live healthfully to avoid infections (as in AGN), to eat balanced diet within the prescribed limit, to take prescribed medications appropriately to maintain follow-up health care, and to report to concerned physician about any exacerbation and signs and symptoms.

Nephrotic Syndrome

The term nephrotic syndrome describes a clinical course that can be associated with a number of disease conditions. Nephrotic syndrome or nephrosis is not a single disease entirely but a constellation of symptoms including albuminuria, hypoalbuminuria, oedema, hyperlipidaemia, and lipiduria. This syndrome causes damage to the glomeruli with resultant proteinuria. It is most often seen in children.

Aetiology

Some of the more common causes of nephrotic syndrome are:

1. *Primary Glomerular Disease*
   - Membranous proliferative glomerulonephritis.
   - Primary nephrotic syndrome.
   - Focal glomerulonephritis.
   - Inherited nephrotic disease.
2. *External Causes*
   i. *Multisystem disease*
      - Systemic lupus erythematous.
      - Diabetes Mellitus.
      - Sickle cell disease.
      - Amyloidosis.

   ii. *Infections*
      - Bacterial (Streptococcal, syphyllis).
      - Viral (herpes zoster, HIV and hepatitis).
      - Protozoal (Malaria).

   iii. *Neoplasms*
      - Hodgkin's disease.
      - Solid tumours of lungs, colon, stomach and breast.
      - Leukaemia.

   iv. *Circulatory problems*
      - Severe congestive heart failure.
      - Chronic constrictive pericarditis.

   v. *Allergic reaction*
      - Insect bites, bee sting and pollen.
      - Drugs (Penicillamine, NSAIDs, Captopril and Heroin).

Pathophysiology

The initial physiological change is nephrotic syndrome is a derangement of cells in the glomerular basement membrane (GBM) resulting in increased membrane porosity and significant proteinuria. As protein continues to be excreted, serum albumin is decreased (hypoalbuminiemia), thus decreasing the serum osmotic pressure. The capillary hydrostatic fluid pressure in all body tissues becomes greater than the capillary osmotic pressure in all body tissues becomes greater then the capillary osmotic pressure and generalized oedema results. As fluid is lost into the tissues, the plasma volume decreases stimulating secretion of aldosterone to retain more sodium and water, which decreases the glomerular filtration rate to retain water. This additional fluid also passes out of the capillaries into the tissue leading to even greater oedema.

Clinical Manifestations

The characteristic manifestation includes peripheral oedema, massive proteinuria, hyperlipidaemia, and hypoalbuminiemia. Characteristic blood chemistries include decreased serum albumin, decreased serum protein, and elevated serum cholestrol. The increased glomerular membrane permeability found in nephrotic syndrome is responsible for the massive excretion of protein in the urine. There is the decreased serum protein and subsequent oedema formation. Ascitis and anasarca (severe generalized oedema) develop if there is a severe hypoalbuminaemia.

The diminished plasma oncotic pressure from the decreased serum proteins stimulates hepatic lipoprotein synthesis which results in hyperlipidaemia. Initially cholestrol and low-density lipoproteins are elevated. Later fat bodies (fatty casts) commonly appear in the urine. Alterations of the humoral and cellular immunoresponse results in infection. Calcium and skeletol abnormalities may occur; results in hypocalcaemia, blunted calcemic response to parathyroid hormone, hypoparathyroidism and osteomalacia. With nephrotic proteinuria loss of clotting factors can result in relative hypercoagulable state i.e., hypercoagulability with thromboembolism is most serious complication.

Management

Treatment of nephrotic syndrome is symptomatic, that is focused on reduction of albuminuria, controlling oedema, and promoting general health. Management of oedema includes the cautious use of angiotensin converting enzynme (ACE) inhibitors, NSAIDs and a low-sodium (2 to 3 g per day), low to moderate-protein diet (0.5 to 0.6 kg per day). Dietary salt restrictions are a key to managing oedema. In some individuals, thiazide or loop diuretics may be needed. If the urine protein loss exceeds 10g/24 per hour, additional dietary protein may be needed. Corticosteroids and cyclophophamide may be used for the treatment of severe cases of nephrotic syndrome.

A major nursing intervention for a patient with nephrotic syndrome is related to oedema. It is important to assess oedema by weighing the patient daily, accurately recording intake and output, and measuring abdominal girth or extremity size. Comparing this information daily provides the nurse with a tool for assessing the effectiveness of treatment. The oedematous skin needs careful cleaning. Trauma should be avoided and the effectiveness of diuretic therapy must be monitored. Measures should be taken to avoid exposure to person with known infections. The nurse should handle the patient properly with their altered body image due to oedema. A sodium-restricted diet is usually prescribed.

The patient and family should be educated regarding:

- The effects of nephrotic syndrome on the kidneys and the possibility of the need for dialysis or renal transplant in the future.
- Medication regimen, name, dose, actions, side effects and the need to complete prescribed antibiotics.
- Nutrition: increased calories, adequate protein and decreased sodium.
- Self assessment of fluid status, including signs and symptoms of hypovolaemia and hypervolaemia.
- Signs and symptoms requiring medical attention: increased oedema, dyspnoea, fatigue, headache and infection.
- Promotion of good health habits to prevent infection, including nutritionally adequate diet, exercise, adequate rest, and sleep and avoidance of source of infection.
- Need for follow-up care to monitor renal function.

Goodpasture's Syndrome

Good pasture's syndrome is an example of cytotoxic (type II) autoimmune disease, is characterised by the presence of circulating antibodies against GBM and alveolar basement membrane (ABM).

Aetiology and Pathophysiology

It is a rare disease that is seen mostly in young male smokers. Although the primary target organ is the kidney, the lungs are also involved. The pathologic nature of the syndrome results when binding of the antibody causes an inflammatory reaction mediated by complement fixation and activation. The causative factors for development of autoantibody production are unknown, although type A influenza viruses, hydrocarbon, penicillamine, and unknown genetic factors may be involved.

Clinical Manifestations

The clinical manifestations include haemoptysis, pulmonary insufficiency, crackles, rhonchi, renal involvement with haematuria and renal failure, weakness, pallor, and anaemia. Pulmonary haemorrhage usually occurs and may precede glomerular abnormality by weeks or months. Abnormal diagnostic findings include low haematocrit and haemoglobin levels, elevated BUN and serum creatinine levels, haematuria and proteinuria, circulating serum anti-GBM antibodies parallel to the activity of the renal disease.

Management

Management consists of corticosteroids, immunosuppressive drugs (e.g. Cyclophosphamide), plasmapheresis and dialysis. Plasmapheresis removes circulating anti-GBM antibody and immunosuppressive therapy inhibits further antibody production. Renal transplantation can be attempted once the circulating anti-GBM antibody titer decreases.

Nursing management appropriate for critically-ill patient who is experiencing symptoms of acute renal failure and respiratory distress. The patient and family need instructions cocnerning current therapy, medications and complications of disease processes. The complication of Goodpasture's syndrome is rapidly progressive glomerulonephritis. (This also occurs as complication of APSGN, SLE and illustrative disease).

Renal Artery Stenosis

Renal artery stenosis is a partial occlusion of one or both renal arteries and their major branches.

Aetiology

Renal artery stenosis can be due to the atherosclerotic narrowing or fibromuscular hyperplasia. It is the cause of approximately 5 per cent of all cases of hypertension. The end result is a narrowing of the lumen of the arteries supplying the kidneys. Obstruction of the renal arteries can be caused by aneurysm, thrombosis and emboli.

Pathophysiology

Renal artery stenosis results in a major reduction in blood flow to the kidneys. This change in renal perfusion causes increased secretion of renin and activation of renin-angiotension-aldosterone system. The end result is acceleration of hypertension, which, if untreated, leads to further pathological changes in the kidneys.

Clinical Manifestation

The clinical manifestation of renal artery stenosis includes:

- Abdominal bruits.
- Hypertension.
- Disparity in kidney size.
- Disparity in kidney shape.
- Delayed appearance of contrast medium in renal anteriogram.
- Hyperconcentration of contrast media in kidneys, calyceal system on intravenous pyelogram.
- Lesion evidenced on renal arteriogram.
- Increased serum creatinine level with captoril challenge.
- Changes in blood flow on duplex doppler ultrasonography.
- Detection of change in blood flow within vessels on MRI.

Management

A renal arteriogram is the best diagnostic tool for identifying renal artery stenosis. The goals of therapy are control of blood pressure, and restoration of perfusion to the kidney. Beta-blocker or angiotension converting enzyme inhibitors are used to manage hypertension. Analgesics are used to manage pain associated with vascular occlusion. Preventing pulmonary embolism is critical in persons with renal vein thrombosis. Anticoagulants are indicated for patients with renal artery occlusion or renal vein thrombosis.

Surgical revascularization of the kidney is indicated when blood flow is decreased enough to cause renal ischaemia or when evidence indicates that renovascular hypertension is present and surgical intervention may result in the patient becoming normotensive. The surgical procedure normally involves anastomosis between the kidney and another major artery, usually spleenic artery or aorta. Percutaneous transluminal angioplasty may be used as an alternative to surgery, especially in older patients who are poor surgical risks. Person with renal artery stenosis and hypertension that does not respond to medication may need a nephrectomy.

Patient should be educated regarding the lower cholestrol including maintaining a diet low in animal fat and increasing aerobic exercises. Patients should be instructed to monitor their blood pressure at home and report any abnormalities to health care provider. If anticoagulant therapy is prescribed, the patient and family should understand precautions to take to avoid injury and signs and excessive bleeding. And patient should be taught to recognize signs and symptoms and report immediately to the concerned health-care provider.

Renal Vein Thrombosis

Renal vein thrombosis may occur unilaterally or bilaterally trauma, extrinsic compression (e.g. tumour, aortic aneurysm), renal cell carcinoma, pregnancy, contraceptive use, and nephrotic syndrome are associated with renal vein thrombosis.

The patient has symptoms of flank pain, haematuria or fever or has nephrotic syndrome. Anticoagulation is an important treatment because there is a high incidence of pulmonary emboli. Corticosteroids may be used in the patient with nephrosis. Surgical thrombectomy may be performed instead of or along with anticoagulation.

Nephrosclerosis

Nephrosclerosis consists of sclerosis of the small arteries and arterioles of the kidneys. There is a decreased blood flow, which results in patchy necrosis of the renal parenchyma. Ischaemic necrosis and destruction of glomeruli with subsequent fibrosis also occurs.

Aetiology

Whereas renal artery stenosis results in hypertension, hypertension causes nephrosclerosis or damage to the renal arteries, arterioles and glomeruli. Hypertension is the major cause of end-stage renal disease.

Pathophysiology

In benign nephrosclerosis, the renal arterial vessels show thickening and narrowing of their lumina, and some glomerular capillaries are sclerosed and collapsed. Renal blood flow can be reduced as the result of these vascular changes. The renal tubules can also be affected, resulting in tubular atrophy signs and symptoms are mild, i.e. mild proteinuria from glomerular damage. Nocturia may occur due to tubular concentrating ability and urinary casts may be present due to tubular injury. Later mild renal insufficiency leads to risk for acute failure.

In malignant nephrosclerosis, the major changes are necrosis and thickening of the arterioles and glomerular capillaries and diffuse tubular loss and atrophy. Gross hamaturia occurs with RBC casts, heavy proteinuria and elevated plasma creatinine. Malignant nephrosclerosis is a medical emergency, and high blood pressure must be lowered to prevent permanent renal damage as well as damage to other vital organs.

Clinical Manifestations
The signs and symptoms of nephrosclerosis are the same as those of chronic renal failure (see page No 741). By the time the signs and symptoms develop, the disease has progressed to an extreme point. Deterioration in renal function progresses gradually. Accelerated or malignant nephrosclerosis is associated with malignant hypertension or complication of hypertension characterized by a sharp increase in blood pressure with a diastolic pressure greater than 130 mm Hg. The patient is usually an young adult, with a male to female ratio 2 : 1. Renal insufficiency progresses rapidly.

Management
Treatment of nephrosclerosis is focussed on early detection and treatment of hypertension. Causative factors are sought and treatment to lower blood pressure is initiated. When significant renal damage exists, stabilizing the person's current level of function or slowing deterioration of the kidney tissue is the goal. Control of hypertension is continued. For hypertensive emergencies, potent vasodilatories such as diazoxide and sodium nitroprusside are used. IV medications usually act rapidly to lower blood pressure. Sodium nitroprusside is given as a continuous IV drip. Monitor the patient continuously for headache, hypotension, muscle twitching, tachycardia, restlessness and retrosternal or abdominal pain. Nursing care of the patient with nephrosclerosis is same as in chronic renal failure (Page No 741). During drug therapy, monitor the patient closely for tachycardia, hypotension, hyperglycaemia, and marked sodium and water retention.

Obstructive Uropathies

Obstruction of the urinary system occurs in any portion of the urinary tract from the urinary calyces in kidney to the urethral meatus. Patients with obstructions have characteristic signs and symptoms, depending on the location and extent of the obstruction. Uncorrected urinary obstruction can lead to renal failure.

Obstruction may be congenital or acquired and due to intrinsic and extrinsic which include:

i. *Intrinsic* causes such as anamolies, diverticuli, tumours or benign growth within the urinary tract, e.g. narrowing of ureteropelvic junction, bladder neck hyperplasia, urethral stricture, BPH and meatal stenosis.
ii. *Extrinsic causes* such as tumours, adhesions, retroperitoneal fibrosis, or prolapsed adjacent organs or functional causes as a result of neurologic or psychogenic factors, e.g. are pelvic and abdominal tumours or prolapsed uterus. Functional causes are vesicosphincter dyssynergia after spinal cord injury and neurogenic bladder secondary to diabetes.

The major causes of urinary tract obstructions according to location are as follows:

i. Lower urinary tract:
   - Bladder neoplasms
   - Urethral strictures
   - Calculi
   - Tumours
   - Benign prostatic hypertrophy (BPH).
ii. Ureteral obstruction
   - Calculi
   - Trauma
   - Nephroptosis (floating or dropped kidney)
   - Enlarged lymph nodes (lymposarcoma reticuli-cell carcinoma, Hodgkin's disease.
   - Congenital anamoly.
iii. Kidney
   - Calculi
   - Ptosis
   - Polycystic kidney disease
   - Pregnancy (usually right-sided).

The common condition of obstructive uropathies discussed are as follows:

Hydronephrosis

Hydronephrosis is the dilation of the renal pelvis and calyces with urine. It may occur either unilaterally or bilaterally. It is due to causes of obstruction of urinary tract.

Pathophysiology
Obstruction of any part of the urinary system from the kidney to the urethra will generate pressure that may cause functional and anatomic damage to the renal parenchyma. When any part of the urinary tract is obstructed, urine collects behind the obstruction, producing dilation of the urine collecting structures. Muscles of the affected area contract in an effort to push the urine around the obstruction. Partial obstruction may produce slow dilation of structures above the obstruction without functional impairment. As the obstruction increases, pressure builds up in the tubular system behind the obstruction causing a backflow of urine and dilation of the ureter (hydrouretor). The urine back-up eventually reaches the kidney causing dilation of the kidney pelvis (hydronephrosis). Pressure build-up in the renal pelvis leads to destruction of kidney tissue and eventually renal failure.

Due to obstruction, urine flow is decreased, even to the point of stagnation. This stagnant urine provides a culture medium for bacterial growth and rarely is obstruction seen without some infection. The specific effects that occur with obstruction depend on the location extent (partial or complete) and duration of the obstruction. Obstruction in the lower urinary tract causes bladder distension. If this is prolonged, muscle fibres become hypertrophied and diverticuli (herniated sacs of bladder mucosa) develop between the hypertophied muscle bands. Since the diverticulum holds stagnant urine, infection often occurs and bladder stones may form.

The obstruction of the upper urinary tract can progress rapidly to hydronephrosis because of the small size of the ureters and kidney pelvis. Increased pressure causes partial ischaemia between the renal cortex and medulla and the dilation of the renal tubules leading to tubular damage. Urinary stasis in the dilated pelvis leads to infection and calculi, which add to the renal damage. Some urine flow back up the renal tubules into the veins and lymphatics as a compensatory mechanism. The unaffected kidney then takes on increased elimination of waste products. With prolonged obstruction, the unaffected kidney hypertrophies may function almost (80 per cent) as effectively alone as both kidneys did before the obstruction. Obstruction of both kidneys leads to renal failure.

Clinical Manifestation

Hydronephrosis occurs without any symptoms as long as kidney function is adequate, and urine can drain. An acute upper urinary tract obstruction will cause pain, nausea, vomiting, local tenderness, spasm of the abdominal muscle, and a mass in the kidney region. The pain is caused by stretching of the tissue and by hyperperistalisis. Because of the amount of pain is proportional to the rate of stretching a slowly developing hydronephrosis may cause only a dull flank pain, whereas a sudden blockage of the ureter e.g. form a stone, causes a severe stabbing (colicky) pain in the flank or abdomen. The pain may radiate to the genitalia and thighs and is caused by the increased peristaltic action of the smooth muscles of the ureter in an effort to dislodge the obstruction and force urine past it. Reflex reaction to the pain causes nausea and vomiting. An extremely dilated kidney may press on the stomach, causing continued gastrointestinal symptoms. This may indicate uremia.

When the bladder is distended from the lower urinary tract obstruction, the person will experience abdominal discomfort and feel the need to void although voiding will not be possible. The bladder may be palpated above the symphysispubis. There may be urge to void usually 250 to 500 ml. nocturia, haematuria and pyuria may also be present.

Management

The diagnosis can be made on complete examination and routine renourogical tests. The medical management is in specific to the cause of the urinary tract obstruction. Treatment centers around re-establishing adequate drainage from the urinary system, such as placing a ureteral catheter above the point of obstruction. Strictures may be successfully dilated.

Surgery is indicated to relieve the obstruction and preserve kidney function. Procedures include pyeloplasty and catheter or stent insertion into the kidney or bladder (nephrostomy, ureterostomy or suprapubic cystotomy). Severe kidney damage may necessitate nephrectomy.

The person with acute obstruction has severe colic, can be treated with narcotics (morphine, mepeuedine) in combination with antispasmodic drugs (Probanthin, balladona prep). General nursing management of urinary obstruction includes pain management, fluid balance assessment, prevention of urinary complications and patient teaching. The patient should be monitored for signs and symptoms of infection. Patients and families should be taught postoperative care of incisions and care and management of indwelling catheters if applicable. Information about medications, diet, fluid restrictions and signs and symptoms of infection and recurrent obstruction should be included in the teaching plan.

Renal Calculi (Stones)

Urinary stones (urolithiasis) may develop at any level in the urinary system but are most frequently found within the kidney (nephrolithiasis). Renal calculi are crystallisation of minerals around an organic matrix such as pus, blood, or devitalized tissue. Most stones consist of calcium salts or magnesium-ammonium phosphate, the remainder are cystine or uric acid stones.

Aetiology

Many factors are involved in the incidence and type of stone formation, including metabolic, dietary, genetic, climatic and occupational influence are as follows:

i. *Metabolic*
   - Abnormalities that result in increased urine levels of calcium, oxaluric acid, uric acid or citric acid.

ii. *Climate*
   - Warm climates that cause increased fluid loss. Low urine volume and increased solute concentration in urine.

iii. *Diet*
   - Large intake of dietary proteins that increases uric acid excretion.
   - Excessive amounts of tea or fruit juices that elevate urinary oxalate level.
   - Large intake of calcium and oxalate.
   - Low fluid intake that increases urinary concentration.

iv. *Genetic factors*
   - Family history of stones formation, cystinuria, gout or renal acidosis.

v. *Life style*
   - Sedentary occupation and immobility.

No demonstrable cause can be found for more than half of the renal stones that occur (idiopathic). However, a major predisposing factor is the presence of UTI. Infection increases the presence of organic matter around which minerals can precipitate and increases the alkalinity of the urine by the production of ammonia. This results in precipitation of calcium phosphate and magnesium-ammonium phosphate. Stasis of urine also permits precipitation of organic matter and minerals. Other factors associated with the development of stones include long-term use of antacids, vitamin D, large doses of vitamin C and calcium carbonate.

Pathophysiology

Most stones are *calcium* (oxalate and phosphate) anything that leads to hypercalciuria is a predisposing factors for renal stones. Factors that contribute to calcium stone formation will include hypercalcaemia and/or hypercalciuria resulting from hyperparathyroidism vitamin D intoxication, multiple myeloma, immobilization, severe bone disease, cancer, renal tubular acidosis, prolonged intake of steroids and increased intake of calcium.

The contributing factors of *uric acid* stone formation are high purine diet, gout renal failure, blood dyscrasiasis, use of thiazide diurectics and alkalysing agents. The factors contributing to *cystine* stone formation are cystinuria resulting from genetic disorder of aminoacid metabolism.

The other important factors in the development of stones include obstruction with urinary stasis and urinary *infection*. With urea-spitting bacteria (e.g. proteus, klebsiella, pseudomonas, and some species of staphylococci). These bacteria cause the urine to become alkaline and contribute to the formation of calcium-ammonium phosphate stones (struvite or triple phosphate stones). Infected stones when they are entrapped in the kidney may assume a staghorn configuration as they enlarge. Infected stones are frequent in the patient with an external urinary diversion and long-term indwelling catheter. Neurogenic bladder or retention of urine.

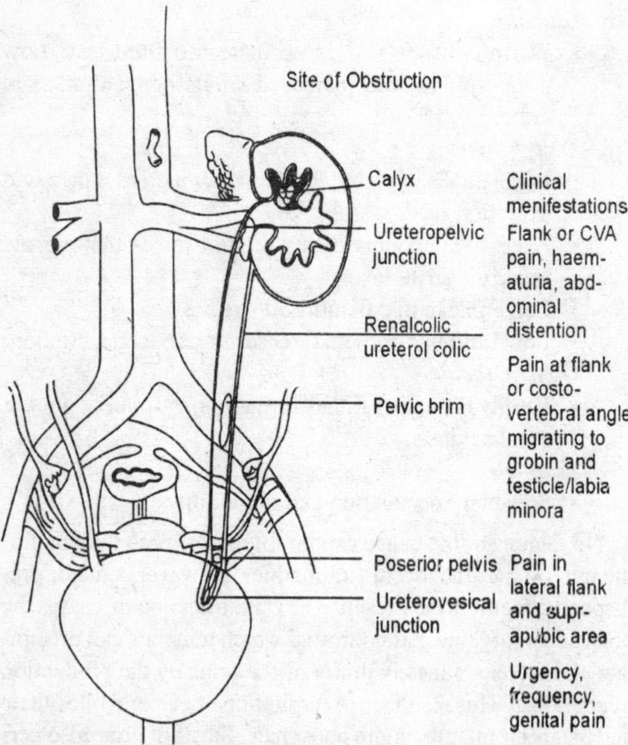

Fig.14.2: Areas where calculi may obstruct the urinary system. The ensuing clinical manifestations depend on the site of obstruction. Stones that have broken loose may obstruct the flow of urine, cause severe pain, and injure the kidney.

Clinical Manifestations

Urinary stones cause clinical manifestation when they cause obstruction to urinary flow, common sites of obstruction are at the ureteropelvic junction (UPJ), in the ureter at the point it crosses the illiac vessels and at the ureterovesical junction (UVJ). Symptoms include abdominal or flank pain (usually severe), haematuria and renal colic. The pain may be associated with nausea and vomiting. If the stone is nonobstructing, pain may be absent. If it produces obstruction in a calyx or at UPJ, the patient may experience dull costovertebral flank pain or even colic. Pain resulting from the passage of a calculus down the ureter is intense and collicky. The patient may be in mild shock with cool, moist skin. As a stone nears the UVJ, pain will be felt in the lateral flank and sometimes down into the testicles, labia, or groin. Other clinical manifestations include the presence of urinary infections accompanied by fever, vomiting, nausea, and chills.

Management

The diagnostic studies performed to determine the presence of renal stones include kidney, ureters and bladder (KUB) X-rays IV or retrograde pyelography; ultrasound; CT; and cystoscopy. Additional studies include urinalysis and serum calcium and serum uric acid levels.

Evaluation and management of patient with renal calculi consists two current approaches. The *first approach* is directed towards management of acute attack. This involves treating the symptoms of pain, infection or obstruction as indicated for the idnividual patient. At frequent intervals, narcotics are typically required for relief of renal colic pain. Many stones pass spontaneously. However, stones larger than 4 mm are unlikely to pass through the ureter. The *second* approach is directed toward evaluation of the aetiology of the stone formation and the prevention of further development of stones. Information to be obtained from the patient includes family history of stone formation, geographic residence, nutritional assessment including intake of vitamins A and D, activity pattern (active or sedentary), history of periods of prolonged illness with immobilization or dehydration and any history of disease or surgery of the GI or GU tract.

Therapeutic measures according to urinary stone are as follows:

i. Calcium oxalate:
   - Increase hydration.
   - Reduce dietary oxalate.
   - Give thiazide diuretics.
   - Give cellulose phosphate to cholate calcium and prevent GI absorption.
   - Give potassium citrate to maintain alkaline urine.
   - Give cholestyramine to bind oxalate.
   - Give calcium lactate to precipitate oxalate in GI tract.

ii. *Calcium phosphate*
  - Treat underlying causes and other stones.

iii. *Struvite or tripla* phosphate stones ($MgNH_4PO_4$)
  - Administer antimicrobial agents, acetohydroxamic acid and antibiotics.
  - Use surgical intervention to remove stone.
  - Take measure to acidify urine.

iv. *Uric acid* stones.
  - Reduce urinary concentration of uric acid.
  - Alkalinize urine with potassium citrate.
  - Administer allopurinol.
  - Reduce dietary purines.

v. *Cystine*
  - Increase hydration.
  - Give alpha-penicillamine and tiopronin to prevent cystin crystallization.
  - Give potassium citrate to maintain alkaline urine.

And adequate hydration, dietary sodium restrictions, dietary changes, and the use of above-stated medication minimise stone formation. High fluid intake at least 3000 ml per day is recommended. Dietary intervention may be important in the management of urolithiasis. Recent research suggests that a high dietary calcium intake, which was previously thought to contribute to kidney stones, may actually lower the risk by reducing the urinary excretion of oxalate, a common factor in many stones. Initial nutritional management should include limiting oxalate-rich foods and thereby reducing oxalate excretion. Foods high in purine, calcium or oxalate contents are as follows:

i. *Purine*
High sardines, herring, mussels, liver, kidney, goose, venison, meat soups and sweetbread.
Moderate: Chickens, almond, crab, veal, mutton, bacon, pork, beef, ham.

ii. *Calcium*
Milk, cheese, ice cream, yogurt, sauces containing milk, all beans (except green beans) lentils, fish with fine bones (e.g. sardines, kippers, herring, salmon) dried fruits, nuts chocolate, cocoa and ovaltine.

iii. *Oxalate*
  - Spinach, rhubarb, asparagus, cabbage, tomatoes, beets, nuts, celery, parsley, runner beans, chocolate, cocoa, instant coffee ovaltine, tea and worcestestrone sauce.

Indication for endourologic, lithotripsy or open surgical removal of stones include the following.

- Stones too large for spontaneous passage.
- Stones associated with bacteriuria or symptomatic infection.
- Stones causing impaired renal function.
- Stones causing persistent pain, nausea and vomiting.
- Inability of patient to be treated medically.
- Patient with one kidney.

Stones in the lower ureter may be removed by endourologic procedure, i.e. cystoscopic manipulation. General anaesthesia may be required, and care is similar to that after cystoscopy.

The percutaneous lithotripsy, extracorporeal shock wave lithotripsy are used to remove stones and the cancel a laser therapy is used to remove stone in the lower ureters. It is pulsed dye laser system designed to break up calculi that have migrated to the lower ureters. The laser probe is inserted through

- Ureterolithotomy
- Pyelolithotomy
- Nephrolithotomy.

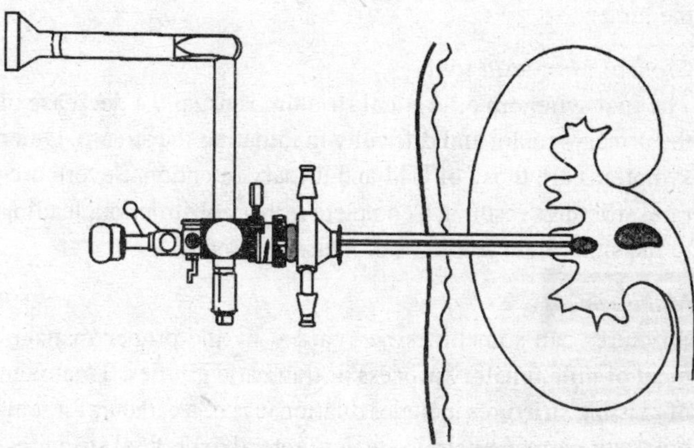

Fig. 14.3: A percutaneous nephrostomy tract permits access to the collecting system of the kidney for removal of kidney stones under direct vision via a nephroscope.

Nursing intervention includes proper assessment and take suitable measure to reduce pain, risk for infection, correcting altered urinary eliminate and reduce anxiety. If any procedure to be performed on the patient, take actions accordingly including health education to patients and family.

Strictures

A stricture is a narrowing of the lumen and is sometimes congenital but is usually acquired. Strictures may occur in the bladder neck, urethra, or ureters.

Aetiology

Strictures of the bladder neck may be congenital or may result from chronic prostatitis in men or cystitis in women. The causes of urethral strictures include trauma from accidents (e.g. those resulting in fractured pelvis), gonorrhoeal infections, and urethral instrumentation. The membranous urethra is a common site of stricture caused by instrumentation, because of its location (the urethral curve just below the prostatic uretnra) and because of the surrounding rhabdospincter muscle prevents easy distension. Meatal stenosis, a narrowing of the urethral opening are common. Ureteral strictures may be caused by severe or chronic infection, radiation therapy, and retroperitoneal abscess formation from inflammatory bowel disease and perforation. Urethral strictures occur more often in men than women because of the length of the urethra.

Pathophysiology

Narrowing of the urethra can result from chronic infection that leads to inflammation of the lining. The inflammation causes a hyperplasia of the lining, and the strictures develop. The truama may completely severe the urethra. When the urethra is anastomosed, stricture frequently occurs at the surgical site. One of the leading causes of urethral stricture is a tumour that puts pressure against exterior of the urethra, resulting in stricture of the lumen.

Clinical Manifestation

The first symptom of urethral stricture is usually a decrease in the urinary stream and difficulty in initiating the stream. Other symptoms are those of UTI and urinary retention. Severe urethral strictures result in a complete urinary obstruction, leading to the signs and symptoms of hydronephrosis.

Management

Strictures can sometimes be avoided by the proper management of inflammatory process or traumatic injuries. Treatment of existing strictures includes dilation, use of a catheter for temporary or permanent drainage, for ureteral or urethral strictures, and surgery. Some patients are taught to dilate urethra themselves between office visits to keep strictural areas open. Nursing intervention includes informing the patient about the procedure, preparing the patient for the procedure, and assessing the patient's need for management, education and follow-up care. Education for the patient and family centers on recognition of early signs and symptoms of a decrease in urine stream and urine retention. Education shouild be focussed on high risk groups.

Renal Tumour

Renal tumour arises from the cortex or pelvis and calyces. Tumour arising from both areas may be benign or malignant.

Aetiology

Exact causes of renal tumour is not known, but certain risk factors have been linked to the disease. The most common risk factor for all concerns of urinary system is cigarette smoking. Occupational exposure to textile dyes, rubber metallurgy, paint, and leather has been implicated in the development of renal cell carcinoma. Other risk factors are the use of phenacetin-containing analgesies and exposure to asbestos, cadmium and gasoline.

Pathophysiology

Renal carcinoma usually develops unilaterally but may occur bilaterlly. In *Stage I*, the margins are well-defined (encapsulated) and compress the kidney parenchyma during growth rather than infiltrating the tissue. The upper pole of the kidney is usually involved and the tumour is usually large at the time of diagnosis. In *Stage II*, the tumour invades the fat surrounding the kidney. *Stage III* consists of local metastasis either through direct extension or through the renal vein or lymphatic (lymph node involvement). Distant metastasis during *Stage IV* are primarily in the lungs or bone; but other areas, such as the liver, spleen, bone, opposite kidney, or brain may also be involved. Prognosis is based on the stage and advancement of the disease at diagnosis.

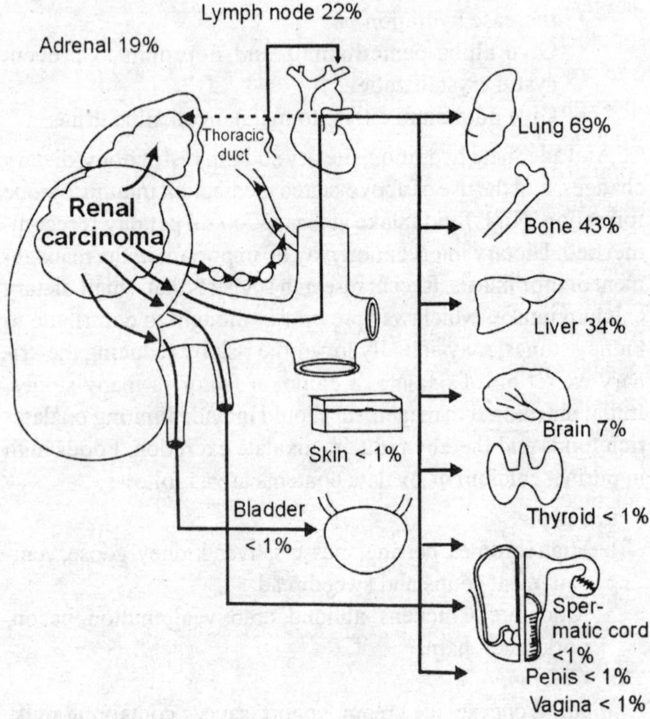

Fig. 14.4: Routes of common metastase from renal carcinoma.

Clinical Manifestation

There are no characteristic early symptoms. Generalized symptoms of unexplained weight loss, fever, weakness and anaemia are the earlier manifestation. The classic manifestation of gross haematurial, flank pain, and flank palpable mass are those of advanced disease. Painless haematuria is the most frequent sign of renal cell carcinoma.

Management

Several studies are used to diagnose adenocarcinoma of the kidney which include IVP, CT scan MRI. Angiography, radionuclide isotope scanning and biopsy.

Unless the person is a poor surgical risk or has extensive metastasis, the diseased kidney is removed (nephrectomy), through a transabdominal, flank, lumbar or thoracoabdominal approach. Radical or partial nephrectomy may be performed accordingly. Radiation is used postoperatively for residual or recurrent tumours and is also beneficial for symptomatic bone metastasis. The use of chemotherapeutic agents in combination with immunomodulating agent has shown some benefits. *Interluckin 2* has shown some promise for the treatment of renal cell carcinoma. The side effects of interleukin 2 can be severe and include severe hypotension rigors and anaphylaxis. Hormonal therapy with progesterone, testosterone and antioestrogen is useful in some patients.

If surgery is the treatment chosen, patient and family teaching will focus on perioperative instructions. Preoperative instructions may include a discussion of the type and length of surgery, type of anaesthesia, and the need for IV Line, catheter, or other drains. Instruction in the use of an incentive spirometer are crucial because inadequate ventilation is frequent problem postoperatively. The patient is informed of the pain medication routine, e.g. management of the patient after nephrectemy is similar to the patients undergoing abdominal surgery and urinary diversion surgery.

Wilm's Tumour

Wilm's tumour is a common renal tumour of infants and children. It is mostly hereditary. The most common manifestation is abdominal swelling, or distension. This distention is often noticed by parents or is found routine examination. Other symptoms include pain, fever, haematuria and hypertension.

These tumours respond well to multimodality therapy which includes surgical and radiation therapy.

Bladder Cancer

The most frequent malignant tumour of the urinary tract is transitional cell carcinoma of the bladder. Most bladder tumours are papillomatous growth within the bladder.

Aetiology

The primary aetiology of bladder cancer is exposure to aniline dyes used in the textile industry. Cigarette smoking is associated with an increase in bladder tumours. Cancer of the bladder is most common between the ages of 60 to 70 years and more in men than women. Risk factors include cigarette smoking, exposure to dyes used in the rubber and cable indsutries, and chronic abuse of phenacitin containing analgesics. Women treated with radiation of cervical cancer and patient who has received cyclophosphomide also have increased risk, but reasons are not known yet.

Pathophysiology

Tumours of the bladder range from small benign papilloma to large invasive carcinomas. Most neoplasms are of the transitional cell type because the urinary tract is covered with transitional epithelium. These neoplasms begin as papillomas. Therefore, all papillomas of the bladder are considered premalignant and are removed when identified. Carcinoma of the bladder graded and staged as follows:

Grades	*Differentiation*
Grade I	Well differentiated
Grade II	Medially differentiated
Grade III	Poorly differentiated
Grade IV	Anaplastic

Stage	*Tissue involvement*
Stage O	Mucosa
Stage A	Submucosa
Stage B	Muscle
Stage C	Perivisicle fat
Stage D	Lymph node

Clinical Manifestations

Gross painless haematuria is the first sign of bladder tumour in most patients. It is usually intermittent, lessening the person's concern and delaying medical care. Haematuria may be accompanied by urgency and dysuria. Some patients are asymptomatic until obstruction occurs. Painless haematuria is seen in renal tumour; so it should be investigated. Cystitis may be first symptom of the bladder tumour, since the tumour acts as a foreign body into the bladder causing inflammation. Symptoms of renal failure result from obstruction of the ureters. Sometime, it causes one to seek medical care. Vesico-vaginal fistula (VVF) may occur before symptoms develop. The presence of renal failure or VVF indicates a poor prognosis because they usually occur after the tumour has infiltrated widely.

Management

When cancer is suspected, urine specimen for cytology can be obtained to determine the presence of cancer cells. Bladder cancers can be detected using IVP, ultrasound, CT or MRI. However, the presence of cancer is confirmed by cystoscopy and biopsy.

Chemotherapy is primarily palliative or used before radiation therapy. CMV (Cisplatin, methotraxate, and vinblantine) with or without doxorubiun hcl is most frequently used therapy. Thiotepa may be instilled into the bladder as a topical treatment for noninvasive bladder cancer. Before instillation of thiotepa, the patient receives 8 to 12 hours of IV hydration. The dwell time for thiotepa is 12 hours after which the drug is drained.

External cobalt radiations of large invasive tumours may be recommended before surgery to retard tumour growth. Super voltage irradiation can be given when the patient physically cannot tolerate include a variety of procedures. Transurethral resection (TUR), with fulguration (electrocautery) is used for

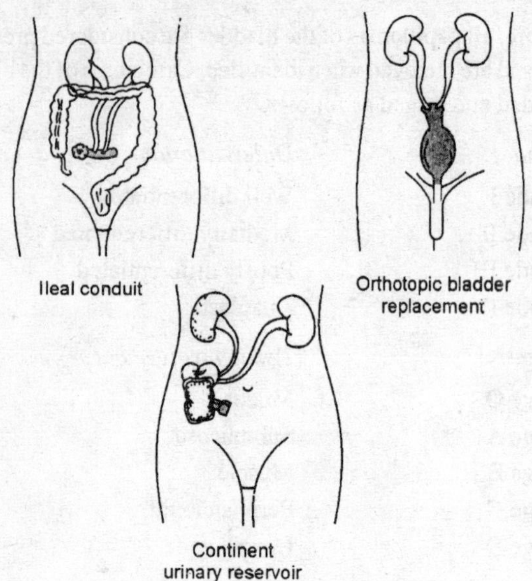

Fig. 14.5: Methods of urinary diversion.

the diagnosis and treatment of superficial lesions with low recurrent rate. This is also used to control bleeding in advanced tumours. Laser photo coagulation, and open loop resection (snaring of polytypes of lesion) with fulguration are also used. Postoperative management as in any surgical procedure is with avoidance of alcoholic beverages, analgesics and stool softener.

Renal Trauma/Trauma of Urinary Tract

Assessing the integrity of the urinary tract must be part of the evaluation of any person with traumatic injury to the lower trunk. A continual increase in the incidence of traumatic renal injuries is related to an increase in the mechanization and speed of transportation and to the increase in violent crimes and injuries. Injuries particularly related to the urinary tract damage include fractures of the pelvis, penetrating blows to the body and blunt trauma.

Aetiology

The majority of incidence occur in men younger than 30 years of age. Blunt trauma is the most frequent cause. Injury to the kidney should be considered in multiple or sports injuries, traffic accidents and falls. It is especially likely when the patient injures the abdomen flank or back. Penetrating injuries may result from violent encounters (e.g. gunshot, or stabbing incidents) or from surgical procedure errors. Pelvic fracture may result in bladder perforation and urethral tearing. A sharp blow to the body particularly to the lower back, may result in contusion, tearing or rupture of a kidney.

Pathophysiology

If trauma of the urinary tract occurs for any reason, urine output may be scant or absent after trauma, urine if present, may be bloody and symptoms of peritonitis may appear. The first symptoms of trauma to the kidney usually are haematuria and pain or tenderness of the upper abdominal quadrant and flank on the involved side. Signs of shock may be present if haemorrhage is extensive.

Management

Clinical findings include a history of trauma to the area of the kidneys. Diagnostic test used to facilitate diagnosis of trauma to urinary tract incldues KUB, cystogram, IVP, renal angiography and CT scan. Laboratory test includes serial urinalysis and haemoglobin, BUN and creatinine levels.

The severity of renal trauma depends on the extent of the injury treatment, range from bedrest, fluids and analgesics to surgical exploration and repair of nephrectomy. Initial treatment includes controlling bleeding, preventing shock and promoting urinary drainage. A cystotomy may be performed to provide urinary drainage when injuries involve the bladder and urethra. Vital signs, fluid balance records, and haematocrit levels are monitored to assess bleeding.

Complaints of pain may indicate ureteral colic, signifying obstruction of the ureter bya clot. Surgery is required to control severe haemorrhages; otherwise the kidney is allowed to heal spontaneously. Bedrest is maintained until gross haematuria resolves; thereafter, activity progress according to tolerance and absence of haematuria. When urethral injuries are suspected, great care must be taken when inserting urinary catheters to prevent further urethral injury.

A kidney may become loosened and 'float' or become displaced (nephroptosis). If symptoms of obstruction occurs, the kidney may be sutured to its anatomical site (nephropexy). Postoperatively the patient's hips are elevated to prevent tension on the suture line. Nephrectomy may be indicated depending on the severity of the trauma.

Nursing interventions vary with type and extent of associated injuries. Specific intervention related to renal trauma include ensuring increased fluid intake, providing comfort, measures, monitoring intake and output, observing for haematuria, determining the presence of myoglobinuria, assessing the cardiovascular status, and monitoring potentially-nephrotoxic antibiotics. Care of the person is similar to nephrectomy or urinary diversion procedures.

Teaching should include preventive strategies such as wearing a seat belt when on automobile, following safety rules, when riding bicycle or walking, and wearing protective equipment when participating in contact sports. Person with one kidney should be cautioned regarding participation in contact sports.

Urinary Retention

Urinary retention is the inability to empty the bladder. The kidneys are producing sufficient urine, but the person is unable to expel the urine from the bladder.

Aetiology

The causes of urinary retention are either mechanical or functional. *Mechanical causes* may be congenital or acquired and include anatomic blockage of urine flow in the lower urinary tract.

- Congenital – Urethral stricture
  – Urinary tract malformation
  – Spinal cord malformation
- Acquired – Calculus
  – Inflammation
  – Trauma
  – Tumour
  – Hyperplasia
  – Pregnancy

Functional causes include impairment of urine flow in the absence of mechanical obstruction which includes:

- Neurogenic bladder dysfunction.
- Ureterovesicle reflux.
- Decreased peristaltic activity of the ureter.
- Detrusor muscle atrophy.
- Anxiety i.e. fear of pain after surgery.
- Medications i.e., anaesthetics, narcotics, sedative, antihistamines, antihypertensives, antiparkinsonism, anticholenergics and antispasmodics.

Pathophysiology

An inability to void results from blockage of the urethra. The end result and primary feature of urinary retention is inability to void. The bladder becomes distended with urine and is sometimes displaced to either side of the midline. Percussion over full bladder produce a "Kettle drum" sound. Discomfort occurs from pressure of the bladder on other organs, and the person has an urge to urinate. Restlessness and diaphoresis also may occur with a full bladder. Voiding 25 to 50 ml of urine at frequent intervals often indicates retention with overflow. The intravesicular pressure increases as the bladder continues to fill with urine.

As the bladder overfills, the restoring capacity of the spincter is taxed. A small amount of urine flows out of the bladder to reduce the intravesicular pressure to the level where the spincter can control the flow of urine once again. The patient may state that the bladder continues to feel full. As the bladder fills again, the cycle is repeated. The urine-specific gravity is normal or high in the presence of retention with overflow because the kidney's ability to produce urine is not impaired.

Management

Urinary retention is urological emergency and if untreated can lead to kidney damage. Intervention for urinary retention is aimed at re-establishing the urine flow. The diagnosis of urinary retention is based on determining the amount of residual urine after voiding attempts. Urine yield of 250 to 300 ml after catheterization is indicative of retention. Routine studies of urorenal systems including a complete history and physical examination with particular attention to GU systems are helpful in identifying retention.

Medications used in urinary retention is determined by the aetiology. Retention due to sensory/neurological problems may be treated with cholenergic drugs. The drugs which stimulate bladder contraction should not be used if obstruction is suspected. Obstruction occurs below the bladder, continuous drainage must be provided to prevent damage to the kidney. One means of providing drainage is by the use of *'cystostomy'* tube (usually Foleys, Malicot, or Pezzor Catheter) which is placed directly into the bladder through a suprapubic incision. If surgery like nephrostomy or pyelostomy indicated can be performed with proper preparation followed by post-procedure care appropriately.

Urinary Incontinence

Urinary incontinence is voluntary unpredictable expulsion of urine from the bladder is encountered in several temporary or permanent conditions, due to cerebral clouding, infection, disturbance of CNS pathways cerebral lesions), disturbance of urethrobladder reflex (upper or lower motor neuron) and tissue damage.

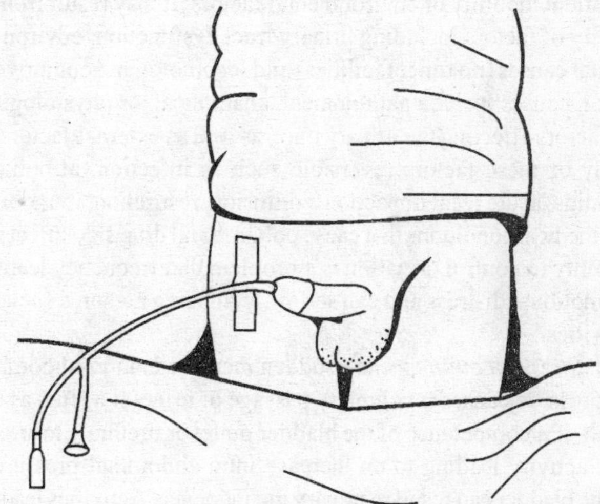

Fig. 14.6: (A) In the male patient, the indwelling catheter is taped to the thigh to straighten the angulation of the penoscrotal junction, thus reducing pressure on the urethra exerted by the catheter.

Aetiology

Anything that interferes with bladder or urethral spincter control can result in urinary incontinence. Causes may be *transient* (e.g.caused by confusion or depression, infection, medications, restricted mobility or stool impaction); *congenital* disorders that produce incontinence include exstrophy of the bladder, epispadias, spinabifides with myelomenigocele, and ectopic ureteral orifice; *acquired* disorder includes functional incontinence, stress incontinence, urge incontinence, overflow incontinence, reflex incontinence, incontinence after trauma or surgery.

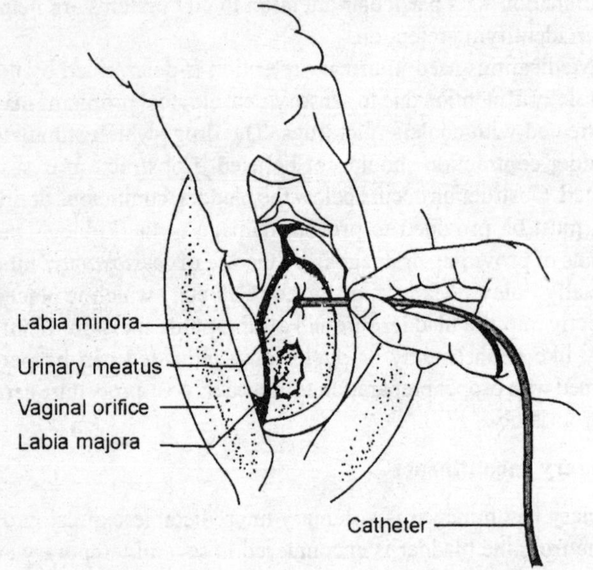

Fig. 14.6: (B) Catheterization of urinary bladder in the female patient.

i. *Functional incontinence* is loss of urine due to problems of patient mobility or environmental factors. It may result from variety of factors including urinary tract dysfunction, environmental causes (no toilet facilities) and locomotor and cognitive factor, causes include pathological, anatomical, or physiological factors affecting the urinary tract, as well as external factors. Many of these factors reversible such as infection, atrophic vaginitis, acute fecal impaction, confusion, restriction, immobility, medical conditions that cause polyuria and drug side effects. Inability to control urination is a problem that frequency leads to emotional distress and can seriously impair a person's social activities.

ii. *Stress incontinence* is a sudden increase in intra-abdominal pressure causes involuntary passage of urine. It occurs as a result of incompetence of the bladder outlet or urethral closure. Any activity leading to an increase intra-abdominal pressure on the bladder can result in urinary incontinence. Activities leading to stress incontinence, including lifting, exercising, coughing and sneezing or laughing.

iii. *Urge incontinence* is the involuntary loss of urine associated with an abrupt and strong desire to void (urgency). It is a condition which occurs randomly when involuntary urination is preceded by warning of few seconds to a few minutes. Leakage is periodic but frequent. Nocturnal frequency and incontinence are common conditions; it may appear with varying severity during psychological stress. *Motor urge* incontinence caused by detrusor muscle instability; *Sensory* urge incontinence caused by hypersensitivity of bladder. The incontinence occurs as a result of uninhibited detrusor contractions. When active detrusor contraction over come urethral resistence, urine leakage occurs. This type of incontinence is seen in patients with multiple sclerosis or after CVA (stroke), Ca, bladder, and other cerebrovascular disorders.

iv. *Overflow (Paradoxic) incontinence.* Involuntary loss of urine associated with overdistension of the bladder is called overflow incontinence. It is a condition when the pressure of urine is overfull, bladder overcomes spincter control. Leakage of small amounts of urine is frequent throughout the day and night. Urination may also occur frequently in small amounts. Bladder is remaining distended and usually palpable. This disorder caused by outlet obstruction (Prostate hyperplasia, bladder neck obstructs in urethral stricture) or by underactive destrusor muscle caused by myogenic or neurogenic factors (e.g. herniated disc, diabetic neuropathy). It may also occur after anaesthesia surgery (haemorroidectomy, herniorraphy, cystoscopy) and neurogenic bladders and after radical pelvic surgery.

v. *Reflex incontinence* is a condition which occurs when no warning or stress precedes periodic involuntary urination. Urination is frequent, moderate in volume and occurs equally during the day and night. It is caused when spinal cord lesion about S.2 interfers with CNS inhibition disorders result in detrusor hyperreflexion and interferes with pathways coordinating detrusor contraction and spincter relaxation.

vi. *Incontinence after trauma or surgery.* Vesico-vaginal or urethro-vaginal fistula may occur in women. Alteration incontinence control in men involves proximal urethral sphincter (bladder neck and prostatic urethra) and distral sphincter (external straited muscle). Fistula may during pregnancy, after delivery of a baby, as a result of hysterectomy or invasive cancer of cervix; or after radiation therapy. Incontinence is found as postoperative complication after transurethral, perineal or retropubic prostatectomy.

Pathophysiology

Bladder sphincter control is necessary for urinary continence. Such control requires normal voluntary and involuntary muscle action coordinated by a normal urethrobladder reflex. As the bladder fills the pressure within the bladder gradually increases. The detrusor muscle within the bladder wall responds by relaxing to accommodate the greater volume. When the bladder has filled to capacity, usually between 400 and 500 ml of urine; the parasympathetic stretch receptors located within the bladder will be stimulated. The stimuli are transmitted through afferent fibres of the reflex once for micturition. Impulses are then carried through the efferent fibers of the reflex are to the bladder, causing contraction of the detrusor muscle. The internal sphincter, which is normally closed, reciprocally opens and urine enters the posterior urethra. Relaxation of the external sphincter and perineal muscles follows, and urine is released. Completion of this reflex can be interrupted and voiding postponed through release of inhibitory impulses from the cortical center, which results involuntary contraction of the external sphincter. If any part of this complex control system is interrupted, urinary incontinence will result. As stated earlier, the causes of urinary incontinence are disturbances of cerebral control, disturbances of urethrobladder reflex, bladder disturbance, relaxed musculation, psychogenic disturbances, etc.

Management

Urinary incontinence can be diagnosed by a variety of urodynamic examinations. A cystomyogram and electromyogram are done to evaluate the detrusor muscle of the bladder as well as sphincter and perineal activity. An ultrasound of the bladder, cystoscopy and IVP are also done to assess the structures and functioning of urinary tract.

Treatments of urinary incontinence can be categorized as behavioural, pharmocological and surgical. A combination of therapies is often used. *Behavioural* techniques include bladder training, timed voiding, prompted voiding, and pelvic muscle exercises. Behavioural therapies help people to regain control of their bladder. Bladder training teaches people to resist the urge to void and gradually expand the intervals between voiding. *Pelvic floor* electrical stimulation uses mild electrical impulses to stimulate muscle contractions.

The common medication for urinary incontinence are as follows:

i. Oestrogens (Premarim, Estratab, Estrace) binds the protein responsible for oestrogen effects; relieves atrophic vaginitis and restores urethral suppleness. Here the nurse has to explain risk of blood clots, review signs of thrombophlebitis and encourage smoking cessation. Examples of oestrogen are quinstrediol and estriol.
ii. Anticholenergic agents such as Pro-Bantine, Oxybutynine, Dicyclomin decrerase the spasticity of bladder, are direct smooth muscle relaxation of bladder. This may cause postural hypertension, for which instruct the patient to change position slowly and assess bowel sounds. These drugs should not be used in patients with glaucoma.
iii. Cholinergic agents such as bethanecol, neostigmines, treat flaccid bladder by stimulating contractions of the bladder. If used, administer medication on empty stomach, monitor vital signs and intake and output and instruct patients to ambulate with caution.
iv. Alpha-adrenergic blocks such as prazosin, phenoxybenzamine, phenylpropanolamine, reduce spasticity of the bladder neck. When administering these drugs, monitor orthostatic vital signs; monitor intake and output and daily weight the patient and instruct patient to avoid OTC medication unless instructed by physician.
v. *Sympathomimetics* such as ephedrine, phenylphrine, increase in bladder neck and urethral tone. During its administration monitor for dysrhythmias, assess vital signs and instruct patient on potential side effects of dizziness, headache or dyspnoea.
vi. *Alpha-adrenergic blockers* such as phenylpropanolamine. Imipramine increases urethral resistance. This should be administered several hours before bedtime. Instruct patient to avoid caffeine containing beverages.
vii. *Calcium channel blockers* such as nifedipine, diltiazine, verapamil, reduce detrusor contractions. When it is used, monitor blood pressure and heart rate and assess for orthostatic hypertension and monitor intake and output.

Surgical approaches vary, depending on the underlying problem. For example, a transurethral resection of the prostate is used to treat BPH. Several surgical procedures help correct anatomic malposition of the bladder neck and urethra that causes female stress incontinence e.g. Vesicourethroplexy. Pre- and postoperative measures are taken accordingly.

The nurse must recognize both the physical and the emotional problems that accompany incontinence. The patient's dignity, privacy, and feeling of selfworth must be maintained or enhanced. Most persons suffering from incontinence can be helped with proper diagnosis and modern therapeutic approaches.

A person with stress incontinence can be taught to do pelvic floor (perineal) muscle exercises (Kegel exercises). The patient should contract the pelvic muscles as though trying to stop the flow of urine, while relaxing the abdomen, thighs and buttocks. Each contraction is held for a few seconds and followed by relaxation for the same period of time. Contraction and relaxation times are gradually increased. These exercises should be repeated in sets of 10 or more contractions and done four to five times each day over several weeks. Consistency and persistence are necessary for success and exercise regimens have to be individualized. Vaginal weights (cones) or biofeedback may help patient gain awareness and control of their pelvic muscles. Vaginal weight training involves holding small weight within the vagina by tightening the vaginal muscles. These exercises should be performed for 15 minutes twice daily for 4 to 6 weeks.

The nurse has a major responsibility to help the patient with incontinence problems in a variety of settings. In the hospital, nursing measures aimed at maintaining urinary continence include: identifying transient causes and assessing patient for signs of bladder infections, foecal impaction, or bladder distention. The nurse should offer the urinal or bedpan or help the patient going to the bathroom every 2 hours or at scheduled intervals. Assuming the usual position for urination (standing for the man and sitting and leaning forward for the woman) or using relaxation techniques often help a patient urinate successfully, particularly in unfamiliar settings. Applying pressure over the bladder area (credes maneuver) may be helpful when bladder outlet distruction is not a problem. The nurse should ensure that the patient has privacy and is not rushed when trying to urinate. Technique to stimulate urination includes running water in the sink, placing hands in water, and pouring warm water over the perinium. Fluid intake patterns monitored and fluids encouraged.

If bladder retaining cannot be achieved, external appliances or intermittent self-catheterization may be indicated. Several external appliances that prevent soiling, decreasing odour, and improved body images are available for men. External appliances for womens are not useful in most situations. However, newly developed inserts, patches, pessaries and bladder neck support devices are useful for some women with stress incontinency. Keeping the skin clean and dry is essential to prevent skin irritation and breakdown.

The nursing responsibilities are often measured for different types of incontinency as follows:

i. Stress incontinence
   - Perineal muscle exercises (e.g. Kegel exercises) i.e.,
     - Tighten the pereneal muscle as if to prevent voiding hold for 3 seconds, then relax.
     - Inhale through pursed lips while tightening perineal muscles.
     - Bear down as if to have a bowel movement. Relax and then tighten perineal muscles.
     - Hold a pencil in the fold between the buttock and thigh.
     - Sit in the toilet with knees held wide apart. Start and stop the urinary stream.
   - Weight loss if patient is obese.
   - Insertion of vaginal pessary, oestrogen vaginal cream.
   - Insertion of condom catheters, or penile clamp, surgery.
   - Urethral inserts, patches or bladder necks support devices to correct underlying problem.

ii. Urge incontinence
   - Treatment of underlying cause.
   - Instructions to have patient urinate more frequently or on time schedule.
   - Anticholenergic drugs, propanthine or imopramine at bed time.
   - Calcium channel blockers, condom catheters, vaginal oestrogen creams.

iii. Overflow incontinence
   - Urinary catheterization to decompress bladder.
   - Implementation of cre's valsalva manoeuver.
   - Alpha-adrenergic blockers i.e. Prazosin to decrease outlet resistance.
   - Bethanechol to enhance bladder contractions.
   - Intermittent catheterization.
   - Surgery to correct underlying problem.

iv. Reflex incontinence
   - Treatment of underlying cause.
   - Decompression to prevent ureteral reflux and hydronephrosis.
   - Intermittent self-catheterization.
   - Alpha-adrenergic blockers (Prazosin) to relax internal sphincter.
   - Diaepam or bacl often to relax external spincter.
   - Prophylactic antibiotics.
   - Surgical sphincteratomy.

v. Incontinence after trauma or surgery
   - Surgery to correct fistula.
   - Urinary diversion surgery to bypass urethra and bladder.
   - External condom catheter.
   - Penile clamp.
   - Placement of artificial implantable sphincter.

vi. Functional incontinence
   - Modification of environment or careplan that facilitates regular easy access to toilet and promote patient safety (better lighting ambulatory assistant equipment, clothing, alteration, timed voiding, different toileting equipment).

Reno-Ureteral Surgery

The most comon indication for nephrectomy are: renal tumour, polycystic kidneys that are bleeding or severely infected, massive traumatic injury to the kidney and the elective removal of a kidney from a donor. Surgery involving the ureters and kidneys is most commonly performed to remove calculi that becomes obstructive, correct congenital anomalies, and divert urine when necessary. Now laparoscopic nephrectomy is also performed to obtain a kidney from a living, related donor to be transplanted into a person with end-stage renal disease.

Preoperative Care

The basic needs/routines of the patient undergoing renal and ureteral surgery are similar to those of any patient who experiences surgery. In addition, it is especially important preoperatively to ensure adequate fluid intake and a normal electrolyte balance. The patient should be told that there will be probably a flank incision on affected side and surgery will require a hyperextended, side-lying position. This position frequently causes the patient to experience muscle aches after surgery. If nephrectomy is planned, the patient must be assured that one working kidney is sufficient to maintain normal renal function.

Postoperative Care

The specific postoperative needs of a patient are related to urine output, respiratory status and abdominal distension.

In the immediate postoperative period, urine output should be determined at least every one to two hours. Drainage from various catheters should be recorded separately. The catheter or tube should not be clamped or irrigated without a specific order. The total urine output should be at least 30 to 50 ml per hour. It is also important to assess for urine drainage on dressing and to estimate the amount. Daily weighing of the patches is important. The same scale, dress should be weighed.

Postoperatively it is important to ensure adequate ventilation. The patient is often reluctant to turn, cough and take deep breath because of the incisional pain. Adequate pain medication should be given to ensure the patient comfort and ability to perform coughing and deep-breathing exercises. Frequently additional respiratory devices such as an incentive spirometer are used every two hours while the patient is awake. In addition, early and frequent ambulation assists in maintaining adequate respiratory function.

Abdominal distention is common in these surgery; may be due to paralytic ileas caused by manipulation and compression of the bowel during surgery. For which, oral intake is restricted until bowel sounds return to normal until IV fluids are recommended.

Urinary Diversion

Urinary diversion may be performed with and without cystectomy. Urinary diversion procedures are performed to treat cancer of the bladder, neurogenic bladder, congenital anomalies, strictures, trauma to the bladder, and chronic infection with deterioration of renal function. Numerous urinary diversion techniques and bladder substitutes are possible including an incontinent urinary diversion, continent urinary diversion catheterized by patient, or an orthotopic bladder so that patient voids urethrally.

- *Incontinent* urinary diversion is diversion to the skin requiring an appliance. The simplest form is the cutaneous ureterostomy, but scarring and strictures led to the use of ileal or colonic conduits, preferably ileal conduit.
  In *ileal conduit* ureters are implanted into part of ileum or colon that has been resected from intestinal tract. Abdominal stoma is created. It helps relatively good urine flow with few physiological alteration. External appliances need to continually collect urine. This procedure is more complex. Postoperative complication may be increased. Reabsorption of urea by ileum occurs. Meticulous attention is needed to care for stoma and collecting device.
- A *continent* urinary diversion is an intra-abdominal urinary reservoir that is catheterizable or with an outlet controlled by the anal sphincter. Continent diversions are internal pouches created similarly to the ileal conduit. Reservoirs have been constructed from the ileum, ileocecal segment or colon. Here, ureters are excised from bladders and brought through abdominal wall and stoma is created. External appliance is necessary because of continuous urine drainage; possibility of stricture or stenosis of small stoma. Periodic catheterization may be required to dilate stomas to maintaining patency.

Nephrostomy may be performed and catheter is inserted into pelvis of kidney. Procedure may be done to one or both kidneys and may be temporary or permanent. It is most frequently done in advanced disease as palliative procedure. There is high risk of renal infection predisposed to calcious formation from catheter. Nephrostomy tube may have to be changed every month. Catheter must never be clamped.

- *Orthotopic* bladder substitutes can be derived from various segments of the intestine. An isolated segment of the distal ileum is often preferred. Various procedures include the hemiKock pouch, studer pouch, and the ilear W-neobladder. In these procedures, the bowel is surgically reshaped to become a neobladder. The ureters and urethra are sutured into the neobladder. Orthotopic bladder substitute allows for natural micturation. Incontinence may be possible problem needing intermittent catheterization.

Preoperative Care

The patient is awaiting cystectomy and urinary diversion must be given a great deal of informations. The nurse must assess ability and readiness to learn and teach the details about the procedure to the patient. The patient's anxiety and fear may be decreased by giving proper information. A discussion of social aspects of living with a stoma (including clothing, changes in body image, and sexuality, exercises and odour) provides the pattern with facts that may lay some fears. The patient who will have continent diversion must be taught to catheterize and irrigate the pouch and be able to adhere to a strict catheterization schedule. Like this; every information should be provided to the patient undergoing surgery.

The basic needs of the patient requiring urological surgery are the same as those of any other surgical patient. Special emphasis must be placed on promotion of ventilation and adequate urine output, prevention of distention and haemorrhage and attention to drainage tubes and dressings.

The care of the person after urological surgery needs emphasis on the following:

i. Promote ventillation
   - Encourage breathing exercises.
   - Encourage self-turning in bed frequently.
   - Encourage ambulation.

ii. Monitor patency and output of urinary catheter.

iii. Prevent complications.
   - Change wet dressings to protect skin.
   - Restrict food and oral fluids if bowel sounds are absent.
   - Encourage fluids to 3000 ml/day when permitted.
   - Monitor for bright red blood on dressing or in urine.

iv. Administer analgesics to control pain.

The following guidelines should be used for changing a urinary pouch.

- Explain procedure to patient, being sure to include sensory information.
- Assemble all supplies.
- Empty the pouch and gently remove the pouch from the skin.

- Cleanse the peristomal skin with mild soap and water. Rinse and pat dry.
- Wash mucus secretions off the stoma gently.
- Measure the diameter of the stoma and cut a corresponding opening in the skin barrier and the pouch or select the corresponding size of percute pouch.
- Apply skin seal around the stoma is desired. Allow the area to dry completely.
- Attach the pouch to the skin barrier. The pouch and skin barrier may be applied to the skin separately or together. In the early postoperative period, it is easier to attach the pouch to the skin barrier and then apply the system in one piece to the skin.
- Apply the pouch and skin barrier around the stoma, keeping the adhesive area free of wrinkles or creases. Press gently and firmly into place. The value at the bottom of the pouch must be closed or attached to drain tubing and collecting bag.

Renal Failure

Renal failure is severe impairment or total lack of kidney function, in which there is an inability to excrete metabolic waste products and water, as well as functional disturbance of all body systems. Renal failure may be acute in onset (developing in hours to days) or chronic (developing slowly and progressively over a course of several years). Renal failure refers to a significant loss of renal function, when only 10 per cent of renal function remains, the person is considered to have end-stage renal disease.

Acute Renal Failure: (ARF)

Acute renal failure is a clinical syndrome characterised by a rapid decline in renal function with progressive azotemia (an accumulation of nitrogenous waste products such as BUN) and increasing levels of serum creatinine. Urine output is generally less than 40 ml/hr (Oliguria) but may be normal or even increased. ARF can be further divided into prerenal, intrarenal or intrinsic and postrenal aetiologies.

Aetiology

i. Prerenal causes consist of outside the kidneys than reduce renal blood flow and lead to decreased glomerular perfusion and filtration. This is caused by intravascular volume depletion, decreased cardiac output, or vascular failure secondary to vasodilation or obstruction.
   - *Hypovolaemia* can lead to decreased renal perfusion, which can be due to:
     - Haemorrhage
     - Dehydration
     - Vomiting
     - Gastric suction
     - Diabetes insipidus
     - Diabetes mellitus
     - Wound drainage
     - Cirrhosis
     - Inappropriate use of diuretics
     - Diaphoresis
     - Burns
     - Peritonitis.
   - Decreased cardiac output
     - Congestive heart failure
     - Myocardial infarction
     - Precardial temponade
     - Cardiac arrhythmias/dysrythmias
     - Open heart surgery
     - Cardiogenic shock.
   - Systemic vasodilation/decreased peripheral resistance
     - Sepsis (Septic shock)
     - Acidosis
     - Anaphylaxis
     - Neurologic injury.
   - Hypotension/hypoperfusion
     - Cardiac failure
     - Shock
   - Renal vascular obstruction
     - Thrombosis of renal arteries
     - Bilateral renal vein thrombosis
     - Embolism.
   - Drugs that may complicate prerenal azosimin include NSAIDS, which block synthesis of vasodilating prostaglandins and angiotensin converting enzyme (ACE) inhibition which blocks synthesis of angiotengiotensin.

ii. *Intrarenal causes*

Prerenal disease can lead to intrarenal disease (tubular necrosis) if renal ischaemia is prolonged. Intrarenal failure is caused by damage to kidney tissues and structures and include tubular necrosis, nephrotoxicity and alteration in renal blood flow.

- Tubule/Nephron damage.
  - Acute tubular necrosis (most common cause)
  - Acute glomerulonephritis
  - Acute pyelonephritis
  - Rhabdomyolosis.
- Vascular changes
  - Coagulopathies
  - Malignant hypertension
  - Taxeamia of pregnancy
  - Systemic lupus erythematous
  - Sclerosis
  - Stenosis.
- Nephrotoxin/Nephrotoxic injury
  - Allergic-antibiotic (Sulfonamide, Rifampin) NSAIDS, ACE inhibitor.
  - Antibiotics- Gentamycin, tobramycin, amphotricin B, Polymyxin B, neomycin, kaneamycin, vancomycin.

- Chemical; Carbon tetrachloride and lead
- Heavy metals: arsenic, mercury
- Iodinated radiographic contrast media (IVP dye)
- Drug-induced intestitial nephritis- NSAIDs, tetracycline furosemide, thizaide, phenyton, penicillin, sulphonamide and cephalosporins.

iii. *Postrenal* causes involve mechanical obstruction of urinary outflow, between the kidney and the urethral meatus, which includes ureteral and bladder neck obstruction due to:
   - Calculi formation
   - Benign prostatis hyperplasia
   - Prostate cancer
   - Bladder cancer
   - Trauma (to back, pelvis or perineum)
   - Strictures
   - Spinal cord disease

Pathophysiology

The kidneys receive approximately one fourth of the cardiac output; therefore, they are very sensitive to alteration in perfusion. Most cases of ARF are caused by ischaemic episode. Ischaemia causes nephron damage, although maintaining of fluid and electrolyte balance is possible 25% of nephron functioning. A urinary output of at least 400 ml/day is necessary for adequate excretion of wastes. The decreased GFR that occurs in ARF is responsible for the increased BUN and serum creatinin levels. The kidneys respond to hypoperfusion in the release of renin and adaptive response to maintain perfusion to the glomerual bed. ARF developes when these adaptive responses are ineffective in maintaining normal kidney function.

The pathophysiology of ARF is not completely understood. Nephrotoxic factors and ischaemia produce acute renal failure (ARF). The possible pathologic process involved in ARF include the following.

- *Renal vasoconstriction:* Hypovelaemia and decreased renal blood flow stimulate renin release, which activates the angiotensin-aldosterone system and results in constriction of the peripheral arteries and the renal afferent arterioles. With decreased renal blood flow, there are decreased glomerular capillary pressure and glomerular filtration rate (GFR) as well as tubular dysfunction and ultimately oliguria.
- *Cellularoedema:* Ischaemia causes an anoxia, which leads to endothelial celloedema. Cellular oedema raises tissue pressure above capillary flow pressure; consequently blood flow through the arterioles may still be altered after treatment of the underlying conditions. Inadequate renal blood flow further depresses the GFR.
- *Decreased glomerular capillary permeability:* Ischaemia alters glomerular capillary permeability. This in turn reduces the GFR, which significantly reduces blood flow and leads to tubular dysfunction.
- *Intratubular obstruction:* When tubules are damaged, interstitial oedema occurs, and necrotic epithelial cells accumulate in the tubules. This accumulated debris also lowers the GFR by obstructing the tubules and increasing intratubular pressure.
- *Leakage of glomerular filtrate.* Glomrular filtrate leaks back into plasma through holes in damaged tubular membranes, which decreases intratubular fluid flow.

Clinical Manifestation

Clinically ARF may progress through phases of onset oliguria, diuresis and recovery. In some situations, the patient does not recover from ARF, and chronic renal failure results.

i. The *onset* is the initial phase of injury to the kidney. Reversal or prevention of kidney dysfunction is possible at this stage by early intervention. In this phase, there is hypotension, ischaemia, hypovolaemia are seen. Symptoms are subtle, which last for hours to days.

ii. *Oliguria* phase follows within one day of the onset. Major problems of the phase include inability to excrete fluid loads, regulate electrolysis and excrete metabolic waste products.

   When urine output is less than 400 ml/24 hours, there is inability to excrete metabolic wastes; increased serum urea nitrogen and creatinine. BUN may increase 20 mg/dl/day. The symptosm include nausea, vomiting, drowsiness, confusion, coma, gastrointestinal bleeding, asterixis, pericarditis. These last for 1-3-weeks, may extend to several weeks in older patients.

   When urine output is less than 30 ml/24 hours, there is inability to regulate electrolytes (hyperkalaemia, hyponatraemia, acidosis, hypocalcaemia, hyperphosphataemia); inability to excrete fluid overload, (fluid overload, hypervolaemia); haematological dysfunction. (anaemia, platelet dysfunction, leukopoenia) cases may require dialysis. The symptoms are nausea, vomiting, cardiac dysrythmias, ECG changes, ku Kussmauls breathing (rapid, deep respirations) drowsiness, confusion, coma, oedema, CCF pulmonary oedema, neck vein distention, hypertension, fatigue, bleeding, infection. The duration also is dependent upon type of toxic injury and duration of ischaemia.

iii. *Diuretic phase.* The diuretic phase begins gradual increase in daily urine output of 1 to 3 litre per day, but may reach 3 to 5 litres or more per day. There is increased production of urine (deficit in concentrating ability of tubule and osmotic diuretic effect of high BUN), slowly increasing excretion of metabolic wastes, hypovolaemia, loss of sodium, loss of potassium, high BUN initially; BUN gradually returns to baseline. Symptoms include, urine output upto 4-5 litres per day, postural hypertension, tachycardia, improving mental alertness and activity, weight loss, thirst, dry mucus membranes and decreased skin turgor. These last for 2-6 weeks after onset of oliguria, but duration may vary accordingly.

iv. *Recovery phase.* The recovery phase begins when the GFR increases so that BUN and serum creatinine levels are starting to stabilize and then decrease. Kidneys are returning to normal functioning, some residual renal insufficiency. Thirty percentage of patients do not attain full recovery of GFR. There is decreased energy levels which last for 3-12-months.

The clinical manifestations of acute renal failure according to body system are:

- Urinary
  - Decreased urinary output
  - Proteinuria
  - Casts
  - Decreased specific gravity
  - Decreased osmolality
  - Increased urinary sodium.
- Cardiovascular
  - Volume overload
  - Congestive heart failure
  - Hypotension (early)
  - Hypertension (after development of fluid overload)
  - Pericarditis
  - Pericardial effusion
  - Arrhythmias.
- Respiratory
  - Pulmonary oedema
  - Kussmauls respiration
  - Pleural effusion.
- Gastrointestinal nausea and vomiting
  - Anorexia
  - Stomatitis
  - Bleeding
  - Diarrhoea
  - Constipation.
- Haematologic anaemia (development within 48 hours)
  - Leukocytosis
  - Defect in plaslet functioning.
- Neurologic
  - Lethargy
  - Convulsions
  - Asterixis
  - Memory impairment.
- Others
  - Increased susceptibility to infection
  - Increased BUN
  - Increased creatinine
  - Increased potassium
  - Decreased pH
  - Decreased bicarbonate
  - Decreased calcium
  - Increased phosphate.

Management

The most important tool for distinguishing prerenal, intrarenal and postrenal causes the history, including a thorough review of recent clinical events and drug therapy. Urinalysis is an important diagnostic test. Urine sediment containing abundant cells, casts or protein suggests intrarenal ATN is associated with abundant urinary casts. Normal urine sediment is possible in both prerenal and postrenal causes. Haematuria, Pyuria and crystals may be associated with postrenal causes. If needed, further tests may be necessary such as CT, MRI, renal ultrasound, retrograde pyelogram and renal scan.

The use of medications in the treatment of ARF is determined by the underlying cause and the presenting symptoms. Hypovolaemia is treated with hypotonic solutions such as OUSI saline. If hypovolaemia is due to blood or plasma loss, packed red blood cells and isotonic saline are administered. Volume replacement's rates must match volume losses on a 1:1 basis. Loop diuretics are used to manage potassium levels. Doses of upto 320 mg/day of fusomide may be required to produce adequate diuretics. Renal failure from nephrotoxin or ischaemia is treated with agents that increase renal blood flow. These include renal-dose dopamine, mannitol and loop diuretics. Inflammatory states as in acute glomerulonephritis are treated with glucocorticosteroids. Patients with impaired renal functions may have altered responses to therapeutic doses of many medications. Uraemia alters the protein-binding sites, absorption, distribution and metabolism of many drugs. NSAIDS and ACE inhibitors are contraindicated in patients with acute renal failure.

When conservative management is not effective, dialysis is required. Dialysis, the process by which waste products in the blood are filtered through a semi-permeable membrane, is indicated. When the patient with ARF is fluid overloaded, and/or has rapidly progressive azotaemia, hyperkalaemia, and metabolic acidosis are used. Three methods are used. Haemodialysis, peritoneal dialysis and continuous renal replacement therapy.

While taking care of the person with acute renal failure following points to be kept in mind which include:

i. Maintaining fluid and electrolytic balance
   - Maintain fluid restrictions.
   - Monitor intravenous fluid carefully.
   - Keep accurate records of intake and output.
   - Weigh patient daily.
   - Monitor vital signs frequently, including postural signs.
   - Assess fluid status of patient frequently.
   - Administer phosphate binding medications as prescribed.
   - During diuretic phase.

- Assess for changes in mental status indicative of low serum levels.
- Assess for presence of irregular apical pulses indicative of hypokalaemia.

ii. Maintaining nutrition
- Provide fluid in small amounts during oliguric phase; gingerable and other effective -scent soft drinks may be tolerated better than other fluids.
- Provide diet.
  - Restricted in protein as prescribed.
  - High in carbohydrates and fat during protein restrictions.
  - Low in potassium during hyperkalaemia, high in potassium during hypokalaemia.
- Take measures to relieve nausea (antiemetic and comfort measure).

iii. Maintaining rest/activity balance
- Maintain bedrest in the acute phase.
- Assist patient with activities of daily living to conserve energy.
- Promote early ambulation when renal status permits.
- Provide for planned rest periods.

iv. Prevent injury
- Assess orientation, reorient confused patient.
- During bedrest, keep side rails raised and use padded rails as necessary.
- When patient is ambulatory, assess motor skills and monitor ambulation and assist patient as necessary.
- Assess patient for signs of bleeding.
- Protect patient from bleeding: instruct patient to use soft tooth brush, perform guaiac test on stool, emesis and nasogastric returns.

v. Preventing infection
- Avoid source of infection: limit visitors to well adults.
- Assess for signs and symptoms of infection.
- Maintain asepsis for indwelling lines or catheters.
- Perform pulmonary hygiene.
- Turn weak or immobile patients every 2 hours and as needed.
- Provide meticulous skin care.
- Bathe patient with superfat soap.
- Administer prescribed antipruritic agents.

vi. Facilitate coping
- Encourage development of nurse-patient relationship to assist patient to express feelings as desired.
- Promote patient independence (autonomy).
- Assist patient to explore alternative way of coping.

In addition, patient and family education to be given to take care of the person with acute renal failure as follows:

- Causes of renal failure and problems with recurrent failures.
- Identification of preventable environmental or health factors contributing to the illness such as hypertension and nephrotoxic drugs.
- Prescribed medication regimen, including name of medication, dosage, reason for taking, desired and adverse effects.
- Prescribed dietary regimen.
- Explanation of risk of hypokalaemia, and reportable symptoms (muscle weakness, anorexia, nausea, vomiting and lethargy).
- Signs and symptoms of returning renal failure (decreased urine output, without decreased fluid intake, signs of fluid retention and increased weight).
- Signs and symptoms of infection, methods to avoid infection.
- Need for ongoing follow-up care.
- Option for the future, explanation of transplantation and dialysis there is a possibility.

Chronic Renal Failure (CRF)

Chronic renal failure involves progressive, irreversible destruction of the nephrons in both kidneys. The disease process progresses until most nephrons are destroyed and replaced by non-functional scar tissue.

Aetiology

Although there are many different causes of chronic renal failure, the end result is a systemic disease involving every body organ. The causes of chronic renal failure includes the following:

i. Glomerular dysfunction
- Glomerulonephritis.
- Diabetic nephropathy.
- Hypertensive nephrosclerosis.

ii. Systemic disease
- Sickle cell anaemia.
- Scleroderma.
- Polyarteritis nodosa.
- Systemic lupus erythematosus.
- HIV-associated nephropathy.
- Vasculitis.

iii. Urinary tract obstruction
- Prostatic and bladder tumours.
- Lymphadenopathy.
- Ureteral obstruction.
- Calculi.

iv. Others
- Chronic pyelonephritis.
- Nephrotic syndrome.
- Polycystic kidney disease.
- Renal infarction.
- Cyclosporin nephrotoxicity.
- Multiple meloma.

(Text Contd... page 747)

Table 14.1: Nursing care plan for the patient with acute renal failure

Problem	*R*	*Objective*	*Nursing Interventions*	*Rationales*
Nursing Diagnosis # 1 Fluid volume deficit: Actual (extracellular dehydration, hypovolaemia). Fluid volume deficit: Actual (intracellular dehydration, hypernatraemia).		(For patient outcomes, see earlier chapter on fluid and electrolyte balance)	• For pertinent information related to total body fluid and electrolyte status, see: Chapter on fluid and electrolyte balance.	
Nursing Diagnosis # 2 Fluid volume, alteration in: Excess (extracellular overhydration, hypervolaemia circulatory overload). Fluid volume, alteration.in: Excess (intracellular overhydration, hyponatraemia).				
Nursing Diagnosis # 3 Electrolyte imbalance, related to: 1. Water deficit. 2. Hypermatraemia. Electrolyte Imbalance, related to: 1. Water excess. 2. Hyponatraemia.		(For patient outcomes, see earlier chapter included the fluids and electrolyte balance).	• For pertienent nursing interventions and their rationales in the care of the patient with sodium imbalance, see: earlier chapter included electrolyte imbalance.	
Nursing Diagnosis # 4 Cardiac ouitput, alteration in: Decreased, related to: 1. Dysrhythmias associated with hyperkalaemia (> 5.5 mEq/liter). 2. Dysrhythmias associated with hypokalaemia (< 3.5 mEq/liter).		(For patient outcomes).	• For pertinent nursing interventions and their rationales in the care of the patient with potassium imbalance, see: earlier chapter on fluid and electrolyte balance.	
Nursing Diagnosis # 5 Acid-base balance, alteration in: Metabolic acidaemia (acidosis).		Patient's condition will stabilize as follows: 1. Arterial blood gases will normalize to baseline values: • pH > 7.35, < 7.45 • $PaCO_2$ optimal level for patient (normal range 35-45 mmHg). 2. Anions will stabilize as follows:	• Monitor neurologic status: Level of consciousness, mental status; cranial nerve function; deep tendon reflexes, seizure activity. • Monitor arterial blood gases. • Monitor serum potassium levels.	• Alterations in neurologic function are commonly associated with severe metabolic acidosis and may include confusion, headache, seizures, coma, and other manifestations. • Reflect effectiveness of ventilatory effort and gas exchange; blood gas levels and pH provide essential data for assessing acid-base and electrolyte balance. • Severe metabolic acidaemia can predispose to hyperkalaemia as excess

Contd...

Contd...

Problem	*R*	*Objective*	*Nursing Interventions*	*Rationales*
		• Bicarbonate (HCO^3) 22-26 mEq/liter. • Chloride 100-106 mEq/liter. • Anion gap 12-15 mEq/liter.		hydrogen ions are moved into cells in exchange for potassium ions, which enter intravascular space (circulation); hyperkalaemia may predispose to cardiac dysrhythmias and cardiac arrest.
		3. Neurologic: Alert, oriented to person, time, place; deep tendon reflexes—brisk.	• Monitor respiratory rate and rhythm.	• Hyperventilation (Kussmaul's breathing): Deep and rapid breating—the body's compensatory response to severe acidemia (pH < 7.20).
		4. Serum potassium level: 3.5-5.5 mEq/liter. 5. Haemodynamic status will stabilize as follows: • Arterial BP within 10 mmHg of baseline. • CVP = mean 0-8 mmHg. 6. Ventilatory effort will maintain blood gas values at optimal level for patient. • Respiratory rate: 12-18/min. • Tidal volume: > 5-7 ml/kg	• For pertinent information related to acid-base abnormalities including definition, pathophysiology, aetiology, clinical presentation, treatment, and nursing diagnoses, see: earlier chapter on fluids electrolyte balance.	
Nursing Diagnosis # 6 Nutrition, alteration in: Less than body requirements.		Patient will: 1. Maintain body weight between 2-5 per cent of patient's baseline. 2. Maintain serum albumin within physiologic range: 3.5-5.0 g/100 ml. 3. Tolerate oral feedings without nausea, vomiting, diarrhoea, or stomatitis.	• Collaborate with nutritionist to perform comprehensive nutritional assessment.	• Provides baseline for planning nutrition that will provide sufficient calories to prevent protein catabolism, and sufficient protein intake to meet body needs while avoiding excess production of urea nitrogen.
			♦ Weigh daily under same conditions.	♦ Body weight is best indicator of fluid gain or loss.
			♦ Monitor intake and output. – Monitor electrolytes closely.	♦ Diligent monitoring of fluid state is essential to prevent fluid excess during oliguric phase, and fluid deficit during diuretic phase.
			• Implement prescribed dietary regimen: ♦ Caloric intake: 2000-3000 calories/24 hr.	♦ The number of calories depends on age, size, and level of activity.
			♦ Low protein intake: ~1 g/kg of body weight/ 24 hr. – Protein sources high in essential amino acids.	♦ Low protein intake helps to control azotemia associated with compromised renal excretion of nitrogenous waste. Goal of therapy: Maintain body weight and prevent protein breakdown.
			♦ Avoid foods high in potassium. – Offer oral high caloric supplements; vitamin and mineral supplements.	♦ Acute renal failure and associated metabolic acidaemia place the patient at risk of developing hyperkalaemia.

Contd...

Contd...

Problem	*R*	*Objective*	*Nursing Interventions*	*Rationales*
			• Implement measures to enhance mealtimes:	
			◆ Provide frequent oral care.	◆ Prevents stomatitis; decreases foul taste; improves appetite.
			◆ Limit fluids with meals; provide more frequent small feedings.	◆ Smaller volume at mealtimes may facilitate gastric emptying and reduce gastrointestinal upsets.
			◆ Encourage family to bring appropriate home-cooked foods; encourage visiting during mealtimes.	◆ Favourite foods may enhance appetite. Helps to provide a mealtime atmosphere conducive to good eating.
			◆ . Encourage rest periods before and after meals.	◆ Avoids undue fatigue.
Nursing Diagnosis # 7 Knowledge deficit: Dietary regimen in renal disease.		Patient will: 1. Verbalize knowledge of prescribed diet; specify dietary restrictions and their significance.	• Initiate patient/family education regarding prescribed diet and meal preparation. Stress those foods permitted versus those foods restricted.	• Compliance with long-term dietary restriction requires that patient/family understand the relationship among renal disease, diet, and medication regimen.
			• Implement alternative approach to providing nutrition as dictated by patient's overall condition: ◆ Nasogastric or enteral feedings. ◆ Total parenteral nutrition.	• Ensures adequate intake of essential amino acids for maintaining and repairing body tissues; sufficient carbohydrate caloric source to reverse gluconeogenesis and catabolic state.
Nursing Diagnosis # 8 Infection, potential for: Depressed immunologic system.		Patient's condition will stabilize as follows: 1. Nonfebrile. 2. White blood count within physiologic range. 3. Patient will verbalize a general feeling of well-being. 4. Absence of infection. ◆ Negative cultures. ◆ Absence of redness, swelling, pain.	• Assess for signs of infection: ◆ Vigilant assessment of all invasive lines and wound dressings is critical. ◆ Observe for redness, pain, swelling at all invasive sites; dressing changes as per unit protocol. ◆ Monitor body temperature, white blood count; obtain cultures as indicated—Sputum, blood, urine, wound.	• Uremic state depresses the body's immunologic defenses and increases patient's susceptibility to infection. ◆ Infection is the most common cause of death in patients with ARF.
			◆ Pulmonary function: Encourage deep-breathing and coughing.	◆ Patient care activities are directed towards prevention of accumulation of pulmonary secretions and atelectasis.
			◆ Auscultate lungs for adventitious sounds of pulmonary congestion or increased secretions; encourage frequent position changes.	◆ Assists in evaluating ventilatory effort; patients with ARF are at high risk of developing pneumonia.
			◆ Urinary function: monitor use of Foley catheter; perform perineal care and cleansing around catheter as per unit protocol; maintain the integrity of the closed drainage system; examine urine for cloudiness or unusual odor.	◆ Use of indwelling Foley catheters in patients with ARF is associated with a high incidence of urinary tract infection (nosocomial infections). If an indwelling catheter is necessary, its insertion and ongoing care require *strict* aseptic technique. ◆ Indwelling catheter should be removed as soon as feasible as determined by the patient's overall condition.

Contd...

Contd...

Problem	*R*	*Objective*	*Nursing Interventions*	*Rationales*
Nursing Diagnosis # 9 Injury, potential for: Uremia-induced gastrointestinal disorders.		Patient will: 1. Tolerate oral feedings. 2. Verbalize having an appetite. 3. Maintain usual bowel routine. 4. Nasogastric secretions and stool negative for occult blood.	• Monitor gastrointestinal function: Assess abdomen for distention, tenderness; bowel sounds in all quadrants. ◆ Monitor for nausea, vomiting, and diarrhoea; test vomitus or nasogastric aspirate and stool for occult blood. ◆ Monitor Hct and Hgb.	• Patients with ARF are susceptible to gastrointestinal upsets, due in part to the chemical irritation caused by bacteria that hydrolyze urea to ammonia in the gut. • Administration of antibiotics or other drugs alters the intestinal flora, placing the patient at increased risk of infection.
Nursing Diagnosis#10 Skin integrity, impairment of: Potential.		Patient will: 1. Maintain intact skin; no breaks, lesions, or infection. 2. Exhibit warm, dry skin, with good turgor and absence of interstitial oedema. 3. Verbalize/demonstrate measures for optimal skin care.	• Maintain skin integrity. ◆ Inspect skin on each shift, especially reddened areas over bony prominences where skin is thin. ◆ Institute measures to prevent skin breakdown: frequent position changes; use of sheepskin or egg crate mattress (pressure relief device); frequent lubrication of skin; active/passive exercises as tolerated. ◆ Teach patient/family the essentials of skin care.	• A comprehensive assessment of skin can assist in early detection of alterations in skin. ◆ Deposition of phosphate crystals in the skin causes troublesome itching, which can lead to excoriation and infection. ◆ Patient/family can be taught to rub a lanolin-base lotion on the skin to avoid scratching and to stimulate circulation.
Nursing Diagnosis#11 Oral mucous membrane, alteration in. Patient will:		1. Verbalize/demonstrate measures for optimal oral hygiene.	• Maintain integrity of oral mucous membranes: Provide oral hygiene; instruct patient/family on measures to enhance oral hygiene.	• Changes in overall health status are often reflected in the status of the oral mucous membranes and the skin. Poor oral hygiene places the patient at risk of developing stomatitis; it decreases the patient's appetite and can seriously curtail oral intake.
Nursing Diagnosis#12 Comfort, alteration in: Pain (pericarditis).		Patient will: 1. Verbalize when in pain. 2. Identify appropriate pain relief measures. 3. Verbalize comfort. 4. Discuss origin of chest pain and significance in ARF.	• Evaluate pain and stress tolerance. ◆ Assess presence of chest pain: Severity, location, duration, quality (type) of pain, influencing factors. ◆ Assess presence of: Fever, chills, pericardial friction rub, gallop rhythm. ◆ Administer analgesic as prescribed, and evaluate its effectiveness in relieving pain. ◆ Instruct patient to lean forward over a pillow or bedside table. ◆ Perform comfort measures: Repositioning; relaxation techniques. ◆ Manipulate the environment and daily routines to provide rest periods. • Identify patients at risk and predisposing factors: Bacterial/viral infections associated with	• Pericarditis is frequently precipitated during the uremic state; fear of "heart attack" on the part of patient/family may complicate therapy and recovery. ◆ Use "SLIDT" tool. ◆ Chest pain associated with pericarditis can be sudden onset, sharp and intermittent, located substernally with radiation to neck and back. ◆ Diligent monitoring is essential because myocarditis and tamponade can lead to cardiac failure. ◆ This positioning frequently relieves chest pain associated with pericarditis. ◆ Comfort measures may decre-ase pain by promoting relaxation. • Prevention and/or prohylaxis is the best treatment.

Contd...

Contd...

Problem	*Objective*	*Nursing Interventions*	*Rationales*
		invasive lines, respiratory and gastrointestinal dysfunction, or wounds; poor dietary intake; depressed immunologic function.	
		◆ Assess for cardiac failure and tamponade.	◆ These complications must be anticipated and can create an acute emergency situation. The focus of diligent, ongoing assessment is to avoid these complications.
		• Discuss underlying cause of pericarditis and its potential impact on patient/family lifestyle.	• An informed patient/family facilitates their participation in the care process.
Nursing Diagnosis#13 Activity, alteration in: Fatigue and anaemia.	Patient will: 1. Verbalize decrease in fatigue. 2 Exhibit willingness to pace activities. 3. Maintain Hct and Hgb within realistic range based on renal function.	• Evaluate activity tolerance—impact of anaemic state:	
		◆ Assess onset, time of day, and duration of fatigue, and clinical circumstances in which it occurs.	◆ Fatigue is a major clinical manifestation attributed directly to the uremic state.
		◆ Monitor laboratory data to determine presence and extent of anaemia: Haematocrit and haemoglobin; complete blood count (CBC), platelet count; blood urea nitrogen (BUN), serum creatinine.	◆ Anaemia is often seen early in ARF and is associated with an inadequate synthesis of erythroprotein factor by the kidneys. Uremia may predispose to bleeding tendencies.
		◆ Assess skin for bruising or petechiae; nasogastric aspirate and stool for occult blood.	◆ Diligent, ongoing assessment is essential to prevent anaemia and/or a major bleeding disorder.
		◆ Minimize iatrogenic blood loss. Draw minimal blood samples for laboratory study; handle patient carefully to prevent bleeding; avoid hypodermic injections.	◆ Efforts to minimize blood loss are essential in the presence of compromised haematologic function associated with uremia.
		◆ Use stool softeners to prevent constipation and haemorrhoidal bleeding; use soft small-lumen nasogastric tube to minimize gastric mucosa irritation; monitor vital signs and watch carefully for signs of anaemia, haemorrhage, and occult bleeding from whatever source.	
		◆ Incorporate rest periods into daily routines. Assist patient/family to set priorities and to pace exercise and other activities alternating with timely rest periods.	◆ Conservation of strength may improve endurance.
Nursing Diagnosis#14 Knowledge deficit, impact of renal disease on patient/family lifestyle when the course of ARF is extended over several weeks or months.	Patient and family will: 1. Verbalize understanding of acute renal failure. 2. Verbalize willingness to make adjustments in lifestyle as necessitated by the course of the illness.	• Knowledge deficit health perceptions.	• ARF may require weeks to months for recuperation and often becomes chronic.
		◆ Assess patient/family baseline knowledge and readiness to learn.	◆ An informed patient/family can participate in care and make adjustments in lifestyle as necessitated by the course of the renal disease.
		◆ Establish a rapport with patient and family.	◆ An environment of mutual respect and trust can enhance the learning process.
		◆ Determine appropriate teaching strategies to facilitate learning:	◆ Learning should occur at a rate that is meaningful and tolerable to patient and family.

Contd...

Contd...

Problem	R	Objective	Nursing Interventions	Rationales
			– Encourage open discussions regarding renal disease: Aetiology, clinical presentation, complications, treatment, and prognosis. – Assist patient/family to relate dietary restrictions and exercise activities to status of renal disease. – Encourage patient/family to verbalize concerns regarding renal disease and expectations of its outcome.	
			♦ Reinforce learning and provide feedback for patient/family progress and achievements.	• Learning is an ongoing process; praise for one's accomplishments stimulates self-motivation, and assists in determining directions for further growth.
Nursing Diagnosis#15 Coping, ineffective individual/family: Potential.		Patient will: 1. Verbalize feelings regarding renal disease. 2. Identify strengths and coping capabilities. 3. make decisions regarding matters of importance to the patient/family. 4. Identify resources available in family and community.	• Evaluate coping capabilities: ♦ Assess patient's ability to solve problems and set priorities.	♦ Problem-solving capability enables patient to assume control and make decisions regarding own actions and behaviours.
			♦ Establish a trusting and caring rapport: Patient advocacy; accessibility to patient.	♦ A definitive, dependable support system assists the patient to assume responsibility for the level of health desired.
			♦ Encourage verbalization of perceptions, concerns, and feelings.	♦ Unexpressed and unresolved fears and concerns may compromise ability to cope effectively.
				♦ Active participation in self-care assists the individual to gain a new sense of dignity and feelings of self-worth.
			♦ Assist patient to identify past coping capabilities. Emphasize strengths; after praise for accomplishments; encourage development of new coping mechanisms.	
			♦ Assist to identify community resources and encourage patient to enlist assistance when necessary.	♦ Additional resources may assist patient to gain increased awareness of self in the interaction among patient, family and environment.

Pathophysiology

Chronic renal failure differs from acute renal failure in which the damage to the kidneys is progressive and irreversible. Progression of CRF is through four stages, decreased renal reserve, renal insufficiency, renal failure and end-stage renal disease (ESRD).

- *Decreased renal reserve*: (Renal impairment). This stage is characterised by normal BUN and serum creatinine levels and an absence of symptoms. 45-75 per cent loss of nephron function and GFR 40-50 per cent of normal.
- *Renal insufficiency:* In this there is 75-80 per cent loss of nephronfunction and 20-40 per cent GFR normal. BUN and serum creatinine levels begin to rise. Easy fatigue, weakness, mild anaemia, mild azotaemia, (which worsen physiological stress), nocturia, polyuria are seen.
- *Renal failure:* In this there are 10-20 per cent GFR normal, increase in BUN and serum creatinine levels, anaemia, Azotaemia, metabolic acidosis. Low urine specific gravity, polyuria, nocturia and symptoms of renal failure are present.
- *End-stage Renal disease (ESRD) or uremia.* In this stage there are more than 85% of loss of nephron, less than 10 per cent of normal GFR, BUN and serum creatinine at high levels. Anaemia, azotaemia, metabolic acidosis and urine-specific gravity are fixed at 1.010 oliguria and symptoms of renal failure appear. It is at this stage where most of the patients face much difficulty in carrying out basic activities of daily living because of the cumulative effect and extent of the symptoms.

Clinical Manifestations

As renal function progressively deteriorates every body

system becomes involved. The clinical manifestations are a result of retained resistances, including urea, creatinine, uremia, is a syndrome that incorporates all the disturbances seen in the various systems throughout the body in chronic renal failure. The body system manifestation in chronic renal failure causes signs, symptoms and assessment parameters as follows:

i. *Haematopoietic system* affected may be due to decreased erythroproteins by the kidney; decreased survival time of RBCs, bleeding, blood loss during dialysis, mild thrombocytopoenia and decreased activity of platelets. The signs and symptoms are anaemia, fatigue, defects in platelet function, thrombocytopoenia, ecchymosis and bleeding. Assessment parameters include haematocrit, haemoglobin, platelet count and observing for bruising, haematemesis or melena.
ii. *Cardiovascular system* affected may be due to fluid overload, Renin-angiotensin mechanism; overload anaemia, chronic hypertension, calcification of soft tissues, uremic toxins of pericardial fluid and fibrin formation on epicardium. These lead to hypervolaemia, hypertension, tachycardia, dysrhythmias, CCF, pericarditis for which monitoring of vital signs, body weight, ECG, heartsounds, electrolytes pain is needed.
iii. *Respiratory system* affected due to compensatory mechanisms for metabolic acidosis, uremic toxins, uremic lung and fluid overload. These lead to tachypnoea. Kussmauls respirations, uremic fetor (or uremic halitosis), tenacious sputum, pain with coughing elevated temperature, hilar pneumonitis, pleural friction rub, and pulmonary oedema, which needs respiratory assessment, arterial blood gas results readings, inspection of oral mucosa, monitoring vital signs and pulse oximetry.
iv. *Gastrointestinal systems* affected may be due to change in platlet activity, serum uremic toxins, electrolyte imbalances and urea converted to ammonia by saliva. This leads to anorexia, nausea and vomiting, gastrointestinal bleeding, abdominal distention, diarrhoea, and constipation, which need monitoring of intake and output, haematocrit, haemoglobin, guaic test for all stools, assessment for quality of stools, assess for abdominal pain.
v. *Neurological system* affected due to uremic toxins, electrolyte imbalance, cerebral swelling, resulting from fluid shifting, which leads to lethargy, confusion, stupor, coma, sleep disturbances, unusual behaviour, asterixis and muscle irritability. This requires monitoring level of consciousness, level of orientation, reflexes, EEG and electrolyte levels.
vi. *Skeletol system* may be affected due to decreased calcium absorption and decreased phosphate excretion. These give rise to renal osteodystrophy, renal rickets, joint pains, retarded growth, it needs assessment of levels of serum phosphorus, serum calcium, and for joint pain.
vii. Skin may be affected due to anaemia, retained pigment, decreased size of sweat glands, decreased activity of oil glands, dry skin, phosphate deposits and excretion of metabolic waste products through the skin. These give rise to pallor, pigmentation, pruritis, ecchymosis, excoriation and uremic frost, which needs observation for bruising, assessment of colour and integrity of skin and observe for scratching.
viii. *Genitourinary system* affected due to damaged nephron. This gives rise to decreased urine output, decreased urine specific gravity, proteinuria, casts and cells present in the urine, and decreased urine sodium, which requires monitoring of intake and output, serum creatinine, BUN, serum electrolytes, urine-specific gravity and urine electrolytes.
ix. *Reproductive system* may be affected due to hormonal abnormalities, anaemia, hypertension, malnutritions and medication. This leads to infertility, decreased libido, erectile dysfunction, amenorrhoea, and delayed puberty which require monitoring intake and output, vital signs, haematocrit and haemoglobin.

In addition, *Psychological changes* including personality and behavioural changes, emotional liability, withdrawal and depression are commonly observed. Fatigue and lethargy contribute to the patient's feeling of sickness. The changes and body image caused by oedema, integumentory disturbances, and access devices (fistulas, catheters) lead to further anxiety and depression.

Management

When a patient is diagnosed as having chronic renal insufficiency, conservative therapy is attempted before maintenance of dialysis begins. Because of the multisystemic effects, chronic renal failure may have serious abnormalities in laboratory values and which are characteristics of person with CRF. Diagnostic measures include identification of reversible renal disease by renal ultrasound, renal scan (if indicated), CT scan (if indicated), haematocrit and haemoglobin levels, BUN, serum creatinine and creatinin clearance level, serum electrolyte, urinalyses and urine culture.

Initial management of patient with chronic renal failure is focussed on controlling symptoms, preventing complications and delaying the progression of renal failure. The treatment goals for the person whose CRF are:

i. Stabilization of the internal environment as demonstrated by
   - Mental altertness, attention span, and appropriate interactions.
   - Absence or control of peripheral and pulmonary oedema.
   - Control of electrolyte balance within the following limits.
     - Sodium 125 to 145 mEq/L
     - Potassium 3-6 mEq/L

- Bicarbonate > 15 mEq/L
- Calcium 9-11 mg/dl
- Phosphate 3-5 mg/dl.
- Serum albumin > 2g/dl.
- Control of protein catabolism and protein metabolic wastes as indicated by following parameters.
  - Urea nitrogen < 100 mg/dl
  - Creatinine < 10 mg/dl
  - Uric acid < 12 mg/dl.
- Absence of joint inflammation and pain.
- Control of anaemia
  Haematocrit ≥ 33 per cent
  Ferritin > 50-100 mg/ml
  Iron saturation > 20 per cent.

ii. Absence of infection.
iii. Absence of bleeding.
iv. Blood pressure controlled at <140/90 mm Hg sitting and < 10 mm Hg postural change in standing.
v. Control of coexisting disease including heart failure, anaemia, dehydration.
vi. Absence of toxicity from inadequately excreted medications.
vii. Nutrient intake sufficient to maintain positive nitrogen balance.
viii. Anorexia and nausea are controlled.
ix. Pruritis controlled.

Medications are used to control blood pressure, regulate electrolytes and control intravascular fluid volume accordingly as prescribed. For example, therapies to lower serum potassium levels are: regular insulin administration intravenously, sodium bicarbonate IV, calcium gluconate, dialysis, kayexalate (Sodicum polystyrone sulffonate) and dietary restriction of potassium (40-50 mEq/L and treatment of concurrent disorders like anaemia, GI disturbances, etc.

While taking care of person with chronic renal failure following points are to be kept in mind.

i. Maintain fluid and electrolyte blance.
- Monitor for fluid and electrolyte excess.
  - Assess intake and output every 8 hours.
  - Weigh patient every day.
  - Assess presence of and extent of oedema.
  - Auscultate breach sounds.
  - Monitor cardiac rhythm and blood pressure every 8 hours.
  - Assess level of consciousness with the interval of every 8 hours.
- Encourage patient to remain within prescribed fluid restriction.
- Provide small quantities of fluid spaced over the day to stay within fluid restrictions.
- Encourage a diet high in carbohydrate and within the prescribed sodium, potassium, phosphorous and protein limits.
- Administer phosphate-binding agents with meals as prescribed.

ii. Prevent infection or injury.
- Promote meticulous skin care.
- Encourage activity within prescribed limits but avoid fatigue.
- Protect confused person from injury.
- Protect person from exposure to infectious agents.
- Maintain good medical/surgical asepsis during treatment and procedures.
- Avoid aspirin products.
- Encourage use of soft tooth brush.

iii. Promote comfort.
- Medicate patient as needed for pain.
- Medicate with prescribed antipruritic use of emollient bath, keep skin moist, and control environmental temperature to modify pruritis.
- Encourage use of damp cloth to keep lips moist, give good oral hygiene.
- Encourage rest for fatigue, however, encourage self-care as tolerated.
- Provide calm and supportive atmosphere.

iv. Assist with coping in lifestyle and self concept
- Promote hope.
- Provide opportunity for patient to express feelings about self.
- Identify available community resources.

In addition, patient and family teaching is needed while taking care of the person with chronic renal failure.

- Relationship between symptoms and their causes.
- Relationships among diet, fluid restriction, medication and blood chemistry values.
- Preventive health care measures: oral hygiene, prevention of infection and avoidance of bleeding.
- Dietary regimen, including fluid restrictions, i.e.
  - Prescribed sodium, potassium, phosphorous and protein restrictions.
  - Label reading and identifying nutritional content of foods.
  - Use of small frequent feedings to maintain nutrient intake when anorexia or nauseated.
  - Fluid prescription and sources of fluid in diet.
  - Avoidance of salt substitute containing potassium.
- Monitoring of fluid excess.
  - Accurate measurements and recording of intake and outputs.
  - Monitoring weight gain and oedema.

- Medication
  - Action, doses, purpose and side effects of prescribed medications.
  - Avoidance of over-the-counter (OTC) drugs, especially aspirin, cold medication and NSAIDs.
- Planning for gradual increase in physical activity including rest periods to conserve energy.
- Measures to control pruritis.
- Planning for following health care.
  - Symptoms requiring immediate medical attention: changes in urine output, oedema, weight gain, dyspnoea, infection, increased symptoms of uremia.
  - Need for continual medical follow-ups.

Add dialysis and kidney transplantation.

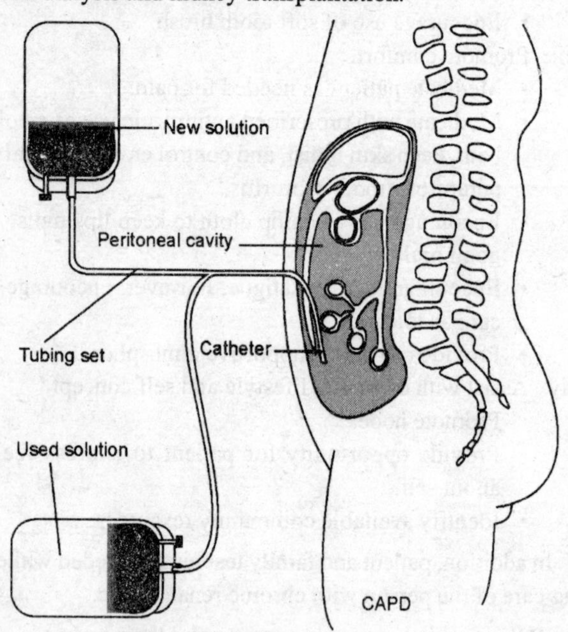

Fig. 14.7: Continuous ambulatory peritoneal dialysis. The peritoneal catheter is implanted through the abdominal wall. Fluid infuses into the peritoneal cavity and drains after prescribed time.

Dialysis Therapy

If complications of ARF become marked (e.g., fluid volume overload with congestive heart failure, hyperkalaemia [>6.0 mEq/liter], and severe metabolic acidemia [pH < 7.20]), aggressive therapy with dialysis may be necessary. An indepth discussion of dialysis therapy, including hemodialysis and peritoneal dialysis, is presented in Table 25-2. (See also Chap. 26).

Continuous Arteriovenous Hemofiltration for Acute Renal Failure

An alternative to peritoneal and hemodialysis in the treatment of critically ill patients with renal failure and/or fluid overload is continuous arteriovenous hemofiltration (CAVH). This technique uses a hemofilter that facilitates removal of water, electrolytes, and small to medium molecular weight molecules from the vascular space, while conserving the cellular and protein contents of circulating blood. The blood enters the extracorporeal circuit by an arterial access, flows through the hemofilter, and returns to the patient by way of a venous access. Blood flow is driven by the hydrostatic blood pressure; no pump is used.

The mechanism underlying hemofiltration involves the use of a transmembrane pressure gradient. This pressure gradient is achieved by the net difference between hydrostatic and osmotic pressures. The hydrostatic pressure consists of two components. These include the arterial blood pressure, which drives fluid across the semipermeable membrane into the ultrafiltrate compartment, and the pressure exerted by the fluid within the ultrafiltrate system, which drives fluid from the fibers into the ultrafiltrate. The pressure opposing the hydrostatic pressure is the colloidal osmotic pressure exerted by the plasma proteins, which do not pass through the semipermeable membrane.

The filter replacement fluid used is determined by the patient's electrolyte values, and the ultrafiltration flow rate is geared to the patient's needs. If the objective is to remove extracellular fluid only, ultrafiltration is regulated at a low rate (approximately 100-300 ml/hour) without subsequent intravenous replacement; if the objective is to clear both extracellular fluid and toxic substances (e.g., urea, potassium), then high ultrafiltration rates and filter replacement fluid are used. The final composition of the ultrafiltrate might include the following: sodium 150 mEq/liter, chloride 114 mEq/liter, potassium 0, bicarbonate 37 mEq/liter, magnesium 1.6 mEq/liter, calcium 2.5 mEq/liter. Clotting of the extracorporeal circuit is prevented by the administration of flow dose heparin. The dose is titrated depending on the patient's coagulation status.

Nursing care of patients undergoing continuous arteriovenous hemofiltration involves patient and equipment preparation, attachment, monitoring of patient and the hemofilter, and termination of hemofiltration. A baseline assessment, including the clinical history, physical examination, and hemodynamic profile, is essential. The hemodynamic profile includes vital signs and measurement of hemodynamic pressures (e.g., central venous, pulmonary artery, pulmonary capillary wedge pressure, and arterial pressures). The patient's weight is ascertained, and baseline laboratory data (e.g., hematology, coagulation, and chemistry profiles) are established.

An access site is established. The most commonly used sites are teh femoral artery and vein; the saphenous or subclavian veins may also be used as the venous access. Scribner-type wrist shunts involving the radial or ulnar arteries and median cubital or basilic vein may also be cannulated. The hemofilter is primed, heparinized, and attached to the patient. The hemofilter must be secured carefully to the patient to prevent accidental disconnection.

Continuous monitoring of the patient's hemodynamic status

is recommended and best achieved using an arterial line. Ideally, use of the pulmonary artery catheter more closely reflects the patient's fluid status. The nurse observes the flow rate every 15 minutes; outputs are recorded hourly. The goal is to remove a large amount of fluid each hour and to replace part of this volume. This results in a net loss of fluid and selected solutes (e.g. urea). The desired hourly fluid balance is specified by the physician. Laboratory values are followed closely to identify trends. It is essential to avoid fluctuations outside the normal range. *Aseptic* shunt care is imperative; monitoring of pulses distal to the access site is essential.

Patient/family educatiaon should include information about the function, purpose, and standard care of patients receiving continuous arteriovenous hemofiltration. Areas of greatest concern include the frequency of patient monitoring and the special equipment involved. The nurse should emphasize that the frequency of care is standard practice for patients receiving this form of therapy.

Table 14.2: Peritoneal dialysis versus hemodialysis: Nursing implications

Objectives	*Peritoneal Dialysis*	*Hemodialysis*
1. Define peritoneal and hemodialysis.	The process of removing metabolic wastes and water from blood by use of the living semipermeable membrane, the peritoneum.	The process of removing metabolic wastes and water from blood by use of a semipermeable membrane of an artificial kidney.
2. State underlying principles used in the dialysis process.	Principles used: A. Osmosis—Movement of water across a semipermeable membrane from an area of lesser to one of greater concentration of solute. B. Diffusion—Movement of molecules from an area of higher concentration to one of lower concentration. C. Filtration—Movement of particles through a semipermeable membrane by means of hydrostatic pressure.	
3. Define ultrafiltration and how it is accomplished.	The removal of fluid (water) by use of an osmotic gradient by the addition of increased concentration of dextrose to the dialysate. Increased dialysis efficiency and ultrafiltration are obtained by using dextrose 4.25 g/100 ml (490-520 mOsm/kg), every sixth exchange.	The removal of fluid (water by use of either positive or negative hydrostatic pressure or a combination of both.
4. State major indications for dialysis.	Fluid overload Electrolyte imbalance Severe acidosis Uremic symptomatology Unavailable vascular access Severe hemodynamic compromise Severe active bleeding Lack of accessible hemodialysis center	Uncontrolled hyperkalaemia Fluid overload Peritonitis Severe acidosis Uremic symptomatology Severe intoxication with a dialyzable substance of low volume of distribution, and low endogenous clearance (e.g., ethanol, ethylene glycol, salicylates, lithium)
5. Discuss primary assessment factors indicating need for dialysis therapy in acute renal failure (ARF).	Primary indications for dialysis therapy in ARF are the presence of: 1. Uremic encephalopathy 2. Pericarditis 3. Bleeding 4. BUN > 100 mg/100 ml 5. Creatining > 10 mg/100 ml 6. Potassium > 6.0 mEq/liter 7. HCO_3^- < 12–15 mEq/liter 8. Severe fluid overload persisting despite maximum conservative therapy Additional factors to be assessed include: 1. Relative risk of complications from dialysis therapy 2. Risk of haemorrhagic or infectious complications of uremia 3. Likelihood of prompt reversal of acute renal failure	
6. Describe major contraindications for dialysis.	Peritonitis Recent abdominal surgery Abdominal adhesions Colostomy/ileostomy	Severe hemodynamic instability (inability to tolerate rapid changes in extravascular fluid volume) Active and severe bleeding Intolerance to systemic heparinization
7. Examine the need for anticoagulation (heparinization) in specific type of dialysis therapy.	Indicated in initial "runs" especially when fibrin clots are observed in the drainage from peritoneal cavity. Heparin is added directly to dialysate solution.	Heparinization (regional) of patient's blood is done prior to the procedure, to keep blood anticoagulated in the dialysis apparatus. *Note:* Patient must be monitored closely for signs of bleeding.

Contd...

Contd...

Objectives	*Peritoneal Dialysis*	*Hemodialysis*
8. Identify advantages of each method of dialysis treatment.	Slower process (36-48 hr) Clears middle molecular weight molecules better (300-800 MW) Little likelihood of disequilibrium syndrome ocurring Safer, simple, less expensive No need for vascular access No need for dialysis technician	More efficient, faster process. Indicated for treatment of uncontrolled hyperkalaemia Clears smaller molecular weight molecules better Preferred treatment for ARF due to: 1. Drug overdose or toxicity 2. Contrast-induced ARF 3. Nonoliguric acute tubular necrosis
9. Consider disadvantages of each method of dialysis.	Risk of peritonitis Does not remove potassium rapidly enough in stage of uncontrolled hyperkalaemia Slow process (36-48 hr) Loss of proteins Cannot be used in presence of abdominal surgery that involves the retroperitoneum Rarely, perforation of bowel or bladder	Requires trained personnel and sophisticated equipment Requires heparinization, which may predispose to: 1. Bleeding 2. Retinopathy (diabetes) Requires maintenance of vascular access Expensive to maintain May precipitate "disequilibrium syndrome" due to rapid removal of fluid
10. Distinguish major complications of dialysis therapy.	Peritonitis (most common) Loss of body protein Hyperglycaemic, hyperosmolar, nonketotic coma Pleural effusion, pneumonia Electrolyte imbalance Dysrhythmias	Hypotension associated with an acute decrease in serum osmolality due to: 1. Removal of urea 2. An acute decrease in intravascular volume from excessive ultrafiltration (hypovolaemia) 3. Acetate accumulation during high clearance dialysis (treated with hypertonic mannitol or saline) Hypervolaemia (hypertension) Electrolyte imbalance Dysrhythmias Dysequilibrium syndrome characterized by: 1. Restlessness, headache, nausea 2. Muscle twitching 3. Disorientation and seizures (severe form) Prevention of dysequilibrium syndrome: 1. Minimize fluid/electrolyte shifts 2. Early and frequent dialysis Hypoxemia may develop partly due to loss of CO_2 into dialysate with consequent reduction in minute ventilation by the patient (treated with bicarbonate solution equilibrated with CO_2 to a partial pressure of 35-45 mmHg, or by increasing fraction of inspired oxygen). Mild thrombocytopenia and leukopenia Bacteremia; cellulitis Thrombosis
11. Describe access sites for each dialysis method.	Stiff peritoneal catheter (acute) Soft Tenckhoff catheter (chronic) These catheters are usually inserted percutaneously in the awake, cooperative patient.	Arteriovenous shunt Arteriovenous fistula Direct arterial stick: Femoral, subclavian
12. Highlight major nursing process considerations in caring for the patient undergoing dialysis therapy. A. Baseline assessment and patient/family preparation.	1. Body weight. 2. Vital signs: Blood pressure lying and sitting; apical/radial pulse; temperature; respirations; rate and rhythm. 3. Neurologic: Mental status; level of consciousness; cranial nerves, sensory-motor function; deep tendon reflexes. 4. Respiratory: Breathing pattern, chest movement, use of accessory muscles; cough; breath sounds; presence of adventitious sounds; presence of pleural friction rub. 5. Cardiovascular; Heart sounds, extra heart sounds, murmur or pericardial friction rub; peripheral pulses; pulse—bounding or thready? Neck vein distention; interstitial oedema. 6. Abdominal exam: Abdominal distention; bowel sounds; palpable liver border, spleen, bladder, abdominal tenderness; Last bowel movement? Costovertebral angle tenderness.	

Contd...

Contd...

<table>
<tr><th>Objectives</th><th>Peritoneal Dialysis</th><th>Hemodialysis</th></tr>
<tr><td></td><td colspan="2">7. Laboratory data: Serum electrolytes, serum glucose, BUN and creatinine; calcium, phosphorus, serum albumin, total protein, CBC, haematocrit and haemoglobin; bleeding and clotting times; arterial blood gases (as indicated).
8. Other studies: ECG, chest x-ray.
9. Patient/family preparation: Patient and/or family should be able to verbalize the need/indication for dialysis therapy, duration, limitation of activity during the procedure, discomfort, risks involved, and expectations of dialysis therapy.</td></tr>
<tr><td>B. Pertinent nursing diagnoses.</td><td colspan="2">1. Fluid volume, alteration in: Deficit (potential).
2. Fluid volume, alteration in: Excess (potential).
3. Comfort, alteration in: Pain.</td></tr>
<tr><td></td><td>4. Injury, potential for: Traumatic insertion of peritoneal dialysis (PD) catheter.
5. Potential for infection (peritonitis).
6. Breathing pattern, ineffective.
7. Bowel elimination, alteration in: Ileus.
8. Skin integrity, impairment of: Potential.
9. Nutrition, alteration in: Less than body requirements.
10. Fear: Unknown procedure.
11. Coping, ineffective: Potential for, individual/family.</td><td>4. Potential for injury (shunt malfunction).
5. Potential for infection (hepatitis).
6. Cardiac output, alteration in: Decreased.
7. Gas exchange, impaired.</td></tr>
<tr><td>C. Planning:
1. Desired patient outcomes.</td><td colspan="2">Patient will:
1. Remain haemodynamically stable: Blood pressure, heart rate optimal for patient; respirations—rate, rhythm, appropriate for patient; lungs clear.
2. Maintain body weight ideal for patient.
3. Maintain serum electrolytes, blood chemistries—BUN and serum creatinine, calcium and phosphorus, serum albumin and total protein, at level ideal for patient.
4. Maintain hematologic studies—CBC, platelets, bleeding/clotting times at level ideal for patient.
5. Maintain body temperature and WBC at levels ideal for patient.
6. Maintain nutrition state in positive nitrogen balance.
7. Verbalize absent to minimal discomfort.
8. Verbalize feelings and concerns regarding dialysis therapy and overall status of renal function.</td></tr>
<tr><td></td><td>9. Experience atraumatic insertion of PD catheter without bowel or bladder perforation.
10. Maintain skin integrity with absent to minimal leakage around PD catheter.</td><td>9. Experience haemodialysis therapy without haemolysis or loss of blood.
10. Maintain a patent shunt/fistula.</td></tr>
<tr><td>2. Nursing interventions</td><td>1. Prepare patient/family.
A. Explain procedure to patient and family.
B. Encourage patient and family to verbalize fears and concerns, and to ask questions.
2. Perform predialysis assessment (see Baseline assessment, above).
3. Assemble equipment at bedside:
A. Dialysate ordered (1.5%, 2.5%, or 4.25%).
B. Add medications to dialysate as prescribed:
• Heparin is added to prevent fibrin accumulation, which could cause a flap valve effect over perforated openings in PD catheter.
• Potassium (dialysate is potassium-free.
• Antibiotics.
• Lidocaine may be added to control local discomfort.
C. Provide masks, sterile gowns and gloves. Aseptic technique must be strictly maintained.
D. Provide additional necessary equipment—tubings, drainage bags, and so forth.</td><td>Shunt care:
1. Assess shunt patency:
A. Palpate for thrill.
B. Auscultate for bruit.
2. Assess for pulsations in tubing and signs of clotting: change of color of blood; separation of blood cells from serum; loss of pulsations.
3. Maintain sterile dressing over shunt access; change daily as per unit protocol.
4. Avoid use of shunt arm to:
A. Take blood pressure.
B. Perform venipuncture.
C. Give injections or intravenous therapy.
5. Instruct patient in self-care of shunt site and emergency measures should shunt separate.
Arteriovenous fistula care:
1. Assess fistula patency:
A. Palpate for thrill.
B. Auscultate for bruit.
2. Avoid restrictive dressing or clothing over fistula site.
3. Note bleeding, skin discoloration, pain, or drainage at</td></tr>
</table>

Contd...

Contd...

Objectives	*Peritoneal Dialysis*	*Hemodialysis*
	E. Have patient void (if producing urine) prior to procedure to reduce risk of bladder perforation. F. Provide assistance with PD catheter insertion. 1. Assist patient during trocar insertion; document how patient tolerated the procedure. 2. Drain initial dialysate "run" to: • Ascertain PD catheter patency. • Determine how much time is needed to fill and drain the abdominal cavity (subsequently dwell period can be adjusted so that entire cycle [instill, dwell, drain] lasts 1 hr).	fistula site, and report immediately. 4. Avoid use of arm with fistula to: A. Take blood pressure. B. Perform venipuncture. C. Give injections or intravenous therapy. *Patient/family preparation:* 1. Explain procedures to patient and family. 2. Encourage patient and family to verbalize fears and concerns and to ask questions. *Perform pre-dialysis assessment* (see Baseline assessment, above). *Implementation:* Haemodialysis requires specially trained personnel.

Peritoneal Dialysis: Procedure

"Up-down" peritoneal dialysis: The first 2-liter dialysate volume may not drain completely; the missing volume is presumably in the gutters of the peritoneal cavity. Failure of the second 2-liter volume to drain completely indicates a mechanical problem. Nursing interventions in this regard include:

A. Altering the patient's position.
B. Ensuring that drainage bag is below the level of the patient.
C. Establishing that there is no airlock. If these maneuvers do not solve the problem, the physician may inject. Gastrografin into the PD catheter, which may reveal kinking or malplacement of the PD catheter.
D. Implementing overall procedure:
   1. Subsequent "runs" include:
      a. Instillation of dialysate—Inflow phase.
      b. Diffusion—Dwell phase.
      c. Drainage—Outflow phase.
   2. Documentation:
      a. Exact time the procedure started.
      b. Amount/concentratiaon of dialysate.
      c. Medications added to dialysate.
      d. Exact time of each phase of the "runs":
         • Instillation: Time started and time completed.
         • Dwell: Total time of dwell phase.
         • Drainage: Time started and when instillation was completed.
      e. Document color of dialysate drainage (drainage may be blood-tinged on first two or three runs).
         • Dialysate drainage:
           Normal—Clear, pale yellow.
           Cloudy—Infection, peritonitis.
           Brownish—Bowel perforation.
           Amber—Bladder perforation.
           Bloody—Initial dialysate drainage may be blood-tinged; persistent bleeding suggests abdominal site or uremic coagulopathy.
      f. Exact amount of total dialysate fluid drained or retained by the patient:
         • Positive balance = fluid gained by patient.
         • Negative balance = fluid lost by patient.

         Thus, fluid retention will create a positive balance, and fluid loss will create a negative balance. The goal of therapy is a negative balance.
      g. Document total intake and output. Include oral and/or intravenous intake, urine output, nasogastric drain age, emesis, diarrhoea, wound drainage, and insensible losses.
         • Diarrhoea occurring after initial runs needs to be evaluated for significant dilution, or blood, which could indicate bowel perforation.
   3. Specific nursing activities:
      a. Monitor vital signs every 15 min initially and subsequently at hourly intervals.
         • A drop in blood pressure or increase in heart rate warns of early shock.

Contd...

Contd...

Objectives	*Peritoneal Dialysis*	*Hemodialysis*

- Notify physician if any signs of bleeding, severe abdominal pain, and/or respiratory distress.
- Respiratory embarrassment can occur as the peritoneal fluid volume limits diaphragmatic excursion.
- Reduction in volume of dialysate exchanges may alleviate compromised ventilatory effort.
- Pleural effusion, if present, may require thoracentesis.

b. Monitor serum electrolytes, blood chemistries, haematology studies.
- Patients receiving 2.5% or 4.25% dialysate solution should have serum glucose determinations at frequent intervals. Hyperglycemic, hyperosmolar, nonketotic (HHNK) coma is a serious complication and must be avoided.

c. Use *strict aseptic technique* with each peritoneal dialysis run to avoid peritonitis.

d. Assess patient frequently for pain/discomfort.
- Pain at catheter placement may respond to changing its position.
- Pain on initiation of peritoneal dialysis may be due to dialysate acidity and is usually relieved by adding lidocaine to the dialysate.
- Dialysate must be warmed prior to instillation for patient comfort.
- Warming also helps to dilate peritoneal blood vessels enhancing the effectiveness of the dialysis treatment.
- Pain at end of drainage phase may be due to suction of the peritoneum against the perforations in teh PD catheter.
- Administer analgesic as necessary.
- Diffuse abdominal pain may herald peritonitis.

e. Assess dialysate drainage: Cloudiness suggests peritonitis.
- Obtain dialysate sample for culture; monitor body temperature.
- Initiate antibiotic therapy as prescribed. Loading dose administered orally or intravenously. Addition of antibiotic to each dialysate instillation at the concentration desired in blood. Exit wound infection may require PD catheter removal.
- Watch for fluid leakage around PD catheter: if it is observed, notify physician.

f. Perform PD catheter site care *(strict aseptic technique).*
- Assess site for signs/symptoms of infection: Redness, swelling, tenderness, induration, purulence.
- Remove dried blood and drainage: Serve as a media for bacterial growth.
- Examine dressings frequently; dressings should not be allowed to remain wet—contamination at PD catheter site can predispose to peritonitis.

g. Perform procedure for dressing change:
- Cleanse exit site gently with povidone=iodine solution beginning around PD catheter where it penetrates the skin and working outward.
- Cleanse entire circumference of catheter with povidone-iodine solution. Allow antiseptic to dry completely to allow for maximum bacteriostatic effect and to prevent gauze dressing from sticking to the skin.
- Secure peritoneal dialysis catheter on sterile gauze pad to avoid skin irritation and decrease risk of catheter contamination from skin.
- Cover site with additional sterile gauze pads and secure dressing. Allow areas of gauze to be exposed to enable skin to "breathe," thus decreasing the risk of anacrobic bacterial growth and preventing bacterial contamination.

Peritoneal dialysis: Major approaches in current use	Major approaches to peritoneal dialysis: • "Up-down" or single bottle manual setup. • "Cycler" peritoneal dialysis apparatus. • Continuous ambulatory peritoneal dialysis (CAPD).	

Reproductive Health Nursing

The reproductive system is inter-related with other systems including the neurologic, endocrine and urinary system and also with general physiologic function. For example, oestrogen (produced primarily in woman's ovaries) influence on bone density and testosterone (produced primarily in a man's testes) influence muscle mass. The reproductive system is also directly related to sexual function and is therefore, intricately interwoven into the complex, sensitive and frequently stress-laden area of psychosocial mores and cultural values regarding sex.

Conditions affecting healthful functioning of the reproductive system of men and women take a high toll in loss of life and acute and chronic physical and emotional stress. Reproductive nursing refers to nursing the disorders of the reproductive system both in men and women. The nurse has a responsibility to assist in general health education to refer patients for appropriate health care, and to understand the treatment available as the nursing care needed when disease develops.

The male reproductive system consists of the external structure—the penis and the scrotum—and the internal structures including prostate gland, the seminal vesicles and several ducts. The female reproductive system consists of the breasts, the uterus, the ovaries, the fallopian tubes and the vagina and the external genitalia (the vulva) as well as ligaments at pelvic bones. A sound knowledge of reproductive system is essential. (For review refer any standard text on "Anatomy and Physiology).

ASSESSMENT OF THE MALE AND FEMALE REPRODUCTIVE SYSTEM

As stated before, reproductive system is inter-related with other systems. Therefore, problems in other systems are often inter-related with problems and stresses within the reproductive system. The nurse must elicit general information as well as information specifically relating to the reproductive system. Reproduction and sexual issues are often considered extremely personal and private. The nurse must develop trust to elicit such information. A professional demeanour is important while taking a reproductive or sexual history which include genitourinary assessment of female and male.

Female Genitourinary Assessment

Every woman who enters the health care system should have a complete gentitourinary health histories which include the urinary system, menstruation, sexual activity, contraceptive use, pregnancies and gynaecological problems or surgeries. In addition, breast health, physical abuse and sexual assault should be screened. The following outline summarises the interview items, symptoms, and health promotion activities to be included in assessment.

1. Current breast health.
2. Problem with breasts.
   - Breast Pain/tenderness.
   - Lumps.
   - Skin dimpling.
   - Lesions or changes in the skin.
   - Discharge from nipples.
3. Current genitourinary health.
4. Urinary symptoms including infections and voiding dysfunction:
   - Dysuria.
   - Frequency.
   - Urgency.
   - Haematuria.
   - Nocturia.
   - True incontinence (loss of urine without warning).
   - Stress incontinence (loss of urine with cough or sneeze).
5. Menstrual history
   - Age at menarchy (first menses).
   - Last menstrual period.
   - Interval of frequency; regular or irregular.
   - Duration.
   - Menstrual flow: light, medium or heavy (number of pads or tampoons used in a specified time period).
   - Menorrhagia (increased amount or duration of flow).
   - Dysmenorrhoea (Pain with menstruation) frequency or severity.
   - Bleeding between periods.
   - Postcoital bleeding (Bleeding after intercourse).
   - Postmenopausal bleeding: essential to assess for any bleeding since menopause to screen for endometrial cancer).

- Postmenstrual syndrome symptoms: irritability, depression, weight-gain, headaches, breast tenderness and breast swelling.

6. Obstetrical history
   - Number of pregnancies (gravida).
   - Pregnancy outcomes:
     - Term: number of births between 37 and 42 weeks of pregnancy.
     - Premature: Number of births before 37 weeks of pregnancy.
     - Living: Number of children living.
     - Abortions: Spontaneous or elective.
   - Types of deliveries: Vaginal, forceps or caesarian.
7. Perimenopausal symptoms
   - Hot flashes/flushes.
   - Headaches.
   - Light sweats.
   - Vaginal dryness.
   - Mood swings.
   - Numbness and tingling.
8. Vulvovaginal problems
   - Discharge, colour, amount and odour.
   - Vaginal itching.
   - Lesions or lumps.
   - Dyspareunia (Pain with intercourse).
   - Vaginisms (spasms of muscles around vagina)
   - History of STDs.
9. Sexual health
   - Sexually active; monogamous versus multiple partners; male/female/both.
   - Satisfaction or problems related to sexual activity.
   - Changes in ability to engage in sex; Vaginal dryness, female sexual disorders, inhibited orgasm; or pain with intercourse.
10. Health promotion practices
    - Contraceptive choice, proper use of method, satisfaction and side effects.
    - Pelvic examination: last pap smear and results.
    - Condom use.
    - Breast, self examination.
    - Vulvo self examination.
    - Mammogram.
    - Personal hygiene; douche, bubble baths, use of tampoon, and feminine sprays.
11. Family history
    - Breast cancer.
    - Cervical, ovarian or endometrial cancer.
    - Diethystilbestrol (DES) use, (Previously used to prevent spontaneous abortion; since it has been associated with cervical adenoses and cervical and vaginal carcinoma and congenital anomalies GU tract. It was banned in 1971).

In addition any history of medication taken in surgeries include dilation and currettage, hysterectomy, oophorectomy, repair of cystocele, repair of rectocele, salpingectomy, tubal sterilization.

Male Genitourinary Assessment

A male genitourinary history includes current health status as well as past medical history, which includes bladder, kidney function, the penis and testes, possible hernias, sexual health and health promotion activities. The following outline summarizes symptoms and health promotion behaviour to be included in the assessment.

1. Current genitourinary health status.
2. Screen for urinary symptoms including infections, voiding, dysfunction or prostate problem.
   - Dysuria (Pain with urination).
   - Frequency.
   - Urgency.
   - Haematuria.
   - Nocturia.
   - Urinary retention.
   - Straining.
   - Hesitancy.
   - Change in force/caliber of stream.
   - Dribbling.
   - History of prostate problems.
   - History of urinary infections.
3. Screen for incontinence.
   - True (loss of urine without warning).
   - Stress (loss of urine with cough/sneeze).
4. Screen for problem with penis such as skin lesions, cancer or STDs.
   - Pain.
   - Lesion or sores.
   - Discharge.
   - History of STDs.
5. Screen for problems with testes such as torsion, cancer or infections and problems with the scrotum such as hydrocele, hernia or varicocele.
   - Lump or swelling in testes.
   - Bulge or swelling in scrotum.
   - Change in size of scrotum.
   - History of hernia.
6. Assess sexual health.
   - Sexually active: monogamous versus multiple partners male/female/both.
   - Satisfaction with or problem related to sexual activity.

Physical Examination

The examination of the external genitalis uses inspection and palpation.

A. *Male genitalia*

An examination should be performed with the patient lying or standing. The standing position is generally preferred. The examiner should be seated in front of the standing patient. Gloves should be used during examination of male genitalia.

- *Pubis:* The nurse observes the diamond-shaped pattern of hair distribution. The absence of hair is not normal. The skin is also evaluated. The pubic hair should be inspected for nits, lice or scabies.
- *Penis:* The nurse notes the size and skin texture of the penis and any lesions, scars or swelling. The lesion caused by chancres, genital warts, herpes or penile cancer. The location of the urethral meatus, as well as the presence of absence of a foreskin should be noted. If present, foreskin should be retracted to note cleanliness and replaced over the gland after observation. The glands are compressed to note any discharge and its amount, colour and odour are present. The nurse also palpates the penile shaft for tenderness, masses and observes the ventral and dorsal aspects.
- *Scrotum and Testes:* The nurse performs a complete skin examination by lifting each testes to inspect all sides of the scrotal sac. The scrotum is inspected for size, symmetry, swelling, inflammation and/or lesions. Palpation of scrotum is done to note changes in consistency or the presence of masses. It is important to note if the testes are distended. The left testes usually hangs lower than the right. Undescended testes is a major risk factor for testicular cancer, as well as a potential cause of male infertility. The patient also be taught TSE (Testes Self-examination).
- *Inguinal region and spermatic cord:* The examiner insepcts the •*Inguinal region* for rashes, lesions, or lymphadenopathy, which may suggest pelvic organ infections. The nurse has to make the patient cough or bear down and notes any conspicuous bulging in the inguinal canals. The nurse also palpates the area for any bulging as the patient again coughs or bears down. The nurse palpates the inguinal and femoral pulses and the local lymph nodes.

The spermatic cord is located posteriously in the scrotal sac. The nurse follows the cord on each side. The inguinal region is gently palpated using the forefinger or small finger and by pushing up through the loose scrotal skin to the abdominal wall along the inguinal region. At this point, the patient again bears down and coughs. The nurse determines whether the strain produces bulging of the intestine through the ring, indicating the presence of hernia a condition which requires follow-up.

- *Anus and Prostate.* The anal sphincter and perineal regions are inspected for lesions, masses and haemorrhoids; A digital examination is required for all patients who have symptoms of prostate trouble such as difficulty in initiating the flow and urge to void frequently.

The prostate gland is palpated by means of rectal examination with the patient standing with the hips flexed over an examination table or in a side-lying position. Before the examination, advise the man that he may feel as though he needs to have a bowel movement. The patient is asked to bear down while a lubricated index finger is gently inserted into the canal and then the rectum. The prostrate and seminal vesicles are palpated. The size, shape and consistency of the lobes and the median sulcus of prostrate are noted. The normal prostate is 2.5 by 4 cm, smooth, heart-shaped, rubbery and non-tender. Rectal examination is most important step in the diagnosis of prostate disease.

- *Male breasts:* The male breast can be easily and quickly examined during routine physical examination. Barring some rare cases, breast cancer does not occur in males, mostly it occurs frequently in the areolar area. The inspection of skin and areolae for the presence of any swelling, retractions or lesions are noted. The breast, areola, and axillae are then palpated for mass.

B. *Female Breasts and External Genitalia*

Physical examination of women often begins with inspection and palpation of the breasts and then proceeds to the abdomen. Examination of the abdomen provides an opportunity to detect pain or any masses that may involve the genitourinary system.

- *Breasts:* In a menstruating women, the ideal time to examine the breast is several days after menstruation, when they are less tender and nodular. Breasts are examined first by visual inspection. The nurse, with the patient being seated, observes the breasts for symmetry, size, shape, skin colour and texture. Vascular patterns and the presence of unusual lesions. The patient is asked to put her arms at her sides, arms over head, lean forward and press hands on hips. The nurse observes for any abnormalities during these maneuvers. The axillae and the clavicle also be examined for any abnormalities.

When the patient assumes a supine position, a pillow is placed under the back on the side to be examined. The patient is asked to put the arm above and behind the head. These maneuvers flatten the breast tissue and make palpation easier. The breast is then palpated in a systemic fashion using a vertical line, a clockwise or a spoke approach. The nurse should use the distal fingers pads for palpation. The tail of spence should be included in the examination because this area and the upper outer quadrant are the areas where most breast malignancies develop. Finally, the nurse should palpate the area around the areolae for masses. The nipple should be compressed to determine the presence of discharge or any masses. The colour, consistency and odour of any discharge should be documented.

- *External genitalia.* The nurse uses gloves for examination of the external genitalia. The monspubis, the labia majora, the labia minora, the perinium and the anal region are inspected for characteristics of skin hair distribution and contour. Lesions, swellings and discharges are noted.

The nurse separates the labia to the maximum to inspect the clitoris, the urethral meatus, the vaginal orifice, the hymen, the preineum, and the anal region. Any inflammation or cysts on Bartholin's gland or Skene's glands are noted.

• *Internal Pelvic Examination*

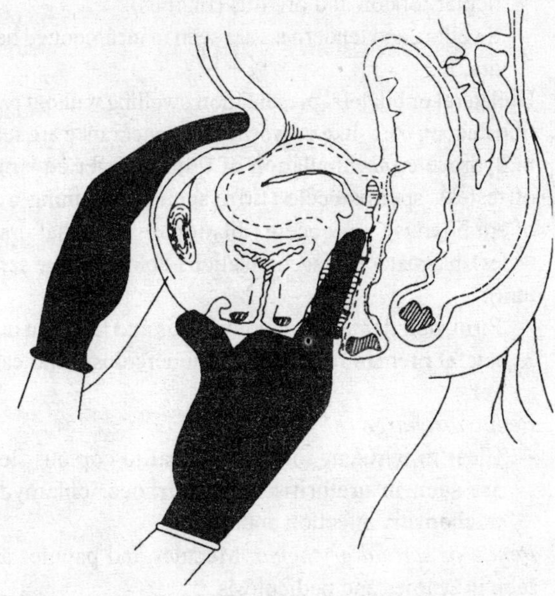

Fig. 15.1: Bimanual Examination of the Pelvic Organs.

Internal Pelvic Examination

Women who are scheduled for pelvic examination should be advised to avoid douching, sexual intercourse and applying any vaginal preparations (medicinal or deodorant) for at least 24 hours before examination. The most common position for the pelvic examination is the lithotomy position. Sim's (lateral position) and knee-chest position also are used sometimes.

During the speculum examination, the nurse observes the walls of the vagina and cervix for inflammation, discharge, polyps and suspicious growths. During this examination, it is possible to take a pap smear and collect secretions for culture and study under the microscope (i.e. wet smears).

After the speculum examination, a bimanual examination is performed to allow assessment of the size, shape and consistency of the uterus, ovaries and tubes. The tubes are not normally palpable. Abdominal palpation is performed to rule out or discover abnormalities. Enlargement of the uterus is detected by palpating in the midline of the lower abdomen. Enlargement of the fallopian tubes and ovaries may be detected by the palpation of the right and left quadrant.

Common Abnormalities of Breast, Female and Male Reproductive Systems

The common abnormalities of breasts, the female reproductive system and the male reproductive system are as follows:

1. *Breasts:*
   - *Nipple inversion or retraction:* Recent onset, erythematous, pain and unilator may be due to abscess, inflammation or cancer. Recent onset (usually within past year) unilateral presentation, lack of tenderness may be due to neoplasm.
   - *Galactorrhoea (in females).*

Nipple Secretions—Milky, no relationship to lactation, unilateral or bilateral or intermittant or consistent presentation is due to drug therapy, particularly phenothiazine, tricyclic antidepressants, methyldopa; hypofunction or hyperfunction of thyroid or adrenal glands; tumours of hypothalamus or pituitary gland; excessive oestrogen; prolonged suckling or breast foreplay.

   - Galactorrhoea (male): Milky, bilateral presentation, as may be due to chorioepithelioma of testes.
   - *Purulent:* Gray-green or yellow colour, frequent unilateral presentation in association with pain, erythema, induration and nipple inversion. It may be due to purpural (after birth) mastitis (inflammatory condition of breast or abcess. Purulent without nipple inversion may be infected sebaceous cyst.
   - *Seron discharge:* Clear appearance, unilateral or bilateral or intermittent or consistent presentation may be due to intraductal papilloma.
   - *Dark green or multicoloured discharge:* Thicky, sticky and frequent bilateral is due to mammary duct-ectasia (dilation of mammary duct).
   - *Serosanguineous or bloody drainage:* Uvulator presentations are due to Papillomatosis (widespread development of nipple-like growths), intraductal papilloma and carcinoma (male and female).
   - *Scaling or irritation of nipple:* Unilateral or bilateral presentation, crusting, possible ulceration. It may be due to Paget's disease, eczema, and infection.
   - *Nodules, lumps or masses*
     - Multiple, bilateral, well-delineated, soft or firm, mobile cyst, pain, premenstrual occurrence, may be due to fibrocytic changes.
     - Rubbery consistency, fluid-filled interior, pain—may be due to mammary duct ectasia.
     - Soft, mobile, well-delineated cyst, absence of pain may be lipoma, and abscesses.
     - Erythema, tenderness, induration are due to infected-sebaceous cyst, abscesses.
     - Usually singular, hard irregularly-shaped, poorly-delineated, non-mobile is due to neoplasm.
2. *Female Reproductive System*
   - Vulvar discharge.
     - Plaque-like consistency, frequent itching and inflammation, lack of odour. It is usually seen in candidiasis (candida or yeast infection, vaginitis).
     - Grayish colour, copious flow, frothy appearance, vulvar irritation. It is usually seen in bacterial vaginosis infection.
     - Purulent odour, grayish-green colour—seen in Trichomonas vaginalis.
     - Bloody colour—seen in chlamydia trachomatis or

Neisseria gonorrhoea infection, menstruation, trauma, cancer.

- *Vulvar erythema*
  - Bright or beefy red colour, itching seen in candida albicans, allergy, and chemical vaginitis.
  - Reddened base, painful vescicles or ulcerations in Genital herpes.
  - Macules or papules, itching is seen in chancroid (STD) contact dermatitis, scabies, pediculosis.
- *Vulvar growths*
  - Soft, fleshy growth; nontender seen in condyloma acuminatum.
  - Flat and warty appearance, nontender seen in condyloma latum.
  - Same as either above; possible pain seen in neoplasm.
  - Reddened base, vesicles and small erosions and pain are seen in lymphogranuloma venerium, genital herpes and chancroid.
  - Indurated firm ulcers, lack of pain and seen in chancre, syphilis and granuloma inguinale.
- *Abdominal pain or tenderness*
  - Intermittent or consistent tenderness is right or left lower quindrane are seen in salpingitis, ectopic pregnancy, rupture ovarian cyst, PID and tubal or ovarian abscess.
  - Periumblical location, consistent occurrence, seen in cystitis, endometritis and ectopic pregnancy.

3. *Male Reproduction System*
   - *Penile growth or masses*
     - Indurated, smooth, dislike appearance, absence of pain; singular presentation are seen in chancre.
     - Papular to irregularly-shaped ulceration with pus, lack of induration are seen in chancroid.
     - Ulceration with induration and nodularity are seen in cancer.
     - Flat, wart-like nodule are seen in candyloma latum.
     - Elevated, fleshy, moist-elongated projections with single or multiple projections are seen in condyloma acuminatum.
     - Localized swelling with retracted tight foreskin, are seen in paraphimosis (inability to replace foreskin to its normal position after retraction and trauma).
   - *Vesicles, erosions, or ulcers*
     - Painful, erythrematous base, vesicular or small erosions are seen in genital herpes, balantitis (inflammation of glans penis) and chancroid.
     - Painless, singular and smaller erosion with eventual lymphadenopathy are seen in lymphogranuloma venereum and cancer.
   - *Scrotal masses*
     - Localized swelling with tenderness, unilateral or bilateral presentation are seen in epididymitis, testicular torsion and orchitis (mumps).
     - Swelling and tenderness are seen in incarcerated hernia.
   - Unilateral or bilateral presentation:swelling without pain translucent, cord-like or worm-like appearance are seen in hydrocele (accumulation of fluid in outer covering of testes), spermatocele (firm, sperm-containing cyst of epididymis), varicocele (dilation of veins that drain testes), haematocele (accumulation of blood within scrotum).
     - Firm, nodular testes or epididymis and frequent unilateral premature are seen in tuberculosis and cancer.
   - *Penile discharge*
     - Clear to purulent colour, minimal to copious flow are seen in urethritis or gonorrhoea, chlamydia trachomatis infection and trauma.
   - *Penile or scrotal erythema.* Macules and papules are seen in scabies and pediculosis.
   - *Inguinal masses:*
     - Bulging, unilateral presentation during straining are seen in inguinal hernia.
     - Shotty, 1-3 cm nodules are seen in lymphadinopathy.

DIAGNOSTIC STUDIES OF REPRODUCTIVE SYSTEM

Many diagnostic tests that are performed to assess problems occurring in other body systems also provide valuable data on the condition of the reproductive system. The following are the most commonly used diagnostic studies in the assessment of the reproductive system and the nurses' responsibility regarding these diagnostic tests. To understand many of the diagnostic studies of the reproductive system, it is important to understand the concepts of sensitivity and specificity. Sensitivity addresses the issue of how well a test identifies people with a particular disease (screening test), specificity testing answers the question of how well a test eliminates those individuals without disease. The goal of sensitivity testing is to avoid false-positive results. It is the nurse's responsibility to ensure that the patient understands the purposes of any test being performed.

Urine Studies

- *Pregnancy testing:* Occurrence of pregnancy is generally validated by measuring outputs of human chorionic gonadotropin (hcG) in the urine by means of an immunologic test. hcG is detected in urine to ascertain whether a woman is pregnant. Hydatidiform mole and chorioepithelioma 'in men and women) may also be detected.

  Nursing responsibility is to obtain through menstrual history from patient, including birth control methods, determine presence or absence of presumptive signs of pregnancy (e.g. breast changes or increased whitish vaginal discharge).

- *Hormone testing*
  - Testosterone level:In the tumours, developmental anomalies of the testes can be detected. For which the nurse instructs patient to collect 24 hours urine specimen. Keep it refrigerated.
  - Follicle stimulating hormone (FSH) assay: This test indicates gonadal failure because of pituitary dysfunction.

Female: Follicular phase	:	2-5 i.u/24 hr.
Mid cycle	:	8-40 i.u./24 hrs.
Leutal phase	:	2-10 i.u./24 hrs.
Menopause	:	35-100 i.u./24 hrs.
Male	:	2-15 i.u./24 hrs.

For FSH assay, patient is instructed to collect 24 hours urine specimen indicates phase of menstrual cycle if menopausal and if an oral contraceptives or hormones.

Blood Studies

- *Prolactin assay:*This test detects pituitary dysfunction that can cause amenorrhoea. In this, nurse observes venipuncture site for bleeding or haematoma formation.
- *Serum hcG assay:* hcg is detected in serum to ascertain whether a woman is pregnant. Here nurse instructs the patient to have blood drawn in laboratory. Elicite where she is in her menstrual cycle, whether she has missed menses and if so how late she is.
- *Serum androgen* and testosterone levels:- These tests ascertain whether elevated androgens are due to adrenal or ovarian dysfunction. Serum testosterone is also drawn to assess cause of amenorrhoea.

  The nurse collects health history to eliminate potential sources of interference with accuracy of results (e.g. use of steroids or barbiturates or presence of hypothyroidism or hyperthyroidism).
- *Serum progesterone:* This test is frequently used to detect functioning corpusluteum cyst. Here nurse observes venipuncture site for bleeding or haematoma formation. Includes last menstrual period and trimester of pregnancy since progesterone level varies with gestation.
- *Serum oestradiol.* This test measures ovarian function. It is particularly useful in assessing oestrogen-secreting tumours and states of precocious female puberty. Normal values depend on laboratory that performs test and should be obtained from that laboratory. It may be used to confirm premenopausal time. Increased serum oestrodiol levels in men may be indicative of testicular tumour. Here the nurse observes venipuncture site for bleeding or haematoma formation.
- *Serum FSH.* This test indicates gonadal failure due to pituitary dysfunction; it is used to validate menopause. In females; follicular phase: 4-30 ml u/ml; Mid cycle: 10-90 ml u/ml; Luteal phase: 4-30 ml u/ml: Menopause 40-250 ml u/ml. In males: 4-25 ml/ml. In this test no food or fluid restrictions are required. State phase of menstrual cycle; if menopausal or if oral contraceptive or hormones.

Syphilis Studies

- *Nontreponimal serologic tests* include: Wasserman (complement fixation), Venereal disease research laboratory (VDRL), (flocculation), Rapid plasma reagin (RPR) (agglutination). These tests are nonspecific antibody test used to screen for syphilis. Positive reading can be made within 1-2 weeks after appearance of primary lesion (chancre) or 4-15 weeks after initial infection.

  Here the nurse tells the patient that fasting is unnecessary,
- Informs the patient that blood sample will be drawn. Observe venipuncture site for bleeding or haematoma formation. Obtain data to determine presence or absence of problems such as hepatitis, pregnancy and autoimmune diseases that may interfere with the accuracy of results.
- *Treponemal Test* fluorescent treponemal antibody absorption (FTAABs). This test detects syphilis antibodies. It also detects early syphilis with great accuracy. It is usually performed if results of nontrepenoma testing are questionable. In this, the nurse tells the same as in venipuncture care.
- *Miscellaneous studies:*
- *Dark field microscopy* is a direct examination of the specimen obtained from potential syphilitic lesion (chancre) performed to detect treponoema. The Nurse has to avoid direct skin contact with open lesion.
- *Wet mounts* is a direct microscopic examination of specimens of vaginal discharge which is performed immediately after collection. This determines presence or absence and number of trichomonas organisms, bacteria, white and red blood cells, and candidal buds or hyphae. Other clues or causes of inflammation or infection may be determined.

In this, the nurse explains the procedure and purpose to patient. Instructs the patient not to douche before examination. Prepare collection of specimens (glass slide, 10-20 per cent potassium hydroxide (KOH) solution, sodium chloride (NaCl) solution, and cotton-tipped applicators).

- *Cultures:* Culture specimens of vaginal, urethral or cervical discharge are taken and used to assess presence of gonorrhoea or chlamydia. Rectal and throat cultures may also be taken depending upon data obtained from sexual history. Here, nurse has to obtain specific contact and sexual history inclusive of oral and rectal intercourse. Instruct against douching before examination. Obtain urethral specimen from men before void. Instruct women who are sexually active with multiple partners to have at least a yearly culture for gonorrhea and chlamydia. Instruct sexually active men to have any discharge evaluated immediately rule out gonorrhoea strains that do not cause classic symptoms of dysuria.

- *Gram's stain:* This presumptive test is used for rapid detection of gonorrhoea. Presence of gram-negative intracellular diplococci generally warrants initiation of treatment. Not highly accurate for women. The nursing responsibility is as in culture.

Cytologic Studies

- *Pap smear:* Microscopic study of exfoliated cells via special staining and fixation technique detects abnormal cells, cells most commonly studied are those obtained directly from endocervix; vaginal pool and endometrial lining of uterine activity.

  In this procedure, instruct women who are sexually active, and who are over age of 18 to have pap smears according to cancer society guidelines. Arrange for smear at mid-cycle time. Instruct patient not to douche for at least 24 hours before examination. Collect careful menstrual and gynaecologic history).
- *Nipple Discharge Test:* Cytologic study of nipple discharge is performed here indicates whether hormonal preparation or other drugs are being taken, breastfeeding or history of amenorrhoea. Instruct patient demonstration of breast-self-examination or examination of breasts that nipple discharge should always be evaluated.

Radiological Studies

- *Soft tissue mammographing:* Low dose X-ray image of breast tissue on photographic film is used to assess breast masses, recent breast enlargement, and nipple discharge to detect malignancy. It is usually an outpatient procedure. For which instruct patient about risks (radiation) and advantages of the examination. Instruct regarding cancer society recommendation.
- *Contrast mammography:* This test is used to evaluate abnormal nipple discharge. It is particularly effective in detecting non-palpable intraductal papillomas. Test consists of injection of radiopaque dye in breast duct. Here determine actual or possible allergy to contrast medium.
- *Ultrasound:* This test measures and records high frequency sound waves as they pass through tissues of variable density. It is very useful in detecting masses greater than 3 cm such as ectopic pregnancies, IUDs, ovarian cysts and hydatidiform moles.

Invasive Procedures

- *Breast biopsy*: Histologic examination of excised breast tissue is performed, either by needle-aspiration or excisional biopsy. Here, prior to surgery, instruct patient about operative procedure, and sedation. After surgery, perform wound care and instruct patient about breast-self-examination.

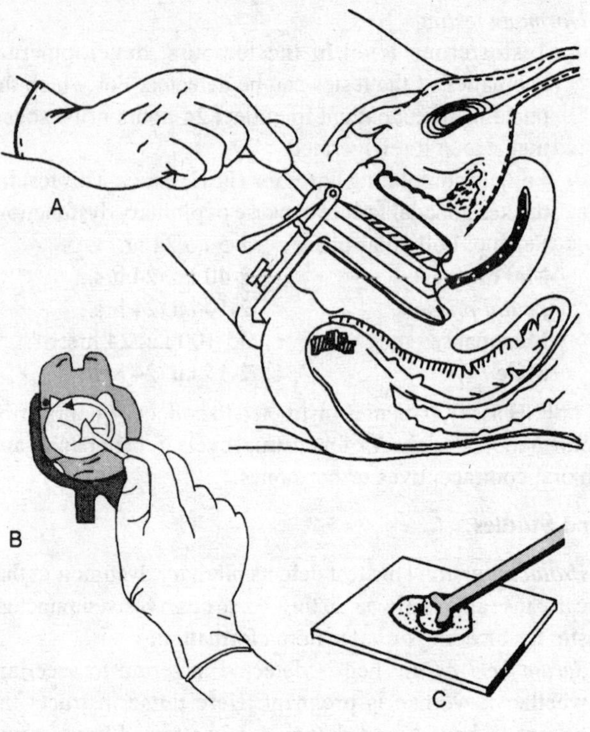

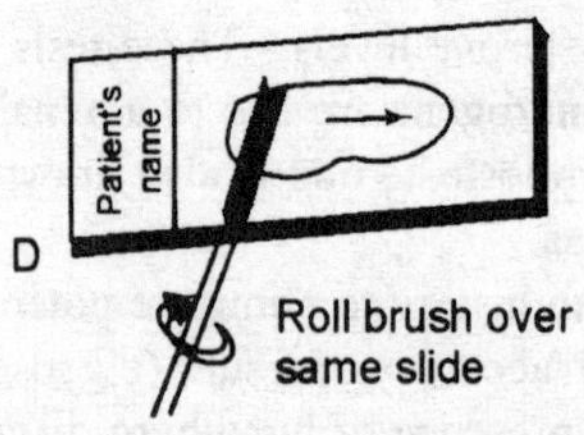

Fig. 15.2: A cervical scrape of secretions for cytology is obtained by using a wooden Ayre spatula. (A) Shows the speculum in place: the Ayre spatula is inserted so that the longer end is placed snugly in the os. (B) A representative sample of secretions is obtained by rotating the spatula. (C) Cervical secretions are gently smeared on a glass slide in a single circular motion. (D) A cytobrush is rotated within the cervical os and smeared onto a glass slide. The slide is placed in the appropriate fixative immediately.

- *Hysterosalpingogram:* This test instillation of radioscopic dye through cervix into uterine cavity and subsequently through and out of fallopian tubes. Spot X-ray images are taken to detect abnormalities of uterus and its adnexa (ovaries and tubes) as dye progresses through them. Test may be most useful in diagnostic assessment of fertility (e.g. to detect adhesions near ovary, an abnormal uterine shape or blockage of tubal pathways).

Here inform patient about procedure and that it may be fairly uncomfortable, especially shoulder pain. Determine possibility of dye allergy.

- *Colposcopy:* Direct visualization of cervix with binocular microscope that allows magnification and study of cellular dysplasia and vascular and tissue abnormalities of cervix. This test is used as a follow-up study for abnormal pap smear and for examination of women exposed to DES in utero. Biopsy of cervix may be taken during colposcopic examination. This test is valuable in decreasing number of false-negative cervical biopsies. The nurse has to instruct patient about the outpatient procedure. Inform patient that this examination is similar to speculum examination. Explain purpose of procedure and prepare patient for it.
- *Conization:*Cone-shaped sample of squamocolumnar tissue of cervix removed for direct study. In this, the nurse explains purposes and method of procedure and that it requires use of surgical facilities and anaesthesia. Instruct patient to rest for at least 3 days after procedure. Also discuss necessity for 3-week follow-up check.
- *Loop electrosurgical excision of transformation zone (LEETZ)*
  It is excision of cervical tissue via an electrosurgical instrument. Here the nurse explains purpose and method of procedure and that it may be done in the physician's office for further diagnostic testing.
- *Loop electrosurgical excision procedure* (LEEP)
  Same as LEETZ.
- *Culdotomy, culdoscopy and culdocentesis: Culdotomy* is an incision made through posterior forni of cul-de-sac and allows visualization of peritoneal cavity (i.e. uterus, tubes, and ovaries).
  Culdascope can then be used to study these structures closely. This technique is valuable in fertility evaluations. Withdrawal of fluid (Culdocentesis) allows examination of fluid characteristics.
- *Laparoscopy* (Peritoneoscopy): This method of entry into the abdomen allows visualization of pelvic structures via fiberotopic scopes inserted through small abdominal incisions. Instillation of carbon dioxide into cavity improves visualization. This technique is used in diagnostic assessment of uterus, tubes, and ovaries. It can be used in conjunction with tubal sterilization.
  In this, the nurse explains purpose and method of procedure. Before surgeon instructs patient about procedure, prepare abdomen, and reassure patient about sedation. Tell patient to rest for 1-3 days after surgery. Inform patient of probability of shoulder pain because of air in the abdomen.
- *Dilation and currettage:* The operative procedure dilates cervix and allows curretting of endometrial lining. This test is used in assessment of abnormal bleeding patterns and cytologic evaluation of lining. In this, instruct the patient before surgery, about the procedure and sedation. Tell patient that overnight hospitalizations is occasionally required. Perform postoperative assessment of degree of bleeding (frequent pad checking first 24 hours).

Fertility Studies

- *Semen analysis:* Semen is assessed for volume (2-5 ml), viscosity, sperm count (Greater than 20 million/ml), sperm motility (60 per cent motil) and per cent of abnormal sperm (60 per cent with normal structures). Here, instruct patient to bring in fresh specimen within 2 hours after ejaculation (may be by masturbation).
- *Basal body temperature assessment:* This measurement indicates indirectly whether ovulation has occurred (Temperature rises at ovulation and remains elevated during secretory phase of normal menstrual cycle). In this, the nurse instructs woman to take her temperature using special basal temperature thermometer. (Calebrated in tenths of degrees) every morning before getting out of bed. Tell the woman to record temperature on graph.
- *Huhner test or Sim's-Huhner:* Mucus sample of cervix is examined 2-8 hours after intercourse. Total number of sperm is assessed to number of live sperms. This test is performed to determine cervical mucus is "hostile" to passage of sperm from vagina to utera. Here nurse must instruct couple to have an intercourse an estimated time of ovulation and be present for test within 2-8 hours after intercourse.
- *Endometrial biopsy.* In this outpatient procedure, small currette is used to obtain piece of endometrial lining to assess endometrial changes common to progesterone secretion after ovulation. Here advise patient that test must be performed postovulation. Explain that procedure should cause only short period of uterine cramping.
- Hysterosalpinogram-same as invasive procedure.
- Serum progesteron-same as blood studies.

REPRODUCTIVE PROBLEMS OF FEMALES/WOMEN

Disease and disorders of the female reproductive system threatens the physical and emotional health of many women, infection process and disorders of menstruation are common and pervasive problem. Malignant neoplasm destroys child-bearing potential and numerous lives.

Vaginitis

Infection and inflammation of the vagina, cervix and vulva tend to occur when the natural defenses of the acidic vaginal secretions (maintained by sufficient oestrogen level) and the presence of *Lactobacillus* are disrupted. The woman's resistance may also be decreased as a result of aging, poor nutrition and the use of the drugs that alter the mucosa organism gain entrance to the areas through contaminated hands, clothing, douche nozzles and during intercourse, surgery and childbirth.

Aetiology

The cause of following infections of vagina are as follows:

- Monilial vaginitis caused by candida albicans (fungus).
- Trichomoniasis caused by Trichomonas vaginalis (Protozoa).
- Bacterial vaginosis caused by gardnerella vaginalis and corynbacterium vaginale.
- Severe recurrent vaginitis caused by candida albicans.
- Foreign body.
- Allergens or irritants.

Most lower genital tract infections are related to the sexual intercourse. Intercourse can transport organisms, injure tissues, and alter the acid-base balance of the vagina. All of these increase risk for inflammation or infections of the vagina. The risk factor associated with infections of the vulva and vagina include the following:

- Pregnancy.
- Age - Premenarche and postmenopause.
- Low oestrogen levels.
- Dermatological allergies.
- Diabetes mellitus-alteration in carbohydrate metabolism.
- Oral contraceptive use.
- Inadequate hygiene.
- Douching.
- Treatment with broad spectrum antibiotics and use of steroids.
- Use of vaginal contraceptives - foams and inserts.
- Intercourse with infected partner.
- Frequent intercourse with multiple partners.
- Tight, nonabsorbent and heat-retaining clothing.

Pathophysiology

The vagina is normally protected from infection by its acid pH and the presence of normal flora such as doderleins bacilus. Any factor that alters the normal vaginal physiology may dispose to infection. If the pH or vaginal mucosa is altered or the woman resistance is decreased by aging-related changes, stress, or diseases and her risk to infection increase. The use of antibiotics which destroys the normal protective flora of the vagina also increases the risk of infection. The risk factors listed in aetiology causes vaginitis.

Clinical Manifestations

The clinical manifestation of vaginitis varies according to its causes which include:

- *Monilial vaginitis:* commonly found in mouth, gastrointestinal tract and vagina. There is white, curd-like, cheesy discharge, characteristic patches on vaginal walls and cervix and foul odour, severe burning, itching, and dyspareunia.
- *Gardnerella-associated bacterial vaginosis.* Grayish-white, hormonous watery discharge with fishy or foul odour; scant amount and may or may not have other symptoms.
- *Foreign body:* Blood-tinged serosanguineous or purulent disease usually with foul odour discharge may be thick or thin.
- *Allergens or irritants.* Increase in usual type and amount of secretions, itching and burning rash.

Management

Genital problems are evaluated by performing a history including sexual history and physical examination and obtaining the appropriate laboratory and diagnostic studies. The diagnosis of vaginitis is made by microscope analysis of vaginal secretions (e.g. KOH analysis, wet smear, or Gram's stain) and culture of the discharge. Serological testing and urine culture may also be used. The management of vaginitis is primarily pharmocological which includes accordingly as follows:

- *Monilial vaginitis.* diagnosed by KOH microscopic examination—pseudohyphase.pH.4.0-4.7 and treated by antifungal agents which includes:
  - clotrimazole (Mycelax, lotriman) applicator intravaginally qHS for 7 days.
  - Micronazole (Monistat) Cream intravaginally qHS for 7 days.
  - Ticonazole 6.5 per cent (Vagistatl) intravaginally qHS for 1 dose.
  - Fluconazole (Diflucan) one tablet orally stat.
  - Nystatin (Mycostatin) suppositories daily or bid for 14 days.
- *Trichomoniasis:* Metronidazole (Flagyl) orally for 7 days or 2 g stat. for both partners symptomatic therapy is suggested.
- *Bacterial vaginosis.* If sexually transmitted; metronidazole (Flagyl) for 7 days and ampicillim 500 mg orally or clindemycin (Cleoun) 300 mg orally for 5 days bid for 7 days: examine and treat both partners. Intravaginal treatment with metro-Gell applicator bid for 5 days; Clindamycin phosphate 2 per cent vaginal cream) applicator qHS for 7 days.
- *Foreign body:* Removal of objects, antibiotic specific to secondary infection.
- Allergens or irritants: Removal of possible allergens or irritant; topical steroid ointment as needed.

Nursing management focusses primarily on the appropriate use of prescribed therapy and measures to prevent reinfection. The nurse instructs the woman to clean the genital area thoroughly with soap and water and dry well before applying any medication. The hands should be washed properly before and after treatment. The nurse advises the woman to remain recumbent for 30 minutes after insertion of suppository or cream to facilitate absorption and prevent loss from vagina. Tampoons should be avoided during treatment. If vaginal drainage is present, the woman is encouraged to wear minipad. Sitz bath can be comforting. The woman is instructed to refrain from intercourse while the infection is being treated and the male partner should use a condom until all symptoms of inflammation have been resolved.

Prevention of infection is an important consideration. The following measures reduces the incidence of vaginal infections which include:

1. Cleanse the general areas thoroughly with mild soap and water daily.
   - Wipe genital area from front to back after bowel movements.
   - Avoid use of vaginal irritants (e.g. harsh deodarants and perfumed soap, deodarant sprays, douches).
   - Do vaginal irrigation as ordered.

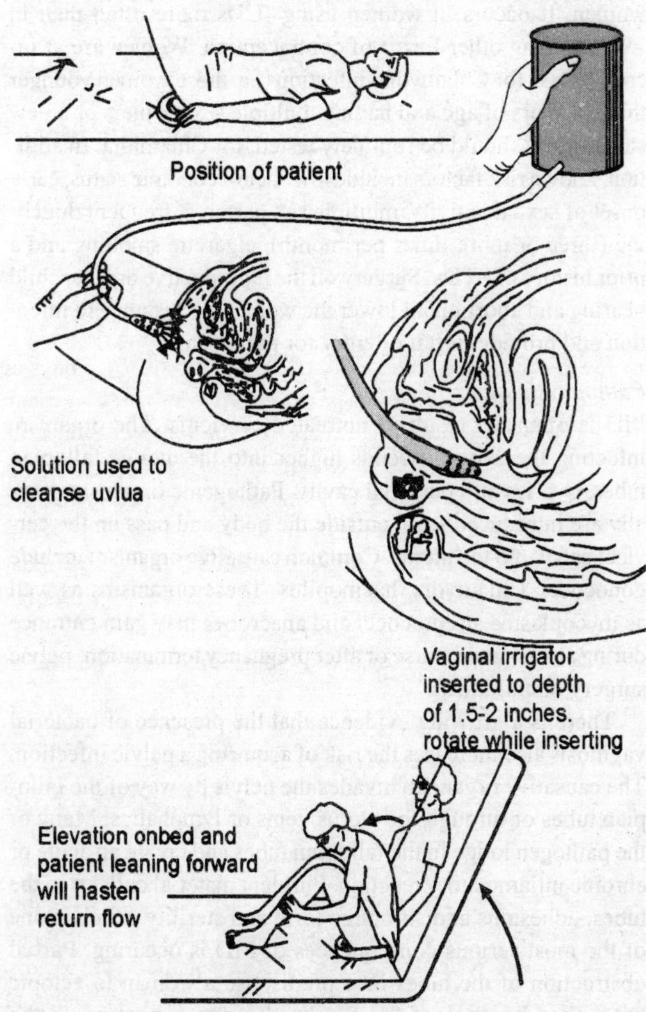

Position of patient
Solution used to cleanse uvlua
Vaginal irrigator inserted to depth of 1.5-2 inches. rotate while inserting
Elevation onbed and patient leaning forward will hasten return flow

Fig. 15.3: Vaginal irrigation. The nurse wears gloves while doing this procedure.

   - Avoid routine douching, which can alter the vaginal pH.
2. Use underwear with cotton crotch and change panties daily; avoid using any clothing that is tight in the crotch or thighs. Avoid wearing underpant while sleeping.
3. Assess sexual partners for any sign of infection (e.g. discharge, lesions, reddened areas on genitalias)
   - Use a barrier method of contraception.
   - Avoid any sexual practice that is painful or abrasive.
   - Avoid anal genital intercourse.
   - Cleanse genital area of self and partner and void before and after intercourse.
4. Change tampoons or napkins frequently during menstruation.
5. Treat athletes foot and "jook itch" with over—the counter-antifungals.
6. Consider using Vitamin C 500 mg per orally (PO) bid to increase the acidity of vaginal secretions.
7. Recognize the signs of infection and respond promptly.

Cervicitis

The term 'Cervicitis' includes number of conditions characterized by inflammation and infection of the cervix. Cervicitis has been linked with cervical cancer.

Aetiology

Chlamydia trachomitis, neisseria gonorrhoea, staphylococus aureas and herpes virus all can cause cervicitis, chlamydia is the most common cause of infection. It is sexually transmitted.

Pathophysiology and Clinical Manifestation

Leukorrhoea may be the only sign and the amount may not be significant. On examination, the cervix is grossly erythematous and oedematous, and there is usually a mucoid purulent discharge. But the amount may be so small that patient does not notice it. There may be the mucopurulent discharge with postcoital spotting from cervical inflammation. The woman commonly has no subjective signs but may report pruritis, burning, lower abdominal pain, or dyspareunia. Symptoms of a urinary tract infection may also be present. Cervical stenosis, salpingitis and infertility are possible sequelae of chronic disease.

Management

Diagnosis is confirmed by the existing signs and symptoms. Vaginitis if present is treated first, the cervix is cultured and appropriate pharmacological therapy is initiated. Gonococcal cervitis is treated with one dose of cephlox IM plus oral doxycycline for 7 days and one dose of oral azithromycin to treat concurrent chlamydial infection. Other organism may be treated as mentioned in the vaginitis. If the woman cervitis does not respond to antibiotics, cryosurgery or laser therapy may be necessary. Treat partners with same drugs.

Cryosurgery is a safe outpatient procedure. Women are told

that a watery discharge is common after treatment but it resolves in several weeks. Healing is usually complete within 6 weeks. Women are also told that they may experience mild to moderate cramping during procedure. Take preventive measure of cervicitis as mentioned in vaginitis.

Bartholinitis (Bartholins Cysts)

Bartholin's cysts are one of the most common disorders of the vulva. They result from obstruction of a duct, which may become infected. Thickened mucous, stenosis or mechanical trauma may initiate the process.

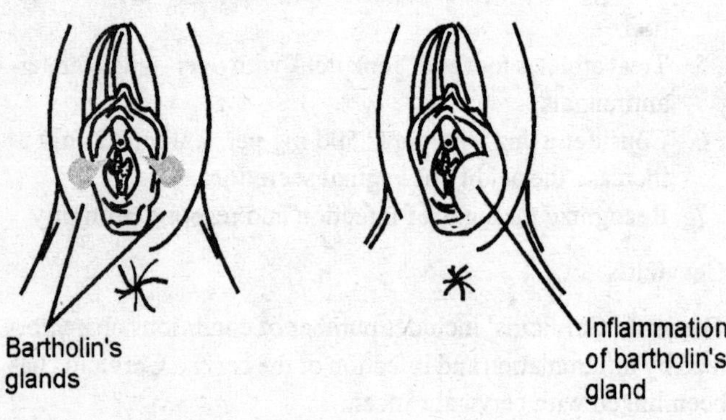

Fig. 15.4: Site and infection of vastibular gland.

Pathophysiology and Clinical Manifestation

The infection is usually unilateral but can be bilateral. Neisseria gonoeroea is the most common infecting organism. The secretary function of the gland continues and the duct fills up with fluid, producing severe inflammation, enlargement of the gland and tissue oedema. The area becomes tender, and even walking may be difficult. The pain is constant, and dyspareunia can be severe. The abscess may rupture, resulting in temporary symptom relief, but usually reforms. Occasionally, the acute inflammation resolves leaving scar tissue that can form a cyst. The cyst usually is nontender but may interfere with ambulation and intercourse.

Management

Cultures are taken and woman is treated for any underlying infection process. If the cysts are symptomatic, incision and drainage may be performed. The cysts tend to recur and a permanent opening for drainage of the gland may need to be constructed by placing a tiny *WORD* catheter through a stab wound into the cyst cavity. The catheter remains in the cyst for 3 to 4 weeks until healing has occurred and a new duct is formed. This procedure is also useful when infection is present. Laser can also be used to remove the cyst. Total gland excision may be performed in older women who have suffered repeated abscesses or when cancer is suspected.

Nursing intervention focusses on comfort. Mild analgesics and sitz baths help relieve pain, yes the most procedures are performed on an outpatient basis, the nurse instructs the woman on the safe use of these interventions at home and reinforces the need to report any signs of infection.

Pelvic Inflammatory Disease (PID)

Palvic inflammatory disease (PID) is a general term that refers to acute subacute, recurrent or chronic infection of the reproductive organs—pelvic peritoneum, veins, or connective tissues. PID is an infectious condition of the pelvic cavity that may involve infection of the fallopian-tubes (Salpingitis), ovaries (oophoritis) and pelvic peritoneum (peritonitis). The infection may be confined to just one structure or be widespread.

Aetiology

PID is rare during pregnancy and occurs at the time of premenarchal, postmenopausal and is found among celibate women. It occurs in women using IUDs more often than in women using other forms of contraception. Women are at increased risk for Chlamydial infection (i.e. those women younger than 24 years of age and having multiple sex partners or a new sex partner) should be routinely tested, for Chlamidia. In addition, known risk factors include low socio-economic status, early onset of sexual activity, multiple sex partners, frequent douching (three or more times per month), cigarette smoking and a prior history of STDs. Surgery on the reproductive organs, child bearing and abortion all lower the women's resistance to infection and provide portal of entry for pathogens.

Pathophysiology

PID is often the result of untreated cervicitis. The organism infecting the cervix ascends higher into the uterus, fallopian tubes, ovaries and personal cavity. Pathogenic organisms usually are introduced from outside the body and pass up the cervical canal into the uterus. Common causative organism include gonococci, Chlamydia, haemopilus. These organisms as well as mycoplasma streptococci and anaerobes may gain entrance during sexual intercourse or after pregnancy termination, pelvic surgery or childbirth.

There is a growing evidence that the presence of bacterial vaginosis also increases the risk of acquiring a pelvic infection. The causative organism invades the pelvis by way of the fallopian tubes or through the uterus veins or lymphatics. Many of the pathogen lodge in the fallopian tubes and create an acute or chronic inflammatory reaction. Purulent material collects in the tubes, adhesions and strictures form and sterility which is one of the most serious consequences of PID is occuring. Partial obstruction of the tubes may predispose a woman to ectopic pregnancy because of the fertilized ovum cannot reach the uterus. Inflammatory adhesions become so severe that surgical removal of the uterus, tubes and ovaries may be necessary. The infection usually remains localized in the lower abdomen and pelvis, although abcesses may form.

Clinical Manifestation

Women with PID usually go to a health care provider when they experience lower abdominal pain. So the clinical manifestation of acute PID includes severe abdominal pain, lower abdominal cramping, intermenstrual bleeding, dyspareunia, fever and chills, malaise, nausea and vomiting. The pain typically starts gradually and is constant. The intensity may vary from mild to severe, and movements such as walking can increase the pain. Pain increases during intercourse. Spotting after intercourse and abnormal vaginal discharge is common. A sensation of pelvic pressure and back pain may also be present, as well as foul-smelling purulent vaginal discharge. Symptoms often appear after the onset or cessation of menses. Abdominal palpation reveals pain and tendency to the lower quadrants of the abdomen, which is confirmed on pelvic examination. Masses may be felt indicating enlargement of the fallopian tubes or ovaries or the presence of an abscess.

Management

PID is a chemical diagnosis based on the patient's signs and symptoms. The diagnosis is based on the data obtained during bimanual portion of the pelvic examination. Diagnostic studies include WBC count and culture of any purulent secretions. A laparoscopy may be done to visualize pelvic structures and accomplish drainage of abscess and lysis of obstructing adhesions. Ultrasonography may be used to evaluate masses.

Treatment is aimed at eradicating the infection and preventing complications. Immediate complication of PID includes septic shock and Fitz-Hugh-Curtis syndrome, which occurs when PID spreads to the liver and causes acute prehepatitis. Long-term complication includes ectopic pregnancy, infertility and chronic pelvic pain PID is usually treated on an outpatient basis. The patient is given a combination of antibiotics such as Cefoxitin) and doxycycline to provide broad coverage against the causative organism. The patient must have no intercourse for 3 weeks. Her partner must be examined and treated. Physical rest and oral fluids are encouraged. Hospitalization may be necessary if the woman is acutely ill. Broad spectrum antibiotics are used until drug sensitivities are determined. Salpingectomy may be necessary if an abscess is found and more radical surgery is needed when all the reproductive organs have been compromised by the infection. If the woman has an IUD, it is removed.

Nursing interventions are largely supportive. Bedrest is a semi-Fowler's position and is recommended to assist pelvic drainage. Heat applied to the abdomen may be comforting, but tube or sitz baths should be avoided during the period of active infection. The vaginal discharge is copious and commonly purulent and may cause pruritis and excoriation. Other nursing measures include managing fever, monitoring vital signs, monitoring intake and output and providing emotional support.

The nurse instructs the woman to cleanse the perineal region every 3 to 4 hours and maintain scrupulous hygiene after urination and defecation. Tampoons should not be used and drainage pads should be changed frequently. A minimum of 3000 ml of fluid is daily recommended. Women treated as outpatients are remained for the seeking of appropriate follow-up because PID can have serious life-long consequence for fertility. The woman's sexual partner may be treated with antibiotics at the same time. The importance of using condoms to prevent reinfection or future infection is stressed.

Problems of Menstruation

Menstrual cycles are influenced by hormones from the hypothalamus gonadotropin-releasing hormone and anterior pituitary (FSH and LH). These hormones influence the development of a dominant follicle and egg within one ovary and resulting production of oestrogen during the follicular phase of the cycle. The oestrogen from the ovary causes the growth of the endometrial lining of the uterus. Following ovulation, the corpus luteum (site of ovulation) produces progesterone that further develops and stabilizes the endometrial lining, building a suitable lining to receive a fertilized egg. The progesterone dominant part of the menstrual cycle is called the luteal phase because of the essential part of the corpus luteum plays. When a fertilized egg does not implant in the endometrial lining, the corpus luteum is not maintained and production of progesterone falls. In response to decreasing level of progesterone, the endometrial lining is shed. This shedding is referred to as "menstruation" or woman's menses or her period. The first day of menses is considered the start of day 1 of the menstrual cycle. Menses may be irregular during first few years after menarche and the years preceding menopause. Once established, a woman's menstrual cycle usually has a predictable pattern. However, considerable normal variation exists among women in cycle length as well as in duration, amount characteristic and menstrual flow.

Almost all women experience problems with their menstrual cycle at some point in their reproductive years. Problems produce a variety of symptoms that may be directly or indirectly related to pelvic organs. Most problems are self-manageable and are rarely brought to the health care provider's attention unless they become severe or persistent.

Premenstrual Syndrome

Premenstrual syndrome (PMS) is defined as a cluster of distressing physical and behavioural symptoms that occur as the second half of the menstrual cycle and are followed by a symptom-free period. PMS constitutes a group of somatic, behavioural, cognitive and mood symptoms distressing enough to impair interpersonal relationships or interfere with urinal activities.

Actiology and Pathophysiology

The aetiology and pathophysiology of PMS are not well understood. But these may the result of a wide variety of hormonal, psychological and nutritional factors. Women with PMS have genetically determined sensitivity to one or more of the neurotransmitter systems such as serotonin. This sensitivity results in heightened response to the normal cyclic fluctuation of the ovarian hormone. Other proposed causes include oestrogen and progesterone imbalances and nutritional deficiency of pyridoxine (Vit B_6) or magnesium.

Clinical Manifestation

PMS is extremely variable in its clinical manifestation. Variations are common between women and for an individual woman, from one cycle to another. Commonly-occurring physical symptoms include, breast discomfort, peripherial oedema, abdominal bloating, episodes of binge, eating and headache. Abdominal bloating and breast-swelling are apparently caused by local fluids' shifts because total body weight does not generally change symptoms of autonomic nervous systems arousal such as heart palpitation and dizziness have been reported. Women may experience anxiety, depression, irritability and mood swings. The symptoms can be grouped on the basis of possible aetiology.

- *Anxiety:* (Nervousness, mood swings, irritability) may be due to high serum oestrogen, low serum progesteron, elevated adrenal androgen and possible disturbance of thyroid axis.
- *Water-related symptoms* (weight gain, swelling of extremities, breast tanderness, abdominal bloating) may be due to high serum aldosterone, retention of sodium and water, decreased colloid osmotic pressure in abdomen.
- *Cravings:* (Craving for sweets, increased appetite) may be due to increased carbohydrate tolerance and low red cell magnesium levels.
- *Depression* (Forgetfulness, crying, confusion, insomnia) due to causes mentioned in the anxiety.

In addition, headache, heart pounding, fatigue, dizziness or faintness may be present.

Management

There is no objective means of diagnosing PMS existance and the diagnosis is primarily established by exclusion. A woman is considered to have PMS if her symptoms interfere with activities of daily living. Symptoms that occur in three consecutive menstrual cycles confirm the diagnosis.

Numerous treatments have been suggested, including both pharmacological and nonpharmocological strategies. But no treatment has been proved to be effective in all cases. The use of oral contraceptive produces symptoms similar to PMS in some women but also relieves symptoms in some women, diagnosed with the disorder. Treatment attempted to reduce number and severity of symptoms and restore the women's psychological health. Treatment strategies for PMS include:

i. *Pharmological Strategies:*
   - Combination oral contraceptives: Used for women with no contraindication.
   - Selective serotonin *Reuptake Inhibitions* (SSRI): Antidepressants—Good relief for mood symptoms.
   - Prostaglandin inhibitors: Administration 2-4 times daily at onset of symptoms.
   - Diuretics: Administration during luteal phase.
   - Tranquilizers, Gonadotrophic inhibitor (Denazol).
   - Evening primrose oil (natural therapy).

ii. *Non-pharmocological Strategies:*
   - Diet: Well-balanced, avoid caffeine, alcohol. Reduce refined carbohydrates and adequate intake of vitamin B_6
   - Stress Management: Relaxation techniques-Abdominal breathing, mental imagery and progressive muscle relaxation.
   - Exercise: Aerobics, walking and swimming.
   - Education and counselling: knowledge of possible causes and treatment daily dairy maintaining Family under-standing, support groups, assertiveness training.
   - Sex and marital therapy.

The nurse helps the woman and her family by teaching following points.

- Teach possible causes of conditions and treatment.
- Teach relaxation techniques.
- Teach patient to do the following.
  - Avoid stressful activities during premenstrual period. Fatigue exaggerate symptoms.
  - Take medication as prescribed.
  - Reduce or eliminate smoking and alcohol consumption.
  - Reduce or eliminate consumption and caffeine.
  - Follow a regular exercise program.
  - Eat well-balanced diet with adequate protein and reduced intake of salts and refined sugars.
  - Incorporate stress-reducing strategies into daily lifestyle.
  - Increase intake of food high in vitamin B and magnesium (green leafy vegetable, legumes and whole grain cereals).

Dysmenorrhoea

Dysmenorrhoea is defined as abdominal cramping or discomfort associated with menstrual flow. It involves uterine pain with menstruation and is commonly called menstrual cramps.

Aetiology

The two types of dysmenorrhoea are primary (when no pathology exists) and secondary (when a pelvic disease or condition in the underlying cause). Primary dysmenorrhoea is not associated with pelvic pathology and occurs in the absence of any organic disease. Its severity usually declines after pregnancy by the age of 30. Secondary dysmenorrhoea occurs in response to organic disease such as PID endometriosis, leimyomas (uterine fistoids) and IUD use.

Pathophysiology

Primary dysmenorrhoea is not a disease. It is caused by either an excess of prostragandin F2Alpha (PGF2Alpha) and/or an increased sensitivity to its neuptors. The sequential stimulation of the endometrium by oestrogen followed by progesterone results in a dramatic increase in prostaglandin production by the endome-trium. With the onset of menses, degeneration of the endome-trium releases prostaglandin. Locally prostaglandin increases myometrial contractions and construction of small endometrial blood vessels with consequent tissue ischaemia and increased sensitization of the pain receptor resulting in menstrual pain. Prostaglandin absorbed into the circulating systems may be responsible for symptoms of headache, diarrhoea and vomiting.

Secondly dysmenorrhoea is usually acquired after adolescence, occurring most commonly in the 30's and 40's. Common pelvic conditions that cause secondary dysmenorrhoea include endometriosis, chronic PID, uterine fibroids and adenomyosis.

Clinical Manifestation

Primary dysmenorrhoea starts 12 to 24 hours before the onset of menses. The pain is most severe. The first day of menses and rarely lasts more than 2 days. Characteristic manifestation include lower abdominal pain that is colicky in nature, frequently radiating to the lower back and upper thighs. The abdominal pain is often accompanied by nausea, diarrhoea, fatigue, headache and light headedness.

Secondly dysmenorrhoea usually occurs after the woman has experienced problem-free periods for some time. The pain which may be unilateral is generally more constant in nature; usually continues longer than primary dysmenorrhoea. Depending on the cause of symptom such as dyspareunia (Painful intercourse) painful defecation, or irregular bleeding may occur at times other than menstruation.

Management

Primary dysmenorrhoea is treated with prostaglandin inhibition which blocks prostaglandin synthesis and metabolism. NSAIDs are effective for many women because these drugs inhibit prostaglandin synthesis. The drugs used commonly are NSAIDS (Ibuprofen, Mefenamic acid (Ponstel), Naproxen, Keto profen. Nursing intervention during drug therapy includes: teach the patient to:

- Take drug on an empty stomach unless GI irritation develops.
- Report the occurrence of any unexplained bleeding (of menorrhagia epistasis).
- Mefenamic acid should be taken with meals, or antacids to decrease GI irritation. It should not be taken for more than 7 days. Treatment of secondary dysmenorrhoea is aimed at the underlying organic cause. Options include both pharmocological and surgical interventions.

Women rarely seek professional help for mild primary dysmenorrhoea. However, women who are consistently unable to engage in normal activities because of menstrual pain should be encouraged to seek medical care. Women often ask nurses what can be done for minor discomfort associated menstrual cycles. They should be advised that during acute pain, relief may be obtained by lying down for short periods, drinking hot beverages, applying heat to the abdomen or back, and taking an anti-inflammatory drug or mild analgeisa. The nurse can suggest noninvasive pain-relieving practices such as distraction and guided imagery.

The nurse instructs the patient that NSAIDS are most effective when taken at the onset of the menses before pain becomes severe, and can be buffered with food or antacid if GI irritation occurs. Other health care measaures can reduce the discomfort of dysmenorrhoea. These include regular exercise, maintenance of proper nutritional habits, avoidance of constipation, maintenance of good body mechanics, and avoidance of stress and fatigue, particularly during the time preceding menstrual periods. Staying active and interested in activities may also help. Women should be taught when dysmenorrhoea occurs as well as how to treat it. Education and supportive therapy can provide women with a foundation for coping with this common occurrence and increase feelings of control and self-reliance. Constipation should be avoided. If pain occurs, the nurse can suggest that the woman—use local heat, which helps dilate blood vessels and relieve ischaemia and use of progressive relaxation strategies.

Amenorrhoea

Amenorrhoea refers to the absence of menstruation.

- Primary amenorrhoea exists if the first menses had not occurred by the age of 16. It usually results from a genetic, endocrine or congenital developmental defect and is often associated with disorders of pubertal development.
- Secondary amenorrhoea exists when a previously menstruating woman ceases to menstruate for more than 3 to 6 months (3 months in a woman with a history of regular menstrual cycle). Skipping an occasional single period is normal. Pregnancy is the most common causes of secondary amenorrhoea.

Aetiology

Anovulation is the most common cause. For missing menses, once pregnancy has been ruled out. Additional causes of secondary amenorrhoea is usually a response to environmental variable, such as altered function of the hypothalamus, pituitary gland, ovaries, thyroid, or adrenal gland. Second amenorrhoea also is a side effects of some medication, and women who take oral contraceptive may experience amenorrhoea for upto 6 months after discontinuing the pill. To sum up, the causes of amenorrhoea are as follows:

i. *Hypothalaemic—Pituitary axis*
   - Reversible CNS—mediated insults (e.g. emotional stress-anorexia nervosa or severe dieting, strenuous exercise, post-pill syndrome and chronic or acute illness).
   - Prolactinoma and other causes of hyperprolactinaemia (e.g. drugs).
   - Cramopharyngioma and other brainstem or parasellar tumours.
   - Congenital conditions (e.g. isolated gonadotropin deficiency).
   - Trauma (e.g. head injury with hypothalaemic contusion).
   - Infiltration process (e.g. Sarcoidosis).
   - Vascular disease (e.g. hypothalaamic vasculitis).
   - Pituitary tumours.
   - Sheehan's syndrome.

ii. *Ovaries*
   - Autoimmune disease (often involving thyroid, adrenal, islet cells).
   - Premature menopause (idiopathic) or resistant-ovary syndrome.
   - Polycystic ovary disease.
   - Congenital or genetic condition (e.g. Turner's Syndrome).
   - Infection (e.g. Mumps, oophoritis).
   - Toxins (especially alkylating chemotherapeutic agents).
   - Radiation.
   - Trauma, torsion (rare).

iii. *Uterovaginal Outflow Tract*
   - Asherman's syndrome (Postcurrettage loss of endometrium).
   - Mulleriah dysgenasis.

iv. *Hormonal Synthesis and Action*
   - Male pseudohermaphroditism (e.g.testicular feminization).
   - 17-Hydroxylase deficiency.

Pathophysiology

Pathophysiology of amenorrhoea is based on the causes. Prolonged secondary amenorrhoea is common among certain groups of conditioned athletes such as gymnasts and long distance runners, because normal menarche is believed to be required approximately 17 per cent of body weight. Weight loss may result in amenorrhoea. The consequences of prolonged amenorrhoea are not fully known.

Clinical Manifestation

Absence of menses and signs and symptoms of underlying causes and effects.

Management

The diagnostic work-up for amenorrhoea includes a detailed history and careful examination of the reproductive system. Pregnancy should be ruled out as a possible cause. The treatment depends on the cause. An organic problem is corrected if possible. Hormone therapy may be required.

The nurse teaches the woman about the problem, its causes and the diagnostic studies are planned. Teaching may include information about weight gain, stress reduction, and reducing the energy drain of strenuous exercise. Women may need counselling and support to deal with feelings of threat to their self-concept and concern overfertility that may be caused by the amenorrhoea.

Dysfunctional Uterine Bleeding (DUB)

Dysfunctional uterine bleeding (DUB) is defined as excessive or irregular uterine bleeding with no demonstrable cause. It can take many forms including excessive flow, prolonged duration of menses and intermenstrual bleeding.

Aetiology

Irregular vaginal bleeding is a common gynaecologic concern. Frequently occurring irregularities include oligomenorrhoea (long intervals between menses), secondary amenorrhoea (cessation of menses for at least 6 months) menorrhagia (excessive menstrual bleeding) and metrorrhagia (irregular bleeding or bleeding between menses).

The causes of DUB during childbearing and postmenopausal years are as follows:

i. *Menorrhagia* (Prolonged profuse menstrual flow during regular periods) is caused by submucous myomas, pregnancy complications, adenomyosis, endometrial hyperplasia, malignant tumours and hypothyroidism.
ii. *Metrorrhagia* (bleeding between periods) is caused by endometrial polyps, endometrial and cervical cancer, exogenous estrogen administration.
iii. *Polymenorrhoea* (increased frequency of menstruations) is caused by anovulation; shortened luteal phase.
iv. *Cryptomenorrhoea* (usually light menstrual flow)—caused by hymenal or cervical stenosis, Asherman's syndrome (uterine synechiae), oral contraceptives.
v. *Menometrorrhagia* (Bleeding at irregular intervals occurs as a result of any conditions causing intermenstrual bleeding; sudden onset is indication of malignant tumours or complications of pregnancy.
vi. *Oligomenorrhoea* (menstrual periods more than 35 days apart) may be caused by anovulation from endocrin causes

(Pregnancy, menopause) or systemic (excessive weight loss); oestrogen-secretory tumours.

vii. *Dysfunctional uterine* bleeding (An abnormal bleeding without known organic cause).

The cause is unknown.

Irregular bleeding may be caused by dysfunction of the hypothalmic-pituitary-ovarian axis such as pituitary adenoma. Changes in lifestyles such as marriage, recent moves, a death in the family, financial stress, and other emotional crises can cause such dysfunctions. (Psychologic factors can influence endocrine function).

Pathophysiology

Dysfunctional uterine bleeding may occur between or during their menstrual periods. When menorrhagia is present, the woman may soak a tampoon or pad every 1 to 2 hours or a week or more. The exact cause of the anovulatory episode is not understood; but it may represent a dysfunction of the hypothalmic-pituitary-ovarian axis that results in continuing oestrogen stimulation of the endometrium. The endometrium outgrows its blood supply, partially breaks down and is sloughed in an irregular manner. Anovulation may also result from thyroid or adrenal abnormalities.

Management

The diagnostic work of DUB starts with a thorough history of the frequency, amount and duration of bleeding. Laboratory test may include blood counts to estimate blood loss, pregnancy tests, thyroid studies, ovulation tests and coagulation studies. Papanicolaou (Pap) smears, pelvic examinations, ultrasonography, endometrial biopsy, and sonohysterography may be employed to assess for structural problems and cancer.

Treatment depends on the nature of the problem (menorrhagia or amenorrhoea), degree of threat to the patient's health and whether children are desired in the future. The cause of bleeding guides medical care. In the absence of an organic cause, the preferred treatment is usually conservative. There are pharmacological options to stop heavy bleeding or reduce it. Further blood loss in subsequent menstrual cycles include the use of oestrogens, progestrins, NSAIDS, antifibrinolytic agents, and gonadotroph in releasing hormona agonists such as danazol. All patients with menorrhagia shouild be assessed for anaemia and treated as indicated.

Surgery may be indicated depending on the underlying cause of the irregular vaginal bleeding. Dilation and Curettage (D and C) was once a common therapy for excessive bleeding or for spotting in perimenopausal woman. Now D and C is used only is extreme cases of bleeding or for older women when endometrial biopsy and ultrasonography provide diagnostic information. Endometrial ablations done by laser or electrosurgical technique has been successful with many 80 per cent cases with uncontrolled menorrhagia. If menorrhagia is caused by uterine fibroids, a hysterectomy may be performed or a *myomectomy* removal of fibroids without removal of the uterus may be performed if the patient wants to preserve her uterus. Hysterectomy may be necessary for those women whose bleeding cannot be controlled with hormones, who are symptomatically anaemic and whose lifestyle is compromised by persistent bleeding.

Mostly care of the DUB cases are provided in the outpatient setting, the nursing role is largely educational. Educating the women about characteristics of the menstrual cycle assists them to identify normal variations. This knowledge can help dispel apprehensions and misconceptions. If the patient's menstrual cycle pattern does not fall within the range of normalcy, the nurse should urge her to visit her health care provider. Myths concerning activities allowed during menstruation are common. The nurse should be prepared to clarify the facts. The patient should be assured that bathing and hairwashing are safe. A daily warm tub bath may actually relieve some of the associated pelvic discomfort. Women can swim, exercise, have intercourse and basically continue that usual daily activities.

The nurse teaches the woman to accurately assess the amount of bleeding in terms of number of pads or tampons, type of pad or tampon and degree of saturation. The nurse helps the woman set up and maintain an accurate record of the bleeding in the form of diary. Frequent changing of tampons or pads meet comfort and hygienic needs during menstruation. The selections of internal or external sanitary protection is a matter of personal preference. Tampons are convenient and make menstruation hygiene easier, whereas pads may provide better protection. Using a combination of tampons and pads and avoiding superabsorbant tampons may decrease the risk of toxic shock syndrome (TSS). TSS is an acute condition caused by toxins of staphylococcus aureus. TSS causes high fever, vomiting, diarrhoea weakness, myalgia, and sunburn-like rash.

The nurse also encourages the woman to express her concerns and fears. Anxiety related to infertility or fear of cancer can be intense but remain unexpressed.

Endometriosis

Endometriosis is the presence of normal endometrial tissue in sites outside the endometrial cavity. The most frequent sites are in or near the ovaries, the uterosacral ligaments, and the uterovesical peritoneum. However, endometrial tissues can be found in many other locations such as the stomach, lungs, intestines and spleen. The tissue responds to the hormons of the ovarian cycle and undergoes mini-menstrual cycle similar to the uterine endometrium.

Aetiology

The aetiology of endometriosis remains unknown. But there are multiple theories and lines of research. The condition may be hereditory because it occurs more often in women whose mothers had the disorder. Theories include the congenital presence of endometrial cells out of their normal locations, the transfer of endometrial cells by means of the blood or lymph system, and menstrual fluid containing endometrial cells up the fallopian tubes and into the pelvic cavity. A more recent theory suggests a possible immune mechanism in the aetiology of endometriosis.

Pathophysiology

With each menstrual period, the seeded endometrial cells are stimulated by ovarian hormones and bleed into the surrounding tissues, causing inflammatory response. Encased blood may lead to palpabie masses known as chocolate cysts. Occasionally the cystes rupture and spread endometrial cells deeper into the pelvis. Repeated inflammation and healing may create adhesions severe enough to fuse pelvic organs or cause bleed of bladder strictures. The ovaries are the most common site of involvement, and the process is usually bilateral. The pelvic peritoneum; the anterior and posterior cul-de-sac; and the uterosacreal, round, and broad ligaments are other common sites. Endometriasis progresses gradually and usually does not produce symptoms until the woman is 30 to 40 years of age.

Clinical Manifestation

The classic feature is menstrual pain and discomfort that becomes progressively worse. Other possible symptoms include abdominal pain, dyspareunia, irregular menses, bowel problems and urinary dysfunction. The most common symptoms are secondary dysnaemorrhoea, infertility, pelvic pain and dyspareunia and irregular bleeding. Less common symptoms include backache, painful bowel movements and dysuria. Pelvic examination reveals a fixed, retroverted uterus that is enlarged, tender and nodular.

When the ectopic endometrial implants "menstruate" the blood collects in cyst-like nodules that have a characteristic bluish black look. Nodules in the ovaries are sometimes called chocolate cysts, because of the thick chocolate-coloured material they contain. When a cyst ruptures, the pain may be acute and the resulting irritation promotes the formation of adhesions, which fix the affected area to another pelvic structures. The adhesions may become severe enough to cause a bowel obstruction, or painful micturition. Adhesion involving the uterus, tubes, or ovaries may result in infertility.

Management

Diagnosis of endometriosis is confirmed by the laparoscopy. The endoscopy is used to carefully map out and describe the extent of disease involvement, and biopsis of suspicious tissue can be obtained during procedure. Ultrasound and MRI may also be used for differentiation of cystic lesion and detecting stage of the disease. Treatment of endometriosis is influenced by the patient's age, desire to get pregnant, symptom of severity, and the extent and location of disease. When symptoms are not disruptive, a watch and wait approach is used. When endometriosis is identified as a possible cause of infertility, therapy will proceed more rapidly.

Drug therapy is used to reduce symptoms. Drugs are selected to inhibit oestrogen production by the ovary so that the endometrial tissue shrinks. The various drugs are used to imitate a state of pregnancy or menopause, since both natural conditions relieve symptoms, continuous use of (for 9 months) combined progestin and oestrogin causes regression of endometrial tissue. Oral contraceptive with minimal oestrogen and high levels of progestins may be used to produce endometrial strophy. Disadvantages to this approach include irregular bleeding and symptoms such as nausea, fatigue and depression.

Drugs with antigonatropic action such as danazol may be used to suppress ovarian activity. Danazol stops endometrial proliferation, prevents ovulation, and produces atrophy of ectopic endometrial tissue. The newest and most expensive therapy is injectable gonadotropin-releasing hormone analog (Leuprolids (lupron)). It causes a hypoestrogenic state resulting amenorrhoea. The side effects include hot flushes, vaginal dryness or emotional lability as in menopause.

Surgical intervention may be necessary if the disorder does not respond to drug therapy. For women wishing to get pregnant, *conservative surgical* therapy is used to remove implants that may block the fallopian tube. Also, adhesions are removed from the tubes, ovaries and pelvic structures. Efforts are made to conserve all tissues necessary to maintain fertility. *Definitive surgery* involves removal of the uterus, tubes, ovaries and as many endometrial implants as possible.

Nurses should educate women about endometriosis with special attention to the common symptoms. The nurse reassures the woman that endometriosis can be treated. The nurse teaches about the prescribed drugs all the management of side effects. Strategies to manage chronic pain are particularly important. The importance of ongoing care and follow-up is reinforced. If surgery is the treatment the nursing care is similar to that of the general preoperative and postoperative care of patient undergoing laparotomy.

Uterine Prolapse

The most commonly occurring problems with pelvic support are uterine prolapse, cytocele and rectocele. The uterus may undergo minor displacement in ways that are considered to be normal variations with little or no clinical effects. Uterine prolapse represents a severe uterine problem in which the uterus protrudes through the pelvic floor apertuor genital hiatus. It is usually associated with a cystocele or rectocele.

Aetiology

Usually vaginal childbirth increases the risk of these problems, i.e. uterine prolapse, cystocele, or rectocele. Uterine prolapse occurs most often in multiparous caucasian women as a resposne to injuries to the muscle and fascia of the pelvis incurred during childbirth.

Women without any children may also have these problems which include the following:

- Systemic conditions such as obesity and chronic pulmonary disease, and local conditions such as ascites and uterine or ovarian tumour are other causes for these problems.
- Chronic coughing, constipation, genetic predisposition and oestrogen deprivation after menopause can also contribute to prolapse. The decrease in oestrogen that normally accompanies the perimenopause also reduces some connective tissue support.

Prolapse usually develops gradually, suggesting that the effects of aging play a major role. As the uterus begins to drop, the vaginal walls become relaxed and the bladder may herniate into vagina (cystocele) or the rectal wall may herniate into the vagina (Rectocele).

Pathophysiology

Variations in the normal position of the uterus or prolapse can result from congenital or acquired abnormalities of the pelvic support structures. Acquired weakness occurs after birth, surgery, and closely-spaced pregnancies and in response to obesity and the loss of tissue elasticity with aging. The severity of the prolapse is designated by degree. In first-degree prolapse, the cervix still rests within the lower part of the vagina. In second-degree prolapse the cervix is at the vaginal opening i.e., cervix protrudes through the introitus, the entire uterus suspended by its stretched ligaments, hangs below the vaginal orifice. Before menopause the uterus hypertrophie's end is engorged and become flabby. The vaginal mucosa thickens and stasis ulcers may develop. Anterior and posterior vaginal wall relaxation often accompany prolapse, allowing for the development of cystocele or rectocele. Older women may have these conditions for years before seeking medical attention.

Clinical Manifestation

Patient with first degree prolapse experiences few symptoms but may report sensations or heaviness or fullness and a feeling that something is falling out or something coming down" of the vagina. In more severe prolapse, when the cervix protrudes at the introitus, the patient may complain of feeling like she is sitting on a ball. With severe prolapse, the woman is clearly aware of the mass. Vaginal bleeding, discharge and infection may be present. Leukorrhoea or menometrorrhagia may develop in premenopausal women with prolapse as a result of uterine engorgement. After menopause discharge and bleeding with prolapse usually results from injection and ulceration.

Women may have dyspareunia, a dragging or heavy feeling in the pelvis backache and bowel or bladder problems if cystocele or rectocele also present. The woman with a cystocele may complain of urinary incontinence (stress incontinence) accompanying any activity that increases the intra-abdominal pressure, such as coughing, laughing or lifting. The patient with rectocele may complain of chronic constipation and develop haemorrhoids. When third-degree uterine prolapse occurs the protruding cervix and vaginal walls are subjected to constant irritation and tissue charge may occur.

Management

Uterine prolapse can be readily identified in pelvic examination. If a cystocele is present, the vaginal outlet is relaxed with a thin-walled smooth bulging mass present in the anterior vaginal wall below the cervix. The mass descends when the patient is asked to bear down. If retrocele is present, palpitation of the vaginal area reveals, a thin-walled rectovaginal septum projecting into the vagina. Many women are found to have both a cystocele and rectocele.

Treatment depends on the degree of prolapse and how much the woman's daily activities have been affected. Pelvic muscle strengthening exercises (Kegel exercises) may be effective for some women. Postmenopausal woman with first degree prolapse are treated with oestrogen therapy to maintain the tone and integrity of the pelvic floor muscle. Exercise therapy is suggested for all women. If pain or bleeding occurs, the uterus may be manually repositioned and supported by the insertion of vaginal pessaries. Pessary is a device that is placed in the vagina to help a support the uterus. A wide variety of shapes exists including rings, arches and balls. They are made of hard rubber or plastic that maintain the uterus in a forward position by exerting pressure on the ligaments attached to the posterior wall of the cervix. When a woman first receivlds a pessary, she also needs instruction for its cleaning a follow-up. Pessaries that are left in place for long periods are associated with erosion, fistulas and increased incidence of carcinoma. Conservative treatment with oestrogen, exercise and a pessary may also be employed for cystocele or rectocele if the woman experiences mild symptoms.

If more conservative measures are not successful, surgery is indicated, surgery to repair cystocele, rectocele and more advanced prolapses is undertaken when symptoms significantly interfere with patient's lifestyle. The procedures designed to tighten the vaginal wall termed 'anterior and posterior colporrhaphy". They are frequently combined with hysterectomy. Cystocele repair may be done abdominally and combined with a uterovesical suspension's procedure called a Marshall-Marchatti-Krantz procedure to correct stress incontinence.

Nurse can assist women to avoid or decrease problem with pelvic support by teaching them how to do exercises to strengthen their pelvic floor muscles. Exercise teaching is an important nursing intervention for any patient with uterine prolapse. The woman is instructed to tighten the muscles of the perineum as if to stop the flow of urine maintain the tension for 5 seconds at a time and repeat the exercise in sets of 10. The exercise is repeated 10 to 12 times daily. Knee-chest exercises are used less often but may be ordererd to stretch or strengthen the pelvic ligament. Corrective exercises for poor posture may also be prescribed.

The nurse encourages obese patients to lose weight to reduce intra-abdominal pressure. Chronic cough and chronic constipation are also corrected, because these conditions contribute to weakness of the muscle wall. Women fitted with a pessary needs to be taught how to insert it and withdraw it if the device becomes displaced or uncomfortable. Pessaries are removed and cleaned once every few weeks or months as recommended.

If vaginal surgery is necessary, the preoperative preparation usually includes a cleansing doucher in the morning of surgery. A cathartic and cleansing enema are usually given when a rectocele repair is scheduled. A perineal shave is done. The below-mentioned guidelines may be followed when the woman undergoing vaginal surgery:

a. Provide perineal care after each voiding or defecation.
   - Poor sterile normal saline over vulva and perineum.
   - Cleanse perineum as needed with sterile cotton balls; cleanse away from vagina towards rectum.
   - Dry perineum as needed with sterile cotton balls.
b. Encourage sitz baths after sutures are removed.
c. If douches are ordered during immediate postoperative period.
   - Use sterile equipment and sterile solution.
   - Insert douche nozzle very gently and rotate carefully.
d. Avoid pressure on suture line
   - Prevent a full bladder; keep urinary catheter patent.
   - Use measures to prevent constipation.
   - Teach patient to avoid the Valsalva's manoeuvre.
   - Keep patient flat or in low Fowler's position in bed.
e. Provide an icepack for perineal discomfort (severel seal plastic bags or glove make an acceptable pack).
f. Encourage leg exercises.
g. Encourage deep breathing.
h. Monitor intake and output.
i. Note characteristics of urine and stool.

The discharge preparation after vaginal surgery, if the patient and family need, following should be advised by the nurses:

- Perform daily douches and tub baths as prescribed.
- Avoid staining at stool.
- Use stool softener and laxative as prescribed.
- Avoid lifting for 6 weeks.
- Avoid sexual intercourse until physician gives permission (usually about 6 weeks).
- Avoid jarring activities.
- Avoid prolonged standing, walking or sitting, continue leg exercises for 6 weeks.

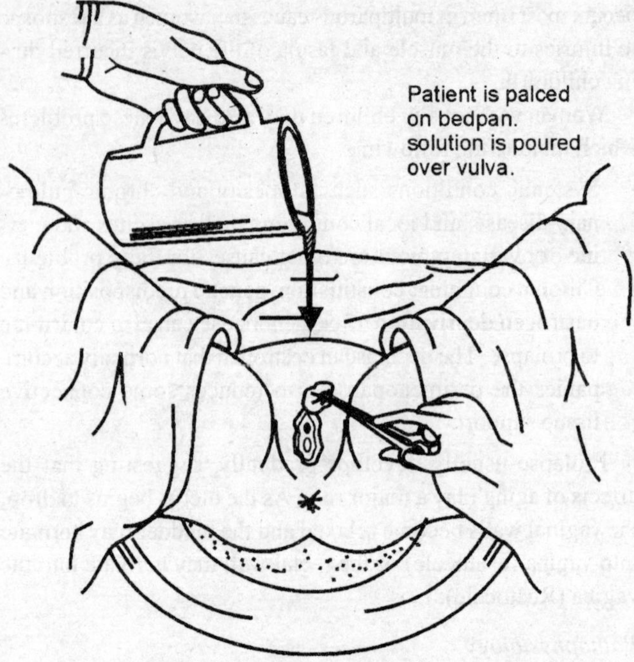

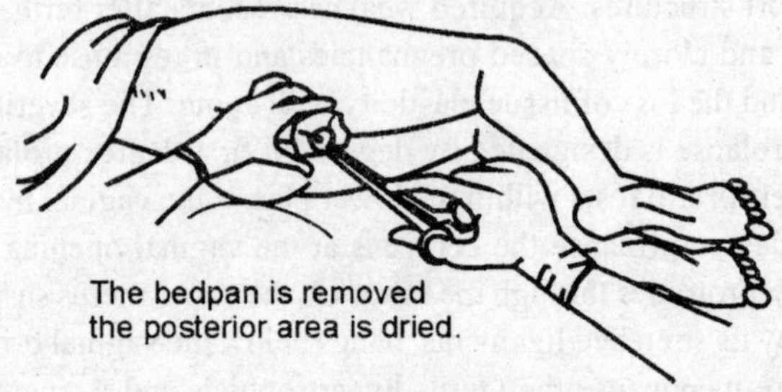

Patient is palced on bedpan. solution is poured over vulva.
Sterile pledgets are used to cleanse; then area is dried.

The bedpan is removed the posterior area is dried.

Fig. 15.5: Perineal Care.

- Vaginal sensation may be lost for several months postoperatively but sensation will return.
- Eat high-fibre diet and drink 300 ml of fluids daily.

Fistulas

A fistula is an abnormal tunnel-like opening between hollow internal organs or between an organ and the exterior of the body.

Aetiology

Fistulas can develop from a variety of causes but usually the result of surgery, childbirth, trauma, carcinoma, radiation therapy. Gynaecologic procedures cause urinary tract fistulas. The name of the fistula indicates the connecting structures. Fistulas can develop between the vagina and the rectum (Rectovaginal), bladder (vesicovaginal) or urethra (urethrovaginal), vescicovaginal fistulas are the most common followed by rectovaginal.

Pathophysiology

Conditions that cause fistulas to form typically compromise

the blood supply and cause tissue damage. Tissue sloughs and a channel gradually develop between the affected tissue and the vagina. The result is a constant leak of urine or escape of flatus or fecal material through the vagina. This is highly distressing to the patient and creates an offensive odour. The drainage excoriates and irritates the vaginal and vulvular tissue.

Clinical Manifestation

When vesicovaginal fistulas (between the bladder and vagina develops some urine leaks into the vagina, whereas with recto vaginal (between rectum and vagina) flatus and feces escape into the vagina. In both instances, excoriation and irrigation of vaginal and vulvalar tissue occur and may lead to severe infections. In addition, wetness and offensive odours may develop causing embarrassment and severely limiting socialization.

Management

Fistulas are diagnosed primarily through pelvic examination. A fistulagram, which involves the inejction of dye into the vagina, may be used to assess the exact location and severity of the fistula.

Small fistulas may heal spontaneously if the tissue is allowed to rest. Surgery is otherwise necessary to close fistula tract. Tissue inflammation and edema must be treated first, and this can take months. Either anterior or posterior colporrhaphy may be used. It may be necessary to temporarily divert the urinary or fecal stream in complex situation. A folley, ureteral or nephrostomy catheter is used to keep the area well drained and is left in place for weeks in some patients. With urinary diversion many urinary fistulas are able to heal spontaneously. Bowel rest contributes to healing rectovaginal fistulas and the patient may be placed on total parenteral nutrition (TPN). A diverting colostomy may also be performed if surgical intervention becomes necessary.

If fistulas are being conservatively managed, nursing interventions focus on comfort and prevention of infection. The nurses teaches woman that a chlorine solution makes an effective deodorizing douche and this solution is also excellent for perineal irrigation. A solution of 5 ml of household bleach to 1 Ltr of water is appropriate. Douching should be performed at low pressure to prevent forcing the solution through the fistula tract. Sitz baths and careful cleaning with mild soap and water is also helpful.

Postoperative care focuses on tissue healing. A small amount of serosanguineous drainage is expected but the patient is carefully monitored for evidence of continued fecal or urinary drainage. Douches may be ordered, and the nurse adminsters gently and at low pressure to protect healing tissue. Bedrest is often enforced for several days, perineal hygiene is great importance. But preoperatively and postoperatively the perineum should be cleansed every 4 hours. Warm sitz baths should be changed frequently. The patient is encouraged to maintain an adequate fluid intake. Encouragement and reassurance are needed in helping the patient to cope with her problems.

Postoperatively nursing care emphasises on avoidance of stress on the repaired areas and prevention of infections.

Postoperative care should be taken on catheters than the indwelling cataheter, usually in place for 7 to 10 days, in drainage at all times oral fluids should be urged to provide for internal catheter irrigation. Minimal pressure and strict asepsis used if catheter irrigation becomes necessary. The first stool after bowel surgery may be purposely delayed or prevent contamination of wound. Later stool softeners or laxatives may be given.

Surgical repair of fistulas is not always effective, even in the best conditions. Therefore, supportive nursing care for patients and her significant others is specifically important.

NEOPLASMS OF THE FEMALE REPRODUCTIVE TRACT

Cervical Polyps

Cervical polyps are benign peudnculated lesion that generally arises from the endocervical mucosi and are seen protruding through the cervicle or during speculum examination. The two main types of cervical polyps are:

1. Endocervical from the canal in the opening of the cervix, and
2. Ectocervical from the lower portion that protrudes into the vagina. Endocervical polyps tend to occur in middle-aged women. Ectocervical polypse are found most often in post-menopausal woman.

Pathophysiology

Most polyps are asymptomatic and discovered on routine pelvic examination. *Endocervical* polyps are usually reddish purple to cherry red, smooth soft growth that may vary in size from a few millimetres to 2 or 3 cm in diameter and length. They are usually attached to the mucosa by a narrow pedicle and may be single or multiple in number. *Ectocervical Polyps* are pale or flesh-coloured, round and elongated and often attach with a broad pedicle. Most polypoidal structures are vascular, and both types of polyps may become infected and necrotic at the tip.

Clinical Manifestation

The classic symptoms is intermenstrual bleeding, particularly after intercourse or douching. Leukorrhoea may be present. The chronic irritation and bleeding can lead to cervicitis, endometritis, or even salphingitis.

Management

Cervical polyps are usually diagnosed direct inspections and can be removed safely in clinic. The procedure causes minimal bleeding, but if bleeding should occur, it can be controlled by electrical or chemical cautery. All the excised tissues are sent for pathological examination. Antibiotics may be given prophylactically particularly if there is any evidence of tissues necrosis or cervicits. Simple removal of polyps is usually curable. The nurse encourages the woman to rest and avoid strenous activities after polyps removal. A prineal pad can be provided to absorb drainage. The nurse instructs the woman to report any significant bleeding or infection. And instruct her to avoid tampon use, douches and sexual intercourse for about a week while healing takes place.

Cervical Cancer

Cervical cancer is the seventh most common type of cancer in women following breast, colorectal, lung, endometrial and ovarian cancers and lymphoma.

Aetieology

Exact cause is unknown, but has a close association existing between early and frequent sexual contact with multiple partners and cervical viral infections, particularly the human papilloma virus (HPV). The HPV has been isolated in the vast majority of precancerous and cancerous changes of the cervix. It is spread predominantly through sexual contact. Studies have found a high incidence of cancer cervix in prostitutes. The rest factors of cervical cancer include the following:

i. *Actual Risk Factors*
- Low socioeconomic status.
- Early age at first coitus.
- Multiple sexual partners.
- History of STD.
- High risk male partner.
- Compromised immunity (HIV, HPV infections).
- Early age at first pregnancy.
- Prostitution.
- Multiparity.

ii. *Potential Risk Factors*
- Heavy use of talc.
- Cigarette smoking.
- Use of oral contraceptives.
- Vitamin A and C-deficiency.
- Derangement of folic acid metabolism.
- Intrauterine exposure to DES.
- Diabetes.
- Nulliparity.
- Frequent douching.

Pathophysiology

Majority of cervical concerns are squamous cell, arising from the epidermal layer of the cervix, cell dysplsia indicates the presence of a precursor lesion, typically called "Cervical intraepithelial neoplasia" (CIN) which has been divided into the following three stages:

CIN I : Mild to moderate dysplasia.
CIN II : Moderate to severe dysplasia.
CIN III : Severe dysplasia to carcinoma in situ.

Women diagnosed with dysplasia may experience disease regression, persistence or a progression to carcinoma. There are usually no signs or symptoms of dysplasia and the diagnosis is based on cytologic findings. Cervical can spread through the blood, by direct extension, a lymph invasion. As the lymph node grows larger, venous blood flow is obstructed and leg oedema, ureteral obstruction or hydronephrosis may occur. Haematogenous spread can occur to the lungs, mediastinum, liver and bone, prognosis based on the stage of the disease, depth of invasion and vascular involvement of the tumour.

Clinical Manifestation

Cervical cancer is asymptomatic in the early stages. As the disease progresses, the woman may experience thin, watery vaginal discharge, and occasional bloody spotting, especially after sexual intercourse or douching. In addition, metrorrhagia, postmenopausal bleeding, polymenorrhoea occurs as early symptoms. With advanced disease, a foul smelling discharge may develop from sloughing of the epithelial tissue. Pain is usually a late sign and can involve pelvic, flank, lower back and abdomen. The growing tumour may place pressure on the rectum and bladder causing irritation and discharge. Haemorrhage is possible with advanced infiltrative tumours, which may also erode the walls of adjacent organs and create fistula. In addition with loss, anorexia, anaemia, dysuria and rectal bleeding also may be present.

Management

Early detection is important to ensure positive outcomes. Routine pap smear screening begins once a woman engages a regular intercourse or turns 18 years old. The pap smear is a screening test but not a diagnostic tool. The diagnosis of cervical cancer can be confirmed only by biopsy. Two most common methods for obtaining cervical biopsy are conization or punch biopsy. Colposcopy allows for microscopic examination of the cervix and improves the accuracy of the biopsy process. In addition to CT scans, IVP, cystoscopy, progestosigmoidoscopy, and barium meal studies of the lower GI tract are based on diagnostic adjuncts.

Chemotherapy has not played a significant role in the management of cervical cancer. Squamous cell cancers tend to be relatively unresponsive to drug treatment. Cervical cancer is treated according to the stage of disease as briefed below.

- *Stage 0:* Carcinoma in site (C IN), intraepithelian carcinoma. Treatment options are cryosurgery, conization, laser surgery, hysterectomy, 5 -year survival rate is 95-100 per cent.
- *Stage 1:* Carcinoma is strictly confined to the cervix (extension to the corpus should be disregarded).

- *Stage Ia:* Preclinical carcinoma of the cervix that is those diagnosed by microscopy. Treatment options are simple hysterectomy or radiation (Cesium implant).
- *Stage I a1:* Minimal microscopically evident stomal invasion.
- *Stage I a2:* Lesions detected microscopically that can be measured. The upper limit of the measurement should not show a depth of invasion of more than 5mm taken from the basis of the epithelium, either surface or glandular from which it originates and a second dimension, the horizontal spread must not exceed 7 mm. Larger lesions should be staged as Ib.
- *Stage Ib:* Lesions of greater dimensions than 1a2, whether seen clinically or not, performed space involvement should not alter the staging but should be specifically recorded so as to determine whether it should affect treatment decisions in future. Treatment options are radiation, and or radical ('Werthem's) hysterectomy. Survival rate is 75 to 85 per cent radiotherapy (external or implant).
- *Stage II:* Involement of the vagina but not the lower third or infiltration of the parametric but not out of the sidewall. Treatment of radical hysterectomy of nodes or radiotherapy.
- *Stage II a:* Involvement of the vagina but no evidence of parametrial involvement.
- *Stage II b:* Infiltration of the parametrial but not out of the side wall.
- *Stage III:* Involvement of lower third of the vagina or exteretion to the pelvic side wall. All cases with hydronephrosis or nonfunctioning kidney should be included unless they are known to be attributable to other cause treatment in radiation.
- *Stage IIIa:* Involvement of the lower third of the vagina but not out of the pelvic side wall of parametrics are involved.
- *Stage IIIb:* Extension on to the pelvic side wall or hydronephrosis or nonfunctional kidney.
- *Stage IV:* Extension ouitside the reproductive tract. i.e., extensions beyond true pelvic or clinical involvement of the mucosa of the bladder or rectum, no state classification with bullous oedema is alone. Treatment options are radiation, surgery (e.g. exenteration) and chemotherapy survival rate is 5-15 years.
- *Stage IVa:* Involvement of the mucosa of the bladder or rectum.
- *Stage IVb:* Involvement of the distant metastasis or disease outside the true pelvis.

Surgical management deals in later part of this chapter.

The guidelines for care of the woman undergoing internal radiotherapy are as follows:

1. *Preimplantation*

   Nursing care before the insertion of the radioactive implant usually includes the following.

   - Provide cleansing enema to empty the bowel.
   - Insert Folley catheter to keep the bladder empty and small during treatment.
   - Provide betadine douche and shake pubic area if ordered.

2. *Implantation period*

   Nursing care during the 24 to 72 hours treatment includes the following:

   - Insert gauze packing into the vagina to separate the rectum and bladder from the irradiated area. One or two stitches may be placed in the labia to support the holder in position.
   - Maintain strict bedrest.
     - Elevate head of bed no more than 20 degrees. Keep the patients as flat as possible.
     - Assist the patient to turn from side to side as needed for comfort.
   - Provide low-residue diet and possibly antimotility agents to prevent bowel distension.
   - Administer analgesic as needed for uterine cramping, which can be severe.
   - Perform routine perineal cleansing if drainage is present, provide room deodarizer if discharge is foulsmelling.
   - Ensure a minimum fluid intake of 2500 ml daily.
   - Visit patient frequently from room door way for emotional support.
   - Provide diversional activities appropriate to activity restrictions.
   - Monitor implant for proper placement; keep long-handled forceps, and lead-lined container in the room in case of dislodgement.
   - Monitor complications:
     - Infection; increased vaginal redness or swelling; increasingly dark, foulsmelling drainage; cloudy urine and fever.
     - Thrombophlebitis: painful leg swelling, positive Horman's sign.

Staff who are involved in internal radiotherapy should follow the following radiation precautions:

- Time at the bedside limited—each contact should last not more than 30 minutes.
- Children and pregnant women/staff should not visit during treatment.
- Staff members should wear a dosimeter during every patient contact to monitor radiation exposure.
- Lead shield may be installed at the side and foot of the bed.
- Staff should use the principles of distance, time, and shielding in all contacts with the patients.
- Implant is always handled by means of long-handled forceps, never with hands. A lead-lined container should be present in the room for use if the implant dislodges.

- A sign that clearly identifies the radiation hazard is pasted on the room door including contact number of radiation safety officer.

The hospitalization period for intracavitary radiotherapy is short, and the patient is discharged soon after the removal of the implant. The woman must learn several self care skills for home management and should be aware of the sign and symptoms of potential complication. Radiotherapy causes fatigue, vaginal stenosis, loss of vaginal lubrication and induced menopause. The nurse should teach the woman regarding careful vaginal douches, techniques and local application of oestrogen cream (to prevent bleeding) and regular vaginal dilation (to prevent vaginal narrowing and fibrosis). If a woman has spouse or sexual partner, regular sexual intercourse usually at least three times per week is one method of minimizing stenosis. Manual oturator can be used to dilate vagina after lubrication. Sexual intercourse may be resumed about 3 weeks after discharge by using proper lubricants. Other selfcare measures include gradually increasing activity, maintaining a liberal fluid intake to prevent *urological* problems and adjusting the diet to prevent bowel problems (e.g. constipation or diarrhoea). The nurse teaches about signs and symptoms that indicate complications. The woman should promptly report unusually heavy discharge, foul-smelling urine, low-grade fever, persistent bowel problems or pain. Radiotherapy can cause fistula in the pelvis. The importance of follow-up care and monitoring is emphasized while teaching.

Uterine Leiomyoma (Fibroids)

Leiomyomas (fibroids, myomas fibromas) are the most common benign tumours of the female genital tract. Leiomyomas are benign tumours of muscle cells origin that contain varying amounts of fibrous tissue.

Aetiology

The exact aetiology is not completely understood. The stimulus for growth is unclear but it is thouight to be related to oestrogen, because leiomyomas are rare before menarche and often decrease in size after menopause. The tumours often enlarge during pregnancy, and with the use of contraceptives. Women who smoke tend to be relatively oestrogen deficient and have been found to have a lower incidence of leiomyomas. Tumours can react enormous proportions weighing as much as 50 pounds.

Pathophysiology

Leiomyomas originate in the myometrium are classified by the anatomical locations. *Submucous myomas* lie just beneath the endometrium and compress it as they grow. They can develop a pedicle and protrude into the uterine cavity or even through the cervical canal. *Intramural* myomas lie within the uterine muscle, and *subserous tumours* lie at the serosal surface of the uterus or may bulge outward from the myometrium. The external tumours also tend to become pedunculated.

Clinical Manifestation

The majority of women with leiomyomas are asymptomatic and may go undetected even when large in size, particularly if the woman is obese. The development of the symptoms depends on the location, size and condition of the tumour. *Menorrhagia* is the most common symptom. Bleeding can result from distortion and congestion of surrounding vessels or ulceration of the overlying endometrium. Bleeding usually takes the form of premenstrual spotting or prolonged light bleeding, after the menses. *Metrorrhagia* is associated with venous thrombosis or necrosis in the surface of the tumour, particularly if it extrudes through the cervix. The blood loss may be significant enough to create an *iron-deficiency anaemia* that does not respond to iron therapy.

Pain is not a characteristic symptom although it can result from tumour degeneration or with myometrial contractions that attempt to expel myoma from the uterus. If the pedicle stalk becomes twisted it can cause sudden, severe pain. Women often report sensation of heaviness in the pelvis or "a bearing down" feeling especially with large tumours. The tumour may cause pelvic circulated congestions and create backache, cosntipation or dysmenorrhoea. The woman even notices and increases in abdominal girth.

Management

Chemical diagnosis is based on the characteristic pelvic findings of an enlarged uterus destorted by nodular masses. Diagnosis confirmed through the use of MRI and CT scan, pelvic sonography, and hysterography or hysteroscopy.

Treatment depends on the symptoms, the age of the patient, her desire to bear children and the location and size of the tumour or tumours. Persistent heavy menstrual bleeding causing anaemia and large or rapidly growing fibroids are indications of surgery. Drug therapy does not play a major role in management of leiomyomas. However, GnRH agonists may be used to reduce the level of circulating oestrogens and shrink the tumour. Leiomyomas are the most common indication for hysterectomy. No diet or activity restricts for leiomyomas.

Endometrial Cancer

Cancer of the endometrium (Uterin corpus) is the most common form of gynaecological cancer and it primarily affects the woman over 50 years of age.

Aetiology

The major risk factor for endometrial cancer is oestrogen in particular unposed oestrogen. Additional risk factors include increasing of age, obesity, diabetes-mellitus, nulliparity, late menopause (after the age of 52) and hypertensions. Obesity is a risk factor because adipose (fat) cells store oestrogen which increases endogenous oestrogen and increases its availability. Pregnancy and birth control pills are protective factors. In addition, the use of oestrogen replacement therapy (ERT) and the use of tamoxifen for breast cancer and other causes of endometrial cancer.

Pathophysiology

Cancer arises from the lining of the endometrium; most tumours are pure adenocarcinomas. The precursor may be a hyperplasic state that progresses to invasive carcinoma. Hyperplasia occurs when oestrogen is not counteracted by progesterone. Direct extension develops into the cervix and through the uterine serosa. An invasion of the myometrium occurs in regional lymphnodes including the paravaginal and para-aortic, become involved. Haematogenous metastases develops concurrently. The usual sites of metastases are lung, bone, liver and eventually the brain. Malignant cells found in the peritonial cavity, presumably by tubal transport, and their presence is included in staging prognostic factors include histologic differentiation, uterine size at time of diagnosis; myometrial invasion, peritoneal cytology, lymph nodes and adenexal metastasis and tumour size. Endometrial cancer grows slowly, metastasizes late and is amenable to therapy if diagnosed early.

Clinical Manifestation

The first sign of endometrial cancer is abnormal uterine bleeding usually in postmenopausal women. Occasionally women have a purulent, blood-tinged discharge. Pain is late symptom and usually occurs with metastatic disease.

Management

Endometrial biopsy may be taken and examined for high risk women to detect early. The other methods for detection of endometrial cancer includes—endometrial aspiration, endometrial washing, dilation and currettage, pap smear, and combination of methods.

Endometrial cancer is treated according to its stages:

Stage I : Confined to corpus.
Stage II : Involves corpus and cervix.
Stage III : Extends outside the corpus but not outside the pelvis (vaginal wall).
Stage IV : Involves bladder rectum or outside pelvis.

The most common treatment is total abdominal hysterectomy with bilateral salpingo-oophorectomy (TAH-BSO). Radiation and surgery are often combined to treat in early-state of the disease. Hormonal therapy (Progestin) and chemotherapy (doxorubicin, cyclopholpomide, cisplatin are often added for stage III and IV diseases).

Nursing care associated with hystrectomy and radiotherapy followed. Nurses play a major role in health teaching about the importance of the careful assessment of all dysfunctions, uterin bleeding in postmenopausal population. Endometrial cancer is treatable disease.

Gestational Trophoblastic Neoplasia (GTN)

Gestational trophoblastic neoplasia (GRN) is the term used to describe choriocarcinoma and related diseases such as hydatid form mole and invasive mole.

The aetiology of GTN is not thoroughly understood. The hydatid form mole often precedes malignant diseases. GTN is an abnormal pregnancy characterized by a degeneration or abnormal growth of the trophoblastic tissue of the placenta, usually in the absence of an intact foetus. It produces a serum marker, human chorionic gonadotropin (HCG) whose levels are directly related to the number of tumour cells.

Early stage of GTN may be similar to normal pregnancy. As the disease progresses, most of the women experience uterine bleeding. Rapid uterin growth occurs. Often accompanied with nausea and vomiting.

Management

The diagnosis of GTN usually accomplished by ultrasonography, aminography, and analysis of HCG levels. Other diagnostic measures may be employed to rule out the presence of metastasis.

Suction currettage is the most common method used for evacuation of molar pregnancy, although hysterectomy may be selected if the woman does not desire future pregnancies. Intravenous ocytocin may be used to assist in expulsion of the tissue, which is then sent for extensive HPE.

Ovarian Cysts

Benign tumours of the ovary are many and varied. The cause of most of them is unknown. For purpose of clarity, they are divided into cysts and neoplasms. *Cysts* are usually soft, surrounded by thin capsules, and are seen mainly during the reproduction years. Follicle and corpus luteum cysts are common ovarian cysts. *Epithelial ovarian* neoplasms are extremely varied. They may be cystric or solid, small or extremely large. Cystric teratomas or dermoids originate from germ cells containing bits of any type of body tissues, such as hair or teeth.

Pathophysiology

Benign cysts and tumours develop from a variety of physiological imbalance. Elevated levels of luteinizing hormone may cause hyperstimulation of the ovaries. Follicular cysts depend on gonadotropins for growth and generally occur during the menstrual years and resolve spontaneously simple cysts occur commonly during menopause.

The characteristics of various type of benign ovarian cysts and tumours are as follows:

1. *Cysts*
   a. *Follicular cysts.*
      - Most common form of cysts.
      - Frequently multiple, range in size from a few mm to as large as 15 cm in diameters.
      - Depend on gonadotropine for growth.

- Occur during menstrual years and usually resolve spontaneously.
- May cause menstrual irregularities if blood oestrogen is elevated.

b. *Corpus luteum cysts*
- Less common variety.
- Associated with normal ovarian function or elevated progesterone.
- Average diameter 4 cm.
- May appear purplish red from bleeding within corpus luteum.
- May cause delayed menstrual bleeding from progesterone secretions.
- Menorrhagia common.

c. *Theca Lutein cysts*
- Least common variety.
- Usually bilateral and produce significant ovarian enlargement upto 30 cm in diameter.
- Develop from prolonged and excessive stimulation by gonadotropins.
- Associated with hydatide form mole 50 per cent of the time and choriocarcinoma 10 per cent of the time.

2. Epithelial Tumours

a. *Serous Tumours*
- Found in all age groups.
- Can be extremely large filling pelvis or abdomen.

b. *Mucinous Tumours*
- Occur in second to third decade of life.
- May be bilateral.
- Can reach spectacular size and largest form.

c. *Endometroid Tumours*
- Small lesions, purplish-blue in colour.
- Large tumours called "chocolate cysts" because they contain chocolate color clots.
- Very low malignancy potential.

d. *Mesonephroid Tumours*
- Usually multifocal.
- Involve peritoneal surfaces and may cause interestinal or urinary tract complications.
- Characterized by papillary proliferation without mitotic activity.

Clinical Manifestation

Ovarian masses are often asymptomatic until they are large enough to cause pressure in the pelvis, constipation, menstrual irregularities, urinary frequency, a full feeling in the abdomen, anorexia and peripheral oedema may occur depending on the size and locations of the tumour. Here there may be an increase in abdominal girth. Pelvic pain may be present if the tumour is growing rapidly, severe pain results when cyst twists in its pedicle (twisted ovarian cyst).

Management

Palpation of the reproductive organs during pelvic examination commonly reveals the presence of any mass or enlargement of the ovary. Any mass palpated in a postmenopausal women requires further investigation which includes ultrasonagraphy and CT scan, etc. and confirm diagnosis.

Many ovarian cysts resolve spontaneously. If the cyst does not decrease in size, oral contraceptive may be prescribed to shrink it. Surgery is usually recommended only when the cyst is larger than 8 cm or occurs after menopause or before puberty. A cystectomy rather than oophorectomy will be performed if possible.

Woman should be educated regarding disease, importance of follow-up care; nurse should reassure the patient who has undergone surgery. If woman goes surgical menopause, oestrogen replacement therapy is initiated.

Ovarian Cancer

Malignant neoplasms of the ovaries occur at all ages including infancy and childhood. It occurs most frequently in women between 55 to 65 years of age.

Aetiology

The aetiology of ovarian cancer is not understood but several factors appear to be associated with it like hereditary, endocrine, environment of the ovarian cancer. Women who have mutation of the BRCA-1 gene have increased susceptibility of ovarian cancer. Incidence rates are high in industrialized areas, which point to environmental influences. Exposure to talc and asbestos, diets high in meat and animal fats and high milk consumption all appear to be linked with the cancer.

Breastfeeding, multiple pregnancies, oral contraceptives use (more than 5 years) and early age at first birth seem to reduce risk of ovarian cancer. It is thought these factors have a protective effect because they reduce the number of ovulatory cycles the women experience. Women who are not exposed to these factors may have risk of getting ovarian cancer.

Pathophysiology

Ovarian cancer is a broad term that can be divided into many categories depending on the cell type of origin. The four main types of ovarian neoplasms are as follows:

- Epithelium: Serous, mucinous and *edometroid.*
- Germ cell: Teratomas (mature and immature) dysgerminoma (occurs less than 20 years)
- Gonadal stroma: Granulosa (theca, serotils, leydig cells)
- Mesenchyma; Fibroma, lymphoma, sarcoma.

Ovarian cancer has two pattern of metastasis: lymphatic and direct. Primary lymphatic drainage of the ovary is through the retroperitoneal nodes surrounding the *renalilium.* Secondary drainage is through the inguinal lymphatics. Ovarian cancer also metastasizes directly to the abdominal cavity.

Clinical Manifestation

In its early stages ovarian cancer is usually asymptomatic. As malignancy grows a variety of symptoms, develops which includes pelvic discomfort, lowback pain, weight change, abdominal pain, nausea, and vomiting, constipation and urinary frequency. Further increase in abdominal girth, bowel and bladder dysfunction, menstrual irregularities, and ascitis can occur. An ovarian malignancy should be considered when abnormal uterine bleeding occurs.

The stages of the ovarian cancer includes the following:

- Stage I : Limited to ovaries.
- Stage II : Involving one or both ovaries with pelvic extentions.
- Stage III : Involving one or both ovaries with intraperitoneal metastasis outside pelvis or positive lymph nodes.
- Stage IV : Involving one or both ovaries with distant metastasis (e.g. liver, lungs).

Management

The early diagnosis of an ovarian cancer usually occurs by chance rather than successful screening. Although no screening test exists today still routine tests like MRI, CT scan and ultrasonography are used. Laparotomy is the primary tool for both diagnosis and staging.

Surgery is the primary therapeutic approach and usually involves TAH BSO. Ascitic fluids or washings are submitted for cytology. All the tissues of the pelivis are carefully assessed, and biopsies of any suspicious tissues are sent for analysis.

Adjuvant therapy is often employed based on the stage of the diseased as follows:

Stage I : Chemotherapy.
Stage II : Instillation of radioactive phosphorous into the peritoneum or combined chemotherapy.
Stage III and IV : Surgical removal of tumour.

The patient receives the standard postoperative teaching appropriate for any major abdominal surgery. Patient teaching concerning the diagnosis, surgery, and adjuvant therapy for ovarian cancer is an integral aspect of nursing care apart from routine surgical nursing measures. Ongoing supportive measures are initiated because of poor prognosis.

Vulvar Cancer

Vulvar cancer is rare and invasive disease; it accounts for the just 5 per cent of malignance of the female genital tract. Similar to cervical cancer, preinvasive lesions are referred to as vulvar intraepthelial neoplasma (VIN) precede invasive vulvar cancer.

Aetiology

Preinvasive disease (vulvar carcinoma in situ) is occurring more commonly in younger women possibly because of factors such as exposure to papilloma virus and HIV. The exact aetiology of this cancer is still unknown. Aetiological factors are believed to include STDs involving the vulva and the use of tight-fitting apparel or nylon undergarments, perineal deodorants, and trauma. Herpes, syphilis and other lesions have all been associated with development of carcinoma. Immunosuppression, diabetes, smoking and hypertension also have been linked. But cause and effect of relationship have not been established.

Pathophysiology

Most of the cancers of the vulva are squamous in 'origin'. The initial lesion often arises, from an area of intraepithelial neoplasia, which can eventually form a firm nodule and ulcerate. The lesion can develop anywhere in the vulva, but 70 per cent of the lesions arise onthe labia. The lesions usually are localized and well demarcated.

Clinical Manifestation

Patient with vulvar neoplasia may have symptoms of vulvular itching or burning, pain, bleeding or discharge.

Management

Diagnosis of vulvar cancer is based on pathology report on the biopsy of the suspicious lesion. VIN managed by eradicatory lesion is medically with 5-fluorouracil (S-Fu) or surgical excision. The standard treatment for invasive carcinoma is radical vulvectomy. It involves excision of the mons pubis, terminal portion of urethra and vagina, excision of portions of the round ligaments in saphenous veins and selected lymphnode dissection.

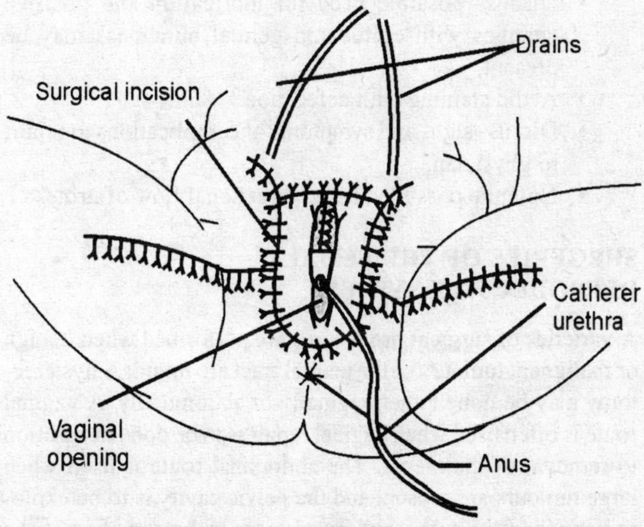

Fig. 15.6: Postoperative appearance after radical vulvectomy.

Nursing care of the woman undergoing radical vulvectomy are as follows:

1. *Preoperative care*
   - Explain treatment and plan of care.
   - Administer enemas and douches as prescribed.
   - Provide emotional support.
   - Teach deep-breathing exercises and leg exercises.
2. *Postoperative care*
   - Maintain bedrest for 72 hours in semi-Fowler's position.
     - Support legs with pillows.
     - Turn every 2 hours.
     - Encourage frequent deep-breathing and use of incentive spirometer.
     - Encourage leg exercises.
     - Avoid stress on suture lines.
     - Assess for signs of complications—atelectasis and deep vein thrombosis.
   - Assess discomfort level and ensure, adequate analgesive.
     - Use PCA pump if possible to allow patient to control dosage.
   - Monitor wound healing
     - Provide perineal hygiene and give sitz baths when ordered; keep perineum dry.
     - Cleanse wound bid and after defecation.
     - Maintain patency of Foley catheter.
   - Provide low-residue diet.
   - Provide diversional activities.
   - Encourage expression of feelings.
3. *Discharge teaching*
   - Use support host for 6 months, elevate legs frequently.
   - Can resume sexual activity in 4 to 6 weeks.
   - Discuss possible need for lubrication and positive changes with coitus and genital numbness may be present.
   - Avoid staining with defecation.
   - Discuss signs and symptoms of complications to report to physician.
   - Note the possible altered directional flow of urine.

SURGERIES OF THE FEMALE REPRODUCTIVE SYSTEM

A varieties of surgical procedures are performed when benign or malignant tumours of the genital tract are found. A hysterectomy may be done either vaginally or abdominally. A vaginal route is often used when vaginal repair is to be done in addition to removal of the uterus. The abdominal route is used when large tumours are present and the pelvic cavity is to be explored or when the tubes and ovaries are to be removed at the same time. The abdominal route can present more postoperative problem because it involves incisions and the opening of the abdominal cavity. The common surgical procedure on the female reproductive tract are as follows:

- Oophorectomy—Removal of an ovary.
- Salpingectomy—Removal of fallopian tube.
- Bilateral Salpinge—oophorectormy (Bil S and O): Removal of both ovaries and fallopian tubes.
- Total hystorectomy—Removal of the entire uterus, including the cervix may be referred to as a TAH (total abdominal hysterectomy). Procedure can be done vaginally or abdominally.
- Subtotal hysterectomy—Removal of the uterus without cervix (Rare).
- Panhysterectomy—(Total abdominal hyperectomy and bilateral salpingo-oopherectomy; Removal of the entire uterus and both fallopean tubes, and ovaries also called TAH-BSO).
- Hystero-ooperectomy—Removal of the uterus and an ovary.
- Hystero-salpingectomy—Removal of the uterus and fallopian tube.
- Radical hysterectomy (Wertheim procedure)—TAH-BSO, partial vaginectomy and dissection of the lymph nodes in the pelvis.
- Vaginectomy—Removal of vagina.
- Pelvic exenteration—Radical hysterectomy, total vaginectomy, removal of the bladder with diversion of urinary systems and resection of bowel with colostomy.
- Anterior pelvic exenteration—Above operation without bowel resection.
- Posterior pelvic exenteration—Above operation without bladder removal.

Nursing care of the woman undergoing hysterectomy are as follows: in addition to routine nursing intervention for any surgery:

Preoperative Care

- Verify patient understanding of the procedure and anticipated care.
- Administer prescribed enemas, laxatives and douches.
- Verify completion of prescribed skin preparation.
- Promote circulation and oxygenation:
  - Apply antiembolic hose.
  - Teach deep breathing-effective coughing-use of incentive spirometer, how to splint abdomen, and how to change position.
  - Teach leg and feet exercises.
  - Teach how to use PCA for pain control.
  - Encourage expression of feelings and concerns.

Postoperative Care

- Promote comfort
  - Administer analgesics and encourage PCA use.
  - Administer antiemetics as needed.
- Promote circulation and oxygenation.
  - Encourage, turning, deep-brerathing, coughing and use of intensive spirometer.

- Encourage leg and feet exercise every hour while in bed.
- Maintain use of antiembolic hose as ordered.
- Encourage frequent ambulation.
- Assess signs and symptoms of thromboembolisms.

• Maintain fluid and electrolytic balance.

- Accurately record all output and drainage.

• Promote elimination.

- Monitor effectiveness of bladder emptying after catheter removal. Catheterize for residual if ordered.
- Monitor signs and symptoms of returning peristalism.
- Encourage frequent ambulation and a liberal fluid intake.
- Teach diet modifications to prevent constipation.

• Provide discharge teach in:

- Teach signs of urinary tract infection.
- Provide teaching regarding incision care.
- Instruct patient to avoid heavy lifting, prolonged sitting and long car drive.
- Tell the patient to refrain from coitus for about 6 weeks and not to douche unless prescribed by her physician. Vaginal bleeding or discharge may persist for upto 6 weeks.
- Help patient to anticipate the occurrence of mood swings and emotional lability during healing.

Infertility

Infertility is the inability to achieve pregnancy after at least one year of regular sexual intercourse without contraception. The problems may be considered primay if the couple has never conceived or secondary if conception was successfully achieved in the past.

Aetiology

Infertility may be caused by either female factors or male factors. The common causes of infertility in men and women are as follows:

1. *Female*
   • Developmental: Uterine abnormalities.
   • Endocrine: Pituitary, thyroid, and adrenal dysfunction, ovarian dysfunction (inhibit maturation and release of ovum).
   • Diseases: PID (especially gonococcus), fallopian tube obstructions. Diseases of cervix and uterus that inhibit passage of active sperm.
   • Other: malnutrition, severe anaemia and anxiety.
2. *Male*
   • Developmental: Undescended testes, other congenital abnormalities (inhibit development of sperm).
   • Endocrine: Hormonal deficiency (pituitary, thyroid, adrenal), inhibit the development of sperm.
   • Diseases: Testicular destruction from disease, orchitis from mumps, and prostatitis.
   • Others: Excessive smoking, fatigue, alcohol, excessive heat (hot baths) use of marijuana.
3. *Both Male and Female*
   • Diseases: STDs, cancer-causing obstructions (inhibit transport of ovum or sperm).
   • Others: Immunological incompatibility (inhibit sperm penetration of ovum) and marital problems.
   • Diethylstilbestrol (DES), exposure in utero (Suggested but not proved as a cause of male infertility).

Pathophysiology

Three basic categories of infertility account for 95 per cent of reproductive dysfunction: anovulation, anatomical defect of the female genital tract and abnormal sperm production. The common cause in male and female explained in aetiology.

The most frequent female causes of infertility include ovulation factor, such as anovulation or inadequate corpus luteum, tubal obstruction, or dysfunction such as endometrosis or damage from pelvic infections, and uterine or cervical factors such as leiomyoma or structural anomalies. Risk factors for infertility include increasing age, tobacco and illicit use of drugs, excessive exercises, severe dietary restriction and specific occupational and environmental exposure.

Clinical Manifestation

In addition to clinical manifestation of the causes of infertility, infertility itself can produce profound psychological effects. When couple find themselves unable to have children, the trauma can affect every aspect of their lives and marriage. The experience of diagnosis and treatment can be an emotional roller coaster of raised expectations and dashed hopes.

Management

A detailed history and general physical examination of the woman and her partner provide the basis for selecting diagnostic studies. The possibility of medical or gynaecologic diseases is explored before tests are performed to evaluate whether the cause is female infertility. These tests include ovulatory studies, tubal patency studies and post-coital studies.

The purposes of an infertility evaluation are to establish the cause of infertility and provide a basis for determining medical or surgical treatment options. The process can be physically painful as well as emotionally and economically stressful. The common diagnostic testing for infertility includes the following:

1. *Male*
   • Semen analysis to determine presence, number and motility of sperms.
   • Testicular biopsy if sperm count is low or absent, the presence of sperm indicates obstruction of vas deferens.

2. *Female*
   - Basal body temperature chart to determine that ovulation is occurring.
   - Postcoital test of cervical secretion, measure the ability of sperm to penetrate cervical mucosa and remain active and determine quality of mucous.
   - Endometrial biopsy: Determine whether ovulation is occurring (if in endometrium).
   - Laparoscopy: Examine the pelvis and determine patency of fallopian tubes.
   - Hysterosalpingiography: Determine patency of uterus and fallopian tubes.
3. *Male/Female*
   - Hormonal tests to determine whether problem is hormonal.

Treatment

Artificial insemination is simple, safe, inexpensive and highly successful infertility treatment when male infertility is the cause. Semen may be deposited by a cervical-vaginal route, intracervically, or intrauterine. A few drops of semen are injected as close to the time of ovulation as possible. Treatment may use the partner's semen (homologous) or donor (heterologous). The fertility donor is carefully determined and the sperms are screened for HIV. This can be an emotional topic for some couples and may induce strong reactions.

Alternative approach to infertility management includes the following:

1. *Invitro Fertilization (IVF) and Embryo Transfer*
   One or more ova are recovered from the ovarian follicles and fertilized with the partners sperm in a Petri dish. Oocyte retrieval is performed by means of ultrasound-guided needle aspiration. The cleaved ova are placed in the patient's uterus through a small catheter about 48 hours after retrieval. Pregnancy rates are related to the number of embryos placed and vary from 18 to 30 per cent.
2. *Gamete Intrafallopian Transfer (GIFT)*
   Oocytes aspirated from follicles are mixed with washed sperm and placed in the uterine tube via laparoscopy. This approach appears to achieve a higher pregnancy rate than IVF. The proembryo travels towards the uterus, following the natural time table for implantation in 4 days.
3. *Zygote Intrafallopian Transfer (ZIFT) and Tubal Embryo Transfer (TET)*
   These procedures are similar to GIFT except transfer to the fallopian tubes occurs at the zygote stage, about 16 to 18 hours after oocyte insemination. TET involves transfer of embryos into the fallopian tube around 40 to 48 hours after oocyte insemination.
4. *Surrogate Mothers*
   Surrogate mothers are women who contract to conceive by artificial insemination and give the baby to the semen donor after delivery. Many social and legal implications with the process have received recent attention through some extremely public law suits over custody of the child.
5. *Ovum Transfer*
   A donor provides the ovum, which is fertilized with the partner's sperm. The embryo is transferred to the infertile woman's uterus after about 5 days via a small catheter. Pregnancy rates have been as high as 25 to 50 per cent.

The management of infertility problem depends on the cause of infertility is secondary to an alteration in ovarian function, supplemental hormone therapy to restore and maintain ovulation may be attempted. Drugs used to induce ovulation include clomiphene citrate (clomid), human menopausal gonadotropin (Pergonal) and bromocriptine (Parlodel).

When a tubal blockage exists, the woman should be referred to a specialist to discuss whether surgical correction (Transcervical balloon tuboplasty-TBT) or IVF is more appropriate. Chronic cervicitis and inadequate oestrogenic stimulation are cervical factors causing infertility. Antibiotic therapy is indicated for cervicitis. Inadequate oestrogen stimulation is treated by administration of oestrogen.

When a couple has not succeeded in conceiving while under infertility management, an option is intrauterin insemination with the husband's or donor's sperm. IVF may be used. Asisted reproductive technologies (ART continue to develop rapidly since the first IVF baby was born in 1978. ARTs include IVF, GIFT, ZIFT, donor gametes, and embryocryo preservation. With the increasing embryocryo preservation assisted hatching, and intracytoplasmic sperm injection, couples have an increased potential for pregnancy. The use of ART poses many ethical, legal, social and financial concerns.

Nurses can assist women experiencing infertility by providing information about the reproductive process and infertility evaluation and addressing the psychologic and social distress that can accompany infertility. Removing or reducing psychologic stress can improve the emotional climate, making it more conducive to achieving a pregnancy.

The nurse has a major responsibility for teaching and providing emotional support throughout the infertility testing and treatment period. Feelings of anger, frustration, grief and helplessness may heighten as more and more diagnostic tests are performed. Infertility can generate great tension in a marriage as the couple exhaust their financial and emotional resources. Recognizing and taking steps to deal with the psychologic factors that surface can assist the couple to cope up in better way with the situation. The nurses also play a role in promoting fertility which includes teaching of prevention of infections, responsibility for infertility, early diagnosis and treatment.

PROBLEMS OF THE BREAST

Breast problems are significant health concerns to women. In a woman's lifetime, there is a one in eighth chance that she will be diagnosed with breast cancer. (Few breast cancers are found in men). Whether benign or malignant, intense feeling of shock, fear and denial often accompany the initial discovery of a lump or change in the breast. These feelings are associated both with the fear of survival and with the possible loss of a breast. Throughout history, the female breast has been regarded as a symbol of beauty, sexuality and motherhood. The potential loss of a breast or part of a breast may be devastating for many women because of the significant psychologic, social, sexual and body image implications associated with it.

Benign Breast Problems

Benign breast disease is common and accounts for about 90 per cent of all breast problems. Because there is no universally-accepted classification system for benign disorders.

Cystic Breast Disease

Fibrocystic changes in the breast constitute a benign condition characterized by changes in the breast tissue. The change includes the development of excess fibrous tissue hyperplasia of the epithelial lining of the mammary ducts, proliferation of mammary ducts and cystic formations. The changes produce pain by nerve irritation from connector tissue, oedema and by fibrosis from nerve pinching.

Aetiology

The underlying cause of cystic breast disease is not fully understood. Changes in the breast are cyclic and thought to be caused by hormonal imbalance or the exaggerated response of breast tissue to ovarian hormone. Breast tenderness is more pronounced during or before the menstruation. Cystic breast disease is most common in nulliparous women between the ages of 40 and 50 years but can occur at any age. Occurrence is least frequent after menopause.

Pathophysiology

Fibrocytic changes do not increase the risk of breast cancer for majority of patients. Masses or nodularities can appear in both breasts and are often found in the upper, outer quadrant, and usually occur bilaterally. Changes once thought be abnormal such as microcysts, apocrine change, adenosis, fibrosis, and varying degrees of hyperplasia are now reorganized as part of the involutional process of breast. These changes include the presence of lumps, of varying size, nipple discharge, and breastpain (mastodynia or mastalgia). Cystic lesions are soft, well-demarcated, and freely movable. The process is almost always bilateral with most lesions located in the left breast. The cyst may contain clear, milky, straw-coloured or yellow to dark brown fluid. Occasionally the contents may be blood-tinged.

Clinical Manifestation

Manifestation of fibrocytic changes include one or more palpable lumps that are usually round, lobular, well-delienated and freely-movable within the breast. Some lumps are fibrous and do not contain cysts. There may be accompanying discomfort ranging from tenderness to pain. The lump is usually observed to increase in size and perhaps in tenderness before menstruation. Cysts may enlarge or shrink rapidly. Nipple discharges associated with fibrocystic breasts is often milky, watery milky, yellow or green.

Management

The woman who discovers a mass or masses in her breast should seek the advice of the health care provider. A needle aspiration generally comprise the presence of cyst. Biopsies in women with fibrocystic disease may be indicated for women with increased risk for breast cancer.

The woman with cystic changes should be encouraged to return regularity for follow-up examination throughout life. She should also be taught *breast self examination (BSE)* to self-monitor the problem. Severe fibro-cystic changes may make palpation of the breast more difficult. Any new lumps or changes in the breasts should be evaluated and changes in symptoms should be reported and investigated.

Many type of treatment have been suggested for a fibrocystic condition. These include the use of a good support bra, dietary therapy (low-salt diet, restriction of methylxanthioses such as coffee, tea, cola, chocolate), vitamin E therapy, analgesics, Danazol (Danocrine), diuretics, hormone therapy, antioestrogen therapy, and surgical therapy (Subcutaneous mastectomy).

The role of the nurse in the care of the patients with benign breast disorders is primarily that of educator and facilitator. The nurse should be knowledgeable about benign conditions, understand their medical management, be able to provide and clarify information and support the patient emotionally and physically through diagnosis and treatment.

A woman with fibrocystic breast, should be told that she may expect recurrence of the cyst in one or both breasts until menopause and that cysts may enlarge or become painful just before menstruation. Additionally she should be reassured that cysts do not "turn into cancer". Any new lump that does not respond in a cyclic manner over 1 to 2 weeks should be examined promptly. The nurse teaches BSE to those women who are not familiar with it and stresses its use every month. Teaching breast models can also be helpful. Women should be taught to recognize through touch their normal breast tissue and the location and size if any lesion is present. They should report significant changes, that differ from the normal cyclic fluctuations or that appear at a different time in the menstrual cycle.

The use of mild analgesics and wearing a firm supportive brassiere may provide comfort and reduce pain. The use of warm

• LOOK FOR CHANGES • FEEL FOR CHANGES•

Hands at side
compare for symmetry.
look for changes in:
• shape
• colour
Check for:
• puckering
• dimpling
• skin changes
• nipple changes

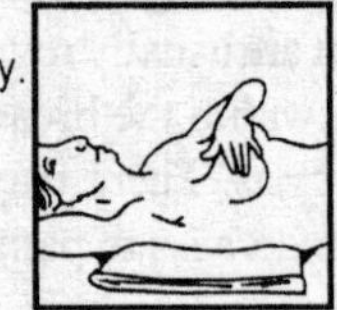

Lie down with
a towel
under right
shoulder;
raise right
arm above
the head.

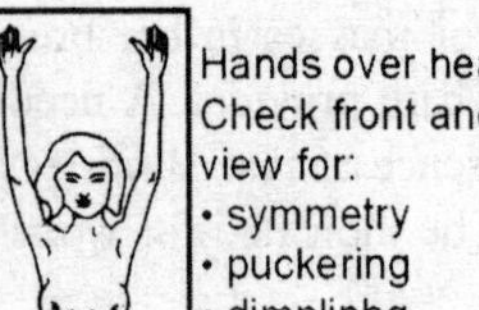

Hands over head.
Check front and side
view for:
• symmetry
• nipple direction
• puckering
• dimplinhg

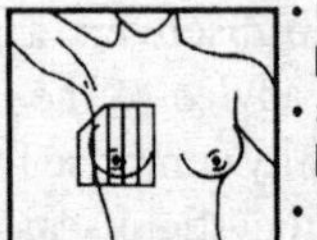

Examine area from
• underam to lower
bra line
• across to brest
bone
• up to collar bone
• back to armpit

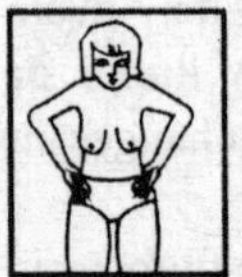

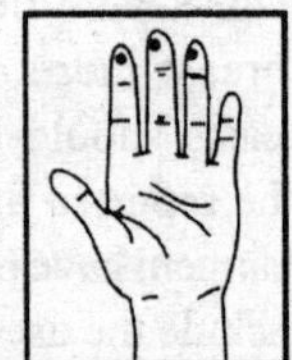

Use the pads
of the three
middle fingers of
the left hand.
Hold hand in
bowed
position.
Move fingers
in dime-
size circles.

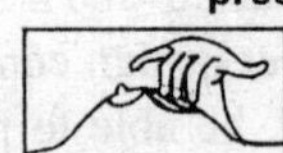

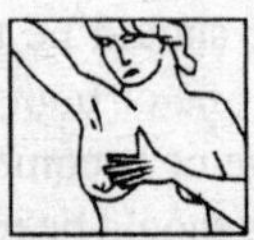

Use three levels of

Examine entire erea
using vertical strip pat-

Now check your left breast
with your right
hand in the same way.
if there are any lumps,

or changes, tell your
doctor right away.

Fig. 15.7: Breast self-exam.

and moist heat may be beneficial to relieve aching pain, eliminating caffeine consumption and decreasing salt content before menstruation to relieve bloating and weight gain can be recommended.

Fibroadenoma

Fibroadenoma is a common cause of discrete benign breast lumps in young women (less than 25 years).

Aetiology/Pathophysiology

The possible cause of fibroadenoma may be increased oestrogen sensitivity in localized area of the breast. Fibroadenoma are tumours of fibroblastic and epithelial origin thought to be caused by hyperestrinisms. They are oestrogen-dependent and associated with menstrual irregularities. Tumours are slow growing and often are stimulated by pregnancy and lactations. Regressions may occur after delivery. Fibroadenomas tend to regress at menopause and become hyalinized. "Giant" fibroadenomas grow very rapidly to 10 to 12 cms in diameter but are not prone to malignant change than smaller lesions. Dimpling or nipple retraction is not associated with fibroadenoma.

Clinical Manifestation

Fibroadenomas are usually small, painless, round, well-delineated and very mobile. They may be soft but are usually solid, firm and rubbery in consistency. There is no accompanying retraction or nipple discharge. The lump is often painless. The fibroadenoma may appear as a single unilateral mass, although multiple bilateral fibrodenomas are reported. Growth is slow and often ceases when size reaches 2 to 3 cm. Size is not affected by menstruation. However, pregnancy can stimulate dramatic growth. Fibroadenomas are rarely associated with cancer.

Management

Fibroadenomas are easily detected by physical examination and are often visible on mammographs. Definitive diagnosis, however requires biopsy and tissue examination.

Surgical removal is the standard treatment of fibroadenoma. Many can be removed under local anaesthesia in a OPD setting. Surgery is not urgent in women under 25 years of age. In women over 35, all new lesions should be examined using an excisional biopsy. Fibroadenoma is not reduced by radiation or are not affected by hormone therapy. The nurse frequently has the opportunity to counsel a young woman with fibroadenoma. During the contact, the benign nature of the lesions should be stressed and follow-up examination and BSE should be encouraged. (See figure 15.7).

BREAST INFECTIONS

Mammary Duct Ectasia

Ductal ectasia is a benign breast disease of perimenopausal and postmenopausal women involving the ducts in the subareolar area. It usually involves several bilateral ducts.

Aetiology

Mammary duct ectasia, also referred to as plasma cell mastitis, is a benign condition of unknown aetiology. Some believe an anaerobic bacteria may be implicated. Another causative factor may be bacterial infections that result from stasis of fluid in the large ducts of the breasts. The primary risk factor is the age between 45 to 55.

Pathophysiology

Mammary duct ectasia involves inflammation of the ducts behind the nipple, duct enlargement, and a collection of cellular debris and fluid in the involved ducts. As the inflammatory response resolves, the ducts become fibrotic and dilated. Nipple discharge usually is bilateral and ranges from serous to thick, sticky or pastelike. Drainage may be green, greenish brown or blood stained. Nipple itching, suggestive of Paget's disease, may accompany transient pain in the subareolar and inner quadrants of the breast. On palpation the areolar area may feel warmlike, the nipple may be red and swollen or flat and retracted. The condition is not associated with breastfeeding.

Clinical Manifestation

Nipple discharge is the primary symptom. This discharge is multicoloured and sticky. Ductal ectasia is initially painless but may progress to burning, itching and pain around the nipple, as well as swelling in the aureolar area. Inflammatory signs often are present. The nipple may retract and the discharge may become bloody in more advanced disease. Ductal ectasia is not associated with malignancy.

Management

Treatment varies depending on the severity of the problem. Because of the chronic nature of the problem, most women are monitored with routine physical examination of the breast. The symptoms of mammary duct ectasia may engender the fear of malignant disease in the patient. Once the benign nature of the chronic condition is affirmed, fears generally are dispelled, and most women are able to deal with their symptoms. Although there is no cure for mammary duct ectasia, antibiotics are prescribed for acute inflammatory episodes, such as the development of an abscess. If the chronic discharge can no longer be tolerated, surgical excision of the retroaereolar ducts is performed.

The nurse must be cognizant of the chronic yet benign nature of this condition and offer support and understanding care. The woman is taught how to cleanse the breast to minimize the risk of infection. Good hand-washing and personal hygiene measures are stressed. Wearing a supportive yet nonconfining brassiere padded with sterile guaze and changing the bra daily or as necessary helps prevent abscess formation. The nurse teaches the woman signs and symptoms indicative of abscess should be reported immediately.

Acute Mastitis and Abscess

Mastitis is an inflammatory condition that occurs most frequently in lactating women. There are two types of mastitis i.e., acute or chronic. The acute form is a rare condition, almost always found in breastfeeding mothers during the first 4 months of lactation. It occurs most frequently from "Staphylococcus aureas or staphylococcus epidermides infection that spreads from a crack in the skin surface of the nipple (cracked nipple) to underlying breast tissue. It may be confined to only one quadrant of the breast. Symptoms include a fissured nipple, fever, chill, localized tenderness and erythema. Purulent discharge from the nipple is usually not observed.

The *chronic* form of mastitis can follow acute mastitis or have a slow and insidious onset. Both acute and chronic mastitis are caused by the same bacterial agents. The chronic form occurs more in older women, and the symptoms can be micro inflammatory breast cancer. The infection usually arises in the sweat or sebaccous glands and spreads in the breast. Symptoms of chronic mastitis include a painful breast mass that involves the nipple and aereola and a low grade fever.

Pathophysiology

In both acute and chronic mastitis there is oedema and congestion of the periodical and inter lobular stromata. The ducts are distended from the accumulation of neutrophils and retained secretions. If an abscess forms its central core may be necrotic and contain creamy, yellow exudate. Fibrosis of the involved tissue can develop after treatment. Both acute and chronic mastitis can mimic breast cancer, but recent lactation usually excludes the acute form forms the need for further assessment.

Clinical Manifestation are explained above in acute and chronic mastitis.

Management

Acute mastitis is easy to diagnose in a nursing mother. Treatment with antibiotics resolves infectious process. In older women, because the conditions have similarities to inflammatory breast carcinoma, surgical incision and drainage of the inflammatory exudate are performed to determine the cause. Antibiotics can then be prescribed.

When acute mastitis is the result of an infection during lactation, most women immediately stop breastfeeding. Breastfeeding should continue unless an abscess in forming or purulent drainage is noted. The infant is not affected by sucking on the involved breast, and antibiotic therapy is not required. Continued breastfeeding is believed to reduce the pain and lessen the volume of milk that can be a source of bacterial growth. If breastfeeding is discontinued, the woman is instructed to keep her breasts as empty as possible by pumping. If the breast is not emptied, it will become engorged and pain will increase. The woman is instructed to complete the entire course of antibiotics and not discontinue them when symptoms are relieved. The older women are more anxious about their diagnosis of cancer. Emotional support and frank discussion are made until biopsy results. Both mastitis require antibiotic theory, rest analgesics, application of local heat.

Breast Cancer

Breast cancer is the most common malignancy, it is second only to lung cancer. It is the leading cause of death from cancer among women.

Aetiology

The underlying cause of breast cancer is still unknown but number of risk factors have been identified, which includes the following:

i. *Age and Gender*
The incidence of breast cancer is increased with age. Nearly two-thirds of breast cancers are found in postmenopausal women usually after 50 years. The reason for the age-related increase is thought to be the increased probability of mutagenic changes occurring over a longer lifespan rather than any instability inherent aging cells. Breast cancer may be inherited (BRCA-I gene) or noninherited.

ii. *Menstrual and Reproductive History*
The risk of breast cancer is increased when menstruation begins at an early age (11-12 years) and extends to a late menopause (about age 55). Nulliparity (childless women) and women who bear their first child near or after the age of 30 years and also family history of mother or sister or both had breast cancer may increase risk.

iii. *Hormones and Oral Contraceptives*
Hormonal replacement therapy at menopause has created a great deal of cancer and controversy, because of the increased incidence of breast cancer associated with it. There is no evidence yet to suggest a causal relationship between oral contraceptives and incidence of and survival from breast cancer.

iv. *Diet and Body Weight*
Animal data and description of epidemiology of breast cancer incidences strongly suggest an association of dietary factors specifically a high-fat diet. With an increased risk of breast cancer. This claim is largely unproved. Body weight, height, obesity and increased body mass have been reported to be associated with an increased risk of breast cancer but still is controversial. In obesity, fat cells store oestrogen.

v. *Benign Breast Disease*
Fibrocystic condition of the breast is not associated with breast cancer. However, biopsy-proven atypical hyperplasia is associated with increased risk.

vi. *Radiation Hazard*
Three groups of women who received low level radiation exposure demonstrated an increased breast cancer risk, which was perticularly notable if the exposure occurred in the early years (less than 30 years), radiation damages DNA.

vii. *Alcohol*
A suggested small increase in risk with moderate alcohol consumption has been reported, although limitation in methodology have been cited, and results require confirmation.

Pathophysiology

Tumours of the breast arise in the epithelial cells either ductal or lobular tissues and are referred to *carcinomas*. A number of histological subtypes also have been identified, but are not commonly seen nor are they invasive as ductal and lobular carcinomas when the tumour is confined within a duct or a lobule and has not invaded surrounding tissue it is considered localized or *in situ carcinoma* of the breast. *Infiltrative* ductal or lobular carcinomas are tumours that have spread directly into surrounding tissues and may have distant metastases if they have penetrated the axillary internal mammary nodes of the systemic circulation.

The breast is divided into four quadrants, upper inner, upper outer lower inner and lower outer. Most breast tumours are located in the upper outer quadrant, but they can occur in any area of the breast of the invasive breast tumours, infiltrative ductal carcinoma is the most prevalant histological cell type followed by infiltrating lobular carcinoma. Brief review of selected histological types of breast cancer their incidence, characteristics and prognosis are as follows:

i. *Infiltrating ductal carcinoma* (Incidence 70 per cent) Characterized by stony hard mass, gritty texture; may appear bilaterally and prognosis is poor, common involvements are in axillary nodes.
ii. Medullary carcinoma (5-7 per cent) characterized by soft mass, often reaches large size, may be circumscribed and prognosis is favourable.
iii. *Mucinous or colloid carcinoma (5 per cent):* slow growing; can reach large size may occur with other tumour type. Prognosis is good if tumour is predominantly mucinous.
iv. *Invasive lobular carcinoma (4 per cent):* Multicentricity is common and may involve both breasts. Prognosis is similar to ductal type.
v. *Paget's disease (3 per cent):* Scaly, eczematoid nipple with burning, itching, discharge, two thirds have palpable underlying mass. Prognosis is related to histological type of underlying tumour.
vi. *Inflammatory breast cancer (lesser than 1 per cent):* Skin red, warm, indurated with obstructive lymphangitis (Pequ d'orange) appearance). Prognosis is poor. Often presents with palpable nodes and evidence of metastasis.
vii. *Lobular carcinoma in situ:* (2.5 per cent) Usually found

in incidental finding in benign breast specimens (high risk for development of invasive cancer). Prognosis is good.

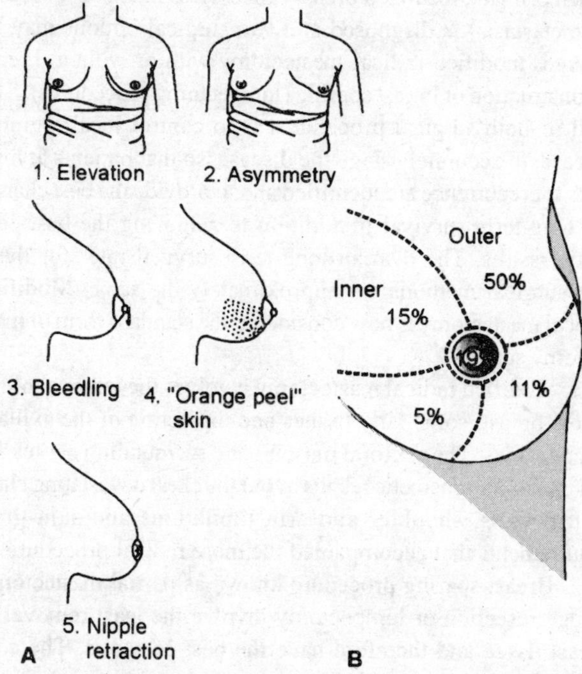

Fig. 15.8: (A) Signs of cancer of the breast. (B) Distribution of carcinomas in different areas of breast.

Clinical Manifestation

Breast cancer is detected in a single lump or mammographic abnormality in the breast and is difficult to differentiate from benign tumours. With more advanced tumours a variety of signs and symptoms are helped in differentiating a benign tumour from malignant tumour. Benign tumours usually have well-defined edges, are encapsulated and are freely movable. The shape of a malignant tumour is more difficult to define and is less mobile on palpation. Usually the result of the tumour becoming 'fixed' and adhering to the chest wall. If palpable, breast cancer is characteristically hard, irregularly shaped, poorly delineated, nonmobile and nontender. As the tumour infiltrates into surrounding tissues, it can cause retraction of the overlying skin and create what is referred to as dimpling. A small percentage of breast cancers cause nipple discharge. The discharge is usually unilateral and may be clear or bloody. Nipple retraction may occur. Plugging of the dermal lymphatics can cause skin thickening and exaggeration of the usual skin markings, giving the skin the appearance of an orange peel (Pseudo-orange) a pseudo-orange breast sign indicates lymphatic obstructive tissue tumour growth with resulting oedema. The breast resembles an orange peel with large prominent pores. These signs are ominous and usually reflect advanced disease. To sum up, clinical manufacture of breast cancers are:

- Lump that is – irregular, star-shaped.
  - firm to hard in consistency.
  - Fixed, not mobile.
  - Poorly defined or demarcated.
  - Usually not tender, but can occasionally cause discomfort.
  - Single.
- Presence of skin or nipple retraction.
- Nipple discharge.
- Pseudo-orange appearance (dimpling) of the skin.

Management

The management of breast cancer is both complex and controversial. Treatment options are ever changing and influenced by new and better surgical techniques, new cytotoxic drug combinations and more accurate knowledge of breast cancer growth and dissemination.

Diagnosis is confirmed on the basis of history including risk factors physical examination of breast and lymphatics. Mammography, ultrasound biopsy, oestrogen-progesterone receptor assays, and other molecular studies (DNA ploidy, sphase, P53, HER-2/ncu). And staging work-up made on the basis of CBC, platelet count, calcium and phosphate levels, LFT sentinelly phnode biopsy, chest X-ray, bone scan, CT scan of chest, abdomen, pelvis and MRI.

At present, there is wide range of treatment options available to both patient and the care providers attempting to make critical decisions about what treatment to select. Many prognostic factors are considered when treatment decisions are made about a specific breast cancer. These factors include lymphnode status, tumour size, histologic classification and the identification of histologic subtypes. All of these enter into the staging of breast cancer. The most widely accepted staging method is AJCC (American Joint Committee on Cancer).

TNM System as given below

Primary tumour (T)

T 0 No evidence of primary tumour.
T is Carcinoma in skin.
T 1 Tunmour less than or equal to 2 cm.
T 2 Tumour greater than 2 cm but less than or equal to 5 cm.
T 3 Tumour greater than 5 cm.
T 4 Extension to chest wall and inflammation.

Regional lymph node (N)

N 0 No tumour in regional lymph nodes.
N 1 Metastasis to movable ipsilateral nodes.
N 2 Metastasis to matted or fixed iphilateral nodes.
N 3 Metastasis to ipsilateral internal mammary nodes.

Distant metastasis (M)

M 0 No distant metastasis.
M 1 Distant metastasis (include spread to ipsilateral supraclavicular node)

Stage grouping

Stage 0	T is	No	Mo
Stage I	T 1	No	Mo
Stage II A	T o	N 1	M o
	T 1	N 1	M o
	T 2	N o	M o
Stage II B	T 2	N 1	Mo
	T 3	N o	M o
Stage III A	T o	N 2	M o
	T 1	N 2	M o
	T 2	N 2	M o
	T 3	N 1 N 2	M o
Stage III B	T 4	Ang N	M o
	Ang T	N 3	M o
Stage IV	Ang T	Ang N	M 1

The role of systemic drug therapy is the treatment of breast cancer (Chemotherapy and endocrine therapy) is either eradicate or impede the growth of micrometastatic disease.

Chemotherapy refers to the use of cytotoxic drugs to destroy cancer cells. The chemotherapy agents and proteol effective for treating breast cancer include the following.

1. *Single agents:* Cyclophosphamide, melphalan, thiotepa, doxorubicin and epirubicin.
2. *Protocols using various agents*
   - CMF – Cycle phosphamide, methotrexate 5 - Fluoracil (5 Flu)
   - CPF – Cyclophosphamide, prednisone.5-Flu
   - CMF/VA – CMF/Vincristine, doxorubicin (A).
   - CMF/VP – CMF/V. prednisone.
   - AC – Doxorubicin cyclophosphamide.
   - FAC – 5 Flu " "
   - FEC – 5 Flu Epirubicine cyclophosphonamide.
   - LMF – Melphalan-methotraxate, 5-Flu-

Hormonal therapy has been a useful treatment modality for breast cancer. Tamoxifen citrate (Nolvadex) is the usual first choice of treatment in postmenopausal oestrogen receptor positive women with or without nodal involvement. Tamoxifen, an antioestrogen drug, blocks the oestrogen receptors sites of malignant cells and that inhibits the growth-stimulating effect of oestrogen. Side effects are minimal including hot flashes, nausea, vomiting, dry skin, vaginal bleeding, menstrual irregularity and other commonly associated with oestrogen.

Radiation therapy used in three situations of breast cancer which:

- As the primary treatment to destroy the tumour or as a companion to surgery to prevent local occurence.
- To shrink a large tumour to operable size and
- As the palliative treatment for pain caused by local recurrence and metastasis. Lumpectomy is always followed by radiation.

Surgery is the main way of breast cancer treatment, especially when the disease is localized without distant metastasis. When primary, localized breast cancer (less than 2 to 4 cm and no metastasis) is disgnosed and two surgical options may be offered: modified radical mastectomy with or without breast reconstruction or breast sparing (lumpectomy procedures). The goal of both surgical procedures is to control local regional disease, to accurately stage the disease, so that patients at high risks for recurrence are identified and to provide the best chance for long-term survival in addition to achieving the best cosmetic results. The ovarian long-term survival rates for these two surgical methods are approximately the same. Modified radical mastectomy is now considered the standard form of mastectomy surgery.

1. Modified radical mastectomy involves the removal of the whole breast, some fatty tissues and dissection of the axillary lymph nodes. The pectoral muscles and surrounding nerves are left intact. The cosmetic results avoid the chest devastating chest wall defects, shoulder and arm limitations and skin graft requirements that accompanied the more radical procedure.

2. Breast-sparing procedure known as partial mastectomy, wedge resection or lumpectomy involve the least removal of breast tissue and therefore have the best cosmesis. The contraindication for use of breast-sparing procedures include the following.

- Pregnancy, first and second timesters preclude the use of radiation therapy.
- Locally-advanced or inflammatory breast cancer.
- Multiple lesions located in separate quadrants of the breast or diffuse malignant or indeterminate—appearing microcalcifications.
- Prior irradiation of the breast.
- History of callagens-vascular disease, which is recognized as having poor tolerance to the effect of radiation therapy.
- Tumour size: large tumour in a small breast, which will not allow adequate resection of tumour.
- Breast size: large pendulous breasts which are difficult to irradiate; small breasts which may result in an unacceptable cosmetic outcome.
- Location of tumour: tumours that are located beneath the nipple necessitate removal of the nipple-areola complex, which has questionable value compared with mastectomy.

NURSING MANAGEMENT OF THE PATIENT UNDERGOING MASTECTOMY

The period between the diagnosis of breast cancer and the selection of the treatment plan is difficult period for the woman and her family. During this period, the woman may be very self-focussed, verbalizing her conflict and indecisions frequently. Appropriate nursing interventions during this period include exploring the women's usual decision-making pattern, helping the woman accurately evaluate the advantages and disadvantages of the options, providing information relevant to the decision and supporting the patient once the decision is made. During this period, the woman may exhibit signs of distress or tension, such as tachycardia, increased muscle tension and restlessness, whenever she focuses on the decision to be made. The nurse should assess the woman's body language motor activity, and affect during periods of high stress and indecision so that appropriate intervention can be carried out.

Irrespective of the surgery planned, the patient must be provided with sufficient information to ensure informed consent. Some patients need extensive and detailed information. For others this only increases anxiety. Sensitivity to individual needs is essential. Preoperative diagnostic studies must be completed. Teaching is the preoperative phase includes instruction in turning, coughing deep-breathing, a review of postoperative exercises, and explanation of the recovery period from the time of surgery until discharge.

The woman who has had a modified radical mastectomy needs specific nursing intervention. Restoration of the functioning of the arms in the affected side after mastectomy and axillary lymph node dissection is one of the important goals of the nursing activities. The woman should be placed in a semi-Fowler's position with the arm on the affected side elevated on a pillow. Flexing and extending the fingers should begin in the recovery room with progressive increase in activity is encouraged. Postoperative mastectomy exercises are isntituted gradually at the surgeon's direction. These exercises are designed to prevent contractures and muscle shortening, maintaining muscle tone, and improve lymph and blood circulation. The difficulty and pain encountered by the woman in performing the previously simple tasks include in the exercise program may cause frustration and depression. The goal of all exercises is return to full range of motion gradually within 4 to 6 weeks.

Postoperative discomfort can be minimized and administering analgesic about 30 minutes before initiating exercises. When showering is appropriate, the flow of warm water over the involved shoulder often has a soothing effect and reduces joint stiffness. Whenever possible, the same nurse should work with the woman so that progress can be monitored and problem can be identified.

Measure to prevent or reduce lymphedema must be used by the nurse and taught the woman. The affected arm should never be dependent even while the person is sleeping. Blood pressure readings, venipunctures, and injection should not be done on the affected arm. Elastic bandages should not be used postoperatively. The woman must be instructed to protect the arm on the operative side from even minor trauma such as pinprick or sunburn. If trauma occurs to the arm, the area should be washed thoroughly with soap and water. A topical antibiotic ointment and a bandage or other sterile dressing should be applied. When lymphedema is acute, an intermittent pneumatic compression sleeve may be prescribed. This device applies mechanical massage to the arm. Manual massage is also effective in mobilizing subcutaneous accumulation of fluid. Elevate the arm, so that it is level with the heart, diuretics, and isometric exercises may be recommended to reduce fluid volume in the arm.

Psychological Management

Throughout interaction with a woman with breast cancer, the nurse must keep in mind the extensive psychologic impact of the disease. All aspects of care must include sensitivity to the woman's efforts to cope with a life-threatening disease. An open relationship in which the woman can express her fears and feelings is essential. The nurse can help meet the woman's psychologic needs by doing the following.

- Assist her to develop a positive but realistic attitude.
- Helping her to identify sources of support and strength to her, such as her partner, family and spiritual practices.
- Encouraging her to verbalize her anger and fears about her diagnosis and impact it will have on her life.
- Promoting open communication of thoughts and feelings between the patient and her family.
- Providing accurate and complete answers to question about her disease treatment options, and reproductive and lactation tissue (if appropriate).
- Offering information about community resources which can help.

Before the discharge, the patient is instructed about wound care management, exercise guideline and sensory change precaution, assessment and management of lymphedema, and prevention of trauma and infection. The following precautions should be taken with the patient after mastectomy:

- Ensure that affected arm is never used for blood pressure, injections or venipunctures.
- Wear no constricting clothing or jewellery, including wrist watch on affected arm.
- Do not carry heavy objects (pocket book, packages) in affected arm.
- Wear rubber gloves when washing dishes.
- Use unaffected arm when removing items from hot oven or protect by wearing a padded glove pot holder.
- Use a thumb when sewing wash needle pricks and cover as necessary.
- Take care when trimming finger nails and cuticles; avoid using scissors for this task.
- Use softening lotion or creams to keep skin in soft and nipple conditions.
- Outdoor activities:
  - Wear gloves when gardening.

- Avoid sunburn-wear protective clothing or use sunscreen liberally.
- Use insect repellent in an area where biting or stinging insects may be located.
- Tend to cuts and scratches immediately by washing and applying protective covering.

Postmastectomy arm exercises includes the following.

- Ball squeezing.
- Pulley motion.
- Handball climbing.
- Elbow pull-in.
- Crossed arm
- Scissors
- Sword of hope.

MALE BREAST PROBLEMS

Gynaecomastia

Gynaecomastia, a transient enlargement of one or both breasts is the most common breast problem in men. It usually occurs in pubertal boys during the time of rapid testicular growth between the ages of 1 to 15 years. This condition is seen in men aged 45 years and older, and also it is seen in obese men because obesity increases the rate of conversion of androgens to oestrogen in patient with cirrhosis of liver, because of the incomplete hepatic clearance of oestrogen. Gynaecomastia may develop in men who are receiving drugs such as oestrogen, cimitedine, certain antibiotics (isonized) antihypertensive agents (reserpine and methyldopa) calcium channel blockers and digoxin.

Pathophysiology

Gynaecomastia is caused by hormonal imbalance. As a result of the large oestrogen secretion, hyperplasia (overdevelopment) of the stromata, and ducts in the mammary gland occurs. The primary cause of gynaemastic in the older man is the aging process may be due to increase of plasma testesterone. Symptoms of gynaecomastia include a firm, circular, disk-like circumscribed, tender mass beneath the areola, it is usually bilateral at onset. In adolescent boys the condition is transient and last for approximately 12 to 24 months.

Gynaecomastia may also be a symptom of other problems. It is seen accompanying developmental abnormalities of the male reproductive organ. It may also accompany organic diseases including testicular tumours, cancer of the adrenal cortex, pituitary adenomas, hyperthyroidism and liver disease.

Management

In suspected clients with gynaecomastia, 'a human chorionic gonadotropin-beta subunit (hcG-B level should be obtained. This finding assists in ruling out malignant testicular germ cell condition, which can manifest with gynaecomastia and an elevated hCG-B level. Chest and mediastinal roentgenogram may be used. In older men biopsy of breast is taken and examined.

Surgery is used for cosmesis only when the gynecomastia persists over a long period of time and is not associated with an underlying disease process.

The nurse who cares for men with gynaecomastia must offer sympathetic understanding. Most men are intensely embarrassed about the condition because breast constitutes a serious assault on male self-image. The condition is visible whenever the man removes his shirt for work or recreation and frequently results in taunts and jokes. Similar problem exists when the person undergoes mastectomy for looking asymmetrical chest. The patients who are treated with hormonal therapy for prostatic cancer should be warned that gynaecomastia is one of the side effects of treatment. The nurse should convince the person by using all his or her skill to cope up with problem associated with gynaecomastia in men.

Male Breast Cancer

Generally, breast cancer has bean found in 1per cent of men. The presentation, diagnosis, and treatment are similar as those for women with the breast cancer. The family history places men at increased risk for breast cancer.

The symptoms are commonly seen at the time of diagnosis include a firm mass directly beneath the nipple in the subareolar area, most frequently in the left breast. A lesion in the upper outer quadrant is the next most frequent location for tumour growth. Bloody nipple discharge with nipple inversion is common. Evidence of Paget's disease of the nipple (eczema), itching, ulceration and local tenderness also may be present. Metastasis may occur to bone, the lungs and the liver.

Management

Treatment for a primary localized tumour is modified radical mastectomy with node dissection. Breast-sparing procedure is usually not used in men. When axillary nodes are involved in the disease process, systemic adjuvant therapy (chemotherapy and hormonal) is advised. CMF and FAC are prescribed.

A man for whom breast cancer is diagnosed faces unique psychosocial stressors that the nurse needs to address on an individual basis. The use of tamoxifen has reduced the need for palliative surgeries such as orchidectomy. The male patient is treated for breast cancer in an uncommon occurrence; however, the nurse will need to be sensitive to his unique needs and tailor the standard surgical care routines to the individual situation.

Male Reproductive Problems

Men's reproductive health care is one dimension of an emerging speciality area in nursing practice. Traditionally, problem of the male reproductive system have been viewed only as problem of urination or fertility. As with women, men have unique biological and social health care need. Often the complexity of the male reproductive system and the multiple psychosocial needs of the patient have been minimized in today's health care system. Consequently, myths and knowledge deficits related to the specifics of sexual function are common in the male population. It is important to provide health care that is sensitive to the unique problems of the male. Problems of the male reproductive system can involve a variety of structures (Penis, urethra, bladder, ejaculatory duct, prostate, prepuce, testis, scrotum, epidymis, vas deferens, rectum), and create anxiety for both the patient and nurse providing care. Anxiety and fear may also cause the patient to delay seeking help for a problem or practising health-promoting behaviours. Our society often does not encourage men to admit or seek help for problems related to their sex organs. The nurse should be particularly sensitive to the possible embarrassment with the male reproductive problems.

Problems of Scrotum and its Contents

The skin of the scrotum is susceptible to number of common skin diseases. The most common condition of the scrotal skin are fungal infection, dermatitis (neurodermatitis, contact dermatitis and seborrhoea dermatitis) and parasitic infection (scabies and lice), are dealt in integumentary nursing or dermatological nursing.

The scrotal sac contains the testes, epididymis, and part of the spermatic cord. Other associated structures include nerve, lymphatic, and vascular networks. These structures are responsible for the production and storage of sperm and provide the pathway for ejaculation. The testes are also involved in hormonal production primarily of testosterone. Consequently, any disorder related to these structures have the potential to affect male fertility adversely as well as interfere with testosteron production. Pathologies of these structures include problems with swelling, twisting cords, trauma, and carcinoma. The testes are particularly sensitive to changes in scrotal environment, such as fluctuation in temperatures and blood flow. Infection is also a common problem.

Epididymitis

Epididymitis is an inflammatory process of epididymis and is the most common intrascrotal inflammation in adult males.

Aetiology

Epididymitis usually secondary to an infectual process (sexually or non-sexually transmitted), with trauma or urinary reflux down the vas deferens. It is most often caused by an ascending infection via the ejaculatory duct through the vas deferens into the epididymis. There are three means of introduction of the infection into the duct system.

i. Infection may be introduced when surgical or diagnostic procedure are performed. The most common organism for contamination is "Escherichia Coli".
ii. Structural malformation or developmental of structural insufficiencies in the child may contribute to problem of urinary reflux. Reflux of sterile or infected urine causes chemical irritation in the epididymis and cause of inflammation.
iii. Adult male between the age 19-35 years, sexual transmission is the most common means of infection. Chlamydia trichomatis and Neisseria gonorrhoea are caused in heterosexual male, E. Coli and H. influenzene are the causes in homosexual males.

Pathophysiology

Epididymitis results from inflammation of the epididymis and scrotal sac. Fluid accumulation in the scrotal sac is an inflammatory response to the infection process. Excess fluid loss into the interstitial space of the scrotal sac leads to diminished blood flow, nerve damage and resultant pain and swelling. Inflammatory fluids also can form pockets of pus called abscesses. Heat generated from the inflammatory process can negatively affect the testicular function of the spermatogenesis. Consequently, complication of epididymitis include testicular infarction, chronic pain from nerve damage, abscess formation and infertility.

Clinical Manifestation

The most common clinical manifestations are severe tenderness, pain in the scrotal area, and noticeable swelling of one or both the sides of the scrotum. The onset of pain may be insidious, gradually increasing over hours or days, the scrotal swelling can cause pain on ambulation and discomfort that is exacerbated by wearing restrictive clothing. Men with epididymitis often walk with type of "waddle" to help spare the scrotum from rubbing up against the thighs or clothing. Elevation of the scrotum will reduce the pain (Prehns signs). Other symptoms include an increase in temperature of the scrotum and symptoms include an increase in temperature. A urethral discharge may also be present, with colour and consistency varying according to the types of causative organism. Urethritis is often associated with epididymitis and associated symptoms include burning on urination, frequency, urgency and general malaise.

Management

Assessment of the patient with symptoms of epididymitis should include a sexual history. For young children, it should include question to determine possible sexual abuse and any history of recent urinary examination or instrumentation. In elderly male, question focuses on history or symptoms of urinary obstruction or recent urinary examination. Urinanalysis, urine and urethral cultures are needed to determine the specific organism and its sensitivity to various antibiotics as well as to provide information for needed medications. Further scrotal ultrasound and radionuclide scanning is performed when diagnosis is questionable.

The nature of the patient's pain is assessed, whether the pain is bilateral or unilateral, and if the pain is of sudden onset or has developed over hours or days. The nurse also notes if pain is relieved by elevating the scrotum. Any symptoms of dysuria are documented such as burning, frequency, urgency, fever and general malaise. A recent history of urethral discharge or change in the discharge is important to help determine the possible type of causative organism. The colour, consistency and amount of any discharge are documented.

The patient is also observed for the classic "Waddle" or a somewhat rolling gait, indicating that the patient is attempting to protect his scrotum. Swelling of the scrotum is documented, as well as whether it is on one or both the sides. Palpation of the scrotum at this time is generally differed to avoid causing severe pain. For patients with chronic recurrent epididymitis, aspiration fluid for the epididymis can be performed.

Treatment of epididymitis usually consists of pain management, medication to treat the infection and supportive care. NSAIDS such as ibuprofen may be used to decrease the inflammation and relieve the discomfort and swelling. If severe pain, narcotics may be used. Stool softners are given to prevent constipation and reduce straining on defecation, which may cause severe pain in the inflammed scrotum. Eradication of infection generally is accomplished by giving oral antibiotics (broad spectrum).

In younger men, less than 35 years of age, the most common cause is through sexual transmission of either gonorrhoea or Chlamydia. The use of antibiotics is important for both partners if the transmission through sexual contact. Patients should be encouraged to refrain from sexual intercourse during the acute phase. If they do engage in intercourse, condoms should be used. Bedrest with the scrotum elevated in towel, application of ice packs, and the use of scrotal supports when the swelling is less severe and it will also help decrease the discomfort caused by the heavy sensation resulting from enlarged scrotum. Bedrest is maintained until the patient is painfree, then a scrotal support is worn for approximately 6 weeks. The patient is instructed to avoid work that would strain the lower abdomen and scrotal area.

Orchitis

Inflammation or infection of the testicle is known as "Orchitis". In this, testes are inflammed, painful, tender and swollen.

Aetiology

Orchitis may be caused by pyogenic bacteria, gonococci, tubercle bacilli or viruses. It generally occurs after an episode of bacterial or viral infections such as mumps, pneumonia, tuberculosis or syphilis. It can also be a side effect of epididymitis, prostatectomy, trauma, infections mononucleosis, influenza, catheterization or complicated urinary tract infection.

Pathophysiology (Clinical Manifestation)

Inflammatory fluid seeks from the testicle into the serus membrane lining the epididymis and the testicle to create unilateral or bilateral swelling. Hydrocele (a collection of fluid within the tunica vaginalis testis) is frequently associated with orchitis. The signs and symptoms of orchitis are the same as those of epididymitis. However, because orchitis is caused by a systemic infectious process rather than a localitized infection, more systemic symptoms are present. Consequently the patient may also have clinical manifestation of nausia, vomiting, and pain radiating to the inguinal canal. As a result of inflammation and fibrosis, some degree of atrophy occurs, which may lead to sterility. Unless both testes are severely involved, infertility is rare. Mumps orchitis is condition contributing to infertility.

Management

Treatment involves the use of antibiotics (if the organism is known) pain medication on bedrest with the scrotum elevated on an ice pack. Any pubertal boy or man who is exposed to mumps usually is given gamma globulin immediately unless he has already had mumps or been vaccinated for the disease. Mumps orchitis could easily be decreased by childhood vaccination against mumps. Broad spectrum antibiotics are given for common bacterial causes. If *hydrocele* is present, the fluid may be aspirated to reduce pressure on the testes. If the hydrocele is surgically trapped within the first 2 days the potential for testicular atrophy is decreased; however, a tap should only be done when oedema is persistent because a chance exists that surgical decompression may exacerbate the inflammation.

Patient education focuses on measures to reduce discomfort from gonodal swelling and alleviate systemic symptoms. During the acute phase of gonadal swelling, the scrotum may be supported with the same method used for the patient with epididymitis. Warm or cold compression may be applied to help reduce swelling and increase comfort. Antibiotics are administered for bacterial causes. Rest and an increased fluid intake are encouraged for all patients. Anti-inflammatory medication is given to help reduce pain and swelling.

Testicular Torsion

Testicular torsion is a condition which involves a twisting of the spermatic cord that supplies blood to the testes and epididymitis in which testicular circulation is acutely impaired.

Aetiology

Testicular torsion is most commonly seen in young males under the age of 20. Torsion may follow activities that put sudden pull on the cremastric muscle, such as jumping into cold water, blunt trauma, or bicycle riding. It may also occur at night when there is less gravitational pull from the testes on the cord allowing more movement and consequent twisting.

Pathophysiology

Torsion interrupts the blood supply to the testes leading to ischaemia and severe unrelieved pain that may be aggravated by manual elevation of the affected side. The scrotum is swollen, tender, and red. The affected side is usually elevated because the twisting and shortening of the cord pulls up the testicle. The cremastric reflex, elecited by stroking the inner aspect of the thigh to cause reflex refraction of the testicle is usually absent on the side of the suspected torsion. Although the scrotum appears infected because of the swelling and redness, both urinanalysis and blood tests are typically normal. Fever is rarely present. Absence of pain after a time may indicate infarction and necrosis. Gangrene may be a serious sequelae.

Clinical Manifestation

The patient experiences severe scrotal pain, tenderness, swelling, nausea, and vomiting. Urinary complaints, fever and WBCs bacteria in the urine are absent. The pain does not usually subside with rest or elevation of the scrotum. Pain is localized to testis and radiates to groin and lower abdomen, severe in nature; similar episodes of self-limiting pains are not unusual. Vomiting is common. Fever, dysuria are rare. On examination, testis may be in elevated position with abnormal lie, testes will be swollen and tender, epididymis also may be tender. Cremastric reflex is usually negative. Pain is constant (Prehn's sign).

Management

Disgnostic studies may include an orchiogram or testicular scan, which qualitatively measures the blood flow to the testis. Doppler studies also help to diagnose torsion.

Detorsion (a process of untwisting the spermatic cord) can be attempted manually. Torsion constitutes a surgical emergency. If manual detorsion is unsuccessful. Unless it resolves spontaneously, surgery to unturn the cord and restore the blood supply must be performed quickly. The torsion causes ischaemia to the testis, leading to necrosis and possible need for removal (orchidectomy). If orchidectomy is performed, a testicular prosthesis is usually inserted. Orchioplexy performs in nongangrenous testicles. As for the nursing care, often orchioplexy and orchiectomy are similar. Ice bags and scrotal elevation may be ordered to reduce swelling. The nurse continues to monitor the patient for signs of testicular necrosis and fever in the case of orchioplexy. A small pentose drain may be placed in the scrotum which will necessitate dressing change.

After surgery the patient should be instructed to limit stair climbing to two flights and not to lift or carry heavy objects for 4 weeks and is instructed to refrain from sexual intercourse/activities for 6 weeks. The use of scrotal support for at least 3 weeks is recommended to control oedema. Sitz baths may help relieve any discomfort.

Body image disturbance may include fears of castration (Orchidectomy) loss of masculinity, sterility and impotence. The nurse provides specific information about the physiological changes resulting from testicular atrophy or surgical removal of testicles. The patient is still able to have an erection after trauma or surgery to the testicles. Fertility may or may not be affected if there is still a remaining healthy testicle. Counselling on alternative means of conception may be suggested. The patient is reminded that the appearance of the scrotum will not be altered if a testicular prosthesis is inserted after orchiectomy.

Other Benign Problems on Testis

The other problems include congenital problem, i.e. cryptoorchidism, acquired problem such as hydrocele, spermatocele and varicocele.

- *Crypto-orchidism* (undescended testes) is failure of the testes to descend into the scrotal sac before birth, which needs surgery to locate and suture the testes to the scrotum.
- *Hydrocelo* is a nontender, fluid-filled mass that results from interference with lymphatic drainage of the scrotum and swelling of the tunica vaginalis that surround the testes, Diagnosis is done by transillumination. No treatment is indicated unless the swelling becomes very large and uncomfortable in which an aspiration or surgical drainage of the mass is performed.
- *Spermatocele* is a firm, sperm-containing, painless cyst of the epididymis that may be visible with transillumination. The cause is unknown, and surgical removal is the treatment.
- *Varicocele* is a dilation of the veins that drain the testes. The scrotum feels worm-like when palpated. The cause is unknown. The varicocele is usually located on the left side of the scrotum as a consequence of retrograde blood flow from the left renal vein. Surgery is indicated if the patient is infertile. Repair of the varicocele may be performed through injection of a sclerosing agent or by surgical ligation of the spermatic vein.

Testicular Cancer

Aetiology

The aetiology of testicular cancer is still unknown. Testicular tumour occurs primarily in men between 20 to 40 years of age. Testicular tumours are more common in males who have had undescended testes (cryptorohidism) or a family history of testicular cancer or anomalies. Other predisposing factors include a history of mumps, orchitis, inguinal hernia, in childhood, maternal exposure to DES, and testicular cancer in the contralateral testis.

Pathophysiology

Testicular tumours may develop from the cellular components of the testis or from the embryonal precursors (germ cell tumour). Testicular tumours are divided into germinal or nongerminal. Germ cell tumours are further divided into two groups; seminomatous and nonseminomatus. The tumours of mixed cell types can also occur. Testicular germ cell tumours are almost malignant. Nongerm cell tumours are rare, usually benign and can occur at any age.

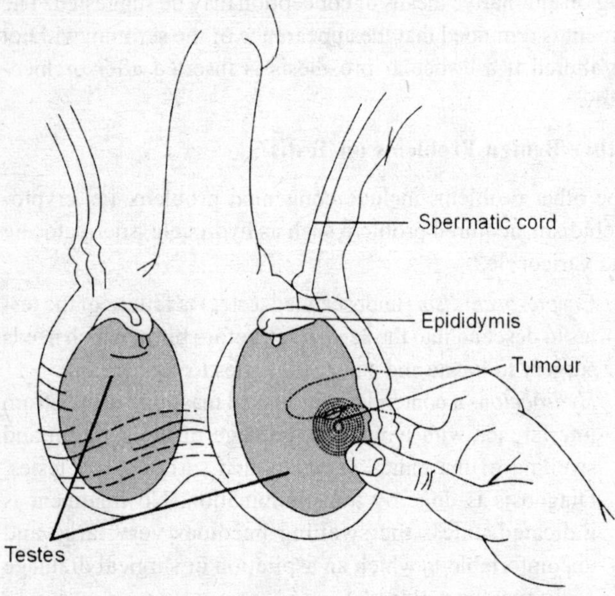

Fig. 15.9: Palpation for testicular tumour. Using the fingertips and thumb, the epididymis, tests, and spermatic cord are located bilaterally.

Clinical Manifestation

Clinical manifestations of testicular cancer are often subtle and go unnoticed by the male until he notices a feeling of heaviness or dragging in the lower abdomen and groin areas. The patient may notice a lump in his scrotum as well as scrotal swelling and a feeling of heaviness. The scrotal mass usually is nontender, painless, very firm and cannot be transilluminated. Other symptoms are nonspecific such as back pain, weight loss and fatigue. Manifestation associated with metastasis to other system include back pain, cough, dyspnoea, haemoptysis, dysphagia (difficulty in swallowing), alteration in vision, mental status, papillodema and seizures.

Management

Palpation of the scrotal contents is the first step in diagnosing testicular cancer. Additional tests that aid in diagnosis include a testicular sonogram and MRI. If testicular tumour is suspected, blood may be drawn to look for the tumour markers of the glycoprotiens, alpha-fetoprotein (AFP) and human chroionic gonadotropin (hCG). Biopsy of the testis is contraindicated because of the highly metastatic character of testicular carcinoma. Testicular cancer is histologically classified as germ cell tumour, i.e., seminos and nonseminomas.

As with many forms of cancer, the survival of the patient is closely associated with early recognition of the tumour. In any suspected case of testicular cancer, the testis is usually removed immediately. *Orchidectomy* consists of enbloc excision of the spermatic cord, the contents of the inguinal canal and the testes with the tunical attached. The adjacent area is explored for metastases. The specimen are then examined to determine the cancer cell type. Staging of the disease as well as pathological findings determine the course of treatment. The staging of the testicular neoplasia is as follows:

- Stage I : No metastasis, confined to testis.
- Stage II : Metastasis to retroperitonal lymph nodes or other subdiaphragmatic area.
- Stage III : Metastasis to mediastinal and supraclavicular nodes or other areas above diaphragm.

Treatment of testicular cancer based on tumour type is as follows:

Stage 0 : Benign form needs surveillance.

Stage I : Seminomatus orchidectomy and radiation therapy.
•Non-seminomatos orchidectomy, modified retroperitoneal lymph node dissection and radiotherapy.

Stage II : •Seminomatus/nonseminomatus orchidectomy, radiation therapy/modified full retroperitoneal lymphnode dissection.

Stage III : Seminomatus/nonseminomatus.
Combination of chemotherapy and full retroperitoneal lymph nods dissection.

Nongerminal testicular tumours treatment consists of four modes of treatment (orchiedectomy, radiation, lymphodenectomy and chemotherapy).

The nurse esplains the effects of orchidectomy and fertility and nurse gives patient teaching, which includes focuses on the planned treatment in its expected effects of surgery, chemotherapy and radiation therapy.

In addition, every male between puberty and 40 years of age should be taught and encouraged to perform monthly testicular self-examination (TSE) for the purpose of detecting testicular tumours or other scrotal abnormalities such as varicoceles and the nurse should teach the patient how to do a self-examination with particular emphasis in males with a history of an undescended testis or a previous testicular tumour. The guidelines for self-examination of the scrotum are as follows:

- During a shower or bath is the easiest time to examine the testes, warm temperature makes the testes hang lower in the scrotum.

- Use both hands to feel each testis. Roll the testes between the thumb and first three fingers until the entire surface has been covered. Palpate each one separately.
- Identify structures. The testis should feel round and smooth like a hard-boiled egg. Differentiate the testis from epididymis. The epididymis is not as smooth as the egg-shaped testis. One testis may be larger than the other. Size is not as important as texture. Check for lumps, irregularities, pain in the testes or a dragging sensation. Locate the spermatic cord, which is usually firm and smooth and goes up towards groin.
- Choose a consistent day of the month such as birth date, that will make it easy to remember for examination of testes. The examination can be performed more frequently if desired.
- Notify the doctor at once if any abnormalities are found.

PROBLEMS OF PROSTATE

Prostatitis

Infections of the prostate occurs infrequently, but it can result in chronic problems that are difficult to eradicate. Prostatitis cause long-term discomfort and problems with fertility.

Aetiology

A number of inflammatory conditions can affect the prostate gland after a male reaches puberty. The four most common forms of prostatitis are acute bacterial prostatis, chronic bacterial prostatitis, nonbacterial prostatitis, and prostatodynia. *Bacterial prostatitis* is frequently associated with an indwelling urethral catheter, urethral instrumentation or trauma. Common causative organisms are Escherichia coli, Psudemonos, Enterobacter, Proteus, Chlamydial trachomatis, Neisseria gonorrhoea and group D streptococci. Chronic bacterial prostatitis should be considered in men with a history of recurrent bacteriuria. *Nonbacterial* prostatitis may occur after a viral illness or it may be associated with other STDs particularly in a younger adult. The aetiology is not known and a culture reveals no causative organism. *Prostadodynia* has the same symptoms as prostatitis (irritation, and pelvic pain on urination), but no evidence of inflammation. The condition is limited to younger men.

Pathophysiology

Bacterial prostatitis generally results from an organism reaching the prostate gland by one of the following routes; ascending from the urethra descending from the bladder, and invasion via the blood stream or the lymphatic channels. The prostate gland becomes swollen, inflammed and painful because of either a bacterial infection or other inflammatory process. The prostate surrounds the urethra and when it becomes swollen it can compress the urethra and cause urinary obstruction. Men

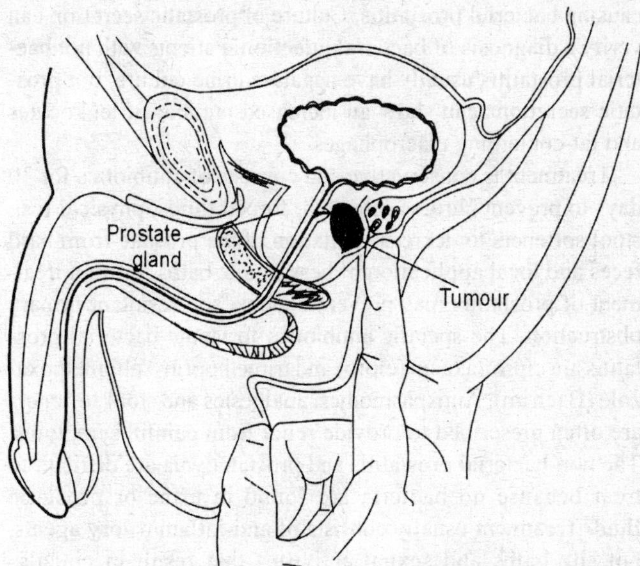

Fig. 15.10: The prostate gland can be felt through the wall of the rectum. The size of the gland, overall consistency, and the presence of any firm areas and nodules are noted.

with prostatitis typically complain of changes in voiding patterns, such as difficulty starting the stream or the need to strain on urination. Low back pain, pelvic pain and perinial pain are other common symptoms. Pain during or after ejaculation may be experienced. In addition, the patients with bacterial prostatitis frequently complain of symptom of UTIs, that can include urgency, frequency, painful urination and haematuria. Bacterial infections cause fever, chills and general fatigue.

Clinical Manifestation

Acute bacterial prostatitis results in manifestation of fever, chills, dysuria, urethral discharge, increased urinary frequency and urgency, low back, rectal, pelvic and perineal pain, and acute cystitis with cloudy and smelly urine. The prostate is extremely swollen, tender, firm and warm to touch. The complication of prostatitis are epidymitis and cystitis. Sexual functioning may be affected as manifested by postejaculatory pain libido problems and erectile dysfunction. Prostatic abscess is a rare complication.

The symptoms of chronic prostatitis may be absent or rare generally milder than that of acute prostatitis. These include backache, perineal pain, ejaculatory pain, mild dysuria, and increased frequency of urination. Factors that may contribute to chronic prostatitis include urethral obstruction, persistent infection above the urethra, and prostatic pathological condition such as congestions, hyperplasia and prostatic calculi. It predisposes the patient to recurrent UTI. The prostate feels irregularly enlarged firm and slightly tender on palpation.

Management

Urine cultures are usually obtained to determine the organisms causing bacterial prostatitis. Culture of prostatic secretion can verify a diagnosis of bacterial infection. Patients with nonbacterial prostatitis usually have negative urine culture, but prostatic secretions can show an increased number of leukocytes and fat-containing macrophages.

Treatment is conservative and consists of antibiotics for 30 days to prevent chronic infection, forced fluids, physical rest, stool softeners to decrease irritation of the prostate from hard feces and local application of heat by sitz baths. Prompt treatment of prostatitis may prevent oedema and resultant urinary obstruction. The specific antibiotics for acute bacterial prostatitis are ciproflaxacin (cipro) and trimethoprim sulfamethoxazole (Bactrim). Antispasmodics, analgesics and stool softeners are often prescribed to provide relief from painful symptoms. The non-bacterial prostatitis and prostatodynia are difficult to treat because no bacteria are found in urine or prostatic fluid. Treatment usually consists of anti-inflammatory agents, hot sitz baths and sexual activities that result in ejaculation. Antibiotics are ineffective against calculi and surgical excision is required. Prostatectomy may be necessary to eradicate infection.

The patient with acute bacterial prostatitis experiences prostate pain when standing, when urinating and during ejeculation. Nursing interventions are aimed at relief of pain and fever, bed rest and maintenance of adequate hydration. The patient with chronic prostatitis should be instructed regarding the long-term nature of the problem. Because the prostate can serve as a source of bacteria, fluid intake should be kept at a high level. Antibiotics may have to be taken for number of months. Activities that drain the prostate, such as intercourse (use a condom to protect the partner from infection), masturbation and prostatic massage are often helpful in the long-term management of this problem. Chronic prostatitis may eventually lead to erectile dysfunction for which the patient may need to seek treatment.

The patient is taught how to take warm sitz bath. Use anti-inflammatory medication and avoid allergy producing foods that may be excerbating the inflammation. The patient should refrain from sexual activity until the antibiotic has started to work, approximately 2 weeks into therapy. After 2 weeks regular ejaculation is encouraged to promote "flushing" of the prostate gland. Complete course of antibiotic should be taken. Abstaining from alcohol and OTC drugs (of decongestants) help exacerbation of the symptom of urinary obstruction. The continued stool softeners can decrease irritation to the inflammed prostate infection.

Benign Prostatic Hyperplasia (BPH)

The prostate gland, located below the bladder, surrounding the urethra and is responsible for contributing to ejaculatory fluid. During puberty the prostate grows rapidly. After puberty, growth tapers off by the age of 30 years. Changes in the size of the gland next occurs after the age of 50, when the gland begins to atrophy and becomes nodular.

Benign prostatic hypertrophy (hyperplasia, BPH) is an enlargement of portions of this gland that eventually cause problems with urination. Parts of the gland may be atrophy, whereas other parts become large and nodular.

Aetiology

BPH is common problem in men over the age of 50. The changes in the size and shape of the prostate are associated with increased androgen levels. Although the cause is not completely understood, it is thought that the primary cause is an increased number of cells resulting from endocrine changes associated with aging process. Excessive accumulation of dihydroxy-testosterons (the principal intraprostatic androgen), stimulation of oestrogen and local growth hormone action are proposed causes.

Pathophysiology

The changes that occur in the prostate gland of older men can create a number of problems with the associated urinary system. When the enlarged nodular tissue of the prostate impinges on the urethra, the urethra elongates and compresses causing obstruction of urinary flow. This can result in a compensatory hypertrophy of the bands of bladder muscle. This in turn increases the trabeculation (contouring) of the bladder wall providing pockets of urinary retention. These trebeculated areas show up on ultrasound. Because of the muscular thickening, the bladder has less capacity. Muscle tone can diminish over time. Consequently, bladder cannot empty completely at each voiding (residual urine); the urine becomes alkaline from stasis and is a fertile medium for bacterial growth.

Clinical Manifestation

In BPH urethral and bladder changes can result in symptoms of urinary obstruction and irritation. Often the symptoms of *obstruction* are gradual and not noticed by the male until acute urinary retention occurs. Symptoms of gradual obstruction include a decrease in the urinary stream with less force on urination and often dribbling at the end of voiding. Other related symptoms include hesitancy, a difficulty in starting the stream, intermittency and inability to maintain a constant stream. The patient may also complain of a sense of incomplete emptying of the bladder. Straining and urinary retention are the symptoms that often convince the patient to seek medical help.

Symptom of *irritation* often accompany the obstructive problems. Nocturia from incomplete emptying is common. Dysuria, urgency, and urge incontinence are symptoms associated with loss of muscle tone in the bladder and changes in the angle of the bladder neck. The patient also has symptoms of UTIs because of incomplete emptying and the increased risk of infection. As the prostate enlarges, so does the vasculature and when straining takes place, these vessels may break and cause haematuria.

To brief the clinical manifestation of BPH, includes prostate gland enlarges, becomes more nodular; straining on urination, hesitancy in starting urine flow; decreased urine stream; postvoid dribbling; nocturia; dysuria, haematuria and urgency.

Other problems that can arise from BPH are kidney disorders caused by backflow of urine. Hydronephritis and pyelonephritis are possible sequelas to urinary obstruction. Anaemia may also occur if blood loss is severe, or as a result of secondary insufficiency. Calculi may develop because of the alkalinization of the residual urine.

Management

Diagnostic test for BPH includes the following.

i. Primary screening.
   - History including symptoms of voiding problems.
   - Physical examination, including digital rectal examination (DRE).
   - Urine analysis with culture.
   - Serum creatinine and blood urea nitrogen.
   - Prostate-specific antigen (PSA)—a blood test to estimate the volume of prostate.
ii. Secondary screening.
   - Urodynamic flow studies—cystourethroscopy, uroflowmetry, IVP.
   - Transrectal ultrasound.
   - Cystoscopy (for surgical candidates).

To primary treatment for BPH is now referred to as "watchful waiting". When there are not symptoms or only mild ones, a conservative noninvasive wait-and-see approach is taken. If the patient begins to have signs or symptoms that indicate an increase in urethral obstruction, further treatment is indicated. The numerous treatment options for BPH can be categorized as pharmocologic, nonsurgical invasive and surgical invasive options.

- *Pharmocologic* hormone manipulation can be used to cause regression of hyperplasic tissue through suppression of androgens. The drugs used for BPH include antibiotics. Finasteride (Proscar), Alpha-adrenergic receptor blocks such as Prazosin (Minipress) Tetrazosin (Hytrin), Tamsulosin (Flomax) Doxazo-sin (cardura) and Herbal medicine extracted from plant (phyto-therapy), i.e., can palmetto have been used.
- *Nonsurgical invasive* can include intermittent catheterization or indwelling catheter can be temporarily used to reduce symptoms and bypass the obstruction. The other non-surgical invasive procedure includes stents and coilsm balloon dilation and heat (Transurethral microwave antenna (Tuma).
- *Surgery* is indicated when there is a decrease in urine flow sufficient to cause discomfort, persistent residual urine, acute urinary retention because of obstruction with no reversible precipitatory cause, or hydronephrosis. Treatment of symptomatic BPH primary involves resection of the prostate. The selection of a surgical approach to remove the tissue depends on the size and position of the prostatic enlargement. The usual surgical procedure for BPH are as follows:
  1. Laser ablation
     - Transurethral, ultrasound guided and laser-induced prostatectomy (TULIP)
     - Visual laser ablation of the prostate (VLAP).
  2. Transurethral resection of the prostate (TURP)-by using resectoscope.
  3. Transurethral incision of the prostate (TUIP).
  4. Suprabubic prostate resection.
  5. Retropubic prostate resection.
  6. Perineal prostate resection.
- *Nursing management*

Nurse is most directly involved with the care of prostate having surgical intervention, the focus on nursing management will be on preoperative and postoperative care.

Preoperative care includes all routine of the person undergoing any surgery. In addition, urinary drainage must be restored before surgery. A urethral catheter such as coude (curved-tip) catheter may be needed to restore drainage-septic technique is important at all times to avoid introducing bacteria into the bladder. Antibiotics are usually administered before any invasive surgical procedures. Any infection of the urinary tract must be treated before surgery. Restoring urine drainage and encouraging high fluid intake (2 to 3L/day unless contraindicated) are also helpful in managing the infection. The patient is often concerned about the impact of the impending surgery on his sexual functioning. The nurse should provide an opportunity for the patient and the partner to express that concerns and proper counselling given by the nurse appropriately.

Postoperative care includes the management of complication of surgery. The main complications of prostatectomy are haemorrhage, bladder spasms, urinary incontinence and infection. Nursing management of the patient following traditional resectoscope and surgery include:

- Promoting adequate urine elimination—Maintain patency of catheter.
- Controlling discomfort from bladder spasms and straining by using narcotics, belladona and opium suppositories and stool softener.
- Preventing infection by using antibiotics—IV or oral.
- Relieving anxiety.

Postoperative nursing care for the person undergoing prostate surgery are as follows:

1. Maintain patency of catheter system.
2. Monitor appearance of urine, red to light pink (24 hrs) to amber (3 days).

3. Monitor patient for signs of water intoxication after TURP (confusion, agitation, warm moist skin, anorexia, nausea, vomiting).
4. Instruct patient not to try to void around catheter, explain feeling of needing to void from pressure of catheter.
5. Avoid use of enemas and rectal thermometers.
6. Give prescribed medication (analgesics, antispasmodics) as needed; tell patients spasm will decrease in intensity and severity within 24 to hours.
7. After catheter removal
   a. Monitor signs of urinary retention.
   b. Monitor for continence, teach perineal exercises if dribbling occurs.
   c. Encourage increased fluids and frequent voiding.
8. Change dressings, frequently around suprapubic wounds after suprapubic prostatectomy to prevent skin maceration.
9. Give patient opportunities to discuss feelings about sexuality and possible incontinence.
10. Teach patient to:
   a. Avoid vigorous exercises, heavy lifting (over 20 pounds) and sexual intercourse for at least 3 weeks.
   b. Avoid driving for 2 weeks.
   c. Avoid straining with defecation using stool softeners or mild laxatives if needed.
   d. Drink at least 2500 ml of fluids per day to prevent urinary stasis and infection and to keep stools soft.
   e. Diet high in fiber facilitates the passage of stool.
   f. Notify doctor if urinary stream diminishes or if bleeding occurs.

Cancer of the Prostate

Cancer of the prostate is the most common cancer in men.

Aetiiology

The cause of prostatic cancer is basically unknown. Prostatic cancer is an androgen-dependent adenocarcinoma. Factors such as sexual activity socioeconomic class, alcohol use have not been shown significant factors. Factors that may affect the development of prostate cancer include hormonal changes and viral infections. Hormonal changes during aging are the reason that prostate cancer is seen almost exclusively in men over age of 40. Positive antibody titers to herpes simplex and cytomagalovirus have been found in men with prostate cancer. Other risk factors include a history of multiple sexual partners, episodes of STDs, the presence of cervical cancers in sexual partners and industrial exposure to cadmium.

Pathophysiology

Cancer of the prostate often starts as a discrete localized hazard nodule in an area of senile atrophy. It is often caused by an adenocarcinoma that arises in peripheral regions of the gland. The growth is generally on the outer portion of the gland, compression of the urethra and subsequent voiding symptoms are not common until late in the disease. The tumour is slow-growing and usually being in the posterior or lateral portions of the prostate. It can spread by three routes. Direct extension is by continuity to the seminal vescicles, urethral mucusa, bladder wall and external sphincter. The cancer later spreads through the prineural lymphatic system to the regional lymphnodes. The vein from the prostate seem to be the mode of spread to the pelvic bones, head of femur, lower lumbar spine, liver and lungs.

Clinical Manifestations

Prostate cancer is asymptomatic in the early stages. Eventually, the patient may have symptoms similar to those of BPH, including dysuria hesitancy, dribbling, frequency, urgency, haematuria, nocturia and retention. The prostate feels hard, enlarged and fixed on rectal examination. The enlargement is usually unilateral, pain in the lumbosacral area, which radiates down to the hips or legs. When coupled with urinary symptoms may indicate metastases. To sum up, clinical manifestation of prostate cancer include:

- Often no symptoms if cancer is confined to the gland.
- Symptoms of urinary obstruction and symptoms of urinary tract infection.
- Low back pain, malaise, aching in legs, a hip pain if cancer has metastatized.

Management

Early recognition and treatment is required to control growth. Primary screening for prostrate cancer consists of palpation of the gland during DRE, a blood test for PSA (a glycoprotein that is detected in the epithelial cells of the prostrate) and TRUS (transrectal ultrasound). Biopsy, needle aspiration, open biopsy, bone screening, grading and staging.

A symptom of staging prostate cancer has been developed to classify the location, size and spread of the tumour and guide treatment decision. *DUKES* system of staging the prostatic neoplasia are as follows:

- Stage A : Microscopic lesions found in prostate gland removed because of benign hypertrophy.
- Stage B : Nodules confined to prostate gland, no capsular adherence, or urethral involvement: normal serum acid phosphatase level.
- Stage C : Carcinoma involving prostatic capsule, seminal vescicles, urethra, bladder and pelvic lymph nodes or a malignant tumour of lesser extent with elevated serum acid phosphatase levels.
- Stage D : Findings as in Stage III plus evidence of extrapelvic lesions or osseous involvement.

Treatment included according to stages as follows:

- Stage A : Continue medical follow-up, observation,

TURP or total prostatectomy and radiation therapy.

- Stage B : TURP, total prostatectomy with or without lymphodectotomy as radiation therapy.
- Stage C : Hormone manipulation: e.g. 2H—releasing hormone analogues) Orchidectomy, radical resection of prostate and radiation therapy.

The types of surgical procedures performed in prostate are:

1. Transurethral resection done when enlargement of the medial lobe surrounding urethra-BPH. No incision, removal by way of urethroscopy.
2. Suprapubic resection performed when extremely large mass of obstructive tissue and prostatic cancer. Low midline abdominal incision through bladder or prostate gland.
3. Retropubic resection-performed when large mass is located high in pelvic area—prostate cancer, low midline abdominal incision into prostate gland (bladder is not incised).
4. Perineal resection, performed when large mass is located low in pelvic area—prostate cancer. Here incision is made between scrotum and rectum.
5. Radical perineal resection is done when mass extends beyond the capsule, includes lymph node dissection—prostate cancer. Here there is large perineal incision between scrotum and rectum.

For all procedures, three-way Foley catheter with 30 ml b uretha is used as drainage tube. The complication of surgical procedures include haemorrhage, water intoxication, incontinence, obstruction, infections, wound infection, impotence and sterility may occur.

Preoperative and postoperative phases of therapy are the same as for BPH. Nursing intervention for patient who undergoes radiation therapy and chemotherapy as in other malignancies (Oncological nursing). If the patient is to have a perineal approach in surgery, he is given a bowel preparation which may include enemas, cathartics and sulfasalazine (Azulfidine) or neomycin preoperatively and only clear fluids the day before surgery to prevent fecal contamination of the operative side.

Additional postoperative care includes:

- Caring for the perineal wound.
- Restoring urinary and bowel continence.
- Promoting sexual function and psychological counselling.
- Dealing with grief.

PROBLEMS OF THE PENIS

Health problems of the penis are rare if sexually transmitted infectious diseases are excluded. Structural problem of the penis is typically related to the head of the penis and the foreskin. The head of the penis is susceptible to diseases caused by irritation, cancer and trauma. Foreskin also is a source of structural difficulties that can affect urinations, cause pain and interfere with blood flow to the penis. Functional problems of the penis primarily involves disorders of erection. Problems of the penis may be classified as congenital, problems of the prepuce, problems with the erectile mechanism and cancer.

Congenital Problem

Hypospadias is a urologic abnormality in which the urethral meatus is located on the ventral surface of the penis anywhere from the corona to the perineum. Hormonal influences in utero, environmental factors and genetic factors are possible causes. Surgical repair of hypospadias may be necessary if it is associated with chordeoc or if it prevents intercourse or normal urination. Surgery may also be done for cosmetic reasons or emotional well-being.

Epispadias and opening of the urethra on the dorsal surface of the penis, is a complex birth defect that is usually associated with other genitourinary tract defects. Corrective surgery to place the urethra in a normal position in the penis is usually done in childhood.

Phimosis and Paraphimosis

Aetiology

Phimosis is a condition in which the opening of the prepuce or foreskin is unable to be retracted behind the glans. The condition may be congenital or acquired as a result of inflammation or infection. It is caused by oedema or inflammation of the foreskin of an uncircumcised male. This results in the foreskin constricting around the head of the penis making retraction difficult. It is generally caused by poor hygiene techniques that allow bacterial and yeast organisms to become trod under the foreskin.

Paraphimosis conversely, is a condition in which the prepuce is retracted over the glans and forms a constriction at the base of the glans. This is usually as a result of manipulation of the foreskin over the glans to infection. Chronic irritation may cause senile carcinoma. Healing of the irritation or infection causes scar tissue formation, which can worsen the acquired phimosis and if the constriction of the foreskin at the head of the penis is severe enough, it causes urinary obstructions and painful urination.

Constriction is also a major problem with paraphimosis. The constriction at the base of the glans usually results in swelling of the glans. If the swelling is not reduced, blood vessels to the glans are compressed, reducing flow. Inadequate blood flow can result in the necrosis of the glans.

Management

Treatment for severe cases of phimosis may consist of incisions in the foreskin to reduce the contracture and widen the opening. Congenital phimosis may be successfully treated by gentle repeated stretching of the foreskin over the glans.

Circumcision may be performed if the prepuce cannot be satisfactorily retracted.

Circumcision, the surgical removal of the foreskin of the penis may be done for religious, cultural or hygienic reasons. Parents are encouraged to make the final decisions after considering all the advantages and disadvantages.

Circumcision is done to prevent recurrence of paraphimosis. When the penis is circumcised, the wound is covered with gauze generously impregnated with petrolatum. Bleeding usually is controlled by applying pressure on dressing that may be bulky and must be removed before the patient can void. It is removed cautiously and replaced after voiding with a fresh petroleum dressing.

Patient education focuses on strategies to reduce the inflammation. Hot soaks and oral antibiotics are often used to treat the swelling and infection that can result from phimosis. Cool compresses are used for paraphimosis. The cool compress is applied to the penis and the penis is elevated for a short period before a gentle attempt is made to reduce the prepuce. Antibiotics, warm soaks and sometimes circumcision or dorsal slit of the prepuce may be required. Careful cleaning followed by replacement of the foreskin generally prevents these problems.

If circumcision has been necessary, the nurse teaches the patient how to change the petrolatum dressing and observe for signs of infection. The nurse also instructs the patient to be alert for signs of bleeding. If severe bleeding occurs, a firm dressing should be applied to the penis and the patient should be taken to medical aid. For the emergency treatment room, an oestrogen preparation may be prescribed for the adult patient for several days after surgery to prevent painful erections.

Cancer of the Penis

Cancer of the penis is rare apart from cancer associated with the STD, human papilloma virus (HPV) and in men who were not circumcised as infants.

Aetiology

The incidence of penile cancer depends greatly on hygienic standards and cultural and religious practices. It almost never occurs in a male who was circumcised at birth. Circumcision after puberty does not decrease the risk of cancer when compared with the incidence among uncircumcised males. Circumcision removes the prepuce or foreskin, which provides a haven for bacteria. The bacteria act on disquamated cells, producing smegma, which is irritating to the tissue of the glans penis and the prepuce. The chronic irritation is considered to be the carcinogenic. Trauma and STDs are thought to be considered as penile cancer rather than causative.

Pathophysiology

Penile cancer starts as a small lesion usually on or under the prepuce and extends until the entire glans and shaft are involved. The initial lesion may assume a variety of forms. It may appear as a small bump, resemble a pimple or wart or occur as a nonhealing ulcer with the edges rolled inward. The latter associated with earlier metastases and a poorer 5-year survival. The most common type of malignancy is squamous cell carcinoma. Phimosis is present in patient with penile cancer, may obscure the lesion. The lesion may then cause erosion through the prepuce, resulting in a foul odour and discharge. Bleeding may or may not be present. Urethral and bladder involvements are rare. Eventually the disease can become autoamputative. If left untreated, death occurs in 2 to 3 years.

Clinical Manifestation

Clinical manifestation of penile cancer includes weakness, fatigue, malaise and weight loss. Men may complain of itching and burning under the prepuce and an occasional foul discharge. A 1-year delay before seeking treatment occurs in 15-50 per cent cases. Biopsy is performed to establish diagnosis. However, benign penile lesions occurs infrequently. Metastasis occurs at the regional femeral and iliac nodes and is associated with significantly worse prognosis. The stages of penile cancer includes the following.

- Stage A : Lesions confined to glans or foreskin.
- Stage B : Shaft or corpora cavernosa invaded by tumour.
- Stage C : Shaft involvement, lymph nodes involved but operable.
- Stage D : Shaft involvement, lymph nodes inoperable and metastases to distant sites.

Management

Treatment is usually surgical. Treatment in the early stages is laser removal of the growth. A radical resection of the penis may be done if the cancer has been spread. Surgery, radiation, or chemotherapy may be tried depending on the extent of the disease, lymph node involvement or metastasis.

Stage 0 : Circumcision.
Stage A : Partial penectomy or amputation of the penis.
Stage B : Total amputation of the penis.
Stage C : Total amputation and lperineal urethrostomy.
Stage D : Hemipelvectomy or hemicorporectormy if scrotum and anus.

The nurse teaches the patient about the potential side effects of radiation in the perineal area. Radiation in this location can cause the skin to become dry, itchy and sensitive. Special gels that are safe to use during radiation may be applied to the affected area. Urethral strictures may develop several months to years after radiation therapy. The nurse informs the patient of symptoms of urethral structure, which includes difficulty starting or stopping the urine flows. Frequent UTI and nocturia and bowel pattern may change during radiation therapy.

The emotional devastation of a diagnosis of penile cancer is difficult to assess. The proposed surgery may be unthinkable to the patient, who is frequently in a state of shock. The scope of support and sexual counselling needed by the patient is beyond the expertise of most nurses. The patient is referred for sexual counselling with experts who can clearly explain the options.

Erectile Dysfunction/Impotence

Erectile dysfunctions is the inability to attain or maintain an erect penis that allows satisfactory sexual performance. Impotence is the inability of a man to have an erection firm enough or sustain an erection long enough for sexual intercourse.

The term *satisfactory* is defined by the couple involved and may vary from couple to couple. The ability to have an erection depends not only on healthy psychological state, but also on adequately functioning neuorological, vascular and hormonal system. The brain is the controlling organ for sexual arousal. The brain perceives sexual stimuli and controls the psychological changes that occur during arousal.

Aetiology

The two fundamental causes of impotence are physical and psychological. Physical cause includes changes in bloodflow to the penis and neurogenic dysfunctions. Diseases such as diabetes, lupus and rheumatoid arthritis can damage blood vessels and cause obstruction of blood flow in the penis. Anaemia and dehydration can cause insufficient blood volumes to maintain an erection. Cardiac diseases and antihypersensitive drugs can interfere with the capillar blood pressure. The risk factors of impotence are as follows:

- Stress.
- Fatigue.
- Drug effects e.g. antihypertensive agents, beta blockers, or alcohol.
- Diabetes mellitus.
- Vascular diseases e.g. hypertension or peripheral vascular disease.
- Neurological disorder e.g. if multiple sclerosis, or spinal cord injury and Parkinson's disease.
- Effects of colorectal, cystectomy or selected prostatectomy procedures.
- Trauma to the perineal area.
- Psychological factors of fear, anxiety, anger, frustrations, performance:
  - anxiety i.e. fear of not performing well during sexual intercourse and fatigue.

Pathophysiology

Inability of the brain to respond to sexual stimuli can interrupt the signals to the para sympathetic nervous system, that release a transmitter substance causing the small arteries in the penis to dilate. The result is insufficient blood flow to fill the network of sinusoids inside the corpora cavernosa (erectile chamber) that cause the penis to enlarge and become firm. When the blood volume in the erectile chamber is inadequate, they cannot create enough pressure to block blood return. Blood drains from the penis and erection cannot be maintained.

The sympathetic nervous system controls both orgasm and ejaculation. The two functions there form can occur without an erection.

After ejaculation or when sexual stimulation diminishes the arteries on the penis constrict, reducing blood flow and the veins expand to allow disengorgement.

Clinical Manifestation

The clinical manifestation of impotence includes the following.

- Inability to have an erection.
- Inability to sustain an erection.
- Inability to have an erection firm enough for penetration. (incomplete erection).

Management of Impotence

Diagnostic tests for impotence include CBC, urinanalysis, BUN, creatinine and fasting blood sugar, cholesterol level, hormonal studies and nocturnal monitoring of penile tumescence. Invasive studies include arteriogram (dye injection to sudy blood flow) and cavernosometry and psychological test is also performed.

Several new medications for impotence are under development. Sildenafil (Viagra) has been released for use and attracted by many persons. Viagra can cause lowering of blood pressure and cardiac arrest. Other side effects are headache and GI disturbances. Topical agents are occasionally used to enhance venous congestion of the penis, e.g. Nitroglycerin ointments—topical vasodilator. Topical and oral agents are often combined with other therapies to treat impotence. Hormonal therapy (Testosterone) increases libido. Vasodilators can induce penile erections by means of increased blood flow, sinusoidal relaxations and increased venous resistance. These generally used drugs are Papaverine and Pentolamine combination injected by a patient into the corpus cavernosum of the penis or inserted into the tip of the penis via suppository. The drug combination may include prostaglandin E (PGE). Many medications have side effects that inhibit erectile function. Modify the dosage or change of drug when needed.

External vacuum devices are sometimes used to achieve an erection for a short time. These devices are cylinders that fit over the penis and use a suction pump to pull blood into the penis. A band is applied to the proximal aspect of the penis when the erection is achieved to impede the venous return. The erection may be maintained for approximately 30 minutes. These devices contraindicated for patients with bleeding disorders, sickle cell anaemia and severe circulatory compromise.

Counselling and sexual therapy classes may be suggested for patients who have identified psychological impotence.

Surgical treatment of impotence include vascular reconstructive surgery, inflatable prosthesis, self-contained inflatable prosthesis and semirigid/malleable prosthesis.

The man experiencing erectile dysfunction requires a great deal of emotional support, for both himself and his partner. The patient needs reassurance and then confidentiality will be maintained. Nurses are in a unique position of conducting routine health assessments on men seeking any form of medical treatment.

Priapism

Priapism is a painful condition, characterized by prolonged erection greater than 4 to 6 hours. Penile ischaemia can result causing permanent impotence or necrosis of the penis.

Aetiology

- Caused by either prolonged venous occlusion or arterial blood engorgement.
- Possible side effects of some impotence therapies.

Treatment

- Treatment is directed as the specific cause.
- Options include administration of alpha antogonists directly into the corpora cavernosa, and IV therapy to re-establish acid-base balance.
- Pain management is a high priority.
(Infertility, vasectomy, male sterilization...).

SEXUALITY TRANSMITTED DISEASES

Sexually transmitted diseases (STDs) are diseases that usually can be transmitted from one person to another with heterosexual or homosexual intercourse or intimate contact with the genitalia, mouth or rectum. Historically they have been referred to as veneral diseases. Although diseases are sexually transmitted there are some notable exceptions to sexual transmission. During pregnancy, the foetus may become infected in utero by placental transmission, and the neonate may acquire congenital syphilis or be stillborn. Infants of mothers with gonorrhoea may contract an infection of the eyes (ophthalmic neonoatarum) during birth, and unless treated it can lead to permanent blindness.

Until the 1980, only five veneral diseases (Syphilis, gonorrhoea, chancroid, lymphogranuloma venerium and granuloma inguinale) were regularly monitored. In 1960s, several diseases were added to the list of STDs. These include "Chlamydia trachomatis, genital herpes, human papilloma virus (HPV), genital myeoplasmas, cytomegalovirus, hepatitis B, vaginitis, enteric infections and ectoparasitic disease. Early in the 1980s the human immuno deficiency syndrome emerged as major STD. We shall discuss some of the important STDs.

Gonorrhoea

Aetiology

Gonorrhoea is caused by neisseria gonorrhoea, a gram-negative diplococcus. Mucosa with columnar epithelium is susceptible to gonococcal infection. This tissue is present in the genitalia (the urethra in men, the cervix in women), the rectum and the oropharynx. The disease is spread by direct physical contact with an infected host, usually during sexual activity. Neonates can develop a gonococcal infection after passage through an infected birth canal. The delicate gonococcus is easily killed by drying, heating or washing with an antiseptic solution. Consequently, indirect transmission of instruments or linen are rare. The incubation period is 3 to 4 days. The disease confers no immunity subsequent to reinfection.

Pathophysiology

In men the gonococcus is introduced into the anterior urethra during sexual activity. Because most men are diagnosed and treated early complications and residual effects of gonorrhoea are uncommon among men. Sterility from orchitis or epididymitis can occur as a residual effect. But this is rare.

The incidence of asymptomatic gonorrhoea in men is believed to be low. However, there is an increasing awareness of the importance of men with asymptomatic infection in the transmission of gonorrhoea.

Gonorrhoea in women, most often begins as asymptomatic cervicitis and the infection can be present for extended periods without causing noticeable signs. Hence there are a high number of infected asymptomatic women. These women do not receive treatment unless gonorrhoea is diagnosed through screening or unless women is identified by a sexual partner and presents herself for treatment. In cases of untreated gonorrhoea, women, the residual effects of chronic PID, infertility and ectopic pregnancies are well known. Other complication of untreated gonorrhoea in both men and women include dermatitis, carditis, meningitis and arthritis.

Clinical Manifestation

The most common signs and symptoms of gonorrhoea are as follows:

A. 1. In *Heterosexual* men there is:
   - Urethritis - often first symptoms.
   - Severe dysuria - especially with first voiding in morning.
   - Purulent discharge from urethra
   - Swelling of the penis and balantitis - rare symptom.

   2. In homosexual and bisexual men, there is
   - Rectal gonorrhoea is common—usually asymptomatic and discovered by rectal culture.
   - Pharyngeal gonorrhoea—usually asymptomatic.

B. *In women*

Women rarely have early distressing symptoms such as men have. When symptoms are present they include the following:

- Slight purulent vaginal discharge.
- Vague feeling of fullness in pelvis.
- Discomfort or aching in abdomen.
- If bladder is involved—burning frequency and urgency usually causes the person to seek medical attention.

The symptoms are so light that they may be ignored.

Management

The most reliable way to confirm gonococcal infection is to isolate the organism in culture. Prevention of gonorrhoea and its complications can be achieved in three stages. The first and most crucial stage is primary prevention that is prevention of the disease. The second stage or secondary prevention involves prevention of complication of the disease such as PID. The third stage or tertiary prevention is reversal of the damage caused by the disease, such as by tubal reconstruction.

Early treatment of infected person is the most effective method of prevention of new infections of sexual partners. Education to acquaint people with the symptoms of gonorrhoeas is efficacy of condoms, and availability of diagnosis and treatment sources. The treatment which necessarily include the following.

- Uncomplicated gonorrhoea: Cefixine (Suprax) 400 mg orally in single dose or Ceftrinaxacin 500 mg orally single dose plus Azithromycin—1 gm orally in single dose or doxyecycline 100 mg orally tid 7 days.
- Follow-up cultures after completion of treatment (usually 7 days).
- Case finding.
- Treatment of contacts.
- Instruction on abstinence from sexual intercourse and alcohol.
- Re-examination if symptoms persist or recur after completion of treatment.
- Repeat serological test for syphilis at one month.

Syphilis

Syphilis is caused by a spirochete, tereponema pallidium that gains entry into the body through either the mucus membrane or skin during intercourse. The organism is readily destroyed by physical and chemical agents including heat, draining and mild disinfectants such as soap and water. The incubation period is usually 3 weeks. However, symptoms can appear as early as 9 days or as long as 3 months after exposure which in case of rectal infection in homosexuals.

Pathophysiology

The signs and symptoms of syphilis developed in four stages as follows:

- *Primary stage*--The duration of stage is 2-8 weeks. There will be a hard sore or pimple on vulva or penis that breaks and forms painless, draining chancre; may be a simple chancre or groups of more than one, may be present also on lips, tongue, hands, rectum or nipples, chancre heals leaving almost invisible scar.

Exudate from lesions and chancre are highly contagious. Duration of stage is 3-8 weeks.

- *Secondary stage:* Appears 2-4 weeks after chancre appears, extends over 2-4-years. Signs and symptoms depends on site, low-grade fever, headache, anorexia, weight loss, anaemia, sore throat, hoarseness, reddened and sore eyes, jaundice with or without heptatitis, aching of joint muscles, long bones; sores on body or generalized fine rash (cutaneous eruptions) condylomatoa auminate (veneral warts) in rectum or genitalia.

Exudates from lesions highly contagious, blood contains organisms. Duration of state is 1-2 years.

- *Latent stage:* No clinical signs—Absence of signs and symptoms. Duration will be 5-20 years. Contagious for about 2 years; not contagious to others after that. Blood contains organism and may be transmitted placentally to foetus. Duration of stage is throughout life or progresses to late stage.
- *Late stage:* Appearance 3-20 years after initial infection. Non-infectious Chronic (without treatment) is possibly fatal. The characteristic finding includes the following.
- *Benign:* Tumour-like mass (Gummas) on any area of the body. They are chronic destructive lesions affecting any organ of the body especially skin, bone, liver and mucus membrane.
- *Cardiovascular:* There will be damage to heart valves and blood vessels aortic valve insufficiency or occular aneurysm of thoracic aorta and aortitis.
- *Neurosyphilis:* Spinal fluid possible contains organism. There will be meningitis, general paresis (Personality changes for minor to psychotic tremors. Physical and mental deterioration). Paralysis, and Taber dorsales (ataxia, areflexia, paresthesias, lightening pains, damaged joints-charcots joints) paresis, insomnia, confusion, delirium, impaired judgement and slurred speech.

Management

Management of syphilis is aimed at eradication of all syphilitic organisms. (Early syphilis (primary, secondary, or early latent) treated with a single dose of Benzathin Penocillin-G (IM) at single visit. Other antibiotics used are Doxycycline, Tetracycline or Erythromycin. Syphilis lasting below 1 year is treated with three weekly injections of Benzathin Penicillin (G) (IM). The symptomatic neurosyphilis is treated by aqueous crystalline penicillin (IV) daily for 14 days followed by penicillin or Benzathin weekly for 3 doses. The other antibiotics such as Doxycyclin, Tetracyclin and Erythromycin are used.

Appropriate antibiotic treatment of maternal syphilis before 10th week of pregnancy prevents infection of the foetus. All patients with neurosyphilis may be carefully monitored with periodic serologic testing, clinical evaluation for 6-month interval and repeat CSF examination for at least 3 years. Specific management is based on the presenting symptoms. Take preventive measures as in gonorrhoea.

Herpes Genitalis

Herpes genitalis (Genital herpes-HSV-2) is caused by infections with Herpes virus hormonis type 2 (HSV-2) HSV-2 can be transmitted from genitalis to mouth through oral-genital contact. Once acquired, herpes genitalis is a 'life-long' disease and carries with it not only intense and recurrent discomfort, but also anxieties about future childbearing malignancy, and sexual and marital function. In early pregnancy, women infected with herpes have an increased change of miscarriage. It endangers the foetus during delivery, caesarian delivery is often necessary. It is also associated with cervical cancer.

Pathophysiology

The incubation period is 3 to 7 days. The primary lesions appear as a vesicle on the external genitalia in men; often on the rectum in homosexual men and on the vagina, cervix or external genitalia of women. These lesions often ulcerate, especially when located on moist surfaces. Following primary herpes, the virus persists in a latent or unrecognized form in most patients. It is believed that latent infections are localized in the ganglia of sensory nerves to the genitalia. When the host factors favour it, the latent infection becomes clinically apparent as recurrent herpes.

Clinical Manifestation

A patient with primary HIV-2 infection may initially complain of burning or tingling at the side of inoculation. Vesicular lesions, which may occur on the penis, scrotum, vulva, perineum, perianal region, vagina, cervix, contain large quantities of infectious viral particles. The lesion scrupture and form shallow, moist ulcerations. Finally, crusting and epitheliazation of the erosions occur. Primary infections tend to be associated with local inflammation and pain, accompanied by systemic manifestations of fever, headache, malaise, myalgia and regional lymphadenopathy.

Urination may be painful from urine touching active lesions. Retention may occur as a result of HSV urethritis or cytitis. A purulent vaginal discharge may develop with HSV cervicitis. The duration of the symptoms is longer and the frequency of complications is greater in women. Transmission of genital herpes, therefore, can occur by sexual contact with an excreter of virus who is free from symptoms. Primary lesions are generally present 17 to 20 days, but new lesions sometimes continue to develop for 6 weeks.

Management

Diagnosis of genital herpes is usually based on the patient's symptoms and history. Other diagnostic measures include viral isolation by tissue culture and cytologic examination of vesicular exudate for multinucleated giant cells.

1. *Primary infection:*
   - Acyclovir (Zovirax) 400 mg orally tid and 7-10 days or
   - Acyclovir 200 mg orally five times a day and 7-10p days or
   - Famiclovir (Famvir) 250 mg orally tid and 7-10 days or
   - Vallyclovir (Valtrex) 1 gm orally twice a day for 7-5 or 10 days.
2. *Recurrent infection*
   - Acyclovir 400 mg orally three times a day and 5 days or.
   - Acyclovir 200 mg orally five times a day x 5 days or.
   - Famciclovir 125 mg orally twice a day x 5 days.
   - Valcyclovir 500 mg orally twice a day x 5 days.
   - Attempt to identify trigger mechanisms).
   - Yearly pap smear.
   - Abstinence from sexual contact while lesions are present. However, it may shed virus without lesions.
   - Provision of symptomatic intervention.
   - Confidential counselling and testing of HIV.

Above drugs are used as daily suppressive therapy for frequent recurrence and severe infection as directed by doctor.

Chlamydial Infections

Chlamydia trachomatis, a gram-negative bacterium, is recognized as a genital pathogen that is responsible for an increasing variety of clinical illnesses.

Aetiology

Chlamydia trachomatis is caused by C. trachomatis, chlamydial infection is recognised as the most prevalent of the STDs. Age, number of sex partners, socio-economic status and sexual orientation are predictors of infection with C. trachomatis.

- *Age:* Infection is rather one, two to three times higher, in sexually active, women under the age of 20 years. The rates of urethral infection are higher teenage males than for adult men.
- *Number of sex partners:* Persons with several sex partners are at higher risk of infection.
- *Socioeconomic status:* Persons at lower socio-economic stratum are at increased risk for infrection with C. trachomatis.
- *Sexual preference:* The prevalence of urethral chlamydial infection among homosexual men is one-third then among heterosexual men. Chlamydial infections can be transmitted

to infants during delivery, causing conjunctivities and pneumonia in many. The incidence of chlamydial is highest in young, promiscuous, indigent, unmarried women who live in the inner city and in those who have had a prior history of STDs.

Pathophysiologym

Chlamydia trachomatis is an intracellular parasite that has specific requirements for adenosine triphosphate (ATP) and amino acids. There are two stages in the life cycle of the organism. In stage I, the infective stage, the elementary body attaches to the host cell and the ingested by phagocytosis. In stage II, the elementary body undergoes metamorphosis to become a reticulate or initial body. This is the metabolic phase of the life cycle. The initial body duplicates by binary fission and changes into elementary body. The host cell, which contains the elementary body, undergoes lysis, liberating infectious organisms that are capable of reinfecting new cells.

The chlamydial infection in males include urethritis, postgenococal urethritis, prostitis, conjunctivitis, pharyngitis and subclicinal LGV. In addition, female cervicitis includes chlamydial infection transmitted to infants by mothers causing conjunctivitis, pneumonia, asymptomatic pharyngeal carriage and gastrointestinal carriage.

The complication in men includes epididymitis, prostratitis Reiter's syndrome, sterility and rectal strictures, and in women, salpingitis, endometritis, perihepatitis, ectopic pregnancy, infertility vulvar/rectal carcinoma and rectal strictures are the complications.

Management

Chlamydial infections respond to treatment with doxycycline (vibramycin) azithomycin (zithromax) or ofloxacin (floxin). It is important that the patient encourages sexual partner(s) to seek care as soon as possible to avoid reinfection of the patient and complications in the partner. Patients who are sexually active should be advised to wear condoms or use of spermicides to prevent reinfection. Social and emotional support of these patients is important as it is with any person with STD.

Lymphogranuloma Venereum

Lymphogranuloma venereum (LGV) is a chronic STD caused by specific strains of C. trachomatis are, i.e. serotype L1, L2 and L3 of C-trachomatis.

The disease is contracted by vaginal, anal or oral intercourses, primary inoculation with the organism may occur at any site involved in closed contact. The incubation period is 3 to 30 days. Lymphadens it is of regional lymph node drainage the site of primary infection occurs and the disease spreads by way of the lymphatic system.

Pathophysiology

The three clinical phases of infection in LGV are:

- Inoculation and appearance of the primary lesion.
- Lymphatic spread and generalized symptoms and
- Late complication.

In individual case, any one of the phases may be absent or unnoticed. The primary lesions which is transient appears as papula, small erosion or vesicle. These are present in the prepuce and glans penis in male and vagina and cervix in females. They are painless. Local oedema may be present. If the rectum is infected, a bloody discharge followed by mucopurulent discharge, diarrhoea and cramping.

Involvement of the lympatic occurs 1 to 4 weeks after the appearance of primary lesion. Penile, vulvar and anal infection can lead to inguinal or femoral lymphadenopathy. Marked inflammation occurs resulting in necrosis, buboes, absesses and inguinal lymph nodes, and infection of surrounding tissue. Healing occurs by fibrosis after several weeks or months and results in scarring which damages lymph nodes and disrupt nodal function.

Constitutional symptoms that occur during the stage of regional lymphadenopathy include fever, chills, headache, meningitis, anorexia, myalgia, and arthalgia. Complication of untreated anorectal infection include perirectal absess, fisutala, in ano, and rectovaginal, rector vesical and ishiorectal fistulas.

Management

LGV is treated with 2-week course of tetracycline, sex partners should also be treated. The patient may require much counselling and teaching as they deal with their disease. Because the fluctuant lymph nodes may be disturbing to the patient self-image, social and emotional support is very much important.

Chancroid

Chancroid is an STD caused by a gram-negative bacillus. "Haemophilus ducreyi: Chancroid has been established as a cofactor for HIV transmission and high rate of HIV infection among patients with chancroid.

Pathophysiology

The initial lesions are acutely tender genital ulcers, lymphadenopathy, and tender buboes. The buboes which are fluctuant, inguinal node masses may suppurate and lead to abscesses. Exudate from the ulcers or aspirate from the buboes is stained and a "shool-of-fish" pattern may be noted on microscopic examination by some one experienced in interpretation. In women, the lesions of the chancroid are most often found in the labia, anus, clitoris, vagina and cervix. Some women do not have lesions but may have mild vaginitis. In men, the lesions appear on the prepuce, glans or shaft of the penis.

Clinical manifestation

The ulcers found in chanceroid are typically ragged and irregular. They are highly infectious and autoimmunity occurs resulting in multiple lesions. The ulcer appears excavated, have a granulating purulent surface and are painful. Often oedema of the surrounding tissue is persistent. The buboes which are most often unilateral, painful and spheric in shape. The skin over the buboes is inflammed. These buboes tend to become softer in abscess form. These abscesses in turn may suppurate and rupture, further spreading infection usually appear when inguinal abscess is formed.

Management

Follow-up is essential, because, treatment failure may occur. The individual is taught to report any sign or symptom that persists or worsen during treatment and abstain from sexual activity until lesions are healed. Proper use of condom should be stressed.

Granuloma Inguinale (Donovanoses)

Granuloma inguinale or granuloma venereum is believed to be most often transmitted by sexual contact, although nonsexual transmission has been reported.

Aetiology

Granuloma inguinale caused by a gram-negative bacillus "Calymmato Bacterium (Donovania) granulomatis" is widely referred to as DONOVAN BACILLUS. The disease is mildly contagious and probably requires repeated exposure for spread of infection. Predisposing factors are poorly understood. The disease is most common in men than women and is particularly common in homosexual men. The incubation period varies from several days to several months.

Pathophysiology

Lesions appear on the genitalia and in the perianal areas. The most common sites of lesions are the prepuce and glans in men and the vagina and the labia in women. The infection first appears with development of subcutaneous nodules. These elevated areas eventually ulcerate, producing sharply defined painless lesions. The ulcers enlarge slowly and bleed on contact. With ulceration, the infection tends to spread along the pubic region. Involvement of the lymph nodes is uncommon but can occur and produce occlusions of the lymphatics resulting in elephantasis.

Management

Treatment with suitable antibiotics and clinician follow-up of anyone diagnosed with granuloma inguinale is extremely important due to the possibility of the treatment failure. All persons should be advised to abstain from sexual activity until all sexual partners complete a course of treatment.

Condylomata Acuminata (Genital Warts)

Condylomota acuminata (Genital Warts) is caused by human papillomavirus (HPV) and highly contagious STD is seen frequently in young, sexually active adults.

Aetiology

Genital warts are sexually transmitted and are the most commonly recognized clinical signs of genital HPV infections. They are important because of their possible role in the development of cervical cancer. The incubation period of the virus is generally 1 to 6 months, but may be longer. The disease is most common in adolescent girls and young women. HPV can remain dormant for decades before recurrences occur.

Pathophysiology

Minor trauma during the sexual intercourse can cause abrasions that allow HPV to enter the body. The epithelial cells infected with HPV undergo transformation, proliferate and form a warty growth. Immunosuppressed persons, pregnant women and diabetics are most susceptible to HPV. Genital warts occur in or around the vulva, vagina, cervix perineum, anal canal, urethra and glans penis. They enlarge during pregnancy and may cause haermorrhage or obstruction during delivery.

Clinical Manifestation

Condylomata acuminatal lesions are discrete single or multiple papillary growths that are white to gray. The warts may grow and coalese to form large cauliflower-like masses. In men, the warts may occur on the penis and scrotum, around the anus and or in the urethra. In women, the warts may be located on the vulva, vagina and the cervix and in preanal area. During pregnancy, genital warts tend to grow rapidly. An infected mother transmits the conditions to her newborn. Bleeding on defecation may occur with anal warts. The genitalis and anorectal region as well as urethra, bladder and oral mucosa may be affected. Research has linked HPV infection with cervical and vulvalar cancer in women and with anorectal and squamous cell carcinoma of the penis in men.

Management

Warts may be confused with condylomata, secondary syphilis, carcinoma or benign tumours. Serologic and cytologic testing should be done. If dysplasia confirmed by pap smear, colposcopic examination and biopsies should be performed. Virapap a test that uses DNA hybridization techniques can be used.

The primary goal, when treating visible genital warts, is the removal of the symptomatic warts. The removal may or may not decrease infectivity. One common treatment is the use of 80 per cent and 90 per cent trichloroacetic acid (TCA) applied directly to the wart surface. Petroleum jelly is applied to the surrounding normal skin to minimize irritation before a small amount of TCA is applied to the wart with a cotton swab. A sharp stinging pain is often felt with initial acid contact, but this quickly subsides. TCA is not washed off after treatment. It can be used in pregnant women.

Podophyllin (10-25 per cent) a cytotoxic agent is recommended therapy for small external genital warts when it is used, it is applied carefully to each wart with normal tissue being avoided, and is then thoroughly washed off in 1 to 4 hours. The substance encourages the sloughing off of skin containing viral particles,. Podophyllin has local (e.g. pain, burning) and sestemic (e.g. nausea, dizziness, leukopoenia respiratory distress), toxic symptoms. It is contraindicated in pregnant women.

Patient managed treatment is also an option. Podofilox liquid and gel are available (condylox and condylox gel). Patient applies solution or gel for 3 successive days followed by 4 days if no treatment can be repeated upto 4 weeks.

If the wart does not regress with any of these therapies, treatment such as cryotherapy with liquid nitrogen, electrocautery, laser therapy 5-Fluoracid, and surgical excision may be indicated.

Prevention of HPV should be stressed. It includes:

Avoiding sexual relationship with persons in known high-risk groups.

- Using latex condoms if having sexual intercourse and
- Avoiding anal intercourse.

Caesarean delviery may be indicated for warts obstructing the pelvic outlet or if a vaginal birth would cause excessive bleeding of the warts.

Trichomoniasis

Trichomoniasis is caused by the protozoan, "Trichomonal Vaginalis". Evidence suggests that the incubation period range between 4 to 28 days. It is most often sexually transmitted by such as towels, toilet seats, and so on. The parasite commonly exists in vaginal or cervical secretions and in seminal fluid. It is estimated that one of five females will have a trichomonal infection during one's life time.

Pathophysiology Clinical Manifestations

Trichomoniasis is commonly viewed as an innoculous infection. Yet there are serious implications for health. During the postpartum period in women who have trichomoniasis, the rate of persistent fever, prolonged vaginal discharge and endometritis is twice as high as in women who do not harbour the organism. Majority of patients with trichomoniasis have cervical rosions and leukorrhoea and has been suggested that chronic irritation may predispose to cervical cancer.

Management

The CDC recommends that both partners be treated simultaneously with metronidazole to prevent reinfection by the untreated partner at a later date. Vaginal inserts of metronidazole in the woman alone are less effective. The drug is known to cross the placental barrier. For this reason it is not given to pregnant women until after the first trimester.

Bacterial Vaginosis

Bacterial vaginosis is the most common vaginal infection among women of childbearing age. Studies have linked it with preterm labour, infections of amniotic fluids, postpartum uterine infections, and PID. It is characterized by an overgrowth of normal flora resulting from introduction of other flora and altered vaginal pH related to sexual activity or poor hygienic practices.

Pathophysiology

Bacterial vaginosis infection characterized by a small amount of homogenous gray or grayish, white discharge. The discharge usually has a disagreeable odour and because it is less irritating than discharge caused by other organism, pruritis is mild or absent. On inspection, the vaginal walls are slightly reddened and the discharge appears to adhere to the mucosal lining.

Management

Self-care measures should be emphasized. These include use of condoms for 4 to 6 weeks after diagnosis, limiting hygienic douching to vinegar and water and wiping from front to back after voiding.

Hepatitis B Virus

Hepatitis B Virus (HBV) is a DNA virus that causes acute or chronic hepatitis, cirrhosis, and hepatocellular carcinoma. There are more than 300 million persons infected world over. The risk of developing HBV infection is greatest in infants at birth and declines with age.

Aetiology

Transmission from mother to neonates if mother is positive for hepatitis B antigen (HBcAg). HSV transmitted sexually and risk factors include multiple sexual partners, a history of STD and homosexuality especially with receptive anal intercourse. It is also transmitted by drug abusers who share needles and by needle sticks by health care workers. It is not transmitted through blood transfusion. Other risk factors include patients on haemodialysis and those who are hospitalized.

Pathophysiology

The hepatitis caused by HBV results in the same symptoms seen in other types of hepatitis. The liver is inflammed and the patient may have jaundice, anorexia, slight fever and gastrointestinal upset, etc.

Management

The centre of disease control of prevent (CDC) recommends vaccination for persons identified as being at high risk, including residents of correctional or long-term care facilities, persons seeking treatment for STD, prostitutes, homosexuals and promiscuous heterosexuals. The CDC also recommends that all children regardless of their exposure to risk stated against

HBV. The vaccine is given at birth, 1 month and 6 months. If serum HBs Ag is not detected after 5 to 7 years, a booster dose of the vaccine should be considered. Vaccination also is recommended for all health care providers/workers possibly by needle sticks. Postexposure prophylactive treatment with hepatitis B immune globules (HBIG) given to the person who had sexual contact with HBV positive partner of HBV carriers.

In addition to those diseases already discussed, pediculosis pubis molluscum conagiosum and scabies are considered to be STDs.

Role of Nurses in Prevention of Control of STDs

The nurses' first responsibility in STD control is to educate person who have sexually transmitted infection or may develop one. Nurses must be knowledgeable about the most prevalent diseases and the signs and symptoms, methods used in diagnosis, treatments and where individual can obtain help and information. Many approaches to curtailing the spread of STDs have been advocated and have met with varying degrees of success. Nurses should be prepared to discuss practices with all patients, not only those who are perceived to be at risk. These 'safe' set practices include abstinence, monogamy, with an uninfected partners, avoidance of certain high risk sexual practices, and use of condoms and other barriers to limit contact with potentially-infectious body fluids or lesions. Sexual abstinence is a certain method of avoiding all STDs, but few adults consider this as feasible alternative to sexual expression. Limiting sexual intimacies, outside of a well-established monogamous relationship can reduce the risk of contracting a STD.

Nurses can exert influence on the community by taking an active role in education programmes. Patient teaching should include the following:

- Explain the importance of taking all antibiotics as prescribed. Symptoms will improve after 1-2 days of therapy, but organism may still be present.
- Teach patient about the need for treatment of sexual partners with antibiotics to prevent transmission of disease.
- Instruct patient to abstain from sexual intercourse during treatment and to use of condoms when sexual activity is resumed to prevent spread of infection and prevent reinfection.
- Explain the importance of follow-up examination and reculture at least once after treatment if appropriate to confirm complete cure and prevent relapse.
- Allow patient and partner to verbalize concerns to clarify areas that need explanation.
- Instruct patient about symptoms of complications and need to report problems to ensure proper follow-up and early treatment of reinfection.

Explain precautions to take, such as being monogamous, asking potential partners about sexual history, avoiding sex with partners, who has IV drugs or who have visible oral, inguinal, genital, perineal or anal lesions, using condoms; voiding and washing genitalia after intercourse (coitus) to reduce the occurrence of reinfection.

- Inform patient regarding state of ineffectivity to prevent a false sense of security, which might result in careless sexual practices and poor personal hygiene.

All sexually active women should be screened for cervical cancer.

HIV INFECTION AND AIDS

HIV infection is one of the most dreadful diseases. Individuals infected with HIV has thus far eventually developed 'Acquired Immuno Deficiency Syndrome (AIDS)'. AIDS severally compromises the body's ability to fight various infections and some forms of cancer. The incidence of HIV infections and AIDS continues to increase steadily worldwide. Therefore, nurses must understand the critical concepts related to this problem. AIDS was considered to be universally fatal until quite recently. Advances in drug treatment, however, are delaying the onset of AIDS for selected persons infected with HIV and are giving new hopes to infected persons.

Aetiology

AIDS is an acquired viral disease. The virus integrates itself into CD4 (T4 helper) cells, causing immune dysfunction and rendering the infected person unusually susceptible to life-threatening infections and malignancies. The causative agent of AIDS is infection with HIV, a human retrovirus that belongs to the Lentivirus subfamily. Several human retroviruses have been identified. Two of them, HIV-1 and HIV-2 have been associated with T4 helper cell depletion, resulting in loss of cellular immunity characterized by AIDS.

The routes for transmission of HIV are well-documented, which includes:

1. Directly from person to person by sexual contact.
2. Direct inoculation with contaminated blood products, needles, or syringes and
3. From infected mothers to her foetus or newborn.

HIV is a fragile virus that can only be transmitted under specific conditions that allow contact with infected body fluids, including blood, semen, vaginal secretions, cerebrospinal fluid, saliva, tears and breast milk. However, blood, semen and vaginal' secretions are the primary routes of infection. Epidemiological studies indicate that transmission through body fluids such as saliva, tears and breast milk is inefficient and unlikely to produce infection.

HIV is not transmitted by casual contacts, including sneezing, coughing, spitting, handshakes, contact with potential secretions on toilet seats, bath tubs, showers, swimming pools, utensils, dishes or lime used by infected persons. Mosquito bites are not a source of infection.

HIV is a blood-borne STD. During any form of sexual intercourse, (anal, vaginal or oral), the risk of infection is considerably greater for the partner who received the semen, although infection can also be transmitted to an inserted partner. The increased risk occurs because the receiver has prolonged contact with the semen; this helps to explain why women are more easily infected than men during heterosexual intercourse. The risk factors for HIV infection are summarised as follows:

i. Sexual practices.
   - Unprotected sex (without condom use).
   - Multiple sexual partners.
   - Anal or oral sexual activity.
   - Improper condom use or condom breakage.
   - Open sore, lesions or irritations in the genital area.
ii. Contaminated blood.
iii. Contaminated needle (For SC or 1M or IV, etc).
iv. Occupational exposure.
   - All health care workers-acute care long-term care, and home care (Doctors, Nurses and others).
   - Dental workers.
   - Correction officers and law enforcement personnel (Police and others).
v. Perinatal exposure (during pregnancy, birth or breast-feeding).

Approximately 25 per cent children of HIV-positive mothers are infected with HIV.

Pathophysiology

The natural history of HIV infection is associated with unpredictable course of disease progression. Many patients undergo a prolonged period of clinically-silent infection, often lasting for more than 10 years. Although the virus is consistently detectable throughout this time, patients typically have only soluble immunological alterations. Once the patient becomes symptomatic, however, decreases in the number of T4 helper cells can be detected and viral replication increases.

The life cycle of HIV is similar to that of the other retroviruses, mature visions interact with specific host receptors and then use the host cell for viral replication. HIV interacts with the CD4 glycoprotein, which occurs on the membrane of the specific cells, primarily the CD4 + (T4) helper lymphocytes. The CD4 protein may also be found on the surface of several other cells as well, including some monocytes, macrophages, glial cells and gastrointestinal cells (GI). Presence of the CD4 and glycoprotein allow the virus fuse to the host cell. The viral core is subsequently injected into the cell cytoplasm, where the viral ribonucleic acid (RNA) genome is translated into dioxyribonucleic acid (DNA) by a retroviral enzyme called reverse transcription. Infection and subsequent viral replication eventually depletes the hosts T4 helper cells, resulting in a dramatics loss of the protective immune response against invading micro-organism.

Many potential co-factors may be associated with HIV disease progression. These co-factors which may be viral, host, or environmental are thought to directly influence the replication of HIV or the severity of its pathogenic effects. *Viral co-factors* that may influence the progression of the disease include herpes simplex virus (HSV) cytomegalovirus) (CMV) Epstein-Barr and (EBV).

Host Co-factors may include variety of cytokines and intracellular mediators. *Environmental* co-factors may induce hyperactivation of the immune system, resulting in an expansion of the pool of HIV, and replicating cells. As viral replication increases and depletes the body of T4 lympocytes, the body's defense mechanism is progressively weekened. Infections that were once disarmed by the healthy immune system are eventually able to cause serious and potentially life-threatening disease. The spectrum of HIV infection ranges from a symptomatic to potentially life-threatening opportunistic infection.

Clinical Manifestation

The early phases of infection with HIV varies from person to person. Some individuals experience symptoms similar to flu or mononucleosis, consisting of fever, fatigue, nausea, vomiting, headache, rash or lymphadenopathy. Symptoms may be mild or serious enough to warrant hospitalization. It is during this time that the viral load (amount of HIV present) is very high, CD and helper cells drop dramatically and the person converts to seropositive HIV status. The initial phase of infection may be followed by a period of latency that may last from several months to 10 years or more. During this time, the person may be completely asymptomatic or experience only mild symptoms such as fatigue. As the immune system becomes further compromised, the symptoms of AIDS develop. Clinical manifestations associated with AIDS are primarily those of opportunistic infections. The common symptoms include the following.

- Chills and fever
- Night sweats
- Dry productive cough
- Dyspnoea
- Lethargy
- Confusion
- Stiff neck
- Seizures
- Headache
- Malaise
- Fatigue
- Oral lesions
- Skin rash
- Abdominal discomfort
- Diarrhoea
- Weight loss
- Lymphadenopathy
- Progressive generalized oedema

The complications of HIV disease present a complex picture of opportunistic infections, neoplasms or condition related to immunodeficiency. If not treated in time, symptoms of opportunistic infection also develop. The common AIDS—Related opportunistic infection includes the following:

- *Bacterial infections:* Mycobacterium avium complex (MAC), Mycobacterium tuberculosis causes fever, diarrhoea and profound wasting.
- *Fungal infections:* Candidiasis (Thrush or vaginal infection), Cryptococcosis (causes meningitis), Histoplasmosis (Associated with fever and weight loss).
- *Protozoal infection:* Cryptosporidium (causes fulminant diarrhoea) Pneumocytis, Carinu (Ac. Resp. failure), Toxoplasma gondii (causes encephalitis).
- *Viral infections* HSV, CMV, (cause Retinitis, blindness).
- *HIV-related cancer:* Kaposis sarcoma, non-Hodgkin's lymphomas, cervical cancer.

HIV can cross the blood-brain barrier, attach to microglial cells and cause encephalopathy or more dysfunction.

Management

HIV infection or AIDS is diagnosed when an individual with HIV has at least one of these additional conditions.

1. CD^{4+T} cell count drops below 200/ml
2. Development of one of the following opportunistic infections (OIs)
   - *Fungal:* Candidiasis of bronchi, trachea, lungs or oesophgus pneumocystis carinu pneumonia (PCP), disseminated or extrapulmonary hissopharmosis.
   - *Viral:* Cytomegalovirus (CMV) disease other than liver, spleen or nodes CMV retinitis (with loss of vision); herpes simple with chronic ulcer or bronchitis, pneumonitis, or esophagitis, progressive multifocal leucoencephalopathy (PML), extrapulmonary cryptococcosis.
   - *Protozoal:* Disseminant or extrapulmonary coccidiomycosis, toxoplasmosis of the brain; chronic intestinal isosporiasis; chronic intestinal cryptosporidiasis.
   - *Bacteria:* Mycobacterium tuberculosis (any site); any disseminated or extrapulmonary mycobacterium including MAC or M. Kansasii, recurrent pneumonia; recurrent salmonella septicemia.
3. Development of one of the following opportunistic cancers: Invasive cervical cancer and Kaposic Sarcoma (KS). Burkitts lymphoma, immunoblastic lymphoma, or primary lymphoma of the brain.
4. *Wasting syndrome occurs:* Wasting syndrome defined as a loss of 10 per cent or more of ideal body mass.
5. *Dementia develops:* The most useful screening test for HIV are those that detect HIV-specific antibodies. The most commonly used test is the enzyme-linked-immunosorbent assay (ELISA). A positive ELISA must be confirmed by the western blot technique. Both depend on antibody formation. The following steps are used in the process of testing blood for antibodies to HIV:

1. A highly sensitive enzyme immunoassay (EIA, ELISA) is done to detect serum antibodies that bind to HIV antigens on test plates; blood samples that are negative on this test are reported as negative.
2. If the blood is LIA reactive, the test is repeated.
3. If the blood is repeatedly EIA reactive, a more specific confirmatory test, such as the western blot (WB) or Immunoflurescence assay (IFA) is done.
   - Western blot (WB) testing used purified HIV antigens electrophoresed on gels. These are incubated with serum samples of antibody in the serum, it is present it can be detected.
   - IFA is used to identify HIV in injected cells. Blood is located with a fluorescent antibody against pH or p^{24} antigen and then examined using a fluorescent microscope.
4. Blood that is reactive in all of the first three steps is reported as HIV antibody positive.
5. If the results are indeterminant, testing should be repeated within 6 months. Consistently in determinant test results require the use of polymerase chain reaction (PCR), viral culture, and other diagnostic measures.
   - PCR analysis DNA extracted from lymphocytes and/ or HIV from serum using an *invitro* amplification procedure.
   - A cell culture system can be used to grow viruses from infected lymphocytes.

Since these tests are expensive and difficult to do, they are usually not used for screening purposes, but may be done in situations where the index of suspicion is high and antibodies are negative. HIV can be classified as laboratory categories as follows: (CDC 1993).

- Category I: Greater than or equal to 500 CD 4 + Cells.
- Category II: 200 to 499 CD4 + Cells.
- Category III: Less than 200 CD4+ Cells.

HIV classification for adolescents and adults according to revised centers for Disease Control and Prevention (CDC 1993) as *Clinical Categories* are as follows:

Category A: One or more of the following conditions are occurring in a adolescent or adult with documented HIV infection. Conditions listed in categories B and C must not have occurred.

- Asymptomatic HIV infection.
- Persistent generalized lymphadenopathy.
- Acute (Primary) HIV infection with accompanying illness or history of acute HIV infection.

Category B: Symptomatic conditions occurring in an HIV

infected adolescents or adult that are not included among conditions listed in category C and that meet at least one of the following criteria.

- The conditions are attributed to HIV infection or are indicative of a defect in cell-mediated immunity.
- The conditions are considered by physicians to have a clinical course or management that is complicated by HIV infection.

Examples of conditions in clinical category B include but are not limited to:

- Bacterial endocarditis, meningitis, pneumonia, or sepsis.
- Candidiasis and oropharyngeal (thrush).
- Cervical dysplasia, severe, or carcinoma.
- Constitutional symptoms such as fever (greater than 38.5°C) or diarrhoea lasting for more than a month.
- Hairy leukoplakia, oral.
- Herpes Zoster (Shingles), involving at least two distinct episodes or more than one dermatome.
- Idiopathic thrombocytopoenic purpura.
- Listeriosis.
- Mycobacterium tuberculosis infection and pulmonary.
- Nocardiosis.
- Pelvic inflammatory disease.
- Peripheral neuropathy.

Category C: Any condition that has occurred, the person will remain in Category C, i.e.

- The conditions clinical category C are strongly associated with severe immunodeficiency, occur frequently in HIV-infected patients and cause serious morbidity or mortality.
- According to proposed classification system, HIV-infected patient would be classified on the basis of both:
  - The lowest accurate (not necessarily the most recent) CD4+ lymphocyte determination and
  - The most severe clinical condition diagnosed regardless of the patients current clinical condition.

Treatment

There are no specific treatment in the early stages of HIV infections. Respiratory treatment may become necessary as the patient's disease progresses. Standard precautions are necessary when the patient is hospitalized or being treated at home. Treatment associated with maintenance and improvement of nutritional status also usually become necessary. Specific treatment related to opportunistic infections are briefly discussed as given below:

Respiratory System

- *Pneumocystis carinil Pneumonea (PCP):* There will be nonproductive cough, hypoxaemia, progressive shortness of breath, fever, night sweat and fatigue. This is diagnosed by chest-X-ray, induced sputum culture and bronchoalveolar lavage. It can be treated by Bactrim, Cleocin Mepron and Crosicosteroids.
- *Histoplasma capsulatum:* In this, there will be pneumonia, fever, cough weight loss, disseminated disease. Diagnosis made by sputum culture, serum or urine antigen assay. This is treated by using amphotericin, B, itoconazole (Sporanax) and fluconazole (Diflucon).
- *Coccidioides immitis:* There will be fever, weight loss, cough, test includes sputum culture, serology, treatment as in histoplasma capsulature.
- *Mycobacteria TB:* There will be a productive cough, fever, night sweats, weight loss, diagnosis by chest X-ray, sputum for AFB and culture. Treated by antituberculosis drugs, INH, Streptomycin, Regampicin.
- *Kaposis sarcoma:* There is dyspnoea, respiratory failure, chest X-ray and biopsy all helps to diagnose. Cancer chemotherapy and radiation are the treatments.

Integumentary System

- *HSV1 and HSV2:* Orolabial mucocutaneous ulcerative lesions (Type 1) genital and perineal mucocutaneous ulcerative lesion (Type 2) Do viral culture and treat with acyclovir, famiclovir valacyclovir (valtrex).
- *Varicell Zoster vira (VZV):* Shingles, erythematous maculopapular rash along dermatromal planes, pain, pruritus are seen. Do viral culture and treat with acyclovir famuclovir (famvir) valtrax and foscarret (foscavir).
- *Kaposis Sarcoma:* Firm, flat, raised nodular, hyperpigmented, multice lesions found in skin, Do biopsy lesions. Treat with cancer chemotherapy, alpha interferon, radiation of lesions.
- *Bacillary angiomatosis:* Erythematus vascular papules, subcutaneous nodules are seen on skin. Do Biopsy and treatment with erythromycin, doxcycline.

Eye

- *CMV retinitis:* Lesions on the retina, blurred vision, loss of vision. Do ophthalmoscopic exam and treat with canciclovir (cytovene) foscarret or cidofovir (vistide).
- *HSV1:* Blurred vision: corneal lesions, acute retinal necrosis, or ophthalmoscopy examination. Treat with acyclovir, famciclovir, etc.
- *VZV:* Ocular lesions, acute retinal necrosis. Do ophthalmoscopy and treat with antiviral drugs.

GI System

- Cryptosporidium muris: Watery diarrhoea, abdominal pain, weight loss, and nausea are seen. Do stool examination, small bowel or colon biopsy. Treat with anti-diarrheals, flaramomycine, azithromycin, asovaquone and sandostatin (Octero tide).

- *CMV:* Stomatitis, oesophagitis, gastritis, colitis, diarrhoea, bloody diarrhoea, pain, weight loss. Do endoscopic visualization, culture, biopsy for ruling out the causes and treat with ganciclovir and antiviral drugs.
- *HSV:* Vesicular eruption on tongue, buccal, pharyngeal or perioral oesophage 1 mucose seen. Do viral culture, administer antiviral drugs.
- *Candida-Albicans:* There will be whitish-yellow patches in mouth, oesophagus, GI tract. Do microscopic examination for scraping from lesion, culture. Administration of flucanozole, nystatin, clotrimazol (lotrimin), itroconazole and amphotericin B are helpful.
- *Mycrobacterium Avium Complex (MAC):* There will be watery diarrhoea, weight loss. Do small bowel biopsy with AFB stain and culture. Administer clarithromycin (Biaxin) rifampin, ciproflaxacin, azithromycin according to culture.
- *Isospora belli:* Diarrhoea, weight loss, nausea, abdominal pain are seen. Do stool examination. Small bowel colon biopsy. Treat with trimethoprim-sulfamethoxazole, pyrimethamine + folinic acid.
- *Salmonella:* Gastroenteritis, fever and diarrhoea. Do stool and blood culture. Administer ciprofloxacin, ampicillin, amoxicillin-Sep.
- *Kaposis Sarcoma:* There will be diarrhoea, hyperpigmented lesions in mouth and GI tract. Do GI series and biopsy. Treat cancer with chemotherapy, alpha-interferon and radiation.
- *nonHodgkin's lymphoma:* There will be abdominal pain, fever, night sweats, weight loss, Do lymph node biopsy and treatment with chemotherapy.

Neurologic System

- *Toxoplasma gondii:* There is cognitive dysfunction, motor impairment, fever, altered mental status, headache, seizures, sensory abnormalities, diagnosis by MRI, CT scan toxoplasma serology and brain biopsy, Treat with pyrimethamine + folinic acid + sulfadiazine, clindamycin azithromycin clarithromycin.
- *JC Papovirus:* Progressive multifocal leukoencephalopathy (PML), Mental and motor declines; diagnosis by MRI, CT scan and brain biopsy; effective antiretroviral therapy may help.
- *Cryptococcal meningitis:* There is cognitive impairment, motor dysfunction, fever, seizures, headache, CT scan, serum, antigen test, CSF analysis and will help to diagnosis. Treatment with amphaterrcin B, flucystosine, flucanozole, helps.
- *CNS lymphomas:* Cognitive dysfunction, motor impairment, aphasia, seizures, personality charges, headache, Do MRI, CT scan. Treat with radiation and chemotherapy.
- *AIDS-dementia complex (ADC):* There is insidious onset of progressive diementia. Do CT scan. Effective antiretroviral therapy may help.

Nursing Management

Health assessment of all patients should include an appraisal of potential risk factors for HIV infection. For obtaining complete, accurate sexual history including past and present sexual activities, skilful interviewing techniques and professional relationship based on trust are required. Nurses need to be able to explain the need for information on intimate sexual activities and phrase questions in appropriate but comprehensive terms.

A major goal of health promotions is to prevent disease. HIV infection is preventable until a vaccine is available; education and behavioural changes are the only effective tools. Educational messages should be specific to the patients' need, culturally sensitive, language appropriate and age-specific. Nurses are excellent resources for this type of education, but nurses must be comfortable with and knowledgeable about sensitive topics such as sexuality and drug use. Risk-reducing sexual activities decrease the risk of contact with HIV through the use of barriers. Barrier should be used when engaging in insertive sexual activity (oral, vaginal or anal) with partner who is known to HIV infected or with partner whose HIV status is not known. The most commonly used barrier is the *male condom.* The major points for correct use of *male condom* are as follows:

- Use only condoms (rubber) that are made out of latex or polyurethane.
  - Natural skin. Condoms have pores that are large enough for HIV to penetrate.
- Store condom: in a cool, dry place and protect them from trauma. The friction caused by carrying them in back pocket, for instance can wear down the latex.
- Do not use condom if the expiration date has been over or if the package looks worn or punctured.
- Lubricants used in conjunction with condoms must be water soluble.
  - Oil-based lubricants can weaken latex and increase the risk of tearing or breaking.
  - Nonlubricated, flavoured condom can provide protection during oral intercourse.
- The condom must be placed on the erect penis before any contact is made with the partner's mouth, vagina or rectum to prevent exposure to pre-ejeculatory secretions that may contain HIV.
- Remove the penis and condom from the partner's body immediately after ejaculation and before the erection is lost.
  - Hold the condom at the base of the penis and remove both at the same time.
- This keeps semen from leaking around the condom as the penis becomes flaccid.
- Remove the condom after use. Wrap in tissue and discard. Do not flush down the toilet as this can cause plumbing problem.

- Condoms are not reusable. A new condom must be used for every act of intercourse.

Now female condoms are also available. Use can be complicated. So careful instructions and practice are required as given below.

- Female condoms consists of a polyurethane sheath with two springs from rings.
  - The small ring is inserted into the vagina and holds the condom in place internally. This ring can be removed if the condom is to be used in anal intercourse. It should not be removed by the condom to be used for vaginal intercourse.
  - The larger ring surrounds the opening to the condom. It functions to keep the condom in place externally while protecting the external genitalia.
- Use only water-soluble lubricants with female condoms.
  - Female condoms come prelubricated and with a tube of additional lubricant.
  - Lubrication is needed to protect the condom from tearing during sexual intercourse and can also decrease the noise that results from friction of the penis against the condom.
- Some men feel that female condom is better than the male condom. Some others like male condoms better. The only way to find out which type of condom works better is to try the both.
- Practice inserting the female condom. The steps shown in figure. Lubrication makes the condom slippery, but do not get discouraged. Just keep trying.
- During sexual intercourse, ensure that the penis is inserted into the female condom through the outer ring. There is a chance that penis will miss the opening, thus making contact with the vagina and defeating the purpose of the condom.
- Do not use a male condom at the time when a female condom is used.
- After intercourse, remove the condom before standing up.
  - Twist the outer ring to keep the semen inside. Gently pull the condom out of the vagina and discard.
  - Do not flush down the toilet, as this can cause plumbing problem.
- Do not reuse female condom.

Cleansing the equipment before use is a risk-reducing activity. It decreases the risk for those who share equipment.

The patient should be taught to recognize clinical manifestation that may indicate progression of the disease so that prompt medical care can be initiated. An overview of the symptoms the patient should report includes the following.

1. Report the following signs and symptoms immediately.
   - Any change in level of consciousness, lethargy, hard to arouse, unable to arouse, unresponsive and unconscious.
   - Headache accompanied by nausea and vomiting, changes in vision, changes in ability to perform coordinated activities, or after any head trauma.
   - Vision changes; blurry or black areas in vison field, new floaters.
   - Persistent shortness of breath related to activity and not relieved by a short rest period.
   - Nausea and vomiting accompanied by abdominal pain.
   - Dehydration, unable to eat or drink, because of nausea, diarrhoea, or mouth lesions; severe diarrhoea or vomiting, and dizziness when standing.
   - Yellow discoloration of the skin.
   - Any bleeding from the rectum that is not related to haemorrhoids.
   - Pain in the flank with fever and unable to urinate for more than 6 hours.
   - New onset of weakness in any part of the body, new onset of numbness that is not obviously related to pressure, new onset of difficulty in speaking.
   - Chest pain not obviously related to cough.
   - Seizures.
   - New rash accompanied by fever.
   - New oral lesions accompanied by fever.
   - Severe depression, anxiety, hallucinations, delusions or possible danger to self or others.
2. Report the following signs and symptoms within 24 hours.
   - New or different headache, constant headache not relieved by aspiring or acetominop.
   - Headache accompanied by fever, nasal congestion or cough.
   - Burning, itching or discharge from the eyes.
   - New or productive cough.
   - Vomiting 2-3 times a day.
   - Vomiting accompanied by fever.
   - New, significant or watery diarrhoea (more than 6 times a day).
   - Painful urination, bloody urine and urethral discharge.
   - New significant rash (widespread, painful, itchy, or following a path down the leg or arm, around the chest or on the face).
   - Difficulty in eating because of lesions.
   - Vaginal discharge, pain or itching.

Nursing Diagnosis commonly used in HIV infections include the following:

- Altered family processes.
- Altered nutrition: less than body requirement.
- Altered oral mucus membrane.
- Altered sexuality problems.
- Altered thought processes.
- Anticipatory grieving.

- Anxiety.
- Body image disturbance.
- Care-giver role strain.
- Chronic low self-esteem.
- Decisional conflict.
- Diarrhoea.
- Fatigue.
- Fear.
- Hyperthermia.
- Ineffective denial.
- Ineffective individual coping.
- Noncompliance.
- Pain.
- Powerlessness.
- Relocation stress syndrome.
- Self-care deficit.
- Situational low esteem.
- Sleep pattern disturbance.
- Social isolation.
- Spiritual distress.

Table 15.1: Nursing care plan for the patient with acquired immunodeficiency syndrome (AIDS): psychologic perspectives

Problem	*R*	*Objective*	*Nursing Interventions*	*Rationales*
Nursing Diagnosis # 1 Fear of death and dying related to: 1. AIDS diagnosis.		Patient will be able to: 1. Verbalize fear regarding AIDS. 2. Identify support systems to deal effectively with AIDS.	• Assess patient's perceived fear as expressed in his own words. • Help to identify factors he feels he has control over, and those he does not.	• Separating those items which are able to be controlled, and those which are not, gives the patient an area where he can focus his energies toward resolution of the fear.
			• Utilize support persons and resources to help patient in sorting out and dealing with fear. ♦ Interview family members and identify those who are positive in their attitude and approach to the patient; encourage their participation in his care. ♦ Investigate patient's background to identify available support resources; contact these resources to help in creating a supportive environment in which the patient can verbalize fear.	• By working within the patient's own framework, support systems and resources can be used more effectively in assisting the patient to deal with his fear.
			• Document patient's questions, and responses in progress notes so as to communicate the patient's goals, progression, as well as regression in working towards goals. • Document any key characteristic behaviour exhibited by patient, and reflective of his underlying fear; use these to help the patient deal effectively with his fear.	• Documentation assists in providing continuity of care.
			• Encourage family participation in patient care activities.	• Clarifying the status of AIDS, including what it is, what can be done to treat it, its prognosis, and expected course for the patient and family members, ultimately will strengthen the effectiveness of the patient-family-health team, support system. • It is essential to be honest and straight-forward.
Nursing Diagnosis#2 Body image, disturbance, related to: 1. Actual bodily changes.		Patient will: 1. Verbalize feelings regarding body changes.	• Assess thoughts and feelings regarding body changes.	• Underlying immune defect of cell-mediated immunity in AIDS places these patients at high risk of developing fungal and other opportunistic infections. Such infections can be

Contd...

Contd...

Problem	*R*	*Objective*	*Nursing Interventions*	*Rationales*
		2. Demonstrate positive attitude regarding self:		physically unsightly, and emotionally difficult for the patient to cope with.
		• Identify strengths. • Express interest in self-care activities. • Involve family in care.	• Ask patient to identify these changes.	• If patient can identify body changes that particularly distress him, the nurse may help him to understand why the infections occur and what can be done to minimize the risk of infection. For example, frequent and meticulous oral hygiene and handwashing.
			• Help patient to become aware of the support systems that surround him and who accept him as he is regardless of body changes.	• By identifying his support system, the patient may begin to realize his acceptance by those caring for him in spite of his body changes; he may realize that his body image in no way threatens their friendship, love, and support for him.
			• Provide personalized nursing care; touch the patient, and care for the patient in a manner you would care for any patient while implementing appropriate precautions.	• Nurses are able to demonstrate their acceptance of him by personalizing care; use of touch therapy is especially reassuring to the patient; furthermore, it sets an example for the family members and significant others to follow. Utilizing this type of approach in caring for the patient reassures him that he is accepted in spite of his own perceptions and self-doubts.
			• Work with family to help them be aware of patient's misgivings about body changes; help them to identify grooming habits important to patient, and to implement a plan of care: Haircut and shave; manicure; use of favourite cologne.	• Involving family in patient's care may enable them to feel positive about contributing in some way. By arranging for special grooming activities, the patient may be made to feel more positive about himself, and his acceptance by others.
			• Document patient's response to care and progress made toward accepting self; update and revise the care plan accordingly.	• Documentation assists in continuity of patient's care as efforts of all health care providers can be focused on identified goals and the achievement of desired patient outcomes.
Nursing Diagnosis #3 Social isolation, related to: 1. Diagnosis of AIDS. 2. Necessary isolation precautions.		Patient will: 1. Explain the reasons for isolation precautions. 2. Inform family and significant others as to need for precautions.	• Explain need for and underlying rationales for instituting isolation precautions.	• Patient, family, and staff must understand what the disease AIDS entails, and implications as to precautions to prevent its transmission to others. This is true not only within the hospital setting, but in daily activities of living.
		3. Demonstrate specific precautions in self-care.	• Implement isolation techniques involving patient and family in performing specific procedures according to hospital protocol.	
			• Assess patient's previous social lifestyle and social interactions.	• If patient has been active socially and enjoys people, this should not change because of AIDS. Patient's preferences should be respected and made known to all who interact with the

Contd...

Contd...

Problem	*R*	*Objective*	*Nursing Interventions*	*Rationales*
				patient. Maintaining some control over his life fosters self-confidence and self-esteem.
			• Maintain socialization process on patient's behalf, and within the patient's activity tolerance. ◆ After conferring with patient, encourage visitors when appropriate. ◆ Keep door to patient room open except when he is sleeping. ◆ Encourage timely use of television and radio to keep abreast of events. ◆ Hang up pictures, cards and other decorations with some meaning to patient.	• Socially withdrawing could lead to a situational depression, or be reflective of depression already present. If patients see the staff as "over-isolating," or perceive a "repugnance" on the part of the staff and/or visitors, they may become depressed, and socially withdraw.
			• Enlist family's help in determining important social situations in patient's life (e.g., birthday, holiday, anniversary, etc.). Work with support system to bring a part of each of these to the patient.	• For patients on isolation, special efforts should be made so that important events or interactions are not left unnoticed.
			• Encourage staff to carry out necessary isolation techniques, but caution not to "over-isolate."	• Patients on isolation precautions sometimes feel they are missing something; such feelings as "being left out" can predispose to a depressive reaction and may delay progress in the patient's improvement.
Nursing Diagnosis # 4 Verbal communication, impaired, related to: 1. CPAP mask. 2. Constant tachypnoea. 3. Fatigue.		Patient will be able to communicate with family, staff and significant others to make his needs known, and to enjoy interacting with others.	• Assess the patient's ability to communicate. ◆ Work with patient to identify the problem underlying his inability to communicate.	• Patients who have had a terminal disease confirmed have a great deal of processing to go through intellectually, emotionally, and psychologically. If the patient needs to verbalize his thoughts and feelings in this regard, an inability to communicate can cause the patient to feel isolated and alone.
			• Work with patient to devise a communication tool to meet his needs: ◆ Use of chalk or alphabet board. ◆ Use of "frequent words used" sheet. ◆ Lip-reading. ◆ Anticipate needs; remain accessible.	• Inability to communicate can be extremely frustrating particularly when it concerns the "small" needs that people in general take for granted. Aggravation associated with small concerns can become exaggerated, and expand into major problems.
			• Document key likes and dislikes so that the entire staff can anticipate patient's needs. For example, ice in water; call bell in left hand.	• If the patient who is already distressed and compromised must use remaining strength and energy requesting the same thing over and over again, or needs to continually make explanations regarding his needs, then the "therapeutic" milieu provided for the patient needs to be reassessed, and a revised plan of care implemented accordingly.

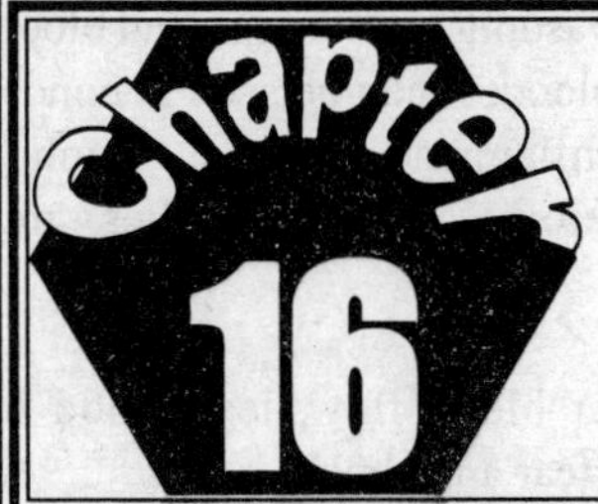

Dermatological Nursing or Integumentary Nursing

INTEGUMENTARY NURSING

Integument or skin is the largest organ exposed to the external environment and provides the first line of defense of the body yet at the same time it is affected by changes in the internal environment. Problems of the skin are often present in difficult management challenges. Clothing and cosmetics can disguise or cover some skin problem, but many a problem cannot be hidden so easily. The emotional impact of skin problem often is more serious than skin problem itself. Dermatology is the study of the skin and its problem. Dermatological nursing is that which deals with all the nursing aspects of dermatological conditions.

Assessment of the Integument or Skin

Assessment of the integument provides data about how the person is affected by and is coping with both external and internal environment. Data obtained in the assessment provide the basis for identification of actual or potential nursing problems related to the skin, infection, fluid and electrolyte balances, nutritional imbalances, or inadequate oxygenation of tissues. Baseline observations are useful for identifying changes that may occur.

Assessment of the skin begins at the initial contact with the patient and continues throughout the examination. Specific areas of the skin are examined during examination of other areas of the body unless the chief complaint is that of a dermatological nature.

Patient's History

The patient's history is an important part of the health assessment and is included with the physical examination. If during a general history, the patient describes a skin problem or skin discomfort itching or superficial pain. Then further data are obtained. The informations will be as follows:

- Usual skin conditions: usual appearance, colour, moisture, texture, or integrity.
- Onset of the problem: Initial sites where changes were first noticed; skin appearance at onset; any other symptoms noted at the time of onset such as pain or itching.
- Changes since onset: changes in location of lesions, changes in appearance, increase in size and new symptoms such as pain or itching.
- Specific known cause: For example contact with poisoning, exposure to known allergen or stress.
- If cause is unknown:
  - Recent exposure to sensitizing substances, such as metals, chemicals, detergents or poisonous plants.
  - Description for a new drug such as penicillin.
  - Occupations that may cause contact with potential skin irritants or hands constantly in water.
  - Recreational activities, for example, painting, camping or gardening.
  - Exposure to sun burn, photosensitivity, or skin cancer or cold frost bite..
- Alleviating factors: physician-prescribed or self-prescribed things.
- Psychological reaction to skin changes; withdrawal from social activities, cosmetics for cover-up; feelings about the problem i.e. body image.
- Previous trauma, surgery or prior disease that involves the skin.

Physical Examination

The skin is an organ that can be examined by direct inspection and observation with no tools but a good light. Palpation is also used in gathering data about certain type of lesions. General principles when conducting an assessment of the skin are as follows:

1. *Be prepared:*
   - Have a private examination room of moderate temperature with good lighting and a room with exposure to daylight preferred.
   - If the lighting is inadequate, lesions may be missed or described inaccurately. If the room temperature is not well controlled, vasoconstriction, vasodilation and papillary erections occur, giving false data.
   - Ensure that the patient is comfortable and in a dressing gown that allows easy access to all skin areas.
2. *Be systemic:*
   - Proceed from head to toe.
   - If only some parts of the skin are inspected, an improved parameter may be omitted or a lesion missed.
3. *Be thorough:*

- Look at all areas carefully. If the person is lying down, ensure to examine the back especially the sacral area.
- Lift folds of tissue, such as under the breasts or gluteal folds.
- The examiner's embarrassment of the examinee may result in inadequate data.
- Do not forget to assess the macus membrane as well.

4. *Be specific:*
   - Perform a general inspection and then a lesion-specific examination.
   - When lesions are identified, describe the lesions using metric system and established parameters colour, size and shape..
5. *Compare symmetrical parts:*
   - Compare the right side with left side.
   - When observing changes in skin colour, or tissue shape, always compare one side of the body with other to differentiate structural from pathological changes as well as symmetry of manifestation.
6. Record the data:
   - Unrecorded data are lost data.
   - Baseline observations indicating normality of abnormality are needed for comparison with subsequent finding.
   - Changes need to be recorded to determine progress toward achieving desired outcomes.
   - Use appropriate terminology and nomenclature when reporting or documenting.
7. *Use appropriate technique:*
   - Palpation is used during physical assessment of the skin.
   - Lesions are palpated for density, induration and tenderness.
   - Standard precautions need to be observed during palpation, and the examiner should determine whether it is appropriate to use gloves.

The objective data to be collected when examining the skin for general health status include skin colour, temperature, moisture, elasticity, turgor, texture, thickness and odour. Brief description of these are as follows:

Colour

Changes in colour are best obtained in the lips, mucous membranes of the mouth, earlobes, finger nails and toe nails and the extremities. The lip shows rapid colour changes. Colour of the skin varies with the amount of melanin in the cells, and with the blood supply. Skin colour may be masked by cosmetics curtaining. Inaccurate assessment of skin colour may be attributed to factors such as conducted in a poorly lit room, room temperature excessive, the presence of oedema, poor hygiene or positioning. The possible colour changes in certain conditions are as follows:

- *Redness* (Erythem) is due to vasodilations more rapid blood flow and more oxygenated blood. It can be seen in conditions like blushing, heat, inflammation, fever, alcohol ingestion, extreme cold, below 15°C. hot flushes, and polycethaemia.
- *Whiteness* (Pallor) due to:
  - Vasoconstriction, slower blood flow, less blood in capillaries, seen in cold, fear and shock.
  - Partially obstructed blood flow, less blood in capillaries seen in vasospasm, thrombus, narrowed vessels and arterial insufficiency.
  - Fluid between blood vessels and skin surgeries seen in oedema.
  - Descreased oxygenation of blood from decreased haemoglobin seen in Anaemia.
  - Loss of melanin seen in vitiligo.
- *Bluish (cyanosis)* is due to deoxygenated haemoglobin, noticed in earlobes, lips, mucous, membranes of mouth, nail beds, seen in heart or lung diseases, inadequate respiration, peripheral blood vessal obstruction, venous disease, cold and anxiety.
- *Yellow (Jaundice)* due to increased bile pigment in blood eventually distributed to skin and mucous membranes and to sclera of eye. This is usually seen in liver disease, obstruction of bile ducts, chronic uraemia and rapid haemolysis.
- *Brown* due to increased melanin deposits; normal in brown black races. This is found in aging, sunburn, anterior pituitary, adrenal cortex, or liver diseases.
- *Dullness* due to:
  - Vasoconstriction in dark skin found in cold, fear, shock.
  - Partially obstructed blood flow in dark skin, found in vasospasm thrombus, narrowed vessels and arterial insufficiency.
  - Fluid between blood vessels and skin surface of dark skin found in oedema.

The colour of the skin indicates degree of blood supplied to and temperature of the skin and oxygen supply and fluid supply to the skin.

Skin is assessed as being dry, moist and oily. *Dry* skin is usually seen in elderly ones because of diseased activity of sebaceous glands. Dry skin is also seen in dehydration: persons with hypothyroidium have thick, dry and leathery skin. *Moist* is caused by the presence of water or sweat in the surfaces. Overheating produces sweating. Hyperthyroidism cases have moist smooth skin. Stressors, shock or any situation stimulate sympathetic nervous system and increase fluid loss through shock gland diaphoresis. In as much as vasoconstriction occurs imulation causes cold, clammy skin. *Oily* skin is seen in adolescence due to excess sebum formation.

The skin is highly elastic and moves freely over most areas. It loses mobility, when it becomes stretched, this occurs with oedema, when the interstitial space becomes filled with fluid, skin becomes rigid in the person with scleroderma. *Turgor* is a tissue tension and is measured by the speed of the skin's return to normal position of fullness after it has been stretched. Decreased turgor may be due to aging or dehydration. The elasticity and turgor tested at the portion of skin over the sternum. Texture and roughness may occur normally on exposed areas, especially elbows and soles of the feet. The skin of an infant is usually soft and smooth, whereas elderly person may roughen and lack underlying tissue substance atrophy. Roughness is seen in hypothyroidism, hypertrophic scarring.

Normal skin is uniformally thin over the body except over the palms and soles. A callus or painless overgrowth of epidermis may develop over these areas as a result of pressure or friction. And normally clean skin is usually free from odour except for areas that contain apocrine sweat glands. Odour occurs because of bacterial composition of protein matter and some draining skin lesions.

In addition to skin assessment, assessment of accessory structures of skin, i.e. hair and nails also is very essential.

Hair growth pattern and distribution are indications of the persons' general state of health. Excessive hair growth is hypertrichosis, usually related to heredity or hormonal changes. Hair loss alopecia is normally with age. Abnormal hair loss may be because of hormonal imbalance, general ill-health, infections of the scalp, typhoid fever, chronic liver disease, stressor and some medication antimetabolite or heparin. Hair should be free from lice and nits. Hair loss on the dorsum of the toes may indicate decreased arterial circulation.

The appearance of the nails' changes with age and with ill-health. Changes in hardness, brittleness, roughness or shape may indicate some metabolic diseases, nutritional imbalances include vitamin deficiency or digestive disturbances. Pale nail beds indicate hypoxia, clubbing of finger is associated with chronic hypoxia. Paronychic an infection of the tissue surrounding the nail characterized by red shiny skin and painful swelling, it may result in psoriasis dermatitis.

Lesions of Skin

When lesions are observed, the following parameters are used for description, type, colour, size, shape and configuration, texture, effect of pressure, arrangement, distribution and variety. The following skin changes are observed in skin lesions.

1. *Changes in Colour or Texture*
   - *Spot:* It is circumscribed; flat; colour change, termed as macule e.g. Freckle, Pimple, Blemish.
   - *Discoloration* reddish-purple: It is bleeding beneath the surface; injury to tissue, termed as "Contusion, e.g. bruise.
   - *Soft whitening* caused by repeated wetting of skin termed as "maceration" e.g. occurs between toes after soaking.
   - *Flake:* Dry cells of surface termed as "scale" e.g. dandruff, psoriasis..
   - *Roughness from dried fluid:* i.e. Dry exudate over lesion termed as "crust" scab. e.g. eczema, impetigo..
   - *Roughness from cells:* It is a leathery thickening of outer skin layer is termed as "lichenification" e.g. callus on foot..
2. *Changes in Shape*
   - Fluid-filled lesions:
     - Less than 1 cm: clear fluid vesicle. e.g. blister, chicken pox
     - Greater than 1 cm. clear fluid bulla. e.g. larger blister, pemphigus.
     - Small, thick yellowish fluid pustule. e.g. Acne..
   - Solid mass-cellular growth.
     - Less than 1 cm papule. e.g. small mole, raised rash.
     - 1 to 2 cm nodule. e.g. enlarged lymph node.
     - Greater than 2 cms tumour. e.g. Benign or malignant tumour..
     - Excessive connective tissue over scar keloid. e.g. overgrown scar.
   - Swelling of tissue.
     - Generalized swelling: fluid between cells oedema. e.g. inflammation swelling and tech.
     - Circumscribed surface oedema, transient; some itching e.g. allergic reaction..
3. *Breaks in Skin Surface*
   - *Oozing, scraped surface:* Loss of superficial structure of the skin abrasion. e.g. "Floor burn scrape".
   - *Scooped out depression:* Loss of deeper layer skin ulcer., e.g. pressure or stasis ulcer.
   - *Superficial linear skin breaks:* Scratch marks, frequency of finger nails excoriations. e.g. scratching.
   - *Linear Cracks or Cleft:* Slit or splitting of skin layer, Fissure. e.g. Athlete's foot.
   - *Jagged cut:* Tearing of skin surface laceration. e.g. accidents, cut by blunt edge.
   - *Linear cut, edges approximation:* cutting by sharp instrument incision. e.g. knife cut.
4. *Vascular Lesions*
   - Small, flat, round, purplish and red spot are due to intradermal or submucous haemorrhage petechia. e.g. bleeding tendency, decreased platelets and vitamin C deficiency.
   - *Spider-like:* red, small, due to dilation of capillaries, arterioles or venules Telengiectasis. e.g. liver disease and vitamin B deficiency.
   - *Discolouration, reddish purple:* escape of blood into fissures ecchymosis. e.g. trauma to blood vessels.

The following terminology is used for lesion configuration and lesion distribution.

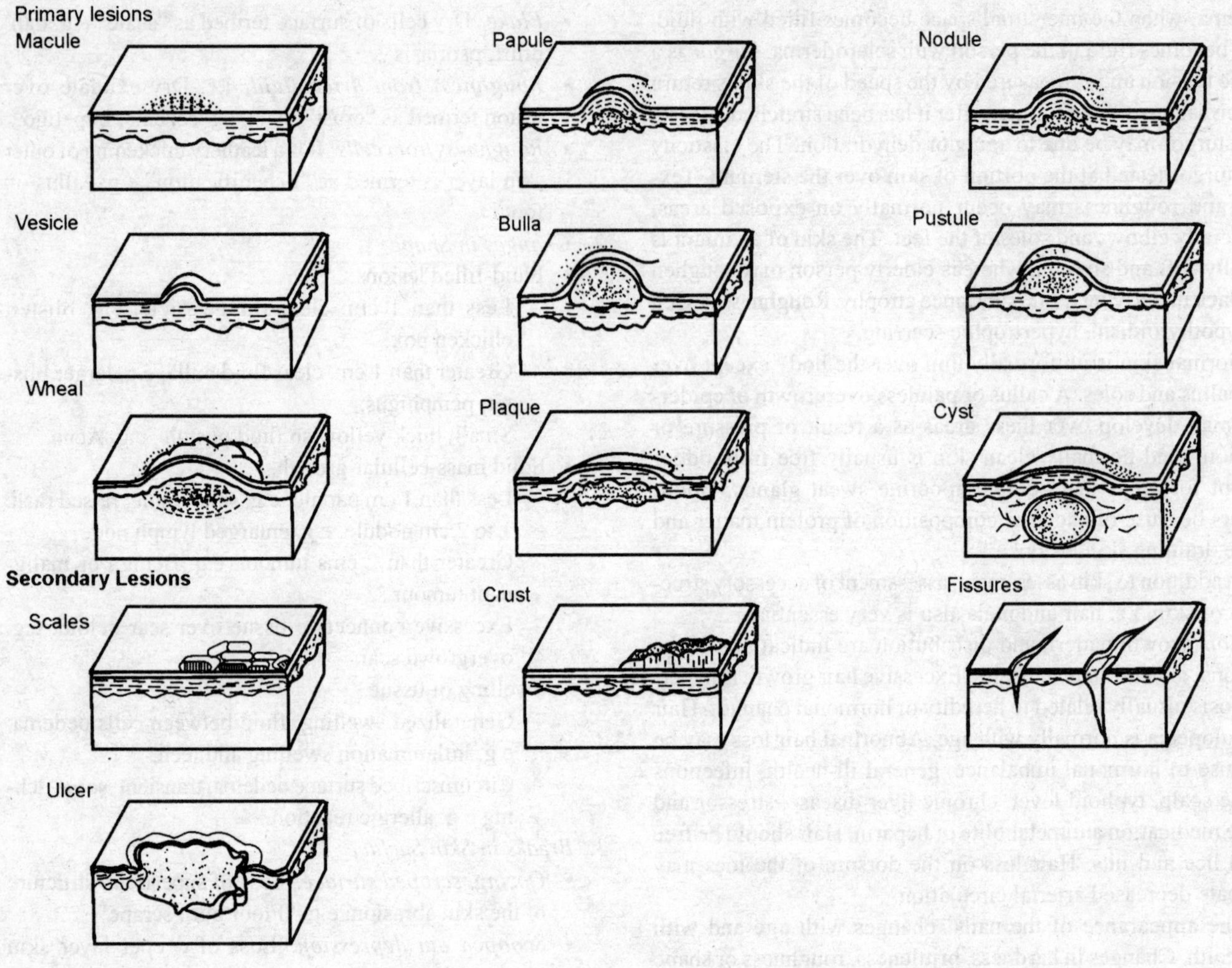

Fig.16.1: Types of skin lesions.

i. *Lesion Configuration*
- Annular—Ring shaped.
- Gyrate Ring—Spiral shaped.
- Iris lesion—Concentric rings or bull's eye.
- Linear—In a line.
- Nummular-discoid-coinlike.
- Polymorptious—Occurring in several forms.
- Punctuats—Marked by points or dots.
- Serpiginous—Snakelike.

ii. *Lesion Distribution*
- Asymmetric—Unilateral.
- Confluent Merging together.
- Diffuse—Wide distribution.
- Discrete—Separate from other lesion.
- Generalized—Diffuse distribution.
- Grouped—Cluster of lesions.

1 • Localized—Limited area of involvement that is clearly identified.
- Statellite—Single lesion and close proximity to a large grouping
- Solitary—A single lesion.
- Symmetric—Bilateral distribution.
- Zosteriform—Band-like distributional song a dermatome area.

Common assessment abnormalities of the integumentary system are as follows:

1. *Alopecia:* is loss of hair localized or generalized. It may be due to hereditary, friction, rubbing, traction, trauma, stress, infection, inflammation, chemotherapy, pregnancy, emotional shock, tineacupitis and immunological factors.
2. *Angioma* is a tumour consisting of blood or lympth vessels. It is due to normal increase with aging, liver disease, pregnancy and varicose veins.

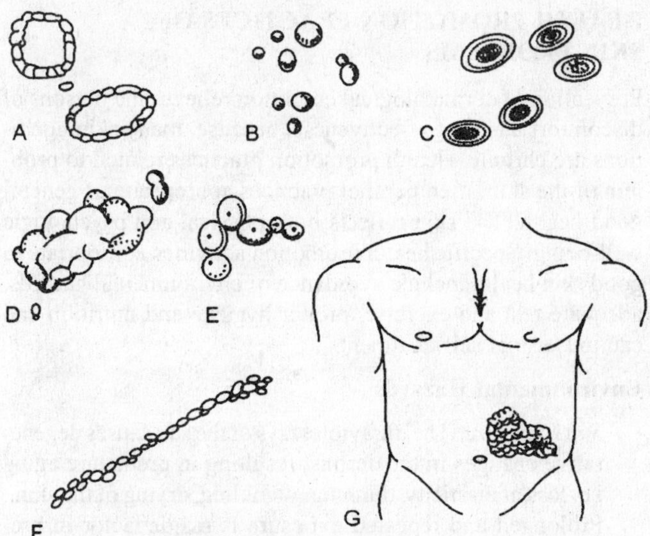

Fig. 16.2: Shape and arrangement of skin lesions: A. annular; B. grouped; C. iris; D. confluent; E. herpatiform; F. linear; G. zosteriform.

3. *Carotenaemia Carotenosis.:* Yellowish discolouration of skin, no yellowing of sclerac, most noticeable on palms and soles. It is due to vegetable containing carotene e.g. carrots, squash and hypothyroidism.
4. *Comedo* black heads and white heads.: Keratin, sebum micro-organisms and epithelial debris within a dilated follicular opening. It is due to acne vulgaris.
5. *Cyanosis:* Slightly bluish-gray or purple discolouration of the skin problems, vasoconstrictions, asphyxiation, anaemia, leukaemia and malignancies.
6. *Cyst:* Sac containing fluid or semisolid material. It is due to obstruction of a duct or gland and parasitic infections.
7. *Depigmentation (vitiligo):* Congenital or acquired loss of melanin resulting in white, depigmented areas. It may be due to genetic chemical and pharmacologic agents, nutritional and endocrine factors, burns and trauma inflammation and infection.
8. *Ecchymosis:* Large, bruise-like lesion caused by collection, collection of extravascular blood in dermis and subcutaneous tissue. It may be due to trauma, and bleeding disorders.
9. *Erythems:* Redness occurring in patches of variable size and shapes. It may be due to heat, certain drugs, alcohol, ultraviolet rays, any problem that causes dilation of blood vessels to the skin.
10. *Excoriation:* Superficial excavations of epidermis. It may be due to pruritis and trauma.
11. *Haematoma:* Extravasation of blood of sufficient size to cause visible swelling. It is due to trauma and bleeding disorders.
12. *Hirsutism* is male distribution of hair in women. It is due to abnormality of gonads or adrenal glands, decrease in oestrogen levels and familial trait.
13. *Intertrigo:* Dermatis of overlying surfaces of the skin. It may be due to moisture, obesity monitor infections.
14. *Jaundice:* Yellow or yellowish-brown discolouration of skin best observed in the sclera secondary to increased bilirubin in blood. It is found in liver disease, REC haemolysis, pancreatic cancer, and common bile duct obstruction.
15. *Keloid:* Hypertrophied scar beyond margin of incision or trauma.
16. *Lichenification:* Thickening of the skin with accentuated skin making. It may be due to repeated scratching, rubbing and irritation.
17. Mole melanocytic nevus.: Benign overgrowth of melanocytes. It is due to defects of development, excessive numbers and large irregular moles and often familial.
18. *Petechae:* Pinpoint, discreate deposit of blood less than 1 mm to 2mm in the extravalcular tissues and visible through the skin or mucous membrane. It is due to inflammation, marked dilation, blood vessel trauma, blood dycrasia that results in bleeding tendencies, e.g. thrombocytopenia.
19. *Telangiectasia:* Visibly dilated, superficial, cutaneous small blood vessels commonly found on face and thighs. It may be due to aging, acne, sun exposure, alcohol, liver failure, corticosteroid medication, radiation, certain systemic diseases, skin tumours and normal variant.
20. *Tending:* Failure of skin to return immediately to normal position after gentle pinching. It is due to aging, dehydration, cachexia.
21. *Varicosity:* Increased prominence of superficial veins. It may be due to interruption of venous return, e.g. from tumour, incompetent values and inflammation.

Diagnostic Studies

Diagnostic studies provide information to the nurse in monitoring the patient conditions and planning appropriate interventions. The common diagnostic studies of the integumentary system are as follows:

i. *Biopsy:*

It is one of the most common diagnostic test used in the assessment of skin lesions. Techniques of biopsy include punch, incisional, excisional and shave subsection.

- *Punch:* Here, special punch biopsy instrument of appropriate size is used. Instrument rotated to appropriate level to include dermis and some fat, suturing may or may not be done.
- *Excisional:* Is useful where good cosmetic results and entire removal desired. Skin is closed with subcutaneous and skin sutures.
- *Incisional:* Elliptical incision made in lesion is too large to excise. Adequate specimen obtained without causing an extensive cosmetic defect.
- *Shave* subsection: Single-edged razor blade used to shave off lesions performed on superficial lesions. Provides full thickness specimen of stratum corneum.

Nursing responsibilities during biopsy include verify that consent form is signed if needed. Assist with preparation of site anaesthesia, procedure and haemostasis. Apply dressing and give postprocedure instruction to patient. Properly identify specimen.

ii. *Microscopic Test:*
   - *Potassium Hydroxide:* Hair, scales or nails examined for hyphae of fungal infection. Specimen is put on a glass slide and 10 to 40 per cent concentration of potassium hydroxide added. In this instruct the patient regarding the purpose of test. Prepare slide.
   - Tzank test (Wrights and Giemsas Stain): Fluid and cells from vesicles or bullae examined. Used to diagnose herpes virus. Specimen put on slide, stained, and examined microscopically. Nurse instructs the patients regarding purpose and use. Use sterile technique for collection of fluid.
   - *Culture:* The test identifies fungal, bacterial, and viral organisms.
     - For fungi, scraping performed if the fungus is systematic involving skin.
     - For bacteria, material obtained from intact pustules, bullae, or abscesses.
     - For viruses, bullae scraped and exudate taken from centre of lesion.

In culture, nurse instructs patient regarding purpose and specific procedure. Properly identify specimen. Follow instruction for storage of specimens if not sent the same to laboratory.

- *Mineral slides:* To check for infestation, scrapings are taken place in slide with mineral oil. Here, nurse instructs patient of purposes of test, prepare slide.
- *Immunofluorescent studies:* Some cutaneous diseases have specific abnormal antibody proteins that can be idealized by fluorescent studies. Both skin and serum can be examined. Here, nurse informs patients of purpose of test and assists in obtaining specimens.

iii. *Other Test*:
   - *Woods light:* Examination of skin with long wave ultraviolet light causes specific substance to fluorescence e.g. Pseudomonal organism, fungal infection, vitiligo. Explain the purpose of examination and inform patient it is not painful.
   - *Diascopy:* Examination of the skin using gentle pressure with a transparent object to check lesion vascularity. Explain the procedure to patient.
   - *Patch Test:* Used to determine whether patient is allergic to any testing material. Small amount of potentially allergenic matter applied under the occlusion, usually skin on back.
   - In this, nurse explains purpose and procedure to the patient. Instructs patient to return 48 hours for removal of allergens and evaluation. Inform patient of revaluation is needed at 96th hour.

HEALTH PROMOTION PRACTICES OF SKIN PROBLEMS

Prevention of dermatological condition relieves the persons of discomfort and cost-effectiveness, because, many skin conditions are chronic. Health promotion practices related to problem of the skin often parallel practices appropriate of general good health. The skin reflects both physical and psychologic well-being. Specific health promotion activities appropriate to good skin health include avoidance of environmental hazards, adequate rest and exercise, proper hygiene and nutrition and cautious use of self treatment.

Environmental Hazards

- *Sun Exposure:* The ultraviolet rays of the sun causes degenerative changes in the dermis, resulting in premature aging i.e. loss of elasticity, thinning, wrinkling, drying of the skin.. Prolonged and repeated exposure is major factor in precancerous and cancerous lesion. Nurses should be strong advocates of safe sun practices. Vitamin D3 is produced in the skin and is necessary for vitamin D synthesis. Few minutes of sun exposure meets this need. The nurse can also inform the patient about the means of protection from the damaging effects of the sun, such as wearing a large brimmed hat, and a long-sleeved shirt of a lightly-woven fabric or carrying an umbrella. Patient needs to know that rays of the sun are most dangerous between 10 am to 2 pm Standard Time or 11 am and 3 pm daylight saving time, regardless of the latitude.

Certain topical and systemic medications potentiate the effects of the sun, even with brief exposure. The nurse should be aware that medication and the photosensitivity of each individual drugs should be examined. The chemicals in these drugs absorb light and release energy that harm cells and tissues. The categories of drugs that may cause photosensitivity are:

- Anticancer drugs e.g. Methotexate
- Antidepressants e.g. Amitriptyline
- Antiarrhythmatic e.g. Quinidine
- Antihistamine e.g. Dipheny
- Antimicrobial e.g. Tetracycline
- Antifungal e.g. Griseofulvin
- Antipsychotic e.g. Chloropromozam, Halperaxal
- Diuretics e.g. Frosemide Lasix.
- Hypoglycaemia e.g. Tolbutamide
- NSAIDS e.g. Diclofenac

Nurses have a role in educating patients who are taking these medications about their photosensitizing effect.

Irritants and Allergens

Patient can present to the nurse with irritation or allergic dermatitis. The nurse should counsel his or her patient to avoid known irritants e.g. ammonia and harsh detergents. The nurse must also be aware that prescribed or over-the-counter (OTC). Topical and systemic medication is used to treat a variety of conditions cause dermatologic reaction.

1. *Radiation*
Although most radiology departments are extremely cautious in protecting both themselves and their patients from the effects of excessive radiation, the nurse should help the patient make intelligent decisions about radiologic procedures.
2. *Rest and Sleep*
Rest and sleep are important health promotion considerations in relation to skin. Rest reduces the threshold of itching and the potential skin damage from the resultant scratching. Sleep is tough to be restorative.
3. *Exercises*
Exercises increase circulation and dilate the blood vessel. In addition to the healthy growth produced by exercise, the psychologic effects can also improve one's appearance and mental outlook. However, caution must be used to avoid or protect the exercising person from overexposure to heat, cold and sun during outdoor exercises.
4. *Hygiene*
Hygienic practices should match the skin type, lifestyle and culture of the patient. The person with oily skin should cleanse the skin with a drying agent more often than with the person with dry skin. Dry skin might benefit from super-fatted soaps and measures to increase moisture, such as the application of moisturizers to the skin. In general, the skin and hair should be washed often enough to remove excess oil and excretions and to prevent odour. Older persons should avoid use of harsh soaps and shampoos because these may result in increasing dryness of their skin. Moisturizers should be used after bath or shower, while the skin is still damp, to seal in this moisture.
5. *Nutrition*
A well-balanced diet adequate in all food groups can produce healthy skin, hair and nails. Certain elements are particularly essential for good skin health. These elements include the following.
   - *Vitamin A* essential for maintenance of normal cell structure, specifically epithelial cells. It is necessary for normal wound healing. The absence of vitamin A cause conjunctive dryness and poor wound healing.
   - *Vitamin B Complex* essential to complex metabolic functions. Deficiencies of Niacin and Pyridoxine manifest as dermatologic symptoms such as erythaema, bullae and seborhoea-like lesions.
   - *Vitamin C* Ascorbic acid-essential for connective tissue formation and normal wound healing. Absence of Vitamin C causes symptoms of scurvy including petechine, bleeding gums and purpura.
   - *Vitamin K deficiency*-interferes with normal prothrombin synthesis in the liver and can lead to cutaneous purpura.
   - *Protein*-necessary in amounts adequate for cell growth and maintenance. It is also necessary for normal wound healing.
   - *Unsaturated fatty acids*—necessary to maintain the function and integrity of cellular and subcellular membranes in tissue metabolism, especially linolec and arachidemic acids.

Obesity has an adverse effect on the skin. This increases in subcutaneous fat can lead to stretching and overheating. Overheating secondary to the greater insulation provided by the fat, occurs an increase in sweating which has an adverse effect on normal or inflammed skin. Obesity has an influence on DM with concomittant skin complication.

6. *Self-treatment*
The nurse needs to increase the patient's awareness of the dangers of self diagnosis and treatment. The wide variety of OTC skin preparation can confuse the consumer. General instructions the nurse can discuss with the patient would stress the duration of the treatment and the need to know and follow package directions closely. If any systemic signs are shown it should be referred immediately.

COMMON SKIN PROBLEMS

Skin problems may result from various causes, such as parasitic infection, fungal, bacterial and viral infections, reaction to substances encountered externally or internally taken new growth.

Parasitic Infections

Pediculosis (Lice Manifestation)
Occurs mostly among children. People on crowded buses. Pediculis Lice are most often found among people who live in overcrowded dwellings with inadequate hygienic facilities.

Pathophysiology
Lice obtain their nutrition by sucking blood from the skin. They leave their eggs or nits on the skin surface attached to the hair shaft and this results in the transfer from one person to another. Three types of lice infest humans; the headlouse, the body louse and pubic louse.

- The head louse pediculus humanus capitis attaches itself to the hair shaft, laying about eight eggs a day. The eggs are firmly attached to the hair or threads of clothing, ova hatch in one week. They may be viewed with a hand lens or flash light and appear as grayish; glistening oval bodies. The head louse usually is confined to scalp and beard. Transmission occurs through use of infected persons' hats, brushes or combs.
- The body louse pediculus humanus corporis resides mainly in the seams of clothing around the neck, waist and thighs. The bite causes minute hemorrhagic points and severe itching. Transmission by direct contact or by way of clothing, bedding and towels.
- The pubic louse Phthirus pubis differs slightly from the head and body louse. It resembles a tiny crab, having claw-like pincers that attach firmly to the pubic hair. Nits are visible in the pubic hair. It is transmitted by sexual contact, bed clothing, towels and occasionally toilet seats.

Clinical Manifestation

Minute, red, noninflammatory, point flush with skin; progression to popular wheat-like lesions. i.e., pin-point erythema, raised macules and pruritis. The bite of the insect with contamination from saliva, head parts and feces-causing intense itching. Scratching may lead to further trauma with the possibilities of secondary infection and enlarged cervical lymph nodes. Secondary excoriations in intracapular region; firmly attached to hair shaft in head and body lice.

Management

Diagnosis is made by physical examination of the appropriate body part. A magnifying glass may be helpful in spotting symptoms and treatment of pediculosis consists of topical application of the pediculicide such as lindane, permethrin, pyrethrin and malathion. When pyrethrin or lindanes are used, a second application of the 7 to 10 days may be necessary. Directions for application differ according to the product and body location. So it should be applied accordingly as per manufacturers' instructions. Contact screening with bed partners. Playmates showed head gear and contacts treated if necessary. Persons with head lice should be instructed to soak comb, brushes and hair utensils in hot water and pediculicide shampoo for 15 minutes. Clothing and bedding should be laundered in hot water and dried on light heat or dry-cleaned.

Scabies

Scabies is caused by the female itchmite (Sarcoptes Scabiei). It is prevalent during periods of overcrowding and occurs in all age groups and socio-economic levels.

Pathophysiology

The female itchmite penetrates the stratum corneum and burrows into the skin. Within several hours of the skin penetration, the itchmite lay a large number of eggs and deposits fecal pellets. The larva mature in 10 to 14 days and move to the skin surface, where the females are impregnated; the cycle then repeats itself. The incubation period varies; but often a long period elapses before symptoms are noted. Delayed hypersensitivity is thought to be a major factor in the lapse between infestation and symptoms. The incubation period in persons with no previous exposure is 4 to 6 weeks.

Clinical Manifestation

The classic symptoms of scabies are intense itching and lesions that resemble wavy brownish, thread-like lines occurring most commonly on the hands especially the interdigital webs., flexer surface of the wrist posterior inner surface of the elbows, anterior axillary folds, nipples in the females, belt line, gluted creasos and male genitalia. The head and neck are rarely involved. Pruritis may be severe, especially at night pruritis thought to be a result of a hypersensitivity reaction. Secondary infection with excoriations and pustule may result from scratching. Scratching destroys burrows. Vesicles are filled with serus fluid may contain mite.

Management

Diagnosis is made on the basis of sign and symptoms and identifying the itchmite under microscope. The goal of therapy is elimination of the itchmite and treatment of complications.

1. Scabies treatment: Patient and all family members.
   a. *Lindane* Kwell, Scabies for with the follow:
      - Apply at bed time in a thin layer over the entire body from neck down.
      - Wash off in 8 to 12 hours.
      - Give a second treatment in 24 hours if prescribed.
   b. *Crotamiton* 10% (Eurax.)
      - It is less effective than lindane.
      - Bathe before initial application and after each treatment.
      - Repeat treatment as prescribed.
   c. *Benzyl Benzoate Emulsion*
      - Give two overnight treatments one week apart as prescribed.
      - Not widely available. Apply as directed by the physician.
2. Treatment for complication from scabies.
   - Postscabies dermatitis with pruritis: topical or oral corticosteroids.
   - Secondary infection with systemic antibiotics.
   - Postscabies papules or nodules treated with coal tar gels.

And teaching the patient with scabies include the following.

- All family members should be treated simultaneously whether or not symptoms present.
- Be sure that all external body areas below the neck covered by the prescribed scabiecide.
- Wash underclothing and bed and bath linen in hot water on the day of treatment; dry in dryer or iron after dry; clothing and bedding that cannot be laundered should be placed in plastic bags for at least one week. Parasite cannot survive longer than 4 days off the human skin.
- Signs and symptoms may not disappear until 1 or 2 weeks after treatment; pruritis of hands and feet may persist for upto 3 months.

FUNGAL INFECTIONS

Fungi are larger and move complex than bacteria. They may be unicellular, such as yeasts, or multicellular such as molds. Many types are pathogenic to humans causing common skin disorders or serious systemic diseases such as blastomycosis. Certain types of fungi cause few symptoms, whereas other produce inflammation or hypersensitivity reaction.

Candidiasis

Candidiasis is caused by candida albicans, a yeast-like fungus, normally inhabits in the GI tract, mouth and vagina, but not usually on the skin. Candidiasis, moniliasis, the inflammation associated with the organism overgrowth on the skin is caused by the toxins that are released. Other predisposing factors are pregnancy, use of birth control pills, poor nutrition, antibiotic therapy, diabetes mellitus and other endocrinal disorder, inhalational corticosteroids and immunosuppressed conditions. Overgrowth of C. albicans causes candidiasis.

Pathophysiology

Candidiasis of the mucous membrane is thrush, the lesions are white spots that look like milk curd on the buccal mucosa and may extend down the oesophagus. Vaginal thrush causes intense itching with a thick, white vaginal discharge. Candidiasis of the skin appears as pruritic, eroded, moist-inflammed areas with vesicles and pastules, and it occurs mostly in body folds such as beneath the breasts, in the inter-gluteal fold or in the groin.

Clinical Manifestaion

The classic clinical manifestation of candidiasis is the presence of satellite lesions on the periphery of the general inflammation. The symptoms and signs of mouth, vagina and skin are as follows.

- *Mouth*-White cheese-like patches leaving erosions when removed.
- *Vagina*-Vaginitis with red,oedemations, painful vaginal wall, white patches, vaginal discharge, pruritus, pain on urination and intercourse.
- *Skin*-Diffuse papular erythematous rash with pin-point satellite lesion around edges of affected area.

Management

Diagnosis of candidiasis at any site made by clinical appearance and microscopic examination and culture.

Treatment aimed at elimination of the precipitating factors. Other measures including keeping the skin dry to avoid maceration; wearing loose absorbent clothing; and using topical medications such as powders, this helps the skin dry. Nystatin myostatis is an antifungal available in tablets, powder or vaginal suppositories and lozenges, amphotericin; cloterimazole, ciclopirox and ketconazol are effective against yeast infections. The sum up measure to prevent candidiasis are:

- Eradication of infection with appropriate medication.
- Skin hygiene to keep it clean and dry.
- Avoidance of lubricants.

Dermatophytoses

There are several different types of dermatophytosa tinea or superficial fungal infection of the skin and its appendages. The most common types are tenia capitis, tinea corporis, tenia cruris and tinea pedis.

1. *Tenia Capitis*

   Tenia capitis is appropriately called ringworm of the scalp; can be caused either by species of "Microsporum or by •Trichophyton fungi. The infection is transmitted readily, especially in crowded condition where poor hygiene exists although many children show a high resistance. Minor scalp trauma facilitates implantation of the spores; therefore, the infection can spread by contaminated barbers' instruments, combs or sharp brushes. It has worldwide distribution, primarily among pre-pubertal children.

The characteristic lesion is round with erythema, a slight scaling, and some postules appearing at the edge of the lesion. Hair loss occurs with the hair shaft broken off at skin level. The hair loss is only temporary because the lesions usually heal without scarring. Usually tenia capitis is noninflammatory, a painful inflammation condition is called "Keroin".

Management

Griseofulvin is an antifungal agent effective in the treatment of all the dermatophytosis. The adult dose of tenia cupitis is 500 mg orally, and absorption enhanced when the drug is administered after a high fat meal. Infection usually resolves within 4 to 6 weeks. A mild antifungal agent, such as tolnaftate or haloprogin may be applied twice daily as ordered. The patients should be advised for shampooing head twice a week, cutting hair short facilitates shampooing. It may cause psychological trauma in children. Therefore, the hair is best left at an acceptable length. Daily shampooing avoids infection.

2. *Tenia Corporis*

   Tenia corporis is dermatophytic infection commonly referred to as ringworm. It occurs in children living in hot and humid climates.

The lesions of tenia corporis occur on non and hairy parts of the body and are flat with an erythmatous scaling border and clearing center. They are typical annular appearance, well-deepened margins with fine cigarette paper scale and *erythmatis*.

Because of the dermatophytoses thrive in moist warm environment, the affected area should be kept clean and dry and overbathing to be avoided. A bland dusting powder can be used to promote dryness. Loose underclothing should be worn.

Mild infections are treated with cold compress; topical antifungals for isolated patches, creams or solution of miconazole Monistat and clotrimazole, Lotrimain. other than topical fungicide. Oral griseofulvin for severe infections.

3. *Tenia Cruris*

   Tenia cruris is dematophytes commonly referred to as 'Jock itch' which occurs most commonly in men, especially who have tenia pedis and those who frequently wear athletic suppress or right shorts. It also occurs in women who wear tight pantyhose or slacks.

Tenia cruris the lesion of. the warm, moist, inter triginous areas of the groin. The lesions are bilateral and extend outward from groin along the inner thigh. The colour ranges from brown to red, scaling is absent and pruritus is unusually present. Lesions are well-defined border in groin area.

Treatment includes topical antifungal cream or solution.

4. *Tenia Pedis*

   Tenia pedis is most common dermatophytosis commonly referred to as "athletes foot". There are several forms of tenia pedis. It is rarely seen in children or women, but is widespread among young men especially those wearing shoes in hot climates. Walking barefoot in gymnasiums or ground swimming pool are susceptible to acquire infection.

The most common form of tenia pedis is intertriginous form. The fungal involvement usually begins in the toe webs, especially in the fourth interspace and may extend to the undersurface of the toe or on the plantar surface.

The person may be asymptomatic or may experience itching and burning in the affected area. The nails may become discoloured, thickened or distorted onychomycosis. There will be interdigital scaling and maceration, erythema and blistering, pruritus and painful.

Treatment includes topical antifungal cream or solution.

The person with tenia pedis needs to be taught meticulous foot hygiene after the toes are dried thoroughly a light dusting of antifungal powder is applied to promote dryness. Caking the powder should be avoided. Socks should be of an absorbant material such as cotton, and may need to be changed more than once daily to promote dryness. A major focus of nursing is to initiate activities that lessen infection, such as wearing sandals, going barefoot, to decrease tissue moisture and using good foot hygiene, which includes washing the feet frequently and drying well between the toes.

5. *Tenia Unguium*

   Tenia unguium is a dermatophytes. In this only few nails on one hand is affected; nails on toes are possibly affected. Fungal scale close to outer margin or lesion, brittle, thickened, broken nails with white or yellow discolouration.

Treatment modalities include:

- Tropical antifungal cream or solution.
- Griscofulvin moderately successful in fingernails.
- Poor response on toe nails.
- Debridement of toe nails to normal contour if problematic.

BACTERIAL INFECTIONS

The skin is covered with numerous micro-organisms especially bacteria. Most bacteria that normally inhabit in the skin are nonpathogenic. The skin provides an ideal environment for bacterial growth with abundant supplies of warmth, nutrients and water. Bacterial infections occur when the balance between the host and the micro-organisms is altered. This can occur on primary infection following a break in the skin. It can also occur as a secondary infection to already damaged skin or as a sign of a systemic disease. The common bacterial infections of the skin are as follows:

1. Impetigo

Impetigo is a common skin infection caused by staphylococci or beta-hemolytic streptococci or combination of both. It can occur at any age group but mostly in children. It occurs during summer or early fall. Factors that promote development of impetigo include tropical climates, uncleanliness, poor hygiene, poor nutrition and poor health.

Impetigo begins as a small thorn-walled vesicle that ruptures, easily and leaves a weeping denuded spot. It becomes pustular and dries to form a honey-coloured crust that appears stuck in the skin. The process, which is superficial may extend below the crust. Usually it is confirmed to face but may occur elsewhere. Clinical management includes vesicelopustular lesions that develop thick, honey-coloured crust surrounded by erythema, pruritic most common in face.

Treatment consists of maintaining cleanliness and applying topical antibiotics. The crusts must be removed and the lesions washed gently two or three times daily to prevent further crust formation. Warm soaks or saline compress may be necessary to soften crusts that adhere firmly. Topical antibiotics are applied thrice a day. Systemic antibiotics such as oral penicillin, benzeathine pencillin I M erythromycin are prescribed.

2. Folliculitis

Folliculitis is usually caused by staphylococcis aureas, but occasionally caused by other bacteria. It may be caused by drainage from other infection. Predisposing factors include uncleanliness, maceration, infection, chemical irritation and injury.

Bacterial infections of the hair follicle may be superficial in the epidermis around the hairfollicle or deep in the tissue surrounding both the lower and upper portions of the hair follicle. Small pustules at hair follicle opening with minimal erythema, development of crusting most common on scalp; beard, extermities in men, tender to touch. Deep folliculitis produces a more severe inflammatory response. Sycoses barbae, barber's itch. is deep folliculitis of the beard, in which hair do not fall out or break such as occurs with tenia barbae. *Hordeolom* Stye is deep folliculitis of the cilia of eyelids. There is usually swelling of the surrounding eyelid, with cursing along the edge of the eyelid.

Treatment of superficial folliculitis includes cleansing with soap and water and supplying topical antibiotics. Warm compresses are applied to encourage resolution of deep folliculities. Topical antibiotics such as neosporin, hasten healing. Healing is usually without scarring and loss of involved hari follicles.

Nursing management focuses on teaching patients about the prescribed therapy and about avoiding predisposing factors.

3. Furuncles and Carbuncles

Furuncles or boils are deep folliculitis that originate either superficial folliculates or as a deep nodule around hair follicle. *Furunculosis* is the appearance of several furuncles. An infection that involves several surrounding hair follicles is termed as *carbuncles*.

Aetiology

The causative organism is usually staphylococcus, but occasionally furuncles can be caused by other bacteria. Both furuncles and carbuncles occur most often in obese poorly-nourished, fatigued, or otherwise susceptible persons whose hygiene may be poor, in debilitated elderly people and in persons with poorly-controlled diabetes mellitus.

Pathophysiology

Local swelling and redness occur together with severe local pain which is decreased by moving the involved part as little as possible. Within 3 to 5 days, the lesion becomes elevated or "points up" the surrounding skin becomes shiny and the center or 'core' turns yellow. A carbuncle has several cores. The boil will usually rupture spontaneously but it may be surgically incised and drained. A drainage occurs, the pain is immediately relieved. The drainage soon changes from a yellow purulent material to a serosanguineous discharge. All drainage usually subsides within a few hours in a few days, the redness and swelling subside gradually.

Clinical Manifestations

In furuncles, there will be tender erythematous area around hair follicle; draining of pus and core of necrotic debris on rupture; they are most likely to occur on face, back of the neck, axillae, breasts, buttocks, perineum, thighs whereas carbuncles are usually limited to the nape of the neck and back. In addition to lesion, malaise, regional adenopathy, and elevated temperature are seen in furunculosis.

Management

For furuncles: Incision and drainage, occasionally antibiotics, meticulous care, of involved skin, frequent application of warm and moist compresses.

For funculosis: Warm compresses; systemic antibiotic after culture and sensitivity study of drainage usually semi synthetic penicillanase-resistant, oral penicillin such as oxacillin. Measures to reduce surface stphylococci include antimicrobial cream to nares, armpits, and groin and antiseptic to entire skin; often recurrent with scarring; incision and drainage of life lesions; prevention or correction of predisposing factors; meticulous hygiene.

For carbuncles: Treatment as in furuncles; often recurrent despite production of antibodies healing slow with scar formation.

Nursing care focuses on preventing this spread of infection. Patients are cautioned to keep their hands away from the discharge to prevent spread of infection.

4. Erysipelas

Erysipelas is a type of cellulitis usually caused by a haemolytic streptococci and *S. aureus*. Elderly people with poor resistance are most often affected. Erysipelas may follow a puncture wound, ulcer or chronic dermatis.

Erysipelas is characterized by localized inflammation and swelling of the skin and subcutaneous tissues, usually of the face, scalp, hands, and genitalia. A bright, sharp line separates the diseased skin from the normal skin. The lesions are hot and red. The infection spreads via the lymphatic system and bloodstream.

Gramstain culture and sensitivity will determine the appropriate antibiotic therapy. Local lesions should be immobilized and elevated to decrease local oedema. Wet-to-dry dressings may decrease pain and dry-up bullous lesions. Moist heat may also be used. If abscess formation occurs, incision and drainage are indicated. Nursing intervention focuses on helping patients assume responsibility for treatment and completing the treatment. It is imperative that the patient completes the course of prescribed antibiotic therapy. Hospitalization is needed in severe cases there will be progression to gangrene if cellulitis is untreated.

General principles of treatment for bacterial skin infection includes cleansing the skin well and applying an antibiotic. The skin is cleansed with soap and water or with hexachlorophene. Water or saline compresses or heat may be used to dry the horny layer of the skin. Topical antibiotics commonly used, include hydroxyquinilones, such as vioform, neomycin, bactiracin, and gentamycin, or erythromycin. Systemic antibiotics are used only when systemic signs such as fever and malaise are present.

VIRAL INFECTIONS OF THE SKIN

Viral infections of the skin are difficult to treat as viral infection anywhere in the body. When a cell is infected by a virus, a lesion can result. Lesions can also result from an inflammatory response to the viral infections. Herpes simplex, herpes zoster and warts are the common viral infections affecting the skin.

1. Herpes Simplex

Herpes simplex occurs on two similar yet serologically different strain type 1 and type 2. Herpes simplex virus (HSV) has a DNA containing core surrounded by a phospholipid covering.

Aetiology

Factors that may precipitate recurrence of herpes simplex lesion include fever, URI, exhaustion and nervous tension. Lesions also are more common during the menses and after direct exposure to the sun rays.

HSV type generally has oral infections, virus remaining in nerve root ganglion and possibly returning to the skin to produce recurrence when excerbated by sunlight, trauma, menses, stress and systemic infections; contagion to those not previously infected; increase in severity with age, transmission by respiratory droplets or virus containing fluid, such as saliva or cervical secretions. The protection against subsequent infection in other areas with episodes of infection in one area.

HSV type 2 is associated with a lesion of the genitalia, that can be transmitted by sexual contact.

Pathophysiology

There are two phases to HSV infections. Primary infection is acquired by direct exposure to virus, usually through macocutaneous contact with an infected individual. After the initial infection, the virus travels to a sensory nerve ganglion and becomes latent. Reactivation of the virus causes disease recurrence. The HSV remains in the cells of the sensory nerves that supply the affected areas and causes recurrent lesions when the person is subjected to stress. The appearance of vesicles is preceded by several hours by a sensation of burning or itching. A cluster of vesicles on an erythematous basic appears at the macocutaneous junction of the lips or nose or an inflammation of the cornea of one eye with photphobia and tearing. The lesion found on the face and mouth (fever, blister, cold sore), eye (keratitis) (encephalitis).

HSV type 2 virus lesions are painful and may crack open. A crust gradually forms and the lesions heal in about 10 days. HSV can be identified by the Tzanck smear.

Clinical Manifestation

In first episode, symptoms occurring 3-7 days or more after contact; painful local reactions, grouped vesicles on erythmematous base; systemic symptom such as fever and malaise are possible or asymptomatic presentation is possible. In recurrent phase, small recurrence is in similar spot; characteristic grouped vesicle is on erythmatous base.

Management

Treatment includes symptomatic medication; soothing, moist compresses petrolatum to lesions, scarring not usual result; antiviral agents such as acyclovir zovinax. *famciclovir* (famvir) and valacyclovir (valtrex). Topical use of acyclovir, idoxuridine or vidarabine has been effective in preventing corneal ulceration and visual impairment in herperetic keratitis. *Acyclovir* is effective in systematically treating primary general herpes simplex and preventing recurrence. Patients with frequent recurrence may benefit from subcutaneous interferon-alfa. Patient education is the primary nursing intervention needed for the patient with HSV infection regarding aetiology, treatment modalities and measures to prevent secondary infection. Topical interferor-alfa, interferor-beta ointment are useful ingenital herpes.

2. Herpes Zoster

Herpes zoster or shingles is caused by the same virus varicella-zoster. that causes varicella (chicken pox). Activation of the varicella zoster virus; frequent recurrence in immunosuppressed patients; potentially contagious to any one who has not had varicella or who is immunosuppressed. It is one of the most persisting and exasperating conditions in elderly persons and leads to discouragement and demoralization.

Pathophysiology

In herpes zoster, clusters of small vesicles usually form in line. They follow the course of the peripheral sensory nerves and often unilateral. Because they follow nerve pathways, the lesions never cross the midline of the body. However, nerves on both the sides of the body can be involved. Two-thirds of persons with herpes zoster develop lesions over the thoracic dermatomes and the remainder show involvement of the trigeminal nerve with lesions on the face, eye and scalp. The rash develops first as macules but progress rapidly to vesicles. The fluid becomes turbid and crusts develop and drop off in about 10 days.

Clinical Manifestation

Linear patches along dermatome of grouped vesicles on erythematous base; usually unilateral and on trunk; burning pain and neuralgia preceding outbreak, mild to severe during outbreak, malaise, fever, itching and pain over the involved area may precede the eruption of lesions. Discomfort from pain and itching is the major problem with herpes zoster. The pain may vary from light burning to deep visceral type pain. Enlargement of the lymph node may occur with rash.

Management

Treatment is symptomatic; antiviral agents such as acyclovir, famciclovir, and valacyclovir; moist compresses, white petrolatum to lesions; analgesia, mild sedation at bed time; Systemic corticosteroids to short course and decrease likelihood of postherpetic neuralgia (PHN), controversal, usual healing without complication but scarring possible postherpetic neuralgia possible.

Analgesic prescribed for pain. Aspirin without codiene for severe pain. Systemic corticosteroid prednisone are useful. Local application of capsaicin cream may give some relief.

3. Verruca Vulgaris

Verruca vulgaris caused by human papilloma virus, spontaneous disappearance in 1-2-years is possible; mildly contagious by autoinoculation, specific response on body part is affected.

Clinical manifestation includes circumscribed, hypertrophic, flesh-coloured papulae to epidermis, painful on lateral compression.

Multiple treatment includes surgery—scoop removal with scissors and currette; liquid nitrogen therapy; blistering agents—cantharidin; Keralytic agents—salicylic acid; CO_2 laser therapy, treatment can result in scarring.

4. Warts

Warts develop from hypertrophy of epidermal cells as a result of a viral infection. Plantar warts is caused by human papilloma virus. It is seen most commonly in older children and young adults.

Pathophysiology

Warts are benign skin growths that grow in variety of shapes.

The common wart is a small circumscribed, painless hyperkeratotic papule usually seen in the extremities, especially the hands. *Filiform* warts are slender finger-like projections occurring mostly on the face and neck. *Plantar* warts grow inward from the pressure on the sole of the feet and may be painful. They are differentiated from calluses by lack of skin lines over the surface. Warts that develop in the anogenital region have a lighter-coloured surface and a cauliflower-like appearance, and they may cause itching. *Anogenital* warts may spread either by sexual activity or by other means. Some genital warts in women may predispose the woman in cancer cervix.

Clinical Manifestation

Plantar warts on bottom surface of foot are growing inwards because of pressure of walking or standing; painful when pressure applied; interrupted skin markings; cone shaped with black dot thrombosed vessels when pared.

Management

The most commonly used therapeutic measures for common warts are electrodessiccation and cryosurgery. In electrodessiccation, the top of the wart is seared gently to soften the keratinized surface and then curretted off and the bleeding points cauterized. This method is not used for plantar warts.

Cryosurgery: consists of freezing the lesion with a substance such as liquid nitrogen. Cauterant chemicals—such as formalin, phenol, nitric acid, canthridin, salicylic acid, or porophyllum may be used. Recalcitrant warts may respond to reciation therapy. Surgical excision is seldom used because of painful scarring may result.

Nursing intervention includes preparing the patient for treatment and assist during treatment.

ALLERGIC CONDITIONS OF THE SKIN

Dermatologic problem associated with allergies and hypersensitivity reactions presents a real challenge to the health care providers. A careful family history and discussion of exposure to possible offending agents provide valuable data. Patch testing involves the application of allergens to the patient skin usually on the back for 48 hours, after which the test sites are examined for erytheme, papules vesicles or all of these. Patch testing is used to determine possible causative agents. This information is valuable to the patient. The best treatment of allergic dermatitis is avoidance of causative agent. The extreme prurits of contact dermatitis is and its potential chronicity make it frustrating problem for the patient, the nurse and the dermatologist.

Dermatitis is a superficial inflammation of the skin, refers to several different conditions resulting in the same type of lesions. Dermatitis is often classified arbitraily according to special features such as cause, pattern, age or type of treatment required. The term *eczema*, is often used synonymously with dermatitis but usually refers to the chronic type.

The common allergic conditions of the skin are in brief as follows:

1. Contact Dermatitis

Contact dermatitis is caused by external agents and may affect various parts of the body. The two types of contact dermatitis are *irritant* and *allergic.*

Aetiology

- Irritant contact dermatitis can occur in any person on contact with a sufficient concentration of an irritant.
  - Mechanical irritation may result from wool or glass fibers.
  - Chemical irritants include acids, alkalies, solvents, detergents and oils commonly found in clearing compounds, insecticides and industrial compounds.
  - Biological irritants include urine, feces, and toxins from insects or aquatic plants. People whose hands and feet are constantly wet often develop irritant contact dermatitis.
- Allergic contact dermatitis is cell-mediated hypersensitivity immune reaction from contact with a specific antigen. Many compounds cause sensitization under specified conditions. Typical antigen includes poison, ivy, synthetics, industrial chemicals, drugs e.g. sulfanilamide or penicillin, and metals e.g. Nichel-chromium.

Common causes of contact dermatitis of different areas are as follows:

i. *Face/Scalp/Ears:* Cosmetics,haircare producers, jewellery cleansers, sunscreen, contact lens solution, metals nickel. glasses.
ii. *Neck:* Perfumes, clothing especially wool.
iii. *Trunk:* Deodarants, clothing, perfumes, laundry products.
iv. *Arms and Hands:*Poison ivy, oak, and sumac, jewellery, nickel, etc. in watch bands, detergents and other cleanser gloves.
v. *Legs/Feet:* Medication for "athletes foot" shoes.

Pathophysiology

Characteristic dermatitis lesions appear sooner in irritant contact dermatitis than in allergic type. Manifestations of delayed hypersensitivity, absorbed agent acting as antigen and sensitization after several exposures, appearance of lesions 2-7 days after contact with allergies.

Clinical Manifestation

Red, hive-like papules and plaques; sharply circumscribed with occasional vesicles; exposed areas are more common; usually pruritic; relation of area of dermatitis to causative agent. e.g. metal allergy and dermatitis on ring finger.

Management

- Weeping uninfected lesions respond rapidly to wet dressings with water or burows solution for 20 minutes four times daily.
- Crusts and scales are not removed but are allowed to drop off naturally as the skin heals.
- Topical corticosteroids for acute extensive exacerbation.
- Systemic antibiotics if infection is present.
- Antihistamines for severe pruritus.
- Plain calamine lotion may be applied for pruritus from poison ivy.
- Elimination of contact allergens.
- Avoidance of irritating affected area.
- Systemic corticosteroid if sensitivity is severe.
- Primary focus of nursing care in prevention includes patient teaching.

2. Urticaria

Usually allergic phenomena, presence of oedema in upper dermis resulting from a local increase in permeability of capillaries usually from histamine.

Clinical manifestation includes spontaneity occurring and rounded elevations, varying size and usually multiple.

Treatment includes removal of source and antihistamine therapy.

3. Drug Reaction

Any drug that acts as antigen and causes hypersensitivity reaction is possible cause, certain drugs more prone to reaction e.g. Penicillin. mediated by circulating antibody.

Clinical manifestation includes rash of any morphology, often red, macular and papular, semiconfluent, generalized rash with abrupt onset, appearance as late as 14 days after cessation of drug, possibly pruritic.

Treatment includes withdrawal of drug if possible, antihistamines, local or systemic corticosteroids are possibly necessary.

4. Atopic Dermatitis

Atopy refers to type I hypersensitivity, which is hereditary and includes asthma, hay fever, eczema and other type of reactions.

Exact cause is unknown, often beginning in infancy and decreasing in incidence with age, association with allergic conditions, costume, hay fever, eczema, elevation, e.g. Ig E levels are common, genetically determined, often family history, decreased itch threshold, stress and increased water contact e.g. frequent hand washing, thumb sucking and other possible agents.

The major symptoms of atopic dermatitis is pruritus, chronic scratching leads to eczematous lesions and subsequent lichenification. There will be scaly, red to redbrown, circumscribed lesions; accentuation of skin marking pruritic and symmetric eruptions common in antecubital and popliteal space in adults. Persons with atopic dermatis are highly susceptible to viral infections Herpes. and bacterial infection staphylococci or bethemolytic streptococci.

There is no cure for atopic dermatitis, but symptoms can be controlled. The focus of therapy in relief of pruritus to break the itch scratch cycle that leads to lesions. For which:

- Topical corticosteroids creams and ointments for localized lesion.
- Topical antibiotic is rarely used.
- Cool compresses with water or burows solution are helpful for acute phases when weeping lesions are present.
- Phototherapy; coaltar therapy, intralesional corticosteroids, lubrication of dry skin.
- Systemic corticosteroids if severe—e.g. eczema.
- Reduction of stress.
- Antibiotic for secondary infection, e.g. penicillin and erythromycin.

Patient education is the major focus of care and should stress prevention of hypersensitivity and control of signs and symptoms. Patient should keep the skin hydrated and avoid temperature extremes and irritating substances. The person with atopic dermatitis will be given education as follows:

- Avoid soap over lesions; soap is an irritant.; use soap minimally over non-affected areas.
- Soak affected areas for 15 to 20 minutes in warm water for hydration; pat skin dry, then immediately apply recommended lotion or cream to seal in moisture.
- Wet wraps may be used in place of soaking; wraps permits evaporation, which cools the skin, thus decreasing pruritus.
- Apply corticosteroids in a thin layer and rub in well; do not use fluonated corticosteroids on the face.
- Avoid wool, furor rough fibers against the skin; they are irritants and cause itching.
- Avoid overheating that increases sweating, leading to itching, wear loose, light clothing in hot weather. Airconditioning promotes comfort sunlight is beneficial to the skin.
- Avoid excessive cold that dries the skin.
- Avoid anything that aggravates the eczema.
- Rinse all garments and bed linen, twice to avoid residue of cleansing agents.
- Consult dermatologist for appropriate laundry agents to prevant irritations from clothing.
- Seek medical care of eczema becomes worse.

5. Other Type of Dermatitis

i. *Lichen Simplex chronicus* LSC is a chronic skin condition that results from repeated scratching. Psychological factors are thought to be involved. It may occur without any cause, LCS is more commonly found on the hands, perineum, legs, and occipital region of the scalp. Once itching starts, the itch scratch cycle is initiated and scratching becomes a habit. The skin becomes excoriated and lichenified plaques resulting. Lesion disappears if scratching ceases, but it is difficult for the person to stop scratching. Itching is often worse at night. Topical corticosteroids are the treatment of choice.

ii. *Seborrheic dermatitis* may occur primarily in areas of increased sebaccan gland activity on the face, ears, scalp, chest and back. The cause is unknown. Mild seborrheic dermatitis is often seen in the scalp in the form of erythema and dandruff and can be controlled easily by shampooing with selenium sulfide (Selsum blue) shampoo. More extensive seborrheic dermatitis leads to red scaly plaques and is treated with topical hydrocortisone.

iii. *Nummulur dermatitis* is chronic condition of uncertain cause occurring most commonly in middle-aged or older men. The lesions of nummular dermatitis are corn-shaped and are found on the dorsum of the hands, the extension surfaces of the extremities and the buttocks. Itching is often severe. The skin is usually dry, therefore, frequent bathing is inadvisable. Exposure to sunlight may be helpful. Treatment consists of topical corticosteroids and antibiotic therapy of lacterin isolated by culture.

iv. *Stasis dermatitis* is a common skin condition of the lower extremities in older person. It is usually preceded by varicosities and poor circulation. With the reduction in venous return from the legs, substances are normally carried away by the circulation remain in the tissue causing irritation. The skin is often reddened and oedematous. Pruritus may be severe. Scratching causes breaks in the skin, which become infected via hands, clothing and other sources. The most important treatment for stasis dermatitis is prevention with careful attention to the treatment of peripheral vascular condition preventing constrictions of the circulation to the extremities. Acute weeping lesions are treated with wet compresses and elevation of the legs.

6. Skin Reactions

Dermatitis Medicamentosa

Dermatitis medicamentosa or drug rash, can be caused by almost any drug. The rash occurs as a result of gradual accumulation of the drug or because of antibodies that develop in response to a component of the medications. Skin manifestations from drug have a nonallergic or an allergic basis. Commonly seen skin reactions include, erythematous rashes, purpura, vesicles, bullae, ulcers, and urticaria. the reactions may occur at any time but the onset is usually sudden.

Most skin reactions are caused by hypersensitivity reaction to drugs. The following reaction may occur.

- Type I Analphylactic urticaria, angioedema.
- Type II Cytotoxic cell injury.
- Type III Immune complex serum sickness.
- Type IV Cell-mediated allergic contact dermatitis, allergic photosensitivity..
- Some drugs have combined reactions. For example, Penicillin may produce type I and type III reaction.

Photosensitivity may occur with certain drugs and may take one of two forms: phototoxicity or photoallergy.

- Phototoxicity may occur in any person taking a photosensitive drug and results from the reaction of the drug chemicals. with radiant energy, particularly ultraviolet light symptoms resemble sunburn erythema, oedema, vesicle..
- Photoallergy reactions are cell-mediated type IV. Hypersensitivity reactions, therefore, affect only a small group of persons after several sensitizing exposures of drug and sunlight. Symptoms resemble eczema.
  Coal tar derivatives, psoralens, tetracycline, nalidixic acid, sulfalim, dectomycin, chloropromazine, certain dyes, diuretics thiazides phenathiazine oral hypoglycaemias and griseofulvin.

The skin reaction to common medications are as follows:

- Antibiotics, sulfonamides, thiazide diuretices barbiturates, phenylbutazone.'
- Purpura Ecchymosis: Petechias., thiazide, sulfonamide, barbiturates, anticoagulants.
- Mucocutanean lesions: Sulfanamides, penicillin, barbiturate, phenylbutazone vesicles, bullae ulcers..
- Urticaria: Penicillin, streptomycin, tetracyclin, insulin, aspirin, dyes, ACTH and antiserum.

Management of dermatitis medicomentosa include stopping the drug and treating the symptoms with cool moist compresses, antihistamines for pruritus, and topical and systematic corticosteroids. Photosensitivity can be prevented by avoiding direct sunlight on the skin when taking drug with photosensitivity effects. Nursing care include patient education regarding skin reaction to drugs and report and take proper remedial measure.

Explorative Dermatitis

Explorative dermatitis is rare and generalized dermatitis. In most cases, cause is unknown, but the disease may be associated with other types of dermatitis or with a lymphoma or it may be result of drug reaction.

The onset of disease may be rapid or insidious and consist of an elevated temperature and generalized erythema, followed by extensive scaling exfoliation. Pruritus may be present and the lesions often become infected. Loss of large amounts of water and protein from the skin leads to hypoproteinaemia, weight loss, and difficulty with temperature control. Heart failure may occur in elderly patient. Death may result from overwhelming infections or circulatory collapse.

Treatment consists of maintaining fluid balance and preventing infection. All drugs are discontinued as potential causative factors although antibiotics may be started after culture and sensitivity tests, and infected lesions. Oral corticosteroids are used for severe case. Daily baths followed by application of patrolatum to the skin promote comfort. Nursing care focuses for management of signs and symptoms and education.

Erythema Multifoma

Erythema multifoma (EM) is self-limiting inflammation of the skin and mucous membranes in genetically suscepticable persons. Although it is mild, it may progress to a toxic epidermal necrolysis type of illness. It can be classified as major and minor. Both forms are thought to be a cell-mediated immune response to relevant antigens.

Some medications trigger EM include phenytoin, carbambazepine, sulfonamides NSAIDS, allopurinol and some antibiotics e.g. cephalosporins. Infection that causes EM include myeoplasmal pneumonia, chicken pox, hepatitis B, infectious mononucleosis and herpes simlex, SLE and leukamia.

Episodes of the disease usually lasts for 1 to 3 weeks. The clinical lesions are characteristically erythematus papulae acrally distributed. The rash is painful and itchy, and it may progress to the bullous variety. The rash occurs on the dorso of the hands, palms, knees, feet and elbows. The oral cavity may be affected by blisters progressing to erosion of the entire oral mucosa and lips. Conjunctivitis may occur it may progress to corneal opacity. If the genital mucosa is involved, adhesions may result as long-term complications. The skin eruptions may be preceded by fever, chest pain and arthralgia. Severe case may be confused with toxic epidermal necrolysis.

A single attack of EM does not usually require treatment. Any suspected triggering agent is discontinued and symptoms treated. Topical steroid may be prescribed to relive itching and burning. Systemic steroids seem to prolong episodes of the disease. A sedatory antihistamine such as hydroxyzine may be of use. The patient with any type of EM needs support and education throughout diagnosic biopsy and treatment as prescribed. Initially other disorders causing blistering must be considered and the patient will require support during this time. Education needed to patient regarding the medication prescribed including administration of dosing and side effects. Nursing intervention is supportive and includes baths, soaks and care.

Infectious Diseases

Skin reactions caused by some communicable diseases such as measle, chicken pox, small pox, scarlet fever, and accompany severe acute rheumatic fever.

- Measles (rubeola) caused by rubeola virus, incubation period is 8-14. days. Rash appears on the face, they will be pink macular-papular rash and lesions coalesce.
- Germal measles (rubella) caused by rubella virus, incubation period 14-21 days. Rash appears on the face, they are pink macular-papular rash, lesions usually discretes and it may coalesce.
- Scarlet fever (Scarlatina) caused by haemolytic streptococcus, incubation period is 1-3 days. Rashes appear on neck and chest. They are bright red scarlet and macules pin point.
- Chicken pox (varicella) caused by varicella zoster virus, incu-bation period is 14-21 days. Rashes appear on back and chest. They are macule papule, vesicle, crust, lesions at different stages.
- Small pox (variola) caused by variola virus, incubation period is 7-21 days. Rashes appear on face and chest. They are macule, papule, vesicle, crust, lesions and all at same stage.
- Typhoid fever caused by Salmonella typhosa, incubation period is 14 7-21. days. Rashes appeal on abdomen. They are macular rash.

Treatment includes treating the diseases.

LUPUS ERYTHEMATOSUS

It is one of the tissue diseases that may result in skin condition. There are two forms, systemic lupus erythematosus SLE and discoid lupus erythematosa DLE. SLE has already been discussed in earlier chapter.

DLE is a chronic relative benign skin that has worldwide presence among all races occurring, most often in fourth decade of life. The precipitating factors include physical trauma and stress.

The lesions of the DLE are well demarcated and erythmatous, have a characteristic scaly border with an atrophied center and vary in size. The more common sites are the cheeks butterfly pattern , nose, ears, scalp and chest, although other parts of the body including mucous membranes may also be involved. DLE occurs in the absence of other signs and symptoms and nuerological abnormalities of SLE.

There is no cure fo DLE. Palliative measures include, topical steroid therapy under occlusive wraps, intralesional steroid therapy, antimalarial therapy with chloroquine, hydroxy chloroquine sulfate or quinacrine hydrochloride. Nursing care is focussed on assisting patients and thus families to live with a chronic incurable disease. Education is necessary regarding palliative and preventive measures. Preventive measures include avoiding physical trauma, using sun screen to prevent sunburn and wearing warm clothing to protect against cold and wind. If stress is a precipitatory factor, measures to reduce stress can be instituted.

PAPULOSQUAMOUS DISEASES

Papulosquamous diseases are characterized by papular, scaly lesions, common disorders are psyriasis, pityriasis rosea and lichen plasius.

Psoriasis

Psoriasis is a genetically determined, chronic, epidermal, proliferative disease. The cause is unknown. There are no specific precipitating factors for the majority of persons. However, some people may develop exacerbations after climatic changes, stressors, trauma, infections, or drugs propronolol, lithium. Pregnant women often experience of remissions of symptoms. It is chronic dermatitis which involves excessively rapid turn over of epidermal cells and family predispositions.

The lesions of psoriasis are elevated, erythematous and sharply circumscribed, with a silvery white scale. Removal of the scale usually results in a characteristic pin-point-bleeding called the 'Auspitz phenomenon'. The primary lesions is a papule; these papules then join to form plaques. Lesions may occur over the entire body but are found more commonly on the scalp, elbows, chins, intergluteal cleft, and trunk. Beefy-red lesions may be observed in an acute flare-up. Nail changes may occur. The nails of persons with psoriasis have characteristic involvement; there may be pitting of the nails, yellowish discolouration, oil drop or salmon patches; leukonychia and whitening of nails, splinter haemorrhage and onycholysis separation of nail from nail bed.

Types of Psoriasis

There are four types of psoriasis viz., psoriasis vulgaris, generalized psoriasis, localized psoriasis and erythematous psoriasis.

- Psoriaris vulgaris may follow streptococcal phanyngitis.
- Generalized postular psoriasis patients require admission to hospital. In generalized and localized postular type, there will be history of plaque type of psoriasis developing pustules on erythmatic base. Other symptoms include fever, chills, arthralgia, hypocalcaemia.
- Erythematous psoriasis produces red colouration of the skin with disquamaline scale over most of the body. It is associated with problems of temperature regulation, hypoalbumenia, pedaloedema, and high output cardiac failure caused by inflammatory vasodilation.

The complication psoriasis is psoriatic arthritis.

Management

Initially the lesions may be treated with topical keratolytic agents salicylic acid, ammoniated mercury. or tropical steroids with occlusive wraps and wet dressing to decrease inflammation. The application of bland emollient petrolatum and mineral oil is important in the treatment of person with psoriasis. These emollients decrease the amount of scale on the psoriatic plaques and the thickness of the plaque. If person is resistent to emollients, coaltar of anthralin products are used. Interlesional injection of corticosteroids for chronic plaques; sunlight, ultraviolet light, alone or with topical or systemic potentiation; no cure is possible, but can be controllable, antimetabolites, methotrexate are used for difficult cases.

The disease is not curable and may wax and wane continuously. Lesions may fade with treatment, only to recur in the same area or elsewhere. Teaching the person with psoriasis will be helpful.

- Nature of psoriasis, non-curable, recurrence of symptoms.
- Reduce episodes of rapidly spreading psoriasis flare-ups. by avoiding skin trauma injuries, sunburn, infections, extremes of temperature, and stress.
- Shampoo hair frequently remove scales of scalps. If scalp has plaques, use a tar shampoo for 10 minutes before rinsing. Press often thick plaques with mineral oil at the night before a morning shampoo; use fine-toothed comb to remove loose scales.
- Avoid self-medication, particularly when receiving prescribed therapy.
- Apply topical medication in a thin layer for most lesions, use a thick layer over plaques.
- Monitor for side effects of medication.
- Seek Medical follow-up during periods of exocerbation.

Pityriasis Rosea

Pityriasis Rosea is a noncontagious skin condition. The cause is thought to be viral. The incidence is higher in winter. The initial symptom is usually a 2 to 10 cm, single, oval lesion herald patch. with a thin scaly border and yellowish centre, appearing most often on the trunk, upper arm or thigh. The herald patch usually precedes other lesions by 1 to 30 days.

A generalized eruptions of multiple erythmatous macule follows the herald patch usually followed by papules. A fine scale is usually present. The distribution of lesions often are in long axes, running parallel to each other on the trunk which creates a "Christmas tree" distribution. The skin usually clears in 6 to 8 weeks and the condition does not recur.

Treatment option consists of tropical steroids and colloid baths. Ultraviolet therapy may be used. Exposure to sunlight to the point of minimal erythema. will speed disappearance of the lesions and itching. The patient should be cautious against sunburn. Nursing care is essentially symptomatic and includes assisting patient with topical steroids and colloid baths if itching is present and educating the patient and family.

ACNE

Acne Vulgeris

Acne vulgaris is an inflammatory disorder of sebacous glands, more common in teenagers but possible development in adulthood. Persistence in adulthood possible. Secondary result of iodides, bromides, cortecosteroids and androgen-dominated birth control pills.

The cause of acne is thought to be multifactorial. Some of the common causes that have been postulated are free fatty acids, endocrine effects, stressors, diet, hereditary and infection.

Pathophysiology

At puberty sabaceous glands undergo enlargement from androgen stimulation. Sebum is released, passed through the follicular canal, and combined with sebacous gland cell fragments, epidermal cells keratin and bacteria. At this time the triglycerides in the sebum and hydrolyzed to glycerol and free fatty acids. The sebum and debris may become plugged in the hair follicle to form an *open comedo* black head., if it is at the surface or *closed comedo* white head.. The dark colour of the blackhead melanin is not dirt and results from passage of melanin from the adjoining epidermal cells. Inflammatory lesions apparently develop from the escape of sebum into the dermis, which then serves as an irritant, causing an inflammatory reaction. Free fatty acids may also be an irritant in the follicle itself.

Clinical Management

Acne occurs mostly on the face and neck, upper chest and back although the upper arms, buttocks and thighs may also be involved. Comedes are the first visible signs, and the skin is characteristically oily. The inflammatory lesions include papules, pustules, nodules, and cysts. Superficial lesions may resolve within 5-10 days without scarring but large lesions last for several weeks and often result scarring. Ice-pickscar..

Management

Treatment of acne may be topical, systemic, intralesional or surgical and includes the following:

i. Topical therapy
   - Basic method therapy.
   - Agents: benzoyl peroxide, vitamin A, acid tretin, antibiotics topical erythromycin., sulfur-zinc lotion.

ii. Removal of comedones with comedo extraction.

iii. Systemic therapy.
   - Used with topical therapy for severe nodular or dystic acne.
   - Isoretinioc acid accutane.
     – A vitamin A acid ana
     – Side affects: dry lips and conjucative on brittle hair tendernege to finger tips and toe trips, hypertriglyceridaemia birth defects.
   - Systemic antibiotics
   - Oestrogen for female patients who have not responded to other therapy.

iv. Intralesional corticosteroid therapy for cystrs of severe acne.

v. Surgery; derm abrasion to remove scars.

Major nursing strategies are counselling and teaching. Stress appears to be one of the causative factors. Therefore, attempts to identify and cope with stressors may be helpful. Acne can be a stressor producing facial disfigurement and sometimes leading to behaviour that is hostile aggressive and anxiouis as well as shy and withdrawn. Psychological counsel is desirable. Knowledge of nature of acne helps the person understand the necessary care. Teaching directed towards general health care of skin with the person with acne are as follows:

i. *Preventive measure*
   - Keep hand and hair away from the face.
   - Avoid constricting clothing over lesions.
   - Shampoo hair and scalp frequently.
   - Avoid exposure to oils and greases.
   - Eat a well-balanced diet and avoid any food that appears to cause skin flare-up.

ii. *General skin care*
   - Keep skin clean; wash face 2 to 3 times daily.
   - Use a medicated soap or agent prescribed by physician.
   - Avoid vigorous rubbing of the skin.
   - Use cosmetics that are water-based, rather than cream-based and avoid those that contain waxesters myristates, palmitates, and stearates..

iii. *During therapy*
   - Follow the prescribed therapy even when immediately improvement is not noted for 2 to 3 weeks.
   - Expect skin desquamation during therapy.
   - Avoid using self-remedies during therapy.
   - Remove cosmetics before applying topical medications.
   - Avoid exposure to direct sunlight if using tretinoin, or taking tetracyclin photosensitivity..
   - Avoid pregnancy if taking accutane possibility of birth defects..

Acne Rosacea

Acne Rosacea is a skin condition that usually affects person over 25 years of age. The cause is unknown. But many causative factors suggested are bacteria, vitamin deficiency, hormonal imbalance, alcohol, caffience, psychological factors and heredity.

Acne rosacea brings with redness over the cheeks and nose, followed by papules, pustules and enlargements of superficial blood vessels. Year of acne rosasea lead to an irregular bulbous thickening of the skin of the distal part of the nose rhinophyma with a red-purple discolouration and dilated follicles.

There is no specific treatment for acne rosacea. Some persons respond to tetracyclin and tropical peeling agents. But there is no specific treatment for the vascular component. Rhinophyma may be treated by plastic surgery.

BULLOUS DISEASES

Pemphigus Vulgaris

Pemphigus vulgaris is characterized by an enormous bullae that appears all over the body and on the mucous membrane. The cause of that disease is thought to have an autoimmune basis.

Rare but worldwidely occurs primarily in persons between the age of 40 and 60.

Tissue injury results from circulating autoantibodies that bind to the structural proteins within the epidermis. Blister formation occurs above in stratum basalis. Healing is commonly associated with the development of postinflammatory hyperpigmentation rather than scarring.

The disease is characterized by *acantholysis* cells slip past one another and fluid accumulates between the cells. By placing the thumb firmly on the skin and exerting lateral sliding pressure, the upper epidermis can be dislodged resulting in erosion or blister (Nikolsky's sign). A Tzanck test will identify acantholytic cells. Injection of the crust produces a foul odour and toxaemia may result. If the disease is untreated, death usually ensues in about 1 year secondary to sepsis.

Hospitalization is usually required for skin care and monitoring of drug effects. The treatment of choice for severe pemphigus is systemic corticosteroids in large doses, the dose is gradually reduced and improvement is noted. Immunosuppressants—such as methotrexate, cyclophosphamide and azathioprine may be given to reduce the corticosteroid dose. Gold therapy gold sodium thiomalate may be given alone or in combination with corticosteroids for chronic therapy.

Nursing care of the person with severe pemphigus can be a challenge. Stryker frames may be used to help the person's change position painlessly and to prevent weight bearing on row surfaces. Air mattress or flotation system may be used to reduce surface pressure on skin and promote comfort. Dakin's solution compresses may be applied to oozing lesions to help controls odour and infection. Infection is major concern because of the immunosuppressive effect of drug therapy. Special mouth care is required for mouth lesions and bland diets are more easily tolerated,. Emotional support and education about general skin lesion care is essential for patient and family.

TUMOURS OF THE SKIN

Skin cell growth may develop from the epidermis, from sebacious or sweat glands, from the melanocyte system or from mesodermal tissue. For example, connective or vascular tissue. Most skin tumours are benign even those are malignant with the exception of such tumours of malignant malenoma.

A. Benign Tumours

The term keratosis refers to any cornification or growth of the horny layer of the skin. Different types of keratosis include corn, and calluses, warts and seborrheic and actinic senile keratosis.

1. *Corns* are due to pressure or ill-fitting shoes. In appearance it will be center core that thickness will be inwardly, pain with pressure usually occur on toes. Treatment includes foot pad with center hole to relieve pressure properly fitting shoes, corn will recur if pressure is not relieved.
2. *Callus* are due to constant pressure on plantar surface of foot. It can also occur on palmar surface of hand. In this thickening of horny layer of skin is soon. Treatment includes relief of pressure, regular massage with softening lotion or creams.
3. *Seborrheic keratosis* are benign, genetically determined growths; this care found in increasing number with age and have no association with sun exposure. Normal aging process rarely develops into malignancy, it must distinguish from actinic keratosis which have malignant potential.

Clinical manifestation includes irregularly round or oval flat-topped papules or plaques, surface is often warty; appearance of being stuck on; increase in pigmentation with age of lesion; usually multiple and possibly itching. Large darkened, greasy warts are usually on trunk, less often on scalp, face and proximal extremities. Sudden increase in number and size may indicate gastrointestinal malignancy.

No treatment except for cosmetic reasons or constant irritation may be removed by currettage, electrodesiccation, or liquid nitrogen cryosurgery. and eliminate source of irritation minimal scarring.

Another condition to similar to seborrheic keratosis is dermatosis papulosa nigra is usually seen in Afro-Americans; there will be a small pedunculated and heavily pigmented lesion. Treatment is also similar to seborrhoic keratosis.

4. *Actinic keratosis* is due to chronic exposure to solar radiation; occur on exposed areas of skin; light-skinned persons are most vulnerable. It is premalignant form of squamous cell carcinoma. It is also known as solar keratosis. The clinical appearance will be round or irregular, red brown to gray in colour with dry scaly appearance. Treatment includes protective clothing, sunscreens, removal of curettage, liquid nitrogen therapy, dermabrasion, electrodesciceation, large lesions application of 1.5 per cent and S-fluorouracil cream.
5. *Skin tags* are common after midlife, appearance on neck, a small, skin-coloured, soft and pedunculated papules. For there is no treatment unless for cosmetic reasons or because of repeated trauma; surgical removal is possible if requested. usually just "clipping off" method anaesthesia.
6. *Lipoma* Benign tumour of adipose tissue, often encapsulated, most common in 40 to 60 year-old age group. It is a rubbery compressible round mass of adipose tissue, single or multiple variable in size possibly extremely large; most common on trunk, back of neck or foreams. For this, usually there is no treatment, biopsy is used to differentiate from liposarcoma, excision usual treatment when indicated.
7. *Vitiligo* Cause is unknown it is genetically influenced, most noticeable is among dark-skinned people and those with summer tan, complete absence of melanocytes the

disease is noncontagious. The clinical manifestations include focal amelanosis complete loss of pigment., macular; variation in size and location, usually symmetric and permanent. Treatment includes attempt at repigmentation of pigmented skin with extensive disease 75 per cent body involved; cosmetics and strains for camouflage and to de-emphasize vitiligonous area..

8. *Lentigo* in which there is an increased number of normal melanocytes in basal layer of epidermis. Senile lentigo liver spots is related to aging and sun exposure. In the hypopigmented it is brown to black, flat-lesions are seen usually on sun exposed areas. Treatment is only for cosmetic purposes, liquid nitrogen, possible recurrence 1-2 years.

B. Premalignant Lesions

Skin lesions that may lead to malignancy include actinic keratitis, leukoplakia, bowens disease and pigmented moles.

1. *Leukoplakia:* The exact cause is unknown. It may be caused by external irritants such as poor-fitting dentures, cheek-biting and pipe and cigarette smoking. Chronic maceration, friction, and senile atrophy may lead to vaginal leukoplakia.

In the mucous membranes develops thickened white patches of keratinized cell, which may eventually lead to squamous cell carcinoma. Erythroplakia red or red and white patches of the mouth has a higher malignancy potential than leukoplakia.

Treatment includes prevention by removal of causative factor; inspection of mouth, mucus membrane, dental care for rough teeth, proper-fitting dentures. Large lesions are usually surgically excised, and a biopsy is performed. Benign lesions may be removed by electrode siccation.

2. *Bowen's disease:* This is due to chemical carcinogens; occurs in old and light-skinned men. It is also called squamous cell carcinoma in situ. Persons affected are at higher risk of developing other malignancies.

The lesions are widely distributed, brown plaques although a single lesion may exist. Treatment includes surgical excision, cryotherapy, curretage and electrodesiccation, carbon dioxide laser therapy and S-fluorouracil cream or solution.

3. *Pigmented nevi* Moles are grouping of normal cells derived from melanocyte like precursor cells. Hereditary predisposition is possible. Most moles are harmless, but others may be dysplectic, precancerous or cancerous.

They appear on most persons regardless of skin colour, may be flat, raised, prominant or hairy. Hyperpigmented areas vary in form and colour. Colour ranges from tank to black. Hyperpigmented areas that vary in form and colour ranges from tan to black. They are flat, slightly elevated haloid, verrucoid, polypoid, dome-shaped, sesile or papillomatous and preservation of normal skin markings; hairgrowth is possible. Dysplastic moles usually occur on the upper back in male and on the legs in females.

Changes in mole that require immediate attention which include:

- Development of a ring of new pigment around the base.
- Development of uneven pigmentation.
- Sudden growth, loss of hair and bleeding.

For moles, no treatment is necessary except for cosmetic reasons, skin biopsy for diagnostic decisions and excision of suspicious lesions. To help remember the characteristics of malignant moles, the American Cancer Society has developed the mnemonic ABCD:-

A. A symmetry of border.
B. Border irregularity.
C. Colour blue-black or variegated.
D. Diameter more than 6 mm.

C. Malignant Lesions

Malignant tumours of the skin exhibit the characteristics of all malignant conditions. However, skin malignancies are generally growing slowly. The presence of a persistent lesion that does not heal in highly suspicious of malignancy and should be biopsied. Adequate and early treatment can often lead to complete cure. The fact that the skin lesions are so visible to increase the likelihood of early detection and diagnosis. Patient should be taught to selfexamine that skin regular.

The risk factors for skin malignancies include having a fair skin type blonde or red hair and blue or green eyes, history of chronic sun exposure, family history of skin cancer, outdoor occupation and exposure to tar and systemic arsenicals and severe sunburns. The brief description of malignant lesions of the skin is as follows:

1. *Squamous cell carcinoma.* The exact cause is unknown;it may arise from acitinic keratoses, Bowen's disease of leukoplakia. This frequently occurres on previously damaged skin e.g. from sun, radiation, scar.. It is malignant tumour of squamous (pricke) cell of epidermis; invasion of dermis surrounding skin and metasis is possible. In early states there is firm nodule with distinct borders with scaling and ulceration and opaque, then later stages, there will be a covering of lesions with scale or horn from keratinization; most commonly found in sun-exposed areas such as face and hands. If precursor was premalignant lesion, the lesion will be indurated and surrounded by an inflammatory base. New lesions appear as firm keratotic nodule with an indurated base. Lip or ear lesion may metastasize to regional lymph nodes. Lesions on hair-bearing areas rarely metastasize.

Treatment includes prevention and early detections.

Removal by excision, curretage with electrode siccation, irradiation, or chemsurgery or chemical caustics For treatment of tumoiur without well-defined borders. A dressing size applied with a fixative paste such as zinc chloride, removal of the dressing remain malignant tissue. Reapplication is usually necessary.

2. *Basal cell carcinoma* is a locally invasive malignancy arising from epidermal basal cells. The exact cause is unknown but most common malignant tumour affecting light-skinned persons over age of 40; primarily occurs over hairy areas that contains pilosebacious follicles.

There will be change in basal cells, no maturation or normal keratonization; continuing division of basal cells and formation of enlarging mass; related to excessive sun exposure, genetic skin type, arsenicals, X-ray radiation, scars and some type of nevi; basal cell possibly pigmented but is absent in nevi.

Clinical manifestation includes nodular and ulcerative–small, slowly enlarging papule; borders semitransulent or "pearly" with overlying telangiectasia, erosion, ulceration and depression of center; normal skin markings, lost. Superficially there will be a erythematous sharply-defined barely elevated multinodular plaques with varying scaling and crusting; similar to eczema but not prurite. Rarely metastatic is treated. If untreated, tumour becomes locally invasive with severe tissue destruction, infection, and haemorrhage. If untreated, metastasizes to bone lung and brain.

Treatment depends on site and extent of tumour; currettage with electrode siccations, excision, irradiations and chemosurgery, electrosurgery, cryosurgery. Ninety-five per cent are slow-growing tumour that invades local tissue.

3. *Malignant Melanoma:* usually develops from a pigmented nevi, although it may arise from healthy skin. Three lesions are considered percurors of melanoma; dysplastic nevi; congenital nevi, and lentigo maligns. Chronic exposure is associated with its developments. There is genetic predisposition to melanoma.

Neoplastic growth of melanocytes anywhere on skin, eyes, or mucous membranes, classification according to major histologic mode of spread. There are lentigo malignamelanoma, nodular melanaoma, superficial spreading melanoma and acral-lentiginous melanoma. There will be a potential invasion and widespread metastasis.

Tumours occur most commonly on the head, neck and lower extremities. The lesions vary considerably in appearance and some with deep pigmentation, irregular borders and surrounding erythema, and others with irregular pigmentation yellow, blue, black and irregular surfaces. The rate of growth varies. Late changes include bleeding and ulceration. The incidence of metastasis from maligned melanoma is high and depends on depth of invasion. Metastasis occurs first to the regional lymph nodes and then haematogenous spread to the lungs, liver and other areas.

As in all malignancies, diagnostic is confirmed by biopsy. Metastatic malignant melanoma is resistant to currently available chemotherapeutic agents. Treatment includes wide excision, full thickness, surgical removal, correlation of survival rate with depth of invasion; poor prognosis unless diagnosed and treated early; spreading by local extension, regional lymphatic vessels and blood stream; adjuvant therapy after surgery may be necessary if lesion is greater than 1.5 mm in depth.

4. *Kapsosis Sarcoma:* The exact cause is unknown. Theories include viral causes, immunosuppression and sexually, transmitted agents, categorized groups affected are elderly men, Jewish and endemic on black Africans., and renal transplant recipients and AIDS related.

Multicentric neoplasm occurs with increasing frequency in HIV-infected individuals; occurs frequently in homosexual men; multiple vascular modules are appearing on the skin, mucous membranes and vescira; severity ranges from minor to fulminant with extensive cutaneous and visceral involvement.

There will be a slowly progressive red, purple or brown plaques or nodules scattered widely over the body on the skin or mucus membranes, especially on the mouth. Lesions have been found in lymph nodes, gastrointestinal tract and lungs. Lesions do not blanch with pressure and are painless.

Diagnosis is based upon biopsy of suspicious lesion. Treatment depends upon severity of lesions and patient's immune status; attempt to avoid treatments to further suppress immune system; possible treatment includes localized radiation, intralesional vinblastine, alpha-interferon combination of cryotherapy and chemotherapy. Patients at high risk should be taught self-assessments for early detection of lesions.

5. *Kerato acanthoma:* occurs on normal skin areas exposed to sun, tar, oils. It is noninvasive and does not metastasize.

They are microscopically similar to squamous cell carcinoma grows rapidly to 1-2 cm, remain quiscent for 2-8 weeks, than regresses spontaneously. Dome-shaped, shiny, pink lesion contain a keratinous plug, which is expelled as the nodule shrinks.

Treatment includes excision and biopsy.

NURSING MANAGEMENT OF DERMATOLOGICAL SURGERY

Treatment of skin lesions by dermatologistic structures include removal of skin lesions. Superficial skin lesions involving only the epidermis which can be removed easily by various means. Deep lesions involving the dermis, such as with some cancers are removed with full thickness and skin excision. The different types of dermatological surgery are:

1. *Tangenital Surgery:* Superficial lesions can be removed by slicing off the lesion with a sharp blade. It is especially

useful for removal of flat lesions. The entire lesion may be removed for diagnosis. Haemostasis is obtained with pressure of gelatin foam.

2. *Currettage:* Currettage is the scraping or scooping out of a superficial lesions with a currette, a spoon-shaped or sharp-edged instrument. A local anaesthetic is usually injected around the lesion before currettage Haemostasis is accomplished with a chemical styptic, such a ferric chloride or monsel's solution, with gelatin foam or by electrocoagulation. Lesions which may be removed by currettage include seborrhoeic keratosis, actinic keratosis, basal cell eptheliema, leukoplakia warts and nevi.
3. *Punch Biopsy:* After the patient received a local anaesthetic, a punch is used to remove deep lesions upto 10 mm in diameter. The tissue is then sent for biopsy. Small punch biopsy may be closed with suture. Larger biopsies are partially closed they then heal by secondary insertion. Haemostasis is obtained with gelatin foam packing.
4. *Cryosurgery:* Tissue can be destroyed by rapid freezing with substance such as liquid oxygen, carbon dioxide snow or gas, liquid nitrogen, dichlorodifluromethane freon or nitrous oxide. The carbon dioxide snow and liquid nitrogen commonly used the rapid freezing causes formation of intracellular ice, which destroys the cell membranous and produces cell dehydration. Cryosurgery is commonly used for removing skin tumours, warts and keloids.
5. *Electrosurgery:* Electric current may be used in dermatological surgery to remove tissue and to control bleeding.
   - Electrodesciccation is drying of tissue by means of monopolar curretage through the needle electrode.
   - Electrofulguration is a form of electrodesciccation in which needle electrode is held close to, rather than inserted into the tissue that spraying area with sparks.
   - Electrocoagulation: Bipolar current is used in which coagulates the tissues, curtailing capillary bleeding and for electrosection, which cuts the tissue.

Preoperative care is as with other patients undergoing any surgery and preoperative teaching about surgery indicated for.

Postoperative care: also includes monitoring and taking measures according to type of surgery. The specific points included are:

After superficial skin surgery, the patient is instructed not to remove the crust scalp which acts as a protective healing occurs under the crust. The crust should be kept as dry as possible if it gets wet, it should be patted dry. Alcohol may be applied and allowed to evaporate. Make-up may be used over the crust. The crust may be left uncovered with an adhesive bandage. Signs of redness, oedema or pain should be reported to surgeon.

After deep skin surgery, the wound is usually bandaged and patient is given specific instruction for care by the surgeon. Aspirin should be avoided for 7 days before and after surgery because of its anticoagulant property it may lead to postoperative bleeding.

Patient and family will require teaching regarding the care of healthy skin and steps to prevent further damages to the skin which includes:

- Avoiding causative agent.
- Cleansing the skin-bathing.
- Avoiding sunlight.
- Taking balanced nutrients.
- Observation of any change in size, colour and any.
- Dangers of self treatment.
- Psychological care.
- Relief of pruritus.
- Temperature control.
- Therapeutic bath and soaks.
- Topical medication.
- Medicated dressing.

Cosmetic surgery on skin may be performed.

Pressure Ulcers

Pressure ulcers is localized area of tissues necrosis caused by unrelieved pressure, tissue layers sliding over other tissue layers, shearing and excessive moisture.

Aetiology

Factors that put a patient at risk for the development of pressure ulcers include impaired circulation, obesity, elevated body temperature, anaemia, contractures, mental deterioration, physical dependence, immobility, incontinence and old age. Systemic illness such as diabetes, collagen diseases, vascular diseases, leprosy, and neurological disorders that affect sensation also result in great risk for ulceration.

Pathophysiology

Unrelieved pressure causes cellular necrosis. The cellular necrosis occurs from vascular insufficiency and causes tissue destruction. Here the pressure is applied to the soft tissue compresses capillaries, distorting structures and occluding blood flow, which leads to ischaemia at first, followed by reactive hyperemia. It compensated by increased shunting of capillary circulation to area under pressure; capillaries increased permeability and leakage of fluids into tissues lead to tissue oedema and inflammation. Then endothelical cells are disrupted, platelets aggregate and thrombi form in capillaries and lead to cellular death. Cellular death leads to tissue necrosis.

Clinical Manifestation

The clinical manifestation of pressure ulcer depend on the stage of the ulcer as follows:

- *Stage I.* In this stage, pressure ulcer is an observable-pressure related alteration of intact skin, whose indications as compared to an adjacent or opposite area on the body may include changes in one or more of the following.

- Skin temperature warmth or coolness., tissue consistency firm or boggy feel., sensation pain, itching..
- The ulcer appears as a defined area of persistent redness in lightly-pigmented skin, whereas in darker skin tones, the ulcer may appear with persistent red, blue or purple hues.

Here nonblanchable erythema, redness that remain present over an area under pressure 30 minutes after pressure source is removed. Epidermis remains intact.

- *Stage II.* In this stage epidermis is broken, superficial lesion, no measurable depth. Partial thickness, skin loss involving epidermis dermis or both. The ulcer is superficial and presents clinically as an abrasion, blister or shallow crater.
- *Stage III.* In this full thickness skin loss down through dermis include subcutaneous tissue may undermine adjacent skin. Full thickness involving damage to or necrosis of subcutaneous tissue that may extend down to but not through underlying fascia. The ulcer presents clinically as a deep crater with or without undermining of adjacent tissue.
- *Stage IV.* Full thickness skin loss extending into suppressive structures such as muscle tendon and bone may underkine and have various sinus tracts.

If the pressure ulcer becomes infected, the patient may display signs of infection such as leukocytosis and fever. In addition, the pressure ulcer may increase in size, odour and drainage, have necrotic tissue, and be indurated, warm and painful. The most common complication in pressure ulcer is recurrence.

Management

Care of the patient with a pressure ulcer requires local care of the wound and support measures such as adequate nutrition and pressure relief. The current trend to keep a pressure sore slightly moist, rather than dry, to enhance reepithelialization. In addition to the nurse and other members of the health team they can provide valuable input into the complex treatment necessary to prevent and treat pressure ulcers. Both conservative and surgical strategies are used in the treatment of pressure ulcers depending on the stage and condition of the ulcer.

A holistic approach to nursing management of the patient with pressure ulcers contain four components.

1. Controlling the contributing factors by reduction or elimination.
2. Supporting the host.
3. Optimizing microenvironments based on principles of wound healing, and
4. Providing education for patients and caregivers.

The Nursing diagnosis are determined from analysis of patient includes.

- Skin integrity, for impaired, related to nutritional deficits, prolonged immobilization and decreased haemoglobin, and serum albumin.
- Risk for infection.
- Impaired physical mobility.
- Tissue perfusion, altered.
- Self-care deficiency.

Nursing intervention to prevent pressure ulcers are as follows:

1. *Incontinence*
   - Cleanse the skin after each episode of incontinence. Check incontinent patients frequently.
   - Assess causative factors of incontinence.
   - Contain urine and feces in absorbent products that control moisture and exposure to skin; plastic-lined products can contribute to the problem.
   - Minimize moisture next to skin from any source.
2. *Nutritional Deficits*
   - Collaborate with dietitian to assess for optimal nutritional support.
   - Assess for symptoms of nutritional compromise decreased appetite and subsequently less oral intake. Serum albumin level of less than 3-3.5 gm/dl; Hgb level of less than 10 gm/dl; signs and symptoms of dehydration, including thirst, poor skin turgor, and dry mucus membrane, elevated haematocrit and serum sodium level.
3. *Skin Care and Early Treatment Measures*
   - Inspect the skin at regular intervals at least daily.
   - Frequency determined by institutional policy, e.g. every shift instead of daily. and patient degree at risk. A head-to-toe inspection should be conducted. With attention to intertriginous areas and bony prominences.
   - Bathing schedule should be developed according to patient's preference, institutional policy, and general skin conditions. Use a mild cleansing agent and avoid water temperature extremes.
   - Assess environmental factors such as temperature and humidity for contribution to skin conditions.
   - Lubricate skin with emollient lotions. Avoid lotion with scents or high alcohol contents.
   - Avoid vigorous massage.
4. *Alteration in Mobility/Activity*
   - Reposition patient at least every 2 hours.
   - Use position pillows or foam wedges to separate skin areas, in contact with each other or to assist with maintaining positions. Use cautiously because these devices can become an additional source of pressure if not properly placed.

- Heels should be elevated off the bed surfaces with supportive pillows. Heel protectors help reduce friction.
- Avoid positioning directly on to trochanter, place patient more appropriately with 30 degree side-lying position.
- Elevating the head of the bed centers all body weight directly over the pelvic triangle. It is best to keep the degree of elevation to less than 45 degrees if possible.
- To reduce friction and shear, use lifting devices to raise patient in bed, rather than dragging patient across the surface of the bed.
- A pressure reduction or relief device should be used for all patients at risk of pressure ulcer formation.
- Patients in wheel chairs and other chairs should be taught to shift weight and have pressure-reducing surfaces on which to sit.

BURNS

Burns are a form of traumatic injury caused by thermal, electrical, chemical or radioactive agents. In other words, injuries that result from direct contact or exposure to any thermal, chemical, electrical or radiation source are termed "BURNS". Burn injuries occur when energy from a heat source is transferred to the tissues of the body. The depth of injury is related to temperature and the durations of the contact or of exposure.

Types of Burns

Burn injuries are categorized according to the mechanism of injury. It may be thermal, chemical, electrical and radiation.

Thermal Burn Injury

Thermal burns are caused by exposure to or contact with flame, hot liquids, semi-liquids steam, semi-solid tar or objects such as:

- Flame : Example: Clothing ignited with fire.
- Flash : Example: Flame burn associated with explosion combustible fuels.
- Scald : Example: –Hot bath water.
  - Spilled hot beverages.
  - Hot grease or liquids from cooking.
  - Steam burns, pressure workers, microwaved food, automobile radiactors.
- Contact: Example: –Hot metal outdoor grill.
  - Hot, sticky tar.

So, the specific examples of thermal burns are those sustained in residential fires, explosive, automobile accidents, scald injuries, clothing ignition and ignition of poorly stored flammable liquids petrol.

Chemical Burn Injury

Chemical injuries are the result of tissue injury and destruction from necrotizing substances. Chemical burns are caused by tissue contact with strong acids, alkalies or organic compounds. The concentration volume, and type of chemical as well as the duration of contact determine the severity of a chemical injury. Chemical injuries to the eyes and inhalation of chemical fumes (e.g. Bhopal Gas Tragedy) are particularly serious.

Chemical burns can result from contact with certain household cleaning agent and various chemicals used in industry, agriculture and the military. More than 25000 chemical products. Chemical can produce respiratory and systemic symptoms as well as skin or eye injuries. For example, when chlorine is inhaled toxic gas produces respiratory distress. Byproducts of burning substances e.g. Carbon are toxic to the sensitive respiratory mucosa. Tissue destruction may continue for upto 72 hours after chemical injury.

As stated earlier, chemical burns are most commonly caused by acids, however, alkali burns also occur. Alkalis are more dangerous than acids,because alkali substances are neutralized by tissue fluids as readily as acid substances. Alkalies adhere to tissues, causing protein hydrolic and liquification. Thus, damages continue even when the alkali is neutralised. An example of alkalies of this type are cleaning agents, drain cleaner and dyes.

Smoke and inhalation of hot air or noxious chemicals can cause damage to the tissues of the respiratory tract. Breathing of hot air may cause damages to the respiratory mucosa. Examples: inhalation injuries commonly occurring are carbon monoxide poisoning, inhalation injury above the glottis and inhalation injury below the glottis.

Electrical Burn Injury

Electrical injury results from coagulation necrosis that is caused by intense heat generated by the electrical energy as it passes through the body. These injuries can result from contact with exposed or faulty electrical wiring or high-voltage power lines. Individuals struck by lightning also sustain electrical injury. It can also result from direct damage to nerves and vessels causing tissues anoxia and death. The extent of the injury influenced by the duration of contact, the intensity of the current voltage, the type of current direct or alternate the pathway of the current and the resistance of the tissues as the electrical current passes through the body. Electrical contact with voltage greater than 40 is potentially dangerous.

Radiation Burn Injury

Radiation burns are the least common type of burn injuries and are caused by exposure to a radioactive service. These types of injuries have been associated with nuclear radiation accidents, the use of ionizing radiation in industry and from therapeutic radiation. A sunburn solar radiation from prolonged exposure to ultraviolet rays is also considered to be a type of radiation burn. The amount of radioactive energy that an individual receives following exposure depends on the strength of the radiative source, the duration of the exposure, the extent of the body area exposed and the amount of shielding between the source and the person. An acute localized injury appears similar to a cutineous thermal injury, and is characterized by skin erythema, oedema and pain. In contrast, the whole body radiation causes radiation sickness that are dose dependent.

Pathophysiology of Burns

Burn wounds occur when there is contact between tissue and energy source on heat, chemicals, electrical current, or radiation. The resulting local effects are influenced by the intensity of the energy, the duration of the exposure, and the type of tissue injured. Immediately after the injury there is an increase in blood flow to the area surrounding the wound. This is followed by release of various vasoactive substances from the burned tissue, which results in increased capillary permeability. Fluid then shifts from the intravascular compartment to the interstitial space producing oedema and hypovolaemia.

The pathophysiologic response that occur immediately following a cutaneous burn injury depends on the extent of size of the burn. For smaller burns, body's response to injury is localized to the injured area. However, with extensive burns, i.e. twenty-five per cent or more of total body surface area (TBSA) the body response to injury is systemic and proportional to the extent of the injury.

Extensive burn injuries affect all major systems of the body. The systemic response to burn injury is topically triphasic, characterized by early hypofunction that is followed later by hyper function of the each organ system.

The physiologic reaction to burns is similar to inflammatory process. Burns may be partial or full thickness. In *partial thickness* injuries involve the epidermis and upper portion of the dermis. Some of the dermal appendages remain, from which the wound can spontaneously re-epithialize. In *full thickness* injuries, all layers of the skin and sometimes, underlying tissues are destroyed. In such cases, grafting is required to close the wound.

In addition to changes in the locally burned area, there are alterations and disruptions in the vascular and other systems of the body. Brief description of those changes are given below:

i. *Fluid and Electrolytic Balance*

Immediately following a burn injury, vasoactive substances i.e.. catecholamines, histamine, serotinin, leukotrienes, kinins and prostaglandins are released from the injured tissues. These substances initiate changes in capillary integrity, allowing plasma to seep into surrounding tissues. Direct heat injury to vessels further increases capillary permeability, which permits sodium ions to enter the cell and potassium ions to exit. Overall, this creates an osmotic gradient, which leads to increase in intracellular and interstitial fluid and further depletes intravascular fluid volume. These substances exert their effect both locally and systematically. The burn injured client's haemodynamic balance, metabolism and immune status are altered.

Haemodynamic alteration leads to inadequate tissue perfusion, which may turn cause acidosis, renal failure, and irreversible burn shock. Hyponatraemia and hyperkalaemia are common electrolyte abnormalities that affect the burn-injured client at different points in the recovery process. Catecholamine release appears to be the major mediator of the hypermetabolic response to burn injury.

ii. *Changes in Cardiovascular System*

In major burn, heart rate and peripheral vascular resistance increases in response to the release of catecholamines and to the relative hypovolaemia, but initial cardiac output falls hypofunction. At approximately 24 hours after burn injury in persons receiving adequate fluid resuscitation, cardiac output return to normal and that increases 2 to 2.5 times normal to meet the hypermetabolic needs of the body hyperfunctions. This change in cardiac output occurs even before circulating intravascular volume levels and are restored to normal. Arterial blood pressure is normal or slightly elevated unless severe hypovolaemia exists.

iii. *Changes in Respiratory System*

Majority of death from the fire are due to smoke and inhalation injury. Without a concomitant inhalation injury, initial findings suggestive of pulmonary insufficiency are rare. Minute ventilation is often normal or slightly decreased early after a burn injury. Following fluid resuscitation and the effects of burn shock on cell membrane potential may cause pulmonary oedema contributing to decreased alveolar exchange. Client may exhibit a rise in minute ventilation or hyperventilation especially if he or she is fearful, anxious or in pain. This hyperventilation is the result of an increase in both respiratory rate and a tidal volume and appears to be the result of the hypermetabolism that is seen after burn injury. Initial respiratory alkosis and respiratory acidosis may associate with hyperventilation and pulmonary insufficiency.

iv. *Changes in Urinary System*

The body responds initially by shunting blood away from the kidneys as a part of the normal neurohormonal stress response, thus decreasing glomerular filtration race and causing oliguria low uring (output). If fluid resuscitation is delayed or inadequate, hypovolaemia progresses and leads to acute renal failure. However, with adequate fluid resuscitation and a rise in cardiac output, renal blood flow will return to normal. Following resuscitation, the body begins to reabsorb the oedema fluid and to eliminate through diuresis. Urine output then increases.

v. *Changes in Gastrointestinal System*

In major burns, blood flows to the mesentric beds is also reduced initially, leading to development of intestinal ileus and gastrointestinal dysfunction. As a result of sympathetic nervous system response to trauma peristalisis decreases, and gastric distension, nausea, vomitting and paralytic ileus may occur. Ischaemia of the gastric mucosa and other aetiological factors put the burn client at risk for duodenal ulcer and gastric ulcer, manifested by occult bleeding and in some cases life-threatening haemorrhage. If the gastrointestinal tract is left untreated and unprotected by antacids, the erosions can progress to ulcer ation i.e. curlings ulcer in burn clients and gastrointestinal bleeding. Following adequate fluid resuscitation, gastrointestinal motility returns, signalled by bowel sounds, flatus, and stool production.

vi. *Changes in Immune System*

In major burn injuries, immune system function is depressed. The loss of the skin barrier and presence of eschare favours bacterial growth. Hypoxia, acidosis, thrombosis of vessels in the wound area impair host resistance to pathogenic bacteria. Depression of lympocyte activity, a decrease in immunoglobulin production, suppression of complement activities and an alteration in neutrophil and macrophage functioning are evident in following extensive burn injuries. In addition, burn injury disrupts the body's primary barrier to infection. Together, these changes result in some degree of immunosuppression, increasing the risk of infection and life-threatening sepsis i.e., systemic septiceamia.

vii. *Changes in Nervous System*

The client injured with burns typically suffers no neurologic trauma. (Example, fall, explosion) impaired perfusion to the brain, hypoxaemia, e.g. close-space fire inhalation injury, e.g. exposure to asphyxiants or other toxic material from the fire., electrical burn injury, or from the effects of the drug present in the body at the time of injury. Burn patient always awake, in hospital. If agitation develops in immediate post-burn period, the patient may be suffering from hypovolaemia or hypoxaemia.

In addition to pathophysiological changes, the burn injured client also shows a myriad of psychological and emotional responses to burn injuries ranging from fear to psychosis. This has been influenced by age, personality, cultural and ethnic backgroiund, extent and location of injuries and the resulting impact on body image.

CLASSIFICATION OF SEVERITY OF BURNS

The treatment of burns is related to the severity of burn injury. The severity of burn injury is classified based on the risk of mortality and the risk of cosmetic or functional disability. Severity of burns is determined by:

- Burn depth.
- Burn size percentage of TBSA burned.
- Burn location.
- Age of burn victim.
- General health of burn victim.
- Mechanism of injury.

i. Burn Depth

Burn injuries are classified as a partial thickness or full thickness.

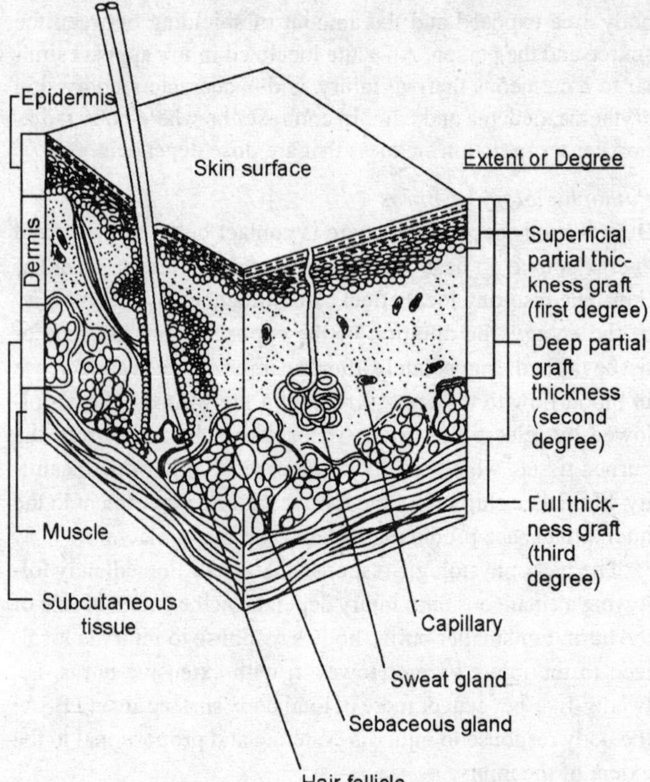

Fig. 16.3: Cross-section of skin depicting blood supply, depth of burn, and relative thickness of skin grafts.

A. *Partial thickness* burn injuries are classified as first and second degree burns or superficial and deep burns.
   - The cause of *Superficial burns* first degree are superficial first degree are superficial sunburn and quick heat flash. Here only superficial devitalization with hyperexaemia is present. Tactic and pain sensation is intact. In superficial burns, clinical appearance will include erythaema, blanching on pressure, pain and mild swelling. The vescicles or blisters although after 24-hour skin may blister and peel. Discomfort lasts 48-72 hours. Desquamation in 3-7 days.
   - The causes of *deep burns* second degree are flame, flash, scald and contact burns. Here epidermis and dermis involved to varying depth. Some skin elements from which epithethelial regeneration can occur remain viable. The clinical appearance of deep burn will include, fluid-filled vescicles that are red shiny, wet if vescicles have ruptured., severe pain caused by nerve inury, there will be a mild to moderate oedema. Superficial burn heals in less than 21 days. Deep burn require more than 21 days to heal. Healing rates vary with burn depth and presence and absence of infection.

B. *Full thickness* burn injuries are classified as 'third' and 'fourth' degree burns. These are caused by flame, scald, chemicals, tar, electric current. Here all skin elements and nerve endings are destroyed. Coagulation necrosis present. The clinical appearances will be dry, waxy white, leathery or hard skin; visible thrombosed vessels insensitivity to pain and pressure because of nerve destructions. There will be possible involvements of muscles, tendons and bones. 3rd degree requires autografting and 4th degree requires autografting or amputation of extremity.

ii. Burn Size Extent.

The size of a burn (percentage of injured skin, excluding first degree burns) is determined by one of the two techniques.

a. The rule of Nines (9s) and
b. An Age-specific burn diagram of Lund-Browder chart.

Burns size or extent is expressed as a percentage of TBSA.

a. *The rule of '9s'* was introduced in the late 1940 as a quick assessment tool for estimating burn size. The basis of this rule is that the body divided into anatomic sections, each of which represents 9% or a multiple of 9% of the TBSA. The method is easy requiring no diagrams to determine the percentage of TBSA injured. Therefore, it has been used in emergency department where the initial assessment occurs.

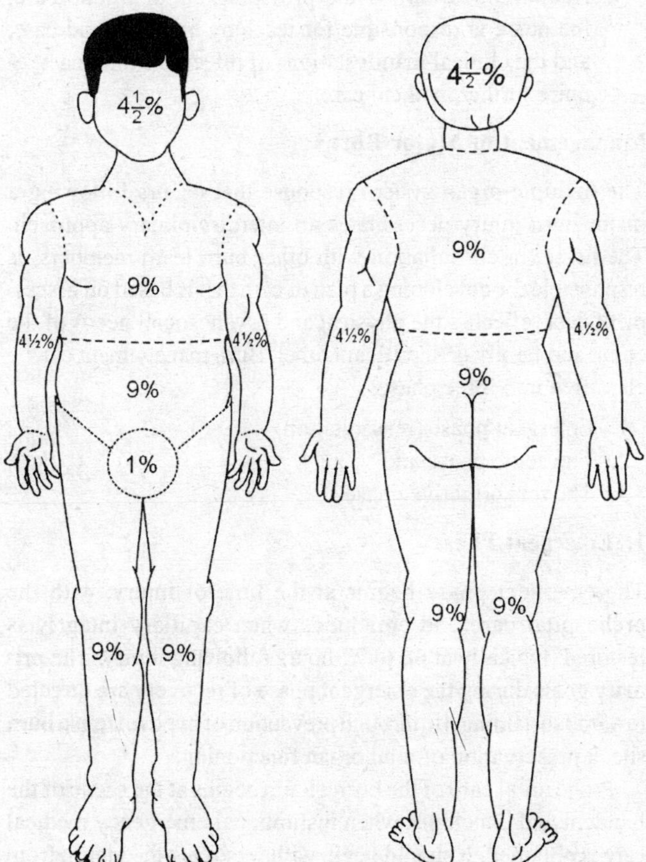

Fig. 16.4: Rule of nines for calculating total burn surface area TBSA.

The Rule of Nine

Head and neck	9%
Arms	9%
Anterior trunk	18%
Posterior trunk	18%
Legs	18%
Perinium	1%
	100%

b. An age-specific burn diagram of Lund-Browder chart—the percentages for body segments according to age and provides a more accurate estimate of burns. Extent of burn injury is most accurate after initial debridement.

iii. Burn Location

The location of the burn wound has a direct relationship to the severity of the burn injury. Burns of the head, face, neck and circumferential burns of the chest are frequently associated with pulmonary complication it may inhibit respiratory function by virtue of mechanical obstruction secondary to oedema or eschar formation. These injuries may also indicate the possibility of inhalation injury or respiratory mucosal damage.

Burns involving the face often have associated with corneal abrasions. Burns of the ears are prone to auricular chondritis and are susceptible to infections and further loss of tissue. Burns of the hands and joints often require intense physical and occupational therapy and have implications for loss of work time and/or permanent physical and vocational disability. Burns of the hands, feet, joints and eyes are of concern because they make self-care impossible and jeopardize later function. Hands and feet are difficult to manage medically because of superficial vascular and nerve supply system.

Burns involving the perineal area are prone to infection due to autocontamination by urine and focus. The burns of the buttocks or genitalia are susceptible to infection and may be source of emotional conflicts because of the pain involved possible disfigurement.

Circumferential burns of the extremeties may produce a tourniquet-like effect and lead to distal vascular compromise i.e., circulatory compromise distal to the burns with subsequent neurologic impairment of the affected extremity. As stated earlier, circumferential thorax burn may lead to inadequate chestwall expansion and pulmonary insufficiency.

iv. Age of the Burn Victim

The client's age affects the severity and outcome of the burn. Mortality rates are higher for children younger than 4 years particularly 0-1 year group, and for clients older than 65 years. Because of an immature immune system and generally poor host defence mechanisms an infant is less able to cope with burn injuries. The older adult heals more slowly and has more difficulty with rehabilitation than a child or younger adult. Infection of the burn wound and pneumonia are common complications of older patient.

v. General Health and Burns

Any patient with pre-existing cardiovascular, pulmonary, or renal disease has poorer prognosis for recovery because of the tremendous demands placed on the body by a burn injury. The patient with diabetes mellitus or peripheral vascular disease is at high risk for gangrene and poor healing, especially with foot and leg burns. General physiological debilitation from any chronic disease, including alcoholism, drug abuse, and malnutrition renders the patient less physiologically competent to deal with a burn injury. In addition, the patient who concurrently sustained fractures, head injuries or other trauma has poorer prognosis for recovery from the burn injury.

vi. Mechanism of Burn Injury

Mechanism of burn injury is an important factor used to determine severity. The special consideration is required for electrical and burn injury or any burn injury associated with an inhalation injury.

As stated earlier, in electrical injuries, heat is generated as the electricity travels through the body resulting internal tissue damage. Here, the voltage, type of current, AC or DC, contact site and the duration of contact are important considerations because they affect morbidity. AC is worst than DC because it is associated with cardiopulmonary arrest, ventricular fibrillation, tetanic muscle contractions and long bone or vertebral compression fractures. There will be risk of acute renal failure due to release of myoglobin.

In chemical burns, systemic to all effects from cutaneous absorption of the offending agent may occur. Organ failure and even death have resulted from prolonged contact and absorption of different chemicals.

Management of Minor Burns

A minor burn injury in the adult is generally considered to be less than 15 per cent of TBSA in the patients younger than 40 years or 10 per cent TBSA in patients older than 40 years without a risk of cosmetic or functional impairment or disability.

Nursing care of minor burn wounds include:

- Wound assessment and initial care of wound.
- Tetanus immunization.
- Pain management.
- Health education.

i. *Wound assessemnt* includes an accurate history of injury i.e., the date and time of accident and the source of the burn and other associated injuries. And also all pertinent pastmedical history which includes drug allergies, medications, illnesses, etc.

Wound care for minor burns includes cleansing, debridement, removal of any damaging agent, i.e. chemical, tar, etc.) and application of an appropriate topical treatments.

Generally burn wounds should be washed with mild soap and rinsed thoroughly with warm water. The wounds may be covered with saline-soaked sponges to lessen the discomfort. Loose nonviable tissue should be carefully trimmed away and any hair should be shaved within all" margin around the burn wound.

A minor chemical burn should be well irrigated with water for at least 20 minutes. Neutralizing agents are not recommended because the neutralizing reaction causes heat, which results in further tissue damage.

ii. *Tetanus immunization:* Burn wound patients are exposed and are prone to get tetanus. To prevent developing tetanus, the current protocol for tetanus immunization is same for clients with minor burns as for clients with any other type of trauma.

iii. *Pain management:* is often achieved with small doses of IV morphine followed by oral analgesia in minor burns.

iv. *Health education:* While providing initial wound care, the nurse is responsible for teaching home wound care, and the clinical manifestations of infections that must require further medical care.

Management of Major Burns

The multiple organ system response that occurs following a major burn injury necessitates an interdisciplinary approach. The nurse, in consultation with other burn team members, is responsible for developing a plan of care that is based on assessment data reflected the physical and psychosocial needs of the client and family or significant other. Burn management can be classified into three phases.

1. Emergent phase (resuscitation)
2. The acute phase and
3. The rehabilitative phase

1. Emergent Phase

The emergent phase begins at the time of injury, with the prehospital care and concludes when capillary integriy is restored, typically at 48 to 72 hours following injury. The primary goals during the emergent phase of recovery are directed towards sustaining life through prevention of hypovolaemia burn shock preservation of vital organ functioning.

Prehospital care of the burn victim begins at the scene of the incident and concludes when institutional emergency medical care is obtained. It should begin with removing the victim from the source of the burn and/or eliminating the source of heat. Prehospital care of the patient with various types of burns are as follows:

i. *Emergency Management of Chemical Burns*

The possible causes of chemical burns are exposure to strong acid alkali, corrosive materials or organophosphorous. So the possible assessment finally may include:

- Burning, degeneration of exposed tissues.
- Discolouration of injured exposed skin.
- Localized pain.
- Oedema of surrounding tissues.
- Respiratory distress if chemical is inhaled.
- Paralysis, decreased muscle coordination if organophosphorous.

When managing such cases the caregiver should:

- Wear appropriate protective garb globe.
- Remove the chemical from contact with patient's body.
- Flush chemical from wound and surroundings area with saline solution or water. Brush off lime and other powders.
- Remove clothing including shoes, watches, jewellery and contact lenses if face is exposed..
- Blot, do not rub, skin dry with clean towels.
- Cover all burned area with dry, sterile dressing or clean dry sheet.
- Monitor airway, if airway is exposed to chemicals.
- Attempt to determine type of chemical exposure.

ii. *Emergency Management of Inhalation Injury*

The possible causes of inhalation burn injuries are exposure of respiratory tract to intense heat, flames, inhalation of noxious chemicals and smoke CO gas. The expected possible assessement findings will include:

- Rapid, shallow respiration.
- Increasing hoarseness.
- Coughing.
- Singed nasal or facial hair.
- Sooty and smoky breath.
- Productive cough, that is black, gray or bloody.
- Irritation of upper airways or burning pain in throat or chest.
- Difficulty in swallowing.
- Restlessness, anxiety.

While managing such cases, the caregiver should:

- Remove patient from toxic environment.
- Establish and maintain airway, anticipates need for intubation of respiratory distress.
- Administer high flow oxygen 100 per cent by nonrebreather mark.
- Be prepared to intubate if respiratory distress occurs.
- Remove patient's clothing.
- Establish IV line with larger-guage needle.
- Monitor vital signs including level of consciousness and oxygen saturation.
- Place patient in a high Fowler's position unless spinal injury is suspected.
- Assess for facial and neck burns or other signs of trauma.
- Prepare for emergency, endotrachial intubation if indicated.

iii. *Emergency Management of Electrical Burns*

The possible causes of electrical burns will be exposure to electric current, i.e. lightening, electric wires, utility wires, etc. The possible findings of such injury may be:

- Leathery and white charred skin.
- Burn odour.
- Impaired touch sensation.
- Minimal or absent pain.
- Dysrhythmias.
- Depth of wound difficult to visualize; assume injury greater than seen.
- Entrance and exit wounds.

When managing such cases, the caregiver should:

- Remove patient from contact with current source by trained personnel first aider.
- Avoid contact with electric current during rescue.
- Assess for patient airway, breathing and circulation.
- Initiate CPR if necessary.
- Establish and maintain airway.
- Maintain cervical spine precautions.
- Administer high flow oxygen (O_2) by nonrebreather mask.
- Establish IV line with large gauge needle.
- Remove patient's clothing.
- Assess burn areas, especially entrance and exit sites.
- Check pulses distal to burns.
- Monitor heart rate and rhythm.
- Cover burn sites with dry sterile dressing.
- Assess for any other injuries e.g. fractures..
- Monitor vital signs including level of consciousness.

iv. *Emergency Management of Thermal Burns*

The possible causes of thermal burns include contact with hot liquids or solids, flash flame, open flame, steam or ultraviolet rays. The possible assessment finding may be:

In case of superficial burns:

- Redness.
- Pain.
- Moderate to severe tenderness.
- Minimal oedema.
- Blanching with pressure.

In case of deep burns:

- Moist blebs and blisters.
- Mottled white and pink to cherry red.
- Hypersensitive to touich or air.

- Moderate to severe pain.
- Blanching with pressure.

In case of severe full thickness burns:

- Shock e.g. tachycaardia, hypotension..
- Dry leathery eschar.
- White, waxy, dark brown, or charred appearances.
- Strong burn odour.
- Impaired sensation where touched.
- Absence of pain with severe pain in surrounding tissues.
- Lack of blanching with pressure.

When managing such cases, caregiver or nurse should:

- Remove patient from environment and stop the burning process.
- Establish and maintain airway; inspect the face and neck for singed nasal hair, hoarseness of voice, stridor, soot in the sputum, anticipate need for intubation.
- Administer fluid.
- Monitor vital signs including level of consciouisness and O_2 saturation.
- Remove clothing and jewellery.
- Examine and treat for other associated injuries e.g. fractured ribs, pneumothorax, etc.
- Determine depth, extent and severity of burn.
- Anticipate need for analgesic and tetanus prophylaxis.
- Cover large burns with dry and sterile dressing.
- Apply cool compresses or immerse in cool water for minor injuries only less than 10 per cent TBSA burn.
- Transport as soon as possible to burn center of hospitals.

In general, the guidelines for prehospital care of burn victims that will be followed are:

1. Remove the victim from the sources of the burn:
   - Flame, extinguish burning clothes.
   - Chemical or scald: remove saturated clothing.
   - Chemical: Brush off any dry chemical and begin to copiously irrigate injured areas with water.
   - Hot tar: Cool the tar with water.
   - Electrical: Turn off electricity or remove the electrical source using dry, nonconductive object e.g. a piece of wood.
2. Assess the ABCs.
   - Establish airway.
   - Ensure adequate breathing 100 per cent O_2 via nonrebreather face mask..
   - Assess circulation.
3. Assess for associated trauma.
4. Conserve body heat.
5. Consider need for IV fluid administration.
6. Transfer to hospital or burn unit.

Nursing of Burn Patient in Hospital

Generally an extensive burn patient is referred to hospital and admitted in burn unit or wards. An initial care of such patients includes the following. This phase is considered as acute phase.

- Reassessment of airway, breathing and circulation and associated trauma.
- Initiation of fluid resuscitation/replacement.
- Placement of an indwelling urinary catheter.
- Placement of nasogastric tube.
- Monitoring vital signs and baseline lab studies.
- Pain management.
- Tetanus immunization.
- Data collection.
- Wound care.
- Psychological support.
- Infection control.
- Nutritional support.
- Physical therapy.

i. *Reassessment of ABCs*

Some intervention performed in emergency phase may be continued in hospital according to that type of burns. The head of the beds should be elevated to facilitate lung expansion if the patient suffers no haemodynamic instability. Oxygen may be administered if necessary.

ii. *Initiation of Fluid Replacement*

For haemodynamic stabilization fluid resuscitation may be initiated immediately on the basis of the percentage of burn injury i.e. more than 15-20 per cent TBSA in adults and more than 10-15 per cent in children and patients with electrical burn. The goal of fluid resuscitation is to give sufficient fluid to allow perfusion of vital organs without overhydrating the patient and risking later complication and circulatory overload.

Generally a crystalloid Ringer's lactate solution is used initially and colloids are used during second day. There, several formulae may be used to determine the amount of fluid to be given in the first 48 hours, which includes the Parkland formula, the Brook's formula and the Evan's formula.

Among them *Parkland formula* is commonly used as follows:

a. First 24 hours: 4 ml of Ringer's lactate X weight in kg of X percentage of TBSA is burned.
   Here one-half amount of fluid is given in the first 8 hours calculated from the time of injury. If the starting fluids is delayed, then the same amount of fluid is given over the remaining time. It should be noted that to deduct any fluids given in the prehospital setting, the remaining half of the fluid is given over the next 16 hours.

For example: Patient weight 70 kg, percentage of TBSA is 80 per cent.

Ist 8 hours = 11,200 ml or 1400 ml/hour.

IInd 16 hours = 11,200 ml or 700 ml/hour.

b. Second 24 hours = 0.5 ml colloid × 70 kg × 80 per cent TBSA/24 hours + 2000 ml 5 per cent dextrose in water run concurrently over the 24-hour period.

For example: 0.5 ml kg × 70 kg × 80 per cent = 2800 ml colloid + 2000 ml 5 per cent D/W i.e. 117 ml colloid/hour and 84 ml 5 per cent D/W per hour.

iii. *Placement of Indwelling Catheter*
An indwelling urethral catheter connected to a closed drainage system should be placed to measure hourly urine production.

iv. Placement of a nasogastric tube for the unresponsive patients or for patients with burns of 20% to 25% of more TBSA to prevent emesis and reduce the risk of aspiration.

v. *Monitoring Vital Signs*
Provide baseline information as well as additional data for determining the adequacy of fluids resuscitation. Baseline laboratory studies should include blood glucost, blood urea nitrogen, creatinine, serum, electrolytes and haematocrit levels, arterial blood gas and COHb levels should also be obtained in case of inhalation injury.

vi. *Pain Management*
The nurse must understand the physiologic as well as the psychologic bases of pain. Allowing the patient to ventilate feelings of anger, hostility and frustration serves to assist the patient in depression of the pain. Pain management is achieved through the administration of intravenous narcotic agent e.g. morpohine.. In adult, small doses are given intravenously and repeated in 5-10-minute interval until pain appears to be under control. Extent of pain relief, blood pressure, pulse, respiratory rate and state of consciousness should be assessed after each dose.

vii. Administration of tetanus toxoid or ATS to prevent tetanus.

viii. *Data Collection* will include all useful information about the incident, time of injury, level of consciousness of patient, any allergies and previous medical history of the patient helps to design the treatment and nursing intervention.

ix. *Wound Care* Care of the burn wound is ultimately aimed at promoting wound healing. Daily wound care involves cleansing,, debridement, of eschar devitalized tissue and dressing of the burn wound. Debridement of burn wound is accomplished through mechanical, enzymatic and surgical means. Wound care also includes typical antibiotic therapy, graft care if done and donor site care. If graft is done, appropriate coverage of the graft, if it is not kept open to air. It should include fine-mesh guage in the closest proximity to the graft before other dressings are applied.

x. *Psychological support:* Since the nurse has the most prolonged contact with the patient and family, it is natural that nurse is to be seen as an important source of emotional support. The nurse must assist the patient in maintaining personal worth and re-esetablishing a satisfactory body image. The nurse must have an almost unlimited supply of patience and understanding. The nurse should involve family members for nursing the burn patient.

xi. *Infection Control:* To prevent infection in the burn patient, nursing care includes vigilant monitoring for clinical manifestation of impending infection, and sepsis, maintenance of clean environment to reduce the reservoir of the microorganisms, use of aseptic technique for all invasive procedures and wound care, and timely administration of prescribed antimicrobial agents systemic and topical.. Universal precautions should be followed when caring all clients with burn injuries. The basic principles for infection control should be followed in burns unit.

xii. *Nutritional Support:* Maintenance of adequate nutrition during the acute phase is essential in promoting wound healing and preventing infection. Based metabolic need may be 40 to 100 per cent higher than normal levels, depending on the extent of the burn. Methods of delivering nutritional support include oral diet restricted in initial stage, till bowel sounds return to normal enteral tube feedings, peripheral parenteral nutrition, total parenteral nutrition and combination of these. The preferred feeding route is oral or enteral; however, the decisions of how to best meet the nutritional needs should be individualized for all clients.

xiii. *Physical Therapy:* The nurse works closely with occupational and physical therapist to identify the rehabilitative needs of the burn clients. An individualized program of splinting, therapeutic, positioning, exercise, ambulation, activities of daily living and pressure therapy should be implemented early in the acute phase of recovery to maximize functional recovery and cosmetic outcome. Patient and family education regarding correct positioning and the need for continued exercise are important.

Table 16.1: Nursing care plan of burn patient

Problem	*Reason*	*Objective*	*Nursing Intervention*	*Evaluation*
1. Fluid volume deficit R/T evaporation, loss, plasma loss, shift of fluid into interstitium secondary to burns.	• Increased capillary leak. • Large shift from intravascular to interstitial space. • Instable vital signs.	• The client will have improved fluid balance as evidenced by • Urine output > 30-50 ml/hr. • Stable vital signs • Clear sensorium, • Sodium and potassium level within range • Systolic BP > 90 mm Hb.	• Assess every 1-2 hours: – Pulses, BP, circulation – Sensation to all extremities – Mental status – Intake output – Pulmonary functions • Assess for hypovolaemia 1 hour × 36 hours • Obtain admission weight. • Establish large bone IV access • Monitor client weight daily • Administer IV fluids and electrolyte replacements as ordered. • Monitor serum electrolytes and haematocrit measurements. • Giver fluids according to patient needs.	(with adequate fluid resuscitation expect fluid balance within 24-36 hours).
2. Potential risk for R/T sympathetic nevous system response to burns.	Fluid deficit.	The nurse will monitor for normoactive bowel sounds, absence of abdominal dissension, flatus, production and normal bowel murmurs.	• Assess need for placement of nasogastric tube. • Assess bowel function: – Auscultate bowel sounds COS – Observe for abdominal dissension – Monitor gastric output and amount, colour, presence of blood and pH.	(Expect bowel sounds to return once fluid volume is balanced).
3. Potential risk for renal failure R/T presence of haemochromogens in the urine due to deep-burn crustingly.	Fluid deficit	• The nurse will monitor or visible urinary haemochromogen and adequate urine output of 70 ml to 100 ml/hr.	• Monitor and document hourly output and urine colour. • Ensure patency of urine catheter. • Administer IV fluids as ordered. • Send urine samples for urine myoglobin/haemoglobin level as ordered.	(once client has diuretics risk reduces).
4. Pain R/T burn injury.	• Exposed nerve endings. • Treatment • Anxiety • Shearing injuries as manifested by demonstration of discomfort and pain.	The client verbalizes satisfaction which level of pain and demonstrates tolerable level of pain.	• Assess the client response to pain with wound care, physical therapy and at rest. • Medicate prior to painful procedures. • Administer IV analgesics as needed to keep pain at tolerable level. • Keep patient warm to promote comfort and prevent energy use caused by shivering. • Evaluate the effectiveness of medication. • Explore relaxation techniques, music therapy, guided imagery, distraction and hypnosis. • Explain all procedures to patient and allow time for preparation. • Talk to the patient while providing care and performing procedure. • Provide emotional support. • Assess for the need of anxielytic drugs. • Reposition patient carefully using lifting sheet as necessary to prevent further damage to skin and minimise pain. • Document the patient's response to prescribed medication and other measures.	Expect level of pain to decrease as burn wounds heal..

Contd...

Problem	Reason	Objective	Nursing Intervention	Evaluation
5. Potential risk for infection R/T impaired skin integrity endogenous flora, and suppressed immune response.	• Loss of skin barrier. • Impaired immune response. • Presence of invasive catheter. • Invasive procedures.	Patient will have wound free of debris and loose necrotic tissue, minimum infection, rapid infection control.	• Administer tetanus prophylaxis Px.n • Maintain infection control technique. – Use good handwashing techniques. – Use sterile technique during topical antibiotic application and dressing changes. – Ensure that hydrotherapy and debridement last for no longer than 30 minutes per session. – Shave appropriate areas to remove possibility of contamination. – Evaluate blisters and devitalized tissues to eliminate medium of bacterial growth. – Cleanse area around eyes with normal saline solution if burned.. • Apply topical antibiotic or sterile dressing. • Before reapplying, cleanse and rinse the burn wound. • Observe wound daily for separations of eschar. • Check wound margins for cilulitis. • Assess for clinical signs of infection. – Discolouration of wounds or drainage – Odour delayed healing – Headache, chills, anorexia nausea and – Changes in vital signs hyperglycoma • Glycosuria, paralytic confusion, restlessness. • Assess signs for infection of catheter insertion. • Monitor vital signs.	
6. Total selfcare deficit R/T functional deficit.	• Deficit in – Grooming – Eating – Bathing – Elimination resulting from the burn injury – Pain – Dressings – Splints – Enforced immobility.	Patient will have less self-care deficits and exhibit optional performance of selfcare.	• Glycosuria, paralytic confusion, restlessness. • Assess signs for infection of catheter insertion. • Monitor vital signs. • Assess the patient's ability to perform selfcare activities to plan appropriate intervention. • Assist or intervene as appropriate. • Encourage the patient to participate no self-care tasks. • Ensure that the patient has adequate time to accomplish tasks. • Provide positive reinforcement when tasks are accomplished. • Assist patient remaining in emotional control to reduce feelings of helplessness.	
7. Impaired physical motility R/T Joint contractures.	• Contractures secondary to pain. • Difficulty in performing ROM. • Pain on movements. • Reluctant to ambulate & participate in selfcare. • Fear of activities that involve joint movement.	• Patient will have maximum potential ROM of all extremities, absence of contractures.	• Assess ROM and muscle strength in blurred areas prone to develop contractures every day and prn. • Maintain burned areas in position of physiologic function with associated injuries, grafting, and other therapeutic devices. • Initiate and encourage passive and active ROM during hydrotheraphy and during waking hours. • Maintain neck, arms legs in extension positions • Keep hands in functional positions. • Help patient to ambulate as tolerated.	

Contd...

Problem	*Reason*	*Objective*	*Nursing Intervention*	*Evaluation*
8. Altered nutrition: Less than body requirement R/T burns.	• Increased metabolic needs for wound healing. – Increased caloric demand. – Inability to ingest increased requirement as manifested by • Weight loss • Low serum alb. level, and • Unwillingness to ingest food.	The patient will have adequate nutrition	• Obtain accurate preburn weight to assess caloric needs. • Assess eating habits/patterns, food preferences, food allergies, within 72 hours admission. • Record caloric intake caloric counts.. • Weight patient daily to follow weight tends. • Provide oral hygiene eash shift prn. • Provide anaesthetically pleasing environment. • Schedule treatments to provide for uninterrupted meal times. • Allow a period of rest prior to meal time if the client has endured a painful procedure or treatment. • Provide aids and devices for eating utensils. • Encourage significant others in family to bring favourite food from home. • Provide nutritious supplements between meals. • Provide positive reinforcement for eating. • Chart caloric intake to monitor adequacy of diet. • Maintain patient NPO with nasogastric tube to low intermittent suction. • Assess return of bowel sounds. • Initiate and monitor hyperalimentation and IV fluid replaced by request.	
9. Impaired gas exchange R/T – Carbon monoxide poisoning – Smoke poisoning – Heat damage to lungs.	Patient has signs of respiratory distress • Dullness • Confusion • Laboured breathing • Tachypnoea • Dyspnoea • Diminished or adventitious breach sounds • Tachycardia • Decrease in PaO_2 and SaO_2 level. • Cyanosis.	Patient will have improved gas exchanges.	• Assess for signs of respiratory distress. • Monitor arterial blood gas and carboxy haemoglobin level as ordered. • Monitor SaO_2 levels. • Administer O_2 therapy as ordered. • Instruct patient on the use of incentive spirometer. • Elevate head of bed. • Monitor need for endotracheal intubation.	(Needs 7 days to reduce)
10. Ineffective Airway clearance R/T burn inhalation injury.	• Signs of tracheal oedema; airway epidermal sloughing; depressed pulmonary ciliary action from intubation injury	Patient will have airway clearance.	• Have client turn, cough, and deep-breaching 1 to 2 ( ) hrx × 24 hours, then 2-4 hours while awake. • Place oral suction device within patient reach for independent use. • Perform endotracheal or nasotracheal suction prn. • Monitor and document character of sputum.	

Contd...

Problem	*Reason*	*Objective*	*Nursing Intervention*	*Evaluation*
11. Altered peripheral tissue confusion R/T constricting circumferential burns		Patient will have adequate peripheral perfusion	• Remove all constricting jewellery and clothing. • Limit use of constricting blood pressure cuff in affected extremity. • Monitor arterial pulse hourly by palpation or ultrasonic flow detector. • Assess capillary refill of unburned skin on affected extremity. • Assess pain level with active ROM exercises. • Elevate affected extremities above the level of the heart to prevent oedema. • Encourage active ROM exercises. • Anticipate and prepare patient for eschartotomy by continuous monitoring.	
12. Anxiety R/T, pain separate from burns.	C/o pain – Separation from family – Guilt associated with injury. – Lack of knowledge about treatment and outcome. – Financial needs.	Patient verbalizes reduction of anxiety	• Administer and evaluate effectiveness of medication and pain before intervention. • Encourage family visits and participation in care to increase feelings of support. • Be open to patient's expressions of feelings about burn event, so patient has opportunity to vent feelings and discuss condition. • Provide information or explanation as assessment indicates. • Describe burn process, signs and symptoms to patient and family on admission. • Explain therapeutic interventions, precautionary measures, gowning, handwashing, and visiting on admission to lent cooperation and reduce anxiety.	
13. Potential for self-esteem disturbance R/T threatened burn.	Actual change in body image	Objective. Patient will develop improved self-esteem	• Determine previoius coping style • Provide atmosphere of acceptance. • Explain projected appearance of burns and grafts during different phases of wound healing. • Allow the client to progress at his/her own pace through stages of denial, grief, and acceptance of enquiry and recovery. • Assess the need for limit setting for maladaptive behaviour to promote patient's self confidence by ensuring continuity of care provider – Discuss all activities and procedures prior to initiation. – Support client role in care and treatment. – Keep client informed by progress. – Provide honest, positive reinforcement. – Help family/significant others to interact with the patient. • Encourage interaction, with others outside. • Help prepare client for social interaction. • Reassure patient and family at every stage to reduce grieving.	
14. Hypothermia R/T epithelial tissue loss	Loss of epithelial tissue and fluctuating ambient air temperature.	The patient will remain normothermic	• Monitor the patient's rectal or cone temperature as indicated. • Limit the amount of body surface exposed during wound care. • Limit hydrotherapy treatment sessions to 30 minutes or less with water temperature 98°F to 102°F. • Use external heat shields/radiated heat lamps. • Keep procedure rooms and surgical suites warm.	

RESPONSIBILITIES OF NURSING PERSONNEL ON BURN PATIENT

A logical extension of the emotional trauma experienced by the patient includes the emotional trauma for the nurse. The nurse must deal with the patient who, at times, is unpleasant and hostile and with the fact that burn therapy is almost always painful. The nurse will sometimes visualize many hours of patient care suddenly destroyed by sepsis and death.

Because of long hospitalizations and intense contact, the relationship between the nurse and the patient can result in strong bonds that can be healthy and healing or destructive and draining. The burn patient can develop demanding or punitive attitudes which may cause the nurse to be reluctant to provide care. The nurse and patient can also develop warm, trusting, mutually satisfying relationships not only during hospitalization but also during long-term rehabilitation. Sometimes the bond can be so strong that the patient has difficulty in separating from the hospital and hospital staff. The frequency and intensity of family contact can also be rewarding as well as training to the nurse. New comers to burn-nursing often find it difficult to cope with not only the deformities caused by burn injury but also the odour, the unpleasant sight of the wound, and the reality of the pain that accompanies the burn.

However, many nurses believe that the care they provide makes a critical difference in helping patients to survive and cope with the severe injury. It is this belief that keeps nurses caring for burn patients and their families. Support services for the burn-nurse in the form of group meeting with members of the medical team. Such meetings help the nursing staff to cope with difficult feeling that may be experienced when caring for the burn patients. The nurse may need the opportunity to ventilate feelings of anger and hostility to an impartial listener. This therapeutic communication process may make the difference between the nurse who can deliver effective nursing care and the nurse who provides mere custodial patient care.

Table 16.2: Nursing care plan for the thermally injured patient

Problem	*R*	*Objective*	*Nursing Interventions*	*Rationales*
Nursing Diagnosis # 1 Impairment of skin integrity related to: 1. Thermal injury: dry/moist heat, chemical or electrical.		The patient has: 1. Had the burning process halted. 2. A skin pH near normal. 3. No complaints of burning on the wound. 4. A decrease in the degree of corneal ulcerations and eye infection.	• Assess burning process. If fire or scald injury and heat are evident on the wound, cool the area with tap water.	• Depth of injury increases due to length of exposure to the burning agent.
			• Remove clothing and jewellery.	• Clothing, jewellery, belts, etc., retain heat and can increase depth of injury.
			• Do not apply ice.	• Vasoconstriction occurs, damaging the surrounding tissues. Core temperature decreases.
			• Cover patient with clean sheet or blanket.	• Prevents excessive heat loss. Body heat is lost through the burned area. • Decreases pain from exposure to air. • Protects from emergency room contamination.
			• Obtain history of the burning agent.	• Provides information on agent as extent and depth of injury are directly related to the concentration, activity, and penetrability of the chemical; also, duration of contact and the resistance of tissues impact on severity of injury.
			• Initiate extensive lavage with cool water for all chemical burns along with simultaneous removal of contaminated clothing. Brush off dry chemicals before lavage.	• Dilution of the chemical and removal of the chemical from the injured tissues will halt the burning process. Although some chemicals create heat when united with water, copious lavage can dissipate that heat away from the body. Health care workers must protect themselves from exposure to chemicals.
			• If eyes are affected, lavage with a minimum of 2-3 liters of NSS. If blepharospasm occurs during irrigation, apply topical ophthalmic anaesthetic agent as prescribed.	• Important to remove all chemicals from the eyes to preserve sight. (Blepharospasm refers to a twitching or spasm of orbicularis oculi muscle).

Contd...

Contd...

Problem	*R*	*Objective*	*Nursing Interventions*	*Rationales*
Nursing Diagnosis # 2 Impaired gas exchange related to: 1. Upper airway oedema. 2. Carbon monoxide poisoning. 3. Smoke inhalation injury. 4. Disruption of alveolar-capillary membrane.		The patient will: 1. Have a carbon monoxide level less than 10 per cent. 2. Maintain a patient airway. 3. Maintain acceptable blood gas parameters: • pH ~ 7.35–7.45. • PaO_2 >60 mmHg (room air) • $PaCO_2$ ~35–45 mmHg 4. Be responsive, awake, and cognizant of the surroundings.	• Assess for signs or symptoms of tracheal obstruction and respiratory distress. • Establish an airway. Administer humidified oxygen at 100 per cent. • Monitor arterial blood gases and carbon monoxide level.	• Upper airway oedema with smoke inhalation can cause a rapid, progressive airway obstruction leading to respiratory arrest. • Carbon monoxide and acute airway obstruction are the greatest threats to life immediately after burn injury. Carbon monoxide level of more than 10-20 per cent is indicative of carbon monoxide poisoning.
			• Assess arterial pH.	• Patient will demonstrate a metabolic acidosis due to decreased tissue perfusion.
			• Assess chest x-ray.	• This may initially be negative but may demonstrate inflammation or pulmonary oedema in 12-24 hours after burn injury.
			• Prepare for endotracheal intubation and mechanical ventilation with positive signs and symptoms of inhalation injury.	• Early intubation prior to the development of airway obstruction is preferred over tracheostomy due to the increased chance of infection from tracheostomy.
			• Assess breath sounds for abnormalities: Wheezing.	• Wheezing is heard across all lung fields due to oedema and inflammation caused by carbon deposits and damage to the airways.
			♦ Rales.	♦ Rales can occur 12-24 hours after injury.
			• Prepare for bronchoscopy. • Administer prescribed bronchodilators as indicated.	• Bronchoscopy will be diagnostic for inhalation injury.
			• Begin vigorous pulmonary toilet.	• Frequent suctioning of smoke inhalation victims is necessary to clear the airway of copious secretions and carbon deposits. ♦ This must be completed aseptically to prevent the lethal complication of pneumonia.
			• Assess chest wall excursion and the use of accessory muscles for breathing.	• For severe burns of the neck and chest, eschar and oedema formation create a splinting effect that prohibits lung expansion.
			• With positive signs of restrictive defect, prepare for escharotomy.	• Eschar is released by cutting the eschar on both sides of the chest and from the zyphoid process and/or sternal notch to the outer chest wall.
Nursing Diagnosis# 3 Fluid volume deficit related to: 1. Capillary leak—loss of plasma proteins. 2. Insensible water loss.		The patient will be maintained with adequate circulating volume and cardiac output as evidenced by: 1. Urine output of 50 ml/hour. If haemochromogens are in the urine, an output of 100 ml/hour is maintained.	• Monitor for signs and symptoms of hypovolaemia including: Hypotension, tachycardia, tachypnoea, extreme thirst, restlessness, disorientation.	• Fluid volume is lost through increased capillary permeability, which begins at the time of injury. Insensible fluid loss through the burn wound contributes to decreasing circulation volume.
			• Administer IV fluids according to fluid resuscitation formulas in Table 65-6. Insert large-bore IV catheter.	• IV placement should be in large vessels for the rapid delivery of fluid.

Contd...

Contd...

Problem	*R*	*Objective*	*Nursing Interventions*	*Rationales*
		2. Adequate blood pressure as evidenced by an arterial systolic pressure approximately 100 mmHg, and urine output is maintained as above. 3. Heart rate: ~100/min. 4. Haemoglobin and haematocrit within normal range.	• Prepare for the insertion of subclavian catheters and arterial lines.	• Difficulty of peripheral IV insertion is due to vasoconstriction and volume depletion. • With the insertion of subclavian catheters, haemodynamics can be more accurately assessed and monitored.
			• Send blood specimens for determination of: Haematocrit and haemoglobin, electrolytes, prothrombin/partial thromboplastin times, blood sugar, BUN, and creatinine.	• Haemodyamic status is also assessed through the laboratory data. • Increased potassium K^+ is due to cellular trauma, which releases K^+ into extracellular fluid. • Sodium is lost from the circulation as oedema forms. • Metabolic acidosis results from the loss of bicarbonate ions with the following.
			• Monitor urine for amount, specific gravity, and the presence of haemochromogens.	• Specific gravity can predict the volume replacement. • Myoglobin is released in the bloodstream from muscle damage, especially in electrical injuries. Haemoglobin is released through the destruction of RBCs. These haemochromogens can cause renal-tubular obstruction. Osmotic diuretics can aid in reversing this process.
			• Administer osmotic diuretics as ordered and monitor response to diuretic therapy.	• Decreased urinary output can be a result of: Decreased renal blood flow; increased secretion of ADH; increased adrenocortical activity.
			• Monitor serum pH. Administer prescribed sodium bicarbonate.	• Correct the metabolic acidosis that results from vasoconstriction and tissue ischaemia.
			• Continue to monitor hourly for the effectiveness of fluid resuscitation.	• Hypervolaemia will lead to increased oedema and pulmonary congestion.
			• Assess gastrointestinal function: Absence of bowel sounds.	• Splanchnic constriction as a result of hypovolaemia leads to paralytic ileus.
			• Insert a nasogastric tube and attach to suction.	• Paralytic ileus occurs in burn victims with a>20-25 per cent total body surface burn.
			• Monitor gastric pH every 1-2 hours. Administer antacids via nasogastric tube as prescribed to maintain a gastric pH>5.	• Antacids help neutralize gastric secretions. Antacids decrease the risk of Curling's ulcer related to stress.
Nursing Diagnosis # 4 Alteration in comfort: pain.		The patient will: 1. Receive assistance in controlling the pain. 2. Verbalize that the pain is tolerable. 3. Receive validation that the pain exists.	• Assess the degree and duration of pain during painful procedures. • Decrease the anxiety of the patient through the use of relaxation, distraction, or music.	• Validate pain during therapeutic modalities, such as wound care and exercise. • Relaxation can reduce intensity. • Acute anxiety can be related to anger or guilt about the accident and the chance of survival.

Contd...

Contd...

Problem	*R*	*Objective*	*Nursing Interventions*	*Rationales*
			• Acknowledge the presence of pain. Explain the causes of pain in burn injury.	• In partial-thickness injury, the presence of prostaglandins and histamines in and around the injured area stimulates peripheral pain receptors and intensifies central perceptions of discomfort. Full-thickness burns initially are painless but as the nerve endings regenerate, pain occurs due to exposure to air.
			• Provide privacy for painful therapies.	• Patients feel a loss of control during painful modalities.
			• Decrease the fear associated with pain and the use of narcotics.	• Patients frequently will not ask for medication for fear of becoming addicted to a drug.
			• Motivate the patient to participate in noninvasive methods to reduce the intensity of pain.	• Patients exhibit wide variability in both pain perception and response to pain, attributed to sociological background and previous pain threshold. ♦ How the injury occurred also contributes to the patient's response.
			• Administer narcotic analgesics as prescribed to provide optimal relief:	
			♦ Administer IV narcotics during the emergent phase.	♦ Due to the capillary leak, IM medications are not absorbed adequately to provide acute pain relief.
			♦ Administer narcotics as often as necessary during the acute phase especially prior to dressing change and exercise.	♦ Inadequate narcotic doses are frequently prescribed due to the fear by the medical professionals of producing respiratory depression or addiction to a narcotic.
			♦ Assess adequate doses of drugs. Assess the patient's response to the medication. Recommend increasing prescribed doses as necessary.	♦ Careful titration of narcotic doses can provide adequate pain relief.
			• Decrease the amount of narcotic analgesia as the burn wound heals.	• At the time of discharge, the patient's pain should be adequately controlled with oral agents.
Nursing Diagnosis # 5 Potential for alteration in peripheral perfusion related to: 1. Circumferential eschar. 2. Compartment syndrome.		The patient will have: 1. Pulses present and of good quality distal to burn area on limbs. 2. Extremities warm to touch. 3. Oedema minimized to prevent vascular compromise.	• Assess pulses on burned extremities every 15 min. Use the ultrasonic Doppler as necessary. Assess capillary refill.	• As oedema forms on circumferential burns, eschar forms a tight constricting band, decreasing the circulation to the limb distal to the circumferential site.
			• Assess for numbness, tingling, and increased pain in the burned extremity.	• Increasing pain in extremities can be predictive of increasing pressure from tight bands.
			• Elevate burned extremities.	• Elevation of the limb promotes venous return and decreases oedema.
			• Apply burn dressing loosely.	• To allow for expansion as oedema forms.
			• Assess muscle compartment pressure.	• Increasing pressure readings from muscle compartments are indicative of decreased tissue perfusion.
			♦ If signs and symptoms of circulatory impairment and inadequate deep tissue perfusion are present, prepare the patient for escharotomy and/or fasciotomy.	♦ These surgical procedures will release constricting eschar bands and improve deep tissue perfusion.

Contd...

Contd...

Problem	*R*	*Objective*	*Nursing Interventions*	*Rationales*
Nursing Diagnosis #6 Potential for sepsis related to: Wound infection.		Table 65-5) The patient will have: 1. Healthy granulation tissue on unhealed areas with <10^5 colonies of bacteria as demonstrated on wound culture. 2. Absence of clinical manifestation of infection (body temperature, WBC). 3. Skin graft sites that have taken. 4. Donor sites that are free of infection.	• Use sterile technique when caring for the burn wound. • Maintain protective isolation with good handwashing technique. • Administer immunosupportive medications as prescribed: Tetanus, gamma globulin. • Perform wound care as prescribed: ◆ Inspect and debride wounds daily; culture wounds 3 times a week or at any sign of infection; shave all burned areas, especially the scalp and perineum; assess carefully any invasive line site for inflammation especially if the line is through a burn area.	• Burn wound is a culture medium for bacterial growth. • Prevent the spread of bacteria from patient to patient. • Immunoglobulins are depressed at the time of severe burn injury. • Quick identification of bacterial wound invasion can decrease the incidence of septic episodes.
			• Monitor the patient constantly for signs and symptoms of sepsis: Temperature; sensorium; vital signs; increase/decrease in bowel sounds; decreased output; fluid translocation; positive blood/wound cultures.	• The burn patient will experience several septic episodes during hospitalization until the burn wound is healed.
			• Administer systemic antibiotics as prescribed and monitor response to therapy.	• Judicious use of antibiotics can decrease the incidence of drug-resistant organism development.
Nursing Diagnosis # 7 Alteration in nutrition related to: 1. Inadequate intake due to inability to eat, therapeutic regimen, or multiple surgeries. 2. Increased metabolic demands.		The patient is: 1. Maintained within 10% of pre-burn weight. 2. Healing burn wound. 3. In a positive nitrogen balance.	• Institute enteral feedings as soon as bowel sounds are present. • Ensure required caloric and protein intake by: ◆ Having a dietitian calculate caloric needs. ◆ Accurate caloric counts; accurate intake and output; daily weights.	• The burn patient may require up to 4000 calories per day. • Formulas have been developed to assess necessary caloric needs utilizing total body surface area burn. ◆ Maintenance of protein mass is critical to survival.
			• If tube feedings are needed to supplement caloric needs: Insert a feeding tubes; assess patency and placement every 4 hours; place patient in a semi-Fowler's position; ◆ Assess for gastric residuals at least every four hours. ◆ Assess bowel sounds every 2-4 hours. ◆ Increase feeding regimen as prescribed. ◆ Monitor for adverse side effects such as diarrhoea or gastric distention. ◆ Accurately document amount of feeding administered.	• Burn victims frequently require more calories than they are able to eat. • Frequent treatment modalities and surgeries interrupt feeding schedules. ◆ Absence of bowel sounds is frequently the first sign of impending sepsis. ◆ If the patient is unable to tolerate enteral feedings, hyperalimentation may need to be considered.
Nursing Diagnosis #8 Impairment of activity related to: 1. Reformation of collagen. 2. Excisional wound therapy. 3. Autografting.		The patient will: 1. Maintain positioning as prescribed during multiple surgeries. 2. Be able to perform activities of daily living. 3. Be ambulatory with no assistive devices. 4. Retain full range of motion of all affected joints.	• Assess the need for positioning and/or splinting. ◆ Consult occupational therapy. ◆ Apply splints and check frequently for fit or areas of pressure. ◆ Clean splints at least every shift. Evaluate the need for continuous splinting or night time use only. ◆ Encourage patient to exercise burned limbs, and to actively participate in as many ADLs as possible.	• Attempt to maintain neutral positioning of burned areas. • Maintain a stretch of skin to decrease the pull of contracture. ◆ As oedema subsides, splints might need revision. ◆ Decrease contamination of the burn wounds.

Contd...

Contd...

Problem	*R*	*Objective*	*Nursing Interventions*	*Rationales*
			• Observe the burn wound closely for any exposed tendons, unresolved oedema, peripheral neuropathies, or points of pressure.	• Rapid identification of problem areas helps to decrease additional injury to burned areas.
			• Assess problem areas:	
			◆ Position patient with neck burns in extension. Use no pillow.'	◆ Prevent the developemnt of neck contractures.
			◆ Inspect ears frequently.	◆ Pressure can cause necrosis and bending can cause chondritis.
			◆ Position patient with axilla burns in 90° shoulder abduction and 10° elbow flexion.	◆ Prevent the formation of scar bands in the axilla.
			◆ Use special skin care and topical agent of choice after each voiding or defecation.	◆ Prevent infection or contamination of the burn wound.
			◆ For facial injuries elevate head of the bed. Lubricate lips every 4 hours.	◆ Decrease oedema formation. Avoid lips that crack and bleed.
			• Inspect the burn wound for early signs of webbing, contracture, banding or keloid formation.	• Quick identification of defects can lead to reversal through the use of splints or pressure.
Nursing Diagnosis # 9 Ineffective coping of individual/significant others related to: 1. Trauma of burns. 2. Family loss. 3. Lack of knowledge of the disease process. 4. Surgical procedures. 5. Expected outcomes.		The patient/significant other will: 1. Demonstrate acceptance of the accident with a decreased level of anxiety. 2. Verbalize fears, grief, and acceptance of an altered body image. 3. Verbalize treatment modalities, process of skin healing and scar/contracture formation. 4. Develop supportive behaviours.	• Assess patient/significant other for level of understanding of burn treatment.	• At high stress times, repetition is necessary for understanding.
			• Describe the pathophysiology of the burn process and what the patient will experience.	• Attempt to enlist the support of the family to help the patient cope with pain and disfigurement.
			• Explain the precautionary isolation of the victim.	
			• Assist and identify the coping mechanisms of both patient/significant other. Provide time for questions and discussion of feelings and fears.	• This event is disruptive to patient/significant other lifestyles, relationships, careers, and finances.
			• Be honest. Do not protect the patient/significant other from necessary emotional experiences.	◆ Frequently there are other injuries or deaths at the scene. Burn victims will ask about the outcome of loved ones. These concerns must be dealt with to enable the patient to cope with his/her injury.
			• Keep patient and significant others informed of the progress of the patient.'	• If the burn is severe, the death and dying process needs to be instituted.
			• Explain all procedures and enlist the patient's cooperation.	• Painful procedures preclude patient cooperation.
			• Develop a contract with the patient/significant other and set realistic short-term goals. Allow the patient to make decisions and choices when possible.	• Allows the patient to have some control over his/her environment.
			• Approach and administer care in a consistent, positive manner. Carry out your part of the contract regardless of the patient's behaviour.	• The patient will be cognizant of the inability to manipulate staff. Burn patients frequently become combative, argumentative and resistant to therapeutic modalities due to the pain.
			• Administer sedatives and analgesics as needed.	
			• Provide adequate rest time.	
			• Encourage discussion of feelings, family, and future plans.	
			• Support and encourage the patient to participate in self-care. Provide assistive devices.	• Patients will experience a positive self-image as ADLs increase.
			• Recommend a psychiatric consult if the patient/significant other need help in order to cope.	• Patient/significant others frequently need help in dealing with body disfigurement and the long-term care needs.
			• Refer the patient/significant other to appropriate resources for aid: burn support groups; social services; rehabilitation centers; financial services.	

Ophthalmic and Otologic Nursing

I. OPHTHALMIC NURSING
[Nursing the Visual Disorder]

Person's orientation to the world is primarily visual. People will learn much about their environment and themselves through their eyes. Practically every behaviour is affected by the visual sense.

Visual systems consist of the internal and external structures of the eyeball, the refractive media, and the visual pathways. The internal structures are the iris, lense, ciliary body, choroid and retina. The external structures are the eyebrows, eyelids, eyelashes, lacrimal system, conjunctiva, cornea, sclera, and extraocular muscles. The entire visual system is important for visual function. Light reflected from an object in the field of vision passes through the transparent structures of the eye, and, in doing so, is refracted (bent) so that clear image can fall on the retina. From the retina, the visual stimuli travels through the visual pathway to the occupital cortex, where they are perceived as an image. Vision contributes meaning and pleasure to the human experience.

ASSESSMENT OF THE VISUAL SYSTEM

Assessment of the visual system is an integral part of the nurse's role, Visual screening is conducted with persons of all ages and in all settings, and most life disorders are identified by nurses, physician, in schools, industry, outpatient clinics or ophthalmologists. Admission to the hospital is usually limited to medical and surgical treatment that cannot routinely be accomplished on an outpatient basis. Because, persons with eye problems usually are managed on an outpatient basis. Visual impairment is usually not the major diagnosis of persons for whom the nurse is providing care. However, visual impairment is frequently present and may be undiagnosed. Therefore, nurses should routinely assess visual ability, especially in persons who have systemic diseases that affect vision or who are taking medication with known visual side effects.

A complete visual assessment consists of a careful patient interview combined with physical assessment of the eye structures. General areas explored during the interview includes the patient assessment of his or her vision and any recent changes in visual acuity, whether glasses for contacts are used on the date of the last professional eye examination. The presence of severeity of common eye symptoms, such as blurred vision, "floaters" dry, scratchy eyes, burning or chronic headaches are explored. The interview allows the nurse also to explore the person's health promotion practices and request to use of protective eye wear, particularly for occupational exposure. Any history of head trauma, loss of consciousness, or direct trauma or infections is important to explore.

Since many eye disorders are inherited, a family history is essen-tial.

Questions are directed especially to a family history of cataracts, glaucoma, diabetes, hypertension, STDs, AIDs, cancer poor vision glasses or blindness. A person's medical that could not be corrected with history is also obtained with particular attention to all medications in current use.

The tissues of the eye are for the most part transparent, making abnormalities easily detectable. Ocular manifestation of systemic disease also can be identified. In addition, the vascular system (retinal vascular system) and cranial nerve (optic nerves) of the eye can be visualized on examination. Assessment includes inspection of the extenal structure and gross measures of visual acuity. A basic assessment of the eye and vision are as given below:

- *Facial and ocular expression:* Prominence of eyes: alert or dull expression.
- *Eyelids and conjunctiva:* Symmetry, presence of oedema, ptosis, itching, redness, discharge, blinking, equality and growths.
- *Lacrimal system:* Tears, swelling and growths.
- *Sclera:* Colour.
- *Cornea:* Clarity.
- Anterior chamber: Depth, presence of blood and pus.
- *Iris and pupils:* Irregularities in colour, shape and size.
- *Pupillary reflex:*
  - *Light:* Constriction of pupil in response to light in that eye (direct light reaction); equal amount of constriction in the other eye (consensual light reaction).
  - *Accommodation:* Convergence of eyes and constriction of pupil as gaze shifts from far to near object.
- *Lens:* Transparent or opaque.
- *Peripheral vision:* Ability to see movement and objects well on both sides of field of vision.

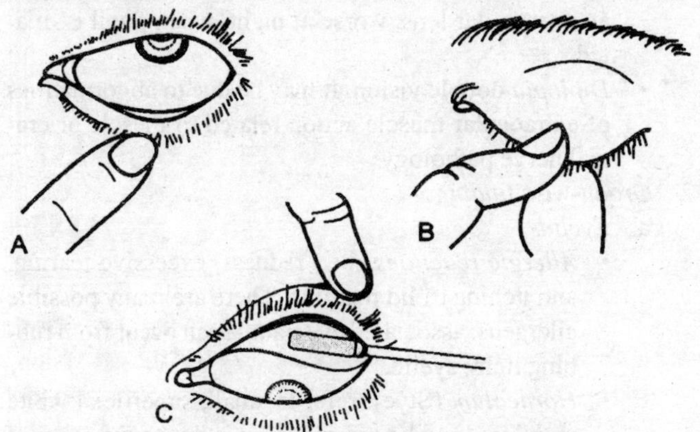

Fig. 17.1: Examining the eye for a foreign particle. (A) Evert lower lid. (B and C) Evert upper lid.

- *Acuity with and without glasses:* Ability to read newsprint, clocks on wall, and name tags and to recognize faces at bedside and at door.
- *Supportive aids:* Glasses, contact lenses, prosthesis.

The normal physical assessment of the visual systems include the following:

- Visual acuity 20/20 ou; no diplopia.
- External eye structures are symmetric without lesions or deformities.
- Lacrimal apparatus is nontender without drainage.
- Conjunctiva clear; sclera white.
- Perrla. Pupil normally equal, round and react to light and accommodation.
- Lense clear.
- EOMI.
- Disc margin sharp.
- Retinal vessels are normal with no haemorrhage or spots.

Common Assessment Techniques: There are related to vision include the following.

1. *Visual acuity testing* is performed to determine patient's distance and near visual acuity. In this, patient reads for Snellen chart and 20 ft. (distance vision test) or Jaoeger's chart at 14 in (near vision test). Examiner notes smallest print patient can read on each chart. Examples of visual acuity measurement are as follows:
   20/20 Normal
   20/40-2 Missed two letters of the 20/40 line.
   10/400 At 10 ft. reads line than normal eye sees at 400 ft.
   CF/2 ft. Counts fingers at 2 feet.
   HM/3 ft. Sees hand movement at 3 feet.
   LP/Proj. Light perception with projection.
   NLP No light perceptions.
2. *Extraocular muscle testing* is performed to determine if the patient's extraocular muscles are functioning in a normal manner, with no underaction or overaction. In this the examiner makes patient follow a light source or other fixation object through a complete field of gaze, in the cover-uncover test, examiner covers patient's eye then uncovers it to see if eye has deviated under the cover.
3. *Confrontation visual field test* is done to determine if patient has a full field of vision without obvious scotomas. Here patient faces examiner, covers one edge, fixates on examiner's face and counts number of fingers that the examiner brings into patient's field of vision.
4. *Pupil function testing* is performed to determine if patient has normal pupillary response. In this, the examiner shines light into the patient's pupil and observes pupillary response, each pupil is examined independently, examiner also checks for consensual and accommodative response.
5. *Tonometry* is to measure intraocular pressure (normal pressure is 10-21 mm Hg). In this applanation, tonometer is gently touched to the anaesthesized corneal surface; examiner looks through ocular of slit lamp microscope, adjusts pressure dial until mires are aligned, and notes intraocular pressure reading.
6. *Slit-lamp microscopy* provides magnified view of the conjunctiva, sclera, cornea, anterior chamber, iris, lens and vitreous. In this the patient is seated with chin placed in chin rest, slit beam illuminate ocular structures, examiner looks through magnifying occular assess various structures.
7. *Ophthalmoscopy* provides magnified view of the retina and optic nerve head. Here examiner holds ophthalmoscope close to the patient's eye, shining light into back of eye and looking through aperture on ophthalmoscope, examiner adjusts dial to select one of the lenses in ophthalmoscope that produces desired amount of magnification to inspect ocular fundus.
8. *Colour vision testing* is performed to determine patient ability to distinguish colours. Here patient identifies numbers or paths formed by pattern of dots in series of colour plates.
9. *Stereopsis testing* is performed to determine patient ability to see objects in three dimensions; to test depth perceptions. From a series of plates patient identifies geometric pattern or figure that appears closer to patient when viewed through special spectacles that provides three-dimensional view.
10. *Keratometry* is done to measure the coreneal curvature often done before fitting contact lenses, before doing refraction surgery or after corneal transplantation.
    The terms describing refractions are:
    - Accommodation-Ability to adjust between far and near objects.
    - Emmetropia-Normal eye, light rays focus on retina.
    - Ametropia-Refractive error, light rays do not focus on retina.

- Myopia-Near sightedness, light rays focus in front of retina.
- Hyperopia-Far sightedness, light rays focus behind retina.
- Presbyopia-Hyperopia from loss of lens elasticity because of aging.
- Astigmatism-Irregular curvature of cornes, light rays do not focus at same point.

Common Assessment Abnormalities found in the Visual System

1. *General findings*
   - *Pain:* i. Foreign body sensation may be due to superficial corneal abrasion, it can result from contact lens wear or trauma; conjunctival or corneal foreign body are usually lessened with lid closure.

     ii. Severe, deep and throbbing pain is due to anterior uveitis, acute glaucoma, infection; acute glaucoma associated with nausea, and vomiting.
   - Photophobia refers to abnormal intolerence to light may be due to inflammation or infection of cornea or anterior uveal tract (iris and ciliary body).
   - Blurred vision is gradual or sudden inability to see clearly. This may be due to refractive errors, corneal opacities, cataracts, retinal changes, (detachment, macular degeneration), optic neuritis, or atrophy, central retinal vein or artery thrombosis, refractive changes related to fluctuations in serum glucose.
   - *Scotoma* refers to blind or partially blind area in the visual field. This may be due to disorders of optic chiasm, glaucoma, central serous choria-retinopathy age and related macular degeneration; injury, migraine headache.
   - *Spots, floaters* i.e., patient describes seeing spots, "spider webs" "curtain" or floaters within the field of vision. The most common cause lies in vitrious liquification (benign phenomenon); other possible causes include haemorrhage into vitreous tumour, retinal holes, or tears, impending retinal detachment, visions detachment, intraocular haemorrohage and chorioretinitis.
   - *Dryness* is discomfort, sandy, gritty, irritation or burning. It is due to decreased tear formation or changes in the tear composition because of aging or various systemic diseases.
   - *Halo around lights* is a presence of a halo around light. It may be due to refractive changes, corneal oedema as a result of a sudden rise in intraocular pressure in angle-closure glaucoma or secondary glaucoma.
   - *Glare* headache, ocular discomfort, reduced visual acuity. It is related to corneal inflammation or to opacities in the cornea, lens, or vitreous that scatter the incoming light; can also result from light scatter around edges of an intraocular lens, worse at night, when pupil is dilated.
   - *Diplopia* double vision. It may be due to abnormalities of extraocular muscle action related to muscle or cranial nerve pathology.
2. *Organ-wise findings*
   a. *Eyelids*
   - *Allergic reactions:* i.e., redness, excessive tearing, and itching of lid margins. There are many possible allergens; associated eye trauma can occur from rubbing itchy eyelid.
   - *Hordeolum* (Stye): refer to small, superficial white nodules along lid margin. This is due to infection of a sebaceous gland of eyelid and causative organism usually bacterial (most commonly staphylococcus aureus).
   - *Chalazion* refers to reddened, swollen area in eyelid, involves deeper tissues than hordeolum can be inflammed and tender. This may be due to granuloma formed around to sebacious gland occurs as a foreign body reaction to sebum in the tissue can develop from a hordeolum or from rupture of a sebacious gland with resulting sebum in the tissue.
   - *Blepharitis* i.e., redness, swelling and crusting along lid margin. It is due to bacterial invasion of lid margins; often chronic.
   - *Dacrocystitis* redness,swelling and tenderness of medial area of lower lid (in region of lacrimal sac). It is due to blockage of nasolacrimal duct and subsequent infection.
   - *Xanthelasma* raised, yellowish plaques on eyelids usually on nasal portion. It may be due to lipid disorders and may be normal fingings.
   - *Ptosis* dropping of upper lid margin, unilateral or bilateral. It is due to mechanical causes as result of eyelid tumours or excess skin; myogenic causes attributable to condition involving the levator muscle or myoneural function; such as myasthenia gravis; neurogenic causes affecting third cranial nerve that innovates the levator muscle.
   - *Entropion* is inward turning of upper or lower lid margin, unilateral or bilateral. It is due to congenital causes resulting in development, abnormalities, involutional entropion related to horizontal eyelid laxity can cause irritation and tearing.
   - *Ectropion* is outward turning of lower lid margin. This is due to mechanical causes as a result of eyelid tumours, herniated orbital fat, or extravasation of fluid; paralytic ectropian occurs when orbicularis muscle functions is disturbed as with Bell's palsy.
   - *Lid lag* slower or absent closing of one lid. It is due to possible involvement in cranial nerve VII.

- *Blepharospasm* increased blink rate when severe spasms occur, it is found unable to open eyelids. It may be due to inflammation, involvement of cranial nerves V and VII, can occur as a response to bright lights.
- *Decreased blink* decreased rate of eyelid closure. It may be due to decreased corneal sensation; possible involvement of CN VII; dry eye and corneal damage may result if blink rate significantly decreased.

b. *Conjunctive*
- *Conjunctivitis:* redness and swelling of conjunctiva may be itchy. It is due to bacterial or viral infection may be allergic response or inflammatory response to chemical exposure.
- *Subconjunctival haemorrhage:* appearance of blood spot on sclera, may be small, it can affect entire sclera. It may be due to conjunctival space caused by coughing, sneezing, eyerubbing or minor trauma, generally it doesn't require any treatment.
- *Pinguecula:* raised area (growth) on conjunctiva, horizontally oriented in medial area of bulbar conjunctiva. This was due to degenerative lesion related to chronic ultraviolet light or other environmental exposure.
- *Jaundice:* yellowish colour of entire sclera. Jaundice is related to liver dysfunction: yellow colour is normal after diagnostic study requiring intravenous fluoresce in injection.

c. *Cornea*
- Corneal abrasion: localized painful disruption of the epithelial layer of cornea can be visualized with fluorescein dye. It may be due to trauma, overwear or improper fit of contract lenses.
- *Corneal opacity:* whitish area of cormally transplant cornea; may involve entire cornea. It may be result of scar tissue formation related to inflammation, infection, trauma, degree of visual acuity deficit depends on location and size of opacity.
- *Pterygium:* triangular, horizontally oriented thickening of bulbar conjunctiva that extends post corneaocleral border onto cornea. It is commonly thought to be or extension of a pinguecula; degenerative lesion is related to chronic ultraviolet light or other environmental exposure; surgical removal is necessary if progression to central cornea.

d. *Globe*
- *Exophthalmos:* Protrusion of globe beyond its normal positionwithin bony orbit; sclera is often visible above iris when eyelids are open. This may be the result of intraocular or periorbital tumours; thyroid eye disease; swelling or tumours of the frontal sinus; dry eye and corneal damage may occur as a result of inability to close eye normally.

e. *Pupil*
- *Mydriasis:* Pupil is larger than normal (dilated). It may be due to emotional influences, trauma, acute glaucoma (fixed middilated), systemic or local drugs and head injury.
- *Miosis:* Pupil is smaller than normal. It may be due to iritis, morphine or similar drugs, glaucoma is treated with miotic agents.
- *Anisocoria:* Pupils are unequal (constricted). It is due to CNS disorders, slight difference in pupil size is normal in a small percentage of the population.
- *Dyscoria:* Pupil is irregularly shaped. It may be due to congenital causes (e.g. iris coloboma); acquired causes (e.g. trauma, iris-fixated intraocular lens implant and posterior synechiae surgery on iris).
- *Abnormal response to light or accommodation:* Pupils respond asymmetrically or abnormally to light stimulus or accommodation. It is due to CNS disorders; general anaesthesia.

i. *Iris*
- *Heterochromia:* Iris are different colours. It is result of congenital causes (Honer's syndrome); acquired causes (Chronic iritis, metastatic carcinoma, diffuse iris nevus or melanoma).
- *Iridokinesis:* Iris appears to shake on movement of eye. It is due to aphakia.

h. *Extraocular muscles*
- Strabismus: Deviation of eye position in one or more directions. It is result of overaction or underaction of one or more extraocular muscles; it can be congenital or acquired; neuromuscular involvement, CN III, IV or VI involved.

i. *Visual field defect*
- *Peripheral:* Partial or complete loss of peripheral vision. It may be due to glaucoma, complete or partial interruption of visual pathway migraine headache.
- *Central:* Loss of central vision may be due to macular disease.

j. *Lens:*
- *Cataract* is opacification of lens, pupil can appear cloudy or white. When opacity is visible behind pupil opening, it is due to aging, trauma, electrical shock, diabetes, chronic system, corticosteroid therapy and congenital.
- *Subluxation or dislocation:* Edge of lens may be seen through pupil. "Setting sun" sign. It is due to trauma and systemic disease (e.g. Marfan's syndrome).

Diagnostic Studies of Visual System

Diagnostic studies provide important information to the nurse in monitoring the patient condition and planning appropriate intervention. The common basic diagnostic studies of vision and their description and nursing responsibilities are as given below:

1. *Retinoscopy* is an objective (though inexact) measure of refractive error, handheld retinoscopy directs focussed light into the eye, refractive error distorts the light. Distortion is neutralized to determine refractive error, useful for the patient unable to cooperate during process of subjective refraction (e.g. confused patients). The procedure is painless, it may need to help patient hold head still. Pupil dilation will make it difficult to focus on nearby objects, dilation may last for 3-4 hours.
2. *Refractometry* is subjective measure of refractive error, multiple lenses are mounted on rotating wheels; patient sits looking through apertures at Snellen acuity chart, lenses are changed; patient chooses lenses then make acuity sharpest; cycloplegic drugs used to paralyse accommodation during refraction process. Nursing responsibilities is as in retinoscopy.
3. *Visual field perimetry* is detailed mapping of the visual field; study uses semicircular, bowl-like instrument that presents patient with a light stimulus in various parts of the bowl. Specific pattern of visual field loss is used to diagnose glaucoma and certain neurologic deficit. Procedure is painless but may be fatiguing, elderly or debilated patient may need rest period; patient must fixate on center target for accurate testing.
4. *Ultrasonography A-scan* probe is applanated against patient's anaesthesized cornea; it is used primarily for axial length measurement for calculating power of intraocular lens implanted after cataract extraction.

   B-Scan probe is applied to patient closed lid; used more often than A-Scan for diagnosis of ocular pathology such as intraocular foreign bodies or tumours, vitreous opacities, retinal detachments. The procedure is painless (Cornea is anaesthized for A-Scan)
5. *Indirect ophthalmoscopy* indirect ophthalmoscopy is worn on examiner's head; light is projected through a handheld lens into patient's eyes, stereoscopic view is larger and provides a better view of peripheral retina, always used when some retinal abnormalities are suspected. Light source is bright, patient may be uncomfortably photophobic especially because pupil is dilated.
6. *Fluorescein angiography* fluorescein (a nonradioctive, noniodine dye) is intravenously injected into anticubital or other peripheral vein, followed by serial photographs (over 10 min. period) of the retina through dilated pupil; provides diagnostic information about flow of blood through pigment epithelial and retinal vessels; often it is used in diabetic patients to accurately locate areas of diabet retinopathy before laser destruction of neovascularization.

   If extravasation occurs, fluorescein is toxic to tissue, systemic allergic reactions are rare, but nurse should be familiar with emerging equipment and procedure, tell the patient that dye can sometimes cause transient vomiting, all nausea, yellow discolouration of urine and skin in normal and transient.
7. *Amsler grid test* test is self-administered using a handheld card printed with a grid of lines (similar to graph paper); patient fixateous center dot and records any abnormalities of the grid lines such as wavy, missing, or distorted areas used to monitor macular problems. Regular testing is necessary to identify any changes in mucular function.
8. *Schirmer tear test* study measures tear volume produced throughout fixed time period; one end of a strip for filter paper is placed in lower lid cul-de-sac; area of tear saturation is measured after 5 minutes is useful in diagnosing keratoconjunctivitis sicca. Test may be done with closed or open eyes.

In addition there are four electrophysiology examinations performed in ophthalmology, electroretinogram (ERG), electro-oculogram (EOG), dark adaptometry, and visual evoked potential. The main purpose of these examinations is to assess the function of the visual pathway from the photoreceptors of the retina to visual cortext of the brain. They are useful in diagnosing retinal vascular occlusions, toxic drug exposure, inherited retinal diseases and intraocular foreign body.

Patient education regarding the purpose and method of testing is a nursing responsibility for all diagnostic procedures.

VISUAL IMPAIRMENT

Visual impairment ranges in severity from diminished visual acuity to total blindness. The patient may be categorized by the level of visual loss.

- Total blindness is defined as no light perception and no usable vision.
- Functional blindness is present when the patient has some light perception but no usable vision.

The patients with either total or functional blindness is considered legally blind and may use vision substitutes such as guide dogs and cones for ampulation and braille for reading. Vision enhancement techniques are not helpful.

Legal blindness is defined as central visual acuity for distance 20/200 or worse in the better eye (with correction) and/or a visual field no greater than 20 degrees in its widest diameter or in the better eye (compared with a normal range of about 180 degree).

Aetiology

Visual impairment has numerous causes and preventable blindness is a major health problem.

- Refractive errors (Myopia, hyperopia, presbyopia, astigmatism) are the most common visual problems, but numerous other nutritional, infections metabolic and systemic disorders adversely affect the function of the eye.
- *Nutritional deficiencies* A lack of vitamin A and B complex can cause changes within the retina, cornea, and conjunctiva. Night blindness is caused by vitamin A deficiency. Optic neuritis can result in vitamin B deficiency especially in alcoholics.
- *Infection* of trachoma, is common cause of visual impairment.
- *Macular degeneration,* is a disease of the aging retina.
- *Cataract and glaucoma*

In addition the eye can also be adversely affected by variety of systemic diseases which include the following:

i. Vascular disorders:
   - *Hypertension:* Persistent uncontrolled hypertension can cause haemorrhage, oedema, and exudates in the retina. Retinal asterics narrow, causing degenerative changes.
   - *Cardiovascular accident:* Depending on the location of the stroke, the patient may experience haemianopsin or blindness.
   - *Sickle cell disease.* This can cause neovascularization, arterial occlusions or retinal haemorrhage.

ii. *Neuological disorders*:
   - *Multiple sclerosis:* Demyelination can result in optic neuritis diplopia and nustagmus.

iii. Endocrine disorders:
   - *Graves disease:* Accumulation of fat and fluid in the retro-ocular tissue can produce exophthalmos (protrusion of eye) and lid retraction.
   - *Diabetic retinopathy*: Retinal capillary walls thicken and develop microaneurysms. Retinal veins widen and become tortuous. Small haemorrhages occur which leave scars that decrease vision. As the disease worsens, neovascularization occurs and the new vessels grow into the vitreous tumour. These vessels are vulnerable to both obstruction and rupture. Vision decreases as "floaters" are perceived in the eye.

iv. Connective disorders:
   - *Rheumatoid arthritis, SLE:* Neovascularizations, inflammations of the cornea, sclera, or uveal tract occur.

v. AIDS-Related Disorders:
   - *Herpes Zoster Ophthalmicus:* Herpes can invade the cornea and create ulceration that is potentially blinding.
   - *Cytomegalovirus (CMV):* CMV affects AIDS patients. It spreads rapidly through the cells of the retina and the blood vessels and can totally destroy the retina.
   - *Kaposis Sarcoma:* The lesions of Kaposis Sarcoma can affect the skin of the eyelids and conjunctiva or the orbit itself.

Pathophysiology

Refractive disorders

Refractive disorders include irregularities of the corneal curvature length and shape of the eye as well as the focusing ability of the lens. The common refractive errors include the following:

- *Myopia:* (near sightedness causes light rays to be focussed in front of the retina. Myopia may occur because of excessive light refraction by the cornea and lens or because of an abnormally long eye. Myopia may also occur because of lens swelling that occurs when blood glucose levels are elevated, as in uncontrolled diabetes. This type of myopia is transient and variable and fluctuates with blood glucose level. During childhood especially during adolescence when the child growth rate increases, myopia may progress rapidly and require frequent changes in the patient's glass. This excessive lengthening of the eye is often attributable to genetic factors.
- *Hyperopia* (far-sightedness) causes the light rays to focus behind the retina and requires the patient to use accommodation to focus the light rays on the retina for near and far objects. This type of refractive error occurs when the cornea or lens do not have adequate focussing power or when the eye ball is too short.
- *Presbyopia* is the loss of accommodation because of age. As the eye ages the crystalline lens becomes larger, firmer and less elastic. These changes decrease the eyes accommodative ability. The accommodative ability continues to decline with each decade of life and by approximately by the age of 70 years, the accommodative power of the lens declines to zero. When this occurs, the patient cannot focus on near objects without some form of visual aid.
- *Astigmatism* is caused by an unequal corneal curvature. This irregularity causes the incoming light rays to be bent unequally. Consequently the light rays do not come to a single point of focus on the retina.
- *Aphakia* is defined as the absence of the crystalline lens. The lens may be absent congenitally or it may be removed during cataract surgery. A lens that is traumatically dislocated results in functional aphakia, although lens remains in the eye.

Macular Degeneration

Degenerative changes occur in the thin layer of blood vessels that arise in the retina and extend into the choroid and their membrane cover. Both neovascular (exudative or wet) and nonneovascular (nonexudative or dry) forms occur. In neovascular degenerations there is a sudden proliferation of new fragile blood vessels in the macular area that tend to leak and damage macula. Scarring occurs and functional losses progress rapidly. It occurs in 5 per cent persons, responsible for 80 per cent severe vision loss. The *nonneovascular* degenerative form of macular degeneration occurs from the deposit of waste products and slow atrophy of the choroid, retina and pigment epithelium.

Clinical Manifestation

In refractive errors/disorders, there is defect of the refracting media of the eye prevents light rays from converging into a single focus on the retina. Defects are the result of irregularities of the cornea curvature, the focusing power of the lens or the length of the eye. The major symptom is blurred vision. In some cases, the patient may also complain of ocular discomfort, fatigue, eye strain or headaches.

Macular degeneration causes a variety of symptoms including visual blurring and distortion and usually causes some degree of central vision loss and a decreased ability to distinguish colours. Early signs and progression of the disease can be readily detected with the use of the Amsler grid. The individual perceives dark spots, missing areas and distorted wavy lines. Intravenous fluorescein angiography may be used to visualize or confirm the extent of neovascularization of vessel leakage is suspected.

Management

Visual impairment caused by refractive errors is usually diagnosed as a part of routine eye examination. The patient with refractive errors uses corrective lenses to improve the focus of light rays on the retina. Eye glasses and contact lenses are widely used to correct common refractive errors and restore visual acuity, includes the following.

i. *Emmetropia:* Normal vision. Light focuses on retina without accommodation for distance vision and with accommodation for near vision. Spectacles and contact lenses are not indicated.
ii. *Myopia*: Spectacle:concave (minus); lens bends light rays outward.
   Contact lens: Rigid, soft, daily wear or extended wear.
iii. *Hyperopia:* Spectacle: Convex (plus) lens binds light rays inward.
   Contact lens: Rigid or soft, daily wear or extended wear.
iv. *Astigmatism*
   Spectacle: Cylinder lens, bends light rays in different directions to align in a focussed point.
   Contact lens: Rigid or soft toric; daily wear or extended wear.
v. *Presbyopia*
   Spectacle: Convex for near vision, can be reading glasses or bifocals with reading correction in lower part of lens.
   Contact lens: Bifocal rigid or soft, monovision (one eye corrected for distance, one for near).
vi. *Aphakia*
   Spectacle: Thick, convex, virtually never used after cataract extraction.
   Contact lens: Rigid, soft, daily wear or extended, not used after cataract extractions.

Refractive surgery, defined as any operative procedure performed for the purpose of elimination of refractive error, it has become an increasingly viable alternative to glasses and contact lenses for persons with visual impairment related to refraction error. The common refractive surgery includes the following:

- Radial keratotomy (RK).
- Incisional keratotomy (IK).
- Photorefractive keratotomy (PRK).
- Laser-in-situ-keratomileusi (LASIK).
- Intraocular lens (IOL) implantation.

All these procedures are performed in ambulatory surgery centres. Careful preoperative teaching is provided to the nurse according to procedure and its advantages. Patients are permitted to gradually resume activities and usually experience a slow improvement of vision over a period of weeks or months. The nurse administers analgesics as needed to keep the patient comfortable and administer antibodies to decrease the incidence of infection.

There is no adequate treatment currently available for the non-neovascular form of macular degeneration. Oral zinc may reduce the progression of the disease. A small percentage of patients with neovascular degeneration can benefit from laser therapy to coagulate the abnormal vessels.

Nurse's Role in Prevention of Visual Impairment

Some forms of visual impairment are preventable and most forms can be slowed or treated with early diagnosis and appropriate therapy. Regular eye examinations by competent professionals are an important health promotion measure throughout life, especially as a person's age advances.

The nurse's role as a health educator with individuals, groups and communities is vital in preventing health problems, that the potential for visual impairment. In addition to health education, the nurse can promote visual health by early recognition of conditions or situations that carry a high risk of visual impairment. The following is information about those adult conditions and situation amenable to nursing interventions.

1. Glaucoma is a significant cause of preventable visual impairment. Early recognition of glaucoma is extremely important in promoting visual health. The nurse can advocate and provide assistance for screening programmes. In addition, nurse should provide health information regarding the importance of regular ophthalmic examination, especially the patient at high risk for this disorder. The nurse can provide this information to an individual patient, groups of patients or the general community.

2. *Ocular* trauma can lead to blindness or severe visual impairment. Many injuries can be prevented by identifying and correcting situations that may lead to eye injuries such as:
   - Failure to properly use eye protection during potentially hazardous work, hobby, or sports activities.
   - Improper handling or storing of chemicals and especially storing alkalies or acids.
   - In appropriate response to ocular injuries, particularly failure to institute prompt, continuous ocular irrigation after exposure to a potentially toxic substance; and
   - Failure to properly use seat belts or infant and child vehicle-restraint devices.

The nurse should take an active role in educating the patient about these potentially harmful situations.

3. As *contact lens* wear becomes increasingly common and contact lens companies continue to market directly to consumers. Many people have become casual about wearing and caring for their lenses. Although contact lenses are generally safe and effective, they can be a significant potential source of ocular problems when the patient does not use or care for the lenses properly. The nurse should promote ocular health by teaching the patient correct wearing and cleaning techniques and recommending appropriate ophthalmic follow-up. Nurse should stress for using only approved contact lens solutions.
4. *Women* of child-bearing age should be immunized against rubella (GM) to prevent congenital blindness in infants, which can result from rubella infection, in the mother during first timester of pregnancy. Person who comes in contact with this group of women especially those who work in health care agencies must be immunized as well.
5. *Genetically* transmitted syndromes and conditions often have ocular manifestations. The nurse working with the patients of child-bearing age should be prepared to make referral for genetic counselling when appropriate.

Eye Infections and Inflammation

Infections and inflammation can occur in any of the eye structures and may be caused by microorganism, mechanical irritations, or sensitivity to some substances. Inflammation of the eye is the most acute condition affecting the eye. The common infection and inflammation of the external eye or extraocular disorder include the following:

1. *Hordeolum* (Sty) is common infection of the sebaceous glands in the lid margins, caused by staphylococcus. It creates a red, swellen, circumscribed and acutely tender postules that gradually resolves or ruptures. The nurse should instruct the patient to apply warm, moist compresses at least four times a day until the abscesses drains. Antibiotic ointment. If severe, incision of postule if it does not resolve spontaneously. If there is a tendency for recurrence, the patient should perform lid scrubs daily. In addition, appropriate ointments or drops may be indicated.
2. *Chalazion* is an inflammation of a sebaceous gland in the lids. It may evolve from a hordeolum or may occur in a primary inflammatory response to the material released into the lid tissue when a blocked gland ruptures. It is sterile cyst located in the connective tissue in the free edges of the eyelid. Lump is small, hard and nontender, but may put pressure on the eye and affect vision. The chalazion appears as a swollen nonpainful reddened area, usually on the upper lid. It may disappear spontaneously become infected or require local excision of impairing vision. Initial treatment is similar to that for a hordeolum.
3. *Trachoma,* a chronic infectious form of conjunctivitis believed to be caused by *Chlamydia trachomatis,* is one of the leading causes of blindness. It can be effectively treated early in the disease with antibiotics, hard to eradicate once chronic.
4. *Keratitis* is an inflammation, or infection of the cornea, it can be superficial or deep, acute or chronic. Staphylococcus and streptococcus bacteria and herpes simplex viruses are common causes. Pain, photophobia or blepharospasm are common. It can result in visual loss. In this, steroids are used to control inflammation, antibiotics, cycloplegies to rest the eye, corneal transplant may be necessary.
5. *Uveitis* is an acute inflammation of the uvea from infection, allergy, toxic agents and systemic disorders. It causes eye pain, swelling photophobia and visual impairment. It may be self-limiting, treatment of underlying cause plus cycloplegics to rest the eye. Warm moist compresses to reduce inflammation and increase comfort.
6. Blepharitis: is a common chronic bilateral inflammation of lid margins. Inflammation of the eyelids frequently begin in childhood and recurs causing redness and scaling of the upper and lower lid at the lash orders. The lids are red rimmed with many scales or crusts on the lid margins and lashes. The patient may primarily complain of itching but may also experience burning, irritation, and photophobia. Conjunctivitis may occur simultaneously.

Daily facial cleaning and shampoo to remove scales, local antibiotics may be helpful. If the blepharitis is caused by a staphylococcal infection, care includes the use of an appropriate opthalmic antibiotic ointment. Seborrheic blepharitis, related to seborrhoea of the scalp and eyebrows is treated with antiseborrheic shampoo for the scalp and eyebrows. Often blepharitis caused by both stapphylococcal and seborrhoeal micro-organism and the treatment must be more vigorous to avoid hordeolum, keratitis and other eye infections. Conscientious hygienic practices involving skin and scalp must be emphasized. Gentle cleansing of the lid margins with baby shampoo can effectively soften and remove crusting.

7. *Corneal ulcer* Infection of the cornea is not common but it can readily lead to ulceration. Ulcers typically cause pain, tearing and spasms of the eyelid. A greyish white corneal opacity is seen with flouorescein evaluation. Minor abrasions heal spontaneously and without scarring; comfort measures critical as the pain can be severe possible need for antibiotics and corticosteroids.
8. *Conjunctivitis* is an infection or inflammation of the conjunctiva. It may result from mechanical trauma such as that caused by sunburn or from infection with organisms such as staphylococcus, streptococci or haemophilus influenzae. Two sexually transmitted agents that cause conjunctivitis are chlamydia trachomatis and Neissaria gonorrhoea. It is often caused by allergic reaction with the body or by external irritants (e.g. poison ivy or cosmetics). Viral agents include human adenovirus and herpes simplex virus. Acute mucopurulent conjunctivitis (pink eye) is usually seen among school children but occur at any age and it is highly infectious.

The symptoms of conjunctivitis may vary in severity. Hyperemia and burning are common initial symptoms that progress rapidly to mucopurulent exudates, which crusts on the base of the eyelashes and easily transfer red to unaffected eye. Viral infections produce minimal exudate. The conjunctiva are grossly reddened and inflammed. Inflammation of the cornea can result in ulceration and even perforation usually in response to virulent organisms such as Neisseria gonorrhoeas. Involvement of the cornea, although rare, is extremely serious and can even result in the loss of the eye. The corneal ulceration is usually identified on slit lamp examination and may be outlined with the use of sterile fluorescein dye.

Treatment of conjunctivitis includes careful cleansing of the eye lids and lashes and the use of topical antibiotics. Warm moist compress may be used to gently remove from adherent crusts from the eyes, especially in the morning. The procedure for applying warm moist compress include the following:

- Use sterile technique when infection or ulceration is present. Clean technique may be used for allergic reactions.
- Use separate equipment for bilateral eye infections.
- Wash hands before treating each eye.
- Temperature of compress should not exceed 49°C (120°F).
- Change compress frequently every 5 minutes as ordered. Always wash hands first.
- Do not exert pressure on the eyeball.
- Sterile petroleum may be used on skin around eyes, if desired to protect the skin.
- If sterile is not required, moist heat may be applied by means of a clean face cloth.
- Since the drainage material is infectious, it should be disposed carefully.

Comon ophthalmic drugs used to treat infection or inflammation includes the following:

1. *Antibiotics and Antiviral Drugs*
   - Polymyxin B. Bacitracin (Polysporin).
   - Polymyxin B, neomycin, bacitracin (Neosporin).
   - Bactracin.
   - Idoxuridine (IDU).
   - Gentamycin sulfate (Garamycin).
   - Chloramphenical (Chloromy.....).
2. *Steroids*
   - Prednisone.
   - Prednisolome acetate.
   - Methyl prenisolone (Depomedrol).
   - Triamcinolone.
   - Dexamethasone.
   - Fluorometholone.
3. *Cycloplegic and Mydriatic Action*
   - Atrophin Sulphate.
   - Cyclopentolate hydrochloride (Cyclogyl).
   - Homatrophine hydrobromide (isopromide).
   - Scopolamine hydrobromide.
   - Tropicamide (Mydriacyl).

The antibiotic may be used in the form of ointment or drop form. Ointment remains in contact with the eye much longer, giving a prolonged effect. There is also less absorption into the lacrimal passages than with eye drops. Eye ointment can, however, produce a film in front of the eye that may blur vision.

The nurse teaches the patient about the disease and its treatment. Since diseases are infectious, avoid crowded environment and to keep the hand away from the eyes. Frequent handwashings are encouraged. The nurse instructs the patient about how to instill the ophthalmic ointment or drops. The ointment is gently placed directly on to the exposed conjunctiva from the inner to the outer canthus. Care should be taken to avoid the eyelashes or any part of the eye that would contaminate the tip of the tube. The nurse warns the patient against possible blurring of vision. If both ointment and drops are used, ointment is applied last. Treatment at bed time minimizes the adverse effects of blurred vision.

Eye Trauma and Injury

Eyes are protected by the bony orbit and by fat pads but sometimes everyday activities can result in ocular trauma. Ocular injuries can involve the ocular adnexa, the superficial structures or the deeper ocular structures. Eye injuries can result in permanent blindness. Most of the injuries are considered to be preventable.

Aetiology

The types of ocular trauma include blunt injuries, penetrating injuries or chemical exposure injuries. Cause of ocular injuries include automobile accidents, accidental occurrences such as falls, sports and leisure activity injuries, assaults, or work-related situation which include the following:

- *Blunt injury:* It is due to hit by fist and other blunt objects. Mechanical trauma can include lacerations of the eyelids as well as direct injury to the eye itself. Contusions can cause bleeding into the anterior chamber (hyphema).
- *Penetrating injury:* It is due to fragments such as glass, metal, wood and knife, stick or other large objects.
- *Chenicak injury:* It can occur in the home, school and industrial setting, and may involve either an acid or an alkali substance. Prompt treatment is essential to prevent permanent eye damage.
- *Thermal injury:* Direct burn from curling iron, or other hot surface. Indirect burn for ultraviolet light (e.g. welding, torch, sun ultraviolet burns are also concerned and may occur from excess sun exposure (skiing, outdoor work, or sunbathing) or the use of heat lamps and tanning beds.
- *Foreign bodies* on the surface of the cornea can cause eye injury, which include particles of glass, wood and metal.
- *Trauma* due to blunt and penetrating objects.
- *Burns* Chemical or thermal injuries already explained above.

Pathophysiology

Although the eyes are vulnerable to trauma, the natural protective mechanism of eyes both prevent and minimize minor eye injuries. The heavy orbit bone protects the eye from most blunt mechanical injuries. The eyes' natural lubricating system is augmented by tears to help flush away chemicals and other foreign bodies and the blink reflex protects from the most low-impact forces.

Acid causes coagulation in the cornea which although produces significant local trauma actually prevents the substance from penetrating and damaging the deeper structures of the eye. Alkaline substance, however, penetrates the corneal epithelium and release proteas and collagenases that can cause corneal necrosis and perforation.

Penetrating injuries or retained foreign bodies can result in sympathetic ophthalmia, a serious inflammation of the ciliary body, iris and choroid that occurs in the uninjured eye. The cause of the acute inflammations is unknown, but it is believed to be some type of autoimmune response. The inflammation can spread rapidly from uvea to the optic nerve. The uninjured edge becomes inflammed, painful and photophobic with a decline in visual acuity.

Clinical Manifestation

After the injury or trauma, the following signs and symptoms are found depending upon the extent of injury or trauma.

- Pain
- Photophobia
- Absent eye movement
- Fluid drainage from eye (e.g. blood CSF, aqueous tumour).
- Redness-diffuse or localized
- Swelling
- Ecchymosis
- Tearing
- Blood in the anterior chamber.
- Abnormal or decreased vision
- Visible foreign body.
- Prolapse bleb
- Abnormal intraoccular pressure.

Management

Prompt professional assessment and care, perhaps, are the most important aspects of management of eye injuries and may protect eyes from serious visual impairment. First aid measures for the injury could be widely taught and posted clearly in all settings in which injuries are significant risks.

1. *Chemical Burns*: are immediately treated with copious flushing of the eye with water. A litmus paper may be applied to the conjunciva to determine the pH if the substance is unknown. Irrigation is continued for at least 15 minutes before the patient is transferred for further evaluation and treatment. The purpose of eye irrigation is to remove chemical irritants, foreign bodies and secretions, and cleanse the eye postoperatively (may be done preoperatively). The eye irrigation procedure is performed as follows:
   - Prepare solutions. Physiological solutions of sodium chloride or Lactated Ringers' solution are most commonly used.
   - Position person comfortably go towards one side so that fluid cannot flow into the other eye.
   - Use appropriate means (e.g. kidney basin, large towel) to catch irrigatory fluid.
   - Use appropriate amounts of solution.
     - If small amounts are needed (cleanse eye postoperatively) sterile cotton balls moistened with solution can be used.
     - If moderate amounts of fluids are needed (removing secretions) plastic squeeze bottle is used to direct irrigating fluid along with the conjunctiva and over the eyeball from inner to outer canthus.
     - If copious amounts of fluids are needed (i.e. for removing chemical irritants) bags of solutions such as intravenous bags along with the tubing to direct the flow onto the eye can be used.
   - Avoid directing a forceful stream onto the eye.
   - Avoid touching any eye structures with irrigating equipment.
   - If there is drainage, wrap a piece of gauze around the index finger to raise the lid and ensure thorough cleansing.
2. *Mechanical trauma:* also requires prompt professional assessment and care. The risk of infection is accompanied by the risk of losing the eye. Antibiotics, wound suture, cycloplegic agents and cold compresses are all possible interventions depending on the exact nature of the injury.

The *first aid* of eye injuries includes the following.

- *Burns, chemical, flame:* Flush eye immediately for 15 minutes with cold water or any available non-toxic liquid; seek medical assistances.
- *Loose substance on conjunctiva, dirt, insects:* Left upper lid over lower lid to dislodge substance, produce tearing, irrigate eye with water if necessary; do not rub eye; obtain medical assistance if these interventions fail.
- *Contact injury; contusion, ecchymosis, laceration:* Apply cold compressor if no laceration is present; cover eye if laceration is present and seek medical assistance.
- *Penetrating objects:* Do not remove object; place protective shield over the eyes (For example paper cup); cover the uninjured eye to prevent excess movement of injured eye and seek medical assistance.

Trauma is often a preventable cause of visual impairment. The nurse's role is individual and community education is extremely important in reducing the incidence of ocular trauma. The efforts concerning eye safety and the first aid for eye injuries should be taken.

The body's natural eye defenses can be appropriately augmented by the use of goggles, shields and safety lenses for sports and high-risk activities. Children need to be taught about the risks associated with BB guns, slingshots, and even rubber bands. The use of protective sunglasses may also be important, depending on the patient's occupation and leisure time sun exposure. The *rules for eyes safety* are as follows:

- Spray aerosols away from eyes.
- Wear protective glasses during active sports such as racquet ball.
- Slowly release steam from ovens, pots, pressure cookers and microwave popcorn bags.
- Gaze at solar eclipses only through adequate filters.
- Wear safety goggles whenever hazardous work is being done or if you are in a work place area where such hazards exist.
- Fit all machinery with safeguards.
- Keep dangerous items and chemicals away from children.
- Store sharp objects safely.
- Pick up rocks and stones rather than going over them with a lawn mower.

Glaucoma

Glaucoma is an eye disease characterized by progressive optic nerve atrophy and loss of vision. It is not one disease but rather group of disorders characterized by:

- Increased intraocular pressure and the consequences of elevated pressure.
- Optic nerve atrophy and
- Peripheral visual loss.

Aetiology

The aetiology of glaucoma deals primarily with the consequences of elevated intraocular pressure (IOP). A proper balance between the rate of aqueous production (referred to as inflow) and the rate of aqueous reabsorption (referred to as outflow) is essential to maintain the IOP within normal limits. The term glaucoma refers to a group of disorders as given below:

- *Primary open-angle glaucoma (POAG):* is chronic or simple usually caused by obstruction trabecular meshwork.
- *Secondary open angle Glaucoma (SOAG)* occur from an abnormality in the trabecular meshwork or an increase in venous pressure.
- *Primary angle-closure glaucoma (PACG)*: narrow angle, acute PACG outflow impaired as a result of narrowing or closing of angle between iris and cornea. Intermittent attacks—pressure normal when angle open, if persistent, acute ocular emergency.
- *Secondary angle-closure*: can result from ocular inflammations, blood vessel changes and trauma.
- *Congenital glaucoma*: is an abnormal development of filtration angle, can occur secondary to other systemic eye disorders.

Pathophysiology

The normal balance of production and drainage of aqueous humor allows IOP to remain relatively constant within the normal range of 10 to 21 mm Hg with a mean pressure of 16 mm Hg. Normal diurnal variations are limited to about 5 mm Hg. Obstruction in any part of the outflow channels for aqueous humor results in a backup of fluid and an increase in IOP. A sustained elevation gradually damages the optic nerve and impairs vision, IOP POAG, the changes occur slowly and the damage is insidious. The process can also occur more rapidly in response to injury or infections or as complications of surgery.

Clinical Manifestation

POG (Primary Open Angle Glaucoma)

- Frequently no signs or symptoms in the early stages.
- IOP typical elevated is greater than 24 mm Hg.
- Slow loss of vision.
- Peripheral vision lost before central.
- Tunnel vision.
- Persistent dull eye pain.
- Difficulty in adjusting to darkness.
- Failure to detect colour changes.

PACG (Primary Angle Closure Glucoma)

- *Acute:* Severe ocular pain, decreased vision, pupil enlarged and fixed-coloured halos around lights, eye red, steamy cornea, may cause nausea and vomiting.
- IOP usually dramatically elevated, may exceed 50 mmHg.
- Permanent blindness if marked increase in IOP for 24 to 48 hours.

Congenital Glaucoma

- Enlargement of eye, lacrimation, photophobia, blepharospasm.

Management

Number of diagnostic tests are used to diagnose and monitor glaucoma. These include:

- Visual acuity measurement.
- *Tonometry:* Measurement of IOP.
- *Tonography:* Estimation of the resistance in the outflow channels by continuously recording the IOP over 2 to 4 minutes.
- *Ophthalmoscopy:* Evaluation of colour and configuration of the optic cup.
- *Visual field permietry:* Measurement of visual function in the central field of vision.
- *Gonicoscopy:* Examination of the angle structures of the eye, where the iris celiary body and cornea meet.
- Fundus photography.

Drug therapy is the foundation of treatment for most forms of glaucoma. The goal of therapy is to keep the IOP low enough to prevent the patient from developing optic nerve damage. Common medication for glaucoma include the following (from a tonic drops or oral).

1. *Miotics* constrict the pupil (miosis) by directly stimulating the spinter muscle (e.g. cholinergics, pilocarpine HCl carbachol). They increase outflow of aqueous humor by ciliary muscle pull on trabecular meshwork. Here nursing intervention includes: evaluate the effectiveness of drug; monitor frequency of use; inform the patient that blurred vision and poor night vision may occur due to a small pupil; other side effectiveness of drug; monitor frequency of use; inform the patient that blurred vision and poor night vision may occur due to a small pupil and other side effects include eye, brow or lid discomfort, burning sensation with drop instillation.
2. *Cholinestarase Inhibition* Constricts ciliary muscle and iris sphincter; iris is pulled away from anterior chamber angle, allowing drainage of aqueous humor and lowering IOP (Ex. Physiostigmine, Isofluorophate, *Demercarium* Bromide, echothiophate iodide). Here Nursing intervention includes advice to avoid use of isofluorophate and demercarium during pregnancy. Inform patient that blurred vision, watering eyes, browache, and change in vision may occur.
3. *Beta Adrenergic Antagonists* decreases aqueous humor production and increase the outflow thereby decreasing IOP (e.g. Timolol maleate, Betaxolol, Levobunolol. Carteolol, Metipronolol). Here evaluate effectiveness, use caution when administering NSAIDS be to patient, who have pulmonary or cardiac disease—can cause spasms.
4. *Carvonic Anydrose Inhibitors:* Decreases aqueous humor production by inhibiting carbonic anhydrase in ciliary processes (an enzyme necessary to produce aqueous humor) (e.g. Acetazolamide Diamox), Ethoxzolamide, Dichlorophenamide, Methazolamide, Darzolamide). In the treatment, evaluate the effectiveness, monitor tingling sensation as extremities, tinnitus, gastric upset, or hearing dysfunction.
5. *Adrenergic Agents:* Reduce aqueous humor formation and increases outflow (e.g. Epinephryl borate, Epinephrin HCl, Epinephrinebitartrate Dipivefrinm Apraclonidine). Here, evaluate the effectiveness, monitor side effects, headache, browache, blurred vision, tachycardia, pigment deposits in cornea, conjunctiva and lids.
6. *Osmotic Agents:* Move water from the intraocular structures, resulting in a marked ocular hypotonic effect, thereby decreasing IOP. (e.g. Glycerine, monitor electrolytes for depletion, monitor glucose levels in patients with type diabetes. Drugs can cause hyperglycemia.
7. *Prostaglandin Agonists*: Increase outflow of aqueous humor. It is used primarily with patient intolerance to or unresponsive to other glaucoma agent (e.g. Latanoprost). Nursing intervention includes monitor renal and hepatic function during treatment. Teach patient about adverse side effects of burning on administration, blurred vision, itching and photophobia.

Surgical intervention indicates when conservative treatments fail to control the IOP. The common surgical procedures are:

- Argon laser trabeculoplasty (ALT).
- Trabeculectomy with or without filtering implant.
- Cyclocryotherapy destruction of ciliary body.

Nursing care for the patient after trabulectomy includes the following.

- Routine postanaesthesia care.
- Protection of operative eye with patch or shield positioning the patient on back or unoperative side and safety measures.
- Maintaining comfort in the operative eye.
- Assessment as appropriate, of the IOP, appearance of the bleb, and anterior chamber depth.
- Administration of medications such as a cycloplegic, a mydriate, and a combination of antibiotic and steroids.

An acute care for PACG includes the following:

- Topical cholinergic agent.
- Hyperosmotic agent.
- Laser peripheral iridotomy.
- Surgical iridectomy.

Postoperative care includes relieving pain, and patient/family education and supporting selfcare including self-administration of eyedrops.

The self administration of eye drops include the following:

- Wash the hands thoroughly before adminstering the medication.
- Tilt the head back and look up towards the ceiling.
- Pull the lower lid gently down and out to expose the conjunctivia and create a sac.
- Bring the dropper from the side and apply the eye drops. Avoid touching the eyelashes, conjunctiva, or surface of the eye with the dropper. Resting the thumb on the forehead can help to stabilize the hand.
- Close both eyes gently. Do not squeeze them tightly to prevent the medication spilling over.
- Apply slight pressure at the inner canthus of the eye to decrease systemic absorption of the medication.
- If more than one drop is to be administered, wait 2-5 minutes before administering the second drop.

Cataract

A cataract is a clouding or opacity within the crystalline lens that leads to gradual painless blurring and eventual loss of vision. The patient may have a cataract in one or both eyes. If present in both eyes, one cataract may affect the patient's vision. The cataracts are third leading cause of preventable blindness.

Aetiology

Cataracts are generally classified as senile (associated with aging), traumatic (associated with injury), congenital (present at birth) and secondary (occurring after other diseases). These include blunt or penetrating trauma, congenital factors such as maternal rubella, radiation or ultraviolet light exposure, certain drugs such as systemic corticosteroids or long-term topical corticosteroids and ocular inflammation. The risk factors associated with cataract include the following:

- Age: The incidence increases dramatically after the age of 65.
- Sex: Cataracts are slightly more common in women than men.
- Ultraviolet light exposure:
  - More common in persons living in warm sunny climates.
  - More common in persons who have worked out door extensively.
- High dose radiation exposure.
- Drug effects: use of corticosteroids, phenothiazines and selected chromotherapeutic agents.
- Poorly-controlled diabetes mellitus accumulation of sorbitol (byproduct of glucose).
- Trauma to the eye.

Cataracts may result from the ingestion of injurious substances, such as dinitrophenol or naphthalene, or systemic absorption of hair dyes. Cataracts may also occur secondary to eye diseases such as uveitis or eye trauma, or with systemic diseases, such as diabetes mellitus, galactosemia, or sarcodiosis.

Pathophysiology

Cataract development is mediated by a number of factors. In senile cataract formation, it appears that altered metabolic processes (decrease in protein, an accumulation of water and an increase in sodium content) within the lens that cause an accumulation and disrupts the normal lens fibre structure. These changes affect lens transparency, causing vision changes. The cause of these pathological changes is not known. Cataracts usually develops bilateally, but at different rate. The primary symptom of cataract is a progressive loss of vision. The degree of loss depends on the location and extent of the opacity. Person with an opacity in the centre portion of the lens can generally be better in dim light when the pupil are dilated. The person with presbyopia may find that reading without glass is possible in the early stages of cataract formation, because the greater convexity of the lens creates an artificial myopia.

Clinical Manifestation

The patient with cataracts may complain of a decrease in vision, abnormal colour perception and glare. There is a gradual painless blurring and loss of vision. Peripheral vision may be affected first. Near vision may initially improve. Glare is due to light scatter caused by lens opacities, and it may be significantly worse at night and in bright light, when the pupil dilates. There will be halos around lights, loss of ability to discriminate between hues and cloudy white opacity on the pupil.

The visual decline is gradual, but rate of cataract development varies from patient to patient. Some patients may complain of a sudden loss of vision because they inadvertently cover their unaffected eye and the decreased acuity of the eye with cataracts becomes "suddenly apparent". Secondary glaucoma can also occur if the enlarging lens causes increased intraocular pressure.

Management

Diagnosis of cataract based on decreased visual acuity or other complaints of visual dysfunction. The diagnostic tests of cataract include the following:

- Visual acuity measurements.
- Ophthalmoscopy (direct or indirect).
- Slit lamp microscopy.
- Blood testing and potential acuity testing in selected patients.
- Keretometrics and A-scan ultrasound (if surgery is planned).
- Visual field perimetry.

Medications do not play a role in the management of cataract. Anaesthetics, anti-inflammatory agents and antibiotics are used after surgery. The presence for cataract does not necessarily indicate a need for surgery, although surgery is the choice of treatment, nonsurgical therapy may postpone the need for surgery, which includes, change, prescription of glasses, strong reading glasses or magnifiers, increased lighting, life adjustment and reassurance.

Surgery is the definitive treatment for cataracts. It is indicated when palliative measures no longer provide an acceptable level of visual function. Common surgical procedure for cataract includes:

- Removal of lens – Phacoemulsification.
  – Extracapsular extraction.
- Correction of surgical aphakia.
- Intraocular lens implantation (most frequent type of correction).
- Contact lens.

Most cataract surgery is performed in the ambulatory surgery centres, few patients require hospitalization. Routines for preoperative care vary with the setting and the eye surgeon. The patient may be asked to perform a face scrub before admission and the eyelashes may be cut. The pupil of the operative eye is dilated and paralyzed before surgery and sedation may be initiated. The drugs used for this purpose are mydriatics (Phenylephrine HCL) and cycloplegics (e.g. Atrophin). The nurse will instil dilating drops and nonsteroidal inflammatory eye drops to reduce inflammation and to help maintain pupil dilation. The nurse ensures that the patient has understood all explanation about the surgery and expected postoperative care and restrictions. The nurse also ensures that plans are in place for someone to transport the patient home and hopefully to assist with patient care during the first ten postoperative days.

Most of the patients are discharged within a few hours. Immediate care of the person after cataract surgery includes the following:

- Position patient on back or unoperated side to prevent pressure in operated eye.
- Keep siderails up as necessary for protection.
- Place bedside table onside of unoperated eye (Patient then turns towards the unoperated side.)
- Place call light within reach.
- Stress avoidance of actions that increases IOP (for example, sneezing, coughing, vomiting, straining, or sudden bending over with the head below the waist).

The nurse instructs the patient to be careful to prevent soap or water from entering the operative eye during face or hair-washing. The nurse also instructs the patient to avoid heavy lifting, active exercises, isometric exercises, or straining during defecation until cleared by the surgeon to prevent abrupt fluctuation in IOP. The nurse reviews plans for following care and provides *patient and family teaching* as given below:

- Teach patient and family proper hygiene and eye care techniques to ensure that medications-dressing, and/or surgical wound are not contaminated during necessary eye care.
- Teach patient and family about signs and symptoms of infection and how to report those to allow early recognition and treatment of possible infection.
- Instruct patient to comply with postoperative restrictions on head positioning, bending, coughing and valsalvas manoeuvre to optimize to visual outcomes and prevent increased IOP.
- Instructs patient to instil eye medications using aseptic techniques and to comply with prescribed eye medications routine to prevent infection.
- Instruct patient to monitor pain and take prescribed medication for pain as directed and to report pain not relieved by prescribed drug.
- Instruct patient about the importance of continued follow-up as recommended to maximize potential visual outcomes.

Retinal Detachment

A retinal detachment is a separation of the sensory retina and the underlying pigment epithelium, with fluid accumulation between the two layers.

Aetiology

Retinal detachment occurs when the outer pigmented layer and the inner sensory layer of the retina separates. Inflammation and bleeding are common contributors to the detachment. The risk factors for retinal detachment includes:

- *High myopia:* Premature, accelerated rate of vitreous detachment, increased incidence of lattice degeneration.
- *Aphakia:* Retinal tears that presumably occur because of surgical disturbance of the vitreous.
- Proliferative diabetic retinopathy: Vitreous remain attached to areas of neovascularization as normal process of vitreal contraction occurs.
- *Retinal lattice degeneration:* Retinal holes common in lattice degeneration, vitreous remains attached to area of degeneration as the normal process of vitreal contraction occurs.
- *Ocular trauma:* Retinal breaks after blunt or penetrating trauma allow fluid to accumulate in the subretinal space.

Pathophysiology

The retina is a smooth unbroken, multilayered surface. Degenerative holes or tears in the retina can allow vitreous humor to pass through and initiate a detachment (rhegamatogenous detachment). The presence of an inflammatory mass, blood clot, or tumour can also separate the retina layers (exudative detachment). The vitreous also undergoes some determination with aging and can fall forward exerting a traction pull on the inner lining of the retina causing detachment (traction detachment).

Clinical Manifestation

Rational detachment may occur suddenly or develop slowly.

Symptoms include floating spots or opacities before the eyes, flashes of light and progressive loss of vision in one area. Patient with a detaching retina describes symptoms that include photopsia (light flashes) floaters and a "cobweb" "hairnet" or ring in the field of vision. The floating spots are blood and retinal cells that are freed of the time of tear, they cast shadows on the retina as they drift about the eye. The flashes of light are caused by the vitreous traction on the retina. The area of visual loss depends entirely on location of detachment.

Once the retina has detached, the patient describes a painless loss of peripoheral or central vision "like a curtain" coming across the field of vision. If the detachment extends to include the macula, blindness results. When the detachment is extensive and occurs quickly, the patients may have sensation that a curtain has been drawn before the eyes but there is no pain associated with the detachment.

Management

The diagnosis of retinal separations is established by ophtholmoscopic examination of the retina to identify the location and extent of the retinal tear. B-scan ultrosonography may be used to improve the accuracy of the diagnosis of the vitreous in opaque. The assistance of nurse is required for diagnosis.

Detachment that compromises vision is repaired surgically. Common surgical techniques to seal retinal breaks and relieve traction on retina includes the following:

- Photocoagulation.
- Cryoretinoplexy.
- Scleral buckling procedure.
- Draining of subretinal fluid.
- Vitrectomy.
- Intravitreal bubble.

In most cases, retinal detachment is an urgent situation and the patient is confronted suddenly with the need for surgery. The patient needs emotional surpport, especially during the immediate preoperative period when preparations of the surgery produce additional anxiety. The nurse administers mydriatics or cycloplegics if ordered. When the patient experiences postoperative pain, the nurse should administer prescribed pain medication and the patient to take the medication as necessary after being discharged. The patient may go home within a few hours after surgery or may remain in the hospital for several days. Patient and family teaching provided as in discussion made earlier after eye surgery.

The nurse attempts to increase the patient's physical and emotional comfort, administering topical antibiotics, topical corticostroids, analgesic, mydriatics as ordered. Follow the positioning and activity as preferred by patient's eye surgeon.

The patient is discharged within a few days. The nurse ensures the patient that family care giver can correctly administer all medications and eyedrops. The nurse reinforces the need to limit activity, avoid bending over below the level of the waist and to avoid constipation and straining. Activities that require close vision such as reading, needle work or writing are limited because they require rapid eye movements and accommodations. Watching television and walking are appropriate, although patients with gas bubbles may still have restrictions on positioning their heads. An eye shield is worn during the sleep for about 2 weeks. The nurse instructs the patient to contact surgeon immediately if acute eye pain develops, eye discharge increases, or turn yellow or green, and if symptoms of detachment recur.

Strabismus

Strabismus is a condition in which the patient cannot consistently focus two eyes simultaneously on the same objective. It is an ocular misalignment that results from an imbalance in the intraocular muscles. One eye may deviate in (estotropia) out (exotropia) up (hypertropia) or down (hypotropia).

Aetiology

The eyes may be misaligned in any direction e.g. esotropia (turning in) extropia (turning out), hypertropia (turning up) and hypotropia (turning down). Strabismus is usually associated with childhood. But it can also be a lifelong disorder. Strabismus in the adult may be caused by thyroid disease, neuromuscular problems of the eye muscles, entrapment of the extraocular muscles in orbital floor fractures, retinal detachment repair or cerebral lesion i.e. brain tumour, head injury, stroke and thyroid ophthalmopathy.

Pathophysiology

The ability to move the eyes in all directions and fixate on an object is the function of the six pairs of extraocular muscles. Stabismus are frequently able to compensate for the confused images and avoid diplopia. Adults with new-onset strabismus are rarely able to compensate. In the adult, primary complaint with strabismus is double vision.

Management

Strabismus is diagnosed through a standard visual field assessment. A variety of treatment options exists.

- Glasses with prisms may successfully realign the eyes and restore binocular vision.
- Eye exercises have been widely prescribed for patients with strabismus to "strengthen" the weak muscles but there is little evidence of their effectiveness.
- Surgical correction is the standard treatment. The extraocular muscles are selectively weakened (recession), tightened (resection) or physically shifted (transposition) to achieve-balanced eye movement. Adjustable sutures can be used to achieve an even more accurate alignment. A slip knot is attached during surgery. Once the anaesthetic has worn off,

the patient ocular alignment is checked and minor correction can be made tightening or loosening the knot.

- Drug therapy with *botulinum nurotoxin* A (Botox) may eliminate the need for surgery or be used in conjunction with surgery. Botox is injcted into the extraocular muscle and interfere with the release of acetylcholine at the neuromuscular junctions. The toxin appear to strengthen the antagonistic muscle and wakens the injected muscle over a period of weeks to months.

Most strabismus surgery is performed on an outpatient basis under either local or geneal anaesthesia. Postoperative care focuses on careful monitoring and preparation of the patient for self-care at home. The eyes may be patched initially for protection, especially if an adjustable suture was used. Patients are instructed to avoid strenous exercises and heavy lifting until approved by the surgeon. Slight redness, swelling and irritation are expected and the nurse instructs the patient to use cold compress for comfort. Dust and heavy pollen can irritate the eye and should be avoided. The nurse instructs the patient to monitor the eye for healing and to promptly report any sign of infection.

EYE TUMOURS

Tumours (benign and malignant) may affect the eye and related structures. They may originate within the eye or metastasize from another primary site.

- Benign neoplasm includes lymphomas, haemangiomas and mucocells from the sinus.
- Malignant tumours threaten both the patient vision and life as extention frequently involves vital structures within the brain.

The eyelids are vulnerable to any of the standard tumours that affect the skin including nevi and xanthelasma (lipid deposits near the corner of the eye). Positive outcomes frequently require early diagnosis and prompt treatment. Treatment usually involves surgical excision but may also include various forms of radiotherapy.

Malignant Melanoma

A melanoma involving the eye is rare, but it is the most common form of intraocular tumour in adults. Retinoblastoma is the most common form of eye tumour, but it is congenital and is typically diagnosed in childhood. Usually melanoma occurs unilaterally.

Malignant melonama occurs in the choroid, ciliary body and iris. They are slow-growing, but they metastasize early due to the vascularity of the choroid. Vision may not be affected until tumour becomes large or affects the macule.

Intraocular malignant melanoma are frequently diagnosed with an ophthalmoscope examination. Ultrasonography and fundus photography may be useful in documenting the size and placement of tumour. Fluorescien angiograpohy may be used to document the vascular involvement the tumour.

Surgery is the primary treatment for an intraocular melanoma. Treatment is based on the exact size, shape and location of the tumour. Every effort is made to preserve the patient's vision if possible. Small tumour that involves the iris may be successfully treated with iridectomy, often with the removal of the ciliary body as well.

Large melanoma of the choroid is usually treated with *enucleation* of the eye, which involves surgical removal of the entire eye including sclera. *Evisceration* is removal of the contents of the eye with retention of the sclera. *Extenteration* involves removal of the entire eye and all other soft tissues in the bony orbit.

Nonsurgical treatment includes radiation therapy, photocoagulation and trachytherapy in which radioactive plaques are sutured into sclera.

Role of Nurse in Enucleation

Enucleation is the removal of the eye. The primary indications for enucleation is blind painful eye. This may result from absolute glaucoma, infection or trauma and ocular malignance.

The diagnosis of the eye malignancy and the need to undergo enucleation create a crisis situation for the patient and family. The virulence of the malignancy may necessitate immediate surgery with little time to prepare for the loss of the eye either physically or emotionally.

The nurse plays an important role in providing support and counselling to the patient during this difficult time. Both the patient and family need to be encouraged to talk about their feelings and concerns and to be helped to adjust their lives when confronted by this serious situation.

The surgical procedure includes severing the extraocular muscles close to their insertion on the globe, inserting an implant to maintain the intraorbital anatomy, and suturing the ends of the extraocular muscles over the implant. The conjunctiva covers the joined muscles and a clear conforming is placed over the conjunctiva until the permanent prosthesis is fitted. A pressure dressing helps prevent postoperative bleeding.

Postoperatively the nurse observes the patient for signs of complications including excessive bleeding or swelling, increased pain, displacement of implant, or temperature elevation. Patient education should include the instillation of tropical ointments or drops and wound cleansing. The nurse should also instruct patient in the method of inserting the conformer into the socket in case it falls out. The patient is often devastated by the loss of an eye. Even when enucleation occurs following a lengthy period of painful blindness, the nurse should recognize and validate the patient's emotional response and provide support to the patient and family.

Approximately 6 weeks following surgery, the wound is sufficiently healed for the permanent prosthesis. The prosthesis is fitted by an ocularist and designed to match the remaining eye. The patient should learn how to remove, cleanse and insert the prosthesis. Special polishing is required periodically to remove dried protein scretions. The measures to take care of *prosthetic* eye is as follows:

- Remove prosthesis, gently depress the lower lid and exert a small amount of pressure under lower edge of prosthesis.
- Wash prosthesis with soap (For example: Ivory) and water. Soap is less irritating than detergents and rinse thoroughly.
- Reinsert prosthesis: place upper portion under upper lids. Pull down lower lid and slip lower edge behind lower lid. With finger or thumb, gently pull down on lower lid and slide prosthesis in place.
- Do not expose the plastic eye to alcohol, ether or any other solvent, they can damage the eye beyond repair.
- If rubbing the eye, rub towards the nose. Wiping away from the nose may cause the eye to fall out.
- Wear a protective patch or goggles when swimming, diving, or water skiing or removal the eye and store it.
- If the eye is left out of the socket, store it in water or contact lens solution.
- Add cornal grafting.

PROCEDURES USED IN OPHTHALMOLOGY

Tonometry

1. Schiotz's tonometry
   a. After instillation of topical anaesthesia the Schiotz's tonometer is gently rested on the eye ball.
   b. The indicator measures the ocular tension in millimeters of mercury (mmHg).
   c. Normal tension is approximately 11 to 22 mm Hg.
2. Applanmon tonometry.
   a. This is the most effective measuring method for determining intracular pressure, however, it requires a biomicroscope and a trained interpreter.
   b. After instillation of topical anaesthesia, the cornea is flattened by a known amount (3.14 mm).
   c. The pressure necessary to produce this flattening is equal to the immecular pressure and counterbalancing the tonometer.
3. Air aptumanon tonometry—This requires no topical anaesthesia and measures tension by sensing deformation of the cornea reaction to a puff of pressurized air.
4. Clinica examination.
   a. Measurement of intraocular tension or pressure.

PROCEDURE 17.1: **ASSISTING THE PATIENT UNDERGOING TONOMETRY*

Equipment: Tonometer

Procedure: *Preparatory Phase*

1. The patient is placed in a tilt-type chair, tilted back and instructed to look upward.

Nursing Action	*Rationale*
Performance Phase	
1. Physician:	
a. Instills a drop of proparacaine 0.5 per cent in each eye.	a. This still produces cornea anaesthesia within a minute.
b. Places a sterile tonometer gently on the center of the cornea for a few seconds.	b. Pressure from one eyeball will be transferred to the sensitive measuring indicator.
c. Repeats for second eye.	
2. Nurse:	
a. Offers the patient an absorbent tissue.	
b. Instructs the patient to pat the closed eyes dry.	
c. Cautions the patient against rubbing the eyes.	c. The cornea is not anaesthetized painful abrasions can result from the natural tendency to rub the eyes because of the unusual numb sensation.

Follow-up Phase

1. Remind patient to have an eye-pressure check at least every 2 years pressure normal.

DIAGNOSTIC TESTS

Radiology/Imaging

There are several imaging studies beyond the basic eye examination that may be done to further evaluate eye disease.

Fluorescein Angiography

1. Introduction of sodium fluorescein intravenously (IV) or by mouth (PO), ophthalmoscopy using a blue filter may be done and/or photographs of the ocular fundus may be obtained.
2. Provides information concerning vascular obstructions, microaneurysms, abnormal capillary permeability, and defects in retinal pigment permeability.

Ultrasonography

Sound waves are used in the diagnosis of intraocular and orbital lesions. Two types of ultrosonography are used in ophthalmoscopy.

1. A-scan—uses stationary transducers to measure the distance between changes in acoustic density. This is used to differentiate benign and malignant tumours and to measure the length of the eye to determine the power of an intraocular lens.

2. B-scan—moves lineraly across the eye increases in accoustic density are shown as an intensification on the line of the scan that presents a picture of the eye and the orbit.

GENERAL PROCEDURES/TREATMENT MODALITIES

1. Instillation of Medications

Refer to procedure 17.2.

Ophthalmic medications may be used for diagnostic and therapeutic purposes.

1. To dilate or contract the pupil.
2. To relieve pain and discomfort.
3. To act as an antiseptic in cleansing the eye.
4. To combat infection: to relieve inflammation.

PROCEDURE 17.2: **INSTILLATION OF MEDICATIONS*

Equipment: Sterile solution of medication (most containers have accompanying dropper).
Small gauze squares or cotton balls.

Procedure: *Preparatory Phase.*

1. Inform the patient of the need and reason for instilling drops.
2. Allow the patient to sit with head tilted backward or to lie in a supine position.

Nursing Action	*Rationale*
Performance Phase	
1. Check the patient's name.	1. For proper patient identification.
2. Check physician's directives and bottle, vial, or tube for the correct medication.	2. To avoid medication error.
3. Check physician's directives designating eye requiring drops. OD (oculus dexter)-right eye OS (oculus sinister)-left eye OU (Oculus uterque)-both eyes.	
4. Wash hands prior to instilling medication.	4. To prevent transfer of microorganisms to patient.
5. Remove cap from container and place on clean surface.	5. To prevent contamination of lid.
6. If eyedropper is used, fill eyedropper with medication but prevent medication from flowing back into bulb end.	6. Loose particles of rubber from bulb end to prevent it slipping from into medication.
7. Using forefinger, pull lower lid down gently.	7. To expose inner surface of lid and cul-de-sac.
8. Instruct patient to look upward.	8. Prevent medication from hitting sensitive cornea.
9. Drop medication into center of lower lid (cul-de-sac).	
10. Instruct patient to close eyes slowly but not to squeeze or rub them. Open eye.	10. Squeezing or rubbing would express medication from eye; closing allows medication to be distributed evenly over eye.
11. Wipe off excess solution with gauze of cotton balls.	11. To prevent possible skin irritation.
12. Wash hands after instilling medication.	12. To prevent transfer of microorganisms to self or other patients.

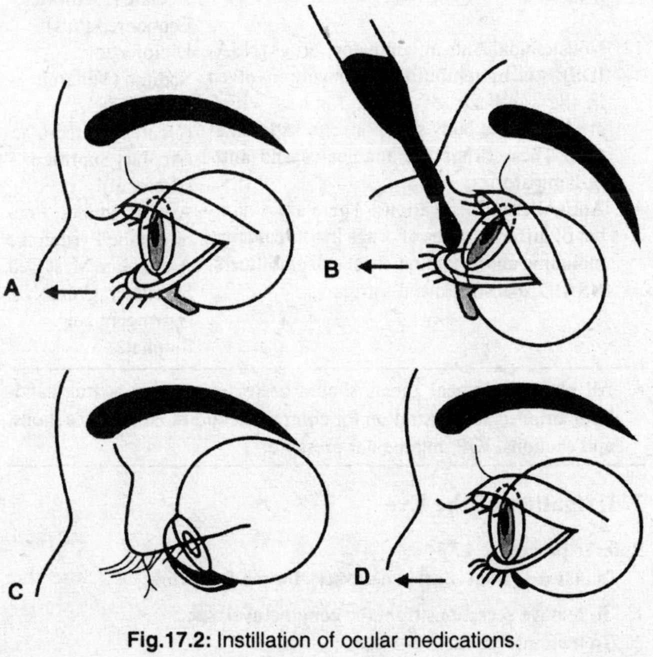

Fig.17.2: Instillation of ocular medications.

Follow-up Phase

Record time, type, strength, and amount of medication and the eye into which medication was instilled.

Patient Education: Self-instillation of Medication

1. Tilt head back.	1. Place eye and lower lid in a horizontal place.
2. Using forefinger, pull lower lid down.	2. Expose inner surface of lower lid.
3. With other hand, hold dropper or container horizontally and facing top of head.	3. Position dropper or container above receiving lid.
4. Look up and instil medication onto lower lid per instructions (i.e. one drop). Continue with steps 10-12 above.	4. Prevents medication from hitting sensitive cornea.

Note: Eye ointment: Ointment from tube is gently squeezed as a ribbon of medication along inner lower lid with care taken not to touch eye with end of tube.
Eye Drops: Wait 5 minutes between each medication.

Ophthalmic Pharmacologic Agents

Pharmacology/Action	*Products*
1. Sympathomimetics: Used in the treatment of glaucoma. Immediate effect is decrease in production of aqueous humor. Long-term effect is an increase in outflow facility. May be used in combination with miotics, beta-blockers, carbonic anhydrase inhibitors or hyperosmotic agents.	Epinephrine epifrin, glaucon epitrate, propine

Contd...

Pharmacology/Action	*Products*
2. Miotics, Direct-Acting: Cholinergic agents that affect the muscarinic receptors of the eye; results include miosis and contraction of the ciliary muscle. In narrow-angle glaucoma, miosis opens the angle to improve aqueous outflow. Contraction of the ciliary muscle enhances the outflow of aqueous humor by indirect action of the trabecular network—the exact mechanism is unknown. Primary use of miotics is in glaucoma but can be used to counter the effects of cyclopletics/mydriatics.	Acetylcholine (Humorsol) Isflurophate (Florpryl) Physostigmine (Isoptoeserine).
3. Miotics, Cholinesterase inhibitors: Inhibit the enzyme cholinesterase, causing an increase in the activity of the acetylcholine already present in the body. Causes intense miosis and contraction of the ciliary muscle. Decrease in intraocular pressure that is seen is a result of increased outflow of aqueous humor. Used for treatment of open-angle glaucoma, conditions where the outflow of aqueous is obstructed postiridectomy problems and accommodative esotropia (inward deviation of one eye).	Demecarin bromide (Humorsol) Isoflurophate (Floropryl) Physostigmine (Isoptoeserine)
4. Beta-Adrenergic-Blocking Agents. Act on the beta receptors of the adrenergic nervous system. Two types of beta sites: B_1 and B_2. B_1 site primarily bronchial and vascular smooth muscle resulting in 1 heart rate and cardiac output. B_2 primarily bronchial and vascular smooth muscle resulting in bronchoconstriction, decreased blood pressure. There are two types of ophthalmic beta-blockers; cardioselective blocker (betoxolol) acts only on B_1 sites and may on rare occasions cause cardiac effects if absorbed systemically. All other nonselective blockers act on B_1 and B_2 sites and cause significant cardiac and pulmonary effects if absorbed systemically. Used for treatment of increased intraocular pressure by decreasing the formation of aqueous humor and causing a slight increase in the outflow facility.	Betaxolol (Betoptic) Levubunolol (Betagan) Timolol (Timoptic) Carteolol (Ocupress)
5. *Carbonic anhydrase inhibitors.* Acts to inhibit the action of carbonic anyhydrase. Suppression of this enzyme results in a decreased production of aqueous humor. It used in combination regime to treat glaucoma and postoperative rise in IOP.	Acetazolamide (Diamox) Methazolamide (Neptazane)
6. Osmotic Diuretics: Osmotic agents used for reduction of IOP is acute attack of glaucoma or before ocular surgery where preoperative reductionof IOP is indicated.	Mannitol (Osmitrol) Glycerin (Glycerol)
7. Mydriatics: Agents that result in dilation of the pupil, vasoconstriction, and an increase in the outflow of aqueous humor. Used for pupillary dilatation for surgery and examination.	Phenylephrine (Ak-Dilate Mydfrin)
8. Cycloplegic Mydriatrics: Block the reaction of the sphincter muscle of the iris and the muscle of the ciliary body to cholinergic stimulation resulting in dilatation of the pupil (mydriasis) and paralyses of accommodation (cycloplegia) used in conditions requiring pupil to be dilated and kept from accommodation.	Atropine Homatropine (Ak-Homatropine) Scopolamine (Isopto-Hyoscine) Cyclopentolate (Cyclogel) Tropicamide (Mydriacyl)
9. Ophthalmic Anti-infectives: Used for treatment of ophthalmic infections. Commercial products intended for treatment of superficial ocular problems, such as conjunctivitis infections, i.e., corneal ulcer, endophthalmitis (intraocular infection).	Antibiotics Bacitracin (Ak-Tracin) Chloramphenicol (Chloroptic) Erythromycin (Ilosone) Gentamycin (Garamycin) Neomycin/polymixin bacitracin (Neosporin) Tobramycin Antifungal: Amphotericin B (Fungizone) Flucanazole Natamycin (Natcyn) Antiviral: Trifluridine (Viroptic) Vidarabine (Vira A).
10. Local Anaesthetics: Block the transmission of nerve impulses. Used topically to provide local anaesthetic for tests, such as tonometry and for procedures of short duration. Injections used in ophthalmology for retrobulbar blocks.	Topical Proparacaine (Ophthaine) Terracaine (Pontocain) Injection: Lidocaine.
11. Ophthalmic Anti-inflammatories-Steroid: Mostly corticosteroids are used topically to relieve pain, photophobia, as well as suppressing other inflammatory processes of the conjunctiva, cornea, lid and interior segment of the globe.	Dexamethasone (Maxidrex, Decadron) Flurometholone (FML) Prednisolone Acetate (Predforte, Econopred Plus)
12. Nonsteroidal Anti-inflammatory drugs (NSAIDS): Act by inhibiting an enzyme involved in the synthesis of prostaglandins which are key in the body's response to inflammation. These drugs are analgesics and anti-inflammatories.	Diclofenac Sodium (Voltaren) Flurbiprofen (Ocufen) Keteorolac (Acular) Suprofen (Profenal)
13. Anti-Allergy Medications: There are a number of different types of drugs in this category including antihistamine, mast cell stabilizers, NSAID anaesthetic and astrigents.	Antihistamines: Phenitramine Pyrilamine Antazoline Mast Cell Stabilizer: Cromolyn. Astringent zinc Sulphate.

Contd...

- All pharmacological agents should be reviewed from a drug handbook prior to administration for contraindications, adverse reactions, and cautions. IOP: intraocular pressure.

2. Irrigation of the Eye

Refer to procedure 17.3.

Ocular irrigation is often necessary for the following.

1. To remove secretions from the conjunctuvak sac.
2. To treat infections.

3. To relive itching.
4. To irrigate chemicals or foreign bodies from the eyes.
5. To provide moisture on the surface of the eyes of an unconscious patient.]

PROCEDURE 17.3: *IRRIGATING THE EYE (Conjunctival Irrigation).

Sterile Equipment: An eyedropper, asepto bulb syringe, or plastic bottle with prescribed solution depending on the extent of irrigation needed.
For copious use, i.e., chemical burns sterile normal saline or prescribed solution and IV set-up with attached tubing.

Preparatory Phase

1. Verify that you have the right patient.
2. The patient may sit or lie in a supine position.
3. Instruct the patient to tilt his/her head towards the side of the affected eye.

STEPS OF PROCEDURE

Nursing Action	*Rationale*
Performance Phase	
1. Wash eyelashes and lids with prescribed solution at room temperature, a curved basin should be placed on the affected side of the face to catch the outflow.	1. Any materials on the lids and lashes can be washed off before exposing conjunctiva.
2. Evert the lower conjunctival sac (If possible, have the patient pull down lower lid with index finger).	2. Exposes inner surfaces of lower lid and conjunctival sac (involves the patient and gives a sense of control).
3. Instruct the patient to look up; avoid touching eye with equipment.	3. Prevents injury to the sensitive cornea.
4. Allow irrigating fluid to flow from the inner canthus to the outer canthus along the conjunctival sac.	4. Prevents solution from flowing toward the lacimal sac, duct, and nose, possibly transmitting infection.
5. Use only enough force to flush secretions from conjunctiva. (Allow patient to hold curved basin near the eye to catch fluid).	5. Prevents eye injury (involves the patient in the treatment).
6. Occasionally have patient close eyes.	6. Allows upperlid to meet lower lid with the possibility of dislodging additional particles.
Follow-up Phase	
1. Pat eye dry and dry the patient's face with a soft cloth.	1. Provides comfort.
2. Record kind and amount of fluid used as well as its effectiveness.	2. Provides documentation for nursing actions.

3. Application of Dressing or Patch

Refer to Procedure 17.4.

One or both eyes may need shielding for the following.

1. To keep an eye at rest, thereby promoting healing.
2. To prevent the patient from touching eye.
3. To absorb secretions.
4. To protect the eye.
5. To control or lessen oedema.

PROCEDURE 17.4: **APPLICATION OF AN EYE PATCH, EYE SHIELD, AND PRESSURE DRESSINGS TO THE EYE.*

Equipment: Eye covering to be used, transparent or adhesive tape, rubber glove, scissors, water.

Nursing Action	*Rationale*
Eye Patch	
1. Instruct patient to close both eyes.	1. It is difficult to close only the affected eye.
2. Place patch over the affected eye.	
3. Secure the patch with three or more strips of transparent tape diagonally from midforehead to below the ear.	3. Transparent tape is easy to remove—use hypoallergenic tape if patient has allergies to tape.
4. For unconscious patient, mois-ten the eye patch.	4. Dry patch can irritate cornea.
Eye Shield (Plastic or Metal)	
1. Apply over dressings or directly over the undressed eye, fastening with two strips of transparent tape.	1. Used primarily to protect the eye. Place tape on outer edges of shield so as not to obstruct vision through holes in shield.
2. For metal eye shields, a guard can be placed around flanged edges before use.	2. Protects skin from metal.
a. Cut 1.2-2.5 cm (1/2-1 in) strip from a rubber glove finger.	a. Covers metal edges of shield or guard.
b. Stretch around perimeter of shield.	b. Two such pieces add cushioning and provide comfort.
Pressure Dressings	
1. Prepare 8-10 adhesive strips by cutting 2.5 cm (1-in) adhesive tape in 35-cm (9-in) lengths. Stretch tape (3M) may also be used.	1. Warming the tape may improve its adhesiveness.
2. Apply two eye patches to the affected eye.	2. Provides pressure dressing bulk.
3. Apply strips from forehead above unpatched eye across dressings to the cheek bone (maxillary prominence).	3. To secure dressing and apply pressure while permitting freedom of movement of the head.

Nursing Focus

Prolonged use of pressure dressing may cause increased temperature in the interior of the covered eye because they act as a moisture chamber. Pressure dressings also may need to be removed periodically for a short time so that air can freely circulate over cornea.

Note: Check for patient's allergies before applying rubber strip tape to guard or to skin.

4. Removing a Particle from the Eye

Refer to Procedure 17.5.

Typically, removing a foreign body from the eye is an uncomplicated first-aid measure. However, if the object appears to be embedded, medical intervention is required, that is, local anaesthetic, antibiotic therapy and clinical expertise in using other instruments. The cornea should be evaluated for abrasion from the foreign body.

PROCEDURE 17.5: **REMOVING A PARTICLE FROM THE EYE*

Equipment: Local anaesthesia
Hand Lens.
Sterile fluorescein strips.
Cotton applicator sticks or tongue blades.
Irrigating saline.
Antibiotic solution.

STEPS OF PROCEDURE

Nursing Action	*Rationale*
1. As patient looks upward, evert lower lid to expose the conjunctival sac.	1. Dust particles are often was-hed by the upper lid.
2. With small cotton applicator dropped in saline, gently remove particle.	2. Wipe gently across lid—inner to outer aspect. Use hand-magnifying lens if necessary.
3. If offending particle is not found proceed to examine upper lid.	
4. Have the patient look downward while you stand in front of the patient.	4. Serves as a safety measure since cornea is away from area of activity.
5. Encourage the patient to relax, move slowly and reassure patient that you will not hurt him or her.	5. Relaxation prevents squeezing the lids shut, a manoeuvre that contracts the obicularis muscle, making eversion of lid impossible.
6. Place cotton applicator stick or tongue blade horizontally on outer surface of upper lid. Apply pressure about 1 cm above lid margin.	6. Because the upper tarsal plate extends 10-12 mm above the lid margin, pressure must be applied at least 1 cm above the lid margin, for easy eversion of lid.
7. Grasp upper eyelashes with fingers of other hand and pull the upper lid outwards and upward over cotton applicator.	7. Particles may be washed under the lid; visual exposure assists in detection. Eyelid will remain everted by itself.
8. Use fluorescein strip to detect corneal abrasion.	8. Green stain will so indicate if abrasion is present.

Examining the eye for a foreign particle (A) Evert lower lid (B and C). Evert upper lid.

Nursing Focus

It is very important to take a patient history. Determine the nature of the particle—Wood? Metal? (What kind magnetic? Copper? Was it projectile?

If particle cannot be removed by the method described above, it may have become imbedded in lens or vitreous, in which case an opthalmologist is required immediately.

Removing Contact Lenses/Prosthesis

Refer to Procedure 17.6.

Because most contact lenses are designed to be worn while awake if a person is injured and incapacitated because of an accident, sickness, or other cause, the lenses should be removed.

Considerations

1. If the injured person is unconscious, or unable to remove lenses, an optometrist or ophthalmologist is called.
2. If professional help is not available and the lenses must be removed, determine the type of lens.
   a. Soft corneal lenses are widely used. The diameter covers the cornea plus a portion of the sclera of the eye. More than 75 per cent of weavers in the United States wear soft contacts.
   b. Rigid or gas-permeable lenses are usually smaller than the cornea of the eye, although some are made to extend beyond the cornea on to the sclera of the eye.
3. Do not remove lenses if the iris is not visible on opening the eyelids; await the arrival of an optometrist or ophthalmologist. If patient is to be transported, note that contacts are in the eyes. (Write out the message and tape it to the patient or send with transporter).

PROCEDURE 17.6: *REMOVING CONTACT LENSES/PROSTHESIS

Equipment: Containers, market, labels normal saline, eye suction cup.

Preparatory Phase

Because the patient will undoubtedly be in the recumbent position, it is acceptable to remove the lens while he or she is in this position.
Wash your hands thoroughly.

Nursing Action	*Rationale*
Performance Phase	
Corneal Lens (Hard Type)	
1. If an eye suction cup is available (as in Emergency Department), simply separate eyelids to expose lens fully; then, place cup over lens and apply slight pressure to cup.	1. The suction produced will permit cup to lift contact lens from cornea.
2. For right eye, stand on right side of patient.	2. Hands will have easier access to eye.
3. Lightly place left thumb on upper eyelid; right thumb on lower eyelid close to the edge and paraller with lids.	3. Thumbs are placed in a lever age position on the eyelids.
4. Gently pull lids apart and observe if contact lens is visible. If contact lens is not visible, wait for an experienced practitioner.	
5. If contact lens is visible, it should slide with the movement of the eyelids while thumbs are still kept at the edges of the eyelids.	
6. Gently open the lids wider beyond the edge of the lens and maintain this position.	

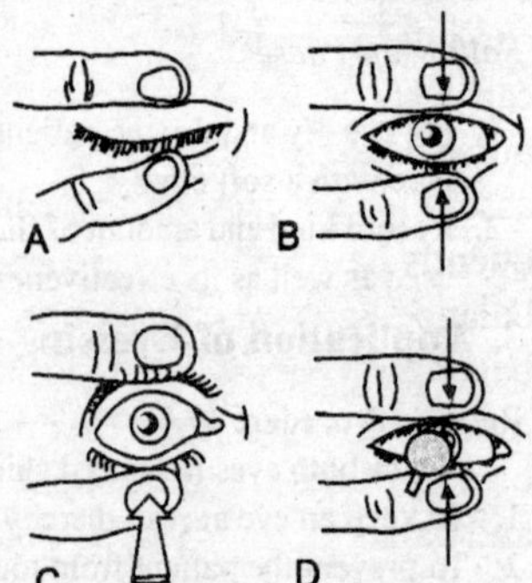

Fig. 17.3: Removing a corneal contact lens.

7. Press gently downwards with right thumb on eyeball.	7. This should cause the contact lens to tip up on the edge.
8. Gently slide the eyelids and thumbs together.	8. This should allow the contact lens to slide out between the lids where it can be taken off.
9. Force should not be used.	9. Cornea may be irreparably damaged.
10. If contact lens can be seen but cannot be removed, gently slide it to the white sclera.	
11. For left eye, move to left side of patient and repeat procedure.	

Soft Contact Lenses

May be removed by gently grasping and pinching contact lens between thumb and forefinger. An ophthalmologist can be called to remove lenses if the patient is unable to do so. Also note, if a contact lens cannot be removed with relative ease, discontinue efforts and wait for the ophthalmologist to remove it.

Disposition of Lenses

1. When lenses are found and removed, please in a case or bottle, label "right" and "left".	1. Since right and left lenses are often different, storing them with proper labels will be appreciated.
2. Store in normal saline solution.	2. This prevents drying and soft lenses must be kept moist.

Note: Extended-wear contacts of disposable contacts worn for more than 1 week may precipitate corneal damage.

II. OTOLOGIC NURSING [Nursing the Disorder of Ear]

Hearing is one of the five senses and both hearing (auditory function) and balance (vestibular function) are important in activities of daily living. Hearing helps us interact with the environment and adds aesthetic pleasure as well as warning danger. Hearing also is essential for the normal development and maintenance of speech. The organs of balance are contained within the ear and relay information about the body's position to the brain.

Nurses are involved in every aspect of the care of the patient with a auditory and vestibular problems including prevention, detection and treatment. Auditory problems are common and can interfere with the person's activities of daily living, which can occur at any age and may require immediate attention. Every nurse needs to be skilful in examining the outer ear and grossly assessing the patient's hearing and equilibrium. Nurses frequently participate in case findings of person with hearing and balance disorders. Detection of hearing impairment and or a balance problem is an important nursing responsibility and the nurse is frequently the first member of the health care team to be approached by the patient regarding problems with hearing and balance.

ASSESSMENT OF AUDITORY SYSTEM

Assessment of the auditory system includes assessment of the vestibular system because two systems are so intimately related. It is often difficult to separate the symptomatology between two systems. The nurse must help the patient describe symptoms and problems in order to differentiate the source of the problems.

Subjective Data

Prior to health history, the nurse attempts to determine if the patient hears well and seeks to validate the patients functional status with the family members or significant others. Generally common behaviour cues suggesting the loss of hearing which include that any adult may exhibit one or more of the following traits:

- Is irritable, hostile or hypersensitive in interpersonal relations.
- Has difficulty in hearing upper frequency consonants.
- Complain about people's mumbling.
- Turns-up volume on television.
- Asks for frequent repetition or misunderstandings.
- Answers questions inappropriately.
- Loses sense of humour, becomes grim.
- Leans forward to hear better, face looks serious and strained.
- Appears aloof and "stuck up".
- Complains of ringing in the ears.
- Has an unusually soft or loud voice.
- Has garbled speech.

The individual may also focus on the speaker's face and lips, rather than making eye contact. If the patient has a hearing loss, it is important for the nurse to face the patient directly and speak clearly. If the patient wears a hearing aid, the nurse ensures that it is in use functioning properly.

The patient should be questioned about previous problems regarding the ears, especially problems experienced during childhood. The frequency of acute middle ear infections (otitis media); perforations of the eardrums, drainage, complications and history of mumps, measles, or scarlet fever should be recorded. Congenital hearing loss can result from infectious diseases (rubella, influenza or syphilis), terotogenic medications or hypoxia in the first trimester of pregnancy. The nurse also assesses the patient for any incidence of pain (earache), drainage (otorrhoea), tinnitus or vertigo. An environmental and work history is also obtained i.e. occupational exposure; history of old trauma (blow to ears or a foreign body).

The nurse completes a thorough medication history as a variety of drugs are potentially ototoxic. Ototoxic agents directly affect the eighth cranial nerve or the organs of the hearing and balance. These drugs can cause symptoms such as tinnitus, headache, dizziness, vertigo, nausea, ataxia, nystagamus or a discernible change in hearing.

The common ototoxic drugs include the following:

- Aminoglycosides: (Gentamycin, chloramycin, streptomycin, amikacin, neomycin and kanamycin).

- Vancomycin, Viomycin, Polymixin B, Polymixin E.
- Loop diuretics: Furosemide, Torsemide, Bumetamide, Ethacrynate acid sodium diamox (acetozolamide).
- Erythromycin.
- Salicilates: Aspirin.
- NSAIDs: Nemocylin.
- Quinine Sulphate: Chloroquin and quinidine.

The patient is questioned regarding self-care of the ears. Determining the frequency of hearing tests are the method and frequency of cleaning the ears, helps the nurse plan appropriate health teaching. Incorrect method of cleaning the ears such as the use of cotton-tripped applicators can lead to impacted cerumens and hearing loss. The nurse asks the patient about any history of ear infection and method of treatment. A history of chronic ear infections alerts the nurse to the possibility of sequelae.

Dizziness hearing loss can have devastating effects on the patient's quality of life. The nurse carefully explores the extent of disruptions of the patients lifestyle caused by the symptoms and evaluates the patient's emotional response to these disruptions. If the ability to communicate is impaired, the patient may feel socially isolated. The nurse carefully explores the nature and effectiveness of the patient coping mechanisms. When either balance or hearing is affected, the patient's risk for injury increases, and safety measure are carefully explored.

Objective Data

The external ear is inspected and palpated before examination of the external canal and tympanum. The auricle, peratricular area, and mastoid area are observed for equality of conformation of both ears, colour of skin, nodules, swelling, redness and lesions. The auricle and mastoid areas are then palpated for tenderness and nodules. Grasping auricles may elicit pain, especially if inflammation of the external ear or otitis.

Visualization of tymphanic membrane is difficult and requires illumination. In addition magnifications allow a more accurate assessment of the ear. An otoscope consists of a handle, a light source a magnifying lens and an attachment for visualizing the ear canal and ear drum. The tymphanum is observed for colour, land marks, contour and intactness.

Assessment of the inner ear for balance is accomplished by observation of gait, the gaze test for nystagmus and the Rombert test.

Diagnostic Studies

Routine blood and urine tests rarely provide significant information related to diseases of the ears. The common diagnostic studies of auditory systems include the following.

1. *Auditory*
   - *Puretone audiometry:* Sounds are presented through earphones in sound proof room. Patient responds nonverbally when sound is heard. Response is recorded on an audiogram. Purpose is to determine hearing range of patient in terms of dB and HZ for diagnosing conductive and sensorineural hearing loss. Tinnitus can cause inconsistent results.
   - *Bone conduction:* Vibrator (Vibrating tuning fork) is placed on mastoid process, and hearing by bone conduction is recorded. It diagnoses conductive hearing loss.
   - *One-syllable and two syllable work lists:* Words are presented and recorded at comfortable level of hearing to determine percentage correct and word understanding.
   - *Auditory evoked potential (AEP).* Procedure is similar to EEG. Electrodes are attached to patient in a darkened room. Electrodes are placed typically at the vertex, mastoid process, or earlobes and forehead. A computer is used to isolate the auditory from other electrical activity to the brain.
   - *Electrccochleography:* Test is useful for uncooperative patient or patient who cannot volunteer useful information. Test records electrical activity in the cochlea and auditory nerve.
   - *Auditory Brainstem Response (ABR):* Study measures electrical peaks along auditory pathways of inner ear to brain and provides diagnostic information related to acoustical neuroma, brainstem problems and CVA.
2. Vestibular
   - *Caloric test stimulus:* Endolymph of the semicircular canals is stimulated by irrigation of cold (68°F or 20°C) or warm (97°F or 36°C) solution into ear. Patient is seated in supine position, observation of type of nystagmus, nausea and vomiting, falling or vertigo produced is helpful in diagnosing diseases of labyrinth.

     Decreased function is indicated by decreased response and indicates disease of vestibular system. Other ear is tested similarly and results are compared.
   - *Electronystagmography (ENG).* Electrodes are placed near patient's eyes and movement of eyes (nystagmus) is recorded in graph during specific eye movements and when ear is irrigated. Study diagnosis diseases of vestibular system.
   - Posturography: Balance test that can isolate one semicircular canal from others to determine site of lesion. Here inform that test is time consuming and uncomfortable; test can be discontinued at any time at patient's request.
   - *Rotatory Chair Testing:* The patient is seated in a chair driven by a moto under computer control. It evaluates peripheral vestibular system.

Hearing Impairment/Loss and Deafness (Hearing Loss)

Hearing loss is one of the main problems. Hearing impairment and dizziness (major symptoms of inner ear problem) can hinder communication with others, limit social activities, and negatively impact employment. Hearing loss diminishes the individual aesthetic enjoyment of major aspects of daily living and can adversely affect quality of life.

Aetiology

Hearing loss is a symptom rather than a specific disease or disorder and can be the result of mechanical, sensory or neural problems. The major types of hearing loss includes the following:

- *Conducting Hearing Loss:* Loss of the ring from mechanical problem.
- *Sensori-neural Hearing Loss:* Loss of hearing involving the cochlea and auditory nerve; bone and air conduction equal but diminished.
- *Neural Hearing Loss:* A sensorineural hearing loss originating in the nerve or brainstem.
- *Fluctuating Hearing Loss:* A sensorineural hearing loss that varies with time.
- *Sensory Hearing Loss:* A sensory neural hearing loss originating in the cochlea and involving the hair cells and nerve endings.
- *Sudden Hearing Loss>:* A sensorineural hearing loss with a sudden onset.
- Central Hearing Loss: Loss of hearing from damage to the brain auditory pathways or auditory center.
- *Functional Hearing Loss:* Loss of hearing for which no organic lesion can be found.
- *Mixed Hearing Loss:* Elements of both conduction and sensorineural hearing loss.

Pathophysiology

Conductive Hearing Loss results from any interference with the conduction of sound impulses through the external auditory canal, the eardrum, or the middle ear. Conductive hearing loss may be caused by anything that blocks the external ear, such as wax, infection or a foreign body, a chickening, retraction, scarring or perforation of the tymphanic membrane; or any pathophysiological changes in the middle ear affecting or fixing one or more of the ossicles.

Sensorineural Hearing Loss results from disease or trauma to the inner ear, neural structure, or nerve pathways leading to the brainstem. Some of the causes of "nerve" deafness are infectious diseases, (measles, mumps and meningitis), arteriosclerosis, ototoxic drugs, neur of cranial nerve VIII, otospongiosis (form of progressive deafness) caused by the formation of new abnormal sponges bone in labyrinth, trauma to the head or ear, or degeneration of the organ of corti occuring most commonly from an advancing age (Presbycusis). Central deafness is also known as central auditory dysfunction, results from the inability of the CNS to interpret normal auditory stimuli may be due to tumour or CVA.

Presbycusis is a hearing loss associated with aging that becomes more common after the age of 50, changes in the delicate labyrinthine structures over the dccades cause a hearing loss predominently in the higher frequencies.

Hearing loss is frequently accompanied by tinnitus, which is defined in a ringing or any other noise in the ear. Tinnitus accompanies most sensorineural hearing losses and is often a warning of impending or worsening hearing loss. Persistent tinnitus is extremely annoying and the only cure for tinnitus is to correct the underlying cause/condition.

Clinical Manifestation

If the hearing loss is congenital and significant, the young child will have significant speech and language problems. Rehabilitation must be started early. Deafness is often called the "unseen handicap" because it is until conversation is started with a deaf adult that the difficulty in communication is not realized. It is important that the health professionals be aware of the need for thorough validation of deaf persons understanding of health teaching. Descriptive visual aids can be helpful. Because of the difficulty in communication, deaf person always or often seeks relationship with other deaf person. The person who develops hearing loss later in life varies in the amount of loss.

Interference in communication and interaction with others can be the source of many problems for the patient and family. Often the patient refuses to admit or may be unaware of impaired hearing. Irritability is common because of the concentration which the patient must listen to understand speech. The loss of clarity of speech in the patient with sensorineural, hearing loss is most frustrating. The patient may hear what is said, but not understand it. Withdrawal, suspicion, loss of self-esteem and insecurity are commonly associated with advancing hearing loss.

Management

Hearing loss is often first detected by a family member rather than by the affected person. All possible hearing test can be performed for knowing the extent of hearing loss.

Hearing aids offers assistance to many individuals with hearing impairments. hearing aids amplify sound in a controlled manner and are used by both hard-of-hearing and deaf persons. Hearing aids make sound louder, but do not improve the ability to hear and the amplication of background noise can be confusing especially in crowded settings.

Regardless of the type, the hearing aid consists of the following parts:

- Microphone to receive sound waves from the air and changes sound waves from the air and changes sounds into electrical signals.
- Amplifier to increase the strength of electrical signals.
- Battery to provide the electrical energy needed to operate the hearing aid.
- Receiver (loudspeaker) to change electrical signals back into sound waves.

Speech reading commonly called lio reading can be helpful in increasing communication. The patient is able to use visual cues associated with speech such as gestures and facial expression to help clarify the spoken message. This helps in verbal and nonverbal communication.

There are three types of implanted hearing devices which are either available for use or underdevelopment. They are cochlear implants, bone conduction devices, and semiplantable heavy devices. Now there are numerous assisting devices available to assist the hearing-impaired persons. Direct amplification devices, amplified telephone receivers, alerting systems that flash when activated by sound, an infrared system for amplifying the sound of the TV and combination of FM receiver and hearing aid are all aids that can be explored by the nurse based on the individual patient needs.

Nursing Interventions/Role of Nurse in Dealing with Hearing Problem

Hearing loss is a major health problem to be concerned. The nurse has an important role in preservation of hearing. To fulfil this role, the nurse has many responsibilities, which include educating the patient about keeping the defects out of ears, environmental noise control, ototoxic drugs, risk for heavy loss and detection of hearing loss.

1. *Keeping the objects out of ears*
   The nurse instructs the patient to keep objects out of the ear. Ears should be cleaned only with a wash cloth and finger. Bobby pins and cotton tipped applicators should especially be avoided. Penetration of the middle ear by a cotton-tipped applicator can cause serious injury to the eardrum and ossicles and may result in facial paralysis as a result of nerve damage. These applicators can also impact cerumen against the eardrum and impair hearing.

   People should be taught to avoid inserting hard articles into the ear canal, obstructing the ear canal with any object, inserting unclean articles or solutions to the ear or swimming in poluted water.
2. *Environmental noise control* Support environmental noise control. Hearing impairment can be caused by an acute loud noise (acoustic trauma), or by cumulative effects of variation intensities, frequencies and duration of noise (noise-induced hearing loss). Sensorineural hearing loss as a result of increased and prolonged environmental noise such as amplified sound is occurring in young adults at an increasing rate. Health teaching regarding avoidance of continued exposure to noise 85 to 95 decibel (dB) is essential. Continued exposure to noise causes some persons to be more irritable and tense. The range of sounds audible to humans are as follows:

   Decibel (dB)

   0: Lower sound audible to the human ear.
   30: Quiet library, soft whisper are the examples.
   40: Living room, quiet office, bedroom away from traffic.
   50: Light traffic at a distance, refrigerator and gentle breeze.
   60: Airconditioner at 20 ft., conversation, sewing machine.
   70: Busy traffic, noisy restaurant. At this dB level, noise may begin to affect hearing if exposure is constant.

   Hazardous Zone for Hearing Loss (Hz)

   80. Subway—Heavy city traffic, alarm clock at two feet, factory noise. These noises are dangerous if exposure to them lasts for more than 8 hours.
   90. Truck traffic—noisy home appliances, shop tools and lawn mowers. As loudness increases, the "safe" time exposure decreases, damages can occur in less than 8 hours.
   100. Chain saw—stereoheadphones, pneumatic drill. Even 2 hours of exposure can be dangerous at this dB level. Such 5 dB increases the safe time is cut in half.
   120. Rockband concert in front of speakers, sand blasting, thunder clap. The danger is immediate; exposure to 120 dB can injure ears.
   140. Gun shot blast, jet plane. Any length of exposure time is dangerous; noise at this level may cause actual pain in the ear.
   180. Rocket launching pad. Without air protection, noise at this level causes irreversible damage;. hearing loss is inevitable.

   The nurse should participate in hearing conservation program in work environment and advise precaution against hearing loss.

   The nurse explores the patient's understanding of the role of the noise in hearing loss and encourage moderation of music levels, especially with the use of headphones. The use of protective ear covers in noisy environments is strongly recommended.
3. *Immunization:* Promote childhood and adult immunization including the measles, mumps and rubella (MMR). Various viruses can cause deafness as a result of fatal damage and malformation affecting the ear. Deafness occurs following exposure to rubella in first trimester of pregnancy. Women should be tested for immunity and taken care accordingly.
4. *Ototoxic drugs* can cause ototoxicity in damage to hearing. Monitor the patient reaction to drugs known for ototoxity as drugs list shown earlier.
5. *Identify the person* who has risk for potential of hearing loss.
6. *Detection of hearing loss* The nurse should be observant of symptoms that indicate hearing loss at all ages.

When communication with the person with hearing impaired, follow the undermentioned guidelines.

1. Get the patient's attention by touching him or her lightly, flickering the room light, or raising an arm or hand.
2. Stand facing the patient with the light on your face; this will help the person's speech (lip) read.
3. Speak slowly and clearly, but do not overaccentuate words.
4. Speak in normal tone; do not shout. Shouting overuses normal speaking movements and may cause distortion. If the person has a conductive loss making the voice louder without shouting may be helpful.
5. If the person does not seem to understand what is said, express it differently. Some words are difficult to "see" in speech reading, such as white and red.
6. Do not smile, chew gum, or cover the mouth when talking to a person with limited hearing.
7. Use phrases to convey meaning rather than one-word answers. Supplement words with body language.
8. Do not show annoyance by careless facial expression. Persons who are hard of hearing depends more on visual cues.
9. Write out proper names or any statements that you are not sure that the patient understood.
10. Encourage the use of hearing aid if the person has one; allow him or her to adjust it before speaking.
11. Avoid the use of the intercom when communicating with the patient.
12. Do not avoid conversation with a person who has hearing loss.
13. Post a note at the bedside and nurse's station alerting personnel that the person is hard of hearing.

The nonverbal and verbal aids for communicating with the patient with impaired hearing are summarized as given below and follow the same:

i. *Nonverbal aids*.
   - Draw attention with hand movement.
   - Have speakers face in good light.
   - Avoid covering mouth or face with hands.
   - Avoid chewing, eating, smoking while talking.
   - Maintain eye contact.
   - Avoid distracting environemnt.
   - Avoid careless expression that patient may misinterpret.
   - Use touch.
   - Move close to better ear.
   - Avoid light behind speaker.

ii. Verbal aids:
   - Speak normally and slowly.
   - Do not overexaggerate facial aggressions.
   - Do not overenunciate.
   - Use simple sentences.
   - Rephrase sentences and use different words.
   - Write name or difficult words.
   - Avoid shouting.
   - Speak in normal voice directly into better ear.

The person with a hearing aid should know how to take care for the aid and what to do if the aid does not work. The nurse must also have basic knowledge of the hearing aid to assist persons who are unable or unwilling to do this when ill. The person is encouraged to use hearing aid and store it safely in its case when it is not in use.

The care of the hearing aid includes the following:

- Turn the hearing aid off when not in use.
- Open the battery compartment at night to avoid accidental drainage of the battery.
- Keep an extra battery available at all times.
- Wash the ear mold frequently (daily if necessary) with mild soap and warm water and use a pipe cleaner to cleanse the cannula.
- Do not wear the hearing aid if an ear infection is present.

When hearing aids fail to work, do the following:

- Check the on-off switch.
- Inspect the earmold for cleanliness.
- Examine the battery for correct insertion.
- Examine the cord plug for correct insertion.
- Examine the cord for breaks.
- Replace the battery cord or both, if necessary. The life of batteries varies according to amount of use and power requirements of the aid.

Batteries last from 2 to 14 days.

- Check the position of the earmold in the ear of the hearing aid.
- Whistles, the earmold probably is not inserted properly into the ear canal or the person needs to have a new earmold made.

Disorders of External Ear

The external ear may be affected by masses, trauma, wax impaction, and infection. Most common disorders of the external ear are as follows:

1. *Masses* Masses may be cysts, exostesis (bony protrusions) infection polyps and malignant tumours.

   Most cysts arise from sebaceous glands. Polyps typically arise from the middle ear or lympatic membrane. Malignant tumours are usually basal carcinomas on the pinna and squamous cell carcinoma in the canal.

   Masses of all types are fairly rare and if treatment is indicated, surgical excisionis performed. Squamous cell carcinoma can invade the underlying tissue and spread throughout the temporal bone and it needs further treatment and follow-up.

2. *Trauma* Both sharp and blunt injuries are common. Penetrating injury can damage hearing but infection and cosmetic appearance are more common concerns. Trauma to the external ear can cause injury to the subcutaneous tissue that may result in a haemotoma. If the haemotoma is not aspirated, inflammation of the membranes of the ear cartilage (Perichondritis) can result. Antibiotics are given to prevent infection. Supportive care and protection from infection are indicated. Cosmetic surgery may be needed.
3. *Foreign bodies* Many options exist. Insects, cotton pieces, nuts and seeds are the most common. Remove carefully aided by microscopic visualization. Insects are removed by filling canal with mineral oil.
4. *Pruritus* This frequent complaint in elders results from sebaceous gland atrophy and dry epithelium. Dry cerumen worsens the itching. Daily application of glycerine or mineral oil drops decreases dryness and softens cerumen.
5. *Impacted Cerumen* This may result from use of cotton-tipped applicator or other object to clean the ear. Age related drying of cerumen increases incidence. Impacted wax is softened and loosened with alternating instillation of glycerine to soften and hydrogen peroxide to loosen the cerumen for removal by warm water irrigation. The clinical manifestation of cerumen impaction includes hearing loss, otalgia, tinnitis, vertigo, cough, cardiac depression (vasal stimulation).
6. *External Otitis*
   External otitis involves inflammation or infection of the epithelium of the auricle and ear canal. The infection begins in the skin lining of the ear canal and can include the canal.

Aetiology

External otitis occurs more frequently in summer than in winter. It may be caused by infection, dermatitis or both. Bacteria and fungi may be cause. The bacteria most commonly cultured are Pseudomonas Aeruginosa, Proteus Vulgaris, Eucherichia Coli, and S. Aureus. The most common fungi are çandida albicans and aspergillus. Fungi are often causative agents of external otitis, especially in warm, moist climates. The warm, dark environment of the ear canal provides good medium for the growth of microorganism. The localised form of the infection is an "ear canal furuncle or abscess. In the presence of a systemic disease such as diabetes, the external otitis can spread wildly through cartilage and bone is then termed as "malignant external otitis". the most common form of external otitis is called "swimmer's ear" because, it is prevalent when water remains in the ear canal. Occasional perichondritis occurs resulting in necrosis of the cartilage and loss of distinctive shape of the auricle.

Pathophysiology

Local trauma, contamination or ongoing exposure to moisture produces an environment conducive to the overgrowth of normal flora. Pain in the external ear is most common symptom,. Painful sites are tender because of the close proximity of the bone (a hard surface), when palpating the ear. A clue to early external otitis is tenderness when gently pulling on the pinna. A frerunner of pain is external otitis itching in the ear canal.

Clinical Manifestation

- Pain (otalgia) is one of the first signs of external otitis.
- Drainage from the ear may be sero-sangineous or purulent. The drainage will be green and have a musty smell.
- Temperature elevation occurs when there is extensive involvement of tissue.
- The swelling of the ear canal can block hearing and cause dizziness.

Management

Diagnosis of external otitis is made by observation with the otoscope light using the largest speculum of the year will accommodate without causing the unnecessary discomfort. Culture and sensitivity studies can be done.

Treatment for an external ear infection depends on the stage of the infection. Local/topical antibiotics are the mainstay of the treatment. If the ear canal is swollen and shut, a "wick" may be inserted to allow the antibiotic drops to penetrate canal. Irrigation may be performed to remove infection and debris. Cotton wicks should be used with caution in young patients, and psychotic patients who may push them farther into the ear. Aspirin or codiene usually controls the pain. Topical antibiotics include polymy in B. colistin, neomycin, and chloromphenicol Nystretin used for fungal infection. Corticosteroids may also be used unless the infection is fungal. If the surrounding tissue is involved, systemic antibiotics are prescribed. Warm, moist compresses or heat may be applied. Improvement should occur in 48 hours but 7 to 14 days are required for complete resolution. In belief, management or external otitis includes:

- Diagnostic : Otoscopic examination, culture and sensitivity
- Treatment by : Analgesics (depending on severity);
  - Warm compress,
  - Cleansing of the canal,
  - Ear wick,
  - Antibiotic otic drops, and
  - Systemic antibiotics.

The nurse instructs the patient/family in the safe administration of ear drops as follows:

- Wash hands before and after procedure.
- Warm the ear drops to body temperature before administration. Dizziness may occur from insertion of drops that are too warm or too cold.
- Instruct the patient to tilt his/her head so that the ear to be treated is up.

- Straighten the ear canal by pulling the external ear up and back.
- Instil prescribed number of drops to run along ear canal.
- Press gently several times on the tragus of the ear to ensure proper instillation or hold the head in position for 2 to 3 minutes.

As an ointment is prescribed to control itching or inflammation it is applied using a cotton-tipped applicator. The applicator is inserted any deeper into the ear than cotton and a new applicator used each time.

The nurse instructs the patient to avoid getting water in the ear plugs or cotton with vaseline. If earplugs are used, thorough cleansing with alcohol or mild detergent between uses is recommended to prevent reinfection. The patient should not go swimming during this time.

PROBLEMS OF MIDDLE EAR AND MASTOID

Infection with its associated complications is the most common disorders of the middle ear, but masses, trauma and other conditions may occur. The less common disorders of the middle ear are perforated tympanic membrane, otostenosis and mastoiditis, the more common disorder is otitis media (acute or chronic).

Perforated Tympanic Membrane

Perforation may occur acutely after trauma or as the result of chronic infection. Damage may extend to the ossicles and worsen the hearing loss.

Acute perforation may heal spontaneously. Infection is treated with appropriate systemic antibiotics. Surgical corrections of the perforations may be performed; myringoplasty for the membrane or tympanoplasty if repair includes the middle ear structures. Crafts may be taken from the muscle fascia, a vein, or perichondrium. Success rate is high.

Otosclerosis

Aetiology

Otosclerosis, an autosomal dominant disease, is the fixation of the foot plate of the stapes in the oval window. It is common cause of conductive hearing loss in youth, especially women and accelerates during pregnancy. It is common finding in children who have a rare disease known as osteogenesis imperfection. Problem involves the stapes, sclerotic bone forms on the stapes limiting its movement and resulting conductive hearing loss. The underlying cause is unknwon.

Pathophysiology

This spongy bone develops from the bony labyrinth, causing immobilization of the foot plate of the stapes, which reduces the transmission of vibration to the inner ear fluids. Although hearing loss is typically bilateral one ear may show greater hearing loss progression. The patient often unawares of the problem until the loss becomes so severe, that communication is difficult. Loss of hearing usually becomes increasingly severe.

Management

Otoscopic examination may reveal a reddish bluish of the tympanum (Schwarz's sign) caused by the vascular and bony changes within the middle ear. Tuning fork tests help identify the conductive component of the hearing loss. On the Rinne test, bone conduction will be better than air conduction if hearing loss is greater than that of 25dB. An audiogram demonstrates good hearing by bone conduction.

A hearing aid may initially be prescribed. Advanced diseases is treated surgically through stapedectomy in which a prosthesis replaces the otosclerotic footplate. The success rate is high.

Nursing management of the patient undergoing stapedectomy is similar to that the patient who has undergone a tympanoplasty. Postoperatively the patient may experience dizziness, nausea, and vomiting as a result of stimulation of the labyrinth intraoperatively. Some patients demonstrate nystagmus on lateral gaze because of disturbance of perilymph. Care should be taken to decrease sudden movements by the patient that may bring on to exacerbate dizziness. Actions (coughing, sneezing, lifting, bending, straining during bowel movements) should also be minimized.

To brief the management of otosclerosis includes:

- Diagnosis by otoscope examination, Rinne Test (512 H2 tuning fork), Weber test, audiometry and tympanometry.
- Treatment by hearing aid, stapedectomy, analyesics, antiemetics, antibiotics and antimotion drugs.

Mastoiditis

Chronic otitis media can result in the extension of the infection into the mastoid cavity. The volume of drainage from the middle ear increases.

Antibiotic therapy is the foundation of care, possibly supplemented by irrigations. Aggressive treatment is appropriate to prevent serious complications. Surgical mastoidectomy may be necessary in rare situations.

Otitis Media

Otitis media is a general term that refers to inflammation of the mucous membranes of the middle ear, eustachion tube and mastoid. The mucous membranes are continuous with those of the respiratory tract and infection can easily ascend to the ear.

Aetiology

Otitis media is caused by various types of bacteria.

- *Acute otitis* media occurs in childhood is associated with colds, sore throat, and blockage of the eustachian tube. The earlier the initial episode, the greater the risk of subsequent episode. Risk factors include young age, congenital abnormalities, immune deficiencies, passive smoke inhalation, eustachean tube damage from viral infections, family history of otitis media, recent upper respiratory infections, male gender, participation in day care, bottle feeding and allergic rhin. Although most patients have mixed infections, bacteria are the predominant aetiologic agents.

- *Chronic Otitis Media* Untreated or repeated attacks of acute otitis media may lead to a chronic condition. This is more common and persons who experience episodes of acute otitis media in early childhood. Organism involved in chronic otitis media include S. aureus, Streptococcus, Proteus mirabilis, P. aeruginoss and E. Coli.
- *Serous Otitis Media* Recurrent infection usually causing drainage and perforation of the tympanic membrane is called chronic otitis media. Between the episodes of infection, fluid may collect in the middle ear (Serous Otitis Media). Blockage in the eustachian tube creates a vacuum that causes fluid formation. When the inflammation accompanying infection subsides and the residual fluid may be too thick to drain.
- *Adhesive Otitis Media* Serous Otitis media is also found in conjunction with upper respiratory infections or allergies. If fluid is present within the ear for a protracted period of time, the tympanic membrane retracts and adhesive otitis media may develop.

  Likewise, any long-term blockage of euttachian tube can also lead to adhesive otitis media and result in hearing loss.

Pathophysiology

Since the middle ear transmits sound from the tympanic membrane to the inner ear, middle ear infection frequently causes conductive hearing loss from pressure behind the tympanic membrane. The hearing loss is usually correctable with resolution of the infection. Common additional symptoms include throbbing pain in the affected ear, inflammation, fever and drainage and bulging of the eardrum with possible perforation. Blood, pus, and other material may be present when perforation occurs. A thick yellow purulent discharge is common finding with chronic otitis media.

Tympanosclerosis. A deposit of collagen and calcium within the middle ear can also result from repeated infection. The deposits can harden around the ossicles and contribute to a worsening of any conductive, hearing loss. Because of the anatomy of the temporal bone, middle ear infection can, in rare cases, lead to a life-threatening brain abscess.

Clinical manifestation

Throbbing pain, fever, malaise, headache and reduced hearing are signs and symptoms of acute otitis media. Chronic otitis media is characterized by clear, bloody or purulent, mucoid or serous discharge accompanied by hearing loss and occasionally by ear pain, nausea and episodes of dizziness. The patient may complain of hearing loss and occasionally by earpain, nausea and episodes of dizziness. The patient may complain of hearing loss, that may be a result of distruction of the ossicles, a tympanic membrane perforation or the accumulation of fluid in the middle ear space. Occasionally, facial palsy or an attack of vertigo may alert the patient to this condition. Chronic otitis is usually painless but if pain is present, it indicates fluid under pressure. Untreated condition can result in perforation of the ear drum and the formation and the formation of cholesteatoma (an accumulation of keratanizung squamous epithelium and the middle ear). It is enlarging tumour behaviour which may destroy adjacent bones including ossicles.

Unless removed surgically a cholesteatoma can cause extensive damage to the structures of the middle ear, can erode the bony protection of the facial nerve, may create a labyrinth fistula, or even invade the dura threatening the brain.

In addition, other complication of the chronic otitis media include, sensorineural hearing loss, facial nerve dysfunction, lateral sinus thrombosis, brain or subdural abscess, and meningitis. In otitis media with effusion, patient complains of a feeling of fullness of the ear, "pluged feeling" or popping and decreased hearing.

Management

The diagnosis of otitis media is usually made based on the patient's symptoms of acute ear pain and fever. Otoscopic examination of the ear canal readily reveals the inflammed bulging tympnic membrane and perforator or drainage if present. Mastoid X-ray may be useful. The aim of treatment is to clear the middle ear infection.

Antibiotic therapy is the key to treatment of otitis media. The common medication for treatment of otitis media include the following:

- *Antibiotics* inhibit cell wall synthesis bacteriocidal (e.g. Amoxicillin trimethoprim sulphate, methoxazole, amoxicillin clavulanate and cefacter). During this treatment, nurse assesses for allergies or sensitivities; instructs patient to take medication round the clock, not to miss any doses and to finish prescriptions completely; assess for super infection.
- *Analgesics* act as CNS depressant, analgesic, antipyretic, anti-inflammatory (e.g. analgesics, antipyretics, narcotic, acetominaphen with codes. Here nurses assess vital signs, especially temperature; caution patient not to drive or operate machinery if taking codeine; also not to take other CNS depressants, including alcohol, while taking medication; teach patient to increase fluid and roughage intake to avoid constipation, take medication with meals to decrease possible nausea; do not increase dose assess effectiveness of pain relief.
- *Antihistamines* (e.g.chlorpheniramine) act on H_1 recepto antagonist, antiemetic, antitursive, anticholeneric, and local anaesthetic action. During this treatment nurse monitors

blood pressure (BP) in hypertensive patients. Avoid driving car or operating machinery until drug effects are determined; caution against alcohol use which may cause an additive effect or drowsiness.

- *Decongestants* (e.g.Pseudoephedrine) is sympathominetic acts directly on smooth muscle; produce little congestive rebound that occurs with nasal sprays. During this treatment the nurse:
  - monitors heart rate, and BP especially in patient with cardiac history.
  - teaches patient not to take medications before bedtime because of stimulant effect.
  - withhold medication if restlessness or tachycardia occurs.
  - teach patient to avoid other over-the-counter medications, which may contain ephedrine.

The systemic antibiotic therapy based on the culture and sensitivity results is initiated. In addition, patient may need to undergo frequent evaluation of drainage and debris in OPDs. Antibiotic ear drops and acetic acid ear drops are also used to reduce infection. When the eustachian tube is chronically obstructed, it may be necessary to remove fluid from the middle ear. Myringotomics, with or without tubes are performed to regain normal middle ear and eustachian tube function. Myringotomy involves making tiny incision in the tympanic membrane through which the fluid can be suctioned. To keep the incision open and prevent reaccumulation of fluid, various types of transtympanic tube can be inserted with incision. These tubes fall out by themselves in 3 to 12 months.

Surgical interventions may be necessary if attempts to control the infection medically are unsuccessful. The ossicles become neurotic. Repairing the damage of middle ear infection requires difficult microsurgical procedure, which includes tympano ossiculoplasty and mastoidectomy. The surgical therapy for chronic ear infected includes:

1. *Myringoplasty:* Surgical reconstruction is limited to repair of tympanic membrane perforation.
2. *Tympanoplasty without mastoidectomy:* An operation to eradicate disease in the middle ear and to reconstruct the hearing mechanism without mastoid surgery, with or without tympanic membrane grafting.

The nurse will assist in all the aspects of management of otitis media which include ear irrigation, instillation of otic drops, powders, acetic acid drops, and administration of analgesics, antiemetics, systematic antibiotics and preoperation and postoperation care for patients who are under grave surgical trauma.

The nurse instructs the patient against having water in the ear during treatment. This includes showering and shampooing as well as swimming. Commercial plugs or other barriers may be used as temporary protections during shampooing. If an ear wash is prescribed, the nurse teaches the patient and designated family caregiver *how to perform ear wash* safely at homes. It should be noted that:

- The procedure should be performed by a family member or significant other if possible. It cannot be performed effectively by the patient alone. The following guidelines are helpful for *performing earwash*.
- Wash hands before and after the procedure.
- Fill a 2 to 3 ounce ear syringe with the solution, warmed to body temperature.
- Position the patient lying on his or her side with the affected ear up.
- Place the tip of the syringe gently into the ear canal. Do not be afraid to insert it into the ear.
- Pump the solution from the syringe back and forth into the ear. Do this vigorously and repeatedly. The fluid must actively move in and out of the ear canal to be effective.
- Assist the patient to lean over the side and let the solution run out of the ear at the end of the procedure.
- Apply ear drops if instructed.
- Continue to use the ear wash solution as instructed for about 2 weeks or until the ear is dry and without drainage.

Most patients undergoing ear surgery have very short-term hospitalization. The nurse teaches the patient what to expect after discharge and how to promote healing during the recovery period. The nurse informs the patient that decreased hearing is expected initially from the presence of swelling and packing in the ear. Cracking or popping noises are commonly heard in the affected ear and are expected. Minor earache and discomfort in cheek and jaw are common, but should be managed effectively with mild analgesics. Dizziness or light-headedness may also be present, initially the patient should be cautious when getting out of the bed and walking. Bleeding and drainage are negligible. A cotton ball frequently provides adequate dressing. In addition, patient teaching after surgery includes the following.

- Sneezing or coughing, with the mouth open or needed for the first week after surgery.
- Blow the nose gently as needed, one side at a time.
- Avoid vigorous activity until approved by the surgeon.
- Change cotton ball dressing as prescribed.
- Report any drainage other than a slight amount of bleeding to the surgeon.
- Keep ear dry for 6 weeks after surgery.
  - Do not shampoo the hair without barrier.
  - Protect the ear when necessary with two pieces of cotton counter piece saturated with petrolatum.
  - Avoid loud noisy environment. Do not fly until approved by surgeon.
- Balance ear pressure as needed by holding nose, closing mouth and swallowing.

PROBLEMS OF INNER EAR

Sensorineural hearing loss is most common. Inner disorder and may occur in conjunction with an identified ear problem or an isolation. The hearing loss usually is incomplete but it is frequently progressive. The loss of discrimination (understanding words) is characteristic feature of sensorineural hearing loss. The inner part of the ear is so delicate that it does not lend itself to surgical correction or repair. Three symptoms that indicate the disease of inner ear are vertigo (whirling), sensorineural hearing loss, and tinnitus (ringing) in the ear. Symptoms of vertigo arise from the vestibular labyrinth, wherein hearing loss and tinnitus arise from the auditory labyrinth. There is an overlap between manifestation of inner ear problems and CNS disorder.

Acoustic Neuroma

Aetiology

It is slow-growing lesion that can occur at any age and usually occurs unilaterally. The tumour typically grows at point where CN VIII enters the internal auditory canal, the temporal bone and may extend to the brainstem. The tumour is more common in women and tends to occur in person between 30 and 60 years of age.

Pathophysiology

The tumour arises from the neurilimmal sheath (sheath of schwann) along the vestibular branch of the nerve and spreads to the cochlear brands. Early diagnosis is important because the tumour can grow and compress the facial nerve and arteries within the ear canal. It is important the tumour should be diagnosed before it becomes intracranial. In rare cases, the pressure of the tumour can become life-threatening symptoms include tinnitus, vertigo, and a progressive unilateral loss of ability to hear high-pitched sound. Disorders of the facial nerve may emerge if the tumour is compressing the structure as well.

Clinical Manifestation

Early symptoms are associated with eighth cranial nerve compression and destruction. They include unilateral, progressive, sensorineural hearing loss, unilateral tinnitus and mild intermittant vertigo. One of the earliest symptoms of an accoustic neuroma is reduced touch sensation in the posterior ear canal.

Management

Diagnostic tests include neurologic audiometric and vestibular tests and CT scan and MRI with gadolinium enhancement. Acoustic neuroma are treated surgically, usually by a neurosurgeon. Surgery to remove small tumours performed through the middle cranial fossa or retrolabyrinthine approach, which preserves hearing and vestibular function. A translabyrinthine approach is usually used for medium-sized tumour and when hearing is minimal. Although hearing is destroyed by this approach, advantages include good access to the tumour and preservation of the facial nerve. Retrosigmoid (suboccipital) or transotic approaches are used for large tumours (greater than 3 cm). It is almost impossible to preserve hearing when the tumour is greater than 2 cm.

Menier's Disease

Menier's disease (idiopathic endolymphatic hydrops) is characterized by symptom caused by inner ear disease; episodic vertigo, tinnitus, fluctuating sensorineural hearing loss and aural fullness. It causes significant disability for the patient because of sudden, severe attacks of vertigo with nausea and vomiting.

Aetiology

Exact aetiology is unknown. A virus believed to play a role in aetiology, but this has not been proven. This disease occurs when the normal fluid and electrolytic balance of the inner ear is disrupted. It may be result in an excessive accumulation of endolymph in the membranous labyrinth.

Pathophysiology

The underlying pathological changes of Menier's disease include overproduction and defective absorption of endolymph, which increases volume and pressure within the membranous labyrinth until distension results in rupture and mixing of the endolymph and perilymph fluids. The two fluids have significantly different compositions and the mixture disrupts the fluid and electrolyte balance within the labyrinth. Then symptoms of disease develop and exhibit.

Clinical Manifestation

The classic Menier's disease attacks last from 2 to 3 weeks approximately; the time is required to close the rupture and restore fluid balance. The symptoms range from mild to incapacitating and include vertigo, tinnitus, and fluctuating sensorineural hearing loss from degeneration of the hair cells. Prodormal symptoms include tinnitus, earfullness and hearing loss. Most of the patients experience vertigo associated with nausea, vomiting and ataxia.

Management

The diagnosis is based on the presence of classic triad of symptoms plus a prodronal symptoms of fullness or pressure in the involved ear. The triad includes episodic true vertigo, sensorineural hearing loss and tinnitus and other disorder can also result in vertigo and balance disturbances. To maintain balance, the brain must integrate data from vestibular visual and proprioceptive system. The glyceral test may help in the diagnosis in Menier's disease.

There is no known cure for Menier's disease and the

management focusses on controlling symptoms. A variety of medication may be used in the management of this disease, primary and the attempt to control disabling symptom which includes the following:

Acute care (One or more)

- Sedatives (diazapam, valium)
- Anticholenergic (atropine).
- Vasodilators.
- Antihistamine (diphenhydramine-Benadryl).

Surgery may be performed when the patient symptoms cannot be satisfactorily controlled with medical intervention, which include:

i. *Conservative surgical interventions*
   - Endolympathic shunt.
   - Vestinodular nerve section.
ii. *Destructive surgical intervention*
   - Labyrinthotomy.
   - Labyrinthectomy.

Nursing Management

During the acute attack, antihistamines, anticholenergics and benzodiazepam can be used as suppressants for the labyrinth. Acute vertigo is treated symptomatically with bedrest, sedation and antiemetics or drugs for lotion sickness administered orally, rectally or intravenously. The patient requires reassurance and counselling that the condition is not life-threatening. Management between attacks may include vasodilation, diuretics, antihistamines, a low-sodium diet and avoidance of caffeine and nicotine, diazepam or antiver used to reduce dizziness. Over a time, patient responds to the prescribed medication.

Diet therapy is frequently quite helpful in controlling the symptoms associated with Menier's disease. The nurse encourages the patient to follow low-salt diet and avoid the excess use of caffeine, sugar, monosodium glutamate and alcohol. The intake of food and fluids over the course of the day, some patients are able to achieve significant symptom improvement from diet modification alone.

Patient needs clear instructions about how to manage in acute attack of vertigo. The nurse instructs the patient to immediately lie down on a firm surface if possible, loosen the clothing, and close the eyes until the acute vertigo stops. Driving and operating machinery should not be attempted during attack. Between the attacks the patient can resume normal activities but should avoid swimming underwater which may cause a loss of orientation.

Loss of balance places the patient with vertigo at high risk for falls. The nurse assists the patient to explore ways to increase the safety of the home environment. The nurse reminds the patient of the importance of sitting or lying down at the onset of dizziness to reduce the risk of falls. The nurse advises the patient to avoid ladders, work on roof or trees or climbing on high places until the vertigo is controlled. Balance therapy can be extremely helpful in supporting the balance network in the brain, and the nurse reinforces the importance of daily practice with these exercises.

Other Vestibular Disorders

1. *Vestibular neuronitis* is the infection of the vestibular nerve with sudden onset commonly caused by virus. First attack of vertigo is most severe and subsequent attacks are less severe.
2. *Labyrinthitis* infection of the labyrinth of inner ear is caused by virus or bacteria. It will have severe vertigo diminishing with time and tinnitus may not be present. There is no permanent sensorineural hearing loss.
3. *Benign Paraxysmal positioned vertigo* is degenerative debris free floating in the endolymph. Many theories suggest the cause is idiopathic, (In this, positional vertigo is with quick head movements or position change).
4. *Presbyastasis (Presbyvertigo)* this is balanced disorders of aging due to degenerative changes of the vestibule. Vertigo attack leads to imbalance when standing/walking, leading to falls and injuries.

Presbycusis of the hearing of old age includes the loss of peripheral auditory sensitivity a decline in word recognition ability, and associated psychologic and communication issues. The cause of presbycusis is related to degenerative changes in the inner ear such as loss of hair cells, reduction of blood supply, diminution of endolymph production, decreased basilar membrane flexibility, and loss of neurons in the cochlear nuclei. Noise exposure is though to be a common factor related to presbycusis.

PROCEDURE 17.7: *IRRIGATING THE EXTERNAL AUDITORY CANAL

Purposes:
1. To remove discharge from the canal.
2. To facilitate removal of cerumen or foreign body.

Nursing Focus

Ask if the patient has a history of draining ears or has ever had a perforation or other complications from a previous ear irrigation. If the reply is "Yes" check with the health care provider before proceeding with the irrigation.

Equipment and Solutions.

- Kind and amount of solution desired (usually warm water).
- Ear Syringe or irrigating container with tubing, clamp and catheter.
- Protective towels.
- Cotton balls and cotton-tipped applicators.
- Solution bowl and emesis basin.
- Bag for disposable items.

Procedure: *Preparatory Phase*

1. After explaining procedure to the patient, place in a position of sitting or lying with head tilted forward and toward affected ear.
2. Position protective towels.

Nursing Action	*Rationale*
Performance Phase	
1. Use a cotton applicator to remove any discharge on outer ear.	1. To prevent carrying discharge deeper into canal.
2. Place basin close to the patient's head and under the ear.	2. To provide a receptacle to receive irrigating solution.
3. Test temperature of solution it should be comfortable to the inner aspect of wrist area.	3. Solutions that are hot or cold are most uncomfortable and may start a feeling of dizziness.

Gerontologic Alert:

Take special care not to irrigate an older adult's ear with cold water, as dizziness may be happened.

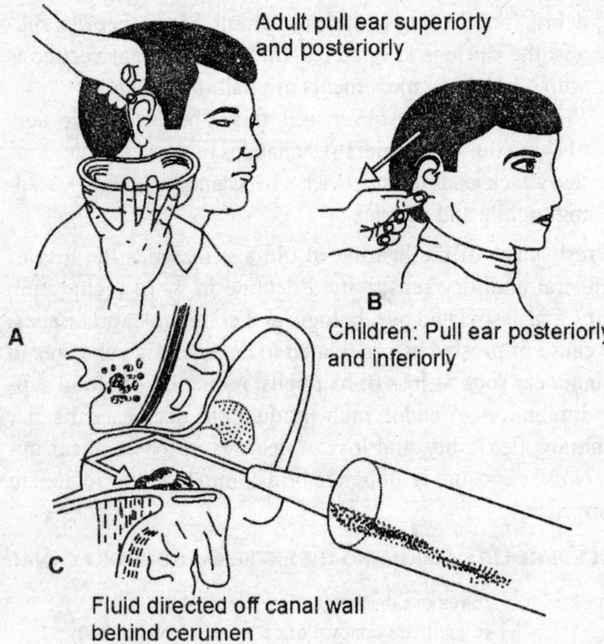

Adult pull ear superiorly and posteriorly
A
B
Children: Pull ear posteriorly and inferiorly
C
Fluid directed off canal wall behind cerumen

Fig. 17.4: Ear irrigation. (A) The external auditory canal in the adult can best be exposed by pulling the earlobe upward and backward. (B) The same exposure can be achieved in the child by gently pulling the auricle of the ear downward and backward. (C) An enlarged diagram showing the direction of irrigating fluid against the side of the canal. NOTE: This is more effective in dislodging cerumen than if the flow of solution were directed straight into the canal.

4. Ascertain whether impaction is due to a foreign hydroscopic (attracts or absorbs moisture) body before proceeding.	4. If water contacts such a substance, it may cause it to swell and produce intense pain.
5. Gently pull the outer ear upward and backward (adult) or downward and outward (child).	5. To straighten the ear canal (See figure).
6. Place tip of syringe or irrigating catheter at opening of ear, gently direct stream of fluid against sides of canal.	6. To decrease direct force of irrigation against eardrum and possibility fo rupturing it.
7. If an irrigating container is used, elevate only high enough to remove secretions or no more than 15 cm (6 in) above patient's ear.	7. To provide safe and effective pressure of fluid, if height is more than 15 cm (6 in) pressure will be too great and may damage tissue.
8. Observe for signs of pain or dizziness.	8. Discontinue treatment if they occur.
9. If irrigating does not dislodge the wax, instil several drops of prescribed glycerin. Carbamide peroxide (Debrox) or other solutions as directed 2 or 3 times daily for 2-3 days.	9. To soften and loosen impaction.

Ear irrigation (A). The external auditory canal in the adult can best be exposed by pulling the realobe upward and backward. (B) The same exposure can be achieved in the child by gently pulling the auricle of the ear downward and backward. (C) An enlarged diagram showing the direction of irrigating fluid against the side of the canal.

Note: This is more effective in dislodging cerumen than if the flow of solution were directed straight into the canal.

Follow-up Phase

1. Dry external ear.
2. Remove soiled equipment and make the patient comfortable.
3. Patient should lie on irrigated (affected) side for a few minutes after procedure to allow any remaining solution to drain out.
4. Record time of irrigation, kind and amount fo solution, nature of return flow, and effect of treatment.

Organ Transplants and Nursing

Organ transplantation has evolved from being a medical experience to a major therapeutic intervention for selected patients. The advances made in organ procurement and preservation, surgical techniques, tissue typing and matching, understanding and management of the immune system, immune suppressive therapy and prevention and treatment of rejection have dramatically increased the demand for organs and tissues for transplantation. Conservative medical management of patients with end stage kidney, liver, heart or lung disease is costly. Although transplant procedures are expensive, the current success rate have made transplantation a cost-effective treatment option compared with traditional medical management. The other financial factors that increase the costeffectiveness of transplantation include the potential earning power of the transplant recipient and the discontinuation of existing disability benefits. Transplantation can restore dignity and quality to the lives of patients and once again become productive member of the society. The transplantations already in practice are allograft transplantation (refers to transplantation of organs/tissue from one member of a species to another member of the same species). The common allograft transplantation includes sold organs like kidney, liver, heart, pancreas and lung and corneas and bone marrow.

ORGAN SOURCES

The sources for organ or tissues for transplantation include living donors, nonheart beating donors (NHBDs), marginal donor, and animals.

Living Donors

In the past, donors were restricted to blood relative (i.e. parents children and siblings). Recently, unrelated donors have been added to the donor pool. These donors are not blood relatives, but have an emotional relationship with the potential recipient (e.g. spouse, step parent, step child and friend. The advantages of live donors include:

- Improved patient and graft survival rates.
- Immediate availability of the organ, no waiting for long periods.
- The ability to schedule the surgery when the recipients in the best possible medical conditions and,
- Immediate functioning of the organ because there is minimal preservation time.

Ethical concern that arise when people donate organs or positions of organs include:

- The risk of surgical complications for the healthy donor.
- The loss of income if the donor is a primary wage earner.
- Uncertain outcomes for the recipient and
- Guilt experienced by the donors must be weighed against the future that organ donors on offers to people with end-stage liver, lung or heart disease who may otherwise die waiting for a cadaver donor with the right match. Respect for autonomy supports the right of the donor assume these risks if the donor's decision is informed, free from coercion and truly autonerons.

Non-Heart-Beating-Donors (NHBDs)

Patients who have been declared dead by traditional cardiopulmonary criteria rather than brain death criteria and other source of transplantable organs. These are NHBD because organ procurement takes place after the heart has stopped beating. Before the institution of brain death criteria these donors were the major sources of transplantable kidneys, but problems with extended ischaemia time leading to cell and tissue damage limited their usefulness.

Recently two different methods for procuring organs from NHBDs have been developed to address this problem: (i) in situ organ preservation immediately after cardiopulmonary arrest, and (ii) procurement from patient who die after choosing to forego life-sustaining treatment.

i. *In-situ organ preservation* involves the infusion of cooled preservation solution through a catheter inserted into the abdominal aorta immediately after death has been declared. This process must be instituted immediately after asystole, unfortunately obtaining family consent for the procedure is difficult, because the family does not have time to adjust to the news of their loved one's death before having to make a decision about organ donation.

ii. *Decision for patient to forego life-sustaining treatment:* The alternative method allowing patients and family the option of donating organs after they have decided to forego life-sustaining treatment has two advantages. *First* because the decision for organ donation is made by the patient and family before death, there is time for them to discuss, reflect and give informed consent before the initiation of any invasive procedure. *Second* the time and place of death are controlled to minimise harm ischaemia time. The patient is taken to the operating room where a surgical team begins organ removal and preservation within minutes of death.

Cadaver Donors/Marginal Donors

The cadaver donors have been liberalized to include increase age (upto 70 years), diabetes, hypertension, some infection, high-risk social history but negative HIV test, some haemodynamic instability, some chemical imbalance and increased organ preservation time. A careful evaluation including histological assessment of the recovered organs is made before transplantation, and careful long-term follow-up is provided to ensure that patient and graft survival rates are comparable to those obtained with traditional cadaver donors. The decision to transplant a marginal donor organ requires not only thorough anatomical and physiological evaluation of the organ, but also a similar evaluation of the recipient including age comor bid condition, and immunological compatibility.

Xenografts

Xenografting, the transplantation of animal organs into humans, has become an attractive option. Potential advantages of xenografting include a readily available organ supply, fewer patient deaths on the waiting list, lower organ procurement costs, a more elective surgical procedure, and size matching for donor and recipients. The major obstacle includes hyperacute rejection and transmission of viral diseases.

ROLE OF NURSES IN DONATION PROCESS

Nurses are commonly the first health care professional to identify a potential organ donor and make the appropriate referral to the local organ procurement organization. Nurses are in the best position to provide compassionate support to families and as well prepared, both educationally and through experience to help the family through this crisis. The nurse can provide both sufficient factual information and the emotional support needed for the next of kin to arrive at a decision about organ and tissue donation, the following *guidelines* will be helpful.

- Make sure that death has been declared and discussed with the family and the family has been given time to assimilate this information.
- Contact the local organ procurement organization to make referral and to determine medical suitability for organ/tissue donation.
- Try to determine the beliefs of potential donor, that is, has a donor card has been signed.
- Identify the legal next of kin and any other family members or significant others who should be included in the discussion.
- Provide a comfortable, private place for discussion between the health team members and the family.
- Ascertain what the family understands about brain death and the hope of recovery.
- Speak slowly, be sensitive, refer to the potential donor by name, and do not be afraid to refer to the potential donor as dead.
- Provide adequate, accurate information on the options available to the family related to discontinuing life support.
- Provide adequate, accurate information on organ/tissue donation, including informed consent, evaluation required and there is no cost to the family.
- Ensure that the family understands the organ/tissue donation will not interfere with the timing of the funeral service or with an open casket service.
- Provide time for the family to discuss the request and make the decision.
- Request written consent only after the family has had time to make the decision and has given an affirmative response.

After procurement of the organ from the donor and transplant to recipient, gifts of organs or tissues are confidential. No one who receives a transplant is told the identity of the donor, and donor families are told only the age and sex of the various recipient and how they are doing after transplantation.

Health care professionals often fear that asking grieving families for organ/tissue donations adds to the family grief. Studies have constantly shown, however, that the strongest advocates of donations are donor families, who view donation as the highest form of charity, giving the ultimate gift, life to another person. Traditionally, one of the biggest obstacles to organ/tissue donation has been the failure to identify potential donors early in the process. Nurses must be knowledgeable about the donor eligibility criteria and knowhow to activate the organ procurement process, which include donor must be free of malignancy, sepsis and communicable diseases including HIV, hepatitis B and C, syphilis and tuberculosis and have no history of intravenous drug abuse.

Selection of Recipient

Since the supply of organ/tissues is limited, appropriate selection is important for both successful outcome and the best use of this scarce resource. Candidacy is determined by a wide variety of medical and psychosocial factors that vary among transplant centers. These factors include disease status, therapeutic benefits of transplantation, age, functional ability and presence of family support. A careful evaluation is completed before transplant to attempt to identify and minimize potential complications after transplant. Contraindications for transplantation include disseminated malignancies, chronic infections, and ongoing psychosocial problems such as non-compliance with medical regimen and chemical dependency.

Tissue Typing and Matching Procedures

Successful transplantation of allografts require manipulation of the recipient immune system. All cells and tissues in the body have markers or antigens on the cell membrane surface. These antigens allow cells to be recognized by other cells as either "self" or nonself. The antigens distributed on the surface of the cells of any one person are unique for that person, except for identical twins, and are controlled by the genes. These cell markers are important in protecting the body from invasions by foreign substances. Because foreign substances have different markers, they can be recognized as nonself by the immune system.

The B and T-lymphocytes of the immune system are the surveillance cells that can recognize the cells membrane markers as foreign (nonself) and non-foreign (self). When the markers on cell membranes are recognized as foreign (nonself), the B and T lymphocytes are activated, they can differentiate, proliferate, and clone to be able to attack and destroy foreign substance. The ability to recognize foreign substances is the result of genetic factors on chromosomes. This region of the chromosome is called the major histocompatibility complex and codes for human leukocyte antigens (HLA), which initiate process of rejection and serve as the targets for immunological attack against the transplanted organ.

In preparation of transplant, some tissue typing and leukocyte crossmatching may be performed. The major tests for tissue typing and matching may be used to establish compatibility between the donor and recipient are as follows:

1. *ABO Compatibility*
   Test surface antigens on RBCs and other tissues, compatibility is same for blood transfusion; recipient would have antibodies to ABO antigens present on donor cells and not on recipient cell
2. *Minor RBC Antigen testing*
3. *Microlymphocytotoxic testing*
   It detects Class I HLA antigens (A, B, C) and matches these antigens between recipient and donor.
4. *Mixed Leukocyte culture or Mixed Lymphocyte Culture* (MLC)
   Lymphocyte or the potential donor are treated to prevent them from responding. In this way, an estimate of the response of a potential recipient (Living Cells) to a potential donor (treated cells) can be made. The MLC is primarily the result of HLA-D differences between donor and recipient. A low response of the recipients cells to the donor's cells is predictive of a successful transplant. This test is helpful in life donor transplants. Because the test takes approximately 7 days to complete, it cannot be used for cadaver transplants.
5. *T-Cell Crossmatch*
   A positive crossmatch occurs when the recipient has demonstrable circulating antibodies against the donors T Cell antigens. These circulating cytotoxic antibodies are detected by incubating donor lymphoid cells in recipient serum and the presence of complement. After a period of incubation, a marker of cells death is added to the suspension and the proportions of dead cells is counted. The presence of significant number of dead cells indicates a positive crossmatch and predicts a poor outcome after transplantation (i.e. hyperacte rejection).
6. *Panel Reaction Antibody* (PRA)
   A blood test using lymphocytoxic antibodies to determine the presence of performed antibodies to HLA antigens. The results range from 0% to 100% and reflect the percentage of antigens on the test panel against which the potential recipient has performed antibodies against which the potential recipient is found to have antibodies against specific HLA antigen, an organ donor carrying those antigens would not be suitable for that recipient because of the increased risk of rejection. A high PRA means that a potential transplant recipient has antibodies against many HLA antigens and finding a suitable donor will be more difficult.

   Still researches are being instituted to have proper testing prior to transplantation.

Prevention of Rejection after Organ Transplantation

Rejection of one of the major problems following organ/tissue transplantation. Rejection can be hyperacute, acute or chronic.

- Hyperacute (antibody medicates) rejection occurs minutes to hours after transplantation.

  Acute rejection most commonly occurs 4 days to 4 months after transplantation.
- Chronic rejection occurs in a process that occurs over month to years and is irreversible.

These rejections can be prevented by using medication. The common medication used for prevention of rejection after organ transplantation are as follows:

1. *Azathioprine (Imuran)* act as an antimetabolite that suppresses proliferation of the rapidly dividing cells including sensitized T and B cells. It can be administered orally or IV. The adverse side effects include bone marrow suppression, (Leukopenia, anaemia, thrombocytopenia), drug-induced hepatitis, oral lesions, increased susceptibility infection, alopecia, malignancies and pancreatis. The nursing intervention included here are:
   - Institute infection control measures.
   - Monitor haemotocrit, WBC count and platelet count.
   - Assess for signs and symptoms of infection or bleeding.

- Administer oral antifungal agent as ordered.
- Decrease dose as ordered.
- Assess for jaundice.
- Monitor serum transuminases, alkaline phosphatase, bilirubin, and coagulation factors.
- Assesses nausea, vomiting and abdominal pain.
- Monitor serum analysis and lipase.
- Inspect oral mucus membrane.
- Assess for hair loss.
- Maintain good oral hygiene.

2. *Mycophenolate mofetil (cellcept)* an antimetabolite that inhibits purine synthesis, which suppresses proliferation of T and B cells. It can be given orally. Side effects include gastrointestinal toxicity (diarrhoea, nausea, vomiting), leukopoenia, thrombocytopoenia. The nursing intervention here includes:
   - Decreased dose as ordered.
   - Monitor GI status (nausea, vomiting, diarrhoea, and. cramps, dyspepsion).
   - Monitor daily weight.
   - Monitor intake output.
   - Administer antiemetic as ordered.
   - Administer antidiarrhoeal as ordered.
   - Institute infection control measures.
   - Monitor white blood cell count.
3. *Corticosteroid (Prednisone, Deltasone, Mehy Prednisone)* can be given orally or IV. These suppress inflammatory response, prevents proliferations of T. cytotoxic lymphocytes. Side effects include, Cushingoid syndrome Peptic ulcer, hypertension, GI bleeding, aseptic necrosis. Sodium and water retention, acne, muscle weakness, fat dystrophy, capillary fragility, delayed healing, hyperglycaemia, mood alterations; bacterial, fungal and viral infection. The nursing intervention includes:
   - Instruct patient about all potential side effects.
   - Administer low sodium diet.
   - Monitor daily weight.
   - Administer low-fat-low cholesterol diet if cholesterol is elevated.
   - Consult dietician.
   - Instruct patient to watch calories intake carefully and eat low calorie snacks between meals.
   - Administer oral corticosteroids with food to minimize GI upset.
   - Administer antacids H_2 receptor blockers as ordered.
   - Perform guiac test stool and emesis.
   - Observe abdominal pain and rebound tenderness.
   - Report complaint of acid indigestion, oesophageal or gastric burning.
   - Monitor blood glucose.
   - Administer insulin as ordered.
   - Instruct patient regarding diabetics, if newly acquired.
   - Inspect skin.
   - Avoid skin trauma and use adhesive tape.
   - Inspect oral mucous membrane.
   - Maintain good oral hygiene.
   - Administer oral antifungal agents.
   - Monitor wound healing.
   - Assess and report complaint of bone or joint pain.
   - Consult physiotherapist.
   - Administer calcium or vitamin D as ordered.
   - Monitor changes in muscle strength.
   - Instruct patient to exercise regularly to counteract muscle weakening.
   - Assess presence of psychosis, euphoria, depression and irritability.
   - Consult psychiatrist if needed.
   - Assess peripheral oedema.
   - Monitor blood pressure.
   - Administer antihypertensive drugs as ordered.
   - Administer diuretics as ordered.
4. *Cyclophamide (Cytoxan)* It is an alkylating agent that interferes with DNA RNA with DNSA and protein synthesis. Cytoxan can be given orally. Side effects are alopacia, leukopoenia, haemorrhage, cystitis. The nursing intervention included are:
   - Institute infection control measures.
   - Monitor haematocrit, WBC count and platelet count.
   - Assess signs and symptoms of infection.
   - Assess for haematuria.
   - Encourage increased water intake with each dose.
   - Assess for hair loss.
   - Reduce dose as ordered.
5. *Cyclosporine (Neoral, Sandimmune)*. Prevents production and release of inteleukin-2, inhibits maturation of T-Cytotoxic lymphocyte precursors. The side effect may be hepatotoxicity, nephrotoxicity lymphomas, infections, hirsutism, hypertension, tremors, gingival hyperplasia, hyper magnesemia and seizures. The nursing interventions included are:
   - Instruct patient about all side effects.
   - Obtain true trough cyclosporine level.
   - Decreased dose is as ordered.
   - Monitor serum creatinine, BUN, potassium, serum, transminase, alkaline, phosphates, bilirubin and coagulation factors.
   - Review medication list of drugs that increase or decrease cyclosporine metabolism.
   - Assess patient for peripheral oedema and high blood pressure.
   - Administer diuretics as ordered.
   - Administer antihypertensive as ordered.
   - Monitor neurological status (tremors, parasthesia) and assure patient that these side effects are dose related.

- Assess for jaundice.
- Instruct patient in use of depilatories if hirsutism occurs.
- Instruct patient to see dentist for teeth cleaning every six months.
- Instruct patient in proper oral hygiene including flossing.

6. *Tacrolimus (Prograf. FK 506)*. Prevents production and release of interlukin-2, inhibits maturation of T-cytotoxic lymphocyte percursors; 100 time more potent than cyclosperine can be administered orally. Side effects are heparotoxicity, nephrotoxicity, neurotoxicity, G.I.toxicity, alopecia, seizures, hypertension, lymphoma. The nursing intervention during the administration includes:
   - Instruct patient about all side effects.
   - Obtain true tough levels.
   - Decrease doses as ordered.
   - Monitors serum create nine BUN, and potassium.
   - Monitor neurological status (headache, confusion and seizures).
   - Assure patient side effects are dose-related.
   - Monitor GI status (anorexia, nausea, vomitting, diarrhoea and weight loss).
   - Monitor daily weights.
   - Monitor intake and output.
   - Monitor blood glucose.
   - Administer insulin or oral hypoglycemic agents as ordered.
   - Educate patient regarding diabetes, if newly acquired.
7. *Muromonab-CO_3 (OKT_3, Orthoclone)*. A monoclonal body that removes circulating T lymphocytes. Side effects are fever, tachycardia, infections, headache, vomitting, chills, joint and muscle pain, diarrhoea, hypertension, bronchospasm, infection, aseptic meningitis, and malignancy. It is administered through IV.

   The nursing intervention during the drug administrations are:
   - Administer prescribed acetaminophen, diphenhydramine and hydrocortisone or time of IV infusion.
   - Administer IV push over 30-60 seconds.
   - Treat symptomatically and provide for patient comfort.
   - Weigh daily (patient should be within 3% of his or her dry weight).
   - Prepare patient for chest radagraphs to assess congestions.
   - Assess for peripheral oedema.
   - Auscultate lungs before the first dose is administered for base line comparison.
   - Administer prescribed diuretics.
   - Monitor GI status (nausea, vomitting, and diarrhoea).
   - Administer IV fluids as ordered.
   - Monitor temperature.
   - Administer acetaminophen as ordered.
   - Report complaints of headache.
   - Administer analgesics as ordered.
   - Report complaints of photophobia and keep room darkened.
   - Arrange for outpatient administration of complete course.
8. *Antilymphocyte globuline (ALG) and Antithymocyte globulin (ATG)* A polyclonal antibody directed against lymphocytes; reduces circulating lymphocytes decreases lymphocyte proliferation. The positive side effects are serum sickness (fever, chills, malaise, joint and muscle pain) leukepoenia, anaphylactic shock, rash, local phlebitis thrombocytopoenia, infection and lymphoma. The nursing intervention includes:
   - Administer medication intravenously.
   - Monitor temperature.
   - Administer acetaminophen/diphen hydramine as ordered.
   - Monitor platelet count.
   - Decrease dose as ordered if platelet is less than 10.
9. *Sirolimus* (Papemycin, Repamune). Suppresses symptocytes, proliferation inhibits B cells from synthexiaing antibodies. The side effects include GI toxicity (diarrhoea, nausea and vomitting). The nursing intervention includes:
   - Administer through central line over 4-6 hours.
   - Monitor gastrointestinal status for nausea, vomiting and diarrhoea.
   - Monitor daily weight.
   - Monitor intake and output.
   - Administer antiemetics as ordered/administer antidiarrheal as ordered.
   - Monitor cholesterol and triglyceride levels.
   - Decrease dose as ordered.
   - Monitor surgical wound for infection and delayed healing.
10. *Chimericant 12-2-Receptor antibody (Simulech) Daclizumas (Humanized) anti TAC zenapax):* are monoclonal antibody against 12-2-receptor, block T-cell activation and proliferation. Side effects is GI toxicity. The nursing intervention includes:
    - Administer by IV infusion over 15-30 minutes through peripheral vein.
    - Arrange for outpatient infusion to complete course of therapy after discharge.

KIDNEY TRANSPLANT

Advances have been made in the art and science of organ transplantation since the first kidney transplant was performed in 1954 in Boston between identical twins. Kidney transplant is the oldest and most common type of transplant procedure.

Indications

Kidney transplant is primarily used to treat patients experiencing end stage renal disease resulting from diabetes, hypertension and glomerulonephritis.

The advantages of kidney transplantation include the reversal of many of the pathophysiological changes associated with renal failure as normal kidney function is restored. It also eliminates the patient's dependence on dialysis and the accompanying dietary restrictions provided the opportunity to return to normal life activities (including employment) and is less expensive than dialysis after the first year.

Management

Kidney transplant is associated with maximal histocompatibility testing, especially in situation involving a live donor ABO compatibility HLA matching, WBC crossmatch and mixed lymphatic crossmatch are all performed.

The patients undergoing kidney transplant will be started and maintained on the full battery of immunosuppressive therapy for life to preserve the transplanted kidney.

Patients awaiting kidney transplant continue on their regular schedule of dialysis right upto the time of transplant. Dialysis is conducted as close to the surgery as possible to ensure that the patient is in the best possible metabolic condition to withstand the rigors of surgery. Living donor kidney is usually beginning to function immediately after surgery. Cadaver kidney may experience delay in functioning and the patient might need to have dialysis resumed after surgery to maintain physiological homeostasis.

Surgical Procedure

The donor kidney is carefully dissected free with its renal artery and vein intact. The ureter is also detected with great care to preserve the periurethral vascular supply. The kidney is removed, flushed with a chilled, sterile electrolyte solution and prepared for transplant into the recipient. The procedure takes about 2 hours.

The transplanted kidney is placed extraperitonically in the iliac fossa. Generally the peritoneal cavity is not entered. The patient's own kidneys are not removed unless they are infected or are the cause of significant hypertension. The patient's kidneys are left intact to maintain erythroprotein production, blood pressure control and prostagland in synthesis and metabolism. Efficient revascularizations is critical to prevent ischaemic injury to the kidney.

The donor uretor is used to the extent possible. If long enough, the donor ureter is tunneled through the bladder submucosa and sutured in place. This allows bladder to clamp down on the ureter as it contracts for micturation, thereby preventing reflux of urine up the ureter into the transplanted kidney. The entire transplant surgery takes about 3 hours.

Nursing Intervention

Nursing care of the patient in the preoperative phase includes emotional and physical preparation for surgery. To prevent rejections, nurse has to be actively involved in immunosuppressive therapy in addition to assisting all required diagnostic testing procedures, and also effectively manage the peritoneal dialysis, preoperative and prepare to continue it postoperatively if indicated.

Postoperative care includes both care of the donor as well as care of the recipient. The postoperative care of the live donor is similar to that provided after a nephrectomy (see ch. page no........). The donor can easily become a forgotten person in the transplant process because most of the attention is focussed on the recipient. The pain of a nephrectomy is significant, and adequate analgesia is essential to ensure comfort, promote ambulation and prevent atelectasis and possible pulmonary complications. Most donors can be discharged within 3 to 5 days and can usually return to work in a month. The majority of donors feel good about the donation because of the improved health of the recipient. Nurses caring for live donor need to acknowledge the precious gift they have given.

The first priority of care of recipient is maintenance of fluid and electrolyte balance and requires nursing measures including monitoring electrolyte imbalances, treating shocks and following measures prescribed by the concerned. Once the patient has recovered from operative procedure nursing care involves ongoing assessment, diagnosis, intervention and evaluation of patient response to the transplant. These include the prevention and treatment of rejection, infection, complication of surgery, and complications of immunosuppression.

Patient education to ensure a smooth transition from hospital to home is an integral part of the nursing care. The first priority for discharge preparations of medication teaching. Patients and their families must be able to explain the action, dosage and potential, adverse effects of all medications. A written list of discharge medication with the administration schedule is supplied for the patient to use at home. The patient should be able to describe the signs and symptoms of rejection and when and how to contact surgeon for further medical help. The signs and symptoms of acute rejection in the renal transplant patient are as follows:

- Decrease in urine output.
- Fever greater than 37.7°C (100°F) may be marked by steroid therapy.
- Pain or tenderness over grafted kidney.
- Oedema.
- Sudden weight gain 2-3 lbs in a 24 hours period.
- Hypertention.
- General malaise.
- Increase in serum creatinine and BUN.
- Decrease in creatinine clearance.
- Evidence of rejection on ultrasound or biopsy.

HEART TRANSPLANT

The first heart transplant was performed in 1967. The procedure has evolved into a viable treatment option for patient with terminal heart disease.

Indications

End-stage cardiomyopathy (dilated CMP) is the pathology in more than 50 per cent of the patients needing heart transplant; inoperable coronary artery disease is the next most common cause of transplant. It is the treatment of choice for patients with end-stage heart disease who are unlikely to survive next 6 to 12 months.

Indication for Heart Transplantation

- Suitable physiologic/chronologic age.
- End-stage heart disease refractory to medical therapy.
- Functional class III or IV status (NYHA).
- Vigorous healthy individual (except to end-stage cardiac disease) who would benefit from procedure.
- Compliance with medical regimen.
- Demonstrated emotional stability and social support system.
- Financial resource available.

Contraindications

- Systemic disease with poor prognosis.
- Active infection.
- Active or recent malignancy.
- Diabetes mellitus type I, with end-organ damage.
- Recent or unresolved pulmonary infarction.
- Severe pulmonary hypertension unrelieved with medication.
- Severe cerebrovascular or peripheral vascular disease.
- Irreversible renal or hepatic dysfunction.
- Active peptic ulcer disease.
- Severe obesity.
- History of drug or alcohol abuse or mental illness.

Donor's availability is serious problem with cardiac transplantation and the waiting period may be prolonged. As the patient's condition deteriorates, extended hospitalization may be required until a suitable donor can be found. These patients are usually physiologically unstable and may require intensive treatment in a critical care setting because of the need for complex drug therapy, intra-aortic balloon pump therapy or the placement of a ventricular assist device.

Once an individual meets the criteria for cardiac transplantation, the goal of evaluation process is to identify patient who would most benefit from a new heart. In addition to the physical examination, psychological assessment of candidates is valuable. A complete history of coping abilities, family support system and motivation to follow through with the transplant and the rigorous transplantation regimen is essential. The complexity of the transplant process may be overwhelming to patient with inadequate support system, and poor understanding of the lifestyle changes required after transplant.

Once potential recipients are placed on the transplant list, they may wait at home and receive ongoing medical care if their medical condition is stable. If their condition is not stable, they require hospitalization for more intensive therapy.

Potential candidates for heart transplants are usually less than 60 years of age and are free of systematic illness or diseases in other organs systems that would limit their changes for long-term survival. Donor and recipient matching is based on body and heart size and ABO type. Tissue crossmatching between donor and recipient generally are not done because of difficulty in obtaining good matches and lack of correlation between match and outcome. Do not match ABO blood group compatibility, negative lymphatic crossmatch and avoidance of a CMV+ve (cytomegalovirus positive) donor if the recipient is CMV+ve. HLA screening is not usually performed and has not proven benefit in light of the scarcity of the donor.

Management

Most donor hearts are obtained at sites distant from the institution performing the transplant. The maximum acceptable ischaemic time for cardiac transplant is 4 to 6 hours.

The recipient is prepared for surgery and cardiopulmonary bypass is used. Heart transplant surgery consists of the removal of the diseased heart (leaving the posterior walls of the recipient, atria to spare the sinoatrial node), followed by anastomosis of the atria, aorta, and pulmonary arteries. The usual surgical procedure involves removing the recipient's heart, except for the posterior right and left atrial walls and their venous connections. The recipient's heart is then replaced with the donor heart, which has been trimmed to match. Care is taken to preserve the integrity of the donor sinoatrial (SA) node so that a sinus rhythm may be achieved postoperatively.

Immunosuppressive therapy usually begins while the recipient is in the operating room. Regimens vary but they usually include azathioprine, corticosteroids, cyclosporine. The patient who undergoes heart transplant receives care similar to that of any patient having open heart surgery. A healthy donor heart usually functions well and the patient's cardiac output stabilizes. Dysr-hythmias are common. The initial postoperative period and hypervolaemia can result from fluid replacement and high-dose corticosteroid therapy. These complications are managed with the same treatments used other cardiac patients. Critical care placement is usually maintained until the patient's condition stabilizes.

There may be possibility of either acute or chronic rejection of endometrial biopsy being performed to confirm the presence of rejection. The potential signs and symptoms of acute rejection of heart transplant includes:

- Fluid retention, peripheral oedema, crackles, jugular vein distention, S_3 gallop.
- Pericardial friction rub.
- ECG changes; dysrhythmias and decreased voltage.
- Decreased cardiac output.
- Hypotension.
- Cardiac enlargement.
- Fever, lethargy, dyspnoea and decreased tolerance of exercises.

The patient showing signs of rejection may be treated with increasing doses of immunosuppressive agents. Additionally, methylprenisolane boluses, lymphocytic immunoglobulin or OKT_3 may be given.The patient needs considerable support during rejection episodes because of the potentially life-threatening nature of rejection and the anxiety associated with the threat of losing the new heart.

Chronic rejection is insidious and is characterized by graft altherosclerosis, which can result in myocardial ischaemia, MI, or cardiac failure. The ischaemia and infarction may not be associated with pain because the transplanted heart is denervated. No effective treatment exists to stop the chronic rejection process or the associated atherosclerosis. Treatment focuses on intervention to improve cardiac function until another heart becomes available.

Since the patient is immunosuppressed, nursing management should involve prevention of infections, which is leading cause of death in this transplant recipient. Nursing care involves a great deal of emotional support and teaching of both patient and the family, because transplantation is the last resort. Preparation for discharge involves the same teaching as discussed for the kidney transplant recipient. Health care measures to improve cardiac fitness, particularly exercises, are reviewed. Patients who have had long waits for donor hearts may have become virtually immobilized before surgery, and they need to vary gradually increase their activity and fitness. The patient and family must understand the plan for repeat cardiac catheterization with biopsies and the timing intervals for these monitoring tests.

LIVER TRANSPLANT

The first human liver transplant was performed in 1963, at the University of Colorado by Thomas Starzl. The procedure has since become a therapeutic option for both adults and children with liver failure. It improves the quality of life for end-stage liver patients and is an accepted treatment modality for those patients.

Indications

Indications for liver transplantation include, congenital bilary abnormalities, inborn errors of metabolism, hepatic malignancy, (confined to the liver), sclerosing cholangitis and chronic end-stage liver disease. Liver transplant is used to treat biliary atresia, fulminant hepatic failure, cirrhosis, hepatitis, metabolic disorders, and primary hepatic malignancy. Cirrhosis of the liver, primarily as a result of hepatitis viruses, is major indication for transplantation in adults. Liver transplants are not recommended for the patient with widespread malignant disease.

Bilirubin concentration is greater than 10 mg/dl., a serum albumin concentration is less than 2.5 mg/dl and a prothrombin time is greater than seconds beyond the control value are clinical features predictive of the need for liver transplant. Other criteria include incapacitating encephalopathy, recurrent variceal bleeding not controlled by scleropathy intractibic ascitis that does not respond to diuretic therapy, or paracentesis, and recurrent bacterial peritonitis.

Management

A liver transplant takes 8 to 12 hours and involves the removal of the recipient's diseased liver followed by implantation of the donor liver allograft. The diseased liver is removed enbloc. A venovenous bypass system may be used to allow normal haemodynamic values to be maintained while the recipient is without a liver. This bypass system helps prevent venous hypertension, circulatory instability and excessive bleeding. The liver transplant procedure is most technically complex of the solid organs because of the intricate vascular and biliary anastomoses that are required.

The major postoperative complications include rejection, infection and occlusion of vessels. The liver is less susceptible to acute rejection than the kidneys, but adequate immunosuppressive therapy is still primary concern. The extensive nature of the surgery and the patient preoperative and liver failure combine to significantly increase the risk of postoperative complication. Cyclosporine is an effective immunosuppressive drug in these cases. Azathiaprine, corticosteroids, OKT_3 are also useful. Other factors in the improved success rate are advances in surgical techniques, better selection of potential recipients and improved management of the underlying disease before surgery.

The patient who had had a liver transplant requires competent and highly-skilled nursing care, either in ICU or in some other specialized unit. Postoperative nursing care includes assessing neurologic status; monitoring signs for haemorrhage preventing pulmonary complications monitoring drainage, electrolytes, and urinay output; and monitoring signs and symptoms of rejection. Constant monitoring of the patient's haemodynamic status and liver function tests including serum transminases, bilirubin, albumen, clotting factors, often show improvement within 24 hours, if a complication does not occur. Immunosuppressive therapy is started before surgery and continued on a regular schedule after the procedure. Worsening liver function, fever, swelling, and tenderness of the liver are all warning signals of a complication. Infection is crucial concern and can be bacterial (gram-negative), viral (HSV-1, VZV, CMV, EBV) or fungal (*C. abbicans* and others Aspergillus fumigatus, Cryptococcus neoformans) and parasites like pneumocytis carinii and toxoplasma gondi.

Common respiratory problems are pneumonia, atelectasis and pleural effusions. The nurse should have the patient use measures such as cough in deep breathing, incentive spirometry, and repositioning to prevent these complications. Drainage from the Jackson-Pratt drain, NG tube, and T-tube should be measured and the colour and consistency of drainage are noted. A critical aspect of nursing care following liver transplantation is monitoring for infection. The first 2 months after the surgery are critical. Fever may be the only sign of infection. Emotional support and teaching the patient and family are essential.

Preparation for discharge involves the same teaching discussed for the kidney transplant recipient. In addition, the patient with alcohilic cirrhosis is counselled that the ongoing involvement with the chemical dependency program is an essential strategy to prevent relapse.

LUNG TRANSPLANTATION

Lung transplantation has evolved as a viable therapy for patients with end-stage lung disease. Improved selection criteria, technical advances, in the methods of immunosuppression have resulted in improved survival rates.

Indications

A variety of pulmonary disorders are potentially treatable with some type of lung transplantation. Indications for lung transplantation include:

- Emphysema.
- α1-Antitrypsin deficiency.
- Idiopathic pulmonary fibrosis.
- Interstitial lung disease.
- Cystic fibrosis.
- Bronchiectasis.
- Pulmonary fibrosis secondary to other diseases (e.g. Sarcoidosis).
- Congenital heart disease with Eisenmenger's complex.

Transplant Options

Various transplant options are available including single-lung transplant, bilateral-lung transplant, heart-lung transplant, and living related lung transplant.

Signle-lung transplantation has been used for restrictive lung disease because decreased compliance and increased pulmonary resistance of the recipient remaining lung results in preferential ventilation and perfusion of the transplanted lungs. Double-lung transplants are typically used in persons with emphysema or cystic fibrosis.

Single-lung transplants are performed through an anterolateral thorocotomy. Some patients require cardiopulmonary bypass, especially those patients with primary pulmonary hypertension. The double-lung transplant procedure has been modified to a bilateral single-lung transplant procedure with individual bronchial anastomoses. Cardiopulmonary bypass is required in the double-lung transplant procedure. When heart-lung procedure are performed with the use of cardiopulmonary bypass, the recipient's heart is first removed and the chronic nerves are isolated. Enough left atrium is removed to allow the donor's right lung to fit into the right pleural space. The lungs are then removed individually by dividing the inferior pulmonary ligaments and transecting the pulmonary hiral structure. The donor heart-lung block is placed into the recipient chest and tracheal anastomesis is completed.

Management

The patient is placed in an intensive care unit after surgery. The most important aspects of care is promoting adequate airway clearance and gas exchange and instituting care to prevent poor gas exchange in a common complication and may be caused by reperfusion oedema of the lung, impaired cough, infections or rejection. Appropriate immunosuppressive therapy is initiated and the patient is monitored closely for rejection.

Infection is an early pulmonary postoperative complications of lung transplantation, initially patient experiences a shallow breathing pattern and difficulty in clearing secretions secondary to denervation of the lung below the trachea, with a resultant decrease in mucociliary clearance and lymphatic drainage. Infection in the transplant recipient is the most significant cause of morbidity and death. The immunosuppressive is necessary to prevent rejection and it makes the recipient susceptible to entering pathogens, including bacterial, viral and fungal and protozoal organisms. Infections are primarily pulmonary and are usually either nosocomial or opportunistic in nature. Aggressive pulmonary clearance measures, including aerosolized bronchodilators, chest physiotherapy, and deep breathing and coughing techniques are necessary to minimize potential complication.

Acute rejection of lung transplants is commonly seen within the first 3 months after transplantation and symptoms include dyspnoea, low grade fever, tachypnoea and chest X-ray findings ranging from infiltrates to consolidation. Treatment of rejection consists of administration of IV methyl prednisolone. One difference in the immunosuppressive regimen for lung transplants is that corticosteroids are not used for the first 7 to 14 days after the transplant. Corticosteroids jeopardize the healing of the tracheal and bronchial anastomosis; therefore, OKT_3 is used instead. Once healing has occurred, immunosuppressive therapy with corticosteroids is initiated.

Bronchiolitis onliterans (obstructive defect that affect the airways, causing progressive occlusion) is the primary manifestation of chronic rejection in lung transplant patients. The onset usually is at least 6 months after transplant is often subacute, with gradual onset of progressive obstructive airflow defect, including enough, dyspnoea, and recurrent lower respiratory tract infection. There is no effective treatment for bronchiolitis obliterans.

Aggressive respiratory care is critical. It is difficult for the patient to clear the airway because the transplanted lung (or lungs) is denervated below the level of the trachea and mucociliary clearance is decreased. Care includes frequent position changes and deep breathing along with postural drainage and coughing. Supplemental oxygen is necessary. The patient with a lung transplant is prone to cardiovascular complication from hypervolaemia or hypovolaemia, myocardial irritability, or decreased contractility. Haemodynamic status is carefully managed to maintain adequate cardiac output without fluid overload that can lead to pulmonary oedema and an elevation in pulmonary vascular resistance. The patient is at risk for dysrhythmias because of the use of cardiopulmonary bypass.

The use of anticoagulants with cardiopulmonary bypass or excessive replacement of blood products puts the patient at risk for bleeding from coagulopathy. Careful monitoring of coagulation studies and blood loss from mediastenum tubes are imperative. Administration of platelets or fresh frozen plasma may be necessary. Additional care needs including nutritional support, comfort measures and promotion of adequate sleep.

Transbronchial biopsies can provide valuable information by helping differentiate among infections, rejection, and lung injury. As with other solid organ transplants, treatment of rejection involves enhancement of immunosuppression.

Preparation for discharge involves the same teaching discussed for the kidney transplant recipient. The importance of adherence to the regimen and regular follow-up are stressed. Any untoward occurrences should be reported needs further investigation and follow-up importance, taught to patient before discharge. Patients are discharged with portable spirometry device to monitor their own pulmonary function.

PANCREAS TRANSPLANTATION

Since the diabetes is the leading cause of end-stage renal disease, pancreas transplants are being performed with increasing frequency and a marked improvement in overall outcomes. Simultaneously transplantation of both the kidneys and pancreas (KP) from the same donor into a patient with type 1 diabetes mellitus and end-stage renal disease.

Indication

The goals of pancreas transplantation are to elimination of the need for exogenous insulin and dietary restriction and to prevent or stabilize the microvascular and neuropathic complications of diabetes. The recipient eligibility criteria for KP transplantation are similar to those kidney transplantations except the age range is more restricted at 18 to 45 years and cardiovascular clearance. It is generally agreed that pancreas transplantation should be offered to a select group of patients who are at low to moderate cardiac risk, highly motivated, and well-informed about the benefits and risks associated with procedure. The risk includes greater morbidity and increased rate of acute rejection and an increased risk of cardiac death.

Management

In the combined KP transplant the recipients own pancreas are left in place and continues to perform its exocrine functions while the transplanted pancreas provide endocrine function. The donor pancreas is placed intraperitoneally in the pubic area. Most centers use a bladder drainage technique to handle the exocrine juices from the donor pancreas. The head of the donor pancreas is anastomosed to the dome of the recipient's bladder with a segment of the donor's duodenum. The donor kidney is placed in the iliac fossa.

The KP transplant recipient has nursing care needs similar to those of any patient after extensive abnormal surgery. Blood glucose levels are monitored closely in the immediate postoperative period as an indicator of graft perfusion. Increasing glucose levels during this time may indicate graft dysfunction as a result of thrombosis, metabolic acidosis may also occur, from the loss of bicarbonate in the exocrine pancreatic juices that are eliminated in the urine. Supplemental sodium bicarbonate may be added to the patient's intravenous infusions or may be administered orally. The extradigestive juices and fluids that are excreted in the urine account for an additional 1000 to 1500 ml of fluid output daily. Consequently, fluid replacement must be adjusted to compensate for these additional losses. The KP recipient may need to drink more than 5 litres of fluid daily to prevent fluid deficits. Changes in kidney function precede signs of rejection and an increase in serum creatinine in an important warning sign. Reversal rejection in the kidney is always associated with preservation of pancreas graft function well.

Many patients find it difficult to maintain an adequate fluid intake because they are so accustomed to the fluid restrictions of dialysis, and they do not have a normal response to thirst. Some patients are discharged from the hospital with venous excess device in place for home intravenous fluid administration. One to two litres of fluid can be administered at night to ensure an adequate fluid balance. In most patients, the exocrine juices produced by the pancreas and excreted in urine significantly decrease after the first 2 months. The patient can then discontinue IV supplementation and maintain fluid balance with oral intake alone. Before discharge, it is critical that KP transplant, recipients be instructed in the signs and symptoms of dehydration including a decrease in weight, dizziness (especially with position changes) increased pulse rate, and generalized weakness. All KP transplant recipients must also be alert to signs and symptoms of metabolic acidosis including weakness anorexia, nausea and vomiting.

If a bladder drainage procedure is used, the patient is also instructed to monitor the urine pH with a dipstick to detect early signs of pancreas rejection. If the patient's vision is impaired, a family member or significant other is taught how to perform test.

BONE MARROW TRANSPLANTATION (BMT)

Bone marrow transplantation (BMT) is used to treat a wide variety of malignant and non-malignant disorders.

Indication

BMT are used for patients with leukaemia, i.e. AML (acute myelogenous leukoaemia, ALL (Acute-lymphocytic leukaemia) and CML (chronic myelogenous leukaemia, lymphomas, and selected solid tumour (malignant). Non-malignant diseases requiring BMT include immunological deficiency disease, aplastic anaemia, and thalassaemia.

In leukaemia, the goal of transplant is to totally eliminate leukaemic cells from the body using combination of chemotherapy with or without total body irradiation. This treatment also eradicates the patient haematopoeitic stem cells, which are then replaced with those of an HLA-matched sibling or volunteer donor (allogenic) with those of identical twin (syngenieic) or with the patients own (autologous) stem cells that were removed (harvested) before the intensive therapy (Bone marrow and peripheral stem cell transplant).

Donors

There are three types of bone marrow donors: (1) *aloogenic:* the use of marrow from an HLA—matched donor; (2) *Syngeneic:* from an identical twin; (3) *autologous:* in which patients serve as their own donors.

The type and extent of disease are the primary determinants of a patient's eligibility for BMT. The risk of relapse after transplantation is reduced if BMT is performed in patients whose disease is in complete remission or those who have minimal residual diseases at the time of transplantation. Additional eligibility criteria include age, the lack of pre-existing organ toxicity or comorbid conditions, and the availability of a suitable marrow donor.

Management

In preparation of BMT, the recipient undergoes intensive chemoradiotherapy to eradicate residual disease, make space in the recipient's marrow for donor cell engraftment, and establish immunosuppression to prevent the rejection of donor marrow in allogenic transplants.

Bone marrow from cells capable of engraftment can be obtained from peripheral blood, foetal liver tissue, foetal umblical cord blood, cadavers, or the sternum or pelvis of a live donor. Most autologous or allogenic bone marrow is obtained by multiple needle aspirations from the posterior iliac crests with the donor under general or spinal anaesthesia. The amount of marrow extracted ranges from 600 to 2500 ml. Complications of bone marrow donation include bruising, bleeding, pain at aspiration sites, infection, transient neuropathies and hypotension secondary to volume loss.

After processing, the marrow is given to the recipient intravenously frozen –140°C or cryopreserved at –196°C and kept for 3 years or more. The bone marrow reinfusion process is technically similar to blood transfusion and takes 2 to 4 hours. The recipient is hydrated with intravenous fluids containing sodium bicarbonate before and after marrow infusion. This ensures adequate renal perfusion and urine alkalinization if red cell haemolysis occurs as a result of incompatibility or trauma. All BMT recipients can expect a red tinge to that urine for upto 12 hours after marrow infusion because of mild intravascular red cell lysis.

The recipient is closely monitored during reinfusion. Many of the common problems seen after transplantation result from the conditioning regimen of radiation and chemotherapy required before transplant. Gastrointestinal complications are the most common problems which include anorexia, nausea, vomiting, diarrhoea, stomatitis and mucositis. Bone marrow suppression can also result in bleeding and infection.

The primary complications of patients with allogenic BMT are graft-versus-host disease (GVHD), relapse of leukaemia especially ALL) and infection (especially interstitial pneumonia). Histocompatibility testing and effective immune suppression are used to prevent or minimize GVHD. Patients can be discharged after BMT when they are afebrile, are able to maintain an adequate oral intake and have met or exceeded specific blood count criteria (Platelet greater than 15000, *boanulocyte* greater than 500 hct 30 per cent. Discharge teaching is similar to kidney transplant. In addition, BMT recipient must be knowledgeable about bleeding precaution and the signs and symptoms of GVHD. Preventing infection is a priority concern.

CORNEA TRANSPLANT

Cornea transplantation is not a life-saving procedure but it has great potential for enhancing quality of life. Most of the visual impairment is resulting from corneal damage. Defective cornea causes blindness.

Indications

The leading causes of corneal damage requiring transplant are keratoconus, Fuch's dystrophy, herpes simplex keratis, pseudophakic hullous keratopathy and chemical burns.

Patients considering cornea transplant must be evaluated for other ocular conditions that can affect visual acuity after transplant. These conditions include strabismus, ambiyopia, retinal disease, glaucoma, and previous cataract surgery. A complete examination of all ocular structures is performed to determine existing conditions that can affect graft survival. The eye is carefully assessed for infection, because corneal transplantation cannot be performed in the presence of infection.

Management

The ideal corneal donor is under the age of 65 years and undergoes enucleation within 6 hours of death. Beyond 6 hours, the supply of glucose in the aqueous humor and endothelium is exhausted and necrosis occurs. In addition, the risk of contamination by bacteria and fungi increases as the interval between death and enucleation lengthens. Donor corneas are usually transplanted within 24 hours, but new preservation methods can extend preservation upto 35 days without significant loss of endothelial cells and ultrastructural integrity.

The type of corneal graft used depends on the depth and size of the damaged area. Corneal transplants or grafts may involve the entire thickness of the cornea (total penetrating), only part of the depth of the cornea (lamellar), or a combination of these, in which the small part of the graft involves the entire thickness of the cornea (partial penetrating). The penetrating graft establishes least well and the surgeon seldom uses a donor eye that is more than 48 hours old.

The patient is permitted out of bed after recovery from the anaesthetic. Discharge takes place within 2 to 4 days. The eye is covered with a sterile pad, and a metal or plastic shield is placed over the pad for extra protection. The patient continues to wear the shield at night for several weeks. Cornea grafts heal very slowly because of the lack of blood vessels in the cornea and require 3 to 6 months for complete healing.

Patient teaching includes instruction about medication and assessment of graft rejection. Patients are usually discharged on cycloplegic, steroid and sulfa eye drops.

Because of the cornea is normally avascular, the recipient immune cells are not exposed to the cornea, and thus immunosuppressive therapy is not required. However, patients are instructed to check graft rejection daily for the rest of their lives. The eye is checked at the same time each day for redness; an increase in redness, irritation or discomfort; a decrease in vision. Any symptoms that persist or increase in severity in a 24 hours period should be reported to the surgeon.

Many persons expect to have their vision restored immediately after the graft. Vision, however, is sometimes poor while the suture remains in place. Once the sutures are removed, vision usually improves remarkably. The sutures may remain in place for at least one year and the patient is evaluated monthly during that time.

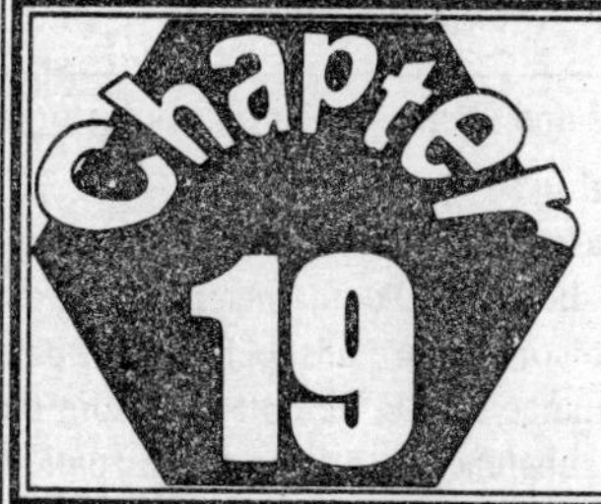

Nursing the Poisoned Client

INTRODUCTION

Poisoning is a major halth problem in the universe resulting in long term disability, major expenditure in health care money and manpower and even death. The causes of poisoning are continually changing due to proliferation of new chemicals and drugs, the reformulation of household products, environmental contamination, as well as to a variety of socio-economic factors such as the stability of the nuclear family, dual career families, job related stress, an aging society, cost containment of health care and a yriad of other factors that may influence that indivudally daily environment. Health care professionals must appreciate the factors that interplay in the problem as a whole, to improve readiness and heighten awareness to deal with this complex issue. The "poisoning" problem requires a multi-disciplinary team approach to manage a diverse set of issues ranging from prevention of poisoning accidents in the home to supporting a critically ill poisoned patient in the intensive care unit. Nursing professionals have played an integral role poisoning and still needs to have an understanding of terminology, resources, assessment, pathophysiology and treatment concept for poisoning is important to enhance the delivery of adequate and appropriate care to the poisoned patient.

Table 19.1: Poisoning exposure: Terminology

Poisoning exposure: Any suspected contact with any substance which when ingested, inhaled, absorbed, applied to, injected into, or developed within the body may cause damage to the structure or disturbance of function to living tissue.

Duration of Exposure

Acute: A single exposure occurring over a relatively short period of time, usually within a period of 8 hours.

Chronic: A repeated exposure to the same substance, or single exposure lasting longer than 8 hours.

Reasons for Exposure

Accidental: An unintended poisoning exposure; commonly involves situations where children gain access to a toxic substance in the home where it is obvious that they did not realize the potential danger of their actions.

Intentional: Implies a purposeful action with an exposure that results from an inappropriate use of a substance for self-destructive, or manipu-

Contd...

Contd...

lative reasons, such as a suicide gesture; ro the improper use of a substance in an attempt to gain a psychotropic effect.

Adverse reaction: An unexpected reaction to a drug, food, or other agent; or the patient experiences an unwanted effect, which is usually due to either an allergic, hypersensitive, or idiosyncratic response at a normal dose, or with normal use of a substance.

Routes of Exposure

Oral: Exposures to substances occurred because they were ingested into the gastrointestinal tract.

Inhalation: Exposure to gascous or vaporized agents into the airways and lungs.

Ocular: Due to substances splashed directly into the eye.

Dermal: Contact with substances that may involve the skin, hair, fingernails, and clothing where direct irritation or percutaneous absorption may occur.

Bites or stings: Exposures resulting from the bite or sting of either an animal or insect, such as a bee, wasp, or hornet.

Parenteral route: An exposure resulting from the injection of a substance into teh body, such as the intravenous administratioan of heroin.

Table 19.2: Common categories of substances involved in poisonings

Substance	*Ranking: % of Total Number of Poisonings*
Cleaning substances Household bleach, ammonia, cleansers, washing and laundry detergents.	9.5%
Plants Within home, in the yard, or in the wild.	8.3
Cosmetics and personal care products Mouthwashes, aftershaves, colognes, perfumes, shampoos, nail polish.	5.8
Bites and envenomations Snakes, spiders and stinging insects.	3.4
Pesticides and rodenticides Agents to kill rodents and insects in the home.	2.9

Contd...

Contd...

environment; highly concentrated industrial agents used by professional exterminators.	
Pharmaceuticals	40.0
Prescription and nonprescription (over-the-counter) drugs (e.g., aspirin, acetaminophen).	

ASSESSMENT OF THE POISON VICTIM

The assessment of the poison victim entails the solicitation of a poisoning history, the physical examination of the poison patient, response to pharmacologic antagonists, as well as analysis of gastric contents, blood, and urine from the poison victim. It should be noted, especially with intentional exposures (drug abuse or suicide gestures), the agent involved in the poisoning is frequently unknown so that all four components of assessment as listed above, must be considered collectively.

History

Often the initial contact with the poisoning will be from the site of the exposure when either the victim or the person managing the poison victim calls either a poison center, hospital, outpatient clinic, or other emergency service. Obtaining a complete and accurate poisoning history will be necessary to assess the immediacy of the situation and the toxic potential of the exposure, to identify medical treatments needed for the poison victim to support the patient's hemodynamic and respiratory systems, and to minimize the extent of the exposure. A thorough poison history is essential to triage decision-making for the poisoned patient. In addition, understanding the basic elements of a poison history will enhance the ability of the health-care professional to interface with the poison control center. Table 3 contains key questions and elements of the poison history.

Physical Examination

The physical examination can determine the necessity for immediate supportive care measures and can confirm evidence of the poisoning. Following the physical examination, the findings must be viewed collectively to define a characteristic constellation of symptoms reflective of a particular toxic substance or group of substances. These characteristic constellations of symptoms are known as "toxidromes." For instance, anticholinergic poisoning from an agent such as atropine will cause a characteristic set of symptoms. A device to remember this toxidrome is: The patient with atropine poisoning will be "dry as a bone," "mad as a hatter," "red as a beet," and "blind as a bat." Table 4 lists the physical finding on examination and the possible corresponding etiologic agents for each listed finding.

Table 19.3: Elements of a poison history

The following include basic questions and elements of a poison history:

1. What was involved in the poisoning?
This information may be difficult to ascertain because the substance involved in the poisoning may not be in the original container, products are frequently reformulated, and many poisonings are unsupervised. If possible, information regarding the substance should be obtained from the label on the container from which the substance was derived. Any patient transported to a hospital should be accompanied by the container with the substance involved in the poison incident.

At the site of exposure, it should be noted whether other substances could have been available to the poisoning victim, any evidence of open medicine containers and household products, or if there were any characteristic smells or odors.

2. Who was involved in the poisoning?
Characteristics of the poisoning victims such as age, weight, and past medical history are important components of the poisoning history. Poisonings involving older children, teenagers, and adults are more likely to be the result of an intentional exposure, in comparison with a victim less than 5 years of age. Weight can also be helpful because, for many toxins, the dose of the toxin in relation to the weight of the patient can be calculated to provide an expected range of toxicity.

3. When did the poisoning occur?
Knowing when the poisoning occurred helps to establish a causal relationship between a poison exposure and symptoms the patient is manifesting, as well as predicting upcoming symptomatology.

4. Where did the poisoning occur?
Knowing where the poisoning occurred is especially important for children, to assist with the determination of what product was involved. For instance, a child found in the bathroom may have access to a set of substances normally found in that aréa of the home such as toilet bowl cleaners, bleaches, medications in the medicine cabinet, versus a poisoning occurring in the yard, or the garage, where substances such as automotive products, pesticides, or garden care products are available.

5. How much of the substance was involved in the poisoning?
This question is important especially when a substance has been ingested. This can provide an estimation of the dose of a toxin that a victim was exposed to, which will allow an estimation of the toxic potential of the poisoning incident.

6. What was the route or routes of exposure?
In addition to ingestions, poisons may also be inhaled, come in direct contact with the eye, splashed on the skin, or be rejected. There are a significant number of poisons that do involve multiple routes of exposure. Each route of exposure requires a specialized decontamination procedure. Also, for each route, those tissues exposed to a toxin may incur direct injury, or may become a route of administration for systemic absorption.

7. What symptoms has the patient had?
Is the patient conscious? Is the patient breathing? Does the patient have a pulse? Are the symptoms likely to be related to the exposure?

8. What was the reason for exposure?
It is important to differentiate between an accidental versus an intentional exposure. As previously noted, many intentional exposures involve multiple drugs, have worse outcomes in terms of morbidity and mortality, and are often accompanied by inaccurate or incomplete histories. Therefore, they may require more aggressive therapy and monitoring.

Contd...

Contd...

9. What first aid has been performed?
It is important to determine whether or not the patient has had an adequate decontamination procedure performed. Many first-aid procedures can complicate the poisoning, such as the use of salt water as an emetic in children, which has resulted in fatalities due to hypernatremia.

10. What current medications is the patient on?
The substances involved in a poisoning may interact with another medication that a patient is chronically administered for a therapeutic purpose. For example, a patient taking an MAO inhibitor who ingests a therapeutic dose of a sympathomimetic or decongestant, such as phenylpropanolamine, could develop a life-threatening hypertensive crisis.[8]

11. What allergies does the patient have?
Some patients are at risk for hypersensitivity reactions to medications, chemicals, and venoms. A patient who has previously been exposed and sensitized to hymenoptera venom may be at greater risk for an acute anaphylactic reaction when stung by a honey bee, wasp, or hornet.

12. What other chronic disease states does the patient have?
Many times, patients with chronic disease states will be at higher risk for severe toxicity to exposures of certain substances. For instance, elderly patients with cardiovascular disease are more sensitive to the effects of and respond poorly to, exposures to carbon monoxide.[9,10]

13. What is the race of the poison victim?
A poison victim with an enzyme deficiency such as a G6PD deficiency, will be at greater risk for an acute hemolytic episode after ingestion of a mothball containing naphthalene than a patient without this enzyme deficiency. It has been determined that certain populations such as blacks, or those of Mediterranean origin, have a higher incidence of this enzyme deficiency.[12]

Laboratory Studies

The laboratory can be a useful adjunct to the other forms of assessment. Qualitative screening tests for drugs and other substances are routinely run on urine samples. Quantitative tests are performed on blood, serum, or plasma samples. Analysis of gastric contents may allow the clinician to determine what was acutely ingested and to confirm exposure to a drug or chemical in some cases before significant systemic absorption has occurred. In some circumstances, a quantitative analysis of substances from the blood of the patient, such as methanol, ethylene glycol, acetaminophen, salicylate, iron, lead, arsenic, and mercury, may be necessary to determine if the substances are at toxic levels in the patient, and if the patient will require specialized therapies. For most other substances, a toxicology analysis is only necessary as confirmatory evidence of the substances ingested. It is of extreme importance to understand what toxicology tests are performed by your institution, as well as the turn around time for their results.

X-ray Examination

An x-ray (radiograph) of the poison patient can provide an assessment of secondary complications from a poisoning episode, such as using a chest x-ray to determine if aspiration has occurred, or using an abdominal x-ray to determine the presence of a radiopaque substance in the gastrointestinal tract. Radiopaque substances may include agents such as chloral

Table 19.4: Expected physical and laboratory findings for poisonous substances

Finding	*Substance*
Blood Pressure	
Hypotension	Sedative-hypnotics (barbiturates, glutethimide), theophylline, iron, cyclic antidepressants, antihypertensives (Aldomet, clonidine)
Hypertension	Amphetamines, cocaine, phencyclidine, anticholinergics (atropine), black widow spider venon.
Respirations	
Slowed rate-apnea	Opiates, alcohols, sedative-hypnotics
Hyperpnea, tachypnea	Salicylates, theophylline, dinitrophenol, CNS stimulants.
Electrocardiogram (ECG)	
Bradyarrhythmia	Beta-blockers, clonidine, organophosphate insecticides, calcium channel blockers (verapamil)
Tachyarrhythmias	Amphetamines, cocaine, caffeine, theophylline, anticholinergics (atropine), cyclic antidepressants, nicotine
Conduction defects (PR, QRS, QT prolongation)	Cyclic antidepressants, quinidine, arsenic, mercury, propoxyphene, propranolol.
Temperature	
Hyperthermia	Salicylates, amphetamine, cocaine, anticholinergics, dinitrophenol, phencyclidine
Hypothermia	Opiates, ethanol, sedative-hypnotics, phenothiazines.
Pupils	
Miosis	Organophosphate insecticides, phenothiazines, chloral hydrate, clonidine, sedative-hypnotics, opiates
Mydriasis	Anticholinergics, cyclic antidepressants, cocaine, LSD, amphetamine
Nystagmus	Phenytoin, barbiturates, phencyclidine.
Bowel Sounds	
Increased	Organophosphate insecticides, sympathomimetics
Decreased	Anticholinergics (atropine, cyclic antidepressants), sedative-hypnotics.
Muscular System	
Muscle tremor	Amphetamines, cocaine, caffeine, theophylline, lithium, alcohol and sedative-hypnotic withdrawal
Muscle flaccid/paralysis	Opiates, clonidine, sedative-hypnotics, botulism.
Muscular System	
Muscle rigidity	Strychnine, tetanus, phencyclidine, haloperidol, methaqualone, phenothiazines.

Contd...

Contd...

Fasciculations	Organophosphate insecticides, nicotine, lithium, phencyclidine
Myoclonus	Cyclic antidepressants, carbamazepine, phenytoin, methaqualone
Integumentary System	
Dry skin	Anticholinergics, vitamin A
Sweaty skin (diaphoresis)	Organophosphate insecticides, nicotine, sympathomimetics
Cyanosis (slate-blue discolorations)	Methemoglobin producers (nitrates, phenazopyridines, aniline)
Alopecia	Thallium, antineoplastic agents
Fingernails (Mees-Aldrich lines; transverse leukonychia)	Arsenic, thallium
Acid-Base Disorders	
Respiratory acidosis	Sedative-hypnotics, opiates
Metabolic acidosis	Salicylates, methanol, paraldehyde, iron, isoniazed, ibuprofen, ethanol, ethylene glycol, carbon monoxide, cyanide
Respiratory alkalosis	Salicylates
Metabolic alkalosis	Sodium bicarbonate

hydrate, heavy metals (i.e., lead, arsenic, mercury, iron), iodide, phenothiazines, cyclic antidepressants, enteric-coated tablets, solvents, and other miscellaneous foreign objects, such as disk batteries, or coins. The x-ray can be used to localize the substance ingested to assist with retrieval from the GI tract.

Diagnostic Trials

The administration fo certain pharmacologic antagonists or antidotes as presumptive therapy, such as naloxone therapy for a suspected narcotic overdose in a comatose patient, may be an extremely useful diagnostic tool in a poisoned patient. If a patient responds to this presumptive therapy (awakens after administration of naloxone), then this becomes a key diagnostic element in the assessment of the poisoned patient. However, a few toxins are antagonized by pharmacologic "antidotes." A list of the more commonly used pharmacologic antagonists with their respective uses is provided on Table 5.

Table 19.5: Pharmacological antagonists used in poisoning

Agent	*Uses*
Antivenin	
(Crotalidae) polyvalent	Pit viper snake bites (rattlesnakes, water moccasins, copperheads)
(Latrodectus mactans)	Black widow spider bites
(Micrurus fulvius)	Coral snake bites
Atropine	Organophosphate and carbamate insecticide poisonings
Calcium gluconate	Calcium-channel blocker (verapamil) poisonings, hydrofluoric acid burns

Contd...

Contd...

Cyanide antidote kit (amyl nitrite, sodium nitrite, sodium thiosulfate)	Cyanide poisonings
Deferoxamine	Iron poisoning
Dimercaprol (BAL)	Arsenic, gold, lead and mercury poisoning
Diphenhydramine	Phenothiazine and butyrophenone-induced dystonias
Edetate calcium disodium (EDTA)	Lead poisoning
Ethanol	Ethylene glycol and methanol poisoning
Fab fragments (Digibind)	Digoxin and digitoxin poisoning
Glucagon	Beta-blocker (propranolol) poisoning
Methylene blue	Drug and chemical-induced methemoglobinaemias
N-Acetylcysteine	Acetaminophen poisoning
Naloxone	Opiate poisoning
Physostigmine	Anticholinergic poisoning
Pralidoxime	Organophosphate insecticide poisoning
Pyridoxine	Isoniazid, hydrazine-containing mushrooms

Pathophysiology and Mechanisms of Toxicity

The mechanisms for toxicity of many toxins are quite varied in nature and involve complex imbalances of physiologic systems. The morbidity and mortality secondary to poisons are often attributed not to the direct mechanism of toxicity of a substance, but to secondary complications from the poisoning, especially those involving the respiratory system. For instance, many sedative-hypnotics may cause a loss of consciousness and the gag reflex in the patient. This may predispose the patient to aspiration of gastric contents, which can result in an aspiration pneumonitis. In addition, patient's who have been either unconscious for a prolonged period of time, develop seizures, or who have suffered crush injuries may be predisposed to destruction of muscle cells resulting in rhabdomyolysis. This releases myoglobin into the urine and may result in acute renal failure.

It is important to realize that any substance could be potentially toxic at a given dose. The famous 15th century Swiss physician and alchemist, Paracelsus, provided a definition of poison: "All substances are poisons; there is none which is not a poison. The right dose differentiates a poison and a remedy." A substance such as table salt may be used on a daily basis without causing any difficulty, but in larger amounts it could result in fatal hypernatremia. In the assessment of acute human poisonings it is best to obtain, if available, the minimum toxic dose of a substance. These are usually derived from individual case histories of poisonings, or case series of poisonings, and may not be available for a wide variety of substances.

Some poisons mediate their toxic effects directly, while others mediate through the production of toxic metabolites, as is the case with methanol, ethylene glycol, and acetaminophen. Poisons may cause immediate effects or damage such as with exposures to alkaline corrosives, resulting in a liquefaction necrosis of tissue within seconds of contact, while others may be delayed in their effects, such as with exposures to the herbicide, paraquat, which can result in pulmonary fibrosis 1-2 weeks following contact. Also, the duration of exposure has a bearing on the toxic potential of many agents in the overall outcome of the poisoning. This is exemplified by chronic salicylism due to repeated intake of high doses of aspirin over a period of days associated with a higher incidence of severe symptoms and death than acute salicylism due to a one-time ingestion.

The following is a list of seven categories of mechanisms of actions of the most common toxic agents. It should be noted that this is not an all-inclusive list and that certain substances may mediate their effects by multiple mechanisms.

1. *Direct surface or cellular injury*—This may be exemplified by agents that cause denaturation of proteins or cellular necrosis upon surface contact. These may include the caustic acids and alkalis or snake and hymenoptera venoms, which mediate their efforts through enzymatic degradation or digestion of tissue.
2. *Enzyme inhibitors*—Most heavy metals, such as arsenic, lead, and mercury, mediate their toxic effects by binding sulfhydryl groups of enzymes, thereby inhibiting enzyme function. Cyanide binds the enzyme cytochrome oxidase, thus inhibiting oxygen utilization and ATP production.
3. *Neurotransmitter potentiation and inhibition*–This is one of the major mechanisms by which various pharmaceutical substances, venoms, and other chemicals mediate their toxic effects. Many effects of these substances can be predicted on the basis of their influence on the autonomic nervous system (the parasympathetic and sympathetic nervous systems; see Chap. 6). The substances may act on one of the following mechanisms:
   a. Blockade of the postsynaptic receptors—The effects of atropine poisoning are mediated by competitive blockade of acetylcholine at muscarinic receptors of the parasympathetic nervous system.
   b. Blocking reuptake of the neurotransmitter into the presynaptic neuron—This results in an excess of the neurotransmitter in the synaptic cleft, and thereby enhances neurotransmission. This is exemplified by the cyclic antidepressants and cocaine. They both result in increased neurotransmission of the sympathetic nervous system by blockade of norepinephrine uptake into the presynaptic neuron.
   c. Increasing the release of the neurotransmitter—Black widow spider venom can cause an increase in the neurotransmitter release in neurons innervating skeletal muscle, resulting in severe neuromuscular symptoms.
   d. Inhibition of the breakdown of the neurotransmitter—This is exemplified by organophosphate pesticides, which inhibit the enzyme acetylcholinesterase, which is responsible for the breakdown of acetylcholine and the termination of neurotransmission. This results in an excess of acetylcholine in the synaptic cleft, which stimulates cholinergic receptors.
   e. The mimicking of the neurotransmitter—This is exemplified by tobacco poisoning through the ingestion of cigarettes. Nicotine is absorbed and can directly stimulate nicotinic receptors of the autonomic nervous system.
   f. Sensitization of the effector tissue to the neurotransmitter—This is exemplified by the effects of halogenated hydrocarbons such as freon. The myocardium may be sensitized to epinephrine after inhalation exposure to freon, which can result in a life-threatening cardiac arrhythmia.
   g. Impaired production of the neurotransmitter—This can be exemplified by isoniazid poisoning, which inhibits the synthesis of GABA (gamma-aminobutyric acid). A decrease in the CNS levels of the inhibitory neurotransmitter, GABA, results in an imbalance of excitatory neuronal activity manifested as seizures in an isoniazid poisoned patient.
   h. Inhibition of release of the neurotransmitter—Botulinum toxin from the bacteria, *Clostridium botulinum*, mediates its effects through inhibition of the release of acetylcholine from the presynaptic neurons that innervate skeletal muscle, resulting in muscular paralysis.
4. *Derangements of metabolic and respiratory processes*—Some toxins compete with normal substrates necessary for respiratory and metabolic processes to produce ATP. This occurs during carbon monoxide poisoning, which has 240 times greater binding affinity for haemoglobin than oxygen, and thus results in oxygen deprivation. Other agents uncouple oxidative phosphorylation, which inhibits ATP production through the electron transport system. Substances such as aspirin and wood preservatives (dinitrophenol) mediate their effects by this mechanism. Patients with poisonings from these agents develop a characteristic hyperthermia because heat is produced as an end-product of metabolism, instead of ATP.
5. *Agents with target organ specificity*—Certain toxins may have a propensity for a particular organ system due to either their avid binding affinity for certain tissues, production of an organ-specific toxic metabolite, or due to the sensitivity of cellular components of an organ system to the toxin. The primary effect of acetaminophen poisoning is hepatocellular damage due to the accumulation of a toxic metabolite within liver cells. The herbicide, paraquat, can result in pulmonary fibrosis, which is often fatal. This may be attributed to the availability of oxygen within pulmonary

tissue, which aids in the production of superoxides and free radicals, resulting in membrane damage and fibrosis of lung tissue.

6. *Alteration fo cellular and/or tissue function*—Some toxins may alter the capability of specialized cells or tissue to perform physiologic functions by inducing structural or chemical alterations. Examples of substances in this category may include a host of methemoglobin producers, which are substances that oxidize the iron core of the hemoglobin molecule from the ferrous (Fe^{+2}) to the ferric form (Fe^{+3}). The newly formed ferric core of methemoglobin is incapable of transporting oxygen, thus rendering a nonfunctional erythrocyte pigment.
7. *Inhibition of anabolic processes*—Some toxins have an effect on cell replication or on the production of various physiologic proteins in the body. These may constitute some of the most toxic agents involved in poisonings. The toxic effects from poisonings with the cyclopeptide mushrooms, of the amanita species, as well as from poisonings of seeds from other plants, such as the castor bean, containing ricin, and the rosary pea, containing abrin, are mediated by inhibition of protein synthesis. This results in severe damage to the liver, kidneys, and in tissues with the highest rate of cell replication, such as the gastrointestinal system.

TREATMENT

In the treatment of the poisoned patient, good, supportive care is of paramount importance and may be most responsible for the decrease in morbidity and mortality secondary to poisonings. Of the supportive care measures, the maintenance of the ABCs (airway, breathing, circulation) is crucial for any severely poisoned patient. Once this has been achieved, then other therapeutic options, such as the use of pharmacologic antagonists, decontamination, and enhancement of elimination, should be considered for the poisoned victim. This discussion will be limited to the decontamination procedures for the poisoned patient.

Decontamination

The general premise for decontamination is to remove the substance involved in the poisoning exposure from the victim to decrease the amount of local tissue damage, as well as limit the amount of the substance absorbed into the body. The decontamination procedure used should be based on the amount of substance involved, its potential for local and systemic toxicity, and the routes of exposure. The routes may include, as previously discussed, the skin, the eye, the lungs, or by ingestion.

Dermal Exposures

Many toxins can cause direct irritation or burns to the skin, as well as be absorbed systemically into the body by this route, which is known as *percutaneous absorption.* For example, a primary route of exposure through the skin is observed with the organophosphate insecticides. Therefore, it is important to decontaminate exposed skin immediately upon exposure to one of these agents to prevent severe systemic toxicity.

In addition, during the decontamination procedure, it is important to protect the decontaminator. Often the persons performing the decontamination may, themselves, become contaminated with the poisonous substance. So, the decontaminator, if using liquid, should wear gloves, an apron, and a mask if necessary when fumes have evolved.

The exposed patient should be washed from head to toe, including the hair and under the nails. Because some agents, such as the organophosphate insecticides, are fat-soluble, they may require special washing solutions, such as tincture of green soap (alcohol-based soap solution), to decontaminate the victim. The patient should be first rinsed with cold water, then with warm water, and finally with hot water. The reason to commence with cold water is to avoid causing peripheral vasodilation, thereby minimizing systemic absorption. It is extremely important to decontaminate a poisoned patient at the site of exposure, rather than "scoop and run." In addition, it is important to remove all clothing from the victim. Certain clothing articles, such as leather products, absorb pesticides and are difficult to decontaminate.

Ocular Exposures

Following ocular exposures to substances, it is important to irrigate the substance from the eye as soon as possible. This should be done, preferably, at the site of exposure. Proper irrigation of the eye or of the affected eye or eyes should consist of a continuous irrigation for a period of at least 15-20 minutes. The irrigation solution may include tap water if at the home, or sterile saline in an emergency room.

Eyedroppers and irrigating syringes are worthless. In the home, the irrigation may be performed on a patient by holding his or her head back over a sink and pouring tap water from a large pitcher, liter bottle, or running faucet at low pressure about 6 inches from the eye. To avoid cross contamination of the eyes, the irrigant should be poured from the bridge of the nose to the outward portion of the eye. Always avoid direct high pressure irrigation. The irrigant can be just poured on the eye, even with children, because the eyes will usually open and close.

In addition, especially in the home setting, it may be useful to wrap a child in a sheet or a towel as a restraint. Other important tips to remember are that the victim should never place any form of medication, such as eyedrops or neutralizers, into an infected eye. Symptoms may not be good indicators of ocular injury, especially in the setting of alkaline corrosive exposures.

Inhalation

Frequently, victims exposed to fumes or gases will also require measures to decrease the amount of exposure and alleviate local irritation. With exposures involving the respiratory tract, measures, such as having the victim breathe fresh air or, in many cases, humidified air, will alleviate local irritation of the mucous membranes and upper airway. If the patient is cyanotic due to asphyxiation or to an impairment of as exchange or delivery of oxygen through the pulmonary system, then oxygen administration to the patient is required. It should be noted that patients exposed to fumes or gases may incur injury to the eyes as well as the upper and lower airways; therefore, it is always important to consider the possibility of multiple routes of exposure, and that the decontamination procedure be targeted towards each route.

Ingestion

The most common route of exposure for poisonings is by ingestion. The approach taken by the clinician to decontaminate the gastrointestinal tract of the poisoned victim has been an issue of ongoing controversy. The premise for GI decontamination is to prevent absorption of a toxin that has a potential for systemic effects. There are many options in the area of gastrointestinal decontamination, such as the induction of emesis, gastric lavage, use of activated charcoal, cathartics, and even in some circumstances, endoscopy and surgery.

Gastrointestinal dilution with water or milk has long been touted as a first-aid procedure for poisonings. This maneuver, if done inappropriately, can complicate a poisoning. For instance, milk used as the dilution fluid may delay the ability to induce emesis with syrup of ipecac, or if a drug has been ingested, oral administration of water may enhance the dissolution of the tablets or capsules, thereby facilitating systemic absorption and possibly resulting in faster onset of toxic effects from the drug. Administration of water is appropriate, though, for a toxic ingestion that produces local tissue irritation or is a caustic. This results in decreasing the contact time between the toxin and the exposed tissue, as well as the concentration of the caustic agent, thereby decreasing the amount or degree of irritation and injury.

The use of neutralizers after acid or alkaline caustic ingestion is not recommended because of the production of heat during the neutralization process. This first-aid charts. A policy statement regarding the gastrointestinal dilution with water as a first-aid procedure in poisoning has been issued by the AAPCC. Their recommendations include the following:

1. Oral dilution with water should *not* be used as a general first-aid measure to treat ingestions of medications.
2. Following the ingestion of a caustic or corrosive substance, the immediate oral administration of water or milk is recommended.
3. Water is the appropriate fluid to administer in conjunction with syrup of ipecac.

It has been demonstrated that the first-aid recommendations on labels of commercial products are often times hazardous, inappropriate, and inaccurate. There are reported cases of patients developing severe toxicity, not from a substance initially involved in the poisoning, but from the first-aid proceduce.

Another modality of therapy is to empty the stomach after ingestion of a poison. Two primary options to accomplish gastric emptying are to induce vomiting or emesis, or with the use of a large-bore orogastric tube to perform gastric lavage. It should be noted that studies assessing the outcome of poisonings have not clearly demonstrated the beneficial effect on patients who are provided gastric-emptying procedures. In fact, many ongoing studies have failed to show a beneficial effect of gastric emptying on the outcome of the poisoned victim. However, it is commonly observed that during these procedures the substance that was ingested is retrieved as evidenced by pill fragments or retrieval of a colored fluid.

In making the decision to perform gastric emptying, the clinician should be cognizant of the pitfalls and contraindications for these procedures, as well as situations in which their use is deemed appropriate. A variety of agents, such as salt water, mustard, and copper sulfate, have been previously used and recommended as emetics in the treatment of poisoning, but most of these are no longer used due to their ineffectiveness or potential hazards associated with their use. Apomorphine, a morphine derivative with central-acting emetic properties, has been considered an effective emetic that produces a rapid onset of emesis. However, this agent has fallen into disuse due to a number of diadvantages: the necessity for parenteral administration, difficulty in preparation of dosage form, its effect on the CNS with the potential for respiratory depression, and its potential ineffectiveness in a patient who has ingested an antiemetic, such as a phenothiazine.

Ipecac syrup, due to its safety, efficacy, and oral route of administration, is considered by most to be the emetic of choice in poisonings. Ipecac is derived from a plant, *Cephaelis ipecacuanha*, and contains a mixture of alkaloids, such as emetine, psychotrine, and cephaeline. Ipecac has both local and central emetic properties. Cardiotoxicity, resulting in fatalities, has been attributed to the use of fluid extract of ipecac, which is 14 times more concentrated than ipecac syrup, and due to chronic abuse (of ipecac syrup) by bulimics. Ipecac syrup is shown to induce emesis in approximately 96% of the patients to whom it was administered, and the onset of emesis will usually occur in 20-30 minutes.

Contraindications to the induction of emesis include those situations in which the risk of pulmonary aspiration in the poisoned patient is high, in the comatose or seizing patient, or after the loss of gag reflex; in which the induction of emesis could precipitate severe gastrointestinal injury, the patient who has ingested a strong acid or base, or solid objects, such as razor blades, or nails; or in patients predisposed to haemorrhagic diathesis, such as patients with cirrhosis and esophageal varices or thrombocytopoenia. As previously noted, removal of the ingested toxin from the GI tract is based on the assertion that there is a significant risk for systemic absorption with significant toxicity once absorbed.

Certain hydrocarbons, such as gasoline, kerosene, or mineral seal oil, may mediate their toxicity primarily through direct aspiration into the lungs (rather than by absorption from the stomach). Therefore, in those settings, it is not advisable to induce vomiting due to the increased risk of aspiration during the procedure, unless the hydrocarbon is aromatic, such as benzene, or halogenated, such as carbon tetrachloride, or is contaminated by another toxic substance, such as a pesticide, because of their potential for systemic absorption and toxicity. Also, due to the delayed onset of emesis with ipecac syrup, an assumption must be made that the clinical status of the patient will not change sufficiently as to contraindicate the induction of emesis during that time period. If substances are ingested that are rapidly absorbed with a fast onset action and that can produce seizures, such as camphor or strychnine, the induction of emesis is not recommended. Other ingestions, such as cyclic antidepressants, may also produce a rapid unpredictable onset of seizures and coma, and, therefore, the induction of emesis in that setting may be hazardous as well.

The other procedure used to empty the stomach is gastric lavage. This requires the use of a large-bore orogastric tube. Lavage should be performed in those situations where induction of emesis with syrup of ipecac is contraindicated, such as the patient who is seizing or comatose. The use of nasogastric tubes to remove contents from the stomach is essentially worthless. The patient must be placed in the left lateral decubitus position, and, if severely obtunded or comatose or if the patient has a loss of teh gag reflex, the airway should be protected with a cuffed endotracheal tube, prior to the lavage procedure. Then a lavage solution, usually saline, in 200-ml aliquots in adults or 10 ml/kg in a child, is instilled into a lavage tube and then removed by aspiration or gravity suction. This should be continued until several liters of lavage fluid have been used or until several liters of lavage fluid have been used or until the lavage fluid is clear. The tube then can be used for the instillation of activated charcoal and cathartic. It should be noted that there are limitations with gastric lavage. Large pill fragments may be unable to travel through the tube, especially those used for children, because of the size of the bore.

Gastric emptying is most effective if performed soon after the poisoning. However, the rate at which a substance is absorbed is quite variable and depends on a variety of patient-related and toxin-related parameters: the presence of food, the patient's intrinsic gastrointestinal motility, the amount of substance ingested, the effect of a substance on gastric emptying time, the time since ingestion, and the physical properties of the substance. Ingestion of substances with anticholinergic properties, which decrease gastric motility and increase gastric emptying time, may be amenable to gastric emptying procedures even a day after ingestion.

Activated charcoal is another useful adjunct to the treatment of poisoning substance that has been provided growing attention and has been identified as the primary line of therapy. Activated charcoal is made from the destructive distillation or burning of organic materials, such as wood, coconut, bones, and rice starch. It is activated by treatment with oxidizing gases such as steam. Activated charcoal, itself, is a fine, black, odorless, and tasteless powder comprised of extremely small and porous particles. This porosity provides a large surface area to adsorb a large quantity of a substance. One gram of activated charcoal has a surface area ranging from 1000-3000 m^2. Substances that are adsorbed by charcoal are those that are unionized and have a large molecular weight. These will include most medications, as well as a wide variety of other chemicals and natural toxins. Other substances poorly adsorbed by activated charcoal include small ionic compounds, such as cyanide and caustic acids or alkalis, or small organic molecules, such as methanol.

Another therapeutic modality used to prevent gastrointestinal absorption of toxins is the administration of cathartics. Cathartics such as magnesium sulfate and citrate, sorbitol, and sodium sulfate have all been used in the treatment of poisonings. It is important that activated charcoal, in most cases, be accompanied by the use of a cathartic to facilitate transport of the charcoal-drug complex. It should also be noted that there is no scientific basis to substantiate the use of cathartics alone. In addition, cathartics are contraindicated and may cause problems in the following situations: small children in whom it may result in fluid and electrolyte imbalances, very old patients, those with preexisting renal disease following the ingestion of nephrotoxic substances and caustics, and patients with recent bowel surgery, absent bowel sounds, hypertension, or congestive heart failrue.

Another method used to decrease absorption of a compound from the gastrointestinal tract is to administer complexation agents, which chemically react with a toxin, resulting in an insoluble, nonabsorbable complex. Examples include the administration of a calcium-containing compound to the patient who has ingested fluoride, which results in an insoluble, neutralized calcium fluoride complex; and the use of bicarbonate for an iron poisoning, where a bicarbonate solution is either administered orally or instilled through a lavage tube following an iron ingestion, which results in the production of insoluble iron salts, such as ferrous carbonate.

Another less frequent mode of removal of a toxic product from the gastrointestinal tract is by endoscopy and/or surgery. Certain products when ingested may either lodge in parts of the gastrointestinal tract or form tenaciously adhering concretions. These are difficult to remove by either lavage or emesis or other methods for GI decontamination and, if left in contact with the GI mucosa, may result in not only systemic absorption, but severe damage to the lining of the gastrointestinal tract. Examples of such substances are: ingestion of iron, especially those with perinatal ferrous sulfate tablets, and disk batteries, both of which can be removed by either endoscopy or surgery.

CASE STUDY WITH SAMPLE CARE PLAN: PATIENT WITH ACUTE POISONING

A 5-year-old boy is brought into the Emergency Department at

6:00 pm by his mother. She is concerned about his "congestion" and sleepiness which began that morning and worsened over the ensuing 9 hours. He was a previously healthy child.

At the triage station of the Emergency Department, it is immediately apparent that the child is obtunded and in respiratory distress. Drooling, stertorous respirations, tachypnea, retraction, and cyanosis were also noted.

The boy's respiration became less labored and the cyanosis disappeared after oxygen was administered with airway positioning and suctioning. On 35% O_2, the patient's arterial blood gases are as follows: pH = 7.34, PCO_2 = 40, PO_2 = 62, and O_2 saturation of 90%. He is responsive only to tactile stimuli as the IV line is placed. The child is then undressed, and a physical examination is performed. The physical examination reveals the following:

VS. T = 36°C
RR = 52/min
HR = 140/min
BP = 148/98 mmHg

General—obtunded, eyes open at times, responds briefly with purposeful movements to painful stimuli, some spontaneous vocalization.

Head—atraumatic.

Eyes—pupils 1 mm, minimally reactive; EOMs full; fundi—not visualized.

ENT—mouth—unremarkable except for copious secretions.

Neck—supple, no adenopathy.

Chest—coarse rhonchi, occasional wheezes and inspiratory rales.

Heart—R R, no murmur.

Abdomen—soft, no organomegaly or mass. Active bowel sounds.

Genitalia—normal; underpants stained with diarrheal stool behind and wet in front.

Skin—profuse sweating.

FIRST AID IN POISONS: Antidotes and Treatment

In a case of suspected poisoning:

1. Send for medical aid, and if possible state in writing the type of poison taken.
2. Prevent any more poison being taken.
3. Give artificial respiration if necessary.
4. If the patient is conscious and is not convulsing and there is no evidence that a corrosive acid or alkali has been taken then vomiting should be induced either by tickling the back of the throat with your index finger, or giving a strong solution of salt and water (one tablespoon of salt to a pint of water).
5. Do not give anything by mouth if the patient is convulsing, unconscious or semi-conscious.
6. Any poison on the skin should be washed away with water.
7. Preserve any urine, vomit, faeces, sputum.
8. Keep any bottles or box which may have contained the poison.
9. Treat the patient for shock. Lie him down and cover him with a blanket.

Table 19.6: First aid in Persons

Poison	*Symptoms*	*Treatment*
Strong acid	Immediate intense burning pain from mouth to stomach. Ulcerated mouth. Vomiting shreds of mucous membrane and altered blood. Dyspnoea due to oedema of the glottis. Shock.	Do not use a stomach tube or an emetic. Give an alkali immediately: ideally lime water, but soap solution in an emergency. Next give milk or olive oil. Strong analgesics to relieve pain. Tracheostomy. Intravenous fluids to combat shock.
Strong alkali and Ammonia	As with acid poisoning but less severe if a weak solution has been taken.	Give dilute acid such as acetic acid, vinegar or lemon juice. Otherwise treat as for acid poisoning.
Antihistamine	Initial drowsiness and lassitude.	Gastric lavage with sodium bicarbonate solution.
	Followed by confusion, coma and convulsions.	Oxygen, artificial respiration and amphetamine if the respiration is depressed. Convulsions are controlled by paraldehyde.
Arsenic	*Acute:* Burning abdominal pain. Severe vomiting and diarrhoea, leading to dehydration and shock. Muscle cramps. *Chronic:* Mild gastroenteritis. Dry cough with a husky voice. Grey skin pigmentation and hyperkeratosis. Jaundice. Peripheral neuritis. Anaemia.	Gastric lavage with copious amounts of water. Dimercaprol (BAL). Morphine to relieve pain. Intravenous fluid to counter dehydration. Remove source, otherwise symptomatic.
Aspirin (salicylates)	Initially, nausea and tinnitus (ringing in the ears), followed by deafness, confusion, restlessness, then coma.	Gastric lavage with water. Intravenous sodium lactate and dextrose saline to counter acidosis and dehydration.
	Profuse sweating leading to dehydration. 'Air junger'. Haematemesis.	Nikethamide if respiration is depressed.
Barbiturates	Initial drowsiness and vertigo.	Gastric lavage with copious amounts of water.

Contd...

Contd...

Poison	Symptoms	Treatment
	There may be hallucinations, followed by coma, which becomes profound with absent reflexes, respiratory depression and fall in blood pressure.	Oxygen and artificial respiration. Stimulants, such as bemegride, amphetamine, picrotoxin and nikethamide.
	Erythematous rashes occasionally occur.	Lumbar puncture. Penicillin.
Belladonna (atropine)	Dry mouth, flushed skin, pupils dilated.	Gastric lavage with very dilute potassium permanganate.
	Rapid pulse and respirations. Restlessness, excitement.	Oxygen and artificial respiration may be required.
	Convulsions and later paralysis and coma.	Convulsions controlled by shortacting barbiturates.
Coal gas (carbon monoxide)	Headache, nausea and giddiness, followed by coma and convulsions.	Artificial respiration. Oxygen with 5% carbon dioxide. Warmth.
	Cherry-pink discoloration of skin and mucosae.	Respiratory stimulants.
Chloral hydrate	Initial drowsiness passing into deep coma with respiratory depression. Low blood pressure and a sub-normal temperature.	Gastric lavage. Stimulants. Oxygen and artificial respiration.
Cyanides	Very rapid unconsciousness followed by convulsions, then flaccid paralysis.	Immediate inhalation of amyl nitrite, and artificial respiration.
	Respirations at first rapid then slow. Strong smell of bitter almonds.	Intravenous injection of sodium nitrite 3%, followed by sodium thiosulphate 50%, then nikethamide. Gastric lavage with dilute potassium permanganate solution. Repeat the injections in one hour.
Ferrous sulphate (tablets containing iron)	Vomiting, diarrhoea and haematemesis. Drowsiness. Shock. 2-4 days later, after apparent recovery, sudden collapse may occur.	Gastric lavage. Give bismuth carbonate 4 hourly by mouth. Vitamin B mixture and tocopherol.
Lead	*Acute:* Vomiting. Intestinal colic. Shock and collapse.	Gastric lavage with dilute sodium sulphate solution, then demulcents such as milk and albumin. Sodium calcium edetate iontravenously.
	Chronic: Tiredness. Constipation.	Symptomatic. Remove from exposure.

Contd...

Contd...

Poison	Symptoms	Treatment
	Anaemia. Blue line on gums. Weakness and palsies. Acute bouts of colic and vomiting. Convulsions and mania.	10% calcium gluconate intravenously for colic. Control convulsions with intravenous barbiturates.
Mercury	*Acute:* Severe abdominal pain. Diarrhoea. Shock. Anuria.	Gastric lavage, followed by egg white. Dimercaprol. Morphine. Warmth.
	Chronic: Gingivitis. Blue line on gums. Tremor. Anaemia. Psychosis.	Remove from further exposure. Symptomatic treatment.
Morphine (codeine, heroin, pethidine)	Euphoria with increasing drowsiness, then profound sleep followed by deep coma. Respirations slow and feeble. Pulse slow. Cyanosis. Pupils: pin-point.	Intravenous nalorphine hydrobromide. Oxygen, artificial respiration. Gastric lavage with dilute potassium permanganate. Stimulants if necessary.
Phenol (lysol)	Immediate burning pain from mouth to stomach. Lips white and hardened. Vomiting. Collapse. Delirium and coma.	Gastric lavage with magnesium or sodium sulphate. Demulcents such as milk or olive oil. Oxygen and artificial respiration, if necessary.
Strychnine	Convulsions. Sweating. Muscular rigidity. Respiratory paralysis.	Thiopentone sodium intravenously or other short-acting barbiturate. Muscle relaxant such as tubocurarine. Gastric lavage with potassium permanganate or tannic acid solution. Oxygen and artificial respiration may be necessary.
Turpentine	Smell of turpentine in breath. Headache, giddiness, drowsiness and sometimes delirium.	Gastric lavage. Demulcent drinks, such as milk and olive oil.
	Pulse thready. Respirations slow. Skin blue and clammy.	Saline purge. Morphia for pain.
DNOC or other derivatives of dinitrophenol, used as weed killer.	Increased metabolic rate. Whites of the eyes may become yellow before symptoms arise. Sweating, fatigue, insomnia. Respiration increased in rate and depth. Tachycardia. Temperature raised.	No specific antidote available. Keep the patient at rest, and give a barbiturate intramuscularly; saline intravenously. Oxygen.

Table 19.7. Nursing care plan for the patient with acute poisoning

Problem	*Reason*	*Objective*	*Nursing Intervention*	*Rationales*
Nursing Diagnosis # 1 Ineffective breathing pattern (tachypnea, stertorous breathing) related to: 1. Altered state of consciousness. 2. Muscle weakness/ paralysis (associated with organophosphate poisoning).		Patient will maintain: 1. Respiratory rate <30/min; regular rhythm and depth. 2. Adequate chest excursion. 3. Tidal volume $>5–7$ ml/kg with spontaneous breathing. 4. Mental status: alert; oriented to name.	• Perform overall assessment. ◆ Assess respiratory function: Respiratory rate, rhythm, depth; chest excursion, tone of respiratory musculature. ◆ Breath sounds/presence of adventitious sounds (crackles).	• Establishes a baseline with which to evaluate the response to therapy. ◆ Organophosphate poisoning can precipitate muscle weakness and paralysis. ◆ Enhanced cholinergic stimulation predisposes to excessive bronchial secretions.
Nursing Diagnosis # 2 Ineffective airway clearance related to: 1. Excessive secretions associated with enhanced cholinergic stimulation caused by organophosphate poisoning.		Patient will: 1. Demonstrate ability to cough and expectorate secretions.	◆ Assess serial arterial blood gases. ◆ Assess neurologic function: Mental status, level of consciousness; sensorimotor function; and deep tendon reflexes. ◆ Assess cardiovascular function: (see Nursing Diagnosis #5, below).	◆ Excessive alveolar and pulmonary interstitial fluid predisposes to impaired gas exchange and hypoxemia. ◆ Disruption of CNS function can be an ominous sign in acute poisoning.
Nursing Diagnosis # 3 Impaired gas exchange related to: 1. Pulmonary alveolar and interstitial congestion.		Patient will maintain arterial blood gases as follows: • PaO2 > 60 mmHg (room air) • PaCO2 ~ 35 to 45 mmHg • pH 7.35 – 7.45	• Implement measures to support alveolar ventilation/ oxygenation. ◆ Initiate endotracheal intubation and mechanical ventilation. ◆ Initiate oxygen therapy. ◆ Teach use of incentive spirometer when indicated. • Implement measures to maintain patent airway: ◆ Timely aseptic suctioning. ◆ Aggressive pulmonary toilet: Postural drainage; chest physiotherapy.	• Patients with acute organophosphate poisoning are at risk of developing hypoxemia. ◆ Altered state of consciousness and neuromuscular impairment compromise respiratory function. • Excessive secretions occur as a result of the enhanced cholinergic response associated with organophosphate poisoning.
Nursing Diagnosis # 4 Potential for poisoning related to inadvertent intake of organophosphate chemical (Dursban).		Patient will recuperate from poisoning episode without any obvious sequelae; patient will maintain: 1. Mental status: Alert; states name. 2. Usual personality (as per parents). 3. Respiratory function within acceptable parameters. Breathing easy; breath sounds clear to auscultation.	• Assess potential/actual poisoning: ◆ What/who was involved in the poisoning? ◆ What was the route of exposure and how much of the agent was taken? ◆ What were the signs and symptoms? ◆ What medications or other emergent actions were taken? • Implement antagonistic treatment as prescribed: ◆ Initiate gastric lavage.	• Thorough assessment including history, physical examination, and laboratory testing are essential to timely diagnosis and treatment (see Table 19.4). • Timely treatment is essential to reverse the effects of the poisoning agent before irreversible pathophysiologic changes occur. ◆ Controversy exists as to the

Contd...

Contd...

Problem	*Reason*	*Objective*	*Nursing Intervention*	*Rationales*
				clinical efficacy of this modality. The decision to initiate lavage therapy is based on the time of exposure; the more recent the occurrence (30 to 60 min), the more effective the outcome. ◆ An inflated cuff will help to prevent aspiration in the comatose patient.
			◆ Assure ET tube cuff is inflated.	◆ Gastric lavage is contraindicated in the scenario of a caustic ingestate (e.g., lye).
			◆ Administer activated charcoal as prescribed and monitor response to therapy.	◆ Activated charcoal decreases toxicity by adsorbing chemical to its surface. Efficacy depends on timing of administration (most effective within 30 to 60 min, but may be effective up to 24 hr). ◆ Activated charcoal si not given if bowel sounds are absent.
			◆ Auscultate for bowel sounds prior to administration. ◆ Monitor gastric pH.	◆ Food in stomach may decrease effect of charcoal.
			◆ Administer prescribed dosage of activated charcoal.	◆ Inadequate dose may induce *desorption**: a reversible process in which an adsorbed chemical is removed from the charcoal causing free chemical to again be available to exert its untoward effects.
			◆ Administer cathartic therapy (e.g., magnesium citrate).	◆ Cathartic maintains bowel motility to hasten elimination of drug/chemical/charcoal complex.
			◆ Administer prescribed anticholinergic (atropine).	◆ Atropine competes with acetylcholine for cholinergic receptor sites tehreby exerting its anticholinergic effect.
			◆ Administer prescribed organophosphate antagonist, pralidoxime.	◆ Pralidoxime reactivates the enzyme cholinesterase, inhibited by the organophosphate; the enzymatic breakdown of acetylcholine reduces the overall cholinergic effect.

Contd...

Contd...

Problem	*Reason*	*Objective*	*Nursing Intervention*	*Rationales*
Nursing Diagnosis # 5 Fluid volume deficit related to: 1. Profuse diaphoresis, lacrimation, salivation, bronchorrhea, associated with enhanced cholinergic stimulation.		Patient will: 1. Maintain stable vital signs. • Blood pressure within 10 mmHg of baseline for patient. • Heart rate < 100/min. 2. Exhibit usual skin color, without cyanosis or mottling; capillary refill brisk. 3. Maintain balanced intake/output: Urine output >30 ml/hr.	• Assess hydration and cardiovascular status: ♦ Heart rate, blood pressure, skin color, temperature, moisture, capillary refill, peripheral pulses. ♦ Assess intake and output. ♦ Weigh daily. ♦ Monitor serum electrolytes and acid-base balance.	• Excessive loss of fluid associated with enhanced cholinergic activity places the patient at risk for hypovolemia. ♦ Assessment parameters should include those indicative of peripheral perfusion. ♦ A meticulous record of intake/output and daily weight provides the best measure as to the patient's hydration status.
		4. maintain body weight within 5% of baseline. 5. Exhibit good skin turgor and moist mucous membranes. 6. Maintain laboratory data within acceptable range: BUN, serum creatinine, serum electrolytes, haematocrit, haemoglobin; urine specific gravity.	• Implement fluid replacement therapy (as per physician).	• Aggressive fluid replacement therapy is necessary to maintain adequate circulating blood volume.
Nursing Diagnosis # 6 Ineffective family coping related to: 1. Feelings of guilt.		Family will: 1. Verbalize feelings about poisoning episode and the circumstances under which it occurred. 2. Verbalize actions to be taken to prevent a recurrence.	• Assess the circumstances within which the poisoning exposure occurred. ♦ Allow the family the opportunity to verbalize their feelings. • Instruct family in precautions that need to be taken to prevent future such crises. ♦ Have family verbalize the telephone number of the local branch of the Poison Control Center. ♦ Have family verbalize emergency measures to be taken if such an episode would inadvertently recur.	• It is essential to evaluate how the poisoning occurred so that measures may be taken to prevent a recurrence. ♦ Verbalizing their feelings may help them to cope with this family crisis. • Family may need to assess how household chemicals are handled in their home setting. ♦ It is essential for all households to have the telephone number of the Poison Control Center. ♦ In the event of an emergency, it is essential that the family not panic, but follow the necessary steps to get help immediately. Minutes can mean the difference between life and death.

Table 19.8: Treatment of specific poisons

Drug	*Toxicity and Excretion*	*Symptoms*	*Treatment*
Acetaminophen (Tylenol, Tempra, Liquiprin)	Potential hepatotoxicity with ingestions of > 8 gm in adolescent and > 2 to 3 gm in child. Hepatotoxicity with serum level > 200 mg/ml 4 hours following ingestion. Major route of excretion— hepatic metabolism	Nausea, vomiting, diaphoresis; 36 to 48 hours following ingestion—jaundice, elevated hepatic enzymes and bilirubin, prolonged prothrombin time; fully reversible or progresses to hepatic failure; renal and myocardial toxicity.	Removal with emesis or lavage, activated charcoal; support for hepatic failure, treatment of hepatic failure, (*N*-acetylcysteine)
Acids (Lysol)	Toxicity related to concentration and duration of exposure.	Corrosive burns of mucous membranes, mouth, oesophagus and stomach; pain in area of burns; circulatory collapse and shock; complications—oesophageal and gastric perforation, glottic edema, pulmonary edema, pneumonia, stricture formation of oesophagus and pylorus.	Emetics and lavage contraindicated; immediate removal from oesophagus with water or milk: neutralization with an alkali not advised; opiates for pain; IV therapy for shock; for further therapy see under Alkali.
Alkali (lye, Drano Saniflush, Clinitest)	Toxicity to esophagus related to concentration and duration of exposure.	Corrosive burns of mucous membranes of mouth and oesophagus; pain in area of burns; circulatory collapse and shock; complications—oesophageal and gastric perforation, glottic edema, pulmonary oedema, pneumonia, stricture formation of oesophagus.	Emetics and lavage contraindicated; immediate removal from esophagus with water or milk: neutralization with an acid not advised; opiates for pain; IV therapy for shock; with evidence of esophageal or gastric burn (clinically, by esophagoscopy or by esophagram), prednisone, 2 to 3 mg/kg/day for 3 weeks and then tapered over 1 week; broad-spectrum antibiotic coverage while on steroids; following therapy, upper GI series for evidence of stricture; dilation of stricture if present.
Ammonium hydroxide (ammonia)	Toxicity to esophagus related to concentration and duration of exposure.	Corrosive burns of mucous membranes of mouth and oesophagus; circulatory collapse and shock; complications include oesophageal and gastric perforation, glottic oedema, pulmonary oedema, pneumonia.	Emetics and lavage contraindicated; immediate removal from oesophagus with water or milk; neutralization with acid not advised; further therapy as outlined under Alkali.
Amphetamines (Benzedrine, Dexedrine, Dexamyl)	Symptoms when therapeutic dose exceeded. Lethal dose in humans estimated at 20 to 25 mg/kg. Major route of excretion—hepatic metabolism and renal excretion.	Nervousness, hyperactivity, mania, psychotic-like state; tachycardia, hypertension, cardiac arrhythmias, hyperpyrexia; convulsions and shock.	Emesis or lavage; activated charcoal; control of seizures with barbiturates or diazepam; support for cardiovascular and respiratory failure; acidification of urine with ammonium chloride to increase excretion of drug; chlorpromazine; phenoxybenzamine or phentolamine for hypertensive emergencies.
Antihistamines and cold medications (Dimetapp, Congespirin, Actifed, Contac, Sudafed, Allerest, Triaminic).	Symptoms when therapeutic dose exceeded Major route of excretion—hepatic metabolism	Excitation, disorientation, drowsiness, coma; anticholinergic syndrome—dry mouth, dilated pupils, fever, flushed skin, tachycardia, absent bowel sounds, urinary retention; hyperten-	Emesis or lavage; activated charcoal; vigorous GI catharsis; treatment of fever; maintenance fluid therapy; support for circulatory and respiratory failure; treatment of seizures with

Contd...

Contd...

Drug	*Toxicity and Excretion*	*Symptoms*	*Treatment*
		sion, hypotension; convulsions; arrhythmias; cardiovascular collapse and respiratory depression.	barbiturates or diazepam, treatment with physostigmine.
Lead	Toxicity by ingestion and inhalation. Symptoms with blood level >40 μg/dl. Danger of encephalopathy with levels greater than 80 μg/dl	Ingestion causes chronic toxicity, inhalation, acute toxicity; abdominal pain, nausea, vomiting; opaque lead particles on x-ray; lethargy, ataxia; encephalopathy; coma	Emesis or lavage; GI catharsis; treatment for renal failure and encephalopathy; calcium EDTA and/or dimercaprol (BAL) or D-penicillamine therapy
Mercury Inorganic	Exposure from inorganic mercury found in rodenticides, mercury amalgam, diuretics	Major toxicity to GI tract, kidneys, and liver; bloody diarrhoea, metallic taste in mouth; abdominal pain; renal tubular damage and anurla; hepatic damage	Emesis of lavage; fluid therapy and transfusion therapy; treatment of liver and renal failure; BAL
Organic	Exposure from manufacturing plants and agricultural urage Major route of excretion—renal and GI tract	Major toxicity to CNS; paresthesias, hypesthesia; weakness, apathy, inability to concentrate, loss of memory; ataxia, tremors, chorea; hearing difficulty; coma, seizures	Penicillamine or *N*-acetylpenicillamine
Naphthalene (mothballs, repellent cakes, deodorizer cakes)	More than 1 tsp is toxic Major route of excretion—hepatic metabolism	Nausea, vomiting, abdominal cramps; convulsions; coma; intravascular hemolysis with G6PD deficiency; oliguria and anuria	Emesis or lavage; control of seizures with barbiturates and diazepam. For intravascular hemolysis, IV fluids and alkalinization of the urine with bicarbonate to prevent precipitation of haemoglobin in tubules. Support for respiratory and circulatory failure; transfusion for anemia.
Narcotic analgesics (morphine, codeine, demerol, methadone, propoxyphene, pentazocine)	Symptoms when therapeutic dose exceeded Major route of excretion—hepatic metabolism	Lethargy, coma; pinpoint pupils; respiratory depression; hypotension; convulsions	Emesis or lavage, activated charcoal, GI catharsis, naloxone hydrochloride, ventilatory support for respiratory failure.
Phencyclidine (PCP, Angel Dust, Peace Pill)	Widespread use. Alleged to be THC, LSD, psilocybin and mescaline Major routes of excretion—hepatic metabolism and renal excretion	Low dose—excitation, paranoid behavior, miotic pupils, nystagmus, increased blood pressure, pulse and respiration; slurred speech, drowsiness. High dose—decreased reflexes, coma, seizures, opisthotonos, hypotension, respiratory depression	Emesis or lavage; continuous gastric suction; reduction of sensory stimull; diazepam, 0.5 mg/kg/day for control of agitation, opisthotonos; acidification of urine with ammonium chloride to enhance renal excretion; support for respiratory and circulatory failure.
Polishes and waxes (Pride, Old English, O'Cedar, Jubilee, Kleer Floor Wax, Bruce Cleaning Wax, Aerowax, Armstrong 1-Step, Pledge Furniture Polish, Stanley Furniture Cream)	Main toxicity is pulmonary, caused by aspiration, CNS signs less severe, secondary to absorption from lungs	Burning of the mouth and esophagus; vomiting and diarrhea; pulmonary involvement—cough, fever, dyspnea, rales, cyanosis, pulmonary infiltrates; infiltrates clear over 1 to 4 weeks.	Do not induce emesis. For pulmonary involvement; oxygen, moisture, antibiotics when clinical course or sputum examination indicates superinfection; supportive therapy for CNS depression and seizures.
Psychedelic drugs (LSD, mescaline, psllocybin, STP, DMT)	Duration and intensity of effect varies from drug to drug and from individual to individual Major route of excretion—hepatic metabolism	Dilation of pupils, tachycardia, mild hypertension, incoordination, visual hallucinations, distortion of sensory perception, exaggerated sense of comprehension	"Talking down" in quiet nonthreatening atmosphere; diazepam, 0.5 mg/kg/day for sedative effect; avoidance of chlorpromazine with STP or DMT.

Contd...

Contd...

Drug	*Toxicity and Excretion*	*Symptoms*	*Treatment*
Detergents, soaps and cleaners	Variable toxicity	Anionic detergents (Tide, Cheer, Ajax, Top Job, Comet, Windex, Mr. Clean, Lestoil, Joy, Spic and Span, bar soap, bubble bath, household detergents) cause mild vomiting and diarrhoea; cationic detergents (pHisoHex, Zephiran, Diaparene) cause nausea, vomiting, convulsions, coma; electric dishwasher and laundry granules cause caustic burns	For anionic detergents—supportive therapy; no removal necessary. For cationic detergents—emesis or lavage, support for coma and respiratory failure, and treatment of seizures with barbiturates or diazepam. For treatment of dishwasher and laundry granule burns, see under Alkali.
Ethyl alcohol (ethanol, isopropyl alcohol, cologne, perfume)	Blood level: 0.05 to 0.15%, mild; 0.15 to 0.3%, moderate; 0.3 to 0.5%, severe; above 0.5%, coma Major route of excretion—hepatic metabolism	Initial excitation, delirium and inebriation; later depression, stupor, coma; alcohol odor on breath; hypoglycaemia; slurred speech and muscle incoordination; respiratory failure.	Emesis or lavage, glucose for hypoglycaemia, maintenance fluids, support for respiratory and circulatory failure, haemodialysis.
Hydrocarbons (kerosene, gasoline, mineral spirits, paint thinner, lighter fluid, barbecue fluid, dry cleaning fluid).	Toxicity to lungs and CNS Major route of excretion—hepatic metabolism	Hydrocarbon smell in mouth and on breath; burning in the mouth and esophagus; vomiting; pulmonary symptoms—cough, fever, bloody sputum, cyanosis, rales, pulmonary infiltrates; CNS—drowsiness, mild coma, seizures.	Removal is not indicated with petroleum distillate hydrocarbon ingestions in children. If very large amounts (10 ml/kg) are taken (as in a suicide attempt), in alert patient, emesis with ipecac syrup is indicated and is a safer method of removal than lavage. For pneumonia, use of oxygen and antibiotics with signs of superinfection, use of steroids not indicated. Supportive therapy for CNS depression and seizures; avoid epinephrine; appropriate support for hepatic, renal, cardiac and bone marrow toxicity.
Chlorinated hydrocarbon insecticides (DDT, dieldrin, lindane)	Variability of toxicity among compounds. Routes of absorption include GI and cutaneous. Variability of absorption from cutaneous route.	Vomiting, excitation, numbness, weakness, incoordination, tremors, seizures, circulatory and respiratory failure.	Decontamination of skin, removal with emesis or lavage, GI catharsis, support for respiratory or circulatory failure, control of seizures with barbiturates and diazepam.
Organophosphate insecticides (parathion, chlorthion, bidrin, Dimetilan, Sevin)	Major route of excretion—hepatic metabolism with metabolites often pharmacologically active.	Blurred vision, sweating, miosis, tearing, sallvation, papilledema, cyanosis, seizures, pulmonary oedema.	Decontamination of skin, removal with emesis or lavage, GI catharsis, support for respiratory or circulatory failure, control of seizures with barbiturates and diazepam, atropine sulfate, pralidoxine chloride.
Iron (ferrous sulfate, ferrous gluconate, ferrous fumarate, vitamins with iron).	Serum level of > 400 μg/dl associated with systemic toxicity. Major toxicities—GI, CNS, liver, and vasculature. Major route of excretion—renal.	Symptoms occur 1/2 to 4 hours post ingestion; vomiting, diarrhea, melena; drowsiness, lethargy, pallor; metabolic acidosis; hepatic damage and coagulation defects; coma and shock; stricture of GI tract; iron tablets radiopaque on x-ray.	Emesis or lavage; bicarbonate or phosphates to precipitate iron and prevent absorption; fluid therapy and expanders for shock. If (a) shock and coma, (b) serum iron level of greater than 400 μg/dl, (c) overdose in lethal range in symptomatic patient, (d) positive provocative chelation, treat with deferoxamine. Haemodialysis or exchange transfusion with renal failure.

Contd...

Contd...

Drug	*Toxicity and Excretion*	*Symptoms*	*Treatment*
Arsenic	Major toxicity—GI, hepatic, renal, and CNS Major route or excretion—renal.	Sweetish metallic taste in mouth; burning sensation in throat; diarrhea, vomiting, dehydration; delirium, convulsions, coma, hyperreflexia, seizures; pulmonary edema; haemolysis; arsenic in GI tract—radiopaque on x-ray; toxic effects on liver, kidney, and marrow.	Emesis or lavage; IV hydration; treatment of liver and renal decompensation; transfusion therapy for hemolytic anemia; dimercaprol (BAL) therapy indicated when unknown amount ingested, with symptoms or when toxic levels exist.
Barbiturates (amobarbital, secobarbital, pentobarbital, phenobarbital)	Potential fatal dose 40 to 50 mg/kg for short-acting barbiturates, and 65 to 75 mg/kg for long-acting barbiturates. Blood levels of 3 to 4 mg/dl for short-acting barbiturates and 10 to 15 mg/dl for long-acting barbiturates found with severe overdose (grades III-IV). Excretion of short-acting barbiturates–hepatic metabolism. Excretion of long-acting barbiturates–renal and hepatic metabolism.	Mental confusion, drowsiness, coma; ataxia, vertigo, slurred speech; decreased deep tendon reflexes, decreased response to pain; hypotension, hypothermia; pulmonary edema with short-acting barbiturates; respiratory failure.	Emesis or lavage; activated charcoal; forced fluid diuresis for long-acting barbiturates; alkalinization of urine for long-acting barbiturates; osmotic agents and diuretics for long-acting barbiturates; maintenance fluids for short-acting barbiturates; support for respiratory and cardiovascular failure; dialysis for long-acting barbiturates.
Bleach (Clorox, Purex, Sani-Chior)	Major toxicities to intestinal mucosa and CNS Major route of excretion—renal.	Irritation and pain of mouth and oesophagus; stricture and perforation do not occur in concentrations presently used; nausea and vomiting; delirium, obtundation, and coma; hypotension.	Removal with lavage if vomiting has not occurred; removal from skin by flooding with water; support for CNS and circulatory failure; treatment as caustic (acid-alkali) nto indicated.
Boric acid	Fatal dose estimated at 0.1 to 0.5 mg/kg Major route of excretion—renal.	Bloody diarrhea and dehydration; erythroderma and exfoliation; lethargy, convulsions; jaundice; hypotension; anuria; coma.	Removal from skin, with ingestion emesis or lavage, IV fluids, treatment of seizures with barbiturates and diazepam.
Camphor (Campho-Phenique, camphor liniment)	Fatal dose for a 1-year-old child is approximately 1 gm. Major route of excretion–-hepatic.	Headache; burning in mouth and throat; camphor odor on breath; nausea and vomiting; feeling of warmth, excitement, irrational behavior, muscle spasms, convulsions, coma; circulatory and respiratory collapse.	Emesis or lavage; activated charcoal; treatment of seizures with barbiturates or diazepam; support for respiratory and circulatory failure.
Carbon monoxide.	Cellular hypoxia as a result of high affinity of carbon monoxide for hemoglobin. Major route of excretion—respiratory.	At 20% carboxyhemoglobin—headache, vertigo, shortness of breath; at 40 to 50% carboxyhaemoglobin—coma, cardiac arrhythmias and ischemia, respiratory failure, irreversible brain damage.	Removal of patient from site of exposure to uncontaminated air; 100% oxygen by mask for 30 min. to 2 hours; with respiratory depression, artificial respiration with 100% oxygen; maintain temperature and blood pressure; recognition and treatment of cerebral oedema.
Carbon tetrachloride	Toxic dose by ingestion is as low as 3 to 5 ml. Causes injury to liver, kidneys, myocardium, CNS. Major exposure—oral or by inhalation. Major route of excretion—hepatic metabolism	Abdominal pain, nausea and vomiting; headache and confusion; obtundation, coma, respiratory depression; circulatory collapse; renal, hepatic and myocardial damage.	Emesis or lavage; maintenance hydration; avoid epinephrine and related compounds; respiratory support; management of renal and hepatic damage.
Cathartics (mineral oil, Ex-Lax, phenolphthalein, Metamucil)	Generally of low toxicity.	Irritation of GI tract causing tenesmus, vomiting, diarrhoea; rarely hypotension, collapse, coma.	With large ingestion, emesis or lavage; milk to decrease GI irritation; if severe symptoms, hydration, medication for pain, treatment of shock.

Contd...

Contd...

Drug	*Toxicity and Excretion*	*Symptoms*	*Treatment*
Salicylates (St. Joseph's, Bayer, Bufferin, Rexall, Empirin, Anacin, Excedrin, Congesprin, Ben Gay).	Symptoms at 150 mg/kg or greater or at serum levels greater than 30 mg/dl; 50 to 80 mg/dl, mild-moderate symptoms; 80 to 100 mg/dl, severe symptoms; greater than 100 mg/dl, potentially fatal. Major route of excretion—renal; minor route—hepatic.	Vomiting, hyperventilation, fever, thirst, sweating, hypoglycemia or hyperglycaemia, prolonged prothrombin time, confusion, delirium, coma, convulsions. In small children, metabolic acidosis; in older children, respiratory alkalosis.	Emesis or lavage; activated charcoal; forced fluid diuresis (1 to 2 times maintenance); colloid for volume expansion; glucose for hypoglycemia; sponging for fever; vitamin K_1 for hypoprothrombinemia; alkalinization of urine with bicarbonate; hemodialysis, peritoneal dialysis or exchange transfusion with (a) levels greater than 100 to 150 mg/dl, (b) anuria, (c) heart disease preventing forced fluid diuresis.
Strychnine (rodenticides)	Fatal dose for an adolescent is 15 to 30 mg. Toxicity due to increased reflex excitability.	Increased deep tendon reflexes with muscle stiffening and opisthotonos; respiratory failure.	Emesis or lavage, control of seizures with barbiturates and diazepam, prevention of peripheral stimuli and enforcement of quiet, support for respiratory and circulatory failure.
Tranquilizers (Mellaril, Equanil, Miltown, Placidyl, Doriden, Noludar, Dalmane, Librium, Valium).	Toxicity when therapeutic dosage exceeded. Major route of excretion—hepatic metabolism.	Sleepiness, weakness, unsteadiness, incoordination, hypotension, cyanosis, respiratory failure, coma.	Emesis or lavage, activated charcoal and GI catharsis, maintenance of an adequate airway and oxygen, support for respiratory and circulatory failure, supportive therapy during coma.
Turpentine and other volatile oils (xylene, toluene).	Predominant CNS toxicity. Major route of excretion—hepatic metabolism.	Nausea, vomiting; CNS excitation, lethargy, coma; pneumonia and pulmonary edema; renal, hepatic and bone marrow toxicity.	Emesis or lavage, treatment of seizures with barbiturates and diazepam, ventilatory support for respiratory failure, treatment of renal, hepatic or bone marrow failure.
Tricyclic antidepressants (impipramine, amitriptyline)	Symptoms when therapeutic dose exceeded. Major route of excretion—hepatic metabolism.	Excitation, disorientation, drowsiness, coma; anticholinergic syndrome—dry mouth, dilated pupils, fever, flushed skin, tachycardia, absent bowel sounds, urinary retention; hypertension, hypotension; convulsions; arrhythmias; cardiovascular collapse and respiratory depression.	Emesis or lavage, activated charcoal, vigorous GI catharsis, treatment of fever, maintenance fluid therapy, support for circulatory and respiratory failure, treatment of seizures with barbiturates or diazepam.

Appendix I
Cardiopulmonary Resuscitation

CARDIOPULMONARY RESUSCITATION (CPR)

Sudden death occurs when heartbeat and breathing stops suddenly or unexpectedly. The major role of CPR is to provide oxygen to the heart, brain, and other vital organs until medical treatment (Advanced Cardiac Life Support - ACLS) can restore normal heart action.

Common causes of sudden death include the following:

- Heart attack
- Electrical shock
- Drowning
- Choking
- Suffocation
- Trauma
- Drug reactions
- Allergic reactions

Two definitions aid in understanding the role of CPR in sudden death.

Clinical Death means that heartbeat and breathing have stopped. This process is reversible when CPR and life-support measures are started during the first few minutes.

Biological Death is permanent cellular damage due to lack of oxygen. Brain cells are most sensitive to the lack of oxygen. This process is final.

Time is critical in starting CPR. If CPR is started within 4 minutes and ACLS within the next 4 minutes, the victim has a good chance of recovery.

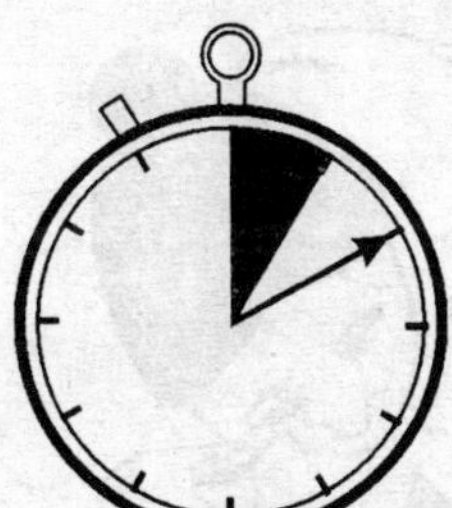

4 Minutes-Brain damage begins

10 Minutes-Brain death certain

In adults, the most common cause of sudden death is due to heart disease. **The best way to save lives is through Prevention.**

The risk of sudden death due to heart disease can be reduced in 3 ways.

1. Reduce risk factors of developing heart disease.
2. Recognize the signs and symptoms of heart attack and implement actions for survival.
3. When needed, perform the proper steps of CPR effectively.

RISK FACTORS FOR HEART DISEASE

Risk Factors that cannot be Changed

- Heredity (Positive Family History)
- Male gender
- Increasing age.

Major Risk Factors that can be Changed or Modified

- Cigarette smoking
- High blood pressure
- High blood cholesterol levels.

Other Risk Factors which can also be Changed or Eliminated

- Diabetes
- Obesity
- Lack of physical activity.

Prudent heart living is a lifestyle which minimizes the risk of future heart disease. This lifestyle includes the following guidelines and recommendations:

- Weight control,
- Physical fitness,
- Sensible dietary habits,
- Avoidance of cigarette smoking,
- Reduction of blood fats, and
- Control of high blood pressure.

Many deaths due to heart attack occur before the victim reaches the hospital. A great number of these deaths could be prevented. The first step is to recognize the signs and symptoms of heart attack.

SIGNS AND SYMPTOMS OF HEART ATTACK

Chest discomfort or pain is the most common signal of a heart attack. People frequently use the following words to describe the pain: uncomfortable pressure, squeezing, fullness, tightness, aching, crushing, constriction, or heaviness.

Location: In the center of the chest behind the breastbone. It may spread to one or both shoulders, arms, neck, jaw, or back.

Duration: The pain of a heart attack will usually last longer than 2 minutes. It may come and go.

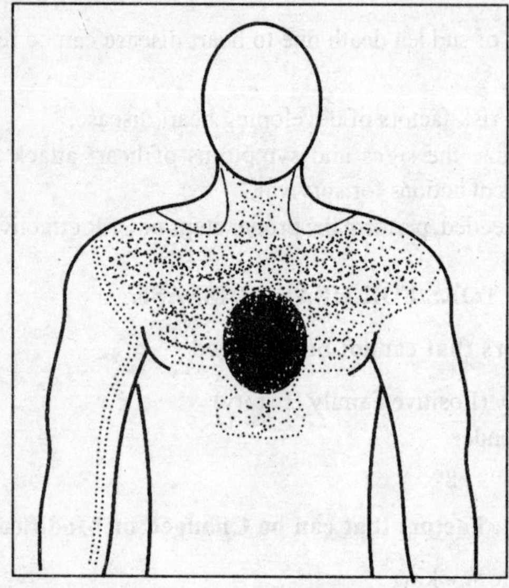

Other Signs and **Symptoms** may include

- Sweating
- Nausea
- Shortness of breath
- A feeling of weakness.

Prompt recognition of the signs and symptoms of heart attack and appropriate medical care can save lives.

ACTIONS FOR SURVIVAL

- Recognize the signs and symptoms.
- Stop activity and sit or lie down.
- If signs and symptoms persist for 2 minutes or longer, call EMS (Emergency Medical Service) or take the person to the nearest emergency room.

INDICATIONS FOR CPR

Respiratory Arrest

Refers to the absence of breathing. When breathing stops first, the heart can continue to pump blood for several minutes. Opening the airway and providing rescue breathing may be all that is needed.

Cardiac Arrest

When the heart stops, there is no pulse. Blood is not circulated and vital stores of oxygen will be depleted in a few seconds. In cardiac arrest, external chest compressions must be started after rescue breathing.

THE ABC's OF CPR

Cardiopulmonary resuscitationis based on 3 basic skill groups.

- Airway
- Breathing
- Circulation

At the beginning of each of the ABC's is an assessment phase. No victim should undergo any step of CPR until the need has been established. Performing chest compressions on someone who has a heartbeat can be harmful.

The basic step of starting CPR are the same for adults, children and infants.

Determine unresponsiveness (Shake and Shout)

A. Open the airway

Determine breathlessness (look, listen, feel)

B. Breathing

Determine pulselessness.

C. Circulation

Begin compressions.

ONE-RESCUER CPR-ADULT

1. **Determine Unresponsiveness**
   Tap or gently shake patient. Shout, "Are you OK?"
2. **Shout for Help!**
3. **Phone EMS for help.**
4. **Position the victim** onto his/her back, on a firm surface. Support the head and neck if you have to turn the victim.

A = AIRWAY

5. **Open the airway.**
   Using head-tilt/chin-lift method, tilt the head back and lift the jaw.

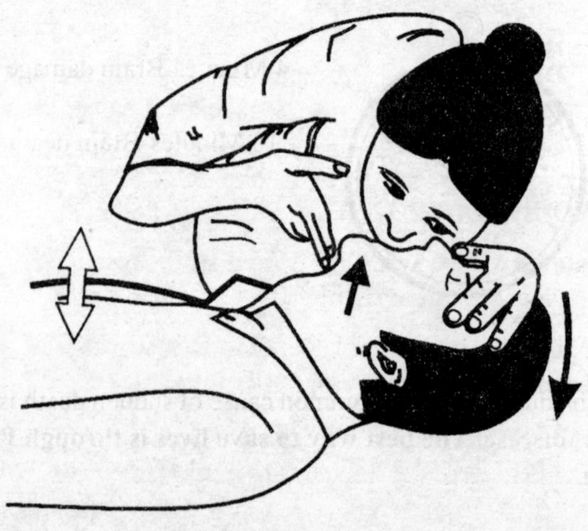

6. **Check for Breathing.** (Time: 3-5 seconds). Look at the chest and abdomen; listen and feel for breathing.

B = BREATHING

7. **Give 2 full breaths.** (Time: 1.5 - 2 seconds per breath) Pinch the nose and cover the mouth with your mouth. Give 2 breaths. Watch for the chest to rise.
8. **Check for a pulse**. (Time: 5-10 seconds) **Feel for the Carotid Pulse.**

C = CIRCULATION

9. **Locate correct hand position.** (Lower 1/2 of sternum)

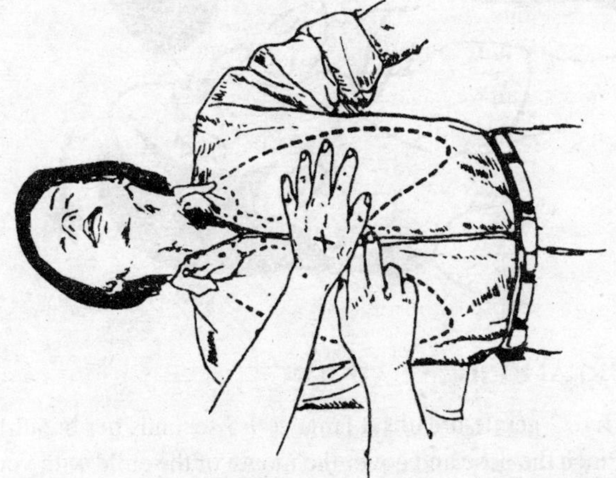

Slide middle and index fingers of hand nearest patient's legs up the rib cage to locate "notch" at lower end of breast bone.

Place heel of hand nearest patient's head on breastbone next to index finger.

Place heel of hand used to locate "notch" directly on top of hand on the breastbone.

10. **Compress** the sternum **1-1/2 to 2 inches** at a rate of **80-100 times per minute**.
11. Do **15 Compressions**.
12. Give **2 Full Breaths**.
13. **Do 4 cycles** of 15 compressions and 2 breaths.
14. **Recheck Pulse.** (Time: 5 seconds) if NO pulse, continue compression/breathing cycles.

TWO-RESCUER CPR

Beginning 2-Person CPR When Both Rescuers Arrive at the same Time

If both persons are available, **One Rescuer should** go to the head of the victim and proceed as follows:

1. Check for unresponsiveness.
2. Position the patient.
3. Open the airway.
4. Check for breathing.
5. Give 2 full breaths.
6. Feel for the Carotid pulse (5-10 seconds). If no pulse, say, "No pulse, begin CPR."

The **Second Rescuer should,** simultaneously:

1. Make sure EMS has been activated.
2. Find the location for external chest compression.
3. Place hands in correct position on chest.
4. Start chest compressions when the first rescuer states no pulse.
5. Give 5 compressions.
6. Stop after the fifth compression and allow ventilator to give 1 breath.

- Ventilator monitors effectiveness of compressions by checking pulse while partner is doing compressions.
- Do 12 cycles of 5 compressions and 1 breath. Ventilator says, "Pulse check, "and feels for the carotid pulse. If no pulse, ventilator gives one breath then says, "no pulse, continue CPR." Second rescuer resumes compressions.

OR

The Addition of a Second Rescuer When CPR is in Progress

When CPR is already being done:

Second Rescuer	Identify yourself as a professional rescuer. **Phone EMS if not done.**
First Rescuer	Complete the cycle of 15 compressions and 2 ventilations.
Second Rescuer	Get into position at patient's chest. Locate landmarks; place hands in correct position.
First Rescuer	Feel for carotid pulse for 5 seconds. If no pulse, Give 1 full breath. Say, "No pulse, continue CPR."
Second Rescuer	Begin chest compressions. (Rate 80-100 per minute) Stop after the fifth compression and allow ventilator give 1 breath.

TWO-RESCUERS-CHANGING POSITIONS

Two-rescuer CPR is best performed with the rescuers on opposite sides of the victim. This permits changing positions without interrupting CPR. The person doing chest compressions directs a change to take place at the completion of the cycle.

Two-Rescuer CPR in Progress

Compressor calls for a change	Say, "*Change*-and, two-and, three-and, four-and, five."

Ventilator	Give 1 full breath.
Rescuers Change Position	Compressor moves to patient's head Ventilator moves to patient's chest.
New Ventilator	Feel for carotid pulse for 5-10 seconds.
New Compressor	Locate landmark and position hands for compressions while the pulse check is being done.
New Ventilator	If no pulse, say, "No pulse, continue CPR."
New Compressor	Give 5 compressions. Pause after the fifth compression to allow ventilator to give one breath.

Rescue Breating—If a pulse is present, the rescuer should check for breathing.

If breathing is absent, rescue breathing should be performed and the pulse and breathing monitored every minute.

Rate of Rescue Breathing:			
	Infant	20 per minute	1 breath every 3 seconds
	Child	20 per minute	1 breath every 3 seconds
	Adult	12 per minute	1 breath every 5 seconds

If the victim has a pulse and is breathing, the rescuer should continue to monitor the victim and maintain an open airway. Place the victim in the *Recovery Position.* This reduces the risk of aspiration and keeps the tongue from blocking the airway.

Recovery Position—Roll the victim onto his or her side so that the head, shoulders, and body move without twisting. Position the victim's arm and leg as shown in the picture below.

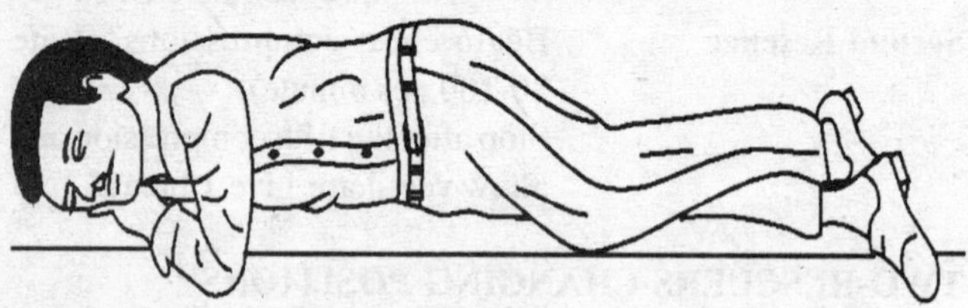

ONE RESCUER CPR—CHILD (1 TO 8 YEARS OF AGE)

1. **Determine Unresponsiveness.**
   Tap or gently shake the child's shoulder. **Shout, "Are you OK?"**
2. **Shout for HELP!**
3. **Position the child** onto his/her back, on a firm surface. Support the head and neck if you have to turn the child.

A = AIRWAY

4. Open the airway. (Head-tilt/Chin-lift) Gently tilt the head back into a slightly extended position; lift chin.
5. Check for breathing. (Time: 3-5 seconds)
   Maintain open airway. Look at the chest and abdomen; listen and feel for breathing.

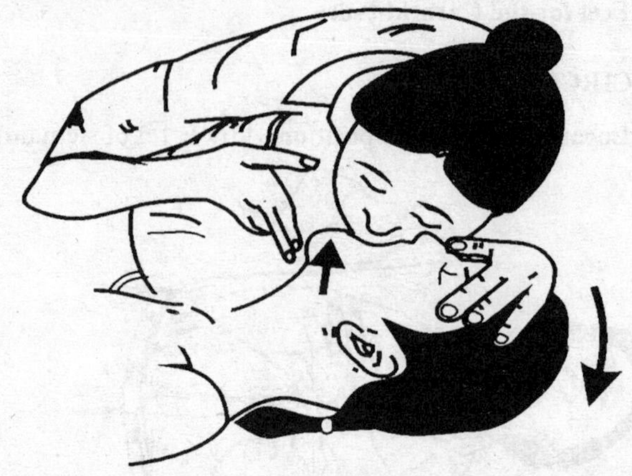

B = BREATHING

6. Give 2 gentle breaths. (Time: 1-1.5 seconds per breath)
   Pinch the nose and cover the mouth of the child with your mouth. Give 2 breaths (enough to raise the chest).
7. Check for a pulse. (Time: 5-10 seconds)
   Feel for the carotid pulse.

C = CIRCULATION

8. To locate correct hand position for chest compression, slide middle finger of hand nearest child's legs up the rib cage to locate the "notch" at lower end of breastbone.

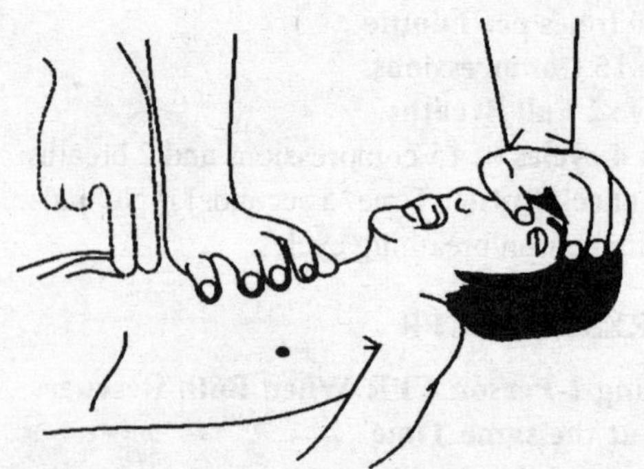

Note: Maintain head-tilt position while checking the pulse and performing compressions.

Place middle finger in "notch" and index finger next to it on the lower end of the breastbone.

Look at where your index finger is placed, then lift fingers off the breastbone.
Place heel of the same hand on the breastbone immediately above where the index finger was placed.

9. Compress the breastbone 1 to 1-1/2 inches at a rate of 100 times per minute. (Use one hand only!)
10. Do 5 Compressions then give 1 breath.
11. Do 20 cycles of 5 compressions and 1 breath.
12. Phone EMS for help. (On a child, perform CPR for 1 minute then phone EMS.)
13. Recheck pulse. (Time: 5 seconds) If no pulse, continue compression/breathing cycles. Recheck the pulse every few minutes.

CPR-INFANT (LESS THAN 1 YEAR OF AGE)

1. **Determine Unresponsiveness.**
   Tap or gently shake infant's shoulder.
2. **Shout for Help!**
3. **Position the infant** onto his/her back, on a firm surface. Support the head and neck if you have a turn the infant.

A = AIRWAY

4. **Open the airway.**
   Using head-tilt/chin-lift method, gently tilt the head back into the "neutral" position.

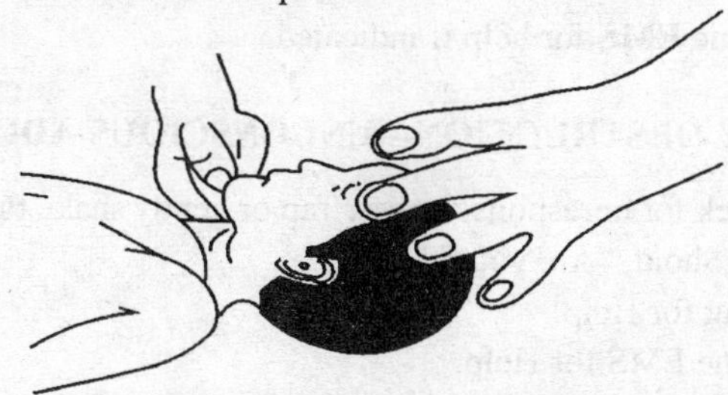

5. **Check for Breathing.** (Time: 3-5 seconds). Look at the chest and abdomen; listen and feel for breathing.

B = BREATHING

6. **Give 2 gentle breaths.** (Time: 1-1.5 seconds per breath) Cover the mouth and nose of the infant with your mouth; give 2 gentle breaths (enough to raise the chest).
7. **Check for a pulse.** (Time: 5-10 seconds)
   Feel for the **Brachial Pulse** on the inside of the upper arm.

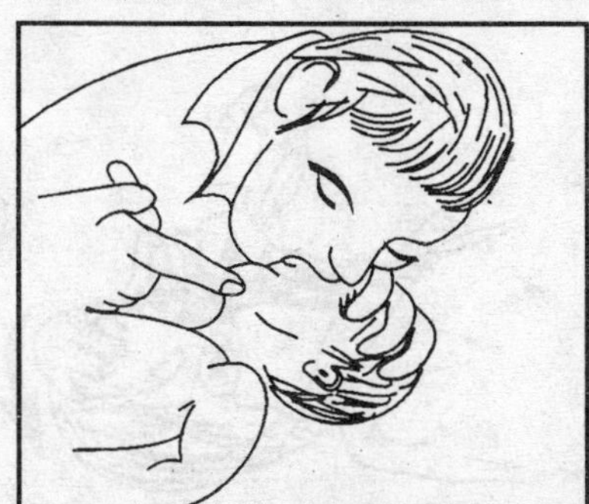

C = CIRCULATION

8. To locate correct hand position, imagine a line is drawn between the nipples.
   Place tip of index finger just below the imaginary line connecting the nipples.
   Place tips of middle and ring fingers next to the index finger.
   Raise index finger.

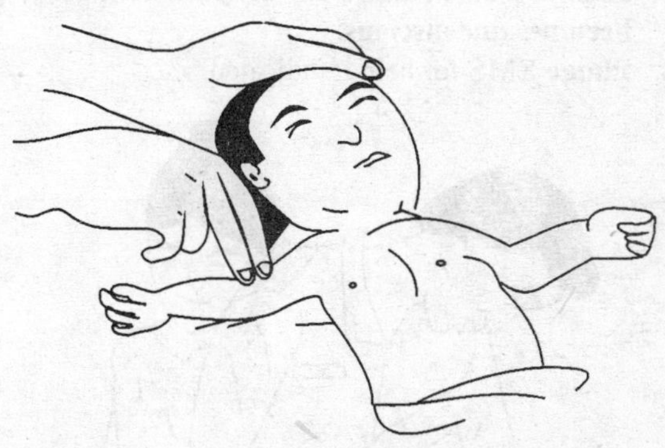

9. **Compress** the sternum **1/2 to 1 inch** at a rate of **at lest 100 times per minute.**
10. Do **5 compressions.**

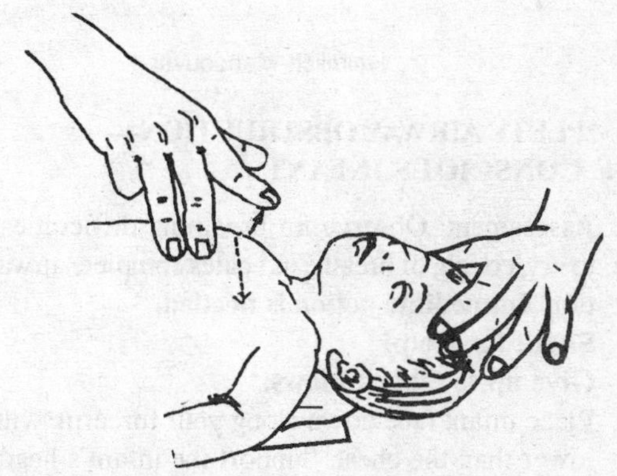

Note: On an infant, perform CPR for 1 minute then phone EMS.

11. Give **1 gentle breath.**
12. Do **20 cycles** of 5 compressions and 1 breath.
13. **Phone EMS** for help.
14. Recheck pulse (Time: 5 seconds) if NO pulse, continue compression/breathing cycles. Recheck pulse every few minutes.

COMPLETE AIRWAY OBSTRUCTION— THE CONSCIOUS ADULT AND CHILD

1. Determine if the patient can cough, speak, or breathe. **Ask, "Are you choking?"** Inability to cough, speak, or breathe indicates complete airway obstruction.
2. **Shout for Help!**

3. **Perform Abdominal Thrusts:**
   Stand or kneel behind patient and wrap arms around patient's waist.
   Place thumb side of one fist against middle of patient's abdomen just above the navel and well below the lower tip of the breastbone.
   Grasp fist with your other hand and press into patient's abdomen with a quick **Upward** thrust.
   Repeat thrusts until obstruction is cleared or patient becomes unconscious.
4. **Phone EMS** for help if indicated.

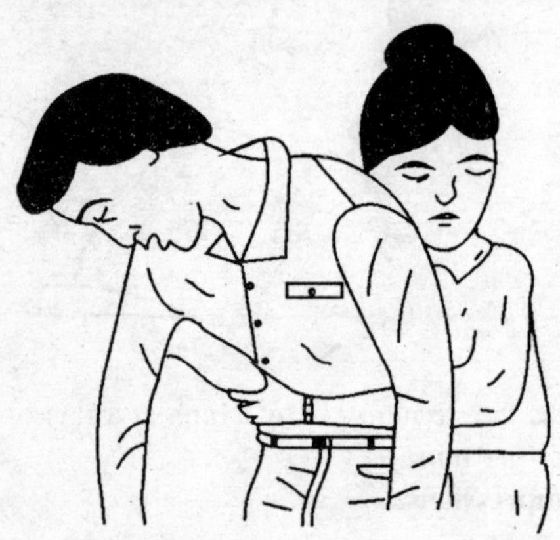

Heimlich Manoeuver

COMPLETE AIRWAY OBSTRUCTION—THE CONSCIOUS INFANT

1. Assessment: Observe for breathing difficulties. Inability to cry, cough, or breathe indicates complete airway obstruction. **Immediate action is needed.**
2. **Shout for Help!**
3. **Give up to 5 back blows.**
   Place infant face down along your forearm, with the head lower than the chest. Support the infant's head and neck by firmly holding the jaw.
   Rest the forearm supporting infant on your thigh.
   Deliver **Back Blows** forcefully between the shoulder blades.

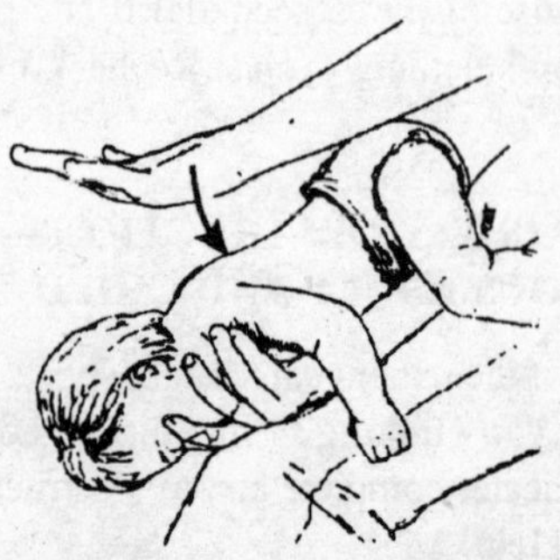

4. **Give up to 5 Chest Thrusts (1/2 - 1 inch)**
   Turn infant as a unit onto his or her back.
   Rest arm supporting infant on your thigh.
   Keep infant's head lower than chest.
   Place tip of ring finger on infant's breastbone just below imaginary line connecting the nipples.

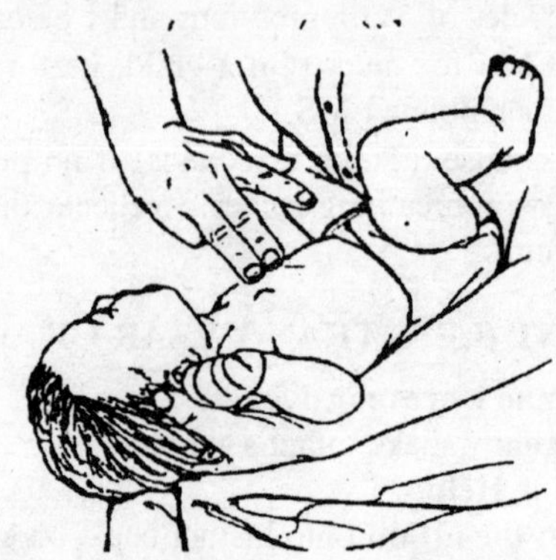

   Place tips of middle and index fingers next to ring finger, then raise ring finger. Note: Pads of the fingers should run down the length of the breast bone.
   Repeat back blows and chest thrusts until obstructionis cleared or the infant becomes unconscious.
5. **Phone EMS** for help if indicated.

AIRWAY OBSTRUCTION—UNCONSCIOUS ADULT

1. Check for unresponsiveness. Tap or gently shake the victim. Shout, "Are you OK?"
2. Shout for Help!
3. Phone EMS for Help.
4. Position the victim onto his/her back on a firm surface. Support the head and neck if you have to turn the victim.

A = AIRWAY

5. **Open the airway.** Using the head-tilt/chin-lift method, tilt the head back and lift chin.
6. **Check for breathing.** (Time: 3-5 seconds)
   Look at the chest and abdomen; listen and feel for breathing.

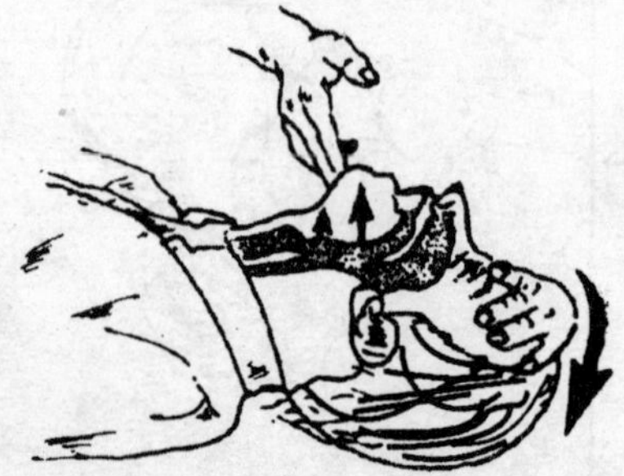

B = BREATHING

7. Give 1-2 full breaths. (Time: 1.5-2 seconds per breath)
   Pinch the nose and cover the mouth with your mouth.
   Note: If unable to breathe into the patient, reposition the head and try again to give 1-2 breaths.

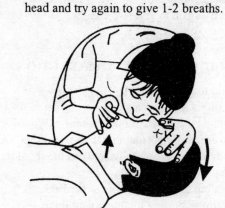

REMOVING THE AIRWAY OBSTRUCTION

8. **Perform 5 Abdominal Thrusts**
   Straddle the victim's thighs.

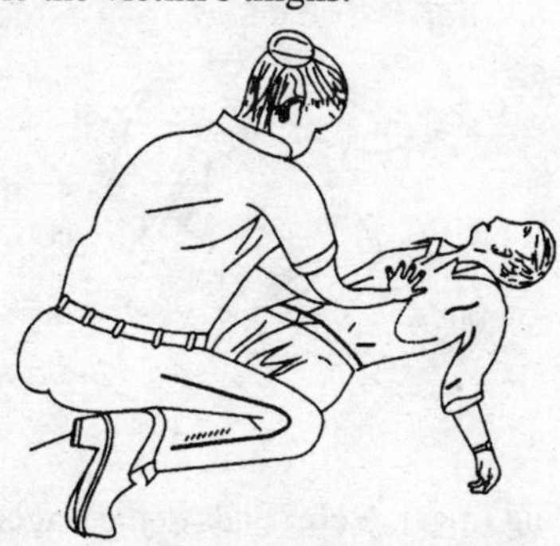

   Place heel of one hand against the middle of the patient's abdomen just above the navel and well below the lower tip of the breastbone. Place your other hand directly on top of the first hand.
   Press into the abdomen 5 times with quick, upward thrusts.
9. **Do a Finger Sweep.**
   Kneel bedside victim's head.
   Open victim's mouth and grasp both the tongue and lower jaw between thumb and fingers of hand nearest patient's legs; lift jaw.

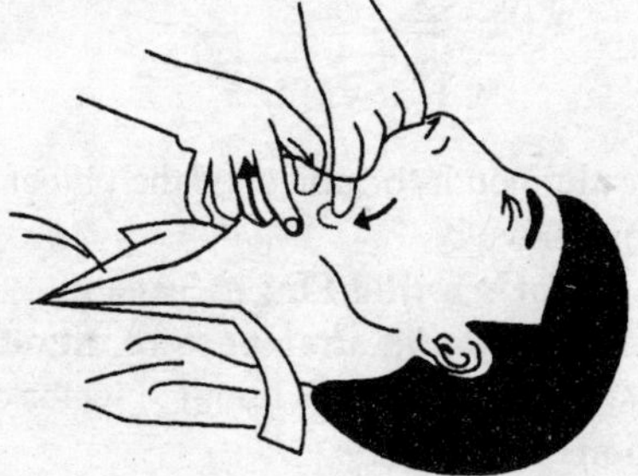

   Insert index finger into mouth along the inside of the cheek and deep into the throat to base of tongue. **Dislodge and remove any object found.**
10. Reposition head and **Attempt to ventilate.**
11. Repeat steps 8, 9, and 10 until object is dislodged and ventilation established.

AIRWAY OBSTRUCTION—UNCONSCIOUS CHILD

1. **Check for unresponsiveness.** Tap or gently shake the child's shoulder. **Shout, "Are you OK?"**
2. **Shout for Help!**
3. **Position the child** onto his/her back. Support the head and neck.

A = AIRWAY

4. **Open the airway.** (Head-tilt/Chin-lift) Gently tilt the head back into a slightly extended position; lift chin.
5. **Check for breathing.** (Time: 3-5 seconds)
   Look, listen, and feel for breathing.

B = BREATHING

6. Give **1-2 gentle breaths.** (Time: 1-1 1/2 seconds per breath).
   Pinch the nose and cover the child's mouth with your mouth.

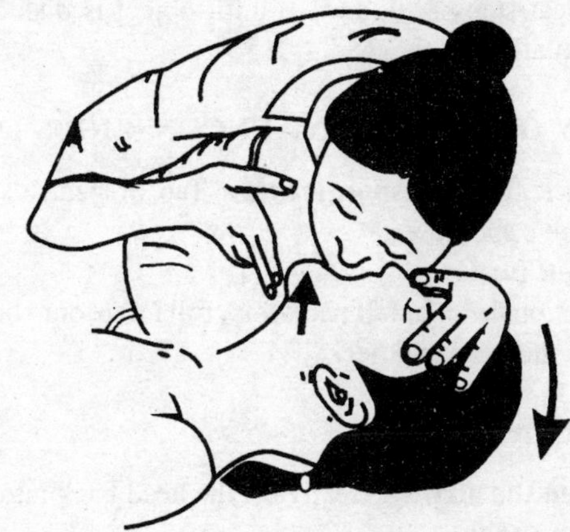

Note: If unable to breathe into the child, reposition the head and try again to give 1-2 breaths.

7. Phone EMS for Help.

REMOVING THE AIRWAY OBSTRUCTION

8. Perform **5 abdominal Thrusts.**
   Kneel at the child's feet. Straddle the thighs of a larger child.
   Place the heel of one hand against the middle of the child's abdomen-just above the navel and well below the lower tip of the breastbone.

Press into the child's abdomen 5 times with quick, upward thrusts.

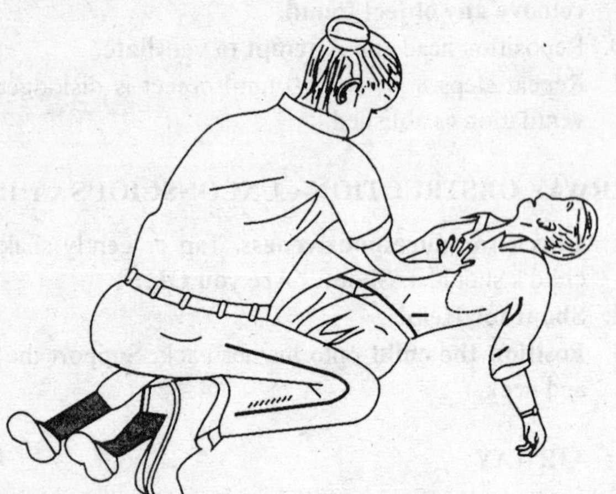

9. **Look inside mouth for object; if the object is visible, attempt to remove it.**
   Kneel beside the child's head.
   Open the child's mouth and grasp both the tongue and the lower jaw between your thumb and fingers of the hand nearest the patient's legs; lift the jaw.
   If the object is visible, attempt to remove it.
   Do not perform a Blind Finger Sweep!
10. Reposition head and **attempt to ventilate.**
11. Repeat steps 8, 9, and 10 until object is dislodged and ventilation established.

AIRWAY OBSTRUCTION—UNCONSCIOUS INFANT

1. Check for **Unresponsiveness.** Tap or gently shake the infant's shoulder.
2. **Shout for Help!**
3. Position the infant. If necessary, roll infant onto back. Support the head and neck.

A = AIRWAY

4. **Open the airway.** Gently tilt the head back into the neutral position.
5. **Check for Breathing.** (Time: 3-5 seconds)
   Look, listen, and feel for breathing.

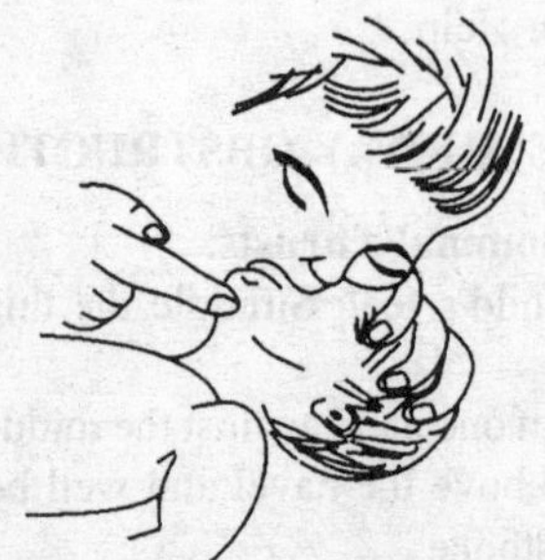

B = BREATHING

6. Give 1-2 gentle breaths. (Time: 1-1 1/2 seconds per breath)
   Cover the infant's mouth and nose with your mouth.

Note: If unable to breathe into the infant, reposition the head and try again to give 1-2 breaths.

7. Phone EMS for Help.

REMOVING THE AIRWAY OBSTRUCTION

8. Give up to **5 back blows.**
   Place infant face down along your forearm, with the head lower than the chest. Support the infant's head and neck. Rest forearm supporting infant on your thigh. Deliver up to **5 back blows** forcefully between the shoulder blades.
9. Give up to **5 chest thrusts.**
   Turn infant as a unit onto his or her back.
   Rest arm supporting infant on your thigh.
   Keep infant's head lower than chest.
   Place pad of ring finger on infant's breastbone just below imaginary line connecting the nipples.
   Place pads of middle and index fingers next to ring finger,

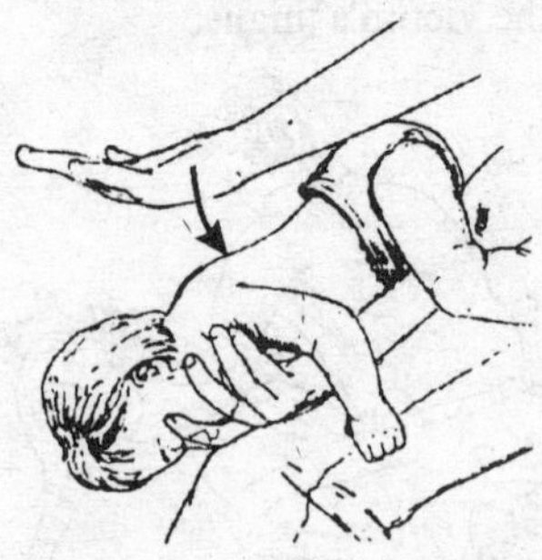

   then raise ring finger. **Note:** Pads of the fingers should run down the length of the breastbone.
   Compress the breastbone 5 times, 1/2 - 1 inch.

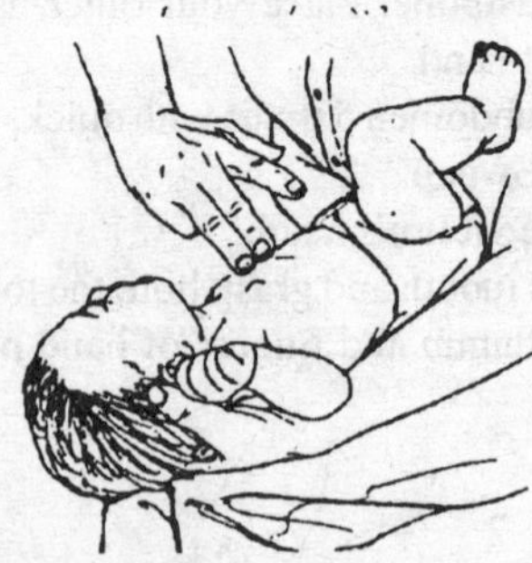

10. Look inside mouth for object; if the object is visible, attempt to remove it.
    Do not perform a Blid Finger Sweep!
11. **Reposition head and attempt to ventilate.**
12. Repeat steps 8, 9, 10, and 11 until object is dislodged and ventilation established.

SUMMARY OF VARIATIONS IN CPR FOR THE INFANT, CHILD, AND ADULT

	Infant *0-1 yr.*	*Child* *1-8 yrs.*	*Adult* *> 8 yrs.*
Location for pulse check	Brachial artery (Arm)	Carotid artery (Neck)	Carotid Artery (Neck)
Compress with	2 Fingers	Heel of one hand	Heel of two hands
Compression depth	1/2" - 1"	1" - 1 1/2"	1 1/2" - 2"
Compressions per minute	At least 100	100	80-100
Rescue Breathing			
Volume	Enough to raise chest	Enough to raise chest	Full Breaths 0.8 L
Length	1-1 1/2 seconds	1-1 1/2 seconds	1 1/2-2 seconds
Rate	20 One every 3 seconds	20 One every 3 seconds	12 One every 5 seconds
Compressions Breaths	5:1	5:1	One-rescuer 15:2 Two-rescuers 5:1

DISEASE TRANSMISSION DURING CPR

Recently, there has been concern about the risk of disease transmission while performing CPR.

Universal Precautions can reduce the risk of disease transmission. Any or all of the following may be necessary:

1. Use of a Laerdal Mask or Ambu Bag instead of performing mouth-to-mouth breathing for all patients.
2. Use of gowns, gloves, masks and eye protection, if needed, when assisting with a Code Blue.
3. Careful handling of all needles and sharps.

ONCE I START CPR, WHEN SHOULD I STOP?

Once started, CPR should only be stopped when:

1. The patient has a pulse and is breathing;
2. Another trained rescuer takes over;
3. The doctor stops CPR and pronounces the victim dead; OR
4. You are too exhausted to continue.

USE OF THE LAERDAL POCKET MASK

The Laerdal Pocket Mask is designed for mouth-to-mask ventilation of a non-breathing adult, child or infant. The mask (or an ambu bag) is to be used in place of mouth-to-mouth ventilation in all Health Care facilities.

Some advantages of the Laerdal Mask:

- Provides a physical barrier between rescuer and patient (Universal Precautions).
- Allows ventilation through mouth and nose simultaneously.
- Promotes an airtight seal to the face even in cases of severe facial trauma.

USING THE LAERDAL POCKET MASK

1. Remove the mask and valve from the container. Push out the mask dome.

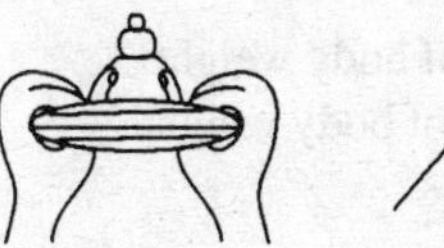
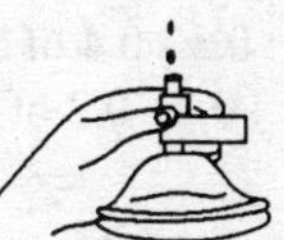

2. Mount the one-way valve on the mask port. Direct exhalation port away from you.
3. Apply the rim of the mask first between the victim's lower lip and chin thus retracting the lower lip to keep the mouth open under the mask. Clamp it with both thumbs on the sides of the mask. Index, middle and ring fingers grasp the lower jaw just in front of the earlobes, above the angles of the jaw, and pull forcefully upward. Open the airway.

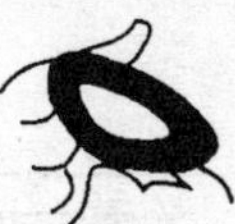
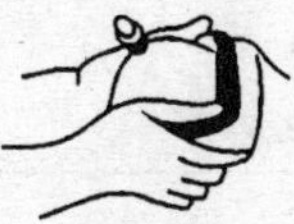

4. Blow intermittently into the mask. Maintain open airway.

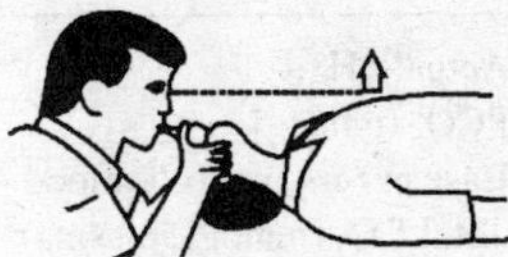

On an Infant

Reverse mask (nose part of mask under the chin of the infant) and apply the mask over the face.

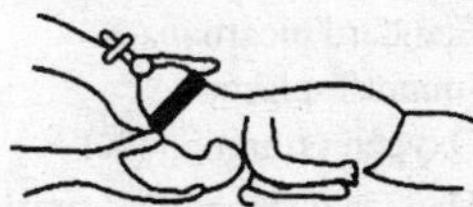

Information and pictures in this Laerdal Pocket Mask summary were adapted from the Laerdal product brochures.

Appendix II
Index of Normal Values

INDEX OF NORMAL VALUES

Body Fluids

Body fluids, total volume : 50 per cent (in obese) to 70 per cent (lean) of body weight

- Intracellular : 0.3 - 0.4 of body weight
- Extracellular : 0.2 - 0.3 of body weight

Blood

- Total volume
- Males : 69 ml/kg body weight
- Females : 65 ml/kg body weight

Plasma volume

- Males: 39 ml/kg body weight
- Females: 40 ml/kg body weight

Red blood cell volume

- Males: 30 ml/kg body weight (1.15-1.21 L/m^2 body surface area)
- Females: 25 ml/kg body weight (0.95-1.00 L/m^2 body surface area).

Blood Acid-Base

	Normal range	
	Arterial	*Venous*
Actual pH	7.35–7.45	7.32–7.42
PCO_2 (mmHg)	35–45	41–51
Base excess (mmol/L blood	0 ± 2.5	–
Total CO_2 (mmol/L plasma)	23–27	26–30
Actual bicarbonate (mmol/L plasma)	22–26	24–28
Standard bicarbonate (mmol/L plasma)	22–26	
Oxygen saturation (%)	96–97	40–70
Oxygen tension PO_2 (mmHg)	80–100	25–40

Cerebrospinal Fluid

Cells	< 5/mm3, all lymphocytes
Chloride	600-700 mg/dl
Glucose	45-75 mg/dl or 60% of serum glucose
pH	7.34 - 7.43
Pressure	50-180 mm H_2O
Protein, lumbar	15-45 mg/dl
Albumin	58%
α1-globulins	9%
α2-globulins	8%
β-globulins	10%
γ-globulins	10% (5-12%)
Protein, cisternal	15-25 mg/dl
Protein, ventricular	5-15 mg/dl

Chemical Constituents of Blood

Antistreptolysin titre	150-200 units/ml
Acetoacetate	0.2-2.0 mg/dl
Acid phosphatase	0.5-12.0 Bodansky units/dl
Acid phosphatase, prostatic	2.5-12.0 IU/L
Aldolase	1.0-6.0 IU/L
Alkaline phosphatase	
Child	5-12 Bodansky units/dl
Adult	1.4-4 Bodansky units/dl
Alpha - 1 antitrypsin	200-500 mg/dl
Ammonia	10-80 μg/dl
Amylase	3-10 Wohlgemuth units/dl
Ascorbic acid	0.4-1.5 mg/dl
Bilirubin	
Adult	0.3-1.1 mg/dl
Newborn	0.4-4.0 mg/dl
At 3 days	1.0-10.0 mg/dl
Carbon dioxide, total	18 ± 3.0 mEq/L
Caeruloplasmin	
Males	36.0 ± 5.6 mg/dl
Females	40.9 ± 6.8 mg/dl
Copper	75-160 μg/dl
Creatinine phosphokinase, Total	0-3.4 micromoles/dl

(Duma modification of Hughes method)

Creatinine phosphokinase isoenzymes	
MM fraction	94-95%
MB fraction	0-5%
BB fraction	0-2%
Creatinine	0.6-1.4 mg/dl
Delta amino laevulinic acid	200 μg/dl
Electrolytes (ISE Analyser)	
Potassium	3.5 - 4.5 mEq/L
Sodium	135 - 140 mEq/L
Chlorides	98 - 110 mEq/L

Calcium (Delhi and Ellingboe)	9 - 10.5 mg/dl
Phosphorus (Fiskee and Subbarow)	
Child	1.1 - 1.65 mmol (2.2 - 3.3 mEq)/L 3 - 4.5 mg/dl
Adult	0.55 - 1.1 mmol (1.1 - 2.2 mEq)/L
Gamma glutamyl transpeptidase (Rosalki's method)	
Male	45 U/L
Female	35 U/L
Gastrin	60 - 200 pg/ml
Glucose, fasting (GOD-POD method)	70 - 110 mg/dl
Glucose 6-phosphate dehydrogenase	5-10 IU/g Hb
G6-PD screen, qualitative	Negative
Immunoglobulin, quantitative (adults)	
IgG	570-1920 mg/dl
IgE	< 0.025 mg/dl
IgA	70-400 mg/dl
IgM	
Males	30-250 mg/dl
Females	30 - 300 mg/dl
IgD (Ramsay's method)	0 - 40 mg/dl
Insulin, fasting	6 - 25 μU/ml
Iron	60 - 140 μg/dl
Iron binding capacity (Ramsay's method)	250 - 450 μg/dl
Lactic acid	5-15 mg/dl
Lipidogram	
Cholesterol	140 - 220 mg/dl
Triglycerides	10-160 mg/dl
Phospholipids	150 - 350 mg/dl
Free fatty acids	< 18 mg/dl
Chylomicrons	Absent
Beta lipoprotein	60 - 75%
Pre-beta lipoprotein	8-20%
Alpha lipoprotein	13-24%
LDH	70-240 IU/L
LDH isoenzymes (Colorimetric method of King)	
LDH1	20 - 34%
LDH2	28 - 41%
LDH3	15 - 25%
LDH4	8 - 16%
LDH5	6 - 15%
Lipase	0 - 160 U/L
Magnesium	1.7 - 2.6 mg/dl
Osmolality	278 - 305 Osm/kg serum water
Phenosulphonphthalein	25% excreted within 15 minutes after injection of 1 ml dye
Phenylalanine	3 mg/dl
Protein, total	6.3 - 7.9 g/dl
Albumin	3.5 - 5.3 g/dl
Globulin	1.8 - 3.6 g/dl
Protein electrophoresis	
Alpha - 1	0.2 - 0.4 g/dl
Alpha - 2	0.5 - 0.9 g/dl
Beta	0.6 - 1.2 g/dl
Gamma	0.7 - 1.7 g/dl
SGOT (AST)	8-40 Karmen units/dl
SGPT (ALT)	0-40 Karmen units/dl
Sulphate	0.5 - 1.5 mg/dl
Urea	15-45 mg/dl
Urea nitrogen	7-21 mg/dl
Uric acid	2.5 - 7.0 mg/dl
Viscosity	1.4 - 1.8 mg/dl (Serum compared to H_2O)
Vitamin A	0.15 - 0.60 mg/dl
Vitamin B_{12}	200 - 850 mg/dl

Function Tests

Circulation

Arteriovenus oxygen difference: 30-50 m/L

Cardiac output (Fick) : 2.5 - 3.6 L/m² body surface area per min

Contractility indexes

- Maximum left ventricular dp/dt: 1650 ± 300 mmHg/s
- Maximum (dp/dt)/p : 44 + 8.4s^{-1}
- (dp/dt)/DP at DP = 40 mmHg : 37.6 ± 12.2s^{-1} (DP = diastolic pressure)
- Mean normalised systolic ejection rate (angiography): 3.32 ± 0.84 end-diastolic volumes per second
- Mean velocity of circumferential fibre shortening (angiography): 1.66 ± 0.42 circumferences per second
- Ejection fraction, stroke volume/end-diastolic volume (SV/EDV): Normal range: 0.55-0.78; average : 0.67
- End-diastolic volume : 75 ± 15 ml/m²
- End-systolic volume : 25 ± 8 ml/m²

Left ventricular work

- Stroke work index : 30 - 110 (g.m)/m²
- Left ventricular minute work index : 1.8-6.6 (kg.m)/m²/min
- Oxygen consumption index : 110-150 ml

Pressures, intracardiac and intra-arterial

- Pulmonary vascular resistance : 2-12 (kPa.s)/L (20-120 (dyn.s/cm²)
- Systemic vascular resistance : 77-150 (kPa.s)/L (770-1500 dyn.s)/cm²)

Gastrointestinal

Absorption tests

D-xylose absorption test: After an overnight fast, 25 g xylose is given in aqueous solution by mouth. Urine collected for the following 5 h should contain 33-53 mmol (5-8g) (or > 20 per cent of ingested dose). Serum xylose should be 1.7 - 2.7 mmol/L Ih after the oral dose (25-40 mg per 100 ml).

Vitamin A absorption test: A fasting blood specimen is obtained and 200,000 units of vitamin A in oil is given by mouth. Serum vitamin A levels should rise to twice fasting level in 3-5 h.

Bentiromide test (pancreatic function): 500 mg bentiromide (Chymex) orally; p-aminobenzoic acid (PABA) measured in plasma and/or urine.

Plasma: 3.6 (± 1.1) mg/L at 90 min
Urine : 50 per cent recovered in 6 h.

Gastric juice

	Conversion factor for SI
Volume	
24 h : 2-3 L	
Nocturnal: 600-700 ml	
Basal fasting : 30-70 ml/h	
Reaction	
pH : 1.6 - 1.8	
Titratable acidity of fasting juice : 4.9 µmol/s (15-35 mEq/h)	0.261
Acid output	
Basal	
Females (mean ± 1 SD) : 0.6 ± 0.5 µol/s (2.0 ± 1.8 mEq/h)	0.2778
Maximal (after subcutaneous histamine acid phosphate 0.004 mg/kg body weight and preceded by 50 mg promethazine or after betazole 1.7 mg/kg body weight or pentagastrin 6 mg/kg body weight):	
Females (mean ± 1 SD) : 4.4 ± 1.4 mmol/s (16 ± 5 mEq/h)	0.2778
Males (mean ± 1 SD) : 6.4 ± 1.4 µmol/s (23 ± 5 eEq/h)	0.2778
Basal acid output/maximal acid output ratio: 0.6 or less	
Gastrin, serum : 40-200 ng/L (40-200 pg/ml)	
Secretin test (pancreatic exocrine function) : 1 unit per kg body weight, intravenously	—
Volume (pancreatic juice): 2.0 ml/kg in 80 min	—
Bicarbonate concentration: 80 mmol/L (80 mEq/L)	—
Bicarbonate output: 10 mmol in 30 min (10 mEq in 30 min)	—

Haematology

Haemogram

Total erythrocyte count	
Males	4.5 - 5.5 millions/cmm
Females	4.1 - 4.8 millions/cmm
Haemoglobin	
Males	14.5 - 16.5 g/dL
Females	12.0 - 14.5 g/dL
Packed cell volume	
Males	38 - 50%
Females	34 - 43%
Mean corpuscular volume	78 - 94 cµ
Mean corpuscular haemoglobin	24 - 33 µg
Mean corpuscular haemoglobin concentration	30-35%
Total leucocyte count	4000 - 11000/cmm
Differential count	
Neutrophils	60 - 70%
Eosinophils	1 - 7%
Lymphocytes	20 - 30%
Monocytes	1 - 6%
Platelets	150,000 - 450,000/cmm
Reticulocyte count	0.5 - 2% of erythrocytes
Erythrocyte sedimentation rate (Westergen)	
Male	0 - 15 mm at end of 1 h
Female	0 - 20 mm end of 1 h
Blood volume	
Average plasma volume	45 ± 5 ml/kg body weight 1487 ± 112 ml/sq meter body surface
Erythrocyte osmotic fragility test	
Increased fragility	Lysis of RBCs seen with over 0.5 per cent of sodium chloride; haemolysis incomplete in 0.3 per cent sodium chloride
Coagulation studies	
Bleeding time (Ivy's method)	1.7 min
Coagulation time (Lee and White)	4 - 8 min
One-stage prothrombin time (Quick)	Control ± 1 sec
Clot-retraction	40 - 65%
Euglobulin lysis time	120 - 240 min
Fibrin degradation products	10 µg/dl
Fibrinogen	200 - 400 mg/dl
Activated partial thromboplastin Time (PTT)	24 - 35 sec
Thrombin time	9 - 10 sec (control + 3 sec)
Whole blood clot lysis time	< 24 hours

Bone marrow study	Normal percentage (range)
WBC reticulum cells	0.2 (0.1 - 2.0)
Blasts	2.0 (0.3 - 5.0)
Promyelocytes	5.0 (1.0 - 8.0)
Myel-neutro	12.0 (5.0 - 21.0)
Myel-eosino	1.5 (0.5 - 3.0)
Myel-baso	0.3 (0.0 - 0.5)
Metamyelocytes	11.0 (6.0 - 17.0)

Stab forms	11.0 (7.0 - 15.0)
PMN neutrophils	20.0 (7.0 - 15.0)
PMN eosinophils	20.0 (0.5 - 4.0)
PMN basophils	0.2 (0.0 - 0.7)
Lymphocytes	10.0 (3.0 - 17.0)
Plasma cells	0.4 (0.0 - 2.0)
Monocytes	2.0 (0.5 - 5.0)
Megakaryocytes	0.4 (0.03 - 3.0)
RBC : Pronormoblasts	4.0 (1.0 - 8.0)
Normoblasts	
Basophilic	1.4 (0.5 - 2.4)
Polychromatophilic	18.0 (7.0 - 32.0)
Orthochromatic	2.0 (0.4 - 4.6)
Unclassified cells	0.3 (0.0 - 0.9)
M : E ratio	3.5 : 1
Haemoglobin studies (normal and abnormal)	
Haemoglobin A,	0.5% of total Hb
Haemoglobin A, C	Up to 6% of total Hb
Haemoglobin A_2	1.5 - 3.5% of total Hb
Haemoglobin foetal	0-2% of total Hb
Haemoglobin plasma	0-5% of total Hb
Haemoglobin, serum	2-3 mg/dl
Methaemoglobin	< 1.8%
Haptoglobin serum	100 - 300 mg/dl
Haemochromogens, plasma	3-5 mg/dl
Haemolysis test	
Acid haemolysis test (Ham)	No haemolysis
Cold haemolysis test (Donath - Landsteiner)	No haemolysis
Erythrocyte lifespan	
Normal	120 days
^{51}Cr-labelled half-life	28 days
Iron turnover rate (plasma)	29-42 mg/24 h
Osmotic fragility	
Haemolysis begins	0.45 - 0.38 NaCl
Haemolysis completed	0.33 - 0.30 NaCl

$$\text{Reticulocyte index} = \frac{\text{Corrected rate}}{2}$$

Reticulocyte index correction factor

$$\text{Corrected rate} = \frac{\text{Observed rate} \times \text{patient's haematocrit}}{\text{Normal haematocrit (45)}}$$

Haematocrit	Correction factor
45	1.00
40	0.71
35	0.52
30	0.38
25	0.28
20	0.20
15	0.13

Note: Reticulocyte index = per cent reticulocytes x correction factor haematocrit and early bone marrow release.

Schilling test : 7-40% of orally administered radiolabelled vitamin B_{12} excreted in urine after 'flushing' with intramuscular injection of B_{12}

Hormones and Metabolites

Adrenocorticotropin (ACTH), serum	15 - 70 pg/ml
Aldosterone, serum	
210 mEq/day sodium diet	
Supine	48 ± 29 pg/dl
Upright (2 h)	65 ± 23 pg/dl
110 mEq/day sodium diet	
Supine	107 ± 45 pg/dl
Upright (2 h)	532 ± 228 pg/dl
Urine	5 - 19 μg/24 h
Calcitonin serum	None detectable
Catecholamines, free urinary	110 ug/24 h
Cortisol, serum	
8 am	5-25 μg/dl
8 pm	5 - 25 μg/dl
Cosyntropin stimulation (30-90 minutes after 0.25 mg cosyntropin intramuscularly or intravenously)	10 μg/dL rise over baseline
Overnight suppression (8 am) (serum cortisol after 1 mg dexamethasone orally at 11 pm)	5 μg/dl
Urine	20-70 μg/24 h
11-deoxycortisol, serum, basal	< 0 - 1.4 μg/dl
Metyrapone stimulation (30 mg/dl orally 8 h prior)	> 1.5 μg/dl

Oestrogens, urine (increased during pregnancy, decreased after menopause)

	Males	*Females*
Total	4-25 μg/24h	5-100 μg/24h
Oestriol	1-11 μg/24h	0-65 μg/24h
Oestradiol	0-6 μg/24h	0-14 μg/24h
Oestrone	3-8 μg/24h	4-31 μg/24h
Oestriocholanolone, serum		1.2 μg/24h

Follicle-stimulating hormone, serum	
Males	6-18 μU/dl
Females	
Follicular phase	5-20 μU/dl
Peak midcycle	12-30 μU/dl
Luteal phase	5-15 μU/dl
Postmenopausal	50 μU/dl
Free thyroxine index, serum	
Adult, fasting	5 ng/dl
Glucose load (100 g orally)	< 5 ng/dl

Levodopa stimulation (500 mg orally in a fasting state) baseline within 2 h

17-hydroxycorticosteroids, urine	
Males	2-12 mg/24h

Females	2-8 mg/24h
5-hydroxyindoleacetic acid	
(5-HIAA), urine	2-9 mg/24h
Insulin, plasma	
Fasting	6-126 μU/ml
Hypoglycaemia	< 5 μU/ml
17-ketogenic steroids, urine	
Under 8 years	0-2 mg/24 h
Adolescent	0-18 mg/24h
Adult males	8-18 mg/24h
females	5-15 mg/24h
Metanephrine, urine	1.3 mg/24h
Norepinephrine, urine	100 mg/24h
Parathyroid hormone, serum	150-300 pg/ml (varies with serum calcium)
Radioactive iodine[131] uptake (RAIU)	5-25% at 24 h (varies with iodine intake)
Renin activity, plasma	
Normal diet	
Supine	1.1 ± 0.8 mg/dl
Upright	1.9 ± 1.7 mg/dl
Low-sodium diet	
Supine	2.7 ± 1.8 mg/dl
Upright	6.6 ± 2.5 mg/dl
Diuretics and low-sodium diet	10.0 ± 3.7 mg/dl
Testosterone	
Total plasma bound	
Adolescent males	100 mg/dl
Adult males	300 - 100 mg/dl
females	25 - 90 mg/dl
Unbound	
Adult males	3-24 mg/dl
females	0.09 - 1.30 mg/dl
Thyroid-stimulating hormone, serum	< 10 μU/ml
Thyroxine (T_4), serum	
Total	4.5 - 11.5 μg/dl
Free	0.8 - 2.4 μ/dl
Thyroxine-binding globulin capacity, serum	15 - 25 μg T/dl
Thyroxine index, free	1 - 4 mg/dl
Tri-iodothyronine (T_3), serum	70-190 mg/dl
T_3 resin uptake	25-45%
Vanillyl mandelic acid (VMA), urine	1-8 μg/24 h

Renal Function Tests

Anion gap	
$Na^{+} - (HCO_3 + Cl)$	10 ± 2 mEq/dl

Osmolality

$$\text{Osmolality (serum)} = 2\,Na^{+}\,(\text{mEq/L}) + \frac{\text{BUN (mg/dl)}}{2.8} + \frac{\text{Glucose (mg/dl)}}{18}$$

Bicarbonate deficit

HCO_3 deficit = body weight (kg) x 0.4 (desired HCO_3-observed HCO_3)

$$\text{Creatinine clearance } \frac{Ucr \times V}{Pcr}$$

= 130 ± 20 ml/min in males

= 120 ± 15 ml/min in females

where

Ucr = Urine creatinine (mg/dl)

Pcr = Plasma creatinine (mg/dl)

V = Urine volume (ml) 24 h

Renal plasma flow

$$RPF = \frac{Upah \times V}{ppah}$$

= 700 ± 100 ml/min in males

= 600 ± 100 ml/min in females

where

Upah = Urine para-aminohippuric acid

V = Urine volume/24 h

ppah = Plasma para-aminohippuric acid

Summary of Values Useful in Pulmonary Physiology

Pulmonary mechanics	Normal values
Spirometry : volume-time curves	
Forced vital capacity	4.0 litres
Forced expiratory volume in 1 s	3.0 litres
FEV_1/FVC	75%
Maximal midexpiratory flow	4.0 litres per second
Maximal expiratory flow rate	8.0 litres per second
Spirometry: flow-volume curves	
Maximal expiratory flow at 50% of expired vital capacity	5.5 litres per second
Maximal expiratory flow at 75% of expired vital capacity	3.0 litres per second
Resistance to airflow	
Pulmonary resistance	< 3.0 cm H_2O/s per litre
Airway resistance	< 2.5 cm H_2O/s per litre
Specific conductance	> 0.13 cm H_2O/s
Pulmonary compliance	
Static recoil pressure at total lung capacity	25 ± 5 cm H_2O
Compliance of lungs (static)	0.2 L/cm H_2O
Compliance of lungs and thorax	0.1 L/cm H_2O
Dynamic compliance of 20 breaths per minute	0.25 ± 0.05 litres per cm H_2O
Maximal static respiratory pressures	
Maximal inspiratory pressure	> 90 cm H_2O
Maximal expiratory pressure	> 150 cm H_2O

Lung Volumes

Total lung capacity	6-7 litres
Functional residual capacity	2-3 litres

Residual volume	1-2 litres
Inspiratory capacity	4.5 litres
Expiratory reserve volume	3.2 litres
Vital capacity	4-5 litres

Gas Exchange (Sea Level)

Arterial O_2 tension	95 ± 5 mm Hg
Arterial CO_2 tension	40 ± 2 mmHg
Arterial O_2 saturation	97 ± 2%
Arterial blood pH	7.40 ± 0.02
Arterial bicarbonate	24 ± 2 mmol/L
Base excess	0 ± mmol/L
Diffusing capacity for carbon monoxide (single breath)	25 ml CO/min/mmHg
Dead space volume	50 ± 25 ml
Physiologic dead space: dead space	≤ 35% VT
Tidal volume ratio (rest)	
(exercise)	≤ 20% VT
Alveolar-arterial difference for O2	< 20 mmHg

Semen

Liquefaction	Complete in 15 min
Morphology	60% normal forms
Motility	75% motile forms
pH	7.2 - 8.0
Spermatocrit	10%
Spermatocyte count	50 million/dl
Volume	2.0 - 6.6 ml

Stool

Bulk	
Wet weight	< 197 g/24 h
Dry weight	< 66.4 g/24 h
Coproporphyrin	12-832 mg/24 h
Fat (on a diet containing 30 g fat/day)	< 7.2 g/24 h or 30% dry weight
Nitrogen	< 2.2 g/24 h
Urobilinogen	40-280 mg/24 h
Water	Approximately 65%

Synovial Fluid

Cells	200 cells/mm³
Polymorphonuclear cells	25%
Crystals	None
Fibrin clot	None
Glucose	Same as serum
Hyaluronic acid	2.45 - 3.97 g/L
pH	7.32 - 7.64
Protein	2.5 g/dL
Albumin	63%
α1-globulins	7%
α2-globulins	7%
β-globulins	9%
γ-globulins	14%
Relative viscosity	300
Uric acid	Same as serum

Urine

Acidity, titrable	20-40 mEq/24h
Ammonia	20-50 mEq/24h
Amylase	25-260 Somogyi unit/h
Bence-Jones protein	None detected
Bilirubin	None detected
Calcium : Normal diet	0.05 - 0.31 mEq/kg body weight/24 h
Low-calcium diet	150 mg/24h
Chloride	120-240 mEq/24h (varies with dietary intake)
Copper	0-32 mg/24h
Creatinine	
Adults	0-200 mg in 24 h
Children	7-11 mg in 24h
Creatinine	1.0 - 1.6 g/24 h or 15-25 mg/kg body weight/24 h
Glucose	
Qualitative	None detected
Quantitative	16-300 µg/24h
Haemoglobin	None detected
Homogentisic acid	None detected
Iron	40-140 µg/24h
Lead	0-120 µg/24h
Myoglobin	None detected
Osmolality	50-1200 mOsm/L
pH	4.6 - 8.0
Phenylpyruvic acid quantitative,	None detected
Phosphorus	0.8 - 2.0 g/24 h
Porphobilinogen	
Qualitative	None detected
Quantitative	0-2.4 mg/24 h
Porphyrin	
Coproporphyrin	50-250 µg/24h
Uroporphyrin	10-30 µg/24h
Potassium	25-100 mEq/24h
Protein	
Qualitative	Non detected
Quantitative	10-150 mg/24 h
Sodium	10-150 mEq/24h (varies with dietary sodium intake)
Specific gravity	1.003 - 1.030
Uric acid	600 - 700 mg/24 h
Urobilinogen	1.0 Enrich units/24 h

Appendix III
Diets in Health and Illness

DIETS IN HEALTH AND IN ILLNESS

Dietetic Requirements

The amount and kind of food each individual requires depends on one's age and sex, the climate of one's country and the sort of work one does, or the life one leads. A man lying in bed needs only 1,700 calories to fulfil his body's requirements, whereas a man doing extremely heavy work may need 5,000 calories—nearly thre times as much.

Diets are made up of: proteins
carbohydrates
fats
water
vitamins
minerals, such as calcium, iron and iodine.

1 gram of protein yields:	4 calories
1 gram of carbohydrate yields:	4 calories
1 gram of fat yields:	9 calories

Calories are the amount of heat needed to raise 1,000 grams of water one degree centigrade. The calorie is used as a unit of measurement in dietetics.

Every diet must contain some protein and the tables show the amount of calories and the weight of protein in grams required by various groups of people. (One ounce is roughly equivalent to 30 grams.)

Total calorie requirements in various conditions of life.
(NB. The proportion of protein required should be noted.)

	Age	*Calories*	*Grams of Protein*
Children	0-1	1000	37
	2-6	1500	56
	7-10	2000	74
	11-14	2750	102
Woman	15-19	2500	93
Man	15-19	3500	130

Requirements of a woman during pregnancy and lactation.

Stage	*Calories*
First half of pregnancy	2500
Second half of pregnancy	2750
During lactation	3000

Calorie requirements of a *Man* and *Woman*

In bed	1750	1500
Sedentary work	2250	2000
Light work	2750	2250
Medium work	3000	2500
Heavy work	3500	3000
Very heavy work	4250	3750
Extremely heavy work	5000	–

Composition of some Comon Foodstuffs per Ounce

	Calories	*Protein grams*	*Fat grams*	*Carbohydrate grams*
Bread	73	2.2	0.2	15.5
Potato	21	0.6	–	4.6
Sugar	108	–	–	26.9
Butter	211	0.1	23.4	
Cheese	117	7.1	9.8	–
Egg	45	3.5	3.3	0.3
Milk	17	0.9	1.0	1.2
Bacon	128	3.1	12.8	–
Beef	89	4.2	8.0	–
Apple	12	0.1	–	3.0
Orange	10	0.2	–	2.2

Diet in Disease

Many diseases are caused by errors in diet. In other cases patients are unable to utilize certain foods and so the treatment is largely dietetic.

The diet is ordered by the physician and the nurse must keep strictly to the physician's orders.

The following specimen diets carry out all the general principles involved and are widely used.

Light Diet

This should consist of easily digested foods, attractively served, so that they stimulate the patient's appetite. Highly seasoned and fatty foods should be avoided.

Avoid rich soups, highly seasoned meats such as sausages, fat meat such as pork, and fried foods.

Do not give fried egg or cheese dishes.

Avoid fried vegetables and gas-producing vegetables such as onions, radishes, green peppers, cucumbers, raw cabbage, dried beans and peas. Raw apples and pears, grapes and melon are all gas-producing and may not be well tolerated.

Avoid pastry and rich puddings and cakes, new bread, fried bread and rye bread.

Do not give effervescent drinks or alcohol.

Low Residue Diet

(For ulcerative colitis, steatorrhoea, diverticulitis, and in acute conditions such as enteric fever and dysentery).

Avoid all pips and skins of fruit (whether raw, cooked or in jam, and currants, raisins and lemon peel in cakes), nuts and all unripe fruit. Fruit juice may be taken. Currants, raisins and figs are particularly undesirable, and all fruit is better stewed than raw. Red currant, apple and other fruit jellies allowed, but no ordinary jams.

Avoid all raw vegetables, whether taken alone (celery, watercress), or in pickles or salad; green vegetables must be passed through a sieve and mixed with butter in the form of a puree. Porridge is only allowed if made with the finest oatmeal.

Avoid alcohol, vinegar, pepper, mustard, curry, chutney, new bread or tough meat.

Reducing Diet

In general, avoid starchy foods, such as bread, cakes, potatoes, etc.; avoid sugary foods and fatty foods.

The diet may contain adequate quantities of lean meat, poultry, lean fish and plenty of green-leaf vegetables and fruit.

N.B. Beer is to be avoided as it contains starch, and fish such as salmon, turbot, herrings, mackerel and sardines are classed as 'fat' fish and are not recommended.

Diet for Constipation

Full diet with the following additions:

Wholemeal bread.

Porridge, made with coarse oatmeal; oatcake.

Vegetables twice a day, especially green vegetables, onions, carrots, parsnips, turnips, tomatoes, watercress and lettuce.

Fruit three times a day, raw or cooked, especially fresh plums and greengages, raspberries, currants, gooseberries, strawberries and figs, pears, apples, oranges and grapes, dried figs, raisins and dates.

Ten stewed prunes for breakfast every morning.

Jam and marmalade with bread and puddings.

Glass of cold water on waking and on going to bed.

Low Purine Diet

(For gout)

It is not generally agreed that the contents of the food have much effect upon gout, but if a low purine diet is advised avoid entirely:

Salmon, halibut, plaice.

Liver, sweetbread, kidney, roe, brain.

Coffee.

Alcohol.

Take sparingly:

Cod, chicken, mutton, veal, beef.

Porridge.

Potatoes, onions, turnips, carrots, parsnips.

French beans, spinach, asparagus.

Dates, figs, rhubarb.

Tea and cocoa.

Cholesterol-Free Diet

(For arteriosclerosis, especially coronary disease)'

Avoid yolk of eggs in any form, including cakes and sweets made with eggs.

Avoid cream.

Avoid cheese.

Avoid kidney, liver, sweetbread, brain.

Avoid duck and goose.

Avoid the fat of meat, pork, suet.

Avoid sausages.

Take as little butter as possible.

Fat-Free Diet

(For liver and gallbladder disease and steatorrhoea.)

Butter should be replaced by honey or golden syrup. No cheese, no nuts, chocolate or cocoa.

Eggs are best avoided, but may not cause nausea if cooked in puddings and cakes.Lean meat is allowed: all fat should be carefully separated by the patient.

Fat meat, ham, bacon and pork to be avoided. No suet. No sausages, liver, kidneys or offal. No fish or meat pastes.

Hadlock, cod, whiting, turbot, brill and plaice are allowed, but no other fish.

The patient should have skimmed milk.

Diabetic Diets

In treating diabetes, the patient's intake of carbohydrates may be restricted or he may be ordered a diet with an ordinary amount of carbohydrate and adequate insulin to cover it. In a fat diabetic patient, a diet containing only 1,300 calories may be ordered; whereas, with a thin diabetic patient, or with a petient who does manual labour, a full diet may be required with sufficient insulin covering it.

Diabetic Diet with 120 grams of Carbohydrate

	grams of carbohydrate
Breakfast	
Egg, bacon, ham or fish	
2 oz. bread or equivalent	30
*Milk	
Butter or margarine	
Coffee or tea	

Mid-Morning
*Milk
Coffee or tea
2 semi-sweet biscuits 10

Lunch
Meat, fish, cheese, eggs
Green vegetables or salad
Small portion root vegetables
3 Oz. potato (i.e. 1 medium potato 15
Fruit (raw or stewed without sugar 10

Tea
*Milk in tea
1 oz. bread or equivalent 15
Butter or margarine
Diabetic jam if desired

Supper
Meat, fish, cheese or eggs
Green vegetables or salad as desired
Root vegetables (small portion)
1 oz. bread or equivalent 15
Butter or margarine
Fruit (raw or stewed without sugar) 10
*Milk

Bedtime
*Milk *Milk taken during the day must not exceed 15 G CHO, i.e. 1/2 pint 15

Total 120

Diabetic Diet with 180 grams of Carbohydrate

grams of carbohydrate

Breakfast
Egg, bacon, ham or fish
2 oz. bread or equivalent 30
*Milk
Butter or margarine
Diabetic marmalade if desired
Coffee or tea

Mid-morning
*Milk
Coffee or tea
2 semi-sweet biscuits 10

Lunch
Meat, fish, cheese or eggs
Green vegetables or salad as desired
Small portion of root vegetables
7 oz. potato (i.e. 2 medium potatoes) 30
or 3 oz. potato and 3 tablespoons unsweetened milk pudding
Fruit (raw or stewed without sugar) 10

Tea
*Milk
1 oz. bread or equivalent 15
Butter or margarine
Diabetic jam if desired

Supper
Meat, fish, cheese or eggs
Green vegetables or salad as desired
Small portion of root vegetables
3 oz. potato (i.e. 1 medium potato) 15
2 oz. bread or equivalent 30
Butter or margarine
Fruit (raw or stewed without sugar 10
*Milk

Bedtime
*Milk *Milk taken during the day must not exceed 30 G CHO i.e. 1 pint 30

Total 180

Diabetic Diet with 230 grams of Carbohydrate

grams of carbohydrate

Breakfast
Egg, bacon, ham or fish
3 oz. bread or equivalent 45
*Milk
Butter or margarine
Diabetic marmalade if desired
Coffee or tea

Mid-morning
*Milk
Coffee or tea
3 semi-sweet biscuits 15

Lunch
Meat, fish, cheese or eggs
Green vegetables or salad as desired
Small portion of root vegetables
6 oz. potato (i.e. 2 medium potatoes) 30
or 3 oz.potato and 3 tablespoons unsweetened milk pudding
Fruit (raw or stewed without sugar) 10

Tea
*Milk in tea
2 oz. bread or equivalent 30
Butter or margarine
Diabetic jam if desired

Supper
Meat, fish,Cheese or eggs
Green vegetables or salad as desired
Small portion of root vegetables
3 oz. potato (i.e. 1 medium potato) 15
2 oz. bread or equivalent 30
Butter or margarine
Fruit (raw or stewed without sugar) 10

*Milk

Bedtime

1 oz. bread or equivalent	15
Butter or margarine	
*Milk *Milk allowance = 30 G. C.H.O. *i.e.* 1 pint a day	30
Total	230

Diabetic Diet with 300 grams of Carbohydrate

	grams of carbohydrate
Breakfast	
Egg, bacon, ham or fish	
4 oz. bread or equivalent	60
*Milk	
Butter or margarine	
Fruit (raw or stewed without sugar)	10
Coffee or tea	
Mid-morning	
*Milk	
Coffee or tea	
3 semi-sweet biscuits	15
Lunch	
Meat,fish, cheese or eggs	
Green vegetables or salad as desired	
Small portion of root vegetables	
6 oz. potato (i.e. 2 medium potatoes)	30
or 3 oz.potato and 3 tablespoons unsweetened milk pudding	
Fruit (raw or stewed without sugar)	10
Tea	
*Milk	
3 oz. bread or equivalent	45
Butter or margarine	
Diabetic jam if desired	
Supper	
Meat, fish, cheese or eggs	
Green vegetables or salad as desired	
Small portion of root vegetables	
3 oz. potato (i.e. 1 medium potato)	15
3 oz. bread or equivalent	45
Butter or margarine	
Fruit (raw or stewed without sugar)	10
*Milk	
Bedtime	
1 oz. bread or equivalent	15
Butter or margarine	
*Milk *Milk allowance = 45 G CHO *i.e.* 1 1/2 pints a day	45
Total	300

Equivalents for Use in Diabetic Diets

Bread: The equivalent to 1 oz. of bread (*i.e.* 15 grams of carbohydrate) is found in the following:

2 Ryvita or Vita-Weat
3 Cream crackers or water biscuits
3 Semi-sweet biscuits
3/4 Cupful cornflakes or other breakfast cereal
3 Tablespoons porridge
1 Medium-sized potato (3 oz.)
2 Tablespoons boiled rice, spaghetti or macaroni
1/2 Pint of milk

Drinks: The following are equivalent to 20 grams of carbohydrate.

- 1 glassful milk (7 oz.) and 2 teaspoons Horlicks, Ovaltine or bourn Vita.
- 2/3 cupful fresh orange jiice (4 oz.) and 2 lumps or 2 teaspoonfuls of sugar.
- Diabetic fruit squash and 4 lumps or 4 teaspoons of sugar
- 1/2 cup milk (3 oz.) in tea or coffee and 1 oz. bread (or equivalent).

Fruit: The following portions of fruits are equivalent to 10 grams of carbohydrate.

apple, dessert	1 small
Apple, stewed	1 1/2 cups
Apricots, dried	6 halves
Apricots, fresh	2 medium
Banana	1 small
Cherries	10 large
Dates	2
Figs, dried	1 small
Figs, fresh	2 large
Gooseberries	6 large
Grapefruit	1 medium
Grapes	12
Greengages	4 medium
Melon	1 slice, 2 in. thick
Orange	1 small
Orange juice	2/3 cup
Peach	1 medium
Pear	1 medium
Pineapple, fresh	1 slice, 1 in. thick
Plums, dessert	2 large
Plums, stewed	3 medium
Prunes	6 small
Raspberries	1 cup
Strawberries	1 cup
Tangerine	1 large

Foods to be Avoided in a Diabetic Diet

The following foods contain a high percentage of carbohydrate, and are therefore to be avoided by the diabetic: Sugar, sweets and chocolate; jam, marmalade, honey or syrup; puddings, cakes and pastries; biscuits (except as equivalants to bread); thickened soups, sauces and gravies; sweetened fruit drinks and minerals.

Foods Allowed at will in a Diabetic Diet

The following foods may be taken as desired by the diabetic: Coffee, tea or soda water; clear broth, Bovril, Oxo or Marmite, and the following vegetables:

Artichokes	chicory	lettuce	radishes
Asparagus	cucumber	mustard & cress	rhubarb
Broccoli	endive	marrow	runner geans
Brussels sprout	French beans	mushrooms	sauerkraut
Cabbage	kale	onions	spinach
Cauliflower	leeks	parsley	swedes
Celery	lemons	pepper-green	tomatoes
			watercress

Distribution of Carbohydrate in the Diet According to the Amount of Insulin taken by the Patient

If no insulin is being taken by the patient, the amount of carbohydrate should be distributed evenly over breakfast,lunch, tea and supper. If protamine zinc and soluble insulin is given, 1/3 of the total carbohydrate should be given at breakfast, 1/3 divided between lunch and tea and 1/3 at supper. With globin insulin, 1/3 carbohydrate should be given at breakfast, 2/5 at lunch, and 2/3 at supper time. When lente insulin is being taken, 1/4 carbohydrate at breakfast, 1/3 at lunch, 1/3 at tea, and 1/4 at supper and 1/20 at bedtime. With isophane insulin, 1/4 carbohydrate should be given at breakfast, 3/16 at lunch, 1/3 at tea time, 1/4 at supper, and about 1/20 at bedtime.

Diet for Patients with Gastric Ulcer

Stage I

All patients have to be given the appropriate medicines, such as magnesium trisilicate, aluminium hydroxide or other alkaline powder, and tinct, belladonna or propantheline before meals, and milk ad. lib.

Patients should avoid soups made with meat stock, meat, fish and poultry, cheese, fried eggs; vegetables, raw fruit, brown and wholemeal bread, cereals and biscuits except plain ones.

Avoid alcohol, strong tea or coffee, Oxo, Bovrill, condiments and seasonings.

Specimen menu giving approximately 2,000 calories:

Breakfast

Strained porridge
Milk
Soft egg (boiled, poached or scrambled)
White bread toasted
Jelly jam, honey or jelly marmalade
Milk drink or very milky tea with sugar.

Mid-morning

Egg flip
Buttered cream crackers

Lunch

Strained cream soup
Melba toast or cream crackers
Milk pudding or pureed fruit
Milk drink or very milky tea with sugar.

Tea

Toast and butter
Jelly jam
Milky tea with sugar.

Supper

Egg custard
Plain cereal pudding or jelly
Milk drink or very milky tea with sugar.

Bedtime

Milk drink
Plain biscuits

Stage II

The patient should have milk ad. lib. and the appropirate medicines.

Avoid soups made with meat stock, highly seasoned meat such as sausages, tinned meat and fish; re-cooked food, pork and bacon; strong cheese, fried eggs, fried vegetables and gasforming vegetables such as onions, green peppers, dried peas and beans; raw vegetables. All cooked vegetables should be sieved.

Avoid fresh fruits except bananas and any cooked fruit with seeds or skins; avoid dried fruits. Do not give pastry, rich puddings or cakes; brown and wholemeal bread, biscuits and cereals.

Avoid strong tea, coffee, Oxo and Bovril, and alcohol. Avoid seasoning and condiments.

Specimen menu giving approximately 2,100 calories.

Breakfast

Cereal (as allowed)
Milk
Soft egg, plain fish or ham (not fried)
White toast or bread
Butter or margarine
Jelly jam or marmalade jelly
Weak tea or coffee with sugar and milk.

Mid-morning

Milk or milky drink
Plain biscuits.

Lunch

Lean meat, fish or poultry (as allowed)
Potato (not roast or fried)

Vegetables (as allowed)
Fruit or milk pudding (as allowed)
Tea or coffee with sugar and milk.

Tea

White bread
Butter or margarine
Jelly or marmite
Weak tea with sugar and milk.

Supper

Meat, fish, cheese or egg dish (as allowed)
Potato ⎤
Vegetables ⎥ as at lunch
Fruit or pudding ⎦
White bread
Butter or margarine
Weak tea with sugar and milk.

Bedtime

Milk or milky drink
Toast and butter or plain biscuits.

Post-peptic Ulcer Regime

Avoid alcohol. Avoid effervescing drinks and coffee.

Avoid all pips and skins of fruits (whether raw, cooked or in jam, and currants, raisins and lemon peel in puddings and cake) nuts and all unripe fruit. For example, an orange may be sucked but not eaten. Currants, raisins and figs are particularly undesirable.

Avoid all raw vegetables, whether taken alone (celery, watercress), or in pickles or salad; green vegetables must be passed through a sieve and mixed with butter in the form of a puree. Porridge is only allowed if made with the finest oatmeal.

Avoid vinegar, lemon juice, sour fruit, spinach, pepper, mustard, curry, chutney, excess of salt, new bread, tough meat.

Take plenty of butter and a tablespoonful of olive oil before each meal.

Eat slowly and chew very thoroughly. An adequate time should be allowed for meals, and rest for at least a quarter of an hour before and after meals. Meals must be punctual.

Don't smoke excessively, no smoking at all if any indigestion.

For six months: A meal or feed should be taken at intervals of not more than two hours from waking till retiring, and again if awake during the night. The feed should consist of a glass of the following mixture, which should be prepared each morning: a quart of milk, and 120 grains of sodium citrate in 1 oz. of water.

After six months of complete freedom: A feed should be taken in the middle of the morning, on going to bed, and again if awake during the night, in addition to the ordinary meals.

A teaspoonful of the 'alkaline powder' should be taken an hour after meals and also directly the slightest indigestion or heartburn is felt.

The bowels should be kept regular by means of magnesia emulsion taken two or three times a day, and, if necessary, liquid paraffin, but no other aperients should be taken.

The teeth shold be attended to by the dentist regularly every six months.

No drugs should be taken in pill or tablet form.

If there is the slightest return of symptoms, the patient should go to bed on a strict diet, and consult his doctor, not waiting for the symptoms to become serious.

High Protein, Low Fat Diet

(For cirrhosis of liver, steatorrhoea, certain cases of nephritis, carcinoma.)

Lean meat, fish, eggs, Cheddar cheese.
White bread, Cornflakes, boiled potatoes, cauliflower, peas.
Small occasional helpings of jam and marmalade.
Baked custards and milk puddings made from skimmed milk.
2 pt. daily of fortified milk consisting of:
2 pt. skimmed milk
2 oz. Sprulac
2 oz. Casilan
1 oz. lactose.

Low Sodium Diet

Avoid adding salt to food at meal times, and only very small quantities may be used in cooking.

The following food should be avoided: Soups made from ham or salt meat; Oxo, Bovril; tinned and preserved meats; smoked and dried products such as ham and bacon; salt fish and offal (though heart and liver may be taken).

The patient should also avoid cheese; beetroot, celery and spinach; puddings made with baking powder or soda; and anything made with self-raising flour.

He should not take meat sauces, pickles, condiments, salad cream or mayonnaise.

Gluten-Free Diet

(This diet is used chiefly to treat coeliac disease and in steatorrhoea. Rye and wheat gluten has to be avoided and special bread, cakes and biscuits are given made of wheat starch).

Breakfast

Oatmeal porridge, cornflakes or other suitable cereals (with milk and sugar)
Egg, bacon, ham, kipper or haddock
Wheat starch bread, toasted if desired
Butter, honey or marmalade
Tea or coffee.

Mid-morning

Tea, coffee or milk
Oat cakes or wheat starch biscuits if desired.

Lunch

Meat, poultry, or steamed, baked or grilled fish
Potatoes
Cooked vegetables or salad
Sago, rice, tapioca, egg custard, blancmange, junket jelly or fruit
Tea, coffee or fruit juice.

Tea

Wheat starch bread
Butter
Jam, honey, syrup or tomatoes
Oat cakes or wheat starch cakes or biscuits
Tea or coffee.

Supper

Meat, fish, cheese or eggs
Potatoes or wheat starch bread and butter
Cooked vegetables or salad if desired
Pudding or fruit as at lunch.

Bedtime

Tea, milk or coffee.

PEPTIC ULCER

Diet I

Haematemesis and Melaena

6.00 am	Milk	1 glass
	with protein supplement	
8.30 am	*Idlies*	–2 nos
	Sambar	–1 cup
	Curd	–1 cup
	Sugar or *Idiappam*	–2 cups
	Milk	–1 cup
	Sugar	
10.30 am	Carrot milk or milk shake or	
	Tender coconut water	–1 cup
12.30 pm	Soft rice	–1 1/2 cups
	Seasoned *dal*	–1 cup
	Vegetable *kootu*	–1/2 cup
	Boiled vegetable saute	–1/2 cup
	Curd	–1 cup
3.30 pm	Milk	–1 glass
	with protein supplement	
	Marie biscuits	–2 nos
5.30 pm	Banana	–1 no
7.30 pm	*Chapati*	–2 nos
	or	
	Rice	–1 cup
	Mixed dal	–1 cup
	Less spicy vegetable curry	–1 cup
	Curd	–1 cup
9.30 pm	Custard with jelly	–1 cup

PEPTIC ULCER

Diet II (During remission from pain)

Peptic ulcer diet I can be followed

Depending upon the tolerance the quantity of food can be increased. Light tea can also be introduced.

DIARRHOEA, DYSENTERY AND CHOLERA AFTER RECOVERY

6.00 am	Tea	–1 cup
8.30 am	*Idlies*	–2 nos
	Bland sambar	–1 cup
	Curd	–1 cup
	Sugar	
	or	
	Oats porridge with very little milk	–1 cup
	Toast	–2 slices
	Jam tea	–1 cup
10.00 am	Tender coconut water	
	or	
	Sweet lime juice	
	or	
	Buttermilk	–1 glass
1.00 pm	Rice/*chapatis*	–2 cups/3 nos
	Dal	–1/2 cup
	Less spicy vegetable curry	–1 cup
	Curd	–1 cup
	Stewed apple	–1 no
4.00 pm	Tea	–1 cup
	Marie biscuits	–2-3 nos
6.00 pm	Orange juice	–1 glass
8.00 pm	Tomato soup	–1 cup
	Kichdi	–2 cups
	Kadi	–1 cup
	or	
	Chapatis	–4 nos
	Dal	–1 cup
	Less spicy vegetables	–1 cup
	Curd	–1 cup
9.00 pm	Jelly	–1 cup

VIRAL HEPATITIS OR OBSTRUCTIVE JAUNDICE

Severe jaundice (Total serum bilirubin over 15 mg/dl)
Protein 40 grams
Fat 25 grams
Carbohydrate 300 grams
Calories 1500

6.00 am	Light tea	
8.30 am	*Idlies*	3 nos
	Bland sambar	
	Curd	

	Sugar	
	or	
	Bread	2 slices
	Jam	
	Oats porridge with 50 ml milk	
	Banana	1 no
	Light tea	
10.30 am	Sweet lime juice	1 glass
	or	
	Orange juice	1 glass
	or	
	Buttermilk	1 glass
1.30 pm	Vegetable soup	
	Rice	2 cups
	Dal or *Sambar*	1/2 cup
	Boiled vegetables with boiled potatoes	1 cup
	Curd	
	Banana	1 no
4.00 pm	Light tea	
	Marie biscuits	
	Orange/apple	1 no
8.00 pm	Tomato soup	
	Rice/*chapati*	2 cups/4 nos
	Sambar/dal	1 cup
	Boiled vegetables with boiled potatoes	
	Buttermilk	
	Fruit salad	

VIRAL HEPATITIS OR OBSTRUCTIVE JAUNDICE

Mild to moderate jaundice (Total serum bilirubin below 15 mg/dl)

6.00 am	Light tea	–1 cup
8.00 am	*Idlies*	–3 nos
	or	
	Idiappam	–3 cups
	Sambar	–1 cup
	Mint chutney	–1 cup
	or	
	Toast	–2 slices
	Jam	–2 tsp
	Dalia porridge	–1 cup
	or	
	Oats porridge	–1 cup
	Light tea	–1 cup
10.00 am	Sweet lime juice	
	or	
	Tender coconut water	–1 glass
1.00 pm	Vegetable soup	–1 cup
	Kichdi	–1 cup
	Palak curry	–1 cup
	Mixed boiled vegetables	–1 cup
	Fruit salad	–1 cup
	Curd	–1 cup
4.00 pm	Tea	–1 cup
	Bread	–3 slices
	Jam	–4 tsp
	or	
	Whole gram sundal	–3/4 cup
8.00 pm	Tomato soup	–1 cup
	Vegetable *upma*	–2 cups
	Rajmah dal	–1 cup
	Curd	–1 cup
	Banana	–1 no
	or	
	Papaya	–200 grams

HEPATIC CIRRHOSIS (NOT IN PRECOMA)

High protein, high carbohydrate, moderate fat, high calorie diet

6.00 am	Skimmed milk	–1 glass
	with protein supplement	–2 tsp
8.30 am	*Idlies*	–2 nos
	Sambar	–1/2 cup
	Poached egg white	–2 nos
	or	
	Bread	–2 nos
	Jam	–3 tsp
	Semolina and green gram dal	–1 cup
	Porridge	–1 cup
	Orange	–1 no
10.30 am	Sweet lime juice	–1 cup
12.30 pm	Rice *dal kichdi*	–1 cup
	Beans *usili*	–1 cup
	Boiled vegetables with lot of peas	–1 cup
	Dal	–1 cup
	or	
	Boiled chicken	–50 grams
	Skimmed milk curd	–1 cup
	Banana	–1 no
4.00 pm	Skimmed milk with	–1 glass
	protein supplement	–2 tsp
8.00 pm	Whole dalia *upma*	–1 cup
	Tomato chutney	–1 cup
	Skimmed milk curd	–1 cup
	Mixed fruit jelly	–1 cup

GALLBLADDER DISEASE

6.00 am	Tea/coffee	–1 cup
8.30 am	*Idlies*	–3 nos
	Tomato chutney	–1 cup
	Sambar	–1 cup

	Orange	–1 no
10.30 am	Buttermilk	–1 glass
12.30 pm	Clear vegetable soup	–1 cup
	Rice	–1 1/2 cups
	or	
	Chapatis	–3 nos
	Thin *dal*	–1/2 cup
	Vegetable *kuttu*	–1 cup
	Vegetable salad	–1 cup
	Buttermilk	–1 cup
	Cut papaya	–1 cup
3.30 pm	Tea	–1 cup
	Marie biscuits	–3 nos
	Tomato soup	–1 cup
7.30 pm	Vegetable *idiappam*	–1 1/2 cups
	Mint chutney	–1 cup
	Sauted mixed boiled vegetable	–1 cup
	Thin butter milk	–1 glass

OBESITY

Mixed diet		
6.00 am	Coffee/tea	–1 cup
	Sugar	–1/2 tsp
8.00 am	*Idlies*	–2 nos
	Tomato chutney	–1/2 cup
	Sambar	–1 cup
	or	
	Toast/bread	–2 slices
	Egg white omelette	–1 no
	Coffee/tea	–1 cup
	Sugar	–1/2 tsp
11.00 am	Thin buttermilk	–200 ml
	or	
	Lime juice with salt	–200 ml
1.00 pm	Vegetable soup	–1 cup
	Chapati/rice	–2 nos/1 cup
	Dal	1 cup
	Chicken curry/fish curry	–50 grams
	Salad	2 cups
	Vegetable curries	–2 cups
	Thin buttermilk	–1 cup
	Apple/orange/sweet lime/guava/papaya	–1 no (100 grams)
4.00 pm	Coffee/tea	–1 cup
	Sugar	–1/2 tsp
	Thin arrowroot/*Marie* biscuits	–2 nos
	or	
	Vegetable sandwich (without butter)	–1 no
	or	
	Whole gram sundal	–1/2 cup
8.00 pm	Vegetable soup	–1 cup
	Chapati/rice	–2 nos/1 cup
	Dal/sambar	–1/2 cup
	Rasam	–1 cup
	Vegetable curry	–1 cup
	Thin buttermilk	–1 glass
	Salad	–2 cups

HIGH BLOOD PRESSURE

6.30 am	Tea	–1 cup
8.30 am	*Idil/chapati/idiyappam*	–3 nos; 1 1/2 cup
	Onion/tomato chutney	
	or	
	dal	–1 cup
	or	
	Plain bread/toasts/cornflakes	–1/2 cup
	Jam	
	Milk	
10.30 am	Fruit juice	–1 cup
	or	
	Milk	–1 cup
1.00 pm	Vegetable soup	–1 cup
	Rice/*chapati*	–1 1/2 cups/3 nos
	Boiled/bland chicken or fish or egg	–50 grams
	Beans/vegetable preparation	–1 cup
	Fruit	–1 No
	Sambar/dal	–1 cup
	Rasam	–1 cup
	Curd	–1 cup
4.00 pm	Tea/coffee/fruit juice	–1 cup
	Biscuits/vegetable sandwich	–1 slice
8.30 pm	Vegetable soup	–1 cup
	Rice/*chapati*	–1 1/2 cups/3 nos
	Green leafy vegetables	–1 cup
	Any other vegetable preparation	–1 cup
	Sambar/dal	–1 cup
	Bland/boiled chicken/fish/egg	–50 grams
	Curds	–1 cup
9.30 pm	Milk	–1 cup

GOUT

6.30 am	Tea/coffee/milk	
8.30 am	*Idlies/Chapatis/Idiyappam*	–1 1/2 cup
	Sugar	
	or	
	Dal	–1 cup
	or	
	Breads/porridge/3/4 cup with milk/cornflakes with milk	–1 cup
10.30 am	Fruit juice/buttermilk	–1 glass
1.00 pm	Rice	–1 1/2 cup
	or	

	Chapatis	–3 nos
	Vegetable preparation	–2 cups
	Dal	–1 cup
	Rasam	–1 cup
	Curd	–1 cup
	Bland/roasted chicken or fish or poached egg cucumber/radish, beet root, salad	
	Sweet lime/apple	
4.00 pm	Tea/coffee/milk	–1 cup
	Marie biscuits	–3 nos
8.30 pm	Vegetable soup	
	Rice	–1 1/2 cup
	or	
	Chapati	–3 nos
	Mixed vegetable preparation	–1 cup
	Ladies finger curry	–1 cup
	Boiled/bland chicken or fish	–1 cup
	or	
	dal	–1 cup
	Curd/buttermilk	–1 cup
9.00 pm	Milk	

ACUTE GLOMERULONEPHRITIS

Approximately
Proteins 30 grams
Fat 60 grams
Carbohydrates 250 grams

Calories	1700	
6.00 am	Tea or coffee	–1 cup
8.00 am	*Idlies* or *Idiyappam*	–3 nos
	Tomato chutney	–1 cup
	Sambar	–1 cup
	Tea	–1 cup
10.00 am	Apple or orange	–1 no
12.30 am	Rice	–1 1/2 cups
	Vegetable *kootu*	–1 cup
	Rasam	–1 cup
	Mixed vegetable curry	–1 cup
	Curd	–1 cup
3.30 pm	Tea	–1 cup
	Marie biscuits	–3 nos
7.30 pm	*Chapatis*	–3 nos
	Dal	–1/2 cup
	Palak curry	–1 cup
	Boiled vegetable saute	–1 cup
	Curd	–1 cup

– Salt and fluid to be followed according to doctor's prescription

NEPHROTIC SYNDROME

Mixed diet
Proteins 120 grams
Fats 70 grams
Carbohydrates 230 grams
Calories 2000

6.00 am	Tea/coffee/milk	1 cup
8.00 am	*Idlies/dosa*	4 nos/3 nos
	phulkas/uppma	4 nos
	Well-cooked vegetables	
	Dal/Sambar	1 cup
	Cooked tomato/onion chutney	4-5 tsp
	Boiled egg/egg omlette	2 nos
10.00 am	Permitted fruits	100 grams
	or	
	Buttermilk	1 glass
1.00 pm	Rice/*chapati*	2 cups/4 nos
	Dal/sambar	2 cups
	Vegetables	2 cups
	Curd	1 cup
	Chicken/fish curry	50 grams
4.00 pm	Milk/tea/coffee	1 cup
	Biscuits	3 nos
	or	
	Bread	2 slices
7.30 pm	Rice/*chapati*	2 cup/4 nos
	Dal/sambar	2 cups
	Vegetables	2 cups
	Curd	1 cup
	Chicken/fish curry	50 grams
Bed time	Milk	1 cup

Protein supplements like soya preparations or proprietary preparations to be liberally included in the diet if vegetarian.

CARDIAC PATIENTS

Stage I

Salt-free, 1800 ml of fluids and 800 calories

6.30 am	Milk-200 ml + 10g skimmed milk powder	
8.30 am	Tender coconut water	–200 ml
10.00 am	Sweet lime juice	–200 ml
12.00 noon	Soup	–200 ml
	Tender coconut water	–200 ml
4.00 pm	Milk 200 ml + 10 g skimmed milk powder	
8.00 pm	Soup	–200 ml
	Tender coconut water	–200 ml
9.00 pm	Milk 200 ml + 10 g skimmed milk powder.	

Stage II

Salt free, 2100 ml fluids and 100 calories

6.00 am	Milk 200 ml + 10 g skimmed milk powder	
8.00 am	Milk	–200 ml
10.00 am	Sweet lime juice	–200 ml
12.00 noon	Soup	–150 ml
	Buttermilk	–200 ml
4.00 pm	Milk - 200 ml + 10 g skimmed milk powder	
	Tender coconut water	–100 ml

8.00 pm Soup –150 ml
rice kanji –200 ml
9.00 pm Tender coconut water –100 ml
9.00 pm Milk - 200 ml + 10 g skimmed milk powder

Stage III

Approximately 40 g protein, salt-free, low-fat, soft diet of 1000 calories

6.00 am Milk - 200 ml + 10 g skimmed milk powder
8.00 am *Iddli* - 2 nos + *Sambar* - 3/4 cup
+ Tomato chutney - 3 to 4 tsp
or
Bread –3 slices
Porridge + milk –3/4 cup
Jam –1 to 2 tsp
+ tender coconut water –200 ml
10.00 am Sweet lime juice –200 ml
12.00 noon Soft *rice/kichdi* –3/4 cup
Plain *dal*
Bland + boiled vegetables
Rasam/khadi
Custard/stewed apple
Buttermilk
4.00 pm Milk - 200 ml + 10 g skimmed milk powder
7.00 pm Soft rice/*kichdi* –3/4 cup
Plain *dal*
Bland + boiled vegetables
Rasam/*khadi*
Custard/stewed apple
Curd

Stage IV

Approximately 1200 calories, 50 g protein, salt-free, low-cholesterol diet

6.00 am Milk - 200 ml + 1 tea bag
8.00 am *Iddli* - 2 nos. *Sambar*, tomato chutney
or
Bread - 2 slices, porridge/cornflakes –1/2 cup
Jam
tender coconut water –200 ml
10.00 am Sweet lime juice –200 ml
1.00 pm Soft rice or *kichdi* –1 cup
Sambar/Dal
2 vegetables
Rasam, curd and fruit
4.00 pm Milk - 200 ml + 1 tea bag + Biscuits –2 nos
7.00 pm *Kichdi*/soft rice –1 cup
Dal/sambar –1 cup
2 vegetables
Rasam
Buttermilk
9.00 pm Milk –200 ml

Stage V diet is approximately 1200 calories, 50 g protein, salt-free, low-cholesterol diet

Stage VI is low-fat, low-cholesterol, low-salt diet.

Note:

Stimulants like coffee and tea are totally avoided.

Raw salads, fruits, vegetables curries and diluted tea may be introduced on the 8th day.

Salt may be introduced in the diet from 6th day and increased to 3-5 grams by the 10th day.

Lean pieces of chicken, fish cooked in minimum of oil or preferably boiled, baked or grilled may be introduced in small quantities after 2 weeks.

Heart patients are advised always to keep their diet low in sodium, energy and cholesterol.

Index

E

F

G

H

I

J

K

L